W9-BIE-447

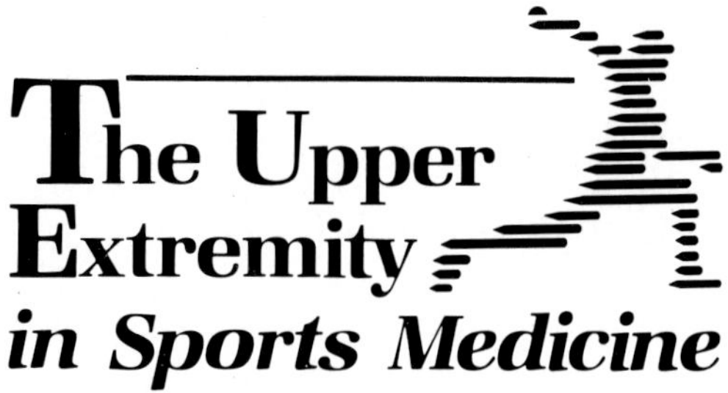

The Upper Extremity in Sports Medicine

Edited by

JAMES A. NICHOLAS, M.D.

Founder and Director
Nicholas Institute for Sports Medicine and Athletic Trauma
Director, Department of Orthopaedic Surgery
Lenox Hill Hospital
Consultant in Orthopaedic Surgery
Hospital for Special Surgery
Team Physician
New York Jets Football Club
New York, New York

ELLIOTT B. HERSHMAN, M.D.

Associate Orthopaedic Surgeon
Department of Orthopaedic Surgery
Consultant, Nicholas Institute for Sports Medicine and Athletic Trauma
Lenox Hill Hospital
Associate Team Orthopaedist
New York Jets Football Club
Team Physician
Hunter College Athletic Program
New York, New York

With

Martin A. Posner, M.D., editor of Hand Section

Associate Clinical Professor of Orthopaedics
Mount Sinai School of Medicine
Chief of Hand Services
Lenox Hill Hospital
Hospital for Joint Diseases and Orthopaedic Institute
Mount Sinai Hospital
Consultant Hand Surgeon for
Nicholas Institute for Sports Medicine and Athletic Trauma
Blythdale Children's Hospital
New York Jets Football Club
New York Knicks Basketball Team
New York Rangers Hockey Team
New York, New York

with 1468 illustrations and 14 color plates

THE C. V. MOSBY COMPANY

St. Louis • Baltimore • Philadelphia • Toronto 1990

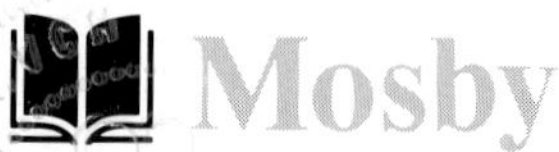

Acquisitions Editor Eugenia A. Klein
Developmental Editor Kathryn H. Falk
Assistant Editor Ellen Baker Geisel
Project Managers John Rogers and Suzanne Seeley
Production Editor Kathy Burmann Wiegand
Design Candace Conner

Printed in the United States of America.

The C. V. Mosby Company
11830 Westline Industrial Drive, St. Louis, Missouri 63146

Library of Congress Cataloging in Publication Data

The Upper extremity in sports medicine/edited by James A. Nicholas, Elliott B. Hershman; with Martin A. Posner.
p. cm.
Companion v. to: The Lower extremity and spine in sports medicine.
Includes bibliographical references.
ISBN 0-8016-3943-3
1. Extremities, Upper—Wounds and injuries. 2. Sports—Accidents and injuries. I. Nicholas, James A., 1921- . II. Hershman, Elliott B. III. Posner, Martin A. IV. Lower extremity and spine in sports medicine.
[DNLM: 1. Arm Injuries. 2. Athletic Injuries. WE 805 U683]
RD557.U67 1990
617.5'7044—dc20
DNLM/DLC

GW/MV/MV 9 8 7 6 5 4 3 2

Contributors

Fred L. Allman, M.D.
Orthopaedic Surgeon
Director, Sports Medicine Foundation of America
Atlanta, Georgia

David W. Altchek, M.D.
Assistant Attending Surgeon
The Hospital for Special Surgery
Assistant Professor of Surgery
Cornell University
New York, New York

Thomas E. Anderson, M.D.
Staff, Department of Orthopaedics
Section of Sports Medicine
Cleveland Clinic Foundation
Orthopaedic Consultant
Cleveland Indians Baseball Team
Cleveland Browns Professional Football Team
Cleveland State University
Cleveland, Ohio

James R. Andrews, M.D.
Clinical Professor of Orthopaedics and Sports Medicine
University of Virginia Medical School
Charlottesville, Virginia
Orthopaedic Surgeon
Alabama Sports Medicine and Orthopaedic Center
Birmingham, Alabama

Jack Andrish, M.D.
Staff, Department of Orthopaedics
Section of Sports Medicine
Section of Pediatric Orthopaedics
Cleveland Clinic Foundation
Consultant, Cleveland State University
Cleveland, Ohio

George H. Belhobek, M.D.
Head, Section of Bone and Joint Radiology
Chairman, Department of Diagnostic Radiology-Clinic
Cleveland Clinic Foundation
Cleveland, Ohio

James B. Bennett, M.D.
Chief, Hand and Upper Extremity Section
Associate Professor
Division of Orthopaedic Surgery
Baylor College of Medicine
Houston, Texas

John A. Bergfeld, M.D.
Head, Section of Sports Medicine
Cleveland Clinic Foundation
Team Physician
Cleveland Browns Football Team
Cleveland Cavaliers Basketball Team
Cleveland Indians Baseball Team
Cleveland, Ohio

George P. Bogumill, Ph.D., M.D.
Professor of Orthopaedic Surgery
Georgetown University Hospital
Washington, D.C.
Consultant in Hand Surgery
Walter Reed Army Medical Center
Department of Orthopaedics
Clinical Professor of Surgery
Uniformed Services University Health Sciences
Bethesda, Maryland

John J. Brems, M.D.
Staff, Orthopaedic Surgery
Section of Arthritis and Joint Replacement Surgery
Cleveland Clinic Foundation
Cleveland, Ohio

T. Pepper Burruss, P.T., A.T.C.
Assistant Athletic Trainer
New York Jets Football Club
New York, New York

Carolyn A. Carlson, P.T.
Director of Rehabilitation Services
Peachtree Sports Medicine Center
Atlanta, Georgia

Vincent J. DiStefano, M.D.
Clinical Professor of Orthopaedic Surgery
Hospital of the University of Pennsylvania
Chairman, Department of Orthopaedic Surgery
Graduate Hospital
Team Physician
Philadelphia Eagles Professional Football Team
Philadelphia, Pennsylvania

Howard J. Ellfeldt, M.D.
Clinical Preceptor
Department of Kansas School of Medicine
Team Physician
Kansas City Chiefs
Kansas City, Missouri

Pierce J. Ferriter, M.D.
Adjunct Orthopaedic Surgeon
Lenox Hill Hospital
Consultant, Nicholas Institute of Sports Medicine and Athletic Trauma
New York, New York

Peter J. Fowler, M.D., F.R.C.S.(C)
Professor of Orthopaedic Surgery
Head, Section of Sports Medicine
University of Western Ontario
London, Ontario, Canada

Ralph A. Gambardella, M.D.
Associate, Kerlan-Jobe Orthopaedic Clinic
Inglewood, California
Assistant Clinical Professor
Department of Orthopaedics
University of Southern California
School of Medicine
Los Angeles, California

Ronald E. Glousman, M.D.
Assistant Clinical Professor
University of Southern California
Associate, Kerlan-Jobe Orthopaedic Clinic
Inglewood, California

Elliott B. Hershman, M.D.
Associate Orthopaedic Surgeon
Consultant, Nicholas Institute for Sports Medicine and Athletic Trauma
Lenox Hill Hospital
Associate Team Orthopaedist
New York Jets Football Club
Team Physician
Hunter College Athletic Program
New York, New York

John A. Hurley, M.D.
Assistant Clinical Professor
University of Medicine and Dentistry
Newark, New Jersey
Attending Orthopaedic Surgeon
Morristown Memorial Hospital
Morristown, New Jersey
Team Physician
Farleigh Dickinson University
Athletic Program
Madison, New Jersey

John F. Jennings, M.D.
Instructor, Orthopaedics
Clinical Fellow in Hand Surgery
Department of Orthopaedics
University of Buffalo School of Medicine
State University of New York
Buffalo, New York

Frank W. Jobe, M.D.
Associate, Kerlan-Jobe Orthopaedic Clinic
Inglewood, California
Clinical Professor
Department of Orthopaedics
University of Southern California
School of Medicine
Orthopaedic Consultant
Los Angeles Dodgers Baseball Team
Los Angeles, California

Vi A. Mayer, OT.R.
Hand Therapist and Instructor
Division of Hand Surgery and Sports Medicine
Department of Orthopaedics
University of Virginia
Charlottesville, Virginia

John R. McCarroll, M.D.
Orthopaedic Surgeon
Methodist Sports Medicine Center
Indianapolis, Indiana
Orthopaedic Consultant for
Indiana University
Athletic Department
Bloomington, Indiana

Frank C. McCue, III, M.D.
Alfred R. Shands Professor of Orthopaedic Surgery and Plastic Surgery of the Hand
Director, Division of Sports Medicine and Hand Surgery
Team Physician, University of Virginia
Department of Athletics
University of Virginia
Charlottesville, Virginia

Charles P. Melone, Jr., M.D.
Clinical Professor of Orthopaedic Surgery
New York University Medical Center
Director, Hand Surgery Service
Cabrini Medical Center
New York, New York

Francis X. Mendoza, M.D.
Adjunct Orthopaedic Surgeon
Chief, Shoulder and Elbow Section
Department of Orthopaedic Surgery
Consultant, Nicholas Institute for Sports Medicine and Athletic Trauma
Lenox Hill Hospital
New York, New York

Karen Middleton, P.T./A.T.,C.
Alabama Sports Medicine
Birmingham, Alabama

Jeffrey Minkoff, M.D.
Associate Clinical Professor of Orthopaedics
Director of Sports Medicine Fellowship
New York University Medical Center
Associate Attending in Orthopaedics
Lenox Hill Hospital
Associate Attending Orthopaedic Surgeon
Hospital for Joint Diseases, Orthopaedic Institute
Team Physician (NHL)
New York Islanders
Orthopaedic Consultant
New Jersey Nets
New York, New York

Lana K. Minnigerode, M.D.
Associate Professor (ret.)
Department of Physical Medicine and Rehabilitation
Research Medical Center
Kansas City, Missouri

C. Alexander Moskwa, Jr., M.D.
Orthopaedic Surgeon
Sports Medicine Princeton
Orthopaedic Associates of Princeton
Princeton, New Jersey

James A. Nicholas, M.D.
Founder and Director
Nicholas Institute for Sports Medicine and Athletic Trauma
Director, Department of Orthopaedic Surgery
Lenox Hill Hospital
Consultant in Orthopaedic Surgery
Hospital for Special Surgery
Team Physician
New York Jets Football Club
New York, New York

Robert P. Nirschl, M.D.
Director of Virginia Sports Medicine Institute
Arlington, Virginia
Clinical Assistant Professor
Georgetown University
School of Medicine
Washington, D.C.

Tom R. Norris, M.D.
Attending Physician
Department of Hand and Orthopaedic Surgery
Pacific Presbyterian Medical Center
San Francisco, California

Patrick F. O'Leary, M.D.
Chief of Spine Section and Associate Director
Department of Orthopaedic Surgery
Consultant, Nicholas Institute for Sports Medicine and Athletic Trauma
Lenox Hill Hospital
Director, Spine Services
Associate Attending Orthopaedic Surgeon
Hospital for Special Surgery
Attending Surgeon
Department of Orthopaedic Surgery
Hospital for Joint Diseases and Orthopaedic Institute
Assistant Clinical Professor
Department of Orthopaedic Surgery
Mt. Sinai School of Medicine
Associate Attending Surgeon
Beth Israel Hospital
New York, New York

James C. Parkes, II, M.D.
Associate Clinical Professor
Orthopaedic Surgery
Columbia University
Team Physician, New York Mets
Consultant, U.S. Tennis Association
New York, New York

Joseph Patten, A.T.C.
Assistant Trainer
New York Jets Football Club
New York, New York

Clayton A. Peimer, M.D.
Associate Professor of Orthopaedic Surgery
Clinical Assistant Professor of Anatomical Sciences and Rehabilitation Medicine
State University of New York at Buffalo
Chief of Hand Surgery
Department of Orthopaedics
Millard Fillmore Hospitals
Buffalo, New York

Jacquelin Perry, M.D.
Chief, Pathokinesiology Service
Rancho Los Amigos Medical Center
Downey, California
Professor of Orthopaedics
University of Southeran California
Los Angeles, California
Consultant, Biomechanics Laboratory
Centinela Hospital
Ingelwood, California

Frank A. Pettrone, M.D.
Associate Clinical Professor
Department of Orthopaedics
Georgetown University Hospital
Washington, D.C.

George Pianka, M.D.
Hand Surgery Fellow
Lenox Hill Hospital
Hospital for Joint Diseases, Orthopaedic Institute
New York, New York
Associate Attending Orthopaedic Surgeon
Elmhurst City Hospital
Queens, New York

Martin A. Posner, M.D.
Associate Clinical Professor of Orthopaedics
Mount Sinai School of Medicine
Chief of Hand Services
Lenox Hill Hospital
Hospital for Joint Diseases and Orthopaedic Institute
Mount Sinai Hospital
Consultant Hand Surgeon for
Nicholas Institute for Sports Medicine and Athletic Trauma
Blythdale Children's Hospital
New York Jets Football Club
New York Knicks Basketball team
New York Rangers Hockey team
New York, New York

Mahvash Rafii, M.D.
Associate Professor of Radiology
New York University School of Medicine
Associate Attending Radiologist
Section of Skeletal Radiology
New York University Medical Center and
Bellevue Hospital
New York, New York

Robert C. Reese, Jr., A.T.C.
Head Athletic Trainer
New York Jets Football Club
Hempstead, New York

Allen B. Richardson, M.D.
Assistant Professor of Surgery
Division of Orthopaedics
John A. Burns School of Medicine
University of Hawaii
Honolulu, Hawaii
Chief Medical Officer
United States Swimming, Inc.
Colorado Springs, Colorado

Andrew Sands, M.D.
Chief Resident
Department of Orthopaedic Surgery
Lenox Hill Hospital
New York, New York

Scott Schemmel, M.D.
Chairman, Department of Sports Medicine
Medical Associates Clinic
Director, Sports Medicine Clinic
Dubuque, Iowa

Lawrence H. Schneider, M.D.
Clinical Professor of Orthopaedic Surgery
Jefferson Medical College of the
Thomas Jefferson University
Philadelphia, Pennsylvania

Michael J. Skyhar, M.D.
Orthopaedic Surgeon
San Dieguito Orthopaedic Medical Group
Scripps Memorial Hospital
Clinical Instructor
Department of Orthopaedics
University of California, San Diego
San Diego, California

Janet Sobel, R.P.T.
Virginia Sports Medicine Institute
Arlington, Virginia
Member, United States Tennis Association
(U.S.T.A.) Sport Science Committee

Howard J. Sweeney, M.D.
Chief, Division of Orthopaedic Surgery
Director, Center for Arthroscopic Surgery
Evanston Hospital
Evanston, Illinois
Head Team Physician
Northwestern University
Associate Clinical Professor of Orthopaedic Surgery
Northwestern University Medical School
Chicago, Illinois

Hugh S. Tullos, M.D.
Head, Division of Orthopaedic Surgery
Baylor College of Medicine
Houston, Texas

Russell F. Warren, M.D.
Chief, Sports Medicine Services
Attending Orthopaedic Surgeon
The Hospital for Special Surgery
Professor of Orthopaedic Surgery
The New York Hospital
Cornell University Medical Center
New York, New York

Keith Watson, M.D.
Teaching Consultant
Department of Orthopaedics
Tarrant County Hospital District
Ft. Worth, Texas

Garron G. Weiker, M.D.
Staff, Orthopaedic Surgeon
Administrative Director
Section of Sports Medicine
Cleveland Clinic Foundation
Cleveland, Ohio

Terry L. Whipple, M.D., F.A.C.S.
Consultant, Hand and Sports Medicine Division
Department of Orthopaedics
University of Virginia School of Medicine
Charlottesville, Virginia
President, Orthopaedic Research of Virginia
Richmond, Virginia

James A. Whiteside, M.D.
Director, Medical Aspects of Sports
Alabama Sports Medicine and Orthopaedic Center
Birmingham, Alabama

E.F. Shaw Wilgis, M.D.
Associate Professor of Orthopaedic and Plastic Surgery
The Johns Hopkins Hospital
Chief, Hand Surgery
Union Memorial Hospital
Baltimore, Maryland

Adolph J. Yates, Jr., M.D.
Instructor of Orthopaedics
Department of Orthopaedic Surgery
The Johns Hopkins University
School of Medicine
Assistant Chief, Orthopaedic Surgery
Francis Scott Key Medical Center
Baltimore, Maryland

John G. Yost, Jr., M.D.
Associate Clinical Professor of Orthopaedic Surgery
Truman Medical Center
University of Missouri
Assistant Team Physician
Kansas City Chiefs
Kansas City, Missouri

To my family for their endless and steadfast enthusiasm, support and understanding.

James A. Nicholas, M.D.

To my parents, who started me on the right road, gave me just enough direction and told me that with diligence and hard work, the path you end up on is the one you desire.

Elliott B. Hershman, M.D.

Foreword

In 1986, Drs. Nicholas and Hershman published two monumental volumes entitled *The Lower Extremity and Spine in Sports Medicine*. In his foreword to these books, Dr. Robert Larson described Dr. Nicholas' treatment philosophy: with any injury there are alterations in the function of adjacent joints and in the athlete as a whole. This "linkage mechanism" serves as a unifying theme to both books. Dr. Nicholas has stressed a multidisciplinary approach to athletic injuries.

The Upper Extremity in Sports Medicine now completes the task of providing the sports medicine practitioner with a comprehensive resource on sports injuries of the musculoskeletal system. The publication of this volume is extremely timely. The explosion of information on the knee in the 1970s and early 1980s was followed by a similar phenomenon for the shoulder in the late 1980s. This book consolidates and clearly presents the new information.

The chapters of this distinguished text reflect the wide experience and acknowledged expertise of the authors. The editors help the reader by summarizing the key points in each chapter throughout the text. Although this work enriches the entire field of sports medicine, the ultimate benefactor will be the individual athlete.

Bertram Zarins, M.D.

Preface

To focus only on the area of injury and its treatment causes us to lose perspective on the injury's broader implications to the body's interrelated systems. In our companion volume, *The Lower Extremity and Spine in Sports Medicine,* we showed that function can be altered in sites distant both distally and proximally from the injury. In this volume on the upper extremity and cervical spine, we continue our efforts to show that all parts of the linkage system work together and therefore can be disrupted together. One must bear in mind that all systems and parts of the body are linked; damage to one system or part has implications for the other systems or parts. In the lower extremity, for example, an ankle injury can cause one to lose strength in proximal segments of muscle far removed from the injury site, such as those that govern hip abduction. When an injury is treated as an entity unto itself, without regard for the other physical systems that may be involved, other problems, such as contractures from disuse and immobilization, may develop. In the upper extremity, injury to the arm, for example, will cause residual disability in scapular and cervical muscle strength, or shoulder or elbow range of motion. Further effects of such weakness and disability can impact on the ability to use and consume oxygen, which will disrupt the economy of motion and impede efficient cardiorespiratory function. One goes on from there to an athlete's stress reactions about inability to perform, which affects his psychologic well-being.

One injury can have wide-ranging effects throughout the body, and disciplines such as anatomy, physiology, pathology, biomechanics, cardiology, kinesiology, and others become united in the sense of each having an answer to the question, "what is wrong?" Therefore in athletic injuries, the whole body must be involved in rehabilitation; power development must not be restricted to just the injured hand, or elbow, or shoulder. It must be a total-body approach, since the body itself is a total and linked system.

Not only the musculoskeletal system is affected by an orthopaedic injury. When muscle weakness causes a person to strain in an activity, the cardiorespiratory system perceives an extra load; this extra load puts maximum demands on the heart and can cause cardiac problems. When the demands of an activity cannot be satisfied, a person can injure himself, even to the point of a heart attack.

We like to conceptualize the comprehensive care of the athlete as the "7 Ps": performer, performance demand, pathology, practice, prescription, practitioner, and prevention. The performer must be aware of the performance demand of his activity, and practice to perfect his performance. As well, the practitioner, through awareness of pathologic conditions both inherent in the human body and peculiar to a particular athlete (history of injury, body type), formulates a prescription for that athlete's safe performance of the sport, and thereby encourages prevention of an injury. This concept recognizes the multidisciplinary aspects of sports medicine, and combines them into a total approach to treatment and rehabilitation.

We at the Nicholas Institute of Sports Medicine and Athletic Trauma, the first hospital-based institute of its kind in the country, have worked for many years to develop the concept of linkage as part of our treatment program. At the Institute, patients are given a program of treatment that encompasses the entire physical system, not just the injury. For example, a hand patient is given strengthening exercises for the arm, shoulder and chest. The body as an integrated system means that the level action in joints such as the elbow and shoulder also involve links in the cervical spine, the upper back, and torso. Motion in the elbow, for example, translates into the shoulder and scapular muscles. Malfunction of any of the links necessarily affects smooth translation, in effect turning a ripple into a tidal wave and disrupting normal movement throughout the linkage. What this means is that an elbow injury that prevents normal elbow movement can cause problems in the scapular region. A whole spectrum of disabilities can flourish throughout the linkage system of the body, caused by one injury affecting one joint in one area. Viewing the body dimensionally as an x y z axis, one can understand how an injury in x can reverberate to y and then into z in linked fashion.

Exercise programs must be tailored to meet the ultimate demands of sport, and rehabilitation must involve the total linkage system, including the athlete's psychologic profile. Such an approach will not only be cost-effective in terms of care, but will also serve the patient well in his daily life.

James A. Nicholas
Elliott B. Hershman

Acknowledgments

Our greatest appreciation and grateful thanks to:

The contributors who found time in their already overscheduled lives to write scholarly, informative, and well-illustrated chapters, making this text a definitive work.

Martin Posner for his able and erudite work and administration of the hand section.

Phil Rosenthal our Administrator, for his managerial acumen, tireless efforts, and constant support.

The Nicholas Institute of Sports Medicine and Athletic Trauma office staff, Pat Guardala, Valeria Burts Jones, and Mary DiRado. Their outstanding typing skills, organizational abilities, and attention to detail made many aspects of organizing this work a simple task.

Peggy Pappas, Karen Heim, and Dawn Williams DeSimone, who organized and adjusted our hectic schedules and responsibilities so that the text could be completed.

Our C.V. Mosby crew, Eugenia Klein, Kathy Falk, Ellen Baker Geisel, and Kathy Wiegand. They displayed great patience, understanding, and untiring support for us and this project.

James A. Nicholas
Elliott B. Hershman

Contents

PART I Cervical Spine

CHAPTER 1 The Relationship Between Cervical Spine Injury and the Upper Extremity

Pierce J. Ferriter
Patrick F. O'Leary

Cervical spine injuries have been associated with all major sports, including water sports,[3] football,[19] skiing,[21] gymnastics,[7] rugby,[12] and ice hockey.[8] Although the incidence of injury to the cervical spine is much lower than injuries incurred to other parts of the body, the impact to the athlete can be much greater.

Sports with cervical spine injury reports

- Water sports
- Football
- Skiing
- Gymnastics
- Rugby
- Ice hockey

The clinical syndrome of acute cervical spine injury with nerve root compression will manifest itself in the upper extremity. The first sign of injury will often be radicular. Discomfort in the shoulder, arm, or hand with or without weakness may be the only symptom of severe cervical injury. Congenital lesions of the cervical spine (those that cause narrowing of the canal) may impinge on the spinal cord. This in turn can cause transient paralysis of the upper and/or lower extremities if unusual demands are placed on the neck during athletic performance.

The purpose of this chapter is to make the physician who treats athletes aware of cervical injuries. The implication of a neck injury is devastating to the patient, family, coaches, and fans alike. This chapter first deals with the epidemiology of cervical injuries and then proceeds to a discussion of the anatomy of the cervical spine. The authors then outline the various injuries that can occur in the cervical spine with their respective mechanisms. The chapter concludes with a discussion of prevention.

EPIDEMIOLOGY

The epidemiology of head and neck injuries was studied when the National Football Head and Neck Injury Registry was established in 1975.[22] To evaluate injury patterns (frequency and associations), comparison was made for two 5-year periods: 1959 to 1963 and 1971 to 1975. Initially, the Registry collected information retrospectively from 1971 through 1975.

During the 5-year period from 1959 to

TABLE 1-1 Comparison of the occurrence of neck injuries between 1959 through 1963 and 1971 through 1975

Source and Year	Cervical Spine Fractures/ Dislocations	Permanent Cervical Quadriplegics
Schneider (1959-63)	56	30
Football Head and Neck Injury Registry	259	99

Torg JS et al: JAMA 241:1477, 1979.

1963, Schneider[19] reported 56 (1.4 per 100,000) injuries that involved a fracture and/or dislocation, and permanent cervical quadriplegia occurred in 30 during that period (0.7 per 100,000). The Registry documented 259 (4.1/100,000) injuries involving a fracture and/or dislocation of the cervical spine in 99 (1.58/100,000) with associated permanent quadriplegia during th 1971 to 1975 seasons. These data reflect an increase in the number of individuals with cervical injuries during the latter 5-year-period (Table 1-1).

These changes reflect the improvements in protective head gear for football players. During the same period of time, the incidence of intracranial injuries decreased dramatically. Since the athletes' heads were protected by the helmets, they were used more for "battering rams" in blocking and tackling. Therefore the number of neck injuries increased dramatically during this time, when the cervical spine was rendered more vulnerable to injuries. As a result of the Registry findings, the National Collegiate Athletic Association (NCAA) and the National Federation of State High-school Athletic Association adopted rule changes intended to control spearing (head-first) techniques. The NCAA Football Rules Committee established these new rules beginning in the 1976 season: (1) no player shall intentionally strike a runner with the crown or top of the helmet; (2) no player shall deliberately use his helmet to butt or ram an opponent; and (3) spearing is the deliberate use of the helmet in an attempt to punish an opponent.

As a result of these rules, Torg[22] demonstrated the decrease in both high school and college levels of cervical spine fractures, dislocations, and subluxations. In 1975, the season before the rule changes, there were 6.5 injuries per 100,000 participants and 29.3 per 100,000 at the high school and college levels respectively. Over the ensuing eight years, the incidence of cervical spine injury gradually declined until there were 1.9 per 100,000 and 6.7 per 100,000 at the high school and college level respectively in 1984. Graphically this decrease is demonstrated as the number of cervical spine fractures, dislocations, and subluxations went from 110 in 1976 to 51 in 1978. This decrease has also been maintained since 1978 to 1984 as shown[22] (Fig. 1-1).

Gymnastics also established patterns of injuries. The National Registry of Gymnastic Catastrophic Injuries was established in 1978. In its first 2 years, the National Registry documented 11 gymnastic injuries involving the cervical spine on the trampoline and mini-tramp across the nation.[4] Nine athletes developed permanent quadriplegia and two patients died (Table 1-2). Most of these participants were skilled, and some were participating under the direction of physical education instructors.

Subsequent to the study by the National Registry, guidelines have been published concerning the use of the trampoline in organized sports activities. The American Academy of Pediatrics has regarded the trampoline as a potentially dangerous apparatus when not used with precautions. The Academy has stated that *the trampoline has no place in competitive sports and should never be used at home or in recreational settings*. These guidelines dramatically decreased the number of serious injuries to participants.

Catastrophic neurotrauma is rare but occurs with some degree of frequency in football and gymnastics. Such injuries occur in other sports, but not with the frequency to allow epidemiologic analysis.

Restructuring of the rules for trampoline use has resulted in a dramatic decrease in spinal injuries from this activity. By the same token, the ruling in 1976 to ban "spearing" and "head-butting" techniques in football tackling has also resulted in a drop in neurotrauma in this sport. The data on hand show that cervical injuries are most likely to result from improper technique and not from the activity itself. Therefore proper education of players, coaches, and teachers will be most effective in controlling serious injuries.

ANATOMY

In the most simple description, the cervical spine is a column of seven vertebral bodies that connect the head to the thorax. Four of the vertebrae are typical (third to sixth) and three are more specialized (first, second, and seventh). The spinal cord is housed in the vertebral canal. A spinal nerve that innervates

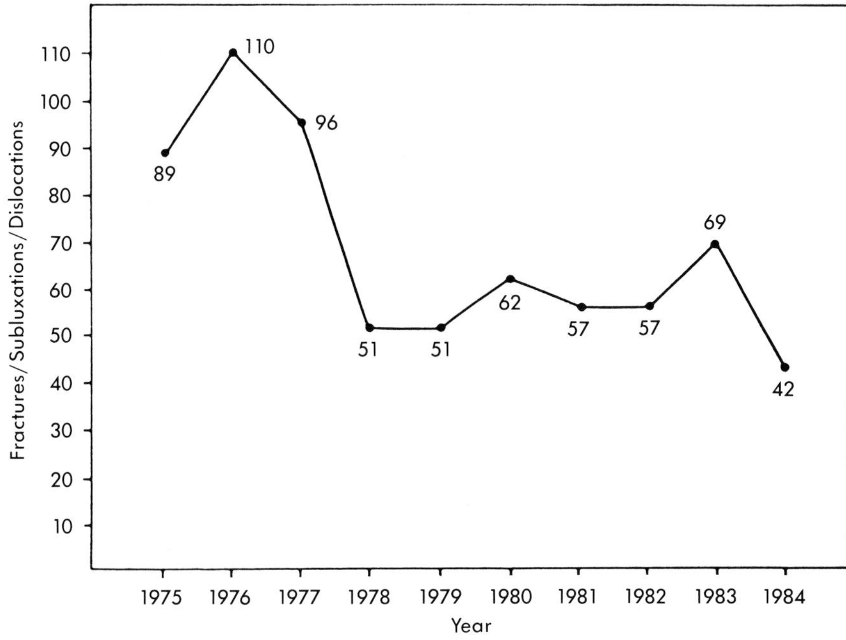

FIG. 1-1. Incidence of cervical spine fractures, subluxations, and dislocations for all levels of participation underwent a dramatic decrease from 1976 to 1978 as a result of the rules change. (Reproduced from Torg JS et al: The National Football Head and Neck Injury Registry. Fourteen-year report on cervical quadriplegia. 1971 through 1984. JAMA 254(24):3439, Dec 27, 1985.)

TABLE 1-2 National incidence of gymnastic injuries, July 1978 through June 1980

Event	Sex	Person	Circumstances	Injury
1. Trampoline	M	Skilled teenager	Practice, gymnastics club	Quadriplegia
2. Trampoline	M	Young boy	Backyard recreation	Death
3. Trampoline	M	Skilled young adult	Backyard game of "horse"	Quadriplegia
4. Trampoline	M	Advanced beginner teen	Military base recreation	Quadriplegia
5. Trampoline	M	College assistant instructor	P.E. class demonstration	Quadriplegia
6. Minitramp	M	College cheerleader	Warmup for football game	Quadriplegia
7. Minitramp	M	High school gymnast	Practice for pep rally	Quadriplegia
8. Minitramp	F	High school cheerleader	Cheerleader practice	Death
9. Tumbling	M	College gymnast	Practicing high-bar dismount	Quadriplegia
10. Unevens	F	High school gymnast	Practicing routine	Quadriplegia
11. Minitramp	M	College cheerleader	Unscheduled practice	Quadriplegia

From Torg JS: Athletic injuries to the head, neck, and face, Philadelphia, 1982, Lea & Febiger.

the upper limb exits through each of the vertebral foramen. Injuries to the cervical spine may produce signs and symptoms related to the upper extremity based on the level of injury, as well as on the amount of nervous tissue affected.

Lower Cervical Segments (C3, C4, C5, C6)

A typical lower cervical vertebrae has a small vertebral body that is concave on its superior surface and convex on its inferior surface (Fig. 1-2) Projecting laterally from the body are the **transverse processes.** The **foramen transversarium** is a canal in the transverse process that transmits the vertebral artery except at C7, where the foramen contains the **accessory vertebral vein.** At the junction of the pedicle and the neural arch are located the **superoarticular and inferoarticular processes.** The articular facets are flat; the superior face dorsally and

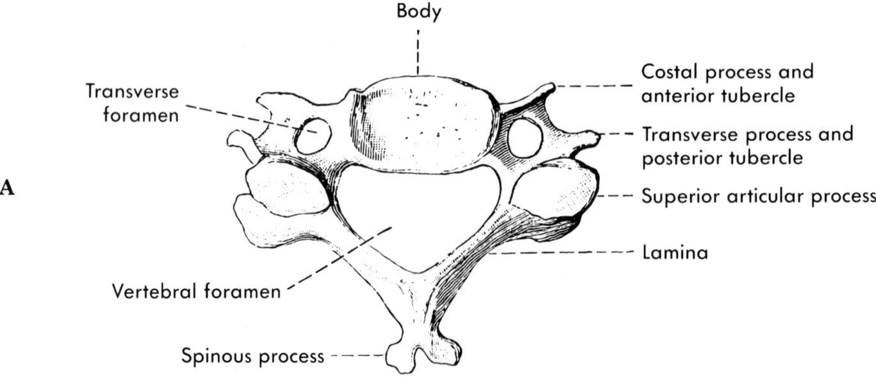

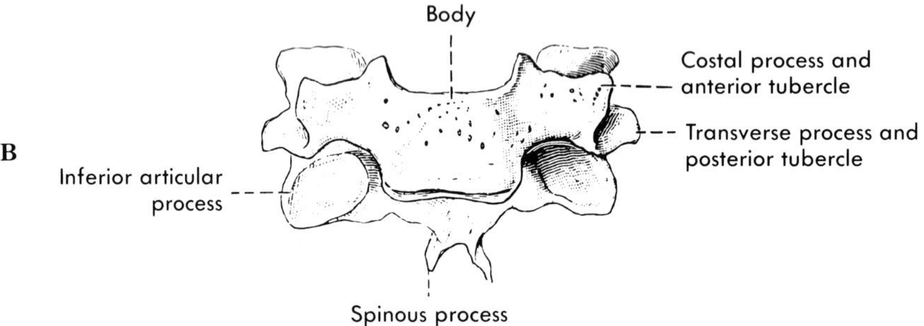

FIG. 1-2. A, Typical cervical vertebrae with its spinous process, lamina, and vertebral body. **B,** Note the articular facets and shape of the vertebral bodies on the frontal view. (Disse J: K von Bardeleben's handbuch der Anatomie des Menschen, Jena, Fischer, vol 1, Section 1, 1896.)

cranially. The inferior facets are directed ventrally and caudally (Fig. 1-3). These articulations form a "shingling" effect that should be preserved in a normal cervical spine. The facet joints of the lower cervical spine are diarthrodial joints with synovial membranes and fibrous capsules. The joint capsules are lax to permit increased motion. When subjected to excessive force, these joints may dislocate, leading to a unilateral or bilateral facet dislocation. The spinous processes of the third, fourth, and fifth cervical vertebrae are usually bifid, whereas those of the sixth and seventh are longer. The distance between the spinous processes is usually constant, and if a line were extended from each tip, they would tend to converge on a central point. Widening of the spinous processes indicates disruption of those ligaments between them and interrupts the converging lines (Fig. 1-4).

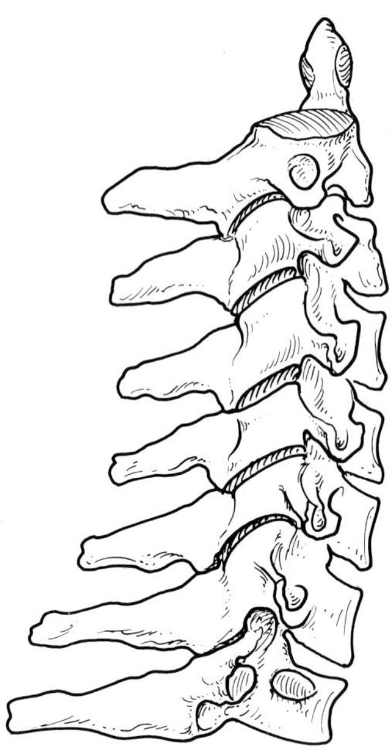

FIG. 1-3. Shingling effect of articular facets. The superior facets are directed dorsally and cranially. The inferior facets are directed ventrally and caudally.

Atlantoaxial Complex (C1, C2)

The first two cervical vertebrae form a unique joint called the **atlantoaxial complex.** The atlas is a bony ring consisting of one posterior and one anterior arch connected

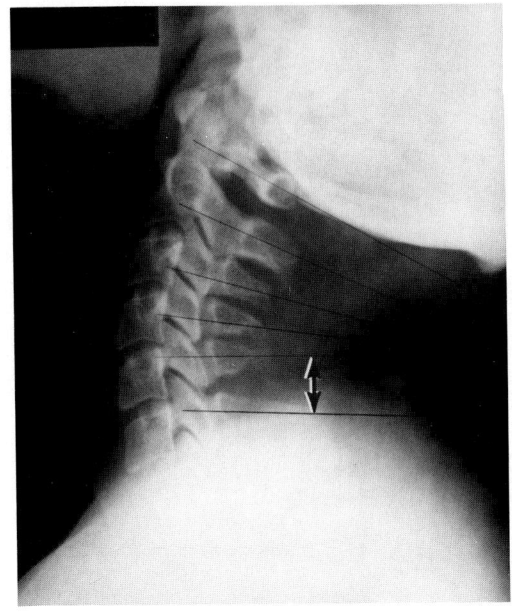

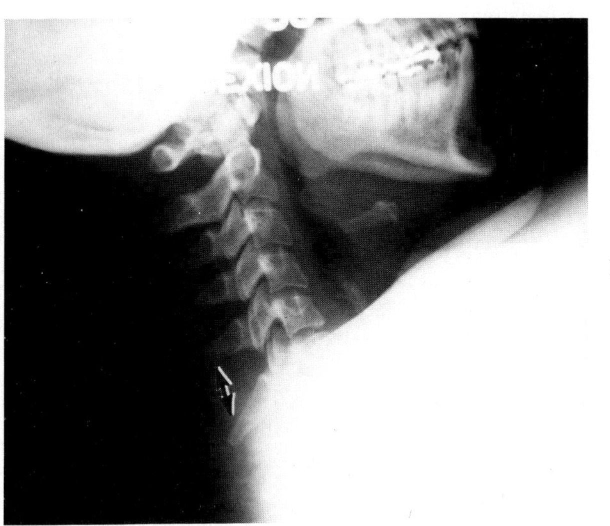

FIG. 1-4. A, Divergence of lines between C-5 and C-6 indicating disruption of the interspinous ligaments. **B,** Accentuated in flexion.

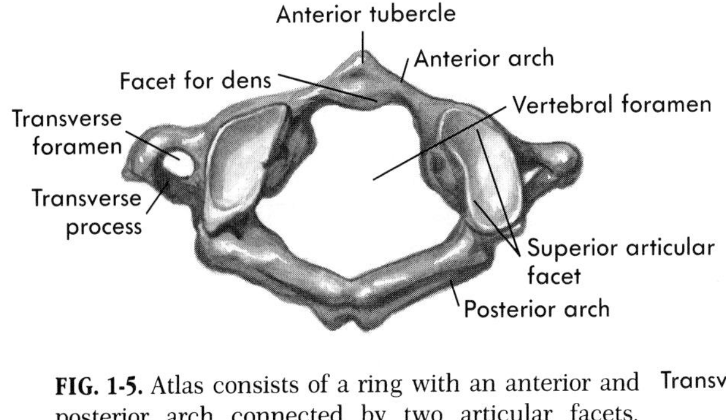

FIG. 1-5. Atlas consists of a ring with an anterior and posterior arch connected by two articular facets. (From Seeley RR, Stephen TD, and Tate P: Anatomy and physiology, St Louis, 1989, Times Mirror/Mosby College Publishing.)

by two lateral masses (Fig. 1-5). The lateral masses bear superoinferior and inferoarticular facets and transverse processes. The superoarticular facets are directed upward for the reception of the occipital condyles. Flexion of the head takes place with these joints. The inferoarticular facets face downward and articulate with the superoarticular facets of the axis.

The second cervical vertebrae, or axis, provides a surface upon which the atlas may rotate. This is the **odontoid process,** or **dens** (Fig. 1-6). The dens represents the body of the atlas. Besides being a pivot joint for the atlas, the dens provides an insertion point for the transverse atlantal ligament.

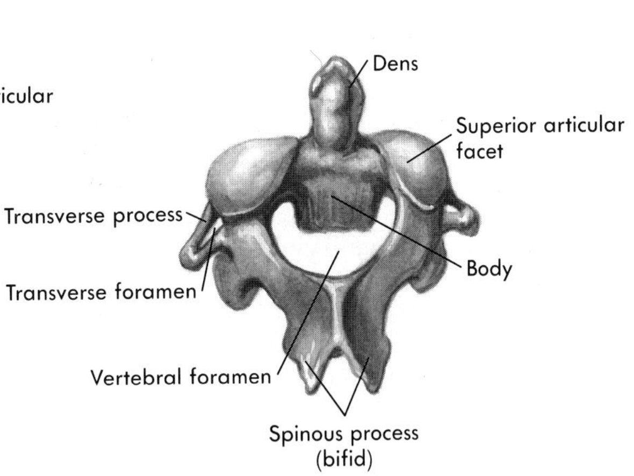

FIG. 1-6. The axis provides a surface from which the atlas can rotate. It contains the bony dens which represents the body of the axis. (From Seeley RR, Stephen TD, and Tate P: Anatomy and physiology, St Louis, 1989, Times Mirror/Mosby College Publishing.)

Transitional Vertebrae (C7)

The seventh cervical vertebra is a transitional vertebra, because it is located between the very mobile cervical vertebral bodies (C1 through C6) and the thoracic vertebral bodies, which are generally much more stable. Its spinous process is longer than that of the other cervical vertebrae and is easily palpable. Its body is proportionally broader than the bodies of the vertebrae above. Because it is at the base of the spine, the seventh vertebra is sometimes difficult to visualize roentgenographically, especially in patients with short necks and muscular chests.

Canal Size

Cervical spinal stenosis is a condition that narrows the spinal canal with the potential of compressing the spinal cord. Several authors[9, 14, 15, 24] have shown that those patients with a narrow canal are much more prone to develop neuropraxias and/or transient quadriplegia when they sustain an acute hyperflexion or extension injury to the neck. Different methods of measuring the spinal canal have been advocated, and these consist of the **direct method**[15] and the **ratio method.**[24] Each author points out that if the spinal canal that is less than 14 mm in diameter or has a ratio of less than 0.80 (which compares the sagittal diameter of the canal to the anteroposterior width of the vertebral body), then the patient is placed at great risk of neurologic injury if the cervical spine is stressed.

Soft Tissue

The ligaments and intervertebral disks maintain the normal alignment of the cervical spine. The **anterior and posterior longitudinal ligaments** are the major stabilizers of the spine and prevent excessive flexion and extension (Fig. 1-7). The anterior longitudinal ligament consists of longitudinal fibers that adhere to the intervertebral disks. It extends from the base of the skull to the sacrum. The posterior longitudinal ligament extends over the dorsal surface of the vertebral bodies within the vertebral canal. The ligament is composed of longitudinal fibers denser and more compact than the anterior longitudinal ligament. It fans out over the posterior surface of the intervertebral disks and prevents posterior extrusion. The intervertebral disk is interposed between adjacent vertebral bodies and forms a strong bond between them. Each disk consists of a gelatinous **nucleus pulposus,** two cartilaginous **endplates,** and the **anulus fibrosis.** The intervertebral disks are important shock absorbers that resist axial loading. Under pressure, the nucleus pulposus becomes flatter and distends the posterior longitudinal ligament.

The articulations of the vertebral arches are secured by the **articular capsule, supraspinous ligaments, interspinous ligaments, and ligamentum flavum.** The facet joints are enveloped by the articular capsules, which are thin and loose. These capsules prevent excessive gliding motion. The ligamentum flavum connects the lamina of each adjacent vertebrae. They consist of strong elastic fibers that are important in resisting excessive flexion of the neck. The interspinous and superspinous ligaments connect the adjoining processes and, along with the ligamentum flavum, resist hyperflexion (Fig. 1-7).

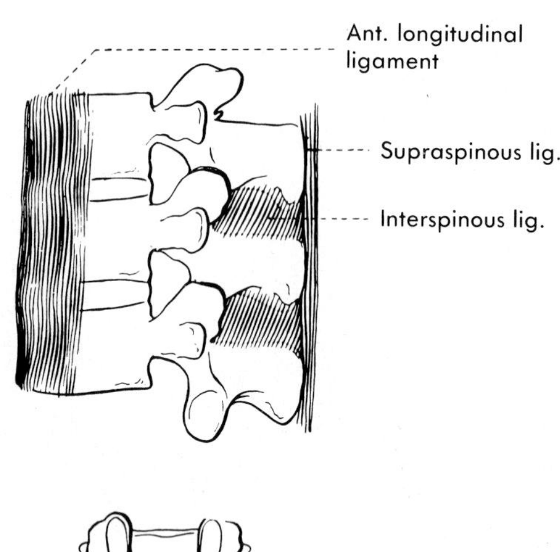

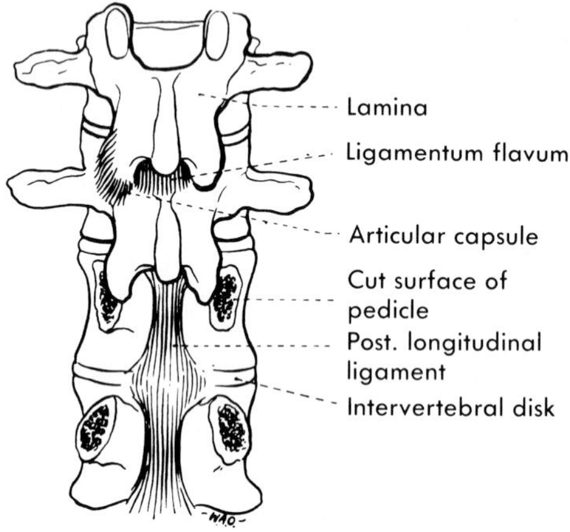

FIG. 1-7. The anterior and posterior longitudinal ligaments of the spine are the major stabilizers of the spine and prevent excessive flexion and extension. The ligamentum flavum connect adjacent lamina. (From Hollinshead WH: Anatomy for surgeons: the back and limbs, Philadelphia, 1982, Harper & Row Publishers.)

Neurologic Anatomy

A general knowledge of the neurologic anatomy of the cervical spine and the upper extremity is necessary for the assessment of neck injuries. Radicular symptoms may be the only finding in cervical fracture, dislocation, and disk herniations. Results of roentgenographic testing may be negative, and the physician must be aware of any neurologic deficit expressed by the patient.

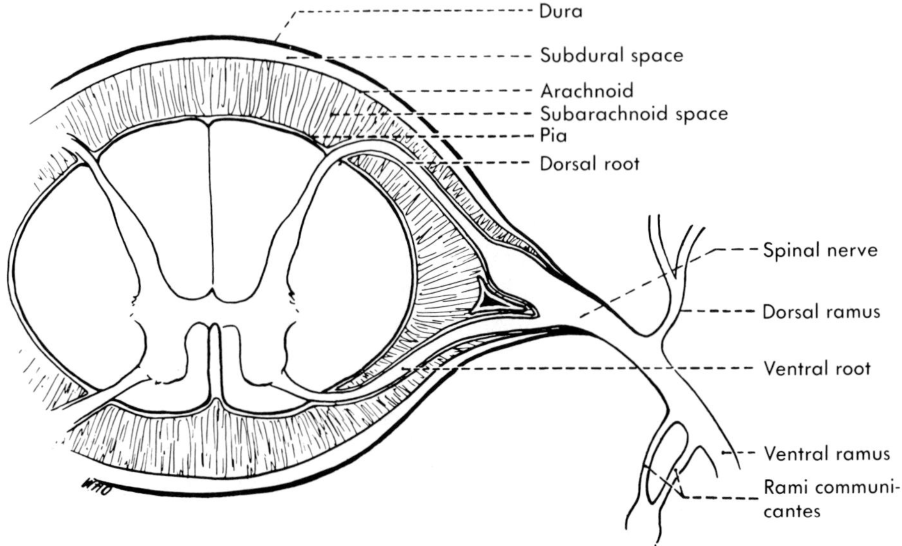

FIG. 1-8. Diagram of a spinal nerve as it exits the intervertebral foramen. (From Hollinshead WH: Anatomy for surgeons: the back and limbs, ed 3, Philadelphia, 1982, Harper & Row Publishers.)

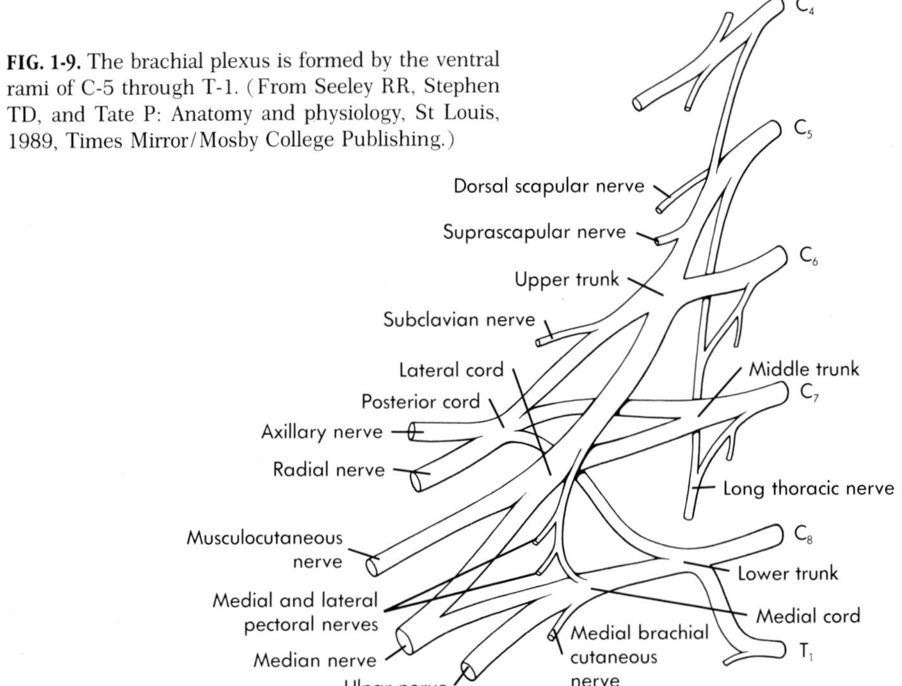

FIG. 1-9. The brachial plexus is formed by the ventral rami of C-5 through T-1. (From Seeley RR, Stephen TD, and Tate P: Anatomy and physiology, St Louis, 1989, Times Mirror/Mosby College Publishing.)

The spinal nerves are formed by the union of the dorsal and ventral roots as they emanate from the spinal cord (Fig. 1-8). Outside the **intervertebral foramen**, the spinal nerve divides into a **dorsal ramus** and a **ventral ramus**. The ventral rami supply the skin and muscles of the upper extremity. The **brachial plexus** is then formed by the ventral rami of the spinal nerves C5 through T1 (Fig. 1-9).

The ventral rami of C5 and C6 fuse to form the **superior trunk.** The C7 ventral ramus forms the middle trunk. The ventral rami of C8 and T form the inferior trunk. Each trunk divides into an anterior and posterior division. The anterior divisions of the superior and middle trunk form the lateral cord. The posterior cord is formed by the posterior division of the tree trunks. The medial cord is formed by the

TABLE 1-3 The segmental sensory distribution of the upper extremity

Spinal Nerve	Dermatomal Distribution
C4	Shoulder pad area
C5	Lateral aspect of arm
C6	Lateral aspect of forearm, hand, and the radial two digits
C7	Middle finger
C8	Ulnar two digits and medial aspect of hand and wrist
T1	Medial aspect of forearm
T2	Medial aspect of arm

From Torg JS: Athletic injuries to the head, neck, and face, Philadelphia, 1982, Lea & Febiger.

TABLE 1-4 The segmental motor innervation in the upper extremity

Spinal Nerve	Area of Innervation
C5,C6	Deltoid and other intrinsic muscles of the shoulder (abduction, hyperextension, and external rotation at shoulder)
C5,C6	Biceps, brachialis, and supinator (elbow flexion and supination of forearm)
C6,C7	Pronators of forearm
C7 (C6,C8)	Triceps and extensors of wrist and of fingers at the metacarpal joints
C8,T1	Intrinsic muscles of the hand

TABLE 1-5 The segmental levels of deep tendon reflexes

Reflex	Corresponding Nerve
Biceps	C5 (C6)
Triceps	C7 (C6)
Radial jerk (Supinator reflex)	C5 (C6,C67)
Ulnar jerk (Pronator reflex)	C6 (C7,C8)

anterior division of the inferior trunk. The cords end by dividing into peripheral nerves. Deficits in the peripheral nerves in the upper extremity alert the examiner to a potential cervical spine injury.

Cervical spine injuries will cause lesions proximal to the plexus at either the spinal cord or the spinal nerve level. The cutaneous and motor functions of the upper extremity follow a segmental pattern of innervation; therefore diagnosis of injuries can be made based on the peripheral nerve deficit. The segmental, sensory, and motor innervation of the upper extremity are noted in Tables 1-3 and 1-4. The deep tendon reflexes also follow a segmental distribution (Table 1-5).

MECHANISMS OF INJURY

The evaluation of cervical spine injuries begins the moment the injury occurs. An understanding of the mechanism of injury can aid in arriving at the proper diagnosis. A variety of mechanisms has been shown to cause significant injury to the cervical spine, causing quadriplegia[23] (Table 1-6). Originally it was thought that in football the helmet acted as a guillotine in the hyperextension injury, severing the posterior cervical spinal cord. Virgin has shown this not to be the case.[25] Carter and Frankel also have shown through static-free body analysis that the impact of the posterior rim of the helmet on the base of the neck is a rare cause of severe cervical spine injury.[1]

A number of mechanisms have been implicated in causing fracture dislocations of the cervical spine. Accidental falls and diving into shallow water (resulting in hyperflexion) have resulted in a number of significant fractures of the cervical spine. On the playing field, however, **axial load** has been the most common mechanism causing cervical fractures. From 1971 through 1975, 52% of all cervical spine quadriplegias resulted from "spearings," when the head was used as a battering ram in football (Fig. 1-10).[22] It must be remembered that during forward flexion of the neck, the cervical spine is straightened, losing its normal cervical lordosis. The resultant straight column of soft tissue, disk, and vertebral bodies must absorb the force. If the energy-absorbing capacity of this column is exceeded, muscle and ligament tears, disk herniation, and fractures can occur. Therefore

TABLE 1-6 Mechanism of injury resulting in permanent cervical quadriplegia (1971-75)

	Injuries Resulting in Quadriplegia, % (n = 73)	Injuries not Resulting in Quadriplegia, % (n = 136)
Hyperflexion	10	11
Hyperextension	3	8
Vertical compression (spearing)	52	39
Knee or thigh to head	15	17
Collision, pileup, or ground contact	11	19
Tackled	7	7
Machine-related	3	0
Face mask acting as lever	0	0

From Torg JS: Athletic injuries to the head, neck, and face, Philadelphia, 1982, Lea & Febiger.

TABLE 1-7 Injury by activity

	Permanent Cervical Quadriplegia, 1971-75		Cervical Fracture Dislocations Without Quadriplegia, 1971-75	
	High School % (n = 77)	College % (n = 18)	High School % (n = 105)	College % (n = 46)
Tackling	72	78	59	49
Tackled	14	22	15	24
Blocking	6	0	7	16
Drill	3	0	5	7
Collision pileup	3	0	12	4
Machine-related	2	0	2	0

From Torg JS: Athletic injuries to the head, neck, and face, Philadelphia, 1982, Lea & Febiger.

it is not surprising that the most vulnerable position of the cervical spine is flexion. In football the highest percentage of injuries occurs in the defensive back position[23] (Table 1-7). The neck is placed under extreme load during a tackle.

INJURIES

A multiplicity of injuries may occur in the cervical spine during athletic competition. The purpose of this chapter is not to identify each injury, but rather to mention the most common injuries and to address how they affect the upper extremity.

In the evaluation of any cervical injury, the physical and roentgenographic findings will be most important in the final treatment. The following are a number of acute cervical injuries that can occur in athletics. Emphasis is placed on those injuries that most commonly cause damage to the upper extremities. Cervical strains and muscle contusions are not addressed here because their clinical findings are most commonly localized to the neck.

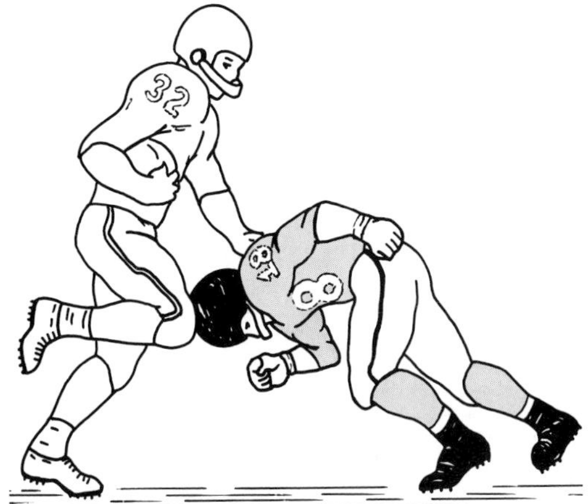

FIG. 1-10. The head is used as a battering ram during spearing. (Originally published in Can Med Assoc J, vol 109, Aug 18, 1973.)

Cervical Burner

The most comon cervical spine injury, which refers symptoms to the upper extremity, is the brachial plexus "stretch" neuropraxia, or **burner.** Clancy has reported a 49% incidence in college football players over their 4-year exposure.[2] He classifies the injuries into three grades, depending on the length of time that symptoms persist and the electromyographic (EMG) findings. The typical history is of a player who develops sharp and

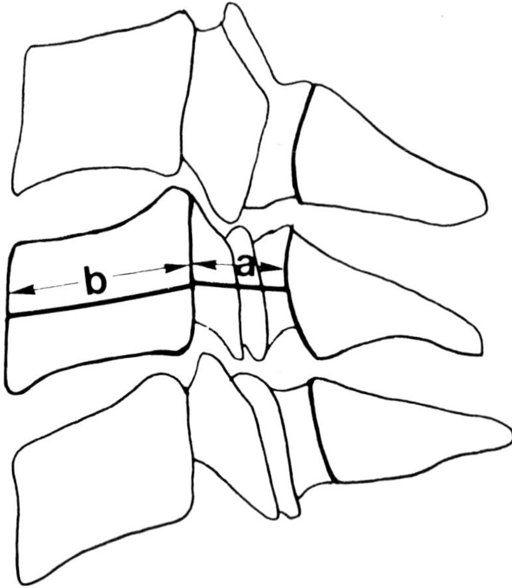

FIG. 1-11. A, The ratio of the spinal canal to the vertebral body is the distance from the midpoint of the posterior aspect of the vertebral body to the nearest point on the corresponding spinolaminar line. **B,** Divided by the antero-posterior width of the vertebral body. (From Torg JS et al: Neurapraxia of the cervical spinal cord with transient quadriplegia, J Bone Joint Surg 68A(9):1354, 1986.)

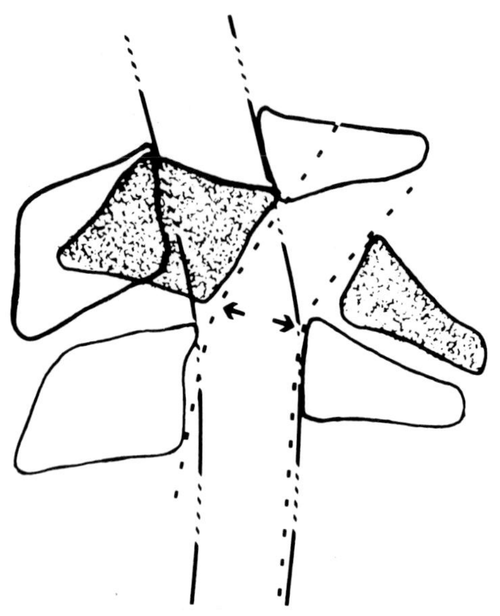

FIG. 1-12. The pinchers mechanism, as described by Panning, occurs between the posteroinferior aspect of the vertebral body and the anterosuperior aspect of the spinolaminar line of the subadjacent vertebra. (From Torg JS et al: Neurapraxia of the cervical spinal cord with transient quadriplegia, J Bone Joint Surg 68A(9):1354, 1986.)

burning pain in the neck that radiates into the arm and hand following contact with the head, neck, or shoulder during a play. There may be associated weakness or paresthesias in the hand. The mechanism of injury is that the athlete's head is laterally flexed away from the site of the injury, and the involved shoulder is driven downward or backward, thus placing traction on the brachial plexus. The clinical manifestations of each grade of injury correspond to Seddon's classification of nerve injuries.[20]

A grade I injury corresponds to a neuropraxia. This results in a transitory loss of motor and sensory function of the upper extremity that may last for minutes or hours. EMG results fail to demonstrate any signs of axonal injury.

A grade II injury is one that produces significant motor weakness and sensory deficit lasting 2 weeks. EMG studies reveal changes consistent with axonotmesis. Most often affected is the upper trunk of the brachial plexus, which causes significant deltoid infraspinatus and supraspinatus, and biceps muscle weakness. Again, the mechanism of injury for the grade II injuries puts a similar stretch on the brachial plexus when the shoulder is driving downward and away from the flexed neck.

A grade III brachial plexus injury corresponds to Seddon's neurotmesis. This injury produces motor and sensory deficits for up to 1 year. Here the mechanism of injury is the same; however, the force is greater. This results in irreversible damage to the nerves, with resulting muscle loss.

Since most of these injuries are transient, no clinical treatment is necessary. For those patients who have more than a temporary loss of motor strength, the treatment consists of rehabilitation and prevention of atrophy of the involved muscles. Players should not involve themselves in contact sports until they have achieved full strength in the upper extremities. A routine cervical spine series should be performed on all patients sustaining a brachial plexus injury to rule out any significant osseous abnormalities.

Transient Quadriplegia

Transient quadriplegia is a neurologic syndrome that has serious implications for the young athlete. The symptoms include burning pain, numbness, tingling, and loss of sensation.[13,24] The extremities may be weak or even completely paralyzed. These findings are transient and usually resolve within minutes. This form of quadriplegia has been caused by hyperflexion and hyperextension, as well as

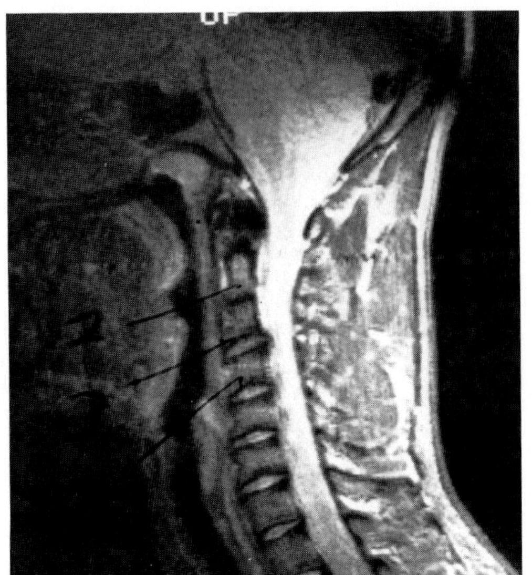

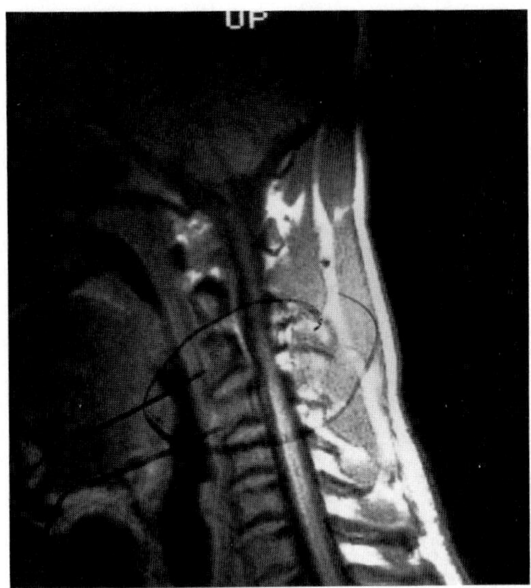

FIG. 1-13. A 19-year-old wrestler who developed temporary quadriparesis during a match. Note narrowing of the spinal canal at C-3 and C-4 by a disk herniation in flexion.

by axial loading injuries to the cervical spine.[24]

The causes of transient quadriplegia have been varied, occurring in individuals with developmental stenosis of the cervical spine, congenital fusions, cervical instability, or protrusion of an intervetebral disk. When any of these entities occur in combination, there is a much higher risk of causing neurologic sequelae by narrowing of the canal diameter. The normal average diameter of the middle part of the cervical spine (between the third and sixth cervical vertebrae) has been reported to be 17 mm.[6,9] The standard method of measurement determines the distance from the midpoint of the posterior aspect of the vertebal body to the nearest point of the corresponding spinolaminar line. Torg (Fig. 1-11) has devised a second method of measurement called the Ratio Method.[24] This ratio compares the sagittal diameter of the spinal canal to the anteroposterior width of the vertebral body. This method compensates for variations in roentgenographic technique. A canal measurement of 14 mm or less at any cervical segment falls below two standard deviations from the norm and puts the patient at risk.

One study reported the association between a narrowed sagittal diameter of the cervical spine and the development of myelopathy. Further compromise of the canal diameter can be caused by osteophytes, vertebral subluxation, or herniated disks. Penning[17] demonstrated the effects of flexion and extension on the sagittal diameter of the cervical spine. He coined the term "pinchers mechanism" when the cord is pinched by the processes of the two opposing bodies, (Fig. 1-12). The degree of pinching is determined by the sagittal diameter of the spinal cord and the degree of extension or flexion (Fig. 1-13).

Patients who evidence clinical symptoms of transient quadriplegia after cervical spinal injury should be regarded with caution. A careful neurologic examination must be performed, recording the onset and resolution of symptoms. Permanent neurologic deficits, quadriplegia, or death may occur if the patient's complaints are ignored and a treatable condition is present. Patients should have an adequate work-up with myelography, since this appears to be the best diagnostic tool at this time to rule out canal narrowing[13] (Fig. 1-14). Torg reported no increased incidence of permanent neurologic damage in 117 athletes who resumed sports activities after sustaining an episode of transient quadriplegia.[24] He warned that patients with other factors contributing to cervical canal stenosis, such as cervical spondylosis, congenital abnormalities, or ligamentous instability, should be treated on an individual basis.

Cervical Spine Fractures and Dislocations

Fractures and dislocations of the cervical spine are common injuries in today's athletic events. They have been documented in skiing, football, trampolining, and rugby. For simplicity's sake, they can be divided into fractures of the posterior elements and fractures of the anterior elements. Because of the proximity of the osseous fragments to the nerve roots and spinal cord, they are often associated with clinical findings referred to the upper

A

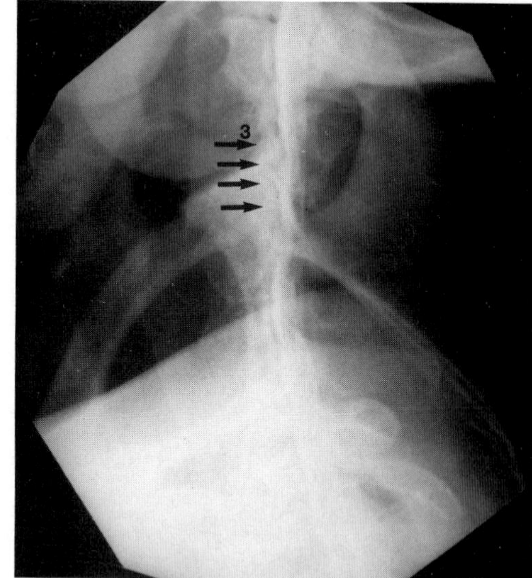

B

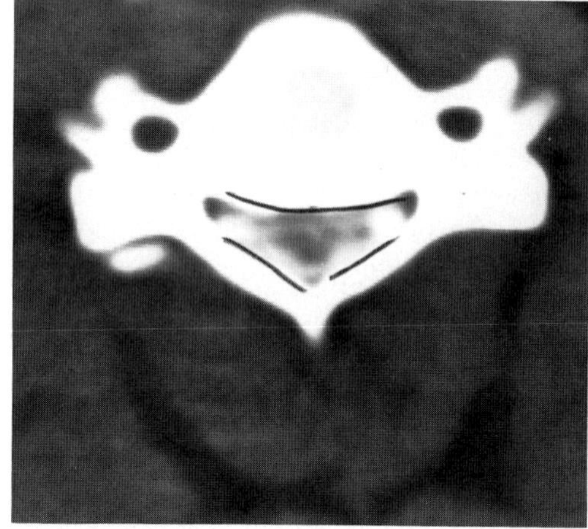

FIG. 1-14. A, Myelogram demonstrates significant narrowing of the dye column caused by spinal stenosis at C-3 through C-5. **B,** Contrast-enhanced CT scan confirms narrowing of the canal.

extremity. Based on the segmental innervation of the sensory and motor elements of the upper extremity, the physician is able to document the level of injury.

Identifying a fracture of the cervical spine is the first step in treating this serious injury. Determining the stability of the fracture and/or dislocation may have far-reaching implications for the health of the athlete. Biomechanical studies have shown that normal ligaments permit very little motion between vertebrae. White[26] has shown that in the stable spine, horizontal displacement of one vertebral body onto another never exceeds 3.5 mm. Angular displacement greater than 11 degrees between each vertebra suggests instability of the cervical spine (Fig. 1-15). Only when ligaments were disrupted did such displacement exist. Therefore, one may reduce displacement of the cervical spine, but it may remain unstable because of loss of the supporting ligaments.

Fractures of the Posterior Elements

Fractures of the neural arch of the second vertebra, or **Hangman's fracture,** occur when a vertical and hyperextension force is applied to the skull and cervical spine (Fig. 1-16). These fractures are usually stable, being adequately treated with a brace that controls flexion.[17] When there is subluxation of the second vertabra on the third, potential instability exists, because of rupture of the anterior and posterior longitudinal ligaments as well as the cervical disks. In these cases, halo immobilization is called for, and surgery may even be necessary when reduction cannot be accomplished. Neurologic symptoms are rare in this injury, since the canal is widened by the fracture.

Another fracture involving the posterior elements of the cervical spine is the **clay shoveler's fracture.** It involves the spinous process of C7, C6, or T1, in decreasing order (Fig. 1-17). Classified as an avulsion fracture, it is caused by distraction of the tight posterior ligaments when the neck is abruptly flexed. The pain is localized to the posterior aspect of the cervical spine; however, it does radiate into the shoulders. These are often difficult to identify on the lateral roentgenogram if the patient has a short neck or broad shoulders. A swimmer's view is often needed. These are stable fractures, and they do well with a short period of collar immobilization.

Dislocations of the cervical spine result from severe flexion and rotational forces. A unilateral or bilateral facet dislocation may occur. A unilateral facet dislocation occurs when the rotational forces tear the facet joint capsule. Lateral roentgenograms demonstrate moderate anterior displacement of the vertebral body (less than 50% of the vertebral body width). On the AP view, the spinous process is deviated toward the locked facet (Fig. 1-18). These are stable injuries but often compress the nerve root as they exit the neural foramen. Motor weakness and sensory loss in the extremities are often associated with these injuries. Careful neurologic examination identifies the level. Treatment involves closed reduction using cervical traction and immobilization with a halo.

Bilateral facet dislocations are more severe injuries, resulting from purely flexion forces. They are often associated with neurologic deficit or complete quadriplegia. The facet capsules, posterior longitudinal ligament, and intervertebral disks are all disrupted. The lateral

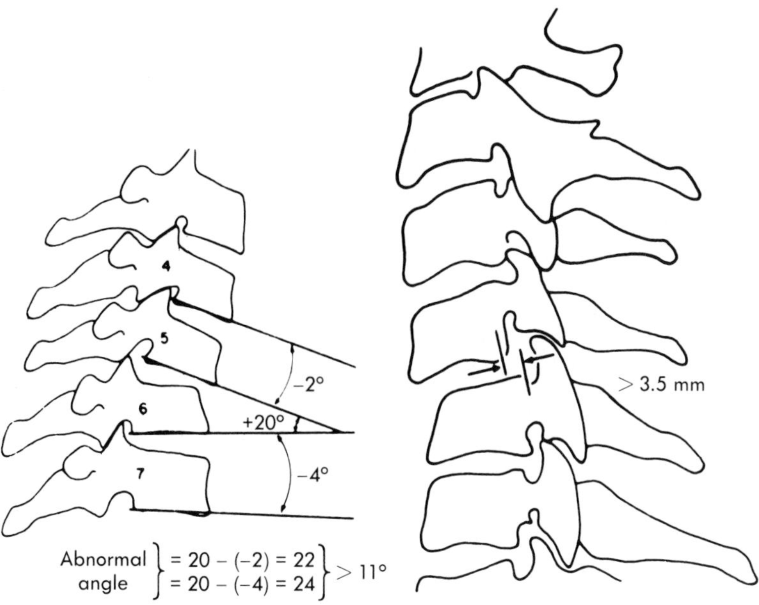

FIG. 1-15. White's criteria for stability. Vertebral body displacement should not exceed 3.5 mm and angular displacement less than 11 degrees. (From White AA, Johnson RM, and Panjabi MM et al: Biomechanical analysis of clinical stability in the cervical spine, Clin Orthop 109:85, 1975.)

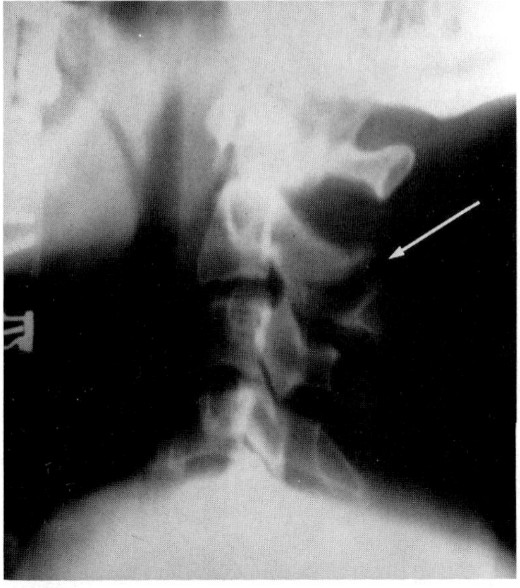

FIG. 1-16. Hangman's fracture through the neural arch of the second cervical vertebra.

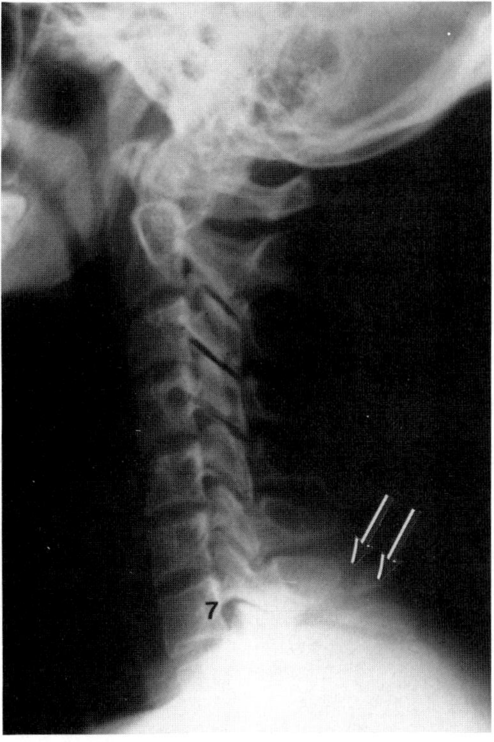

FIG. 1-17. Clay shoveler's fracture involves an avulsion of the spinous process of C-7.

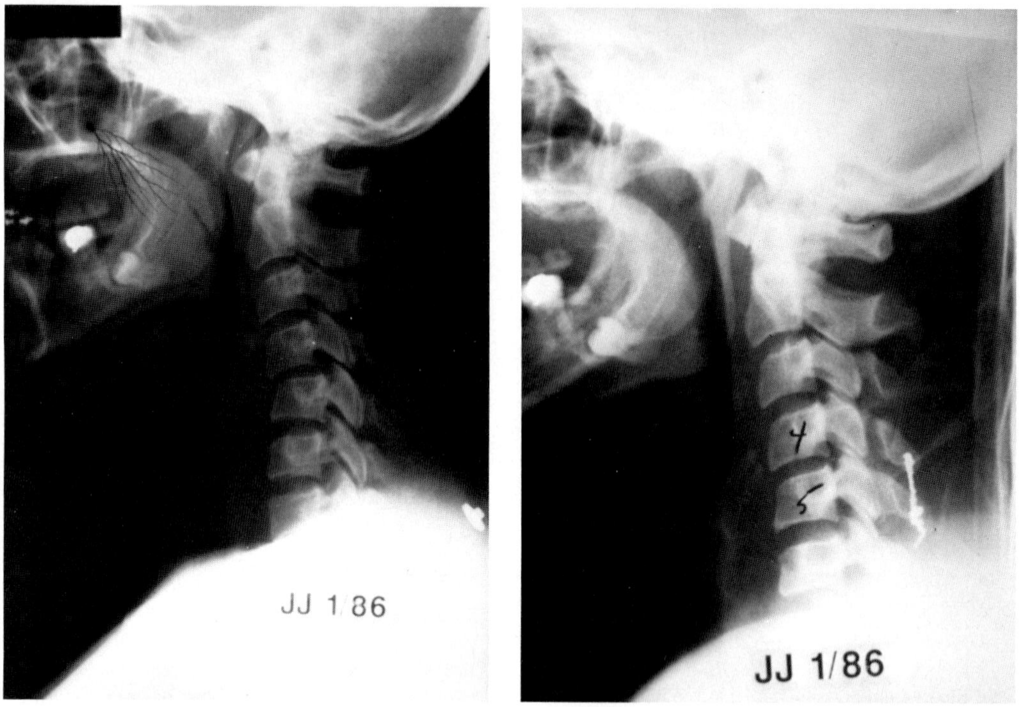

FIG. 1-18. Unilateral facet dislocation of C-4 on C-5. Note displacement is less than 50%.

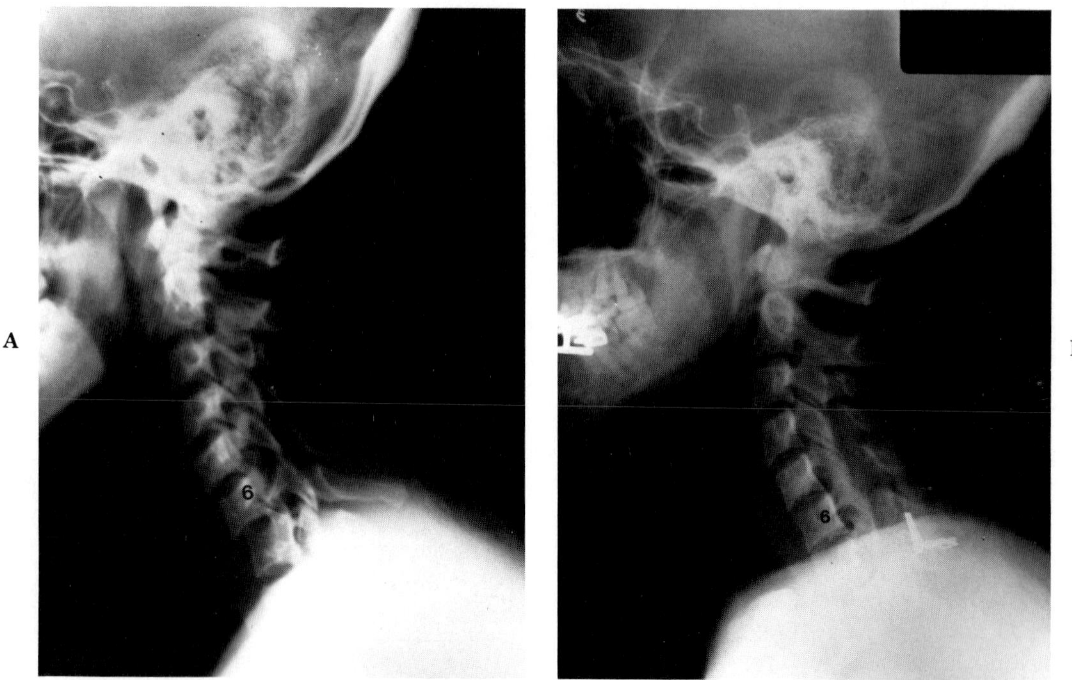

FIG. 1-19. A, Bilateral facet dislocation of C-6 on C-7. **B,** Solid posterior fusion 1 year later.

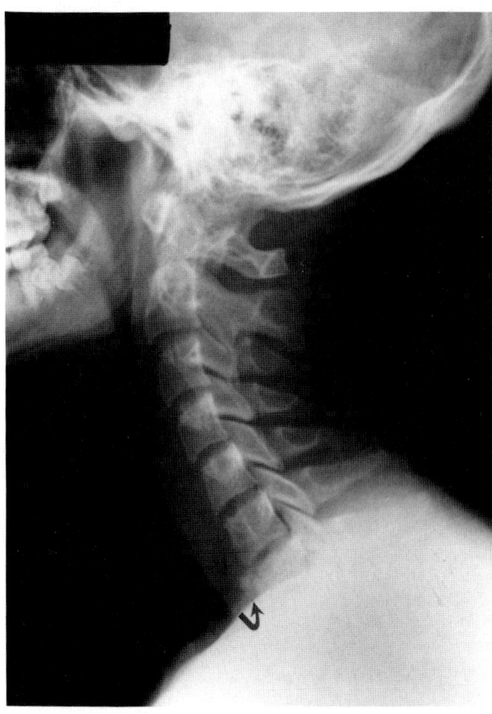

FIG. 1-20. Type II fracture of C-7 in a gymnast.

view demonstrates anterior displacement of the involved vertebra greater than 50% of the AP width (Fig. 1-19). Because these injuries are unstable, they require reduction and posterior fusion.

Fractures of the Anterior Elements

Fractures of the anterior portion of the vertebral bodies are caused by axial loading as well as flexion forces. The pattern of the fracture and extent of disruption of the vertebral body depend on the amount of force applied to the neck at the moment of impact. Compression fractures are classified into four types based on the amount of bony disruption. Type I is the tear-drop fracture, which ruptures the cortical endplate and breaks a chip off the anterior lip of the vertebral body; type II occurs when the fracture involves the upper half of the vertebral body, and a larger fragment may be broken off anteriorly; type III is a fracture of both the superior and the inferior endplates, with the fracture lines running throughout the vertebral body (the posterior cortex is intact); type IV is a fracture of the vertebra likened to a burst fracture of the lumbar spine; this destroys the entire vertebral body with retropulsion of the fragments into the spinal canal. Types III and IV fractures are often associated with neurologic compromise (Fig. 1-20).

Types I and II fractures are treated with immobilization and do well. Types III and IV fractures are more serious; therefore treatment is often surgical. Flexion and extension roentgenograms are often necessary to detect instability, as measured by White's criteria. Computed tomography (CT) scanning and myelography detect bony fragments in the spinal canal (Fig. 1-21). If surgery is necessary, based on instability or neurologic injury, an anterior approach is necessary, since the fracture is located anteriorly in the cervical spine. Decompression and fusion of the appropriate level will be necessary.

Cervical Disk Herniation

Acute cervical disk herniation resulting from athletic injuries is a rare but reported event.[2] Roaf[18] has shown that compressive loading results in vertebral endplate fracture with extrusion of the nucleus pulposus into the vertebral body. If asymmetric compression occurs, the pressure will tear the anulus, expressing the nucleus into the vertebral canal and foramen.

Cervical disk herniations that compress the nerve root characteristically cause neck, shoulder, and arm pain. The pain is often associated with motor weakness and sensory disturbances in the upper extremity, based on the segmental nerve distribution. A decreased reflex may also be noted. Conservative care is the rule. The athlete ceases competition and is placed at rest with a soft cervical collar and appropriate medications. When the symptoms persist or a significant neurologic deficit is present, a more detailed work-up is necessary. Magnetic resonance imaging (MRI) has proved to be an excellent way to screen and detect cervical disk herniations. The extent of the herniation can be documented (Fig. 1-22). Myelography with CT scanning has stood the test of time and is also an excellent diagnostic tool, as well as a test done before surgery (Fig. 1-23). Cervical disk excision with fusion has lead to excellent results when necessary[5] (Fig. 1-24.) Return to athletic participation after disk excision and fusion is decided on a case-by-case basis, based on age, activity level, and neurologic recovery.

INJURY PREVENTION

America has been enveloped by the fitness movement, with millions actively participating in some sport or exercise daily. Associated with this is a corresponding increase in the number of athletic injuries involving the cervical spine. Prevention of cervical spine injuries begins with education of the treating

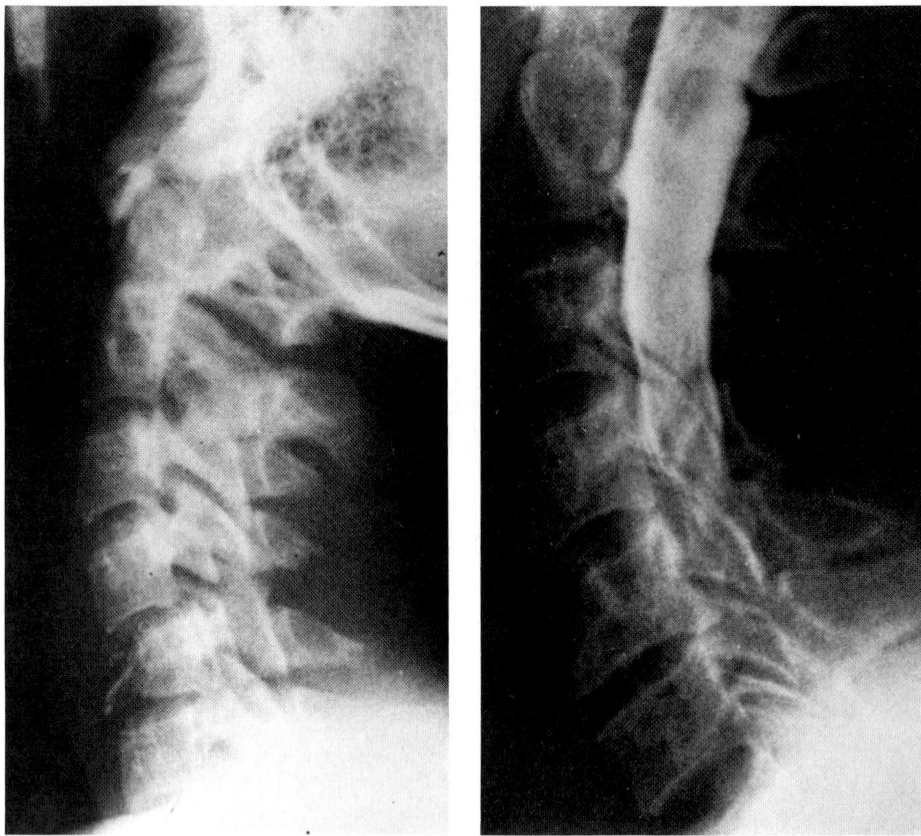

FIG. 1-21. Displaced anterior body fracture of C-5. Myelogram demonstrates complete block of the dye column at C-5. (From Weidner A: The cervical spine research society editorial committee, In: The cervical spine, Philadelphia, 1989, JB Lippincott Co.)

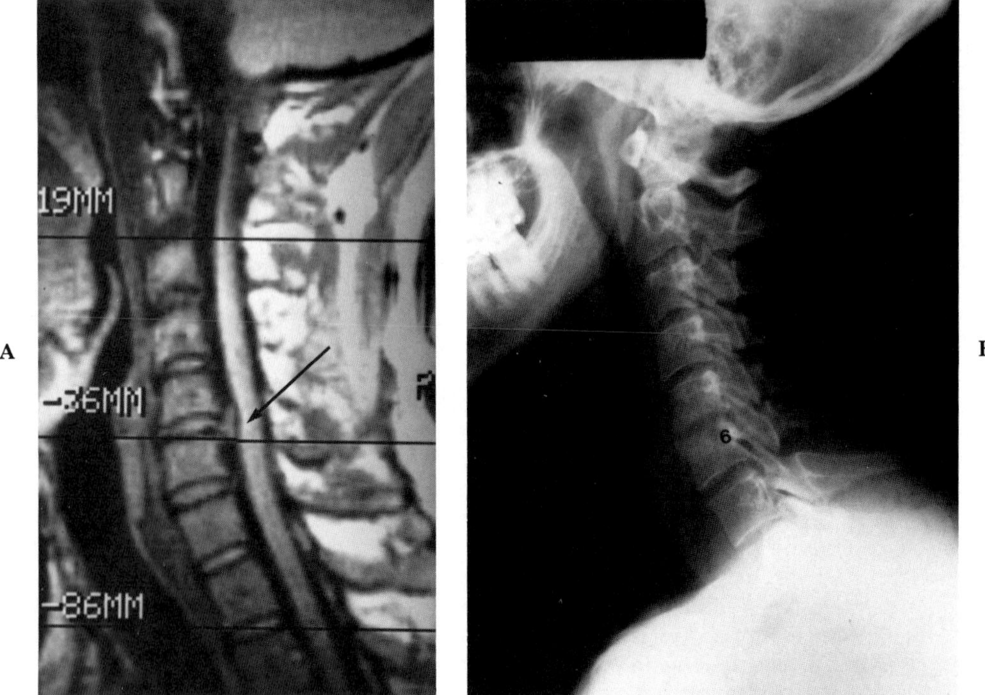

FIG. 1-22. A, MRI demonstrates cervical disk herniation at C5-6. **B,** Cervical fusion at 10 weeks.

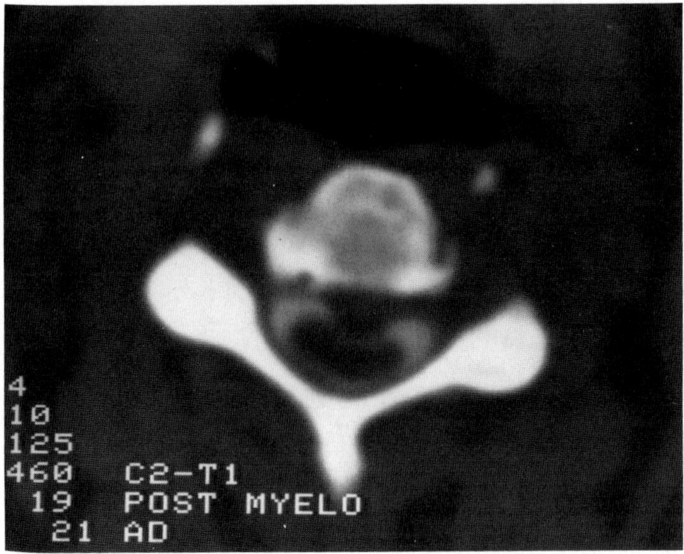

FIG. 1-23. Myelogram and CT scan demonstrates herniated cervical disk at C3-4.

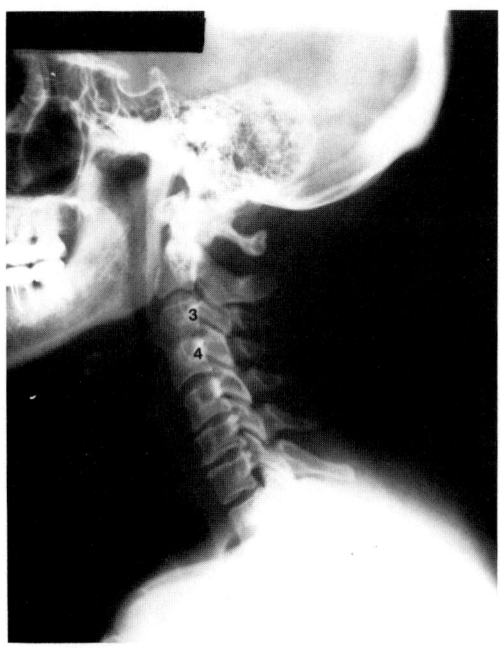

FIG. 1-24. Solid fusion at C3-4 1 year later.

physicians, coaches, and players alike. It has been shown that modifying techniques and providing closer supervision during athletic events promotes reduction of serious injuries.

Coaches have an important role in the prevention of serious injuries, since they come into daily contact with the players and supervise their activities. It has been shown that modifying sports techniques has produced dramatic reduction of serious cervical injuries in football. It is up to the coaches to enforce these techniques among their players. Closer supervision during activities such as diving and gymnastics has also been demonstrated to lessen the chances of significant cervical injuries.

And finally education must involve the players. They must understand the proper techniques involving their sport. They must wear protective equipment when necessary, and they should be educated to the dangers of their sports, such as spearing in football and improper techniques in diving, because of the high risks of injuries involved in these activities.

If such awareness exists among all personnel involved, a continuing decrease in severe injuries will follow.

SUMMARY

The physician must be aware of the variety of injuries that can occur in the cervical spine. Treatment of a patient with a cervical spine injury begins with the initial evaluation. A meticulous neurologic evaluation should be carried out to document evidence of paralysis, either sensory or motor. This examination must be repeated over hours and days to observe for recovery. If symptoms do not resolve, the physician will have to search for the cause with various tests, as outlined in this chapter. The physician's hardest role will occur when significant pathologic damage exists in the spine, whereupon the athlete may be advised to cease participation. Surgery will be a career-ending procedure for most athletes, since further injury could be devastating.

When significant neurologic injury exists, however, surgery could become a necessary event to alleviate symptoms.

A missed or improperly treated cervical spine injury can lead to a lifetime of severe disability for the athlete. The purpose of this chapter has been to present information about a variety of injuries that can occur in the cervical spine, along with their mechanisms and clinical presentations. Since the upper extremity is linked via its neurologic anatomy to the cervical spine, many injuries will manifest themselves as pain, weakness, or sensory loss there. The physician who recognizes and understands this can prevent serious injury.

REFERENCES

1. Carter DR, and Frankel VH: Biomechanics of hyperextension injuries to the cervical spine in football, Am J Sports Med 8:302, 1980.
2. Clancy WG, Jr, et al: Upper trunk brachial plexus injuries in contact sports, Am J Sports Med 5:209, 1977.
3. Clarke KS: A survey of sports-related spinal cord injuries in schools and colleges, 1973-1975, J Safety Res 9:140, 1977.
4. Clarke K, et al: First annual gymnastics catastrophic injury report, Washington DC, 1980, U.S. Gymnastics Safety Association.
5. Cloward RB: Acute cervical spine injuries, CIBA Clincal Symposia 32(1), 1980.
6. Edwards WC and LaRocca H: The developmental segmental sagittal diameter of the cervical spinal canal in patients with cervical spondylosis, Spine 8:20, 1983.
7. Ellis WG, et al: The trampoline and serious neurological injuries: a report of five cases, JAMA 174:1673, 1960.
8. Feriencik K: Trends in ice hockey injuries: 1965 to 1977, Phys Sportsmed 7:81, 1979.
9. Gant TT, and Puffer J: Cervical stenosis: a developmental anomaly with quadriparesis during football, Am J Sports Med 4:219, 1976.
10. Goss CM: Gray's anatomy of the human body, ed 29 (American), Philadelphia, 1973, Lea & Febiger.
11. Hollinshead WH: Anatomy for surgeons: the back and limbs, ed 3, Philadelphia, 1982, Harper & Row, Publishers, Inc.
12. Hoskins T: Rugby injuries to the cervical spine in English schoolboys, Practitioner 223:365, 1979.
13. Ladd AL, and Scranton PE: Congenital cervical stenosis presenting as transient quadriplegia in athletes, J Bone and Joint Surg 68A (9):1371, ?
14. Moiel RH, et al: Central cord syndrome resulting from congenital narrowness of the cervical spine canal, J Trauma 10:502, 1970.
15. Murone I: The importance of the sagittal diameters of the cervical spine in relation to spondylosis and myelopathy, J Bone Joint Surg 56B (1):30, 1974.
16. Edwards WC, and LaRocca H: The developmental segmental sagittal diameter of the cervical spinal canal in patients with cervical spondylosis, Spine 8:20, 1983.
17. Penning L: Some aspects of plain radiography of the cervical spine in chronic myeolopathy, Neurology 12:513, 1962.
18. Roaf R: A study of the mechanics of spinal injuries, J Bone Joint Surg 42B:8, 1960.
19. Schneider RC: Serious and fatal neurosurgical football injuries, Clin Neurosurg 12:226, 1966.
20. Seddon H: Surgical disorders of the peripheral nerves, Edinburgh, 1972, Churchill-Livingstone.
21. Shields CL, Jr, Fox JM, and Stauffer ES: Cervical cord injuries in sports, Phys Sportsmed 6(9):71, 1978.
22. Torg JS, et al: National Football Head and Neck Injury Registry: Report and conclusions 1978, JAMA 241:1477, 1979.
23. Torg JS: Athletic injuries to the head, neck and face, Philadelphia, 1982, Lea & Febiger.
24. Torg JS, et al: Neurapraxia of the cervical spine cord with transient quadriplegia, J Bone Joint Surg 68A (9):1354, 1986.
25. Virgin H: Cineradiographic study of football helmets and the cervical spine, Am J Sports Med 8:310, 1980.
26. White AA, et al: Biomechanical analysis of clinical stability in the cervical spine, Clin Orthop 109:85, 1975.

PART II Shoulder

CHAPTER 2 Anatomy of the Shoulder

John A. Hurley

To describe the anatomy of the shoulder joint, one may be more accurate by using the term "the shoulder joint *complex*." There are really four joints composing the shoulder joint complex—the glenohumeral, the acromioclavicular, the sternoclavicular, and the scapular thoracic articulation—rather than just the shoulder joint, which many people interpret as being just the glenohumeral joint (Fig. 2-1). The shoulder joint complex is unique in that it connects the axial skeleton and the remainder of the upper extremity. The concerted action of these four joints enables one to use the remainder of the upper extremity with efficiency and accuracy. The shoulder joint complex, because of its bony configuration, flexibility, and gliding motions, gives one the ability to use the upper extremity in a multitude of positions and motions. If for any reason one of these joints is injured, this can alter one's ability to use the remainder of the upper extremity with any degree of precision.[51]

DEVELOPMENT OF THE SHOULDER JOINT COMPLEX

The development of the shoulder joint complex has been studied by several authors. It begins in utero from a number of ossification centers.* (Fig. 2-2).

Humerus

The humerus begins to ossify in early intrauterine development somewhere between the fourth and ninth weeks of gestation.[13,24,29,31] The ossification centers that represent the humeral metaphysis as well as the diaphysis are ossified at time of birth, while those of the proximal and distal epiphysis remain unossified.[24,68] The proximal humerus

*References 10, 24-26, 29, 37, 47, 48, 64.

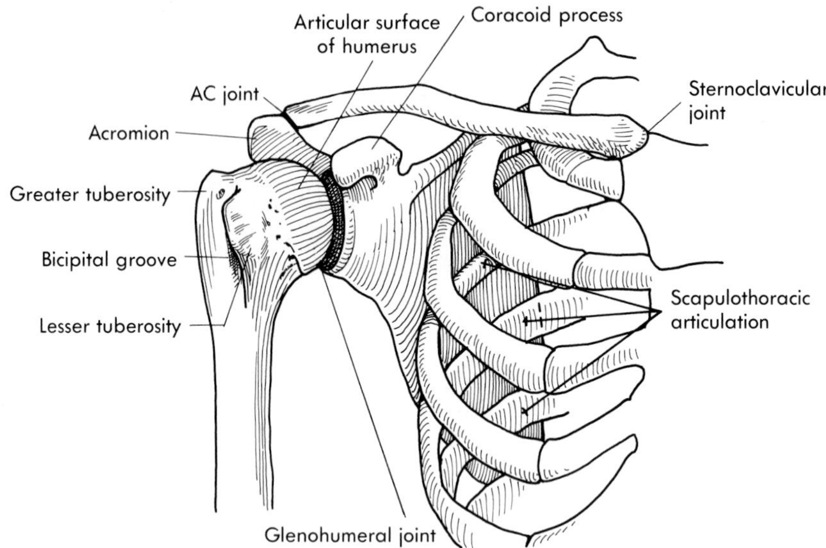

FIG. 2-1. The shoulder joint complex: the acromioclavicular joint, sternoclavicular joint, glenohumeral joint, and scapulothoracic articulation.

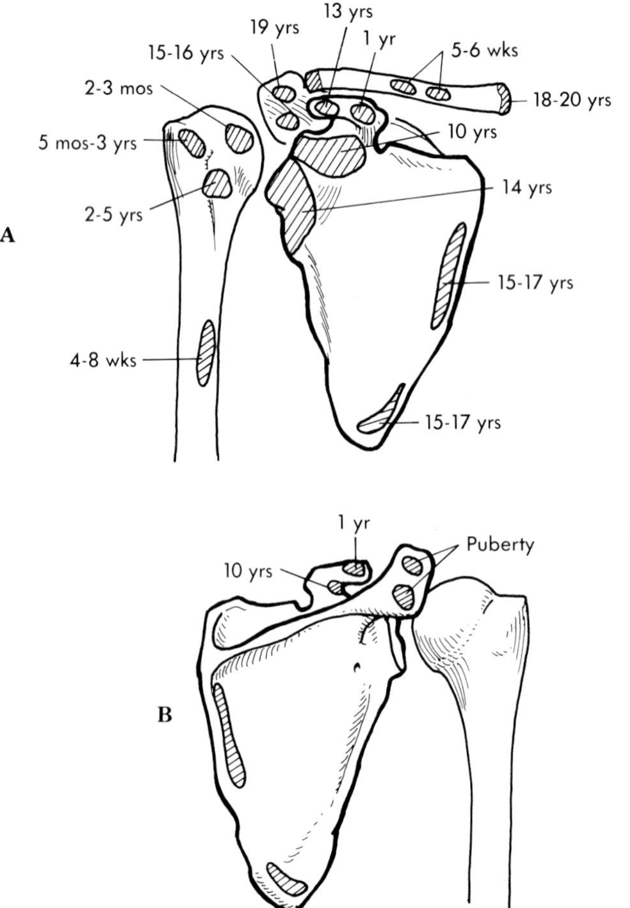

FIG. 2-2. Ossification centers. **A**, Scapula and humerus. **B**, Clavicle.

develops from three separate centers of ossification, the first one being for that of the head and the other two being for the greater and lesser tuberosities. The ossification center for the humeral head appears at approximately 2 to 3 months after birth but at times may not be visualized until approximately the sixth month of postnatal development.* Approximately 20% of newborn infants will demonstrate roentgenographic evidence of ossification of the proximal humeral epiphysis at birth.[48,68] The ossification center for the greater tuberosity does not develop until some time between the fifth month and third year of life; the center for the lesser tuberosity, appearing approximately 2 years after that for the greater tuberosity, usually appears some time in the third year of life.[11,19,48,62] The greater tuberosity then fuses first to the lesser tuberosity, and these coalesce with the ossification center for the humeral head at approximately the fifth to the seventh year of age roentgenographically.[62] Ogden has noted microscopic evidence of fusion at an earlier stage.[48] The proximal humerus fuses with the humeral shaft during the late teens for females and approximately 1 year later for males. In addition, the proximal humerus accounts for approximately 80% of the growth of the entire humerus, with the distal epiphysis accounting for the remaining 20%[19,68]

Clavicle

The development of the clavicle also begins in the early fetal stage and is the first bone to ossify.[25,27,68] The clavicle develops from intramembranous bone, with the primary center for ossification occurring from two separate areas in the central portion of the shaft of the clavicle.[47] These fuse quite rapidly during early fetal development, somewhere between the fifth and sixth week of gestation. Epiphyses then appear at either end of the clavicle, with the medial or sternal epiphysis appearing at approximately 18 to 19 years of age (range 12 to 22 years) and usually fusing with the remainder of the clavicle during the early to middle twenties.[19,27,31,47] The medial or sternal growth plate contributes most to the longitudinal growth of the clavicle, accounting for approximately 80% of the entire length; the lateral or acromial growth place account for the other 20%.[47] The lateral epiphysis, although rare in occurrence, has been noted to appear at approximately 19 to 20 years of age; however, it fuses quite rapidly after its appearance with the remainder of the clavicle and therefore may not be as readily detectable roentgenographically as many of the other ossification centers.[64,68]

*References 11, 19, 24, 37, 48.

Scapula

The development of the scapula also begins in utero beginning at approximately 2 months' gestation, with the scapular body being the only portion that is well ossified at the time of birth.[13,19,27,68] However, complete ossification of the scapula does not occur until well into the early twenties. The scapula develops from multiple ossification centers; one of the earliest ones is that of the middle portion of the coracoid process, which appears as early as 4 months of age, but may not be apparent until 15 to 18 months of age[13,59,62,68] The second ossification center appears at the base of the coracoid process, which becomes apparent at approximately age 10 to 11; this ossification center also contributes to the formation of the superior 25% of the glenoid fossa. The coracoid may also have several other ossification centers. One appears at the tip of the coracoid process during the middle teens. It resembles a shell-like pattern at the coracoid tip, which roentgenographically may be mistaken for an avulsion fracture.* (Fig. 2-3).

The acromion also has two to five multiple ossification centers appearing during the early to middle teens. These have been named by various authors as the preacromion, mesoacromion, metaacromion, and basiacromion; they usually fuse first with each other and then with the remainder of the body of the scapula during the early to middle twenties.[19,31,59,68] However, at times they may remain unfused, leading to a condition known as "os acromiale," which was originally noted by Liberson in 3% of the cases he studied, with bilateral involvement in 60%. Other authors have noted an incidence of somewhere between 7% and 15%.[40,41,45,68] (Fig. 2-4).

Other ossification centers originating during scapular development appear along the vertebral border of the scapula and along the inferior angle of the scapula. Both of these appear during puberty and fuse with the remainder of the body during the late teens to early twenties. The final ossification center to be discussed in regard to the scapula, and perhaps most important, is that for the remainder of the glenoid. This is formed from a horseshoe-shaped epiphysis that forms the

*References 13, 19, 37, 58, 68.

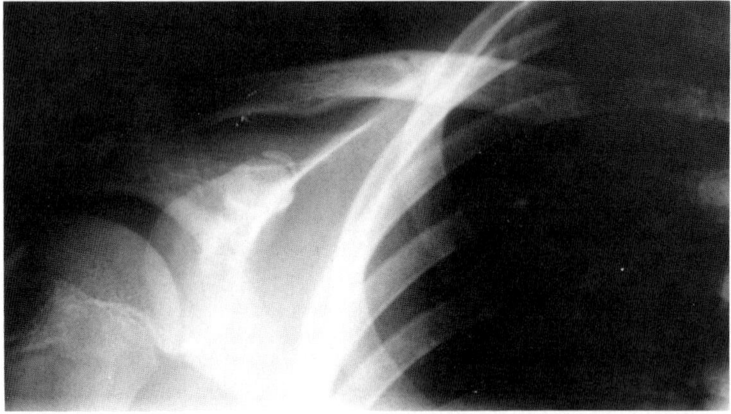

FIG. 2-3. Roentgenogram demonstrating ossification center at the tip of the coracoid, which may be interpreted as an avulsion fracture.

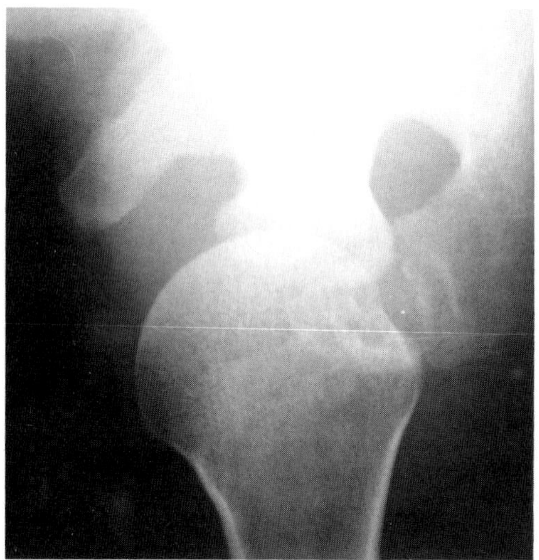

FIG. 2-4. Roentgenogram of os acromiale demonstrating failure of fusion between mesaacromion and metaacromion.

inferior three fourths of the glenoid fossa. This center appears at puberty and fuses with the remainder of the scapula during the late teens to early twenties.[59,62]

▪ ▪ ▪

Being aware of these many ossification centers and the time frames during which they appear and fuse may be quite helpful to one in evaluating roentgenograms of adolescents sustaining trauma, as well as in evaluating certain developmental deformities that may be congenital, secondary to growth arrest, or a maldevelopment of one these ossification centers.

OSTEOLOGY OF THE SHOULDER JOINT COMPLEX

Clavicle

The initial bone to note in a discussion of the bony architecture of the shoulder joint complex is the clavicle, because it serves as the connection between the axial skeleton and the appendicular skeleton of the upper extremity. The clavicle has an S-shaped configuration with a convex anterior border medially and a concave anterior border laterally. It has a cylindrical configuration medially, being somewhat thicker, while laterally it becomes flattened and narrow. The S-shaped configuration of the clavicle gives it some inherent stability and mobility during elevation of the upper extremity.

Sternoclavicular Joint

Medially, the clavicle articulates with the sternum as well as with the first rib, forming a synovial articulation. Laterally the clavicle articulates with the acromion to once again form a synovial joint. The articulation between the clavicle and the sternum medially and with the first rib is a relatively incongruent joint, with only 50% of the clavicle articulating with the manubrium and first rib and the remainder being prominent superiorly.[19]

Acromioclavicular Joint

A similar situation occurs laterally where the clavicle articulates with the acromion. This is a somewhat incongruous articulation. The clavicle serves as the origin and insertion for several muscles about the upper extremity that support it, with roughened surfaces ap-

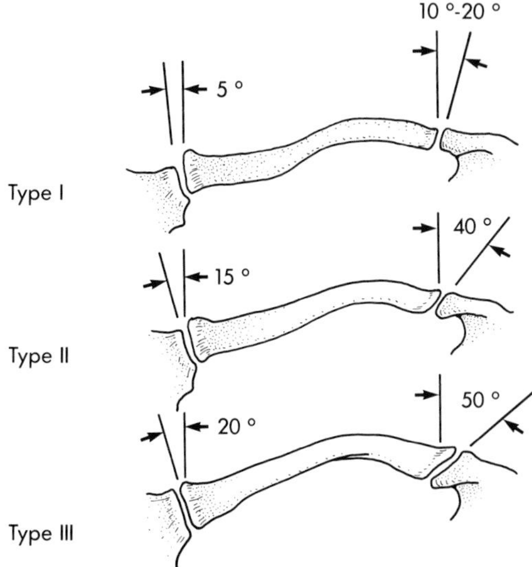

FIG. 2-5. Variations in the acromioclavicular and sternoclavicular articulations.

pearing on both the superior and the anterior borders of the clavicle, which serve as attachment sites for these muscles. DePalma described varying morphologies to the lateral end of the clavicle with regard to both its torsion and its articulation with the acromion.[16,18,19] These could basically be broken down to three types: type 1 has a relatively vertically oriented joint; type 2 has a more oblique configuration sloping medially at its inferior surface; and type 3 has an almost horizontal angulation between the acromion and clavicle (Fig. 2-5). Moseley also described a variety of articulations between the lateral clavicle and acromion.[43] One type of articulation overrides the place where the clavicle is superior to the acromion, similar to DePalma's type 2. One has a vertical incongruency similar to DePalma's type 1. A third type has an underriding articulation where the clavicle articulates on the undersurface of the acromion. The clinical significance of these according to DePalma was the fact that the majority of patients with degenerative changes at the acromioclavicular joint had type 1 clavicles, which he felt was secondary to the increased shear forces acting on the articular surface in this type of joint. Also the type 1 joints were smaller in comparison to the types 2 and 3, thereby increasing their contact forces.

Scapula

The scapula is the other bone that makes up the shoulder joint complex. It is composed of the scapular body, the scapular spine, the acromion, the scapular neck, the glenoid fossa, and the coracoid process.

Scapula components

- Body
- Neck
- Spine
- Glenoid
- Coracoid

Body

The body of the scapula is a large, flattened, triangular area situated on the posterior lateral aspect of the upper thorax between the second and seventh ribs, oriented 30 to 45 degrees anterior to the coronal plane of the body.[6] The costal surface is concave and is known as the "subscapular fossa," whereas the dorsal surface is convex and divided by the spine of the scapula into a supraspinous and infraspinous fossa, with these latter two communicating by way of the spinoglenoid notch. At the superior border of the supraspinous fossa is the supraspinous notch through which travels the suprascapular nerve. The notch is turned into a closed space by the suprascapular ligament, which travels from the superior corners of the notch. Above the ligament travels the suprascapular artery (see Fig. 2-12). The suprascapular nerve can become entrapped as it travels through the notch by thickening of the ligament secondary to trauma or fracture, or on occasion ganglia have been reported to cause compression of the nerve as it travels through the notch.[22,53]

Coracoid Process

The coracoid process is a bony projection off the anterior surface of the scapula just medial to the scapular neck (see Fig. 2-1). The coracoid projects anteriorly and laterally and has a hooked configuration; it serves as the origin and insertion of several muscle and ligaments that will be discussed later. The coracoid process lies near the junction of the lateral and middle thirds of the clavicle and can generally be easily palpated along the medial border of the deltoid muscle. It serves as an important landmark in surgical procedures about the shoulder, because the neurovascular structures travel along the inferior medial surface of the coracoid.

Acromion

The acromion has received a great deal of attention in regard to its configuration and orientation and the effect it has on various pathologic conditions that affect the shoulder. The slope of the acromion has been studied to evaluate its association with pathologic conditions of the rotator cuff.[2,7,42,46] Several investigators have examined the slope of the acromion by obtaining lateral roentgenograms of the scapula. They measure the angle formed by a line joining the posteroinferior aspect of the acromion and the anterior margin of the acromion with a line formed by joining the posteroinferior aspect of the acromion and the inferior tip of the coracoid process. From these measurements a system to classify the various **angles of inclination of the acromion** has been developed: type 1 acromions have a relatively high angle or flat undersurface; type 2 have a downward curve and a decreased angle of inclination; and type 3 have almost a hooked-shape configuration along the anterior portion of the acromion and a further reduction of the angle of inclination. According to these authors, the lower the angle of inclination the higher the association with pathologic conditions of the rotator cuff.

Glenoid Fossa

The glenoid has also been investigated once again to determine whether any abnormalities exist in the configuration of the glenoid that may lead to the development of shoulder disorders.* The glenoid has a comma-shaped appearance, with the tail superior and the head inferior. Several investigators have evaluated the version of the glenoid to see whether an abnormal glenoid version existed in patients with instability patterns about the shoulder. Das, Saha, and Roy were some of the earlier investigators, and they found the normal version of the glenoid to be retroverted approximately 2 to 12 degrees.[15] Studies by this author and others using computed tomography (CT) scans have noted a mean retroversion of between 2 and 7 degrees in a normal patient population.[14,33,39,54] Saha found that patients with anterior instability tended to have an increased anteversion of the glenoid; however, this has not been substantiated by other investigators.[14,15] Studies on posterior instability of the shoulder have also focused on the version of the glenoid, with one author noting an increased retroversion of −15 degrees on plain roentgenograms of his patient population, with posterior instability of the shoulder. Studies by this author noted an increased retroversion in his patient population of between −9 and −10 degrees as determined by CT scans.[9,33] Therefore it appears that the glenoid may have varying version angles that may contribute to instability patterns about the shoulder, especially in patients with posterior instability.

*References 14, 15, 33, 39, 54.

Proximal Humerus

The final bone in discussing the shoulder joint complex is the proximal humerus, which consists of the head, the anatomic neck, which is a slight constriction lateral to the articular surface, and the greater and lesser tuberosities.

Tuberosities

The **greater tuberosity** is the most lateral structure on the superior aspect of the humerus and projects superiorly as well as posteriorly; the **lesser tuberosity** is situated along the anterior margin of the proximal humerus. The tuberosities are separated by the intertubercular groove through which passes the biceps tendon. The proximal end of the humerus connects with the shaft of the humerus, via the surgical neck.

Glenohumeral Articulation

The humeral head that articulates with the glenoid has been studied by several investigators once again to determine normal vs. abnormal anatomy. It has been found that the humeral head has a slight retroversion in relationship to the humeral epicondyles measuring approximately 20 to 35 degrees, whereas the angle formed by the humeral head and shaft was found to be between 130 and 150 degrees.[14,19,34,61] Abnormalities in the version of the humeral head have not been found in conjunction with shoulder instability problems.[14,39,54] As previously mentioned, the proximal end of the humerus articulates with the glenoid in what one would assume be a perfect sphere. However, Saha has noted a relative incongruency in this articulation. He noted three different types of glenohumeral articulation being based on the relative size of the humeral head in comparison to the glenoid, with the size of the humeral head being smaller, equal to, or larger than the corresponding radius of curvature of the glenoid.[60,61] This may have some significance in relationship to patients with instability patterns, as noted by one study in which patients with recurrent dislocations were noted to have a smaller glenoid diameter in relationship to the humeral head, which therefore decreased the effective contact surface and made a somewhat more unstable configuration.[14,54,60]

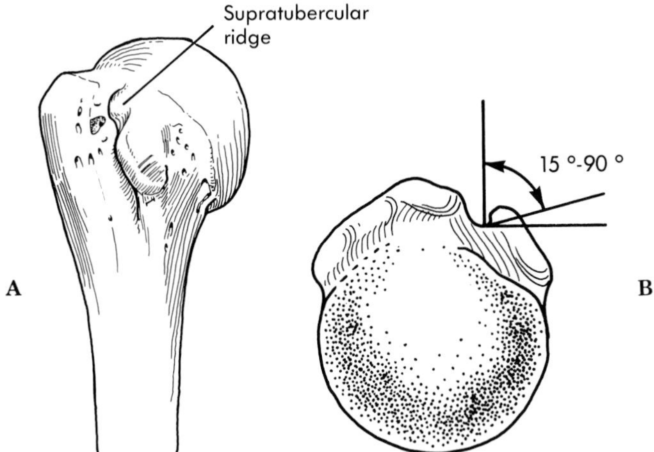

FIG. 2-6. A, Bicipital groove with supratubercular ridge. **B,** Angle of inclination, of medial wall.

Bicipital Groove

Finally, as previously mentioned, the bicipital groove travels between the greater and lesser tuberosities and lies along the anterior aspect of the surface of the humerus. The bicipital groove may demonstrate varying configurations, as noted by Hitchcock, depending on the height of the medial wall of the groove, which is formed by the lesser tuberosity. (Fig. 2-6).[19,30] In 70% of the specimens he studied, the medial wall had a height of about 60 to 90 degrees in relationship to the floor of the groove, with the remaining specimens having a lower medial wall. DePalma has also noted this, as well as the presence of a supratubercular ridge of bone in the superior portion of the groove, which projects from the lesser tuberosity. He thought that a combination of a supratubercular ridge and a decreased height of the medial wall may predispose an individual to instability of the bicipital tendon within the groove.[19]

CAPSULAR AND LIGAMENTOUS SUPPORTS OF THE SHOULDER JOINT COMPLEX

The joints that make up the shoulder joint complex are relatively unconstrained and rely heavily on the surrounding soft tissue structures for stability.

Sternoclavicular Joint

The sternoclavicular joint, as noted previously, is composed of two relatively incongruent surfaces, the medial end of the clavicle and the posterior lateral aspect of the manubrium and first rib (Fig. 2-7).[16] With only the inferior portion of the clavicle articulating with the manubrium and first rib, the presence of a **fibrocartilaginous disk** between these two surfaces serves to improve the articular congruency of these two surfaces. The fibrocartilaginous disk divides the joint almost completely in half and attaches superiorly to the upper medial end of the clavicle and passes downward between the articular surfaces to attach to the first costal cartilage.[5,16-18] In a small percentage of the specimens studied by DePalma, there was a perforation within the substance of the disk.[17] He thought that the disk acted as a buffer in protecting the joint from degenerative change, as well as in stabilizing the sternoclavicular joint.[17] Degenerative changes in the sternoclavicular joint were not noted to significantly occur until somewhere in the seventh decade. The joint is further supported by the capsule, anterior and posterior sternoclavicular ligaments, interclavicular ligament, and costoclavicular ligaments. The **costoclavicular ligaments** extend from the undersurface of the proximal end of the clavicle to the superior surface of the first rib and are composed of an anterior and posterior fasciculus.[5,12,18] The anterior bundle travels upward and lateral from the first costal cartilage to the proximal end of the clavicle, while the posterior bundle travels upward and medially. These two bundles become unified along their lateral margins and there is a bursa between the two bundles.[12,18] The **interclavicular ligament** runs across the superior aspect of the manubrium to join the medial ends of both clavicles. Bearn[5] studied the anatomy of the sternoclavicular joint and assessed the various ligaments in regard to their stabilizing effect on the joint and in maintaining clavicular poise. He identified the capsule, the interclavicular ligaments, costoclavicular ligaments, and the fibrocartilaginous disk and did selective cutting studies to determine the effect each ligament had on maintaining the clavicular poise. He found that it was not until he cut the capsule of joint that he found complete downward depression of the lateral end of the clavicle, and therefore he thought that this was the main supporting structure of this joint, whereas cutting the remaining ligaments had little effect on clavicular poise. Cave,[12] on the other hand, thought that the costoclavicular ligaments were important in maintaining clavicular stability in the studies that he did.

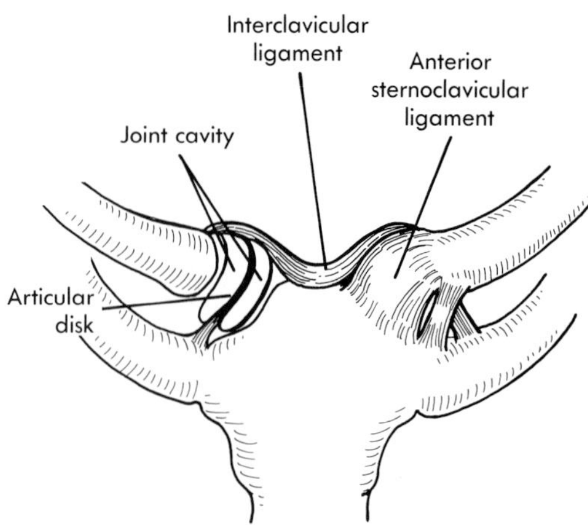

FIG. 2-7. Sternoclavicular joint with interposed fibrocartilaginous disk and surrounding ligaments.

Sternoclavicular joint supporting structures

- Capsule
- Anterior sternoclavicular ligament
- Posterior sternoclavicular ligament
- Costoclavicular ligament
- Interclavicular ligament
- Sternohyoid muscle
- Sternothyroid muscle
- Sternocleidomastoid muscle

The sternoclavicular joint is further supported by the sternohyoid and sternothyroid muscles, which attach immediately behind the sternoclavicular joint and the sternocleidomastoid muscle, which attaches in front. These muscles also act as important barriers to the great vessels that lie directly behind them.

Acromioclavicular Joint

The acromioclavicular joint is formed by the lateral end of the clavicle and acromion (Fig. 2-8). This articulation is also a relatively incongruent one for which nature, once again, has provided an intraarticular **fibrocartilaginous disk** to improve congruity. DePalma noted that the disk undergoes degeneration and found a significant amount of disk degeneration as well as articular cartilage changes in the bone as early as the second decade, with the disk almost completely degenerated by the fourth decade.[16] The acromioclavicular joint is reinforced by the surrounding capsule and ligaments, containing an anterior, posterior, superior, and inferior component, in addition to the coracoclavicular ligaments, which are composed of two individual ligaments, the **conoid and trapezoid ligaments.** The acromioclavicular ligaments extend from the acromion to the clavicle circumferentially around the joint, while the conoid and trapezoid ligaments extend from the undersurface of the clavicle to the tip of the coracoid process and function mainly as suspensory ligaments for the upper extremity. The conoid ligament is cone shaped and attaches on the posteromedial aspect of the coracoid, with its base being attached to the undersurface of the clavicle. The trapezoid ligament extends from the anterior lateral base of the coracoid to insert onto the undersurface of the clavicle also. The coracoclavicular ligaments attach along the posterior curve of the clavicle and are very important in helping to rotate the clavicle on its long access with overhead activity.[19] Several investigators have studied the stabilizing effects that each set of ligaments has on the acromioclavicular joint.[21,58,67] Urist, one of the original investigators, found that the coracoclavicular ligaments are important in controlling vertical stability while the acromioclavicular ligaments function primarily in restraining posterior translation of the clavicle.[67] Fukuda et al, in biomechanical studies on the ligamentous system of the acromioclavicular joint, have confirmed Urist's findings and have also determined the important influence the acromioclavicular ligaments have on controlling posterior axial rotation of the clavicle in addition to posterior displacement.[21] They

Acromioclavicular joint supporting structures

- Acromioclavicular ligaments
- Coracoclavicular ligaments

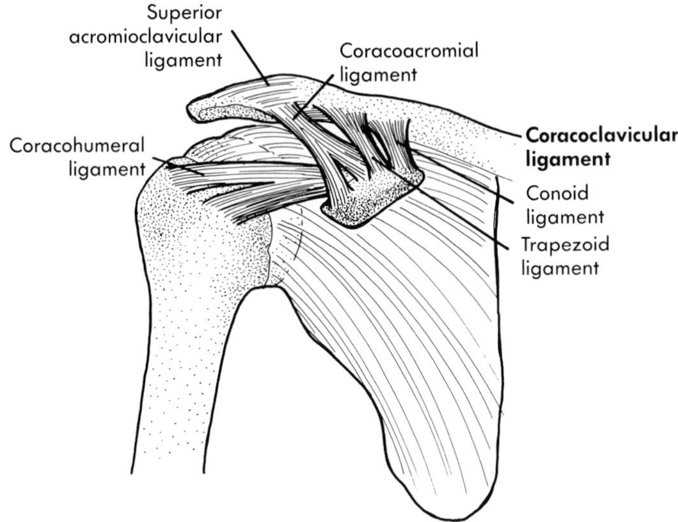

FIG. 2-8. The acromioclavicular joint with surrounding ligaments, including the coracoclavicular, coracoacromial, and coracohumeral ligament.

also found that the conoid ligament was the primary restraint to anterior and superior displacement of the clavicle.

Glenohumeral Joint

The glenohumeral joint can be compared to a golf ball sitting on the tee with minimal restraints. It relies on the surrounding joint capsule and ligaments to provide static stability and also the surrounding muscles, that is the rotator cuff, to provide dynamic stability. The glenoid only articulates with approximately 30% of the humeral head, whereas this contact surface is increased to approximately 75% by the glenoid labrum.[50,61]

Labrum

The labrum was once thought to be a fibrocartilaginous structure surrounding the glenoid and providing further stability; however, studies by Moseley and Overgaard have demonstrated it to be a redundant fold of capsular tissue with a minimal fibrocartilaginous component near its transitional zone.[24,44] The labrum, in and of itself, does not appear to provide much stability to the glenohumeral joint.[44,68] The labrum is continuous with the articular cartilage of the glenoid; it centrally and laterally functions as the insertion site for the glenohumeral ligament. DePalma has shown in cadaver dissections that the superior portion of the labrum dissociates from the underlying glenoid with advancing age.[20] Other authors have noted this phenomenon in throwing athletes; this has been attributed to the pull of the biceps tendon during the throwing arc.[1]

Glenohumeral Ligaments

The glenohumeral ligaments have been studied by many investigators and have been described in Gray's *Anatomy* as being capsular thickenings.* The capsule of the glenohumeral joint is two times the surface area of the humeral head, which provides one with the ability to move the arm throughout a large arc of motion that is unique to the glenohumeral joint.[36] Studies on the strength of the glenohumeral joint capsule have shown it to be twice as strong as that of the elbow, as well as having a greater stretching capacity.[36] As previously mentioned, the ligaments insert onto the labrum and glenoid neck. Reeves has shown in his studies that the weakest point of this attachment site in the young is at the labral site, while in the elderly the capsule and subscapularis tendon tear laterally in a dislocating shoulder.[57]

Three ligaments have been defined anteriorly and are referred to as the **superior, middle, and inferior glenohumeral ligaments** (Fig. 2-9). Superiorly, the **coracohumeral ligament** also provides stability to the shoulder. The coracohumeral ligament extends from the base of the coracoid process to the top of the bicipital groove on the greater tuberosity. It covers the interval between the supraspinatus and subscapularis and has been found to provide stability to the joint when the arm is in a dependent position.[4] Underneath the coracohumeral ligament is the superior glenohumeral ligament, which orig-

*Reference 13, 27, 36, 44, 49, 57, 65, 66, 68.

inates from the upper segment of the glenoid labrum at the supraglenoid tubercle and base of the coracoid process to insert onto the upper segment of the lesser tuberosity at the anatomic neck. The middle glenohumeral ligament originates from the anterosuperior portion of the glenoid labrum down as far as the junction of the middle and inferior thirds of the glenoid and is directed slightly downward in an oblique direction to insert along the medial aspect of the lesser tuberosity.[66] The middle glenohumeral ligament lies underneath the subscapularis muscle and tendon; this relationship is well demonstrated during arthroscopy.

The inferior glenohumeral ligament is the thickest of the ligaments and reinforces the inferior capsule.[49,66] The inferior glenohumeral ligament originates along the inferior border of the glenoid labrum and glenoid rim to attach onto the inferior neck of the humerus. The anterior superior edge is slightly thickened and has been referred to as the superior band of the inferior glenohumeral ligament, while the inferior portion of the ligament is somewhat thinner and has been referred to as the axillary pouch.[66] Tuerkel et al[66] have done studies on the stabilizing effect of the various ligaments about the shoulder, and they found the superior band of the inferior glenohumeral ligament to be the major stabilizer of the glenohumeral joint when the arm is in 90 degrees of abduction and external rotation. These authors also noted that in the neutral position the subscapularis muscle and the middle glenohumeral ligament provided the majority of the stability to the shoulder. With further degrees of abduction, for example, 45 degrees, the stabilizers became the subscapularis, the middle glenohumeral ligament, and the superior portion of the inferior glenohumeral ligament. With further abduction, the subscapularis was positioned superior to the humeral head, uncovering it somewhat anteriorly and inferiorly, thereby providing little stability in this position. Posteriorly, the capsule is rather thin in comparison to the anterior capsule, therefore providing little restraining force to glenohumeral movement posteriorly.

Synovial Recesses

The anterior ligaments can insert directly onto the labrum or their insertion can occur further medially along the scapular neck, forming synovial recesses. These recesses were described by both DePalma and Moseley and can have varying sizes, depending on how far medial along the neck of the scapula the ligaments insert and also depending on their occurrence.[20,44] These authors described several types of recesses, with type 1 occurring above the middle glenohumeral ligament, type 2 occurring as one synovial recess below this middle glenohumeral ligament, type 3 appearing as one above and one below the middle glenohumeral, and type 4 occurring as one large recess above the inferior glenohumeral ligament with the middle glenohumeral being absent. These recesses are clinically important in that they represent a discontinuity in the anterior capsule mechanism and ligamentous structures, which may predispose the shoulder to recurrent instability.[19] In addition, according to DePalma, these recesses prevent the subscapularis tendon from coming into close proximity to the underlying scapular neck, therefore diminishing the dynamic stability provided anteriorly by the subscapularis. The most common of the recesses is that above the middle glenohumeral ligament. In addition to these recesses, many times an interval occurs between the superior and middle glenohumeral ligament. This serves as the entrance to the subscapularis bursa from the glenohumeral joint and may be of variable size and occurrence. It has been implicated as a possible cause for recurrent instability.[13,19,20,44]

Synovial recesses

- Above middle glenohumeral ligament
- Below middle glenohumeral ligament
- Above inferior glenohumeral ligament

CORACOACROMIAL ARCH

The coracoacromial arch is formed by yet another ligament about the glenohumeral joint, that being the **coracoacromial ligament** along with the acromion process (see Fig. 2-8). The coracoacromial ligament is a triangular band containing two fascicles originating from the lateral border of the coracoid from its tip to its base; these then converge laterally to insert on the anterior aspect of the acromion just lateral to the acromioclavicular joint. The ligament extends posteriorly along the acromion to the lateral border of the acromial process.[31] The function of the coracoacromial ligament has not been clearly defined. The coracoacromial arch is a relatively unyielding structure that protects the humeral head from trauma as well as providing

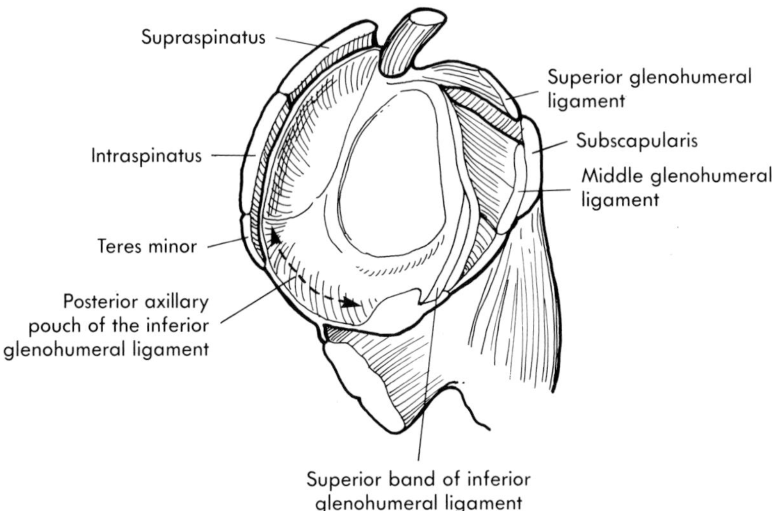

FIG. 2-9. Lateral view of glenoid with surrounding ligaments and muscles.

some stability against superior migration of the humeral head. Between the coracoacromial ligament and the underlying rotator cuff is the subacromial bursa, which is one of the larger bursae about the shoulder complex and gives the shoulder some inherent gliding ability. The bursa extends from the coracoid process medially to the greater tuberosity laterally with further extension posteriorly and anteriorly. There are numerous other bursae surrounding the shoulder joint complex that improve the gliding mechanics of the shoulder and can generally be found between tendons and the underlying bones.

MUSCLES OF THE SHOULDER COMPLEX

The muscles surrounding the shoulder joint complex provide one with the ability to generate motion while at the same time providing dynamic stability to the glenohumeral joint.* Muscles about the shoulder joint complex can basically be broken down into three categories, those attaching to the scapula with their origin from the axial skeleton; those that have their origin from the scapula and insert onto the humerus; and those that have their origin from the axial skeleton and inserting onto the humerus.

Axial Skeleton to Scapula

The first group of muscles, those attaching to the scapula with their origin from the axial skeleton, include the trapezius, levator scapula, rhomboid major and minor, and serratus anterior (Fig. 2-10). The **trapezius muscle** originates from the superior nuchal line and the external occipital protuberance of the skull, the spinous processes of the seven cervical vertebrae, and the spinous processes of all the thoracic vertebrae and their intervening supraspinous ligaments. The upper fibers run obliquely downward to insert along the distal third of the clavicle, whereas the fibers of the lower cervical and upper thoracic region travel laterally to insert onto the acromion, with the fibers from the lower thoracic region traveling laterally and upward to insert along the spine of the scapula. The trapezius is innervated by the spinal accessory nerve, which travels along its undersurface. Lying beneath the trapezius are the levator scapula, rhomboid major and minor, and the serratus anterior.

Scapula to spine muscle attachments

- Trapezius
- Levator scapula
- Rhomboid major
- Rhomboid minor
- Serratus anterior

The **levator scapula** originates from the posterior tubercles of the transverse processes of the first through fourth cervical vertebrae. It inserts into the superior angle of the scapula and along the medial border of the scapula to approximately the level of the scapular spine. It receives its innervation from the cervical plexus and occasionally from the dorsal scapular nerve.

The **rhomboids** also lie deep to the trapezius, with the rhomboid minor arising from

*References 3, 32, 34, 35, 50, 60, 63.

the spinous processes of the seventh cervical and thoracic vertebra and the intervening supraspinous ligament. It inserts along the medial border of the scapula near the base of the scapula spine. The rhomboid major starts from the spinous processes of the second through fifth thoracic vertebrae and their respective supraspinous ligaments, and it also inserts along the medial border of the scapula just below the insertion of the rhomboid minor. Both rhomboids are supplied by the dorsal scapular nerve, which travels on the deep surface of each of these respective muscles close to their scapular insertion.

The **serratus anterior** arises from the outer surface of the first eight ribs and follows the curvature of the ribs to insert along the medial aspect of the scapula on its costal surface. The upper portion of the muscle inserts along the medial border of the scapula, whereas the lower portion inserts at the inferior angle of the scapula, which is thought to be where this muscle has its main action. The serratus anterior is supplied by the long thoracic nerve that travels along the superficial portion of the muscle.

These five muscles act to move the scapula with some of them having more than one function because of the multitude of fibers that make up each muscle.[31,34] The trapezius acts to elevate as well as retract the scapula. The rhomboids and levator scapula primarily retract and rotate the scapula downward. The serratus anterior acts to rotate the scapula upward as well as to protract the scapula. The function of the serratus can be appreciated when there has been injury to the long thoracic nerve, because one will notice winging of the scapula. The most important function of the serratus is to rotate the scapula upward, which happens because of its insertion along the inferior angle of the scapula. Upward rotation of the scapula is also brought out by the trapezius by virtue of its fibers inserting onto the acromion. The concerted action of these two muscles therefore becomes important in rotating the acromion away from the humerus in forward elevation of the upper extremity, thereby avoiding impingement.

The next muscle is the **pectoralis minor,** which is an anterior muscle originating from the axial skeleton in general from the second to fifth rib, with some variability between these and the third through the sixth rib. The pectoralis minor inserts onto the medial aspect of the coracoid process and is covered by the pectoralis major. It serves to protect the neurovascular structures that travel on its inferior surface. The pectoralis minor muscle is innervated by the medial and lateral pectoral nerves.

Scapular motion

- **Trapezius**
  Elevate scapula
  Retract scapula
- **Rhomboids**
  Retract and rotate scapula downward
- **Serratus anterior**
  Rotates scapula upward
- **Levator scapula**
  Retract and rotate scapula downward

Axial Skeleton to Humerus

The next set of muscles, the latissimus dorsi and pectoralis major, begin from the axial skeleton and insert onto the humerus.

Latissimus dorsi

The **latissimus dorsi** starts from the spinous processes of the lower six thoracic vertebra and all of the lumbar and upper cervical vertebrae. It also takes origin from the posterior iliac crest and the lower three ribs; the fibers of the muscle then converge to insert along the anterior surface of the proximal humerus between the pectoralis major and teres major at the crest of the lesser tubercle and the floor of the intertubercular groove. It receives its innervation from the thoracodorsal nerve, which travels on its undersurface; its main function is to adduct, medially rotate, and extend the arm.

The other muscle in this group is the **pectoralis major,** which begins at the medial third of the clavicle, lateral aspect of the manubrium, body of the sternum, and cartilages of the first six ribs. The upper fibers travel in a lateral direction while the lower ones travel up and under the upper fibers, twisting as they go under the upper fibers to insert on

Axial skeleton to humerus

- **Latissimus dorsi**
  Adducts
  Medially rotates
  Extends
- **Pectoralis major**
  Adducts
  Medially rotates

the inferior border of the greater tuberosity at the lateral lip of the intertubercular groove. The pectoralis major is innervated by the lateral and medial pectoral nerves and serves to adduct and medially rotate the arm.

Scapula to Humerus

The next set of muscles originates from the scapula and inserts onto the humerus. The most superficial muscle in this group is the deltoid, while the deeper muscles include the rotator cuff (i.e., supraspinatus, infraspinatus, subscapularis, and teres' minor) and the teres' major.

Deltoid

The deltoid originates from the lateral third of the clavicle, the acromion, and the spine of the scapula, and inserts into the deltoid tuberosity along the anterior lateral aspect of the proximal humerus. The middle portion of the deltoid that arises from the lateral aspect of the acromion is the most powerful portion of the muscle because of its interposed tendon-like septa that serve as both the origin and the insertion of numerous muscle fibers, giving the deltoid muscle a multipennate configuration. The deltoid receives its innervation from the axillary nerve, which winds around the humeral neck and then travels along the undersurface of the deltoid at approximately the level of the inferior aspect of the glenohumeral joint.

Scapula to humerus muscles

- Deltoid
- Supraspinatus
- Subscapularis
- Teres major
- Teres minor
- Infraspinatus

Rotator Cuff

Functional anatomy. The rotator cuff muscles act to dynamically stabilize the shoulder. This has been studied by many investigators in patients with recurrent instability of the shoulder.* The subscapularis muscle in particular has been identified as the cause of recurrent instability by the fact that it becomes attenuated through repeated dislocations.[63] Jobe has noted on electromyogram (EMG) analysis a misfiring of the subscapularis muscle in patients with anterior instability.[28] Others have noted the ability to decrease the incidence of recurring instability with a rehabilitative program focused at strengthening the internal rotators, especially the subscapular.[3] Cain et al showed the importance of the posterior shoulder muscles (i.e., the infraspinatus and teres minor) in controlling external rotatory forces about the shoulder, thereby decreasing the strain on the inferior glenohumeral ligaments and adding a restraining force to anterior dislocation.[11] Basmajian has noted the importance of the supraspinatus muscle and superior capsule in preventing downward subluxation of the humeral head with respect to the glenoid.[4,32] It therefore becomes apparent that the function of all the rotator cuff muscles is extremely important in dynamically stabilizing the glenohumeral joint.

Vascular anatomy. The blood supply to the rotator cuff has also been studied by various investigators noting an arterial supply to the tendons of the rotator cuff coming from their respective muscle bellies; the supraspinatus is noted to have a relative area of avascularity approximately 1 cm from its insertion to the greater tuberosity. This was rather consistent in all the specimens at all ages studied by Rathbun and MacNab.[55] This zone of relative avascularity has been implicated as the cause for degeneration of the supraspinatus tendon and as a cause of rotator cuff tears.

Subscapularis muscle. The subscapularis muscle arises from the costal surface of the scapula, with its muscles converging into an anterior tendon that inserts onto the lesser tuberosity of the humerus. It is innervated by the subscapularis nerve.

Supraspinatus. The supraspinatus muscle arises from the supraspinous fossa and passes laterally under the coracoacromial arch to attach to the greater tuberosity. It is supplied by the suprascapular nerve and vessels that travel on its undersurface.

Infraspinatus. The infraspinatus muscle arises from the infraspinous fossa and travels laterally to insert on the posterior aspect of the greater tuberosity. It is also supplied by the suprascapular nerve and vessels.

Teres minor. The teres minor muscle arises from the central third of the lateral border of the scapula below the scapular neck to pass behind the long head of the triceps and insert onto the lower posterior aspect of the greater tuberosity.

Teres major. Finally, the teres major muscle arises from the lower third of the lateral border of the scapula and travels around the anterior aspect of the humerus and in front of the long

*References 3, 4, 11, 28, 35, 51, 52, 60, 63.

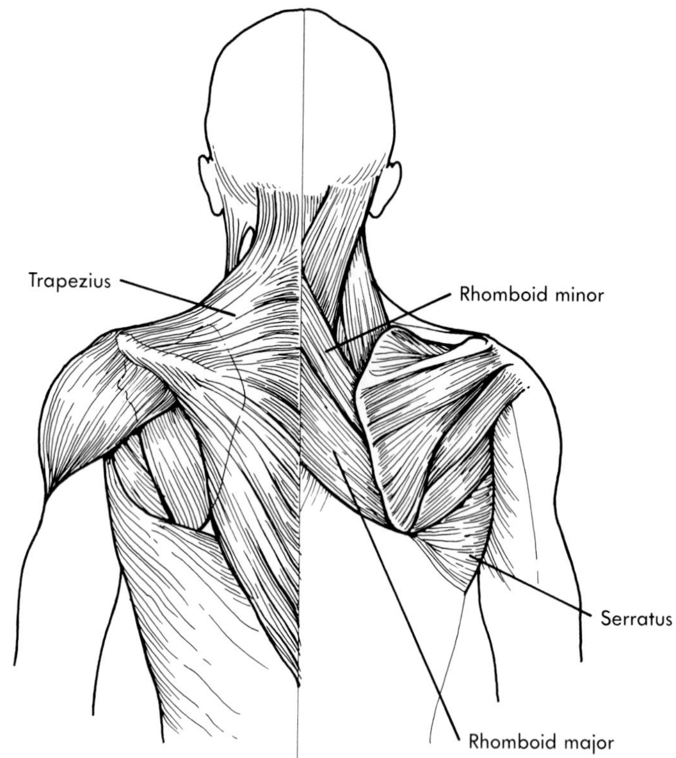

FIG. 2-10. Posterior view of superficial and deep muscles connecting the axial skeleton to the scapula.

head of the triceps to insert onto the crest of the lesser tubercle. The lower border of the teres minor posteriorly corresponds to the lower border of the subscapularis muscle anteriorly.

The upper border of the teres major along with the lower border of the teres minor and the long head of the triceps form a space called the **triangular space,** through which travel the scapular circumflex vessels (Fig. 2-11).[13,27,31,68] Lateral to this is the **quadrangular or quadrilateral space** formed by the lower border of the teres minor, the upper border of the teres major, the lateral border of the long head of the triceps, and the medial border of the humerus, through which travel the axillary nerve and the posterior humeral circumflex artery.* The teres minor and deltoid receive their innervation by the axillary nerve, whereas the teres major is supplied by the lower subscapular nerve.

Biceps

The last muscle tendon unit of the shoulder joint complex to discuss is that of the biceps and biceps tendon. The biceps originates via its long head at the superior border of the labrum and by its short head from the coracoid process. These portions converge distally and finally insert into the bicipital tuberosity of the radius. The intercapsular portion of the biceps is tendinous; it travels distally to enter the intertubercular groove as it exits the glenohumeral joint. The synovial lining of the glenohumeral joint accompanies the biceps tendon as it exits into the intertubercular groove.* Because of its attachment to the superior labrum, it has been implicated as being a deforming force in causing superior labral tears in the throwing athlete.[1] Its function is thought by some to act as a depressor of the humeral head when the arm is in external rotation, because in this position it travels over the top of the humeral head.

*References 13, 27, 31, 56, 68.

NEUROVASCULAR SUPPLY TO THE SHOULDER JOINT COMPLEX

Arterial Supply

The arterial circulation to the shoulder joint complex is derived mainly from the axillary artery, which is a continuation of the subclavian artery into the axilla. As it continues into the arm, it becomes the brachial artery and

*References 13, 19, 27, 31, 68.

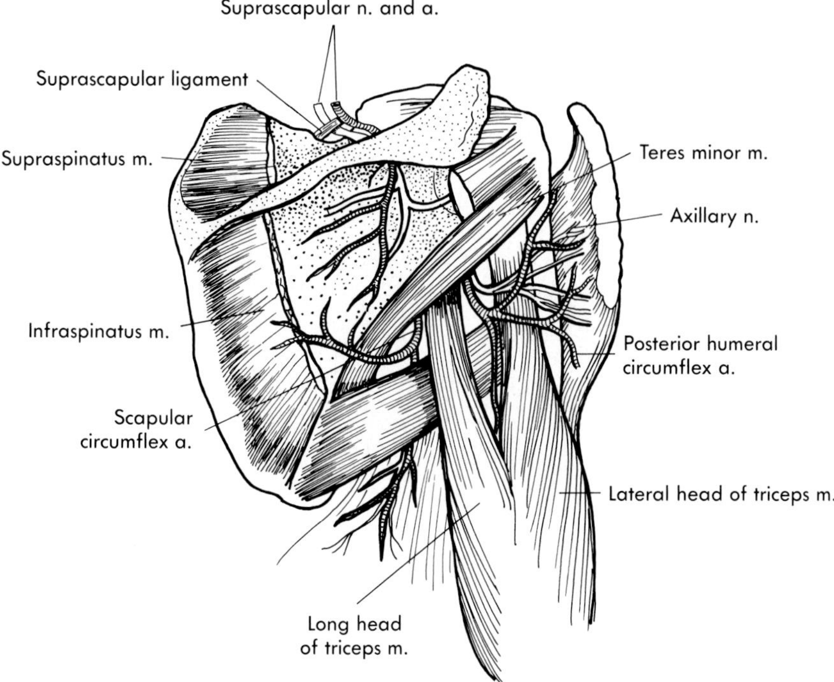

FIG. 2-11. Posterior view of shoulder with quadrangular space containing the axillary nerve and posterior humeral circumflex artery; and triangular space containing the scapular circumflex artery.

Axillary artery branches

- Superior thoracic artery
- Thoracoacromial artery
- Lateral thoracic artery
- Subscapularis artery
- Anterior humeral circumflex artery
- Posterior humeral circumflex artery

finally divides into its two terminal branches, the radial and ulnar arteries. The axillary artery gives off six main branches to supply the shoulder joint complex: the superior thoracic artery, the thoracoacromial artery, the lateral thoracic, the subscapularis, and the anterior and posterior circumflex humeral vessels (Fig. 2-11).[27] Proximal to the axillary artery in the region of the subclavian division, a branch is given off called the thyrocervical trunk; from this arises the suprascapular artery, which supplies the supraspinatus and infraspinatus muscle. The main arteries traveling toward the shoulder joint complex itself are those composing the acromial branch of the thoracoacromial artery, which passes above the coracoacromial ligament. It is important to be aware of this branch when dissecting in this area during surgery that requires release of the coracoacromial ligament, because it may lead to excessive bleeding if cut. The anterior and posterior humeral circumflex arteries arise at the lower border of the subscapularis muscle and can be injured in surgical dissections for recurrent dislocations, fractures, or joint replacement. The ascending branch of the anterior circumflex humeral artery is the main source of blood supply for the humeral head.[38] It enters the bone at the upper end of the bicipital groove and gives off branches to the greater and lesser tuberosity. The blood supply to the glenohumeral joint arises primarily from branches of the suprascapular, subscapular, and both humeral circumflex arteries.

Venous System

The venous system about the shoulder joint complex in general accompanies the arteries. Its termination is in the axillary vein, which is a continuation of the basilic vein. The cephalic vein enters into the axillary vein proximally and reaches the axillary vein by passing between the deltoid and the pectoralis major

Venous drainage systems

- Axillary vein
- Basilic vein
- Cephalic vein

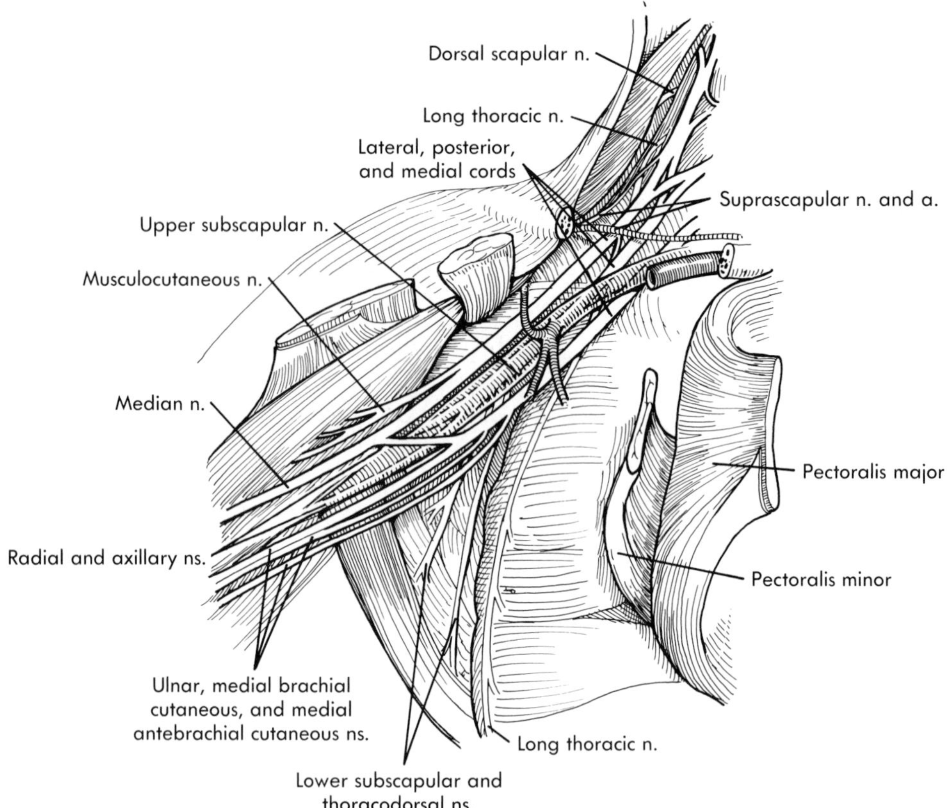

FIG. 2-12. The neurovascular supply to the shoulder joint complex.

muscles, which once again is an important landmark in anterior surgical approaches to the glenohumeral joint.

Nerve Supply

The nerve supply to the shoulder joint complex (Fig. 2-12) arises mainly from the fifth through the seventh cervical nerve root via its formation into the brachial plexus. The plexus is formed by the fifth, sixth, seventh, and eighth cervical nerves and the first thoracic nerve. It then forms an upper, middle, and lower trunk, from which arise anterior and posterior divisions. These then realign into forming cords, which are named lateral, medial, and posterior because of their relationship to the axillary artery.

The important branches in regard to the shoulder joint complex are those of the lateral cord, which includes the lateral pectoral nerve, and the musculocutaneous nerve, which leaves the axilla by passing through the coracobrachialis several centimeters below its insertion. The musculocutaneous nerve is subject to injury during retraction of the conjoint tendon during anterior shoulder surgery.

The posterior cord gives off the remaining important branches in regard to the shoulder joint complex. These are the upper subscapular nerve, which supplies the subscapular muscle, the thoracodorsal nerve, which travels along the lateral border of the scapula and supplies the latissimus dorsi, and the lower subscapular nerve, which gives off a branch of the subscapularis muscle and then continues along to innervate the teres major.

Finally, the axillary nerve travels along the inferior portion of the subscapularis muscle and then winds around the shoulder joint capsule and humeral neck, where it divides into an anterior and posterior branch. The anterior branch travels around anteriorly to supply the middle and anterior deltoid, and the posterior branch supplies the posterior deltoid as well as the teres minor. The axillary nerve, as previously mentioned, is quite susceptible to injury during surgery about the shoulder, and studies by Tullos et al have noted the close relationship of the axillary nerve during surgical procedures about the shoulder.[8] They found the nerve to be within 0.5 to 2.5 cm of a posterior arthroscopic portal; between 0.65 and 0.9 cm of an anterior shoulder approach; and within 0.32 cm of the incisions in the capsule during a capsular shift procedure.

The other important nerves about the

shoulder joint complex include the long thoracic nerve, which travels along the medial wall of the axilla to supply the serratus anterior, and the suprascapular nerve, which arises from the upper trunk to travel along the superior border of the scapula in the suprascapular notch. The suprascapular nerve may be compressed by the transverse ligament, on top of which travels a suprascapular artery to go on to innervate the supraspinatus and infraspinatus muscles. The nerve supply to the glenohumeral joint arises primarily from the axillary nerve, suprascapular nerve, and lateral pectoral nerves.[23]

REFERENCES

1. Andrews JR, Carson WG, and McCleod W: Glenoid labrum tears related to the long head of the biceps, Am J Sports Med 13:337, 1985.
2. Aoki M, Usui and Ishii M: The slope of the acromion and rotator cuff impingement. Presented to the Society of American Shoulder and Elbow Surgeons Second Open Meeting, New Orleans, 1986.
3. Aronen JG, and Regan K: Decreasing the incidence of recurrence of first time anterior shoulder dislocations with rehabilitation, Am J Sports Med 12:283, 1984.
4. Basmajian JV, and Bazant FJ: Factors preventing downward dislocation of the adducted shoulder joint, J Bone Joint Surg, 41A:1182, 1959.
5. Bearn JG: Direct observations on the function of the capsule of the sternoclavicular joint in clavicle support, J Anat 101:159, 1967.
6. Bechtol C: Biomechanics of the shoulder, Clin Orthop 146:37, 1980.
7. Bigliani LJ, and Morrison DS: The morphology of the acromion and its relationship to rotator cuff tears. Presented to the Society of American Shoulder and Elbow Surgeons Second Open Meeting, New Orleans, 1986.
8. Bryan WJ, Schauder K, and Tullos H: The axillary nerve and its relationship to common sports medicine shoulder procedures, Am J Sports Med 14:113, 1986.
9. Brewer B, Wubben R, and Carrera G: Excessive retroversion of the glenoid cavity, J Bone Joint Surg 68A:724, 1986.
10. Camp JO, Cilley EI: Diagrammatic chart showing time of appearance of the various centers of ossification and period of union, Am J Roentgenol 26:905, 1931.
11. Cain PR et al: Anterior stability of the glenohumeral joint: a dynamic model, Am J Sports Med 15:144, 1987.
12. Cave AJE: The nature and morphology of the costoclavicular ligament, J Anat 95:170, 1961.
13. Clemente CO: Gray's Anatomy, ed 13 (American Edition), Philadelphia, 1985, Lea & Febiger.
14. Cyprien JM et al: Humeral retrotorsion and glenohumeral relationship in the normal shoulder and in recurrent anterior dislocation (scapulometry), Clin Orthop 175:8, 1983.
15. Das SP, Saha AK, and Roy GS: Observations on the tilt of the glenoid cavity of scapula, J Anat Soc India 15:114, 1966.
16. DePalma AF: Degenerative changes in the sternoclavicular and acromioclavicular joints in various decades, Springfield, Ill., 1957, CC Thomas.
17. DePalma AF: The role of the disks of the sternoclavicular and acromioclavicular joints, Clin Orthop 13:222, 1959.
18. DePalma AF: Surgical anatomy of acromioclavicular and sternoclavicular joints, Surg Clin N Am 43:1541, 1963.
19. DePalma AF: Surgery of the shoulder, Philadelphia, 1983, J.B. Lippincott, Co.
20. DePalma AF, Callery G, and Bennett G: The variational anatomy and degenerative lesions of the shoulder joint, Instr Course Lect 6:255, 1949.
21. Fukuda K et al: Biomechanical study of the ligamentous system of the acromioclavicular joint, J Bone Joint Surg 68A:434, 1986.
22. Ganzhorn RW et al: Suprascapular nerve entrapment: a case report, J Bone Joint Surg 63A:492, 1981.
23. Gardner E: The innervation of the shoulder joint, Anat Rec 102:1, 1949.
24. Gardner E: The prenatal development of the human shoulder joint, Surg Clin North Am 43:1465, 1963.
25. Gardner E: The embryology of the clavicle, Clin Orthop 58:9, 1968.
26. Gardner E, and Gray DJ: Prenatal development of the human shoulder and acromioclavicular joints, Am J Anat 92:219, 1953.
27. Gardner E, Gray DJ, and O'Rahilly R: Anatomy, Philadelphia, 1975, W.B. Saunders Co.
28. Glousman R et al: Dynamic EMG: analysis of the throwing shoulder with glenohumeral instability. Presented to the Society of American Shoulder and Elbow Surgeons Third Open Meeting, San Francisco, 1987.
29. Gray DJ, and Gardner E: The prenatal development of the humerus, Am J Anat 124:431, 1969.
30. Hitchcock HH: Painful shoulder: observation on role of tendon of long head of biceps brachii in its causation, J Bone Joint Surg 30A:263, 1948.
31. Hollinshead WH, and Rosse C: Textbook of anatomy, ed 4, New York, 1985, Harper & Row, Publishers, Inc.
32. Howell AB et al: Role of the supraspinatus muscle in shoulder function, J Bone Joint Surg 68A:398, 1986.
33. Hurley JA et al: Posterior shoulder instability: results of operative vs. non-operative treatment. Presented to the American Academy of Orthopaedic Surgeons, San Francisco, 1987.
34. Inman VT et al: Observations on the function of the shoulder joint, J Bone Joint Surg 26:1, 1944.
35. Jobe FW et al: An EMG analysis of the shoulder in throwing and pitching, Am J Sports Med 11:3, 1983.
36. Kaltsas DS: Comparative study of the properties of the shoulder joint capsule with those of other joint capsules, Clin Orthop 173:20, 1983.
37. Kohler A, and Zimmer EA: Borderlands of normal and early pathologic in skeletal roentgenology, ed 11 (American Edition), New York, 1968, Grune & Stratton.
38. Laing PG: The arterial supply of the adult humerus, J Bone Joint Surg 38A:1105, 1956.
39. Laumann U, and Kramps HA: Computer tomography on recurrent shoulder dislocation. In Bateman JE: Surgery of the shoulder, St. Louis, 1984, The CV Mosby Co.
40. Liberson R: Os acromiale: a contested anomaly, J Bone Jone Surg 19:683, 1937.
41. McClure JG, and Raney B: Anomalies of the scapula, Clin Orthop 110:22, 1975.
42. Morrison DS, and Bigliani LU: The clinical sig-

nificance of variations in acromial morphology. Presented to the Society of American Shoulder and Elbow Surgeons Third Open Meeting, San Francisco, 1987.
43. Moseley HF: The clavicle: its anatomy and function, Clin Orthop 58:17, 1968.
44. Moseley HF, and Overgaard B: The anterior capsular mechanism in recurrent anterior dislocation of the shoulder, J Bone Joint Surg 44B:913, 1962.
45. Mudge K et al: Rotator cuff tears associated with os acromiale, J Bone Joint Surg 68A:427, 1984.
46. Neer CS, and Poppen NK: Supraspinatus outlet. Presented to the Society of American Shoulder and Elbow Surgeons Third Open Meeting, San Francisco, 1987.
47. Ogden JA, Conologue GS, and Bronson ML: Radiology of post-natal skeletal development: the clavicle, Skeletal Radiol 4:196, 1979.
48. Ogden JA, Conologue GJ, and Jenson P: Radiology of post-natal skeletal development: the proximal humerus, Skeletal Radiol 2:153, 1978
49. Ouesen J, and Nielsen S: Stability of the shoulder joint, Acta Orthop Scand 56:149, 1985.
50. Perry J: Anatomy and biomechanics of the shoulder in throwing, swimming, gymnastics and tennis, Clin Sports Med 2(2):247, 1983.
51. Poppen NK, and Walker PS: Normal and abnormal motion of the shoulder, J Bone Joint Surg 58A:195, 1976.
52. Poppen NK, and Walker PS: Forces at the glenohumeral joint in abduction, Clin Orthop 135:165, 1978.
53. Post M, and Mayer, V: Suprascapular nerve entrapment: diagnosis and treatment, Clin Orthop 223:126, 1987.
54. Randelli M, and Gambrioli, PL: Glenohumeral osteometry by computed tomography in normal and unstable shoulders, Clin Orthop 208:151, 1986.
55. Rathbun JB, and MacNab I: The microvascular pattern of the rotator cuff, J Bone Joint Surg 52B: 540, 1970.
56. Redler M, Ryland L, and McCue F: Quadrilateral space syndrome in a throwing athlete, Am J Sports Med 14:511, 1986.
57. Reeves B: Anterior capsular strength of the shoulder, J Bone Joint Surg 50B:858, 1968.
58. Rockwood C, and Green D: Fractures in adults, Philadelphia, 1984, J.B. Lippincott Co.
59. Rockwood C, Wilkins K, and King R: Fractures in children, Philadelphia, 1984, J.B. Lippincott Co.
60. Saha AK: Dynamic stability of the glenohumeral joint, Acta Orthop Scand 42:491, 1971.
61. Sarrafian SK: Gross and functional anatomy of the shoulder, Clin Ortho 173:11, 1983.
62. Silverman F: Caffey's pediatric x-ray diagnosis, ed 8, Chicago, 1985, Yearbook Medical Publishers, Inc.
63. Symeonides PP: The significance of the subscapularis muscle in the pathogenesis of recurrent anterior dislocation of the shoulder, J Bone Joint Surg 54B:476, 1972.
64. Todd TW, and DeErrico J, Jr: The clavicular epiphyses, Am J Anat 41:25, 1928.
65. Townley CO: The capsular mechanism in recurrent dislocation of the shoulder, J Bone Joint Surg 32A:370, 1950.
66. Turkel SJ et al: Stabilizing mechanisms preventing anterior dislocation of the glenohumeral joint, J Bone Joint Surg 63A:1208, 1981.
67. Urist MR: Complete dislocation of the acromioclavicular joint: the nature of the traumatic lesion and effective methods of treatment with an analysis of 41 cases, J Bone Joint Surg 28:813, 1946.
68. Warwick R, and Williams PL, (editors): Gray's Anatomy, ed 35 (British Edition), Philadelphia, 1973, W.B. Saunders Co.

CHAPTER 3 History and Physical Examination of the Shoulder

Tom R. Norris

The effective management of an athlete's painful shoulder most importantly requires an accurate diagnosis. This is determined on the basis of an extensive knowledge of extrinsic and intrinsic causes of shoulder pain, combined with a detailed history, a complete physical examination, and judicious use of ancillary testing. An understanding of shoulder anatomy, kinematics, biomechanics, and familiarity with specialized use of the shoulder and arm in specific sports will assist in identification of the complex derangements that can interfere with optimal shoulder function.

ETIOLOGY OF SHOULDER PAIN

Unfortunately, multiple problems may exist in the same athlete. It is common to see a combination of bone, muscle, tendon, ligament, and, more rarely, nerve and vascular injuries in the evaluation of shoulder dysfunction. Acromioclavicular arthritis may coexist with cervical radiculopathy. Shoulder impingement and rotator cuff tearing, commonly seen in the middle-aged or aging athlete,[66] are now being recognized from overuse in the younger athlete with shoulder instability.[79] Failure to appreciate these complex interrelationships may result in incomplete or ill-conceived treatments and thus impede the athlete's return to optimal function.

Extrinsic Problems

The neck is the most common source of extrinsic pain radiating to the shoulder. This pain may be gradual in onset or result from acute trauma.

In football, a spearhead tackle may fracture the cervical spine, leading to quadraplegia. A tackle that forces the head away from the shoulder with associated "burners" and "stingers"[132] stretches the upper cords of the brachial plexus and results in transient shoulder and arm weakness. Repeated episodes or more severe injuries cause permanent weakness.[140]

The brachial plexus is at risk with any falls that force the head and shoulder apart. The athlete is susceptible to these hard falls in gymnastics, wrestling, and higher-speed sports such as bicycling, motorcycle racing, skiing, and hockey.

Cervical arthrosis with spondylosis, foraminal osteophytes, herniated disks, and more distal nerve entrapment syndromes should be considered in the neurologic evaluation, with screening ancillary tests performed as necessary. Electrodiagnostic studies, roentgenograms, computerized tomography, magnetic resonance imaging, and noninvasive vascular studies each have a role.

Extrinsic causes of shoulder pain

- Brachial plexus injury
- Cervical spondylosis
- Cervical disk herniation
- Syringomyelia
- Thoracic outlet syndrome
- Diaphragmatic irritation
- Lung tumor
- Brachial neuropathy
- Myocardial ischemia

The presentation of an athlete with a C5-6 disk will be similar to that of a suprascapular nerve entrapment or a rotator cuff tear with spinatii atrophy and shoulder external rotation weakness.

The history of spinal cord injury in the cervical or even thoracolumbar region may be followed years later with shoulder pain and apparent arthritic dissolution of the humeral head. Although it has been stated that syringomyelia does not usually cause pain in the shoulder, the posttraumatic syrinx associated with advanced shoulder arthritis occurs in patients who initially manifest severe shoulder pain. Screening tests, with aspirations and cultures to rule out infection of the glenohumeral joint, and MRI have allowed identification of the previously missed posttraumatic syrinx. The treatment was altered to provide adequate syrinx shunting rather than local shoulder surgery.[121]

Shoulder pain can be misconstrued as primary neck pathology. If for any reason an athlete has shoulder pain, there will be a tendency to immobilize or protect the arm with adduction, internal rotation, and slight elevation of the shoulder. Muscle fatigue and spasms, primarily in the posterior trapezius and levator scapular insertion, result in secondary neck pain.

Thoracic outlet syndrome with proximal compression of the nerves and arteries is much less common than cervical radiculopathy and is more difficult to diagnose. Leffert reports that a history of trauma is present in approximately 40%.[89] Women of childbearing age are predilected in a ratio of 3.5:1 compared with men. The pain classically radiates to the medial arm and forearm, and occasionally to the ring and small fingers, causing inability to use the arm above shoulder level because of fatigue. These same symptoms may be the initial symptoms with recurrent transient subluxations of the glenohumeral joint.[91, 145, 147] The differential is important. Repairing a subluxing or dislocating shoulder can eliminate the numbness, tingling, and positional fatigue in the combined clinical setting.

The history of onset is important. The atraumatic slow loss of the ability to raise the arm may occur from a viral plexitis. An arthrogram is normal and the electromyographic is helpful in making the diagnosis, whereas after sudden traumatic loss of the ability to raise the arm, the differential diagnosis would indicate either a neck or brachial plexus injury with rotator cuff tear or fixed dislocation of the shoulder. That these can also occur in combination emphasizes the need for thorough evaluation, even if only one cause may have been identified.[81]

Identification of the primary cause of shoulder pain is not always easy. Referred pain to the shoulder girdle region occurs from mul-

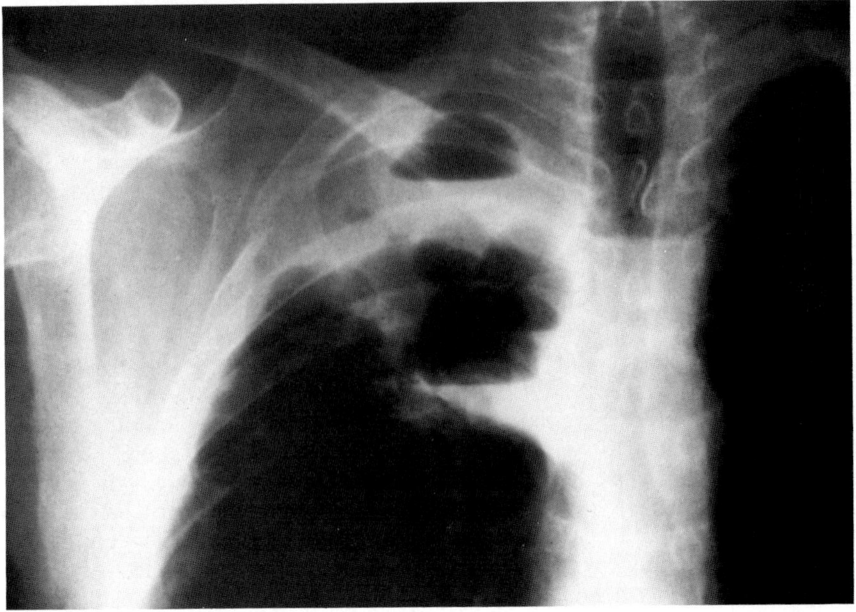

FIG. 3-1. Pancoast tumor. First symptom was shoulder pain.

tiple sources other than the neck. With diaphragmatic irritation, pain is referred along the phrenic nerve to the supraclavicular region, the trapezius, and superomedial angle of the scapula.[27] Pulmonary infarction may irritate the diaphragm. A subphrenic abscess or ruptured abdominal viscus, gallbladder, and hepatic parenchymal disease may be present with epigastric pain, as well as pain over the top of the shoulder, with concomitant tenderness and scapular pain. Gastric and pancreatic diseases may refer to the interscapular region.

The rare superior sulcus lung tumor or Pancoast tumor, occasionally coincident with Horner's syndrome, may have shoulder pain as its initial symptom[88] (Fig. 3-1).

Prolonged vigorous aerobic and anaerobic exertions in long-distance running, causing myocardial ischemic pain, may also cause pain to radiate at the base of the neck in the clavicular region, through the shoulder, and down the ulnar border of the left arm. The transverse and descending aortic diseases classically radiate to the left shoulder, whereas those of the ascending right side of the arch radiate to the right shoulder.

Many times the cause of the referred shoulder pain cannot be established. Early on, objective findings in the shoulder are absent, whereas over time the shoulder stiffness that develops becomes a cause of pain in and of itself, with secondary ipsilateral neck and scapular muscle fatigue.

Intrinsic Problems

Intrinsic causes of shoulder pain in the athlete fall into six basic groups:

1. Instability—subluxations and dislocations of the glenohumeral, AC, and SC joint
2. Impingement lesions—rotator cuff tears and ruptures of the long head of the biceps
3. Fractures of the proximal humerus, scapula, and clavicle
4. Arthritis—SC, AC, and glenohumeral joints
5. Miscellaneous—calcific tendonitis, myositis ossificans,[93] adhesive capsulitis, tumors, and nerve or vessel injury

Intrinsic causes of shoulder pain

- Instability
- Impingement
- Fractures
- Arthritis
- Calcific tendonitis
- Myositis ossificans
- Adhesive capsulitis
- Tumors
- Neurovascular injury
- Psychologic disturbance

6. Psychologic presentations with abnormal posturing, "painful subluxations," or other painful symptoms grossly in ex-

cess of physical findings with nonorganic or functional causes

Pain or injuries may occur in an isolated group or in combination.

MECHANISMS OF INJURY AND THEIR ROLE

The Throwing Motion

Second only to running injuries, athletic injuries affecting the shoulder joint are the next most common. Throwing is the most common motion used in sports.[117] The overhead throwing motion has been extensively analyzed for the baseball pitcher.* With minor variations, its biomechanics are similar to those used in football, shotput and hammer throw, all racket sports, and three of the four swimming sports, namely the freestyle, backstroke, and butterfly.[130] The throwing mechanism involves a set sequence of body motion, beginning with pelvis, upper trunk rotation, upper arm, forearm, and hand.[10] It has been divided into five stages: preparation and windup, early cocking, late cocking, forward acceleration, and follow-through with deceleration.† Skilled throwers seldom use more than 90 degrees abduction; however, the arm rapidly moves from the extremes of external to internal rotation.[42] Preliminary electromyographic analysis has elucidated the shoulder and elbow function in throwing,[130,155] tennis strokes,[1,148] and swimming.[110,126,159]

These throwing motions share the common need for upper and lower body positioning and proper timing to decrease stress on the glenohumeral joint and provide power.[117] Analysis of the throwing arm angles; the mechanics of the lead shoulder, arm, and foot; the gloved arm; and the rhythm have demonstrated predictable injuries to the shoulder and elbow.[2] Poor mechanics can cause shoulder and elbow injuries.[2,56] A stiff front leg causes trunk vaulting when rotation is needed. "Closing off," or getting the arm ahead of the body before significant trunk rotation increases the load on the shoulder. "Rushing" or "opening up"[76] too soon gets the body ahead of the throwing arm, thereby increasing the stress on the anterior glenohumeral and medial elbow ligaments.[60,77,79] During the rapid change from maximal external rotation in the late cocked position to full internal rotation of the follow-through phase, the medial elbow is placed under tension with a valgus stress. The ulnar collateral ligament can be stretched or ruptured. Ulnar nerve entrapment from overuse, stretching, and fibrosis develops.[77] The lateral elbow is subjected to repeated compression.[83,92]

In the adolescent, osteochondritis dissecans of the capitellum and elbow loose bodies develop.[83,159,161] The pull of the subscapularis and longitudinal tension along the humerus serve to widen the proximal humeral epiphyseal plate that has a stress fracture.[36,64,92]

Maximal stretching in the external rotation cocking phase directly about the humeral head on the posterior glenoid rim while stretching or avulsing the anterior ligamentous and labral attachments results in recurrent anterior inferior subluxations. The force and torque pitching with the strong muscle contractions have been reported to fracture the humeral shaft.[57,92] The rapid deceleration in the follow-through places traction on the posterior and superior capsular and tendonous structure. Two lesions described by Bennett,[16,17] namely ossification of the triceps long-head origin at the inferior glenoid and ossification at the posterior glenoid rim,[12,94] are thought to occur as a result of the traction during deceleration in pitching (Fig. 3-2). Posterior abutment of the maximally externally rotated humerus in cocking is postulated as being another cause of the posterior glenoid rim ossification and posterior humeral head defects that are separate from Hill-Sachs defects.[78] Whereas detachment of the anterior superior labrum is attributed to the pull of the long head of the biceps during the deceleration phase,[4,106] detachment of the anterior-inferior labrum is one of instability from repeated stresses from extreme external rotation and abduction.

The "Dead Arm Syndrome," with transient numbness and arm weakness following a hard throw, has become a commonly accepted historical symptom indicative of shoulder subluxations.[144,147] The overuse syndromes, with subacromial impingement termed "throwers and swimmers shoulders" with increasing frequency, are associated with recurrent shoulder subluxations.[65,107] That glenohumeral instability can cause secondary shoulder impingement has important therapeutic implications. It explains why coracoacromial ligament release, alone or in conjunction with anterior acromioplasty,[82] often has failed to relieve the impingement symptoms, whereas treatment directed to restoring joint stability, with repair of detached ligaments or reducing the joint volume in multidirectional instability with capsular shift procedures, have been successful.[60,79,113]

*References 5, 7, 79, 101, 105, 149, 157.

†References 56, 60, 78, 80, 83, 158, 160.

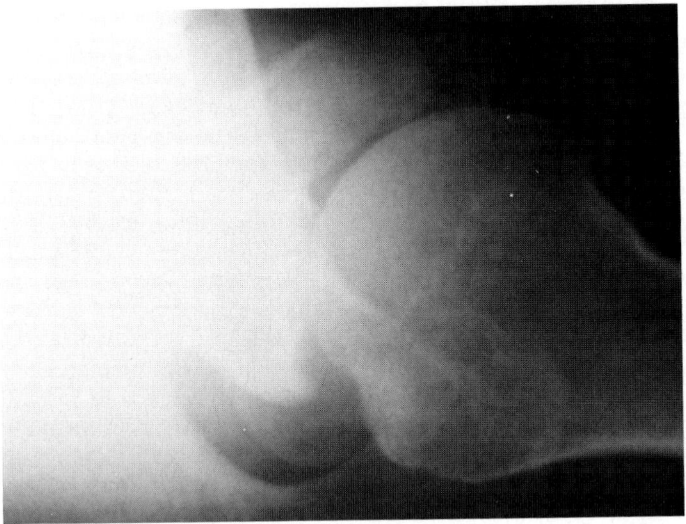

FIG. 3-2. Bennett lesion. Posterior glenoid rim fracture ossification in a 53-year-old man who pitched from age 9 until age 22, at which point pain ended his overhand throwing career.

Types of Shoulder Injury

Albright et al[2] reported that throwing injuries are directly related to the duration of exposure and intensity of participation. Clancy[37] recognized the role of tissue overuse in athletic shoulder injuries. Previously, injury mechanisms have been expanded from traumatic and atraumatic to include repetitive microtrauma and others.

Macrotrauma

An acute forceful direct or indirect injury causing fracture dislocation or soft tissue disruption can be defined as macrotrauma. An acute strain or ligament tear will become a chronic situation if an early diagnosis is not made, followed by adequate rests, splinting, repair, and reconditioning before return to the same activity.[42] Rotator cuff tears in the younger athlete are rare, but when they occur are from violent injuries with large avulsions. In patients over age 30, acute tears may be superimposed on more chronic degenerative impingement lesions, with or without previous cuff tearing. The initiating trauma for tearing lessens with advancing age.[104]

Classification of injury types

- Macrotrauma
- Repetitive microtrauma
- Atraumatic

Repetitive Microtrauma

Chronic overuse syndromes with repetitive stretching, as in rowing, swimming, or throwing, are injuries of repetitive microtrauma. These may be associated with lack of or improper conditioning for the sport performed. Frequently there are deficiencies in one muscle group (most commonly the shoulder external rotators), lack of flexibility, or longer than normal sessions.[79,80]

Warming up is necessary for safe stretching. Without stretching for complete range of motion before beginning competition, the muscles are more susceptible to extrinsic overload, with disruption of attachments or intrinsic muscle tearing.[31] The healing sequence after tissue overload includes edema with inflammation, fibrin and granulation tissue deposition, and tissue calcification or ossification.[42] If the healing process is repeatedly interrupted, the process itself may become pathologic. The tissue then responds with different mechanical properties that decrease performance or lower threshold for new injury. An example might be the Bennett shoulder lesions, with posterior glenoid calcification that eventually interferes with pitching.[16,17,94]

Atraumatic

Atraumatic disorders are generally those of shoulder instability in patients with generalized ligamentous laxity or congenital hypoplasia of the glenoid. When an individual experiences pain in the absence of traumatic or overuse syndromes and with normal roentgenographs, the psychologic stresses and motivation may need evaluation.[14,15,61,62,143,146]

Impact Versus Nonimpact Injuries

Whereas general mechanisms of injury may be associated with specific injuries, the condition of the athlete's tissue influences the ease with which these injuries may occur.

Impact injuries may be divided into direct and indirect trauma.[74] Nonimpact injuries occur from overuse syndromes and muscle strains, ruptures, and avulsions. In cases of direct trauma, the injury force is in direct contact with the shoulder complex. Indirect forces injuring the shoulder usually pass up through the hand, wrist, or elbow and result in a rotational or longitudinal force directed along the humerus.

Examples of direct trauma include the following:

1. Posterior dislocations of the sternoclavicular joint[168]
2. Acromioclavicular subluxations or dislocations after a fall on the posterior superior shoulder[59,135,168]
3. Direct blows to the supraclavicular brachial plexus at the base of the neck or axillary nerve as it courses under the deltoid
4. Clavicle fractures
5. Muscle contusions

Indirect trauma results in muscle, tendon, ligament, and brachial plexus stretch, strain, rupture, and bony fractures. Glenohumeral subluxations are usually from indirect forces. Anterior dislocations occur from abduction and external rotation of the arm, whereas traumatic posterior dislocation occurs from a forward fall on the adducted, internally rotated arm, with the posterior force directed through the hand or elbow along the humeral axis. The violent muscle contractures produced by an epileptic seizure or electric shock flex, adduct, and internally rotate the humerus, forcing it posteriorly.

Although Bankart believed the prime mechanism of anterior dislocations was a direct blow to the posterior humerus, this is not common. When it does occur, the direct compression of the humeral head into the anterior glenoid rim is more likely to fracture the glenoid (Fig. 3-3). This results in an unstable joint after reduction in 80% of these fractures.[72] Similarly, a direct blow to the anterior shoulder can drive the humerus posteriorly, resulting in a locked posterior fracture-dislocation (Fig. 3-4).

Fractures of the proximal humerus occur from both direct and indirect forces. Direct blows and falls can fracture the humerus. Indirect or rotational forces with the forearm used as a lever, as in shotput[150] and wrestling,[169] can fracture the humerus. Recently, a patient was seen who fell from his bicycle, landed on his elbow, and, through this longitudinal force travelling up the humerus, sustained a midshaft clavicle fracture.

Repetitive compression or impact loading may injure the joint surface. While this has long been associated with capitellar osteochondritis with pitchers[83,159] and osteolysis of the outer clavicle in weight lifters, (Fig. 3-5),[19,33,35] it has more recently been described in the humeral head in a tennis player who hit 1000 tennis backhands a day using a ball machine.[75]

Nonimpact injuries with muscle ruptures occur when the muscle-tendon unit is forced beyond its physiologic limit. Hoyt[74] ascribed this to excessive use beyond its fatigue limits, a sudden powerful contraction against resistance initiated by the muscle antagonists, or by external force working against a muscle contraction. Examples include ruptures of the subscapularis[22] or humeral shaft from arm wrestling, rupture of the pectoralis insertion from weight lifting[87] or extreme muscle tension resulting from hanging by the arm.[102] Wrestlers, on the other hand, are predilected to rupture at the sternocostal origin rather than at the musculotendinous junction or tendinous insertion.[44,102]

Fractures at the base of the coracoid have been reported in rugby with an unknown mechanism,[99] in trapshooting as a stress fracture,[29] and in tennis as an avulsion fracture from the recurrent pull of the pectoralis minor.[18] An unusual example of muscle pull causing a comminuted scapular body fracture has occurred during pushups.[45] Hematoma in a scapular fracture preventing use of the supraspinatus can be confused clinically with a rotator cuff tear. Good roentgenographs in three right-angle planes will allow differentiation of the "pseudo cuff tear."

SPECIFIC PROBLEMS

Instability

Glenohumeral instability is the most common shoulder problem in the younger athlete, yet its varied presentations can make it one of the more difficult conditions to accurately diagnose, especially since ligamentous laxity, in and of itself, may not be the cause of an athlete's shoulder pain.

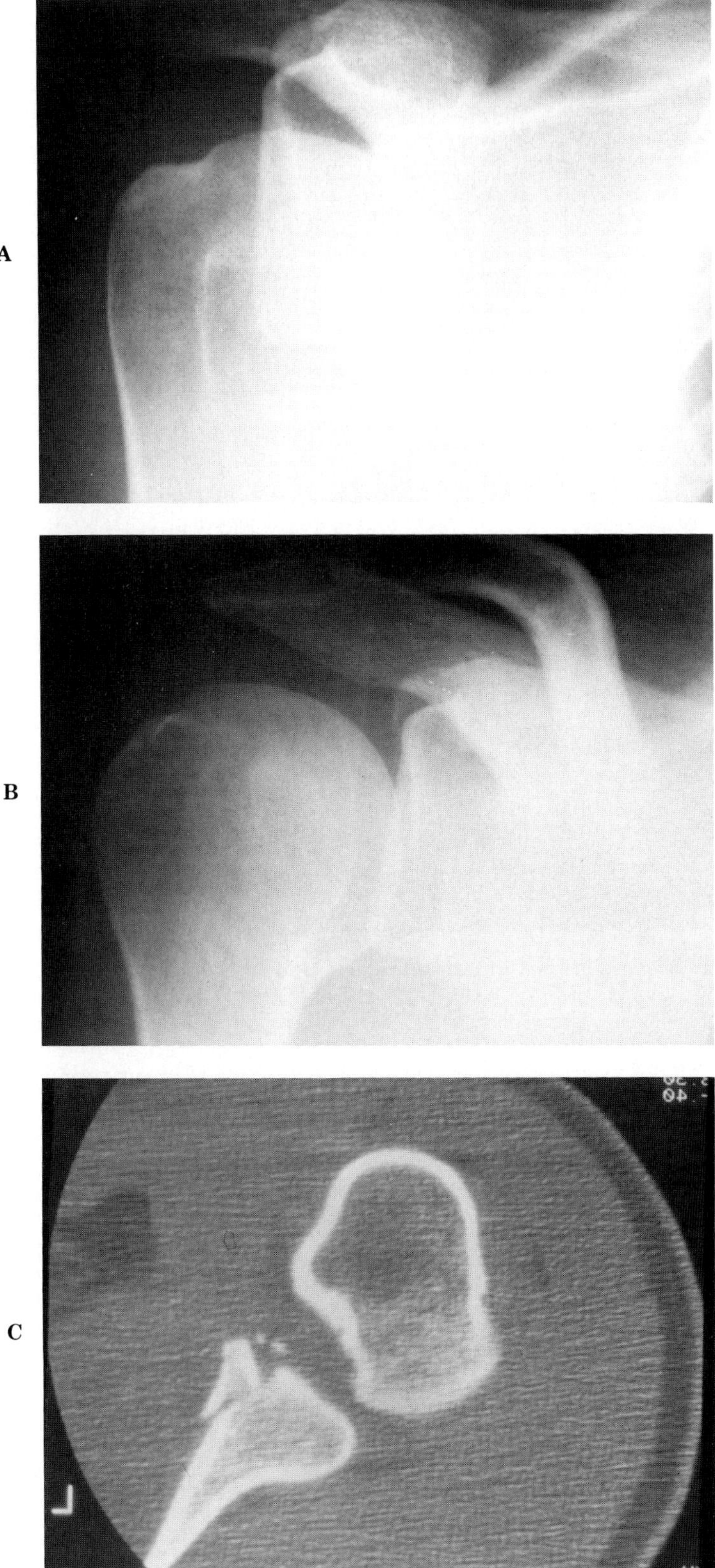

FIG. 3-3. A, Anterior humeral head dislocation from a direct blow to the posterior shoulder. **B,** Following reduction, a large anterior-inferior glenoid rim fracture is evident. **C,** CT scan accurately documents the extent of glenoid involvement.

A

B

C

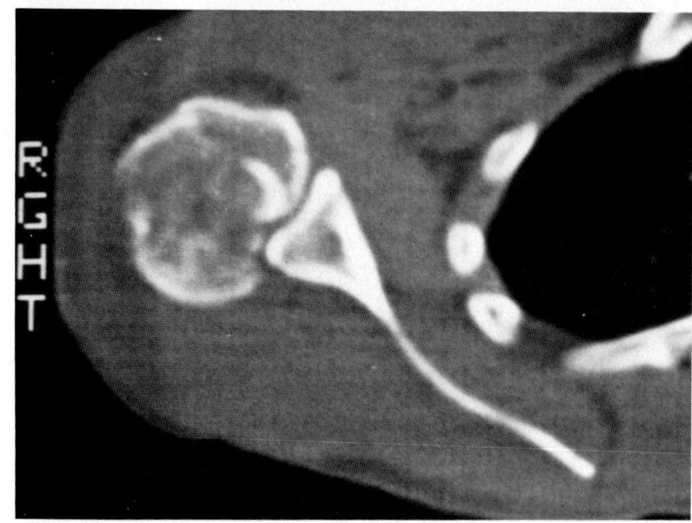

FIG. 3-4. Locked posterior shoulder dislocation from direct trauma of a tree branch striking shoulder as automobile went off the road. **A,** The long axis of the humerus is directed posteriorly proximally. The coracoid is prominent. The anterior humeral head area is depressed. A fullness is noted posteriorly. **B,** True A-P view of glenohumeral joint in the scapula plane demonstrates an overlap of the head with the glenoid. **C,** CT scan demonstrates the locked posterior dislocation with an anterior humeral head impression fracture (reverse Hill-Sachs lesion).

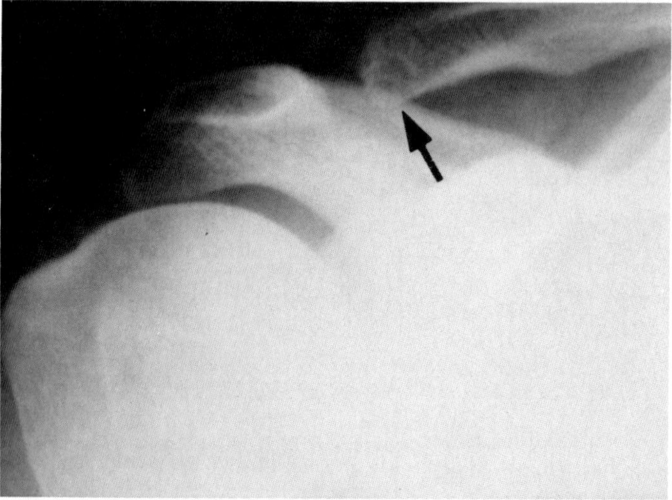

FIG. 3-5. Early osteolysis of the outer clavicle with subcortical cystic lesions in a weight lifter.

Anatomic Considerations

The shoulder anatomy is unique and is the body's most mobile and versatile joint. The glenoid cavity is shallow. Its articular surface is relatively flat compared to the humeral head. Only 25% to 30% of the humeral head articulates with the glenoid at any one time. The shallow cavity is functionally deepened by the intact labral and ligamentous attachment at its perimeter. The inferior glenohumeral ligament complex is the prime static stabilizer for anterior,[162] posterior,[53,127] and inferior[113] stability (Fig. 3-6). The middle glenohumeral appears to have a role secondary to the inferior glenohumeral ligament in anterior stability.[127]

The rotator cuff actively centers the humeral head in the glenoid cavity except when the arm is in extreme abduction and external rotation.[73,79] Then an obligatory posterior translation occurs. Shear forces over the articular cartilage and labral attachments occur with the forward acceleration in pitching as the humeral head glides anteriorly. Abnormal translation occurs in those with ligamentous detachments.[133,134] Once the anterior labrum has been detached, it no longer serves as a buttress to anterior subluxation or a tether to

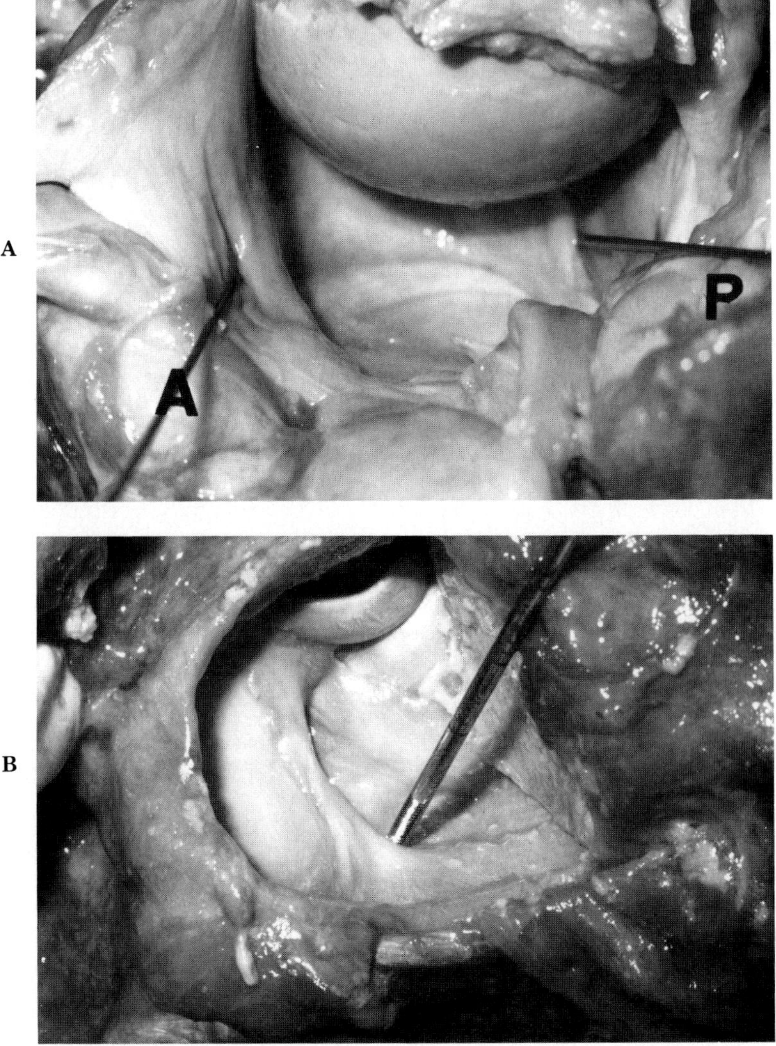

FIG. 3-6. The inferior glenohumeral ligament complex provides the prime stabilizer for anterior, inferior, and posterior stability. **A,** As seen from above, thickenings of the complex form anterior *(A)* and posterior *(P)* inferior glenohumeral ligaments that pass from the humeral calcar up each side of the glenoid rim to blend with the labrum. A small inferior recess is normally between the two ligaments. **B,** The anterior inferior glenohumeral ligament as seen in a right shoulder (from behind with the humeral head removed) becomes confluent with the anterior labrum. It is the strongest glenohumeral ligament and the prime stabilizer when the arm is abducted and externally rotated.

posterior instability. Increased subluxation in both directions can occur.[125,152]

The scapular rotators—namely the trapezius, rhomboids, and serratus anterior—function by positioning the glenoid for optimal stability.[78]

Classification

Shoulder instability is defined in terms of the following:

1. *Directions*. Anterior, posterior, inferior, anterior-superior, and multidirectional
2. *Degree*. Dislocation (humeral head escapes the glenoid cavity)
   Subluxation—passive translation with more than 50% of the humeral head over the glenoid rim without complete dislocation[118,119,127]; active translation more than 4 mm from the center of the glenoid cavity[73]
3. *Timing*. Acute, recurrent, chronic, or fixed
4. *Etiologic force*. Trauma—major injury. Microtrauma—repetitive stretching. Atraumatic—congenital ligamentous laxity
5. *Motivation*. Voluntary—muscle contracture or positional, with or without abnormal secondary psychologic gain
   Involuntary—positional or with trauma
6. *Anatomy*. Bony architecture—dysplasia, hypoplasia, aplasia of glenoid or humeral head
   - Glenoid rim fracture (see Fig. 3-3)
   - Humeral head impression fracture
   - Anteriorly from posterior dislocation (see Fig. 3-4)
   - Posteriorly from anterior dislocation (Hill-Sachs defect) (Fig. 3-7)
   - Ligamentous, labral, and muscle integrity, that is, labral detachment (see Fig. 3-7), Subscapularis avulsion, or cuff tear
   - Neurologic status—Erb's palsy, plexus injury, or CVA

Anterior Instability

Anterior instability from acute trauma (as in football) or from repetitive stretching (as in pitching) occurs in an anterior-inferior direction. In up to 85% of such injuries, the labrum has been detached from the anterior-inferior glenoid rim.

The optimal time for postreduction immobilization for the first dislocation is thought to be between 3 and 6 weeks.[84,115] Recurrence in the athlete is probable.[42,69] The younger the athlete, the more likely a recurrence will occur; however, it does not occur as frequently in the nonathlete or if adequate immobilization and rehabilitation take place before the return to sports.[154]

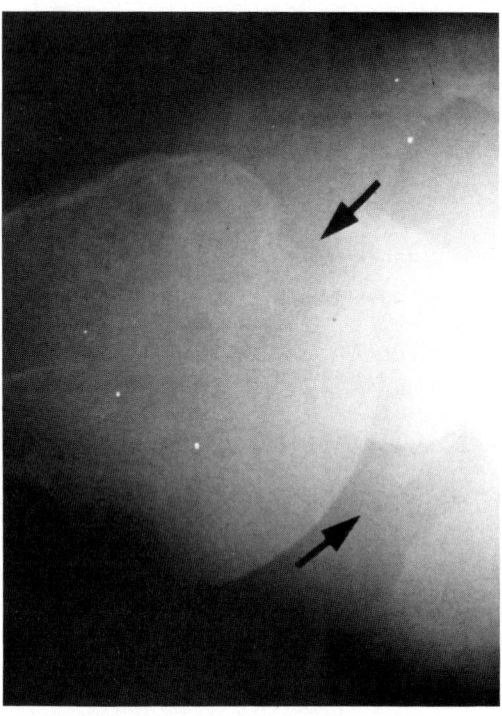

FIG. 3-7. West Point axillary view. Ectopic calcification of the anterior inferior glenoid is pathoneumonic for a labral detachment and anterior instability. The posterior lateral humeral head Hill-Sachs impression fracture is the pathoneumonic roentgenographic sign often seen in anterior dislocations after reduction.

The major diagnostic efforts are to ascertain whether the glenoid labrum and inferior glenohumeral ligaments are secure. The clinical evaluation, specialized oblique axillary roentgenographs (see Fig. 3-7),[142] CT arthrotomography,[11,103,107,128,153] and, if necessary, arthroscopy[78] can provide this information before operative repair begins.

Anterior dislocations require assistance with their first and often subsequent reductions. Roentgenographs confirm the direction and degree. Blazina and Saltzman[24] reported on recurrent anterior subluxation and advanced the understanding of more subtle forms of instability. The humeral head may dislocate or sublux over the anterior inferior glenoid rim when the arm is in the throwing position of abduction, external rotation, and extension. With hard throwing, the subluxation may manifest itself as a "dead arm."[147] Transient neurologic symptoms radiate down the arm and forearm and usually to the ulnar side of the hand. For a few minutes, the athlete is unable to use the arm, but then recovers with residual aching. Popping, catching, and fear that the arm will slip in the provocative position are commonly reported.

Labral tearing, with subluxation manifesting as clicking, has been identified in the anterior inferior glenoid in pitching[128] and in swimming.[107] Loose bodies seen in roentgenographs of the shoulder are an indication of recurrent shoulder dislocations.[119]

Whereas other forms of instability are thought to be capsular in origin, anterior-superior instability is seen postoperatively after a rotator cuff or greater tuberosity dehiscence. The humeral head cannot be fixed in the glenoid cavity. It rides superiorly with the pull of the deltoid when the force couple action of the supraspinatus and long head of the biceps no longer serves as a head depressor (Fig. 3-8).

Posterior Instability

Posterior shoulder instability is classified as acute posterior dislocation, with or without a head impression fracture; chronic locked posterior dislocation (often originally missed)[67]; and recurrent posterior shoulder subluxation.

The **acute posterior dislocation** without a head impression fracture is rare, but if not reduced and immobilized in external rotation with the arm at the side, it will become recurrent. Both the acute posterior dislocation and the posterior locked (head impression fracture) dislocation occur in sports from a fall on the elbow or outstretched hand when the arm is flexed forward, adducted, and internally rotated. The same injury can occur—although not usually in sports—from electric shock, epileptic seizure, or alcoholic withdrawal seizures. Up to 80% of these are missed by the first examining physician. Although most of these result from violent muscle contractures or trauma directed along the axis of the humeral shaft, I have seen a case in which a tree limb went through a car windshield, knocking the shoulder backwards with a direct blow as the car went off the road (see Fig. 3-4). The history, a high index of suspicion, and an axillary roentgenograph or CT scan will prevent missing this lesion in an individual with limitations of forward flexion, external rotation, and forearm supination (Fig. 3-4, *C*).

Chronic recurrent posterior subluxations are frequently demonstrable by the patient either in arm position or selected muscle contracture.[122] It may be unilateral after trauma, or bilateral with pain only on one side, with or without a precipitating traumatic event. Hawkins and McCormack[68] classify four subsets as: (1) voluntary habitual (emotionally disturbed), (2) voluntary, (3) not willful (muscular control), and (4) involuntary positional and involuntary unintentional (not demonstrable by patient).

The usual history is one of gradual onset in which both shoulders can sublux posteriorly either by contracture of the anterior deltoid

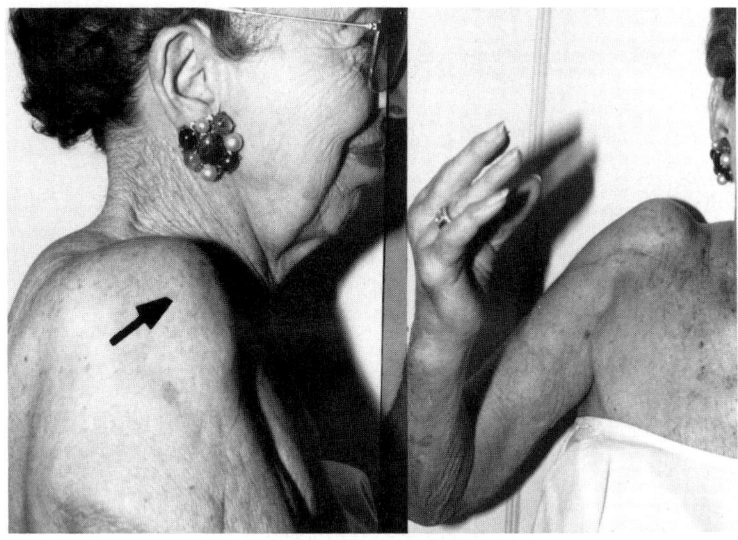

FIG. 3-8. Anterior superior ascent of the humeral head with a large cuff tear as in this rheumatoid or tuberosity avulsion. The supraspinatus and long head of the biceps can no longer fix the humeral head in the glenoid as the deltoid attempts to elevate the arm. Following failed surgery, this is exacerbated by loss of the coracoacromial ligament as an anterior superior restraint.

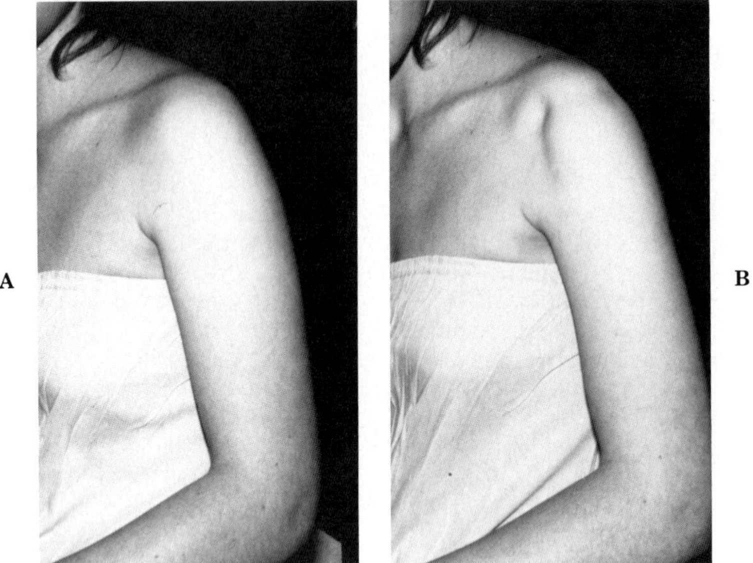

FIG. 3-9. Voluntary posterior inferior shoulder subluxation. **A,** Reduced. **B,** Subluxed and fixed by muscle contractures of the anterior deltoid and pectoralis with simultaneous relaxation of the posterior deltoid and external rotators.

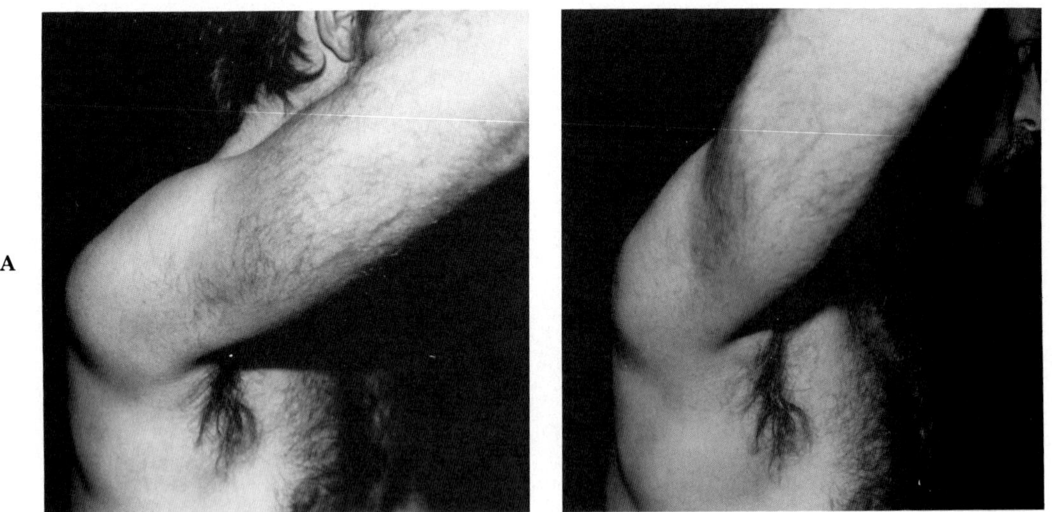

FIG. 3-10. A, Positioned posterior subluxation. **B,** Reduction with snap. This could be confused with anterior instability if the shoulder were mistakenly thought to be reduced in the first position *(a)*.

and pectoralis (Fig. 3-9) or by arm position with the arm forward flexed (Fig. 3-10, *A*). Extension of the arm causes a sudden snap with a concomitant reduction (Fig. 3-10, *B*). If the shoulder subluxes posteriorly unintentionally with forward flexion, pain may interfere with the sport. Although it is easy to demonstrate, the athlete may not know what is happening, and the physician often does not consider it in the differential diagnosis for shoulder pain. While apprehension is common for anterior instability, it is not reliable for posterior instability.

Athletes with recurrent posterior subluxations aggravate their shoulder problem with sports that stress the posterior capsule. In my practice, these have been more common in butterfly swimmers, rowers, archers,[55] and weight lifters, who feel pain on bench pressing. As a result of excessive stretching, recurrent subluxations may be associated with rotator cuff tendonitis.[68] External rotational

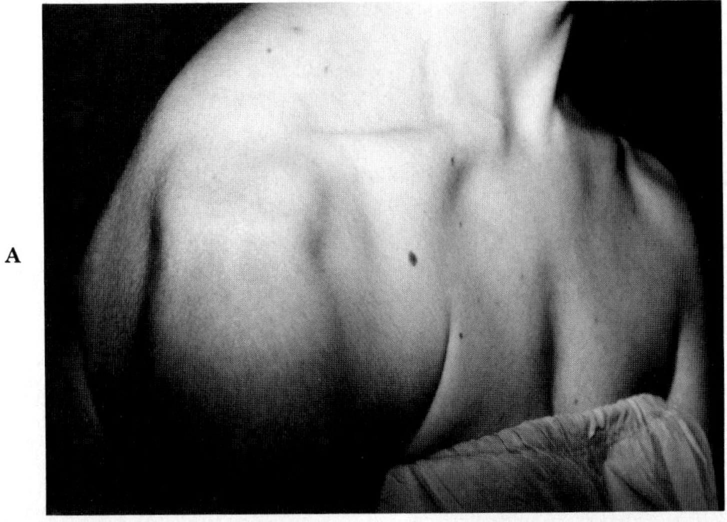

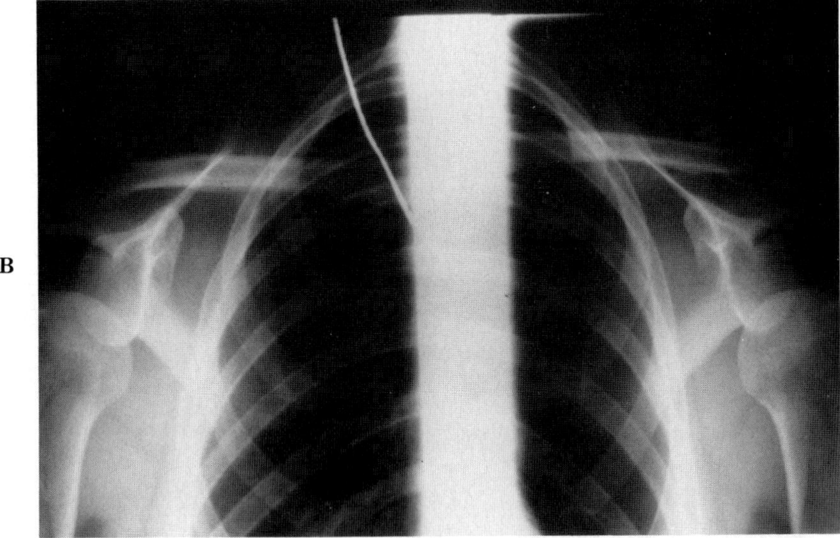

FIG. 3-11. Inferior subluxation of the glenohumeral joints. **A,** A sulcus develops between the acromion and humeral head. **B,** Roentgenograph demonstrating inferior capsular laxity with a 20-pound weight strapped to each forearm.

strengthening, with the arms at the side and avoidance of posterior capsular stress, have been moderately effective in alleviating patients' symptoms. For those who had a specific traumatic onset and unsuccessful conservative exercises, Froncek et al[53] report encouraging results using posterior capsular shift procedures in returning athletes to their former sports.

Multidirectional Instability

In 1980, Neer and Foster[113] identified the hallmark of multidirectional shoulder instability as abnormal inferior glenohumeral laxity in the absence of labral detachments. The typical occurrence is in an athlete with generalized ligamentous laxity without appreciable trauma. Vague aching or recurrent slipping of the shoulder with increasing disability are common with weight lifting or sports that require repetitive overhead arm movement, such as in pitching or swimming. Multidirectional subluxations might be suspected in a swimmer who reports pain in the pull-through phase in the water and recovery phase out of the water.[6] Secondary rotator cuff tendonitis may occur with normal acromial morphology in a young athlete. Transient pain and paresthesias, radiating distal to the elbow, are common with arm use, and yet neurologic evaluation is normal.

At the time of examination, both shoulders can be pulled inferiorly to create a sulcus between the humeral head and acromion (Fig.

3-11, *A*). The shoulders also can be subluxed anteriorly, posteriorly, or in both directions simultaneously with the aid of mild inferior traction. Roentgenographs, with 20-pound weights strapped to both forearms, may reveal excessive bilateral inferior laxity[119] (Fig. 3-11, *B*), but pain may preclude relaxation and thereby the inferior subluxation on the symptomatic side. Correlating the patient's pain and ability to relax during the test assists in interpretation of otherwise confusing roentgenographs. Shoulder arthrography may demonstrate an enlarged inferior capsular pouch (Fig. 3-12, *A* and *B*), CT arthrotomography (Fig. 3-12, *C*) and arthroscopy reveal normal labral and ligamentous attachments.

Evaluation of other joints for laxity may demonstrate hyperextension of the elbows and knees, thumbs that can touch the forearms with wrist flexion, and ballerina-type hip

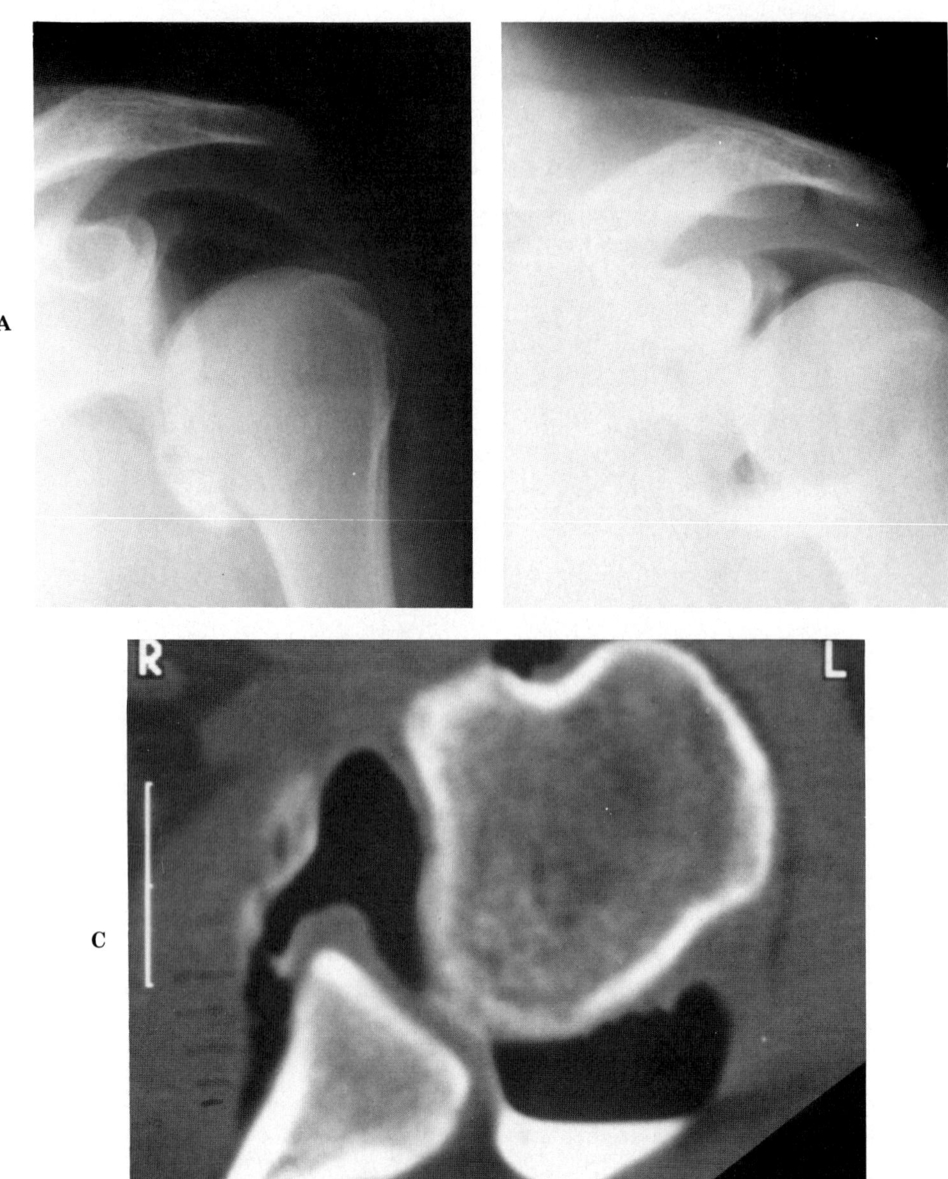

FIG. 3-12. Air-contrast arthrogram in athlete with multidirectional shoulder instability. **A,** Enlarged inferior capsular pouch. **B,** Traction obliterates inferior pouch as humeral head subluxes inferiorly. **C,** CT-assisted air-contrast arthrogram is normal. Dye extravasates into the subscapularis recess. Air outlines the triangular-pointed anterior labrum and more blunted posterior labrum. The margins of the labrum are intact without evidence of tearing, detachment, or abnormal straining with contrast. Positive contrast is seen in the posterior capsular pouch.

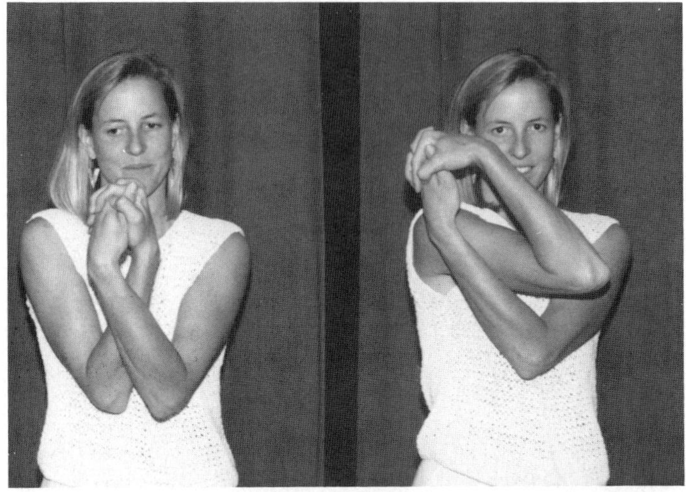

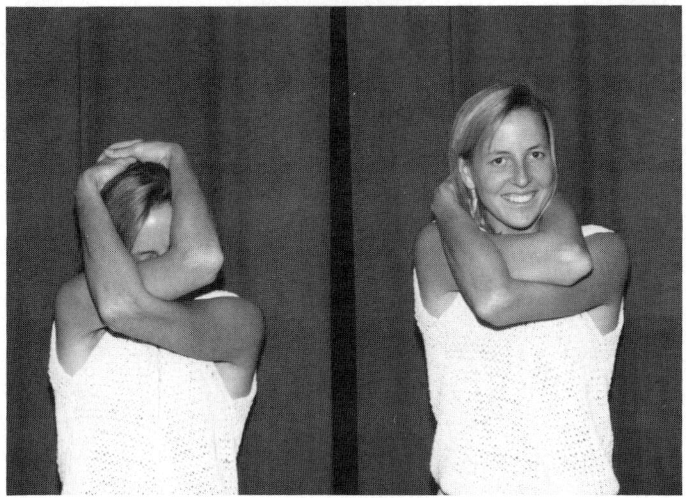

FIG. 3-13. Bilateral generalized upper extremity laxity of shoulders and wrists is required to perform this series of maneuvers. Once the symptomatic right shoulder was repaired, these maneuvers could not be repeated.

laxity, if the feet can be placed over the head behind the neck[113,119] (Fig. 3-13).

Pitfalls to be avoided in the diagnosis and treatment of multidirectional instability (MDI) include the following:

1. Traumatic labral detachment allows for increased motion in all directions on examination. Repair of the labrum is sufficient; additional capsular shifting serves to overly tighten the shoulder.
2. Failure to repair labral detachments with anterior, posterior, or combined procedures may still allow for residual inferior instability and thereby mimic MDI.
3. In an athlete with MDI, overly tight anterior repairs (Putti-Platt, Magnuson-Stack, Bristow) may displace the head to the opposite side of the joint. Early arthritis with pressure necrosis of the head and glenoid results when the capsular restraints on all three sides of the joint have not been balanced, yet iatrogenically hold the head in a fixed subluxed position (Fig. 3-14).

Matsen[100] attempted to simplify the instability considerations with two pneumonics:

TUBS Traumatic etiology
Unidirectional
Bankart ligamentous detachment
Surgical repair

AMBRI Atraumatic etiology
Multidirectional
Bilateral
Rehabilitation with rotational strengthening exercises as primary treatment; effective in approximately 80% of patients.
Inferior capsular shift is the surgical treatment for failed exercises

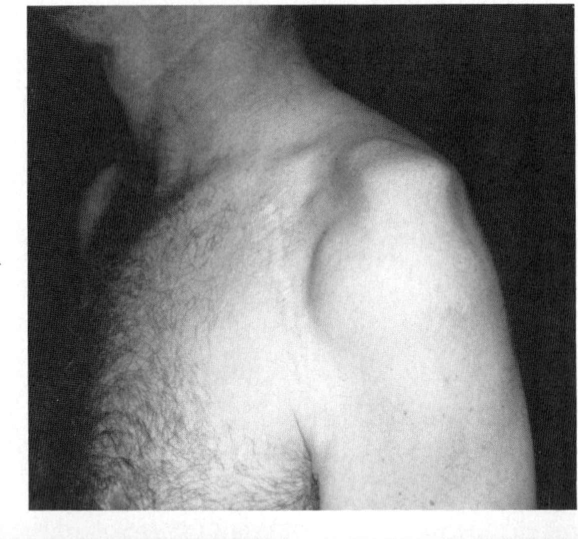

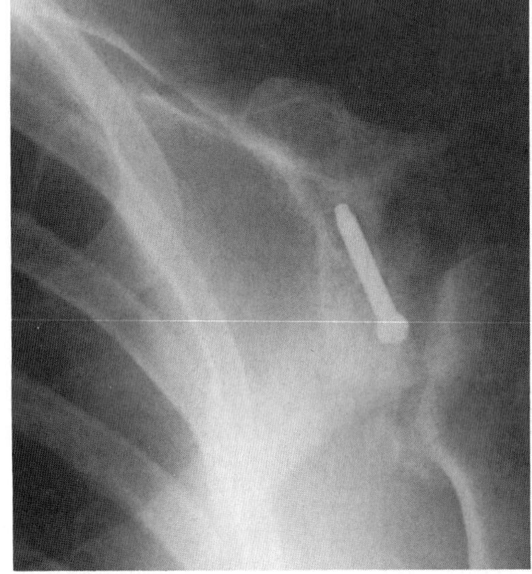

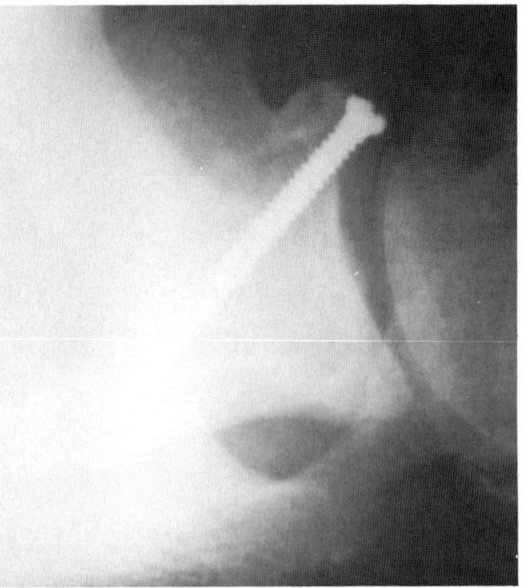

FIG. 3-14. Failed anterior instability repair. Unrepaired anterior labrum with unidirectional repair resulted in fixed posterior humeral head subluxation. Transfer of the coracoid muscles under the axillary nerve resulted in permanent paralysis even though the epineurium was intact. A prominent bony block with hardware and fixed posterior subluxation resulted in degenerative arthritis. **A,** Clinical loss of the deltoid. **B** and **C,** Hardware impingement excavates the anterior humeral head and contributes to the fixed posterior subluxation.

Impingement

The terminology for impingement lesions has led to confusion. In 1834, Smith described rotator cuff tears as a pathologic entity. In 1934, Codman,[38] in the first book dealing with the shoulder, recognized the continuing pain and dysfunction caused by the neglected rotator cuff tear and recommended its repair. Many names and causes for this continuum have been sited for these lesions, including bursitis, tendonitis, acute trauma, overuse, instability, aging, tendon degeneration, vascular deficiencies, and mechanical impingement. McLaughlin[104] noted "that the rotator cuff is the only tendon situated between two bones . . . is compressed by every motion of the shoulder until it succumbs to the ravages of attrition long before most other tendons." Neer unified these concepts when he recognized the wear centered on the supraspinatus, just posterior to the long head of the biceps, as it passed underneath the anterior acromion, acromioclavicular joint, and coracoacromial ligament.[111] Secondarily, the long head of the biceps and infraspinatus may become involved. Four stages of impingement include: phase I—termed "edema and swelling," is now correlated with the overuse ten-

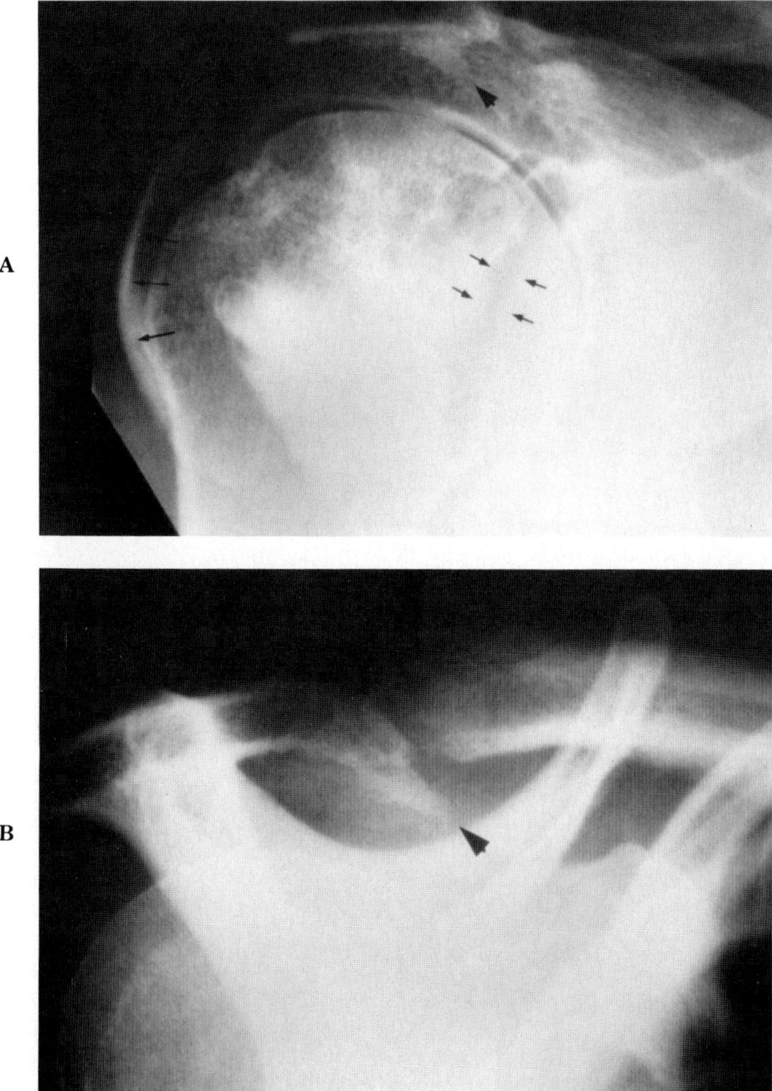

FIG. 3-15. Rotator cuff tear with stage III impingement. **A,** The positive contrast from the shoulder arthrogram has extended beyond the normal attachment of the greater tuberosity, indicating a rotator cuff tear. The small arrows medially mark the long head of the biceps, demonstrating its integrity. If the arm was in external rotation and if dye were to extend down its sheath, the appearance should not be confused with a rotator cuff tear. Calcification extends into the coracoacromial ligament. **B,** In the lateral scapula view the supraspinatus outlet is compromised by an inferior projection of the anterior undersurface of the acromion. Calcification is seen extending into the superior portion of the coracoacromial ligament. This type III hooked acromion (by the Bigliani-Morrison classification) is the most frequent shape associated with tearing of the rotator cuff.

donitis from sports requiring repetitive overhead arm action; phase II—thickening and fibrosis is correlated with incomplete thickness rotator cuff tears, as seen by ultrasonography, arthography, and arthroscopy; phase III—complete thickness tearing and bone changes consisting of sclerosis or spurring along the anterior acromion, with excrescences on the greater tuberosity with subcortical cystic lesions (Fig. 3-15). Phase IV—cuff tear arthropathy[112] may occur in a small percentage of neglected cuff tears (Fig. 3-16). Over time, the humeral head subluxes superiorly.[166] In some instances, the combination of superior and anterior instability and loss of nutritional factors with the persistent cuff tear lead to softening of the head and rotator cuff tear arthropathy. The humeral head then erodes into the undersurface of the AC joint in its superiorly subluxed position, without a stable fulcrum for the glenoid. At this advanced stage, except for sports that in-

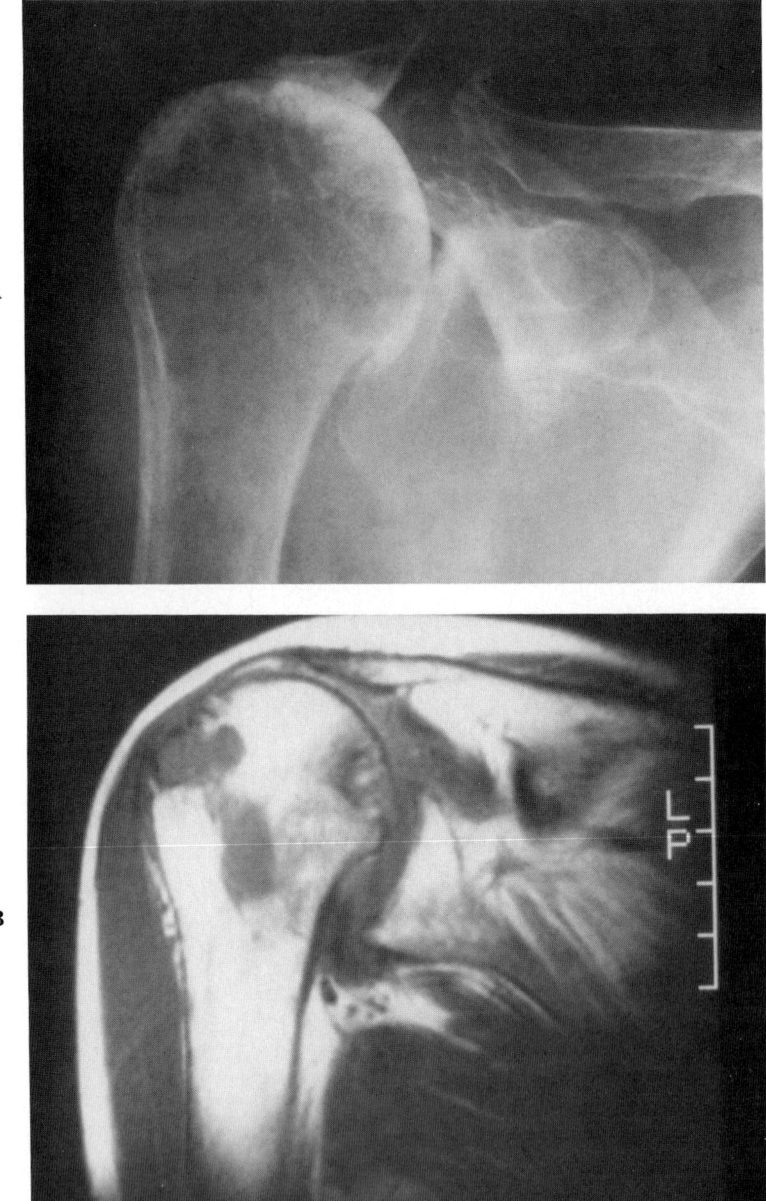

FIG. 3-16. Rotator cuff tear arthropathy with loss of supraspinatus and superior migration of the humeral head. **A,** The humeral head thins out the acromion as a new facet is formed superiorly. The humeral head can no longer be fixed within the glenoid for adequate elevation or use of the intact deltoid. **B,** An MRI in this patient following failed cuff surgery demonstrates roughening and necrosis of the subchondral bone.

volve underhand throwing, like horseshoes, an athlete's career has ended.

The clinical presentations with impingement syndrome are recognized in young athletes involved in sports using repetitive overhead arm motion. They become sore, and at times a swimmer will not be able to continue swimming because of the pain that accompanies use of the arm at the level of the shoulder.[65,82,131,138,139] Use of resistive paddles have served to hasten the symptoms.

The athlete may report fatigue involving the rotator cuff. It is thought that muscle imbalance contributes to poor coordination for the repetitive activities. The external rotators, consisting of the infraspinatus and teres minor, are much weaker as compared with the pectoralis major, latissismus dorsi, teres ma-

A

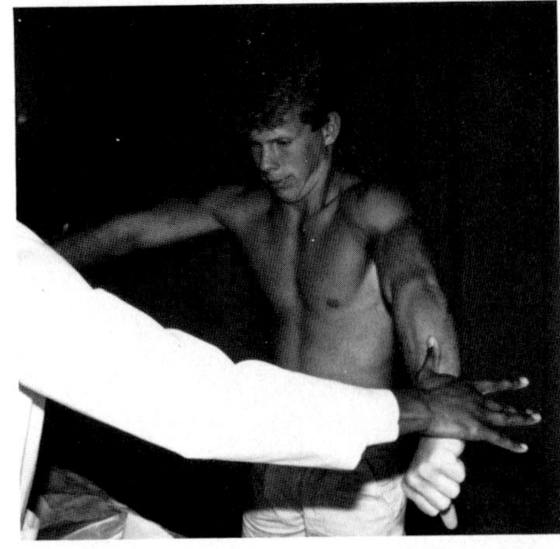

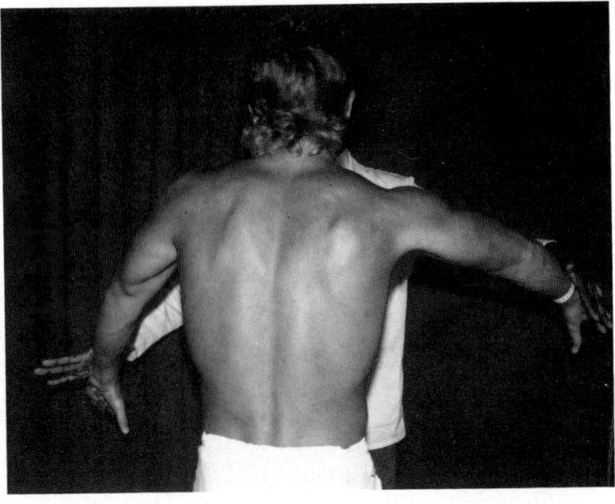

B

FIG. 3-17. Isolated testing of the supraspinatus begins with the arms in 90 degrees abduction and 30 degrees forward flexion and internal rotation with the thumbs pointing downward. This athlete is unable to resist the examiner's downward force on the left side.

jor, subscapularis, and anterior deltoid. Abnormal rhythm has also been implicated if there is either reduced shoulder motion with a stiffness involving the posterior capsule or, alternatively, increased joint laxity from repetitive capsular stretching. The positive clinical signs include subacromial crepitus with rotation in 90 degrees of abduction and a painful arc of motion on actively lowering the arms between 120 degrees and 170 degrees; catching often accompanies this motion. The arm may suddenly drop or need to be supported by the other arm. Weakness of the external rotators is determined by testing the arm at the side. Isolated supraspinatus weakness may be found when the arm is tested against a downward force once placed in 90-degree abduction, 30-degree forward flexion, and full internal rotation (Fig. 3-17).

Temporary pain relief follows a 10-cc subacromial injection of xylocaine.[32,115] With incomplete thickness tears, strength returns to normal for the duration of the effects of the xylocaine.

Ruptures of the long head of the biceps may occur at the musculotendinous area in the very young athlete, but in the middle-aged or aging athlete, this is usually at the top of the biceps groove and associated with an impingement lesion[21,88] (Fig. 3-18).

The differential diagnosis of rotator cuff impingement is adhesive capsulitis, nerve compression (C5-6 disk [Fig. 3-19], suprascapular neuropathy, or other brachial plexus lesions), and shoulder instability. The provocative tests to demonstrate a positive impingement overlap with anterior apprehension in testing instability or the pain produced by stretching a partially frozen shoulder.

Calcific Tendonitis

Calcific tendonitis can occur at any age during adulthood. It has a predilection for the middle-aged athlete involved in repetitive activities. It can occur in any of the tendons of the rotator cuff, although it is more frequently seen in the supraspinatus, 1 to 2 cm from the tendon insertion in the greater tuberosity. The athlete may manifest impingement-like symptoms, with aching and pain exacerbated by activities requiring overhead arm motion. There is no correlation between the size of the deposit and the symptoms.[167] If the pain is longstanding, then there is a tendency for secondary shoulder stiffness to develop in the athlete.

The second presentation is the more severe form, with exquisite pain at rest, inability to sleep, and additional aggravation by motion. The athlete holds the arm as if it were a piece of Steuben glass. The common findings in the evaluation are point tenderness over the calcific deposit and increase in pain when the involved muscle is actively used or if the examiner stretches against the end-range stiffness. Full but guarded motion may be present. Assistance may be requested in getting the arm down to the midthoracic level on internal rotation testing.[167] It can be diagnosed under penetrated (35% to 40%) anterior and posterior roentgenograph views, in internal and external rotation, and by a lateral scapula view to determine the precise location of the deposit (Fig. 3-20).

Seven percent of individuals with shoulder

A

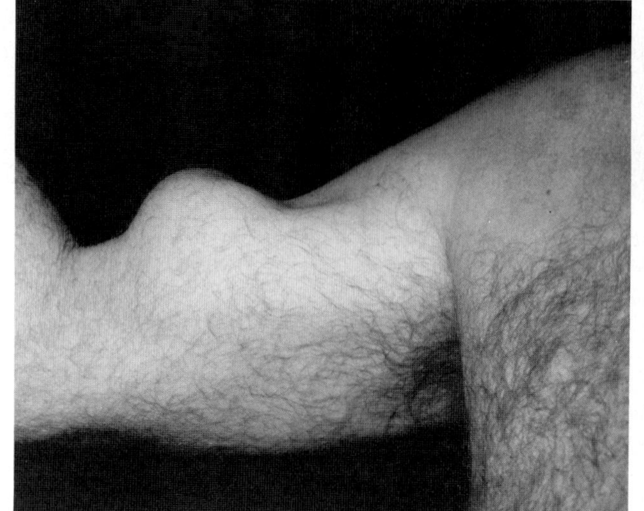

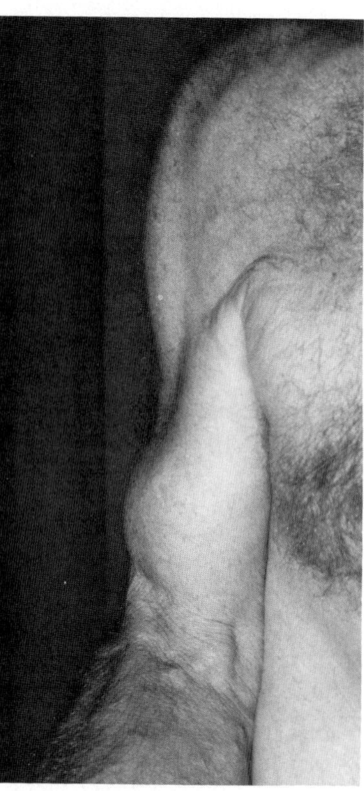

B

FIG. 3-18. Proximal rupture of the long head of the biceps. **A,** At the musculotendinous junction in the young athlete. **B,** At the biceps groove in this 69-year-old athlete.

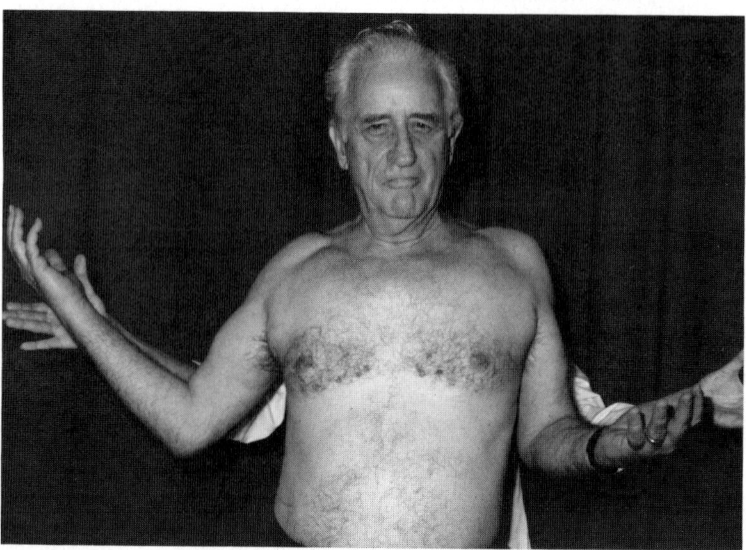

FIG. 3-19. Herniated C5-6 disk resulting in external rotation weakness mimics rotator cuff tear of the left shoulder. Once the arms are released the left arm falls in towards the stomach, demonstrating passive but not active external rotation.

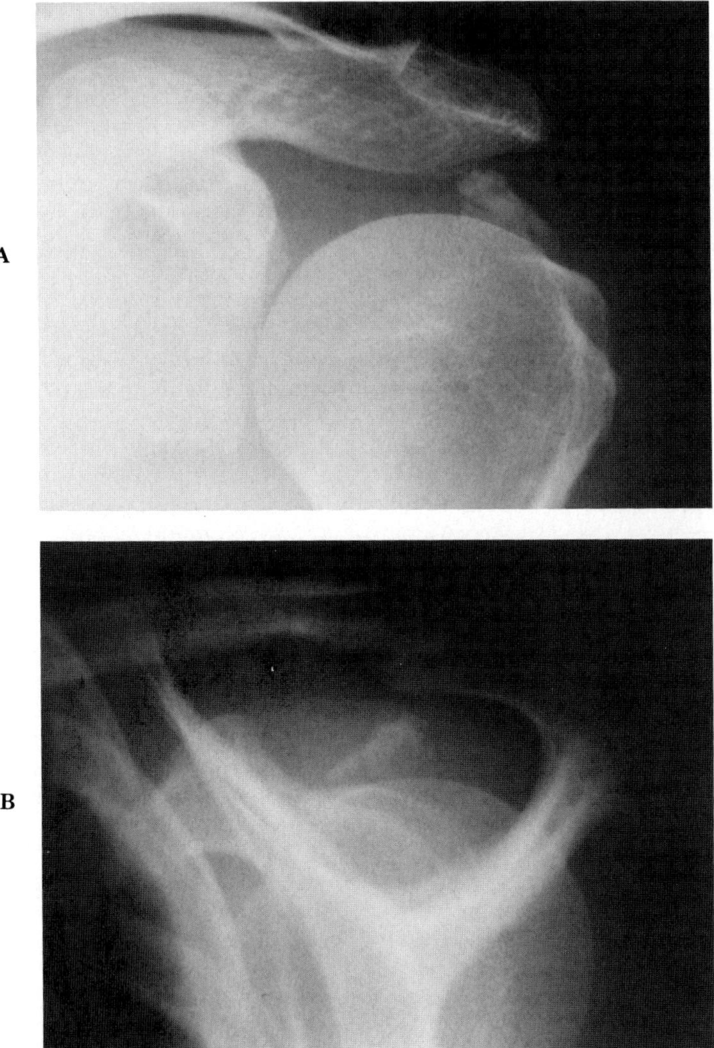

FIG. 3-20. Calcific tendonitis in the supraspinatus 1 cm from its insertion. **A,** External rotation view. **B,** Lateral scapula view.

pain have symptomatic calcific tendonitis.[50] Approximately 3% of asymptomatic patients will demonstrate calcification in the rotator cuff.[137] Thirty-five to forty-five percent of the asymptomatic individuals will eventually become symptomatic.[28] Although the etiology is uncertain, Uhthoff et al[163] proposed tissue hypoxia as the initial event leading to hydroxyapatite deposition, followed by macrophage adsorption and collagenous reconstitution.

Two types of deposits may be seen: the well-circumscribed, gritty, sand like deposit is consistent with the chronic phase, whereas the amorphous deposit of toothpaste consistency is characteristic of the resorptive healing phase. The latter phase is associated with the exquisite pain; the former phase may be present on an incidental x-ray film without symptoms with other chronic aching symptoms. Corticosteroid injections, and more likely the needle puncture of the deposit in the acute resorptive phase, allow the deposit to escape into the subacromial space and resorb. Calcific deposits are seen less frequently now by the treating orthopaedic surgeon than 30 years ago. It is not clear whether this is a change in the natural history of the disease or whether the deposits are more often adequately treated by the primary care physicians.

Adhesive Capsulitis ("Frozen Shoulder")

Although there are many causes of shoulder stiffness, perhaps the most perplexing is that of adhesive capsulitis resulting in a markedly restricted joint capsule.[167] There is a strong predilection for women in the menopausal and early postmenopausal age group. It is rarely associated with tearing of the rotator cuff. Its cause is unknown. Neviaser[116] reported dense adhesions in the capsule, whereas Lundberg[95] found no adhesions at surgery, with fibrosis of the deep layers on biopsy. Bland et al[23] postulated that an autonomic dysfunction results in impaired circulation, secondary fibrosis, and stiffness. This hypothesis satisfactorily explains the lack of adhesions within the joint when the shoulder is examined arthroscopically or visualized at open surgery.

Clinically, many orthopaedists ascribe the onset to episodes of shoulder immobilization. Stiffness follows protection of the arm in adduction, internal rotation, and slight elevation of the shoulder. The precipitating cause could be placement of the arm in a sling after a Colles' fracture, cervical radiculopathy, angina, intrinsic calcific tendonitis, or failure to mobilize the arm after a stroke. Frequently the precipitating cause is not found. The treatment goal is restoration of the inferior capsular pouch by stretching, exercises, manipulation under anesthesia, or open release. Shoulder stiffness invalidates many of the other diagnostic maneuvers for impingement and instability testing. Unfortunately, the missed posterior fracture dislocation may present as a frozen shoulder. An axillary roentgenograph eliminates this confusion.

Precipitating cause of adhesive capsulitis

- Forearm, wrist, and hand fractures/injuries
- Cervical radiculopathy
- Angina
- Calcific tendonitis
- After CVA
- Unknown

Neurologic Problems

Neurologic problems occur in the amateur or young athlete more frequently than in the professional.[13] They often manifest radiating pain, burning, and numbness in the shoulder or extending down the arm, with local stunning and inability to lift the arm, forearm, or wrist. Primary shoulder pathology will not be associated with pain extending beyond the elbow. Spinal cord injuries and cervical spine fractures, although infrequent, still occur with spearhead football tackles or hard falls when the head and shoulder are forced apart. Common mechanisms for this include forward falls in gymnastics and skiing or being thrown over the handle bars of a speeding motorcycle or bicycle.

Paralysis of the entire limb and severe burning is a sign of nerve root avulsion; fractures of the first rib, clavicle, and coracoid are associated with severe brachial plexus stretching.[90] Those injuries caused by a hockey stick or other sharp object to the neck can result in weakness of the trapezius, with a dragging, aching sensation in the shoulder.[13] The athlete may be unable to shrug the shoulder and may later report secondary impingement symptoms with attempted overhead arm extension.

Wearing a heavy backpack or falling with a backpack has been associated with **serratus anterior palsy.** Loss of the serratus anterior with traction to the long thoracic nerve of Bell has been reported in overhead weight lifters[156] and in the discus thrower, who presumably tears the scapula fixators that allow for stretching of the nerve with subsequent scapula winging.[63]

Compression or traction of the **suprascapular nerve,** with pain and weakness in hitting a backhand or in serving, has been seen in suprascapular nerve entrapment as well as in occult ganglions pressing the suprascapular nerve. This being the highest structure coming off the plexus, it is also susceptible to direct blows in contact sports.[13]

Isolated infraspinatus atrophy has occurred with traction, trauma, and ganglions (Fig. 3-21). Loss of the suprascapular nerve branch to the infraspinatus at the level of the spinoglenoid notch or distal has been reported in injuries caused by stretching.[47,51,108] The isolated infraspinatus palsy was a common finding in Italian volleyball spikers.[51] Another mechanism that caused weakness and posterior shoulder pain involved severe stretching of the infraspinatus muscle after a violent throw.[148] As seen on MRI, the infraspinatus was replaced with fatty tissue.

The relationship of the **axillary nerve** to the glenohumeral joint makes it particularly prone to injury during shoulder joint trauma.[39] The axillary nerve is susceptible to stretching with an anterior dislocation or direct contusion by a backwards fall on the quadrilateral space or a blow to the deltoid.[13,40] The nerve is found to be injured in 20% to 30% of glenohumeral dislocations and humeral neck fractures when it is assessed by EMG 2 to 3 weeks after injury.[40] In those over 50 years of age, it is as high as 50%.[25,48,129] Unfortunately, sensibility testing in the axillary nerve distribution of the lateral arm has not proved reliable.[25]

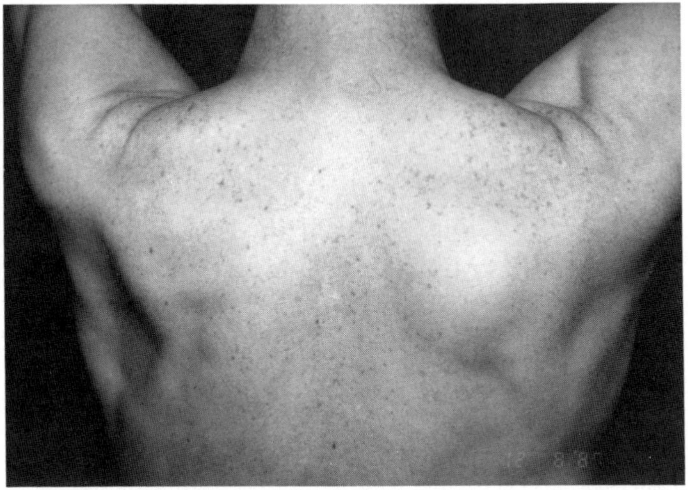

FIG. 3-21. Isolated infraspinatus atrophy of the left shoulder.

The **musculocutaneous nerve** is susceptible to direct frontal blows. Athletes will report numbness in the lateral forearm to the base of the thumb and have a weak to absent biceps.

Sports injuries account for 2.9% to 5.7% of all the peripheral nerve system injuries.[71,85] The radial, ulnar, peroneal, and axillary nerves are the peripheral nerves most frequently injured in sports.[71] The axillary and musculocutaneous nerves are the most likely to be injured in athletic reconstructive procedures about the shoulder[34,40,123] (see Fig. 3-14).

Scapulothoracic Problems

The scapulothoracic articulation is a gliding joint between the thoracic rib cage and the scapula. It is separated by filmy bursa. Problems in this area occur from muscle paralysis, snapping scapula, and rib fractures. In the group of muscle paralyses, winging from a serratus anterior palsy and scapular ptosis or drooping from a trapezius palsy hamper the athlete because of fatigue pain and inability to adequately place the scapula under the glenoid. With a serratus anterior palsy, the scapula cannot be fixed to the chest wall as the arm is elevated (Fig. 3-22). The winging is accentuated by contracture of the rhomboids and pectoralis minor muscles.[164] Increasing pain develops and the athlete is unable to lift with power or push. In trapezius palsies, impingement is aggravated with arm abduction. The shoulder droops and is subject to easy fatigue.

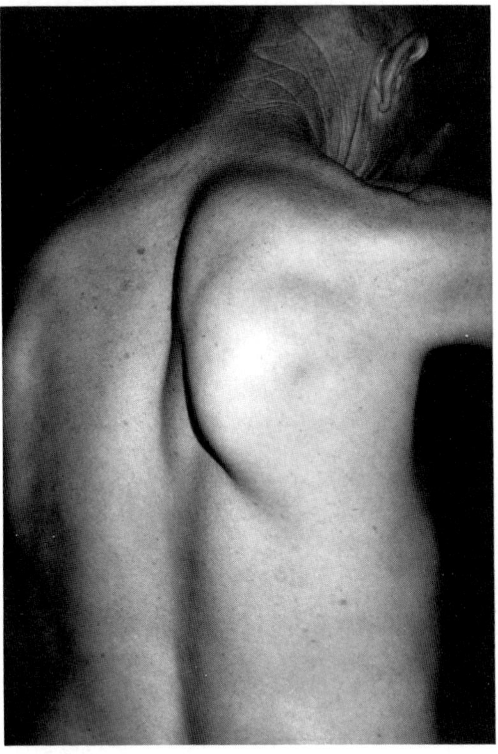

FIG. 3-22. Winging of the right scapula with serratus anterior paralysis.

Scapulothoracic crepitus, or a snapping scapula palpable at the superior medial border of the scapula, is not a well-understood entity. Rarely, an osteochondroma on the undersurface of the superior medial border of the scapula will account for the crepitus. Alternatively, a malunion after multiple rib fractures will interrupt the gliding motion of the scapula on the chest wall. More commonly, there is no known cause of the crepitation and grinding that can be produced by moving the scapula up and down against the chest wall. Snapping and pain are localized to the superior medial border as it articulates with the thorax. Modification of activities, strengthening of the subscapularis and serratus anterior, and occasionally a corticosteroid injection in the scapulothoracic bursa are sometimes successful in treatment of what can be an intermittently painful syndrome. If psychologic problems can be excluded, a subperiosteal excision of the superior medial pole through a muscle-splitting incision relieves the pain and snapping in eight of nine cases.[8] The procedure had to be repeated in one patient who was skeletally immature at the index procedure.

Arthritis

Arthritis of joints of the shoulder girdle include the sternoclavicular, acromioclavicular, and glenohumeral joints. Sporting activities which can produce arthritis include direct trauma with fractures, dislocations, or repetitive loading.

Sternoclavicular Joint

Arthritis of the sternoclavicular joint may occur from direct trauma with a rare posterior dislocation or indirect trauma with the more frequent anterior subluxation and dislocations. Arthritis of this joint is rarely sports-related[135] and is gradual in onset in postmenopausal women.[30] In a 27-year period, Thorndike found few sternoclavicular joint injuries in organized college athletics at Harvard.[135] The few severe injuries to the sternoclavicular joint are high-kinetic injuries from bicycles, motor vehicles, polo, snowskiing, and, occasionally, football.[135]

Acromioclavicular Joint

Weight lifters' shoulders describes a condition with repetitive loading at the acromioclavicular joint resulting in degenerative arthritis and (at times) an osteolysis of the outer clavicle.[33,35]

Glenohumeral Joint

Glenohumeral osteoarthritis with eccentric wear of the posterior glenoid has been observed in weight lifting as well as in many other sports in which the strong rotator cuff muscles are intact and function well. The athlete may report aching and fatigue pain, or bone-on-bone grinding noises that are accentuated with resistive muscle testing with sharp pain. The diagnosis is confirmed with roentgenographs. Other causes of glenohumeral arthritis to consider in the patient's history include an arthritis occurring after recurrent dislocations[119,121,122] or occurring after fixed humeral head displacement to the opposite side of the joint in repairs for instability that are too tight[113,114,123] or in which the humeral head abuts on metal in or near the joint.[124,170]

PSYCHOLOGIC FACTORS IN SHOULDER PAIN*

When the orthopaedic history and examination, together with any indicated special studies, are unsuccessful in clearly suggesting an anatomic diagnosis, functional causes of pain must be considered. Indeed, even when shoulder pain has an anatomic basis, psychologic factors may result in a clinical presentation which, on first regard, seems more serious than is actually the case. Although the terms **anatomic** (organic) and **functional** (nonorganic) and their variations are commonly used to describe pain, it should be understood that this dichotomy is an artificial one. Most pain—especially chronic pain—has both organic and psychologic underpinnings.

Clinicians are frequently unable to relinquish the notion that pain must always originate in peripheral receptors and nowhere else. Association pathways in the brain link peripheral pain (afferent) pathways with the limbic system, through which emotions are processed. Pain is a final common pathway that can signal disturbance in either or both the physical and the psychologic domain.

Nonorganic (or functional) causes of pain must always be included in the differential diagnosis of chronic pain. The differential diagnosis of functional pain includes depressive and anxiety spectrum disorders (including major depression, dysthymia and generalized anxiety disorder), adjustment disorders, somatoform disorders, factitious disorders, and malingering. Sometimes chronic pain may be a manifestation of a psychotic disorder, such as schizophrenia.

Functional causes of pain

- Depression
- Anxiety disorders
- Adjustment disorders
- Somatoform disorders
- Factitious disorders
- Malingering
- Psychosis

Functional pain is not (and should never be) regarded as a diagnosis of exclusion. Certain individuals, because of events and cir-

*References 9, 14, 15, 46, 49, 52, 97.

cumstances during the formative years, are prone to pain. They are particularly vulnerable to development of chronic pain in response to events and circumstances of their adult lives that resonate (frequently at an unconscious level) with the situations in their formative years, which rendered them prone to pain in the first place. More often than not, they do not understand the dynamics involved. Not realizing its origin in the psyche, they seek an organic explanation for their pain. Their conviction (which may reach delusional proportions) is that the pain is not only organic, but that (reinforcing the delusion) it results because of a specific "target incident" or "injury." Many such injuries are "red herrings" that serve as a smokescreen to obscure the emotional situation responsible for and underlying the chronic pain. In the case of shoulder pain, the underlying situation often has to do with *shouldering* a burden or with *shouldering* responsibility or with *bearing up* in the face of personal or financial loss.

Depressed individuals invariably have lowered tolerance of pain. They may perceive as disabling or incapacitating pain that for healthy individuals would be, at worst, an annoyance. The depressed individual uses chronic (nonorganic) pain at an unconscious level to legitimize his or her dependency (primary gain) and to secure caretaking (secondary gain) from the environment. Many young persons are driven to almost superhuman lengths to achieve athletically in an unconscious search for parental acceptance or approval. For some, the only way out without losing face is to be "forced," because of a painful orthopaedic condition, to curtail their activities. Their pain bespeaks a conflict between *consciously* wanting to continue the striving for athletic achievement on the one hand, and *unconsciously* wanting to lessen the incessant pressure to achieve, on the other. Similarly, in the individual whose emotional neediness is concealed by a façade of independence and self-sufficiency (often since a young age), a chronic pain syndrome is evidence of the conflict between consciously wanting to continue shouldering responsibility and providing, on the one hand, and unconsciously wanting passively to be taken care of and to receive the emotional nurturing denied earlier in life, on the other. In these situations the chronic pain syndrome legitimizes the curtailment of activity by the patient, who can then become passive and less dependent *without losing face*. It is this face-saving dynamic, an internal mechanism to preserve self-esteem, that is termed "primary gain." The primary gain usually far outweighs the *secondary gain* in terms of its overall importance and should be recognized as the *raison d'etre* for the functional pain.

Pain, depression, and anxiety are frequently observed in association with one another. At times, chronic pain may be an early manifestation of a depressive disorder. It is common for the patient to conclude that the chronic pain caused the depression. In most cases of functional pain, it is the other way around: the pain is an early manifestation of an unrecognized or so-called masked depression that is smoldering beneath the surface.

How is the orthopaedist to recognize the patient with chronic shoulder pain in whom functional factors are of primary importance? Typically such pain has been precipitated by and reflects not physical, but emotional injury. A careful history will usually reveal a circumstance or event, such as separation from close ones (spouse, children, parents, siblings) material or financial loss (including job loss) or increased responsibility, in close temporal proximity to the onset of functional pain. In athletes, precipitants may be particularly important athletic contests or events.

Somatization is the expression in physical terms of emotional pain. Somatists use denial and repression, and they usually externalize blame. They usually do not volunteer the precipitating psychosocial stressors that brought on their physical symptoms because they do not understand the connection. Indeed, they often resist inquiry into the important psychosocial arena with anger and the question, "What's that got to do with my shoulder pain?" It is therefore particularly important to remain mindful that individuals who, in their developmental years, have been emotionally shortchanged (by parental fighting or divorce, emotional or physical parental absence, parental alcoholism, family poverty, and the need, at an early age, to shoulder major breadwinner responsibilities, or who have been physically or sexually abused) are particularly vulnerable to somatization. It is to the benefit of the orthopaedist to spend a few minutes during the history to inquire appropriately.

The "MADISON" pneumonic outlines the behavioral indicators that suggest psychogenic pain.[61,62]

M—Multiple complaints

Patient manifests a variety of symptoms, often unrelated to the pain that brought them into the office. For example, a patient with shoulder pain will also discuss pain in the knees, gastrointestinal pain, headaches, etc. Particularly significant is that the reports of pain are related to multiple systems in the body and are clearly unrelated to one another.

A—Authenticity
The patient "doth protest too much." In this case, the patient uses overkill to convince the physician of the authenticity of the pain. There may be some preamble related to other physicians who have not believed the patient. This is especially significant in those instances in which the patient attempts to "head the doctor off at the pass" to prevent the physician from forming his or her own opinion. The patient is engaged in an argument long before the doctor has arrived at that juncture.

Behavioral indicators that suggest psychogenic pain

- M—Multiple complaints
- A—Authenticity
- D—Denial
- I—Interpersonal variability
- S—Singularity
- O—Only you
- N—Nothing works

D—Denial
This refers to inappropriate affect about the pain, as well as the denial of affect about other aspects of the patient's life. Doctors are attuned to the patient who complains too much, but they should also be concerned about those who deny negative effect from their injuries. The stoic or compliant patient may be easier to deal with in the office, but there is also the possibility that he or she is using the pain in some way to get a greater reward. Hence the absence of negative affect about the sequelae of the injury.

Along these lines, be careful about the patient who denies any negative effect from the impact of the pain on the rest his or her life. An essential question in an examination is, "How do you feel about your injury?"

I—Interpersonal variability
The patient who is more psychogenic will vary his or her report of pain according to the person interacted with. Hence, office staff will get one level of discomfort and the doctor another. It may vary in either direction. That is, doctor getting more or less than his or her staff. Some variability is normal and appropriate. Excessive variability is indicative that there are more variables, other than the organic ones that need to be considered.

S—Singularity
The patients report their symptoms in a manner that indicates "only they" have this kind or degree of pain. Any attempts to put them into a category—"people who have your kind of injury"—are met with resistance. Their reqquest for "special" consideration should be heard as a warning signal.

O—Only you
The doctor is placed on a special level that indicates that the patient sees him or her as the only one who can help them. This is particularly seductive, as it plays to the doctor's ego needs. It should serve as a warning to remember that, with many of these patients, there were several doctors who have preceded them who have also been "special", until they failed, in the patients' eyes that is. This is a problematic area, as the "only you" is often used as a way of engaging the doctor to behave in some way out of the ordinary; that is extra medication, more frequent visits, disability certification, etc.

N—Nothing works
For the patient who is more psychogenically involved, literally "nothing works." The emphasis here is on the "nothing" part of the statement. Medication, which should have some effect—however minimal—is said to be *totally* ineffective. The same is true for physical therapy and all of the other varieties of treatments. In other words, the absoluteness and the uniformity of the intransigence are the issues here. Reinforcing this is an often benign indifference that the patient has toward the doctor's "failure" to resolve the problem. It suggests that there is some other agenda that may need to be resolved before the patient is willing to allow any treatments to have an impact.

Although it is not the task of the orthopaedist to establish precise psychiatric diagnosis, it is important that functional problems not be overlooked because of failure to consider the appropriate history. It is the task of the psychiatrist and the clinical psychologist, working collaboratively, to establish the precise diagnosis. Although obtaining an MMPI with a computerized interpretation may identify *some* problems as functional, the diagnostic precision from such an approach is not great. An analogy would be for the orthopaedist to rely solely on roentgenographic and other imaging findings out of context in diagnosing a shoulder problem. The results of the MMPI and of other diagnostic measures are best interpreted against the backdrop of a thorough history and physical and mental status examinations.

Persuading a patient to undergo psychologic evaluation can be problematic. It is almost axiomatic that the more the patient resists, and the more angry he or she becomes, the more likely it is that a relevant psychiatric diagnosis will be discovered. There are ways to convince the recalcitrant individual to be evaluated:

1. Some orthopaedists make such evaluation a part of their workup in every case of chronic shoulder pain. Increasingly, physicians are including psychiatric screening of candidates for organ transplantation and for other major surgery. Such screening proves cost-effective in that it can identify patients who, with special preoperative or postoperative help, will have smoother courses than they might otherwise.
2. Sometimes a patient will volunteer that stress makes the pain worse. Such information can provide good reason for psychologic evaluation to understand how the individual copes with stress and to consider techniques to manage stress optimally.
3. When chronic pain is the manifested problem, it can be helpful to explain to the patient that everyone has an emotional reaction to pain and that if pain is longstanding, the emotional reaction can result in excess pain after surgery or in other postoperative morbidity. Patients should see the evaluating psychiatrist as a physician with particular understanding of chronic pain, rather than as a doctor who treats crazy persons.

However it is done, the referral should be made in a manner that reflects an acknowledgement of the validity of the patient's pain. Pain is pain and, whether of organic or functional origin or both, it hurts, and it is unpleasant. Only when the psychologic dimensions of chronic shoulder pain are understood can a rational treatment plan (with a reasonable chance of success) be devised.

PHYSICAL EXAMINATION

The shoulder evaluation begins with the patient seated. The female's gown is placed above her breasts, below the axilla, and is tied in the back. Bra straps are lowered. The male is undressed above the waist. This allows observation of the front and back, symmetry of motion, muscle atrophy, and bony prominences. By standing behind the seated patient, the examiner begins with the cervical spine. Flexion and gentle rotation are evaluated first. In the absence of rheumatoid arthritis or other significant cervical spine disease, this serves as a beginning psychologic screening test. Exaggerated reports of pain or parathesias in nonanatomic distributions alert the examiner to possible overly anxious or hysterical responses. This provides an early basis for interpretation of subjective symptoms.

Foramenal closure maneuvers, with hyperextension and lateral bending of the neck, are used to screen for cervical radiculopathy. Mild pain in the cervical spine or radiating to the levator scapula insertion is not uncommon, whereas pain radiating to the shoulder and more distal in the upper extremity suggests that additional neurologic workup be considered.

Sternoclavicular Joint

This joint is evaluated for sprains, anterior and posterior subluxations and dislocations, arthritis, fractures, and in the child, physeal injuries that may simulate as a dislocation.

Observation

The patient is observed both from the front and behind for prominences, depressions, or abnormal asymmetric motion when the arms are elevated.

Palpation

The medial ends of the clavicle can be evaluated with the physician standing behind the patient. A finger can be placed in the superior sternal notch to palpate the medial clavicle above the articulation with the sternum. Direct pressure over the sternal costal articulation elicits pain if there is arthritis or a recent capsular sprain with associated swelling.

Posterior dislocations of the sternoclavicular joint are rare. Clinically they can be palpated as a depression between the sternal end of the clavicle and the manubrium. In the acute setting, pulses are palpated for a great vessel injury. The airway is assessed to ensure there is no difficulty in breathing.

Anterior subluxation or dislocation is the more common direction of instability (Fig. 3-23). The sternal end of the clavicle can be grasped between the examiner's fingers and moved cephalad or caudad. With abduction and extension of the shoulders, it will retract more laterally. The subluxation may be reduced, but is usually unstable. Hypertrophy and degenerative arthritis are not uncommon in postmenopausal women on the dominant arm.[26,30,141]

Provocative Tests

If the patient has reported clicking or instability, motion of the arm is encouraged to reproduce the symptoms. Grasping the sternal end of the clavicle to compress it or attempt to sublux it is another means of testing the stability of the joint. Adduction of the arm

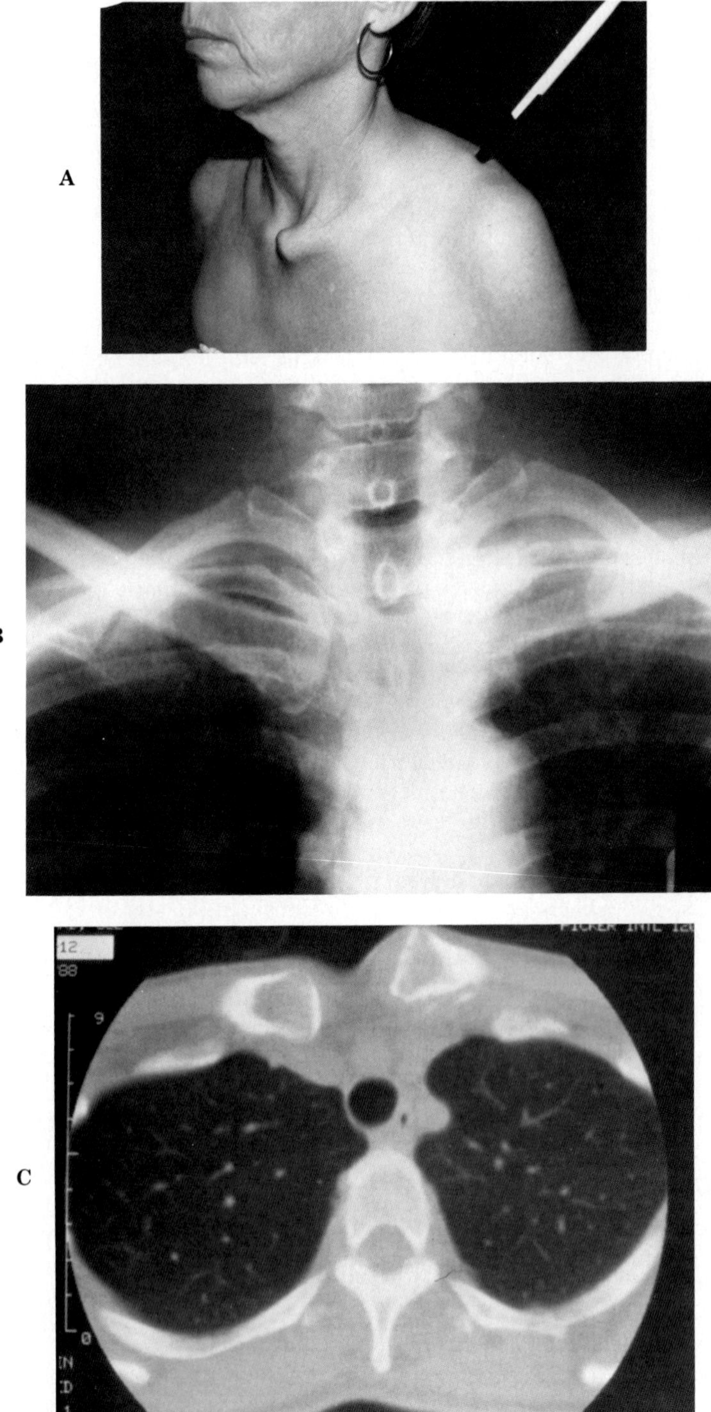

FIG. 3-23. Bipolar clavicle dislocation with anterior sternoclavicular joint dislocation and type IV posterior acromioclavicular joint dislocation. **A,** The prominent left sternoclavicular joint is the more clinically obvious, but the posteriorly displaced distal clavicle is the more symptomatic secondary to supraspinatus impingement. **B,** Anterior-posterior roentgenographs of the sternoclavicular joints demonstrate more high-riding left clavicle. This combined with a 15-degree cephlad tilt would exaggerate the difference. **C,** CT scan documents the anterior dislocation of the left as compared with the right sternoclavicular joint.

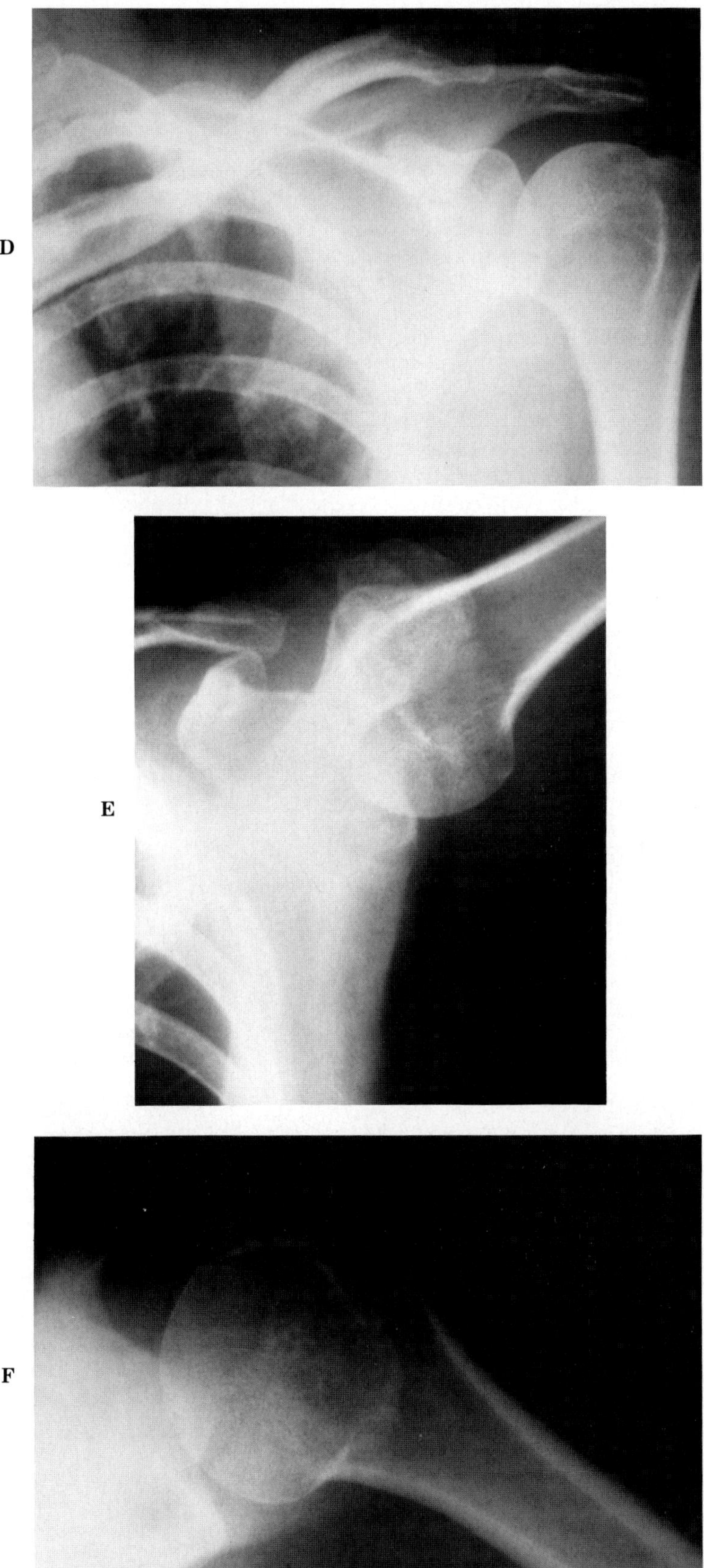

FIG. 3-23 con't.d **D,** The anterior-posterior roentgenograph of the type IV acromioclavicular posterior dislocation shows widening at the acromioclavicular joint. **E,** The Stryker notch view. **F,** The axillary view. Both of these views demonstrate the posterior displacement of the distal clavicle relative to the acromion.

across the chest can compress the involved joint. This might increase pain if there is traumatic or degenerative arthritis.

Acromioclavicular Joint

The acromioclavicular joint is a diarthrodial joint between the lateral end of the clavicle and the medial aspect of the acromion. Coracoacromial ligaments control anterior and posterior translation of the outer clavicle, whereas coracoclavicular ligaments, consisting of the trapezoid and conoid ligaments, hold the shoulder girdle up to the outer end of the clavicle. This joint is evaluated for arthritis and ligamentous disruption with instability. Allman originally described three classes of acromioclavicular joint injuries.[3] Rockwood has expanded the classification to six types.[141]

Type I. Sprain of acromioclavicular ligaments without displacement of the joint.

Type II. Disruption of acromioclavicular ligaments, sprain of coracoclavicular ligaments, and slight upward displacement of the clavicle compared with the shoulder.

Type III. Disruption of acromioclavicular and coracoacromial ligaments with relative upward displacement of the outer clavicle and an increase of the coracoclavicular space by 25% to 100%. The deltoid and trapezius muscles have been detached from the outer clavicle (Fig. 3-24).

Type IV. Acromioclavicular ligaments disrupted, coracoclavicular ligaments partially or completely disrupted, posterior dislocation of the clavicle into the trapezius with detachment of the deltoid and trapezius from the distal clavicle (see Fig. 3-23).

A

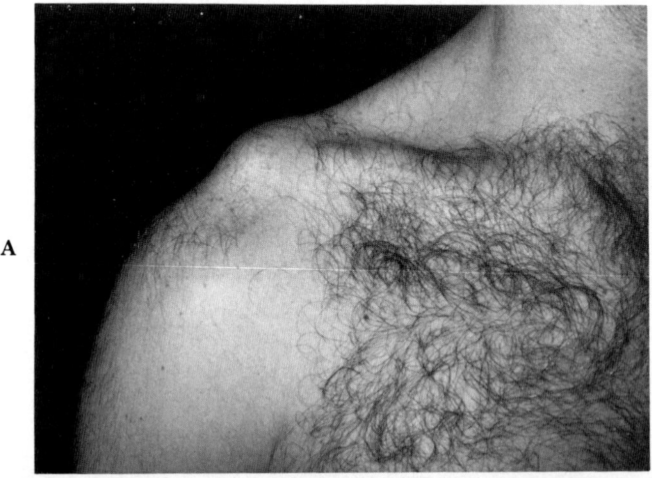

B

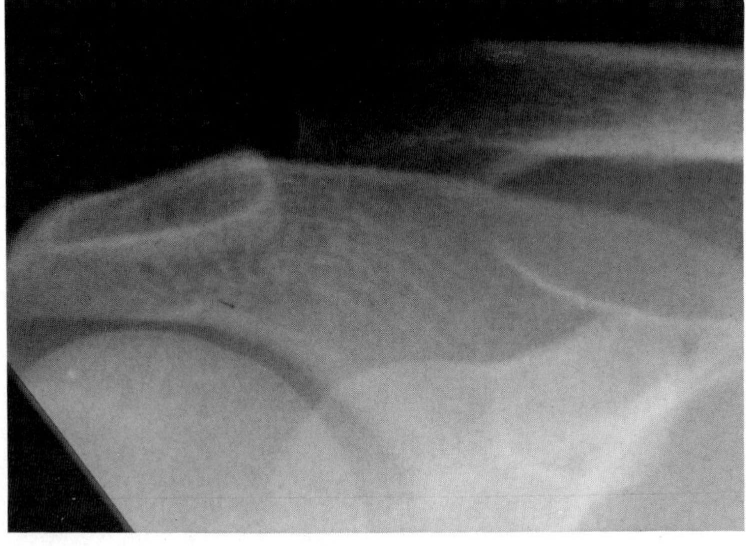

FIG. 3-24. Grade III acromioclavicular separation. **A,** Clinical prominence of the outer clavicle is demonstrated as the shoulder girdle subluxes inferiorly. **B,** Roentgenographic appearance.

Type V. Severe version of type III, with coracoclavicular interspace increased 100% to 300%, compared to normal. The clavicle is displaced towards the base of the neck; the deltoid and trapezius have been detached from the outer half of the clavicle.

Type VI. Acromioclavicular ligaments are disrupted, coracoclavicular ligaments may be intact or disrupted, and the clavicle is dislocated inferiorly or under the acromion or coracoid process.

With this classification in mind, the acromioclavicular joint is evaluated.

Observation

The outer clavicle is viewed to determine whether it is prominent, relative to the acromion, or displaced in one of the directions consistent with an acromioclavicular joint injury. While it is often described as upward displacement of the outer clavicle, the shoulder girdle displaces downward from the clavicle, which is normal position with coracoclavicular ligamentous disruptions.

The outer clavicle warrants careful evaluation in the presence of an obvious sternoclavicular joint dislocation. Bipolar dislocations of the clavicle are visually objectional at the sternal end, but clinically painful at the acromial end, with impingement on the supraspinatus when posteriorly displaced into the trapezius (see Fig. 3-23).

Palpation

The acromioclavicular joint is located by palpating the base of a V formed between the spine of the scapula and the posterior clavicle, as it articulates with the acromion. The anterior and posterior aspects of the acromion are then identified. The lateral acromion is palpated and its position is confirmed by rotating the humerus when longitudinal traction is placed in the line of the humerus. Once the acromial margins can be identified, then the acromioclavicular joint is palpated from posterior to anterior. Direct pressure over the acromioclavicular joint is painful in acute injuries with swelling and degenerative arthritis. Gentle ballottement confirms the joint location. Crepitus may be illicited with arthritis or instability.

The coracoid and the coracoclavicular ligaments are palpated for evidence of tenderness, indicative of a sprain, in the event that there is either no displacement of the joint seen with roentgenography or a tear when displacement is encountered. With types III and V acromioclavicular joint injuries, there is a prominent step off at the outer end of the clavicle.

Provocative tests

With pressure over the outer end of the clavicle, an upward force placed along the lines of the dependent humerus will reduce suspected acromioclavicular joint subluxation or dislocation. Forward flexion of the arm with adduction across the chest will accentuate a type V acromioclavicular joint injury, tenting the skin over the outer clavicle as it comes close to tickling the ear.

Adduction of the arm across the chest also serves as a provocative compression of the intact acromioclavicular joint. This would be painful with acromioclavicular arthritis or osteolysis of the outer clavicle and needs to be differentiated from posterior capsular tightness and other more severe forms of shoulder stiffness.

In a type IV posteriorly displaced distal clavicle, the signs and tests for an impingement syndrome will be positive. The outer clavicle may be more difficult to palpate because it is buried in the trapezius and supraspinatus.

Glenohumeral Joint

Observation

The muscles about the glenohumeral joint are observed for atrophy or bulges. The supraspinatus and infraspinatus are best viewed from behind and from the side. With a C5-6 disk or with a long-standing rotator cuff tear, infraspinatus atrophy can be appreciated. Ruptures of the long head of the biceps can be viewed as a more distal enlargement of the lateral half of the biceps in the arm and later accentuated with external rotation–resistance testing or biceps muscle strength testing.

Normally the long axis of the humerus passes up through the anterior acromion. The acromion superiorly covers the posterior half of the humeral head rather than extending over the entire humeral head. When the coracoid is prominent and there is a depression anteriorly, then a posterior or locked posterior fracture dislocation must be suspected. Alternatively, psychiatrically disturbed individuals may intentionally or unintentionally hold their arm in a posteriorly subluxed position, with the elbow positioned slightly forward through a strong contracture of the pectoralis and anterior deltoid (see Fig. 3-9).

Inferior subluxation of the humerus with atrophy of the deltoid may be noted after a birth injury or other brachial plexus injury, a cerebral vascular accident, or a dislocation of or iatrogenic injury to the axillary nerve. A sulcus is present between the acromion and humeral head. An acute anterior dislocation of the shoulder in an athlete or a chronic fixed anterior dislocation (more commonly seen in an alcoholic) will present with a humeral head prominence anteriorly, usually in the subcoracoid region, with a depression at the upper portion of the posterior deltoid under the acromion.

Lastly, an anterior-superior position of the humeral head tenting the skin is noted after a massive rotator cuff tear or a cuff dehiscence after a surgical repair. Attempted forward flexion increases the proximal migration of the humeral head (see Fig. 3-8).

Palpation

The bony prominences, including the coracoid, the acromioclavicular joint, the acromion, are palpated to determine whether the humeral head is located in the glenoid cavity. The cuff insertion may be tender, with calcific tendonitis or rotator cuff tears. Rotating the humerus with the finger in one position can often bring the area of the calcific deposit underneath the examining finger. The long head of the biceps tendon can be palpated in the intertubercular groove directly anteriorly when the arm is in 10 degrees of internal rotation. Firm pressure over the biceps tendon almost uniformly causes discomfort; therefore, this has not been a very helpful sign for evaluating a tendonitis. The contour of the biceps is palpated for symmetry within each individual arm and in comparing the two arms. Ruptures of the long head of the biceps are far more common than ruptures of the medial head of the biceps. Dimpling in the upper part of the long head of the biceps, with an increased girth in the lower half of the muscle on the lateral side, is indicative of a proximal rupture at the musculotendinous junction in the young, and through the tendon in middle-aged and older athletes[21] (see Fig. 3-18).

Palpation of the supraspinatus and infraspinatus is done with the arms at the side. A hollow depression can often be appreciated in the body of the muscle if it has ruptured or if a nerve injury has occurred (Fig. 3-25). It is later palpated at the time of muscle strength testing to determine whether there are active contractures.

Range of Motion Testing

Active range of motion is measured with the patient sitting (Fig. 3-26). This is to avoid confusion that might otherwise occur with abnormal position through the knees or trunk. As proposed by the American Shoulder and Elbow Surgeons, total elevation is measured as the angle between the elevated arm and

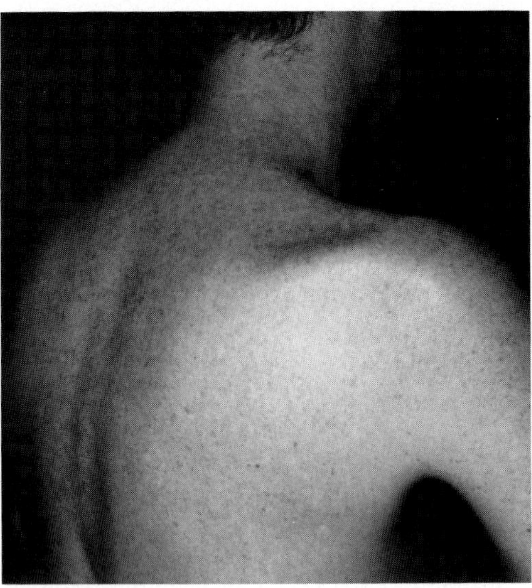

FIG. 3-25. Atrophy of the supraspinatus and infraspinatus following a difficult arthroscopic access to the glenohumeral joint and injury to the suprascapular nerve.

the thoracic rib cage (see the form on page 73 and 74). External rotation is measured with the elbows flexed to 90 degrees and the arms at the side, then again with the arms in 90 degrees of abduction. Active internal rotation is measured behind the back to the highest vertebral level that the patient can bring his or her hitchhiking thumb up the lumbar or thoracic spine.

Passive supine range of motion includes forward elevation with the arm close to the head, external rotation with the arms at the side, and again in 90 degrees of abduction (Fig. 3-27). With the examiner's hand placed on the scapula to prevent it from rolling forward, internal rotation in 90 degrees of abduction is measured. Testing for rotation in 90 degrees of abduction has been the most reliable method of testing glenohumeral motion as opposed to scapulothoracic motion. Thus, adhesive capsulitis or a locked posterior fracture-dislocation has minimal if any motion once the scapulothoracic motion has been eliminated by bringing the arm to 90 degrees of abduction. The difference between the active and passive motion is noted. For example, a patient with a rotator cuff tear or nerve injury will frequently have full passive motion, but may lack active external rotation or elevation.

Muscle Strength Testing

Shoulder muscle strengths are graded on the orthopaedic grading scale: 5 is normal, *4* is good, *3* is fair, *2* is poor, *1* is trace, and *0* is paralysis. All three divisions of the deltoid, the

AMERICAN SHOULDER AND ELBOW SURGEONS

EXAMINATION DATA FORM

Evaluation date:

Name: Chart # Dominance:

List findings as Involved/Univnolved: (R/L) (L/R) Bilateral?

Diagnosis:

Previous surgery:

Number of steroid injections:

I. Pain: / *(5 = none, 4 = slight, 3 = after unusual activity, 2 = moderate, 1 = marked, 0 = complete disability)*

II. Shoulder Motion:

A. Patient sitting:

1. Active total elevation of arm: / degrees
2. Active external rotation with arm at side: / degrees
3. Active rotation - 90 degrees abduction: / degrees
4. Passive internal rotation (segment reached) / *

**1 = Less than trochanter*	*5 = L5*	*9 = L1*	*13 = T9*	*17 = T5*
2 = Trochanter	*6 = L4*	*10 = T12*	*14 = T8*	*18 = T4*
3 = Gluteal	*7 = L3*	*11 = T11*	*15 = T7*	*19 = T3*
4 = Sacrum	*8 = L2*	*12 = T10*	*16 = T6*	*20 = T2*

B. Patient Supine:

1. Passive total elevation of arm: / degrees*
2. Passive external rotation with arm at side: / degrees
3. Passive external rotation - 90 degrees abduction: / degrees
4. Passive internal rotation - 90 degrees abduction: / degrees

**Total elevation of arm measured by viewing patient from side and using goniometer to determine angle between arm and thorax.*

C. Impingement:

1. Painful arc of motion: /
2. Relieved by subacromial xylocaine injection: /
3. Crepitus: /

III. Strength: *(5 = normal, 4 = good, 3 = fair, 2 = poor, 1 = trace, 0 = paralysis)*

A. Anterior deltoid: / E. Trapezius: /
B. Middle deltoid: / F. Triceps: /
C. External rotation: / G. Biceps: /
D. Internal rotation: /

IV. Stability: *(5 = normal, 4 = apprehension, 3 = rare subluxation, 2 = recurrent subluxation, 1 = recurrent dislocation, 0 = fixed dislocation)*

A. Anterior: / C. Inferior: /
B. Posterior: / D. Superior: /

V. Function: *(4 = normal, 3 = mild compromise, 2 = difficulty, 1 = with aid, 0 = unable)*

F1.	/	Use back pocket	F9.	/	Sleep on shoulder
F2.	/	Rectal hygiene	F10.	/	Pulling
F3.	/	Wash opposite underarm	F11.	/	Use hand overhead
F4.	/	Eat with utensil	F12.	/	Throwing
F5.	/	Comb hair	F13.	/	Lifting
F6.	/	Use hand/arm @ shoulder	F14.	/	Do usual work
F7.	/	Carry 10-15 lbs./arm @ side	F15.	/	Do usual sport
F8.	/	Dress			

VI. Patient Response: / *(3 = much better, 2 = better, 1 = same, 0 = worse)*

VII. Roentgen Assessment:
(Circle findings, denote side)
Plain roentgenogram______ Fluoroscopy______ MRI______
Tomography______ CT Scan______ Stress roentgenogram______

A. No abnormalities______

B. Arthritis: 4 = none
3 = mild
2 = moderate
1 = severe

Glenohumeral______
Acromioclavicular______
Sternoclavicular______

1.______ Avascular necrosis
2.______ Cuff tear arthropathy
3.______ Cysplasia
4.______ Metabolic
5.______ Neuropathic
6.______ Osteoarthritis
7.______ Post-traumatic
8.______ Recurrent dislocations
9.______ Rheumatoid
10.______ Septic

C. Impingement:
1. Anterior acromial spur______ Sclerosis______
2. Bone reaction greater tuberosity______
3. Inferior spurs A-C joint______
4. Superior displacement humeral head: calcar/inferior glenoid
5. Humeral head/acromion level______ mm ______ mm
6. Arthrogram: cuff tear: yes______ no______
   a. Complete thickness______
   b. Incomplete thickness______
7. Sonogram: cuff tear: yes______ no______
   a. Complete thickness______
   b. Incomplete thickness______
8. Unfused acromial epiphysis:
   pre______ meta______ meso______ basi______

D. Instability: Anterior/Inferior/Posterior
1. Glenohumeral dislocation
2. Glenohumeral subluxation
3. Inferior subluxation with weights
4. Hill-Sachs defect
5. Glenoid rim:
   fracture______ bone reaction______ anterior/posterior______
6. Glenoid wear: anterior______ posterior______
7. Loose body

E. Trauma/Fractures:

Proximal humerus
1. Two part
2. Three part
3. Four part
4. Articular split
5. Humeral shaft

Scapula
1. Glenoid
2. Other

A-C Joint
1. Separation
   Grade I II III

Clavicle
1. Proximal 1/3
2. Middle 1/3
3. Distal 1/3

S-C Joint
1. Separation
2. Intraarticular fracture

F. Follow-up HHR or TSR
1. Humeral prosthesis: (1 = no abnormalities, 2 = lucent line, 3 = drift, 4 = loosening, 5 = fracture, 6 = ectopic cement)
2. Glenoid prosthesis: (1 = no abnormalities, 2 = lucent line [see below], 3 = wear, 4 = loosening, 5 = fracture, 6 = ectopic cement)
   Lucent lines: complete, incomplete, loosening, progressive
3. Position of implants: (1 = normal, 2 = subluxation, 3 = dislocation) (A = anterior, P = posterior, S = superior, I = inferior)
4. Ectopic bone: (1 = none, 2 - mild, 3 = moderate, 4 = severe)

A

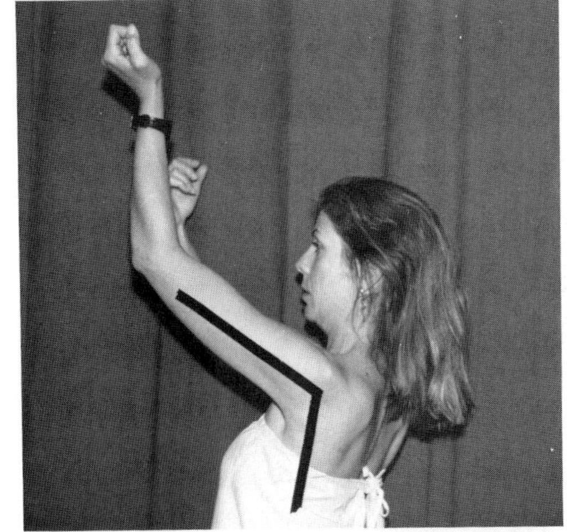

B

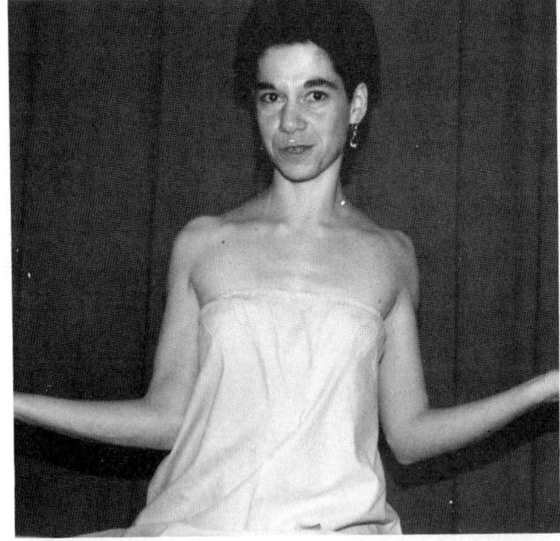

C

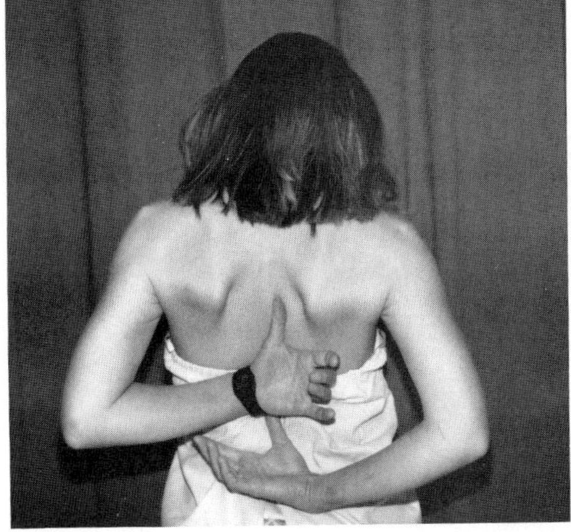

FIG. 3-26. Active range of motion. **A,** Active elevation measured in forward flexion compares the axis of the arm with that of the thorax. **B,** External rotation is measured with the arms both at the side and in 90 degrees abduction. **C,** Internal rotation is measured as the patient actively brings the thumb up the midline of the spine. The nondominant arm can normally reach 2 vertebral levels higher. T7 to T8 correlates with the inferior pole of the scapula.

external rotators, the internal rotators, biceps, triceps, the trapezius, and serratus anterior are routinely tested.

Motor Examination

Deltoid. The three divisions of the deltoid are tested by placing the arm in slight flexion, slight lateral abduction, and slight posterior extension, respectively (Fig. 3-28). The patient is then asked to resist the examiner's force, which would push the lower arm back to a neutral dependent position. Pushing at the distal humerus is preferable to pushing on the hand or wrist. This avoids the effect of active flexion or extension at the elbow that occurs when the examiner pushes on the hand or wrist.

At times there is concern that the deltoid might have ruptured from its origin, either from traumatic injury or from dehiscing after a surgical procedure in which it was detached and then repaired. To test the anterior deltoid, the arm is passively placed in 30 degrees forward flexion, the patient's arm is supported, and he or she is asked to relax. The deltoid muscle is palpated at its acromial and clavicular origins. The patient is then asked to maintain the arm in this position. If the deltoid muscles fibers—and not an upwardly subluxing humeral head—push the fingers outward, then the integrity of the muscle and its attachments can be assured. Other causes of weakness might be a large tear of the rotator cuff. Other divisions of the deltoid can be tested in a similar manner.

Internal rotators. The internal rotators are tested by placing the hands in internal rotation across the abdomen (Fig. 3-29). The patient is asked to resist an external rotation force. Care is taken to ensure that the patient does not use the triceps and biceps and thereby convert a test of internal rotation muscle strength to one of the elbow flexion-extension group. The pectoralis and latissismus dorsi muscles are tested by placing the arm in 30 degrees of abduction and asking the patient to both adduct the arm against the chest wall while attempting to internally rotate it. The pectoralis is palpated over the anterior chest wall and in the anterior axillary fold for muscle contractures and possible ruptures. The latissismus dorsi is palpated over the posterior chest wall and in the posterior axillary fold for its muscle strength and integrity.

External rotators. The external rotators consist of the infraspinatus and teres minor. They are tested with the arms at the side, while the arms are in slight external rotation. The elbows are flexed to 90 degrees. An attempt is

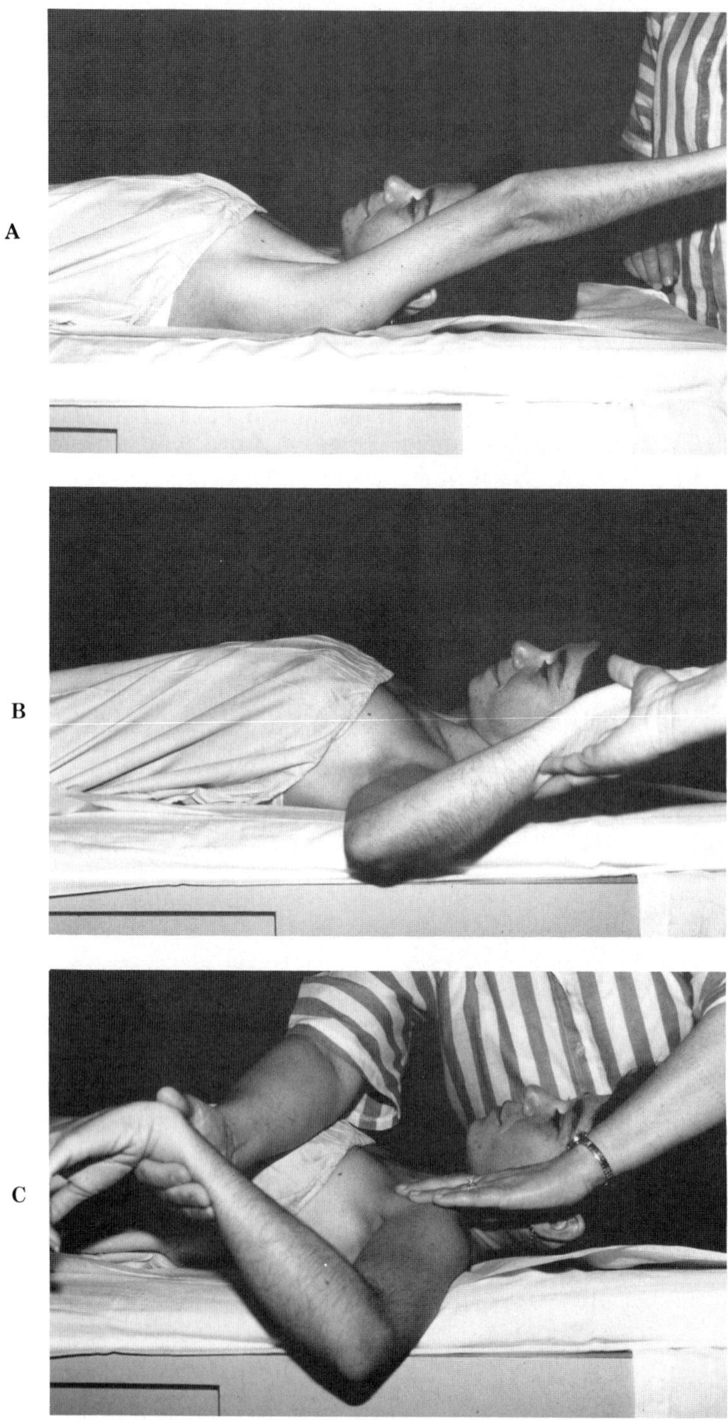

FIG. 3-27. Passive range of motion. **A,** Supine elevation. **B,** Supine external rotation in 90 degrees abduction. **C,** Internal rotation in 90 degrees abduction with a hand to stabilize the scapula from riding upward permits reproducible results. The arms are also measured for passive external rotation at the side.

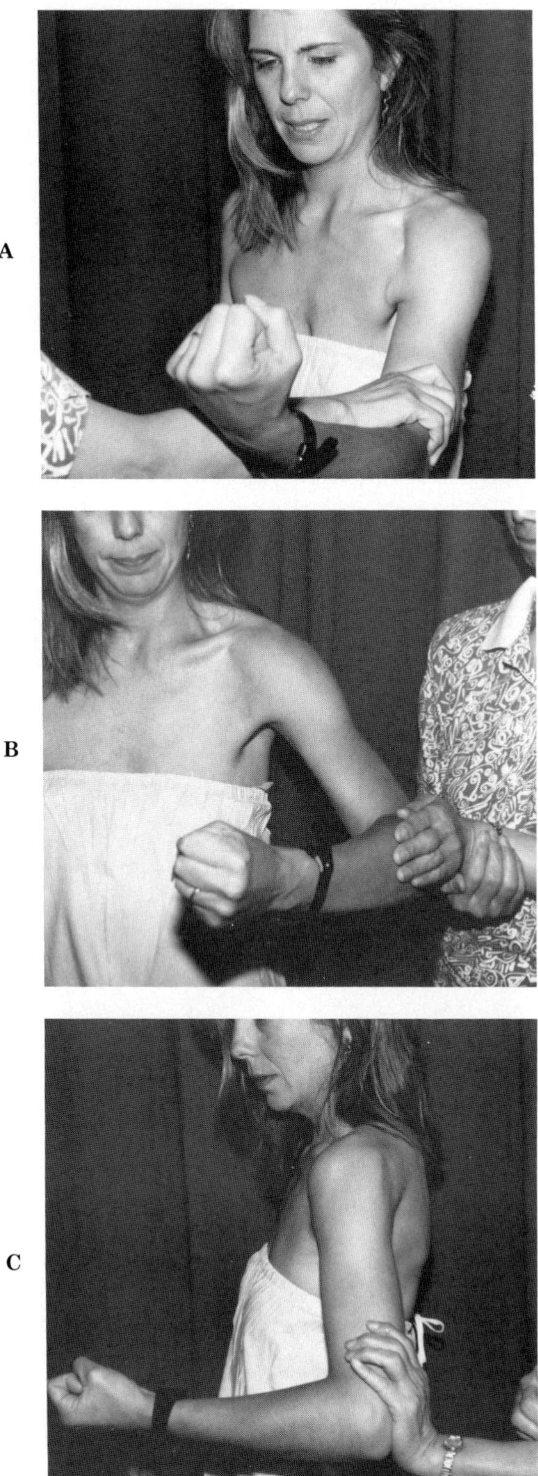

FIG. 3-28. The three divisions of the deltoid are tested for strength and appearance. **A,** Anterior. **B,** Lateral. **C,** Posterior.

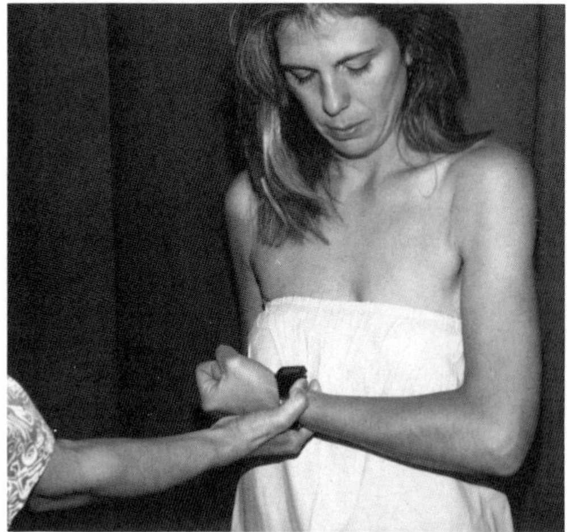

FIG. 3-29. Internal rotation strength is tested with the arm at the abdomen as the athlete resists an external rotation force.

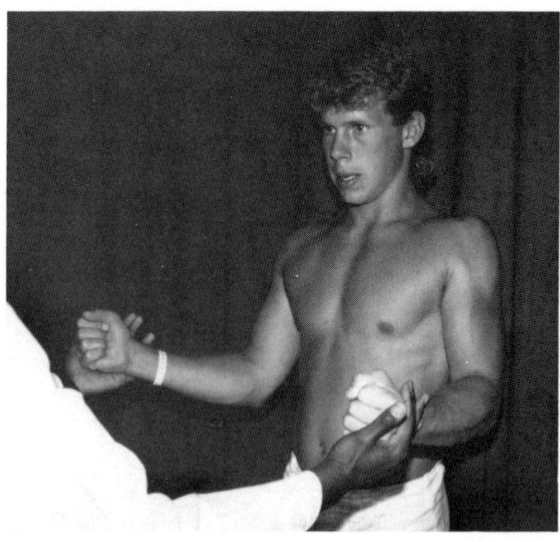

FIG. 3-30. External rotation strength testing with the arms at the side.

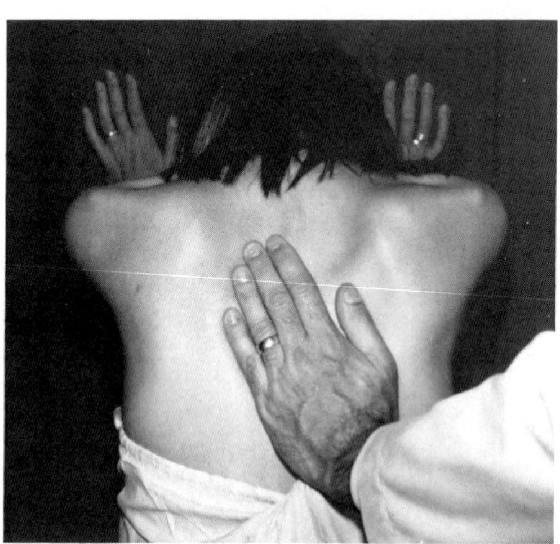

FIG. 3-31. Testing the serratus anterior to determine if winging of the scapula occurs.

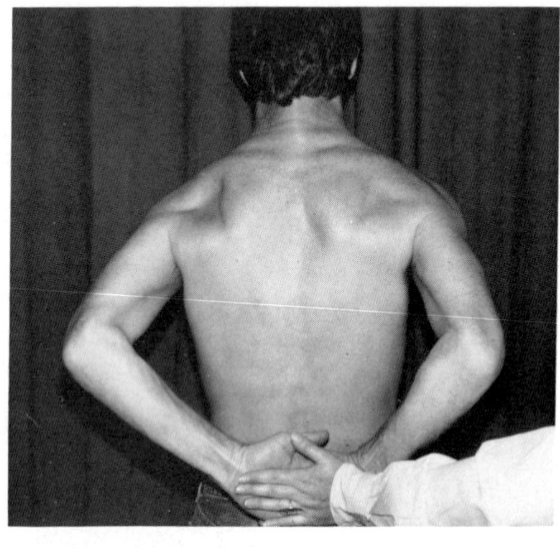

FIG. 3-32. Rhomboids and teres minor can be visualized when the athlete extends his or her arms behind his or her back against a resistance.

made by the examiner to push both hands together as the patient resists (Fig. 3-30).

If the patient cannot hold the arm in slight external rotation, then significant weakness from detachment or nerve injury is anticipated. These individuals will try to comply with the test by placing the forearm on the stomach, extending the arm with the posterior deltoid, and bringing the hand to the side, but not away from the body.

Supraspinatus. The supraspinatus is isolated by pushing downward on the wrists of the arms after they have been placed in 90 degrees abduction, 30 degrees of forward flexion, and internal rotation, with the thumbs pointing downward (see Fig. 3-17).

Serratus anterior. The serratus anterior is tested by pressing forward on the thoracic spine when the individual rests both arms in front leaning on a wall with the elbows in full extension. The muscle is intact if no significant winging occurs (Fig. 3-31).

Rhomboids/teres minor. Visualization and palpation of the rhomboids and the teres minor can be achieved by having the patient place both hands behind his or her back, at the level of the buttocks, and push posteriorly to extend the arms against resistance (Fig. 3-32).

Trapezius. The trapezius is tested by asking the patient to shrug both shoulders toward the ears (Fig. 3-33).

Special Tests

Impingement

The following methods are used to evaluate impingement. Subacromial crepitus can be palpated while the arm is actively or passively rotated when in 90 degrees of abduction. Painful arc of abduction, between 120 degrees and 70 degrees, may occur as the patient gradually lowers the arm from full elevation to the side. This may be further exacerbated if the patient slightly resists a downward pressure while going through this same motion. A catch or sudden giving away of the arm at midrange reproduces Codman's "drop arm test." A positive *impingement sign* occurs when the patient experiences pain on forceful abduction of the internally rotated arm against the acromion (Fig. 3-34).

The *impingement injection test* is relief of more than half of this painful arc of abduction pain after placing 10 cc of xylocaine in the subacromial space. In instances in which impingement pain may preclude a full muscle strength testing or when there is a partial thickness rotator cuff tear, the subacromial xylocaine injection test will relieve enough pain so that the patient has normal strength on the isolated supraspinatus test. For those with complete thickness rotator cuff tears, weakness is still present. The impingement sign is not a valid test in the face of a partially frozen shoulder. Even the subacromial injection of xylocaine does not relieve the stiffness pain.

Biceps

Pathologic processes implicating the long head of the biceps include tendonitis, rupture, and instability. The pain from tendonitis or a partial thickness tearing may be exacerbated with a test of the biceps tendon gliding in its groove against resistance. This is tested by asking the patient to flex the shoulder with the elbow extended, the forearm supinated against the examiner's resistance. Production of pain in the intertubercular groove is considered a positive test.

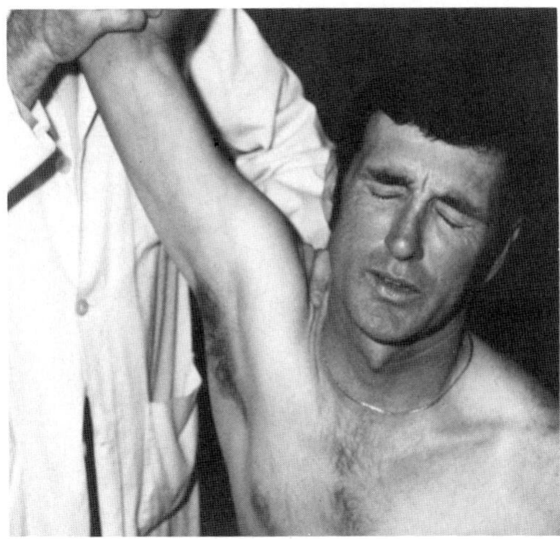

FIG. 3-34. A positive impingement sign is pain on forceful abducton of the internally rotated arm against the acromion.

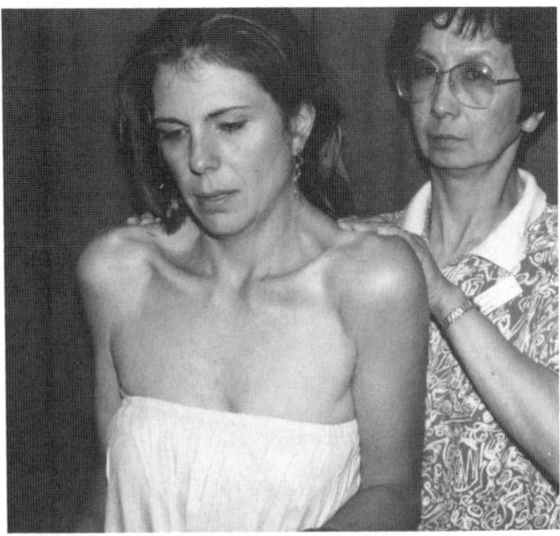

FIG. 3-33. The trapezius is tested as the individual attempts to shrug both shoulders upwards.

Subluxation of the long head of the biceps may occur with large rotator cuff tears in which the transverse humeral ligament has been worn through in the impingement process, or in individuals with fractures involving the greater tuberosity that extends into the biceps groove. Recurrent subluxations of the long head of the biceps in young athletic patients has been an erroneous diagnosis in an athlete who actually has glenohumeral instability.

Instability

The patient is first asked to voluntarily sublux his or her shoulders to demonstrate their laxity (see Fig. 3-9). Then provocative maneuvers to reproduce glenohumeral subluxations or dislocations can be done with the patient sitting, supine, or standing.[58,119,165] With the patient sitting, the examiner can stabilize the scapula by placing one finger on the coracoid and resting the body of his or her hand and forearm on the scapula. With the other hand, the index and middle fingers grasp the anterior humeral head and the thumb grasps the posterior head. Then a variation on the load shift test for knee instability is performed. A force is directed anteriorly and inferiorly (Fig. 3-35). Subluxation of the head over the anterior inferior glenoid rim is esti-

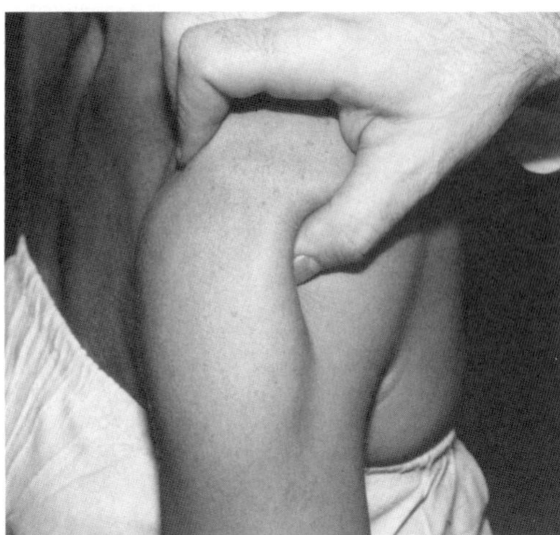

FIG. 3-35. Anterior inferior subluxation creates a void under the posterior acromion and a slight bulge below the coracoid.

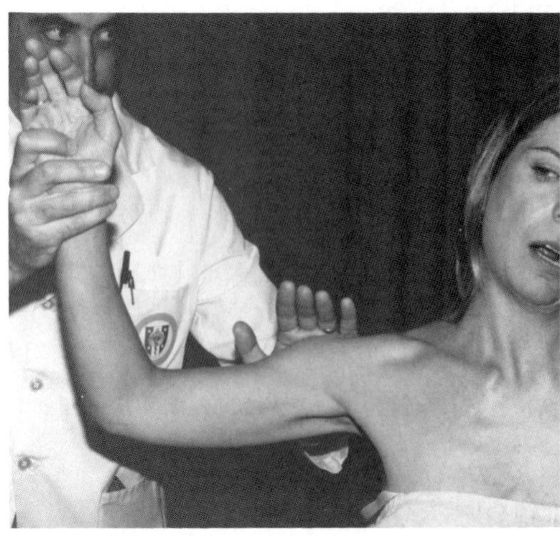

FIG. 3-36. Positive apprehension test. Attempts to anteriorly inferiorly sublux the abducted and externally rotated arm are exacerbated by forceful pressure on the proximal posterior humerus directed anteriorly.

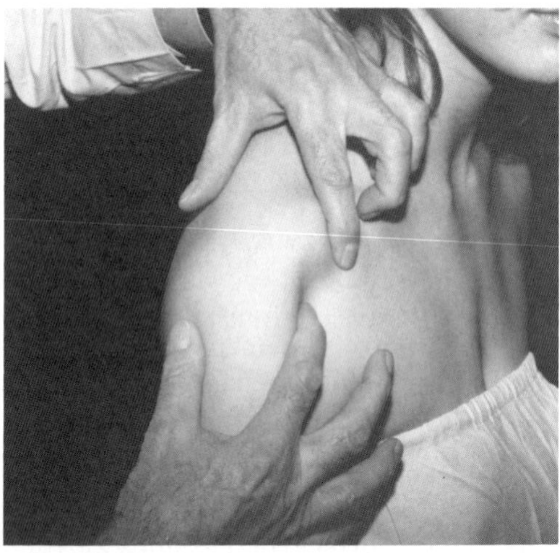

FIG. 3-37. Posterior subluxation with the scapula stabilized is considered abnormal when more than 50% of the humeral head can be translated in a posterior direction.

mated as to degree. Pain may preclude this testing.

With the patient seated, abduction and external rotation of the involved arm and a force directed in an anterior inferior direction from behind may cause a palpable subluxation, labral crepitation, or frank dislocation (Fig. 3-36). The patient is most apprehensive and will resist this maneuver when the arm is abducted to approximately 120 degrees and externally rotated. The patient's subjective apprehension that the shoulder may slip out of joint is considered a positive apprehension finding, whether or not the joint actually subluxes. The differential diagnoses in this position are impingement and a partial frozen shoulder.

Variations of this test may be done while the patient is sitting or supine, with longitudinal traction on the arm in the axis of the slightly abducted humerus, with a force in an anterior inferior direction from behind on the proximal humerus.[58,118,119,125]

Posterior instability testing involves static translation of the humeral head posteriorly, with the thumbs placed on the scapular spines bilaterally. Pressure over both humeral heads, from anterior in a posterior direction, may cause posterior translation (Fig. 3-37). Translation up to 50% of the humeral head diameter is considered normal.[118]

The patient may demonstrate posterior subluxation by muscular control, or either the examiner or patient may demonstrate posterior instability by positioning the arm in forward flexion, internal rotation, and directing a posterior force along the axis of the humerus (Fig. 3-38). For an individual with lax recurrent posterior subluxations, mere elevation of the arm in slight forward flexion without internal rotation may cause a subluxation. The humerus slips out posteriorly, unnoticed except as a slightly posterior bulge. The diagnosis is confirmed with extension of the arm posteriorly to the coronal plane of the scapula, which is accompanied by a quick snap (see Fig. 3-10). Reduction is more easily palpated than the subluxation. Apprehension may be present, but is much less reliable than in anterior instability.

Inferior instability is tested with a downward traction of both arms at the side. A sul-

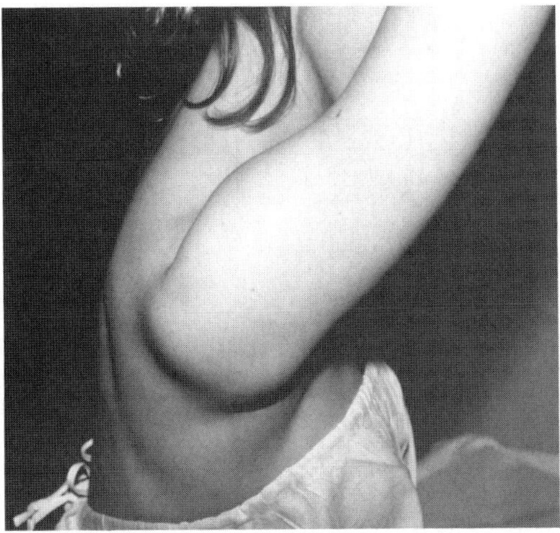

FIG. 3-38. Posterior subluxation of the humeral head is increased with a longitudinal force on the internally rotated and adducted humerus.

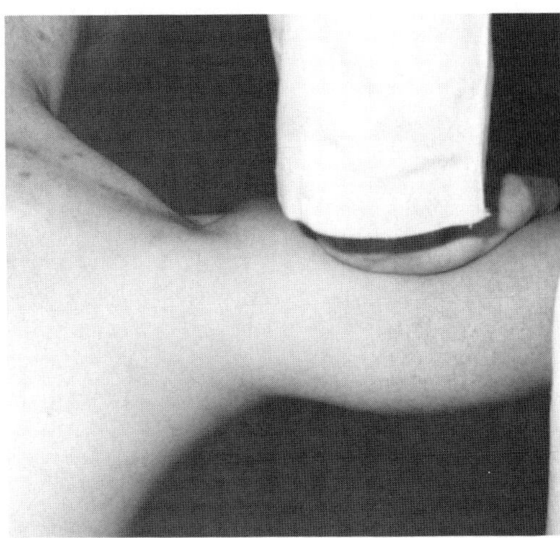

FIG. 3-39. Inferior subluxation tested in a variation of the Feagin maneuver is associated with a palpable bounce and pain.

cus will develop between the top of the humeral head and the undersurface of the acromion in lax individuals (see Fig. 3-11). If this test is painful, then by the time roentgenographs are obtained in this provocative position, some patients resist the downward pull and do not reproduce the previous clinical findings.

In the Feagin maneuver-variation on the anterior-inferior instability testing,[119] the examiner places the patients arm at 90 degrees of elevation. The patient's elbow is resting on either the examiner's shoulder or the examiner's belt. Then, with both hands over the top of the proximal humerus, the arm is pulled downward with a quick motion. Reproduction of the subluxation or palpable bounce is considered a positive finding (Fig. 3-39).

Reproduction of the pain, or fear that the shoulder is going to dislocate, is a variation of anterior apprehension. For multidirectional instability, the shoulders can often be subluxed anteriorly, posteriorly, and inferiorly. All directions are tested. An estimation is recorded as to the percentage of the humeral head diameter that can be slipped over the glenoid rim. Crepitation over the labrum is common. In the absence of labral tearing, the subluxation is less painful than in traumatic anterior-inferior instability lesions. Posterior apprehension is less reliable than is anterior.

Scapulothoracic Joint

Observation

Both scapula are observed to ensure that they appear symmetrical on the chest wall, both when at rest (with the arms at the sides) and through full ranges of motion. Abnormal rhythm, with greater scapular than glenohumeral motion, occurs when there is shoulder stiffness.

Palpation

Muscles inserting into the scapula are palpated for tenderness or muscle spasm. Frequently the middle and posterior trapezius and the levator scapula are tight when the patient has protected the arm with adduction, internal rotation, and slight elevation of the shoulder. The common differential diagnosis is between primary cervical and painful shoulder lesions.

Range of Motion

Range of motion is evaluated in combination with the glenohumeral motion. The superior medial angle of the scapula is palpated for snapping or crepitus. The muscle strength and integrity of the rhomboids, trapezius, and serratus are evaluated. Any scar on the neck from an office node biopsy with trapezius weakness raises the suspicion of an iatrogenic spinal accessory nerve injury.

SPECIAL TESTS AND THEIR CLINICAL SIGNIFICANCE

Roentgenographs

Routine tests for shoulder pathology begin with five screening views. The first three right-angle trauma views in the scapular plane include a true anterior-posterior of the glenohumeral joint (Fig. 3-40), a lateral scapula (Fig. 3-41), and an axillary view.[119] The true anterior-posterior of the glenohumeral joint assesses the integrity of the cartilage,

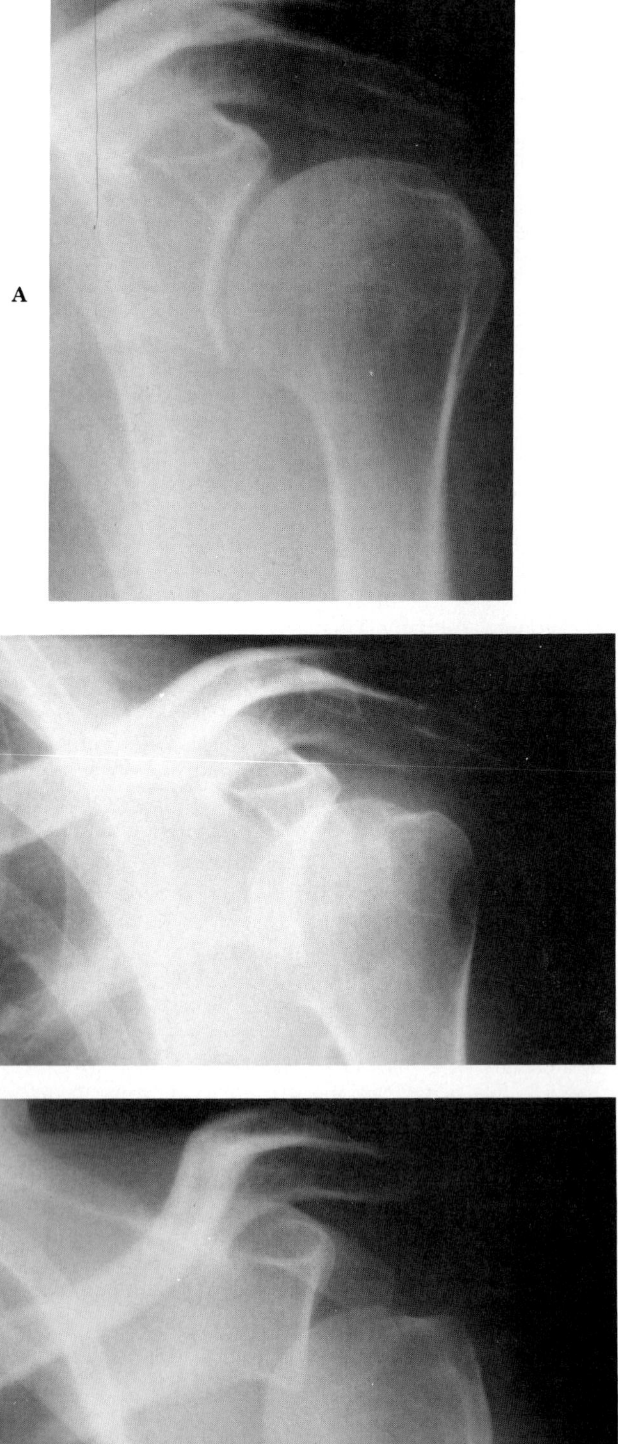

FIG. 3-40. True anterior-posterior view in the plane of the scapula. **A,** Reduced glenohumeral joint with articular space visible between the head and the scapula. **B,** Posterior dislocation with overlap of the head from the glenoid in the same patient as in **A. C,** Anterior dislocation with the humeral head in a subcoracoid inferior position that slightly overlaps the glenoid.

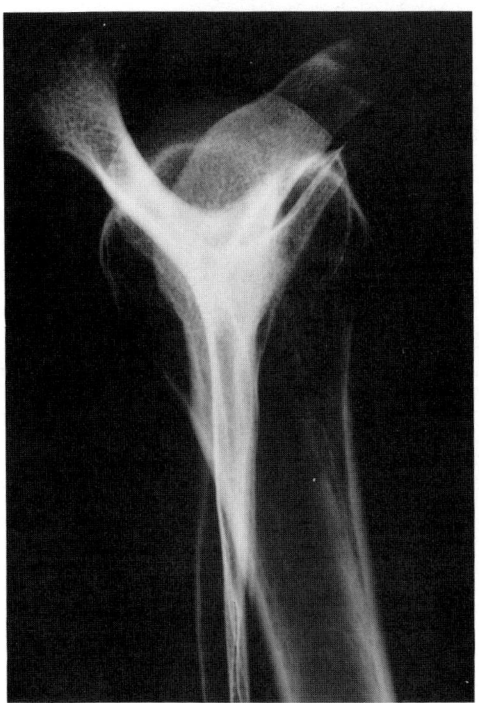

FIG. 3-41. In the normal lateral scapula view, the humeral head is centered on the Y formed by the coracoid, spine of the scapula, and body of the scapula. Anterior displacement is more easily recognized than posterior displacement. Slight obliquity may exaggerate or diminish the prominence of the humeral head posteriorly in a locked posterior fracture-dislocation and thus allow the examiner to miss the diagnosis.

concentric reduction without the overlap of the humeral head to rule out an anterior or posterior dislocation or fracture dislocation. Loose bodies found in 10% of recurrent dislocations may be seen in the inferior capsular recess.

In the lateral scapula view, the head covers the small glenoid. It is at the center of the Y formed by the acromion, spine, and body of the scapula. Displacement of the humerus anteriorly, posteriorly, and inferiorly in respect to the scapula denotes instability or dislocation. Calcific deposits in the rotator cuff are localized as to which tendon is involved, then compared with other views. The three shapes of the acromial undersurface with a type I flat, type II curved, and a type III hooked acromion require 10 degrees to 35 degrees caudal projection so that the medial portion of the scapula and supraspinatus fossa do not project over the acromial outline. An acromial spur or calcification extending into the coracoacromial ligament is seen in some with longstanding impingement.

The acromial morphology is further examined in the axillary view for failure of ossification of either the preacromial or mesoacromial epiphyses. The unfused acromial epiphysis has a high correlation with rotator cuff tears and long biceps ruptures after a patient is more than 30 years of age.[123] This is the most important view to diagnose a posterior fracture dislocation, estimate the size of the humeral head defect, and evaluate eccentric glenoid wear (Fig. 3-42). The diagnosis, classification, and treatment recommendations for fractures of the proximal humerus are based on the above three trauma series views.

The two classic views to rule out calcific tendonitis are anterior-posterior views, with the arm in internal and external rotation. Thirty-five to forty percent under penetrated views will visualize the calcific deposits, whereas the calcium will be burned out on the standard darker views.

In internal rotation, the Hill-Sachs posterior lateral humeral head impression fracture after an anterior dislocation is seen as a straight line inside the most lateral portion of the head[70] (Fig. 3-43). The Stryker notch view, a supplemental view, images the defect when the patient places a hand on top of his or her head. An anterior posterior view is taken with a 10-degree cephalad tilt.

The external rotation view allows evaluation of cystic changes in the greater tuberosity, excrescences, localized osteopenia, sclerosis, and loss of the normal contour of the greater tuberosity with more advanced rotator cuff tears. The missing greater tuberosity in this view represents an avulsion. If the greater tuberosity fragment is not seen over the top of the head, then it is usually hidden in the anterior-posterior view, behind the humeral head and glenoid, but will be visualized either on the lateral scapula view or axillary view (Fig. 3-44). These five views are usually sufficient for calcific tendonitis, chondrocalcinosis, degenerative arthritis, trauma, metabolic diseases, and inflammatory arthritis.[151]

Additional tests to evaluate shoulder instability include the weighted views, with 20 pounds of weight strapped to each forearm. Care is taken not to have the patient hold the weights, in an effort to avoid reduction of passive subluxation by active use of the deltoid. Bilateral inferior subluxation denotes generalized shoulder capsular laxity. Unilateral subluxation is significant on the involved side; it may represent guarding from pain, if present only on the asymptomatic side, in an otherwise lax individual.[119]

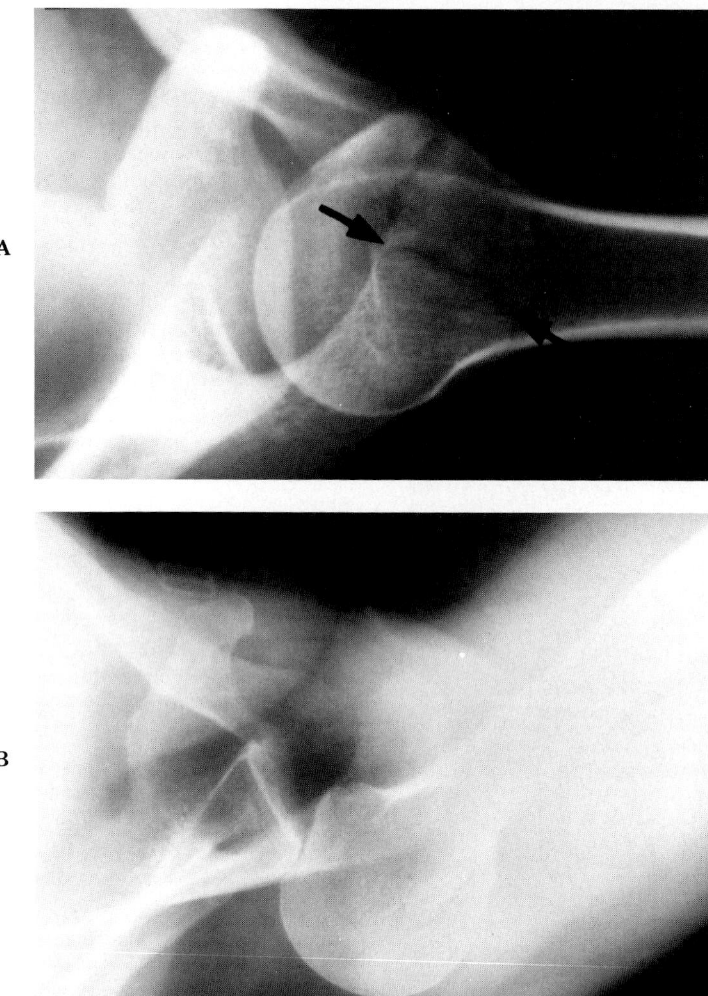

FIG. 3-42. The axillary lateral view is the third and most important view to correlate with the others to evaluate fractures of the humeral head, glenoid, unfused acromial epiphyses, cartilage wear, and coracoid stress fractures. **A,** This patient with an unfused mesoacromion has an associated rotator cuff tear. **B,** Posterior dislocation without a humeral head impression fracture in the axial plane corresponding with Fig. 30-4, *B*.

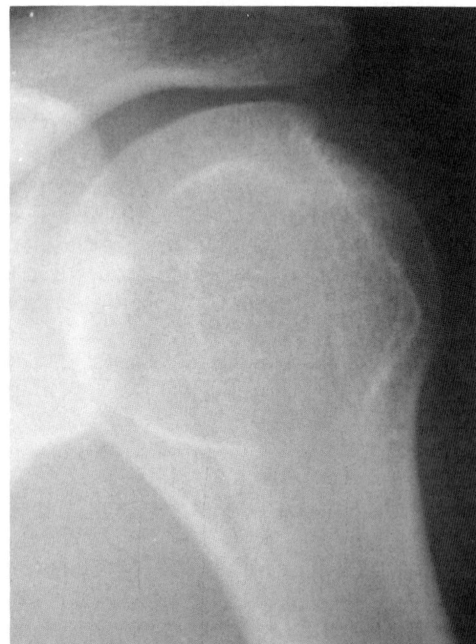

FIG. 3-43. The Hill-Sachs posterior lateral humeral head defect often is seen as a straight line on an internal rotation anterior posterior view.

The West Point axillary view[142] is obtained to evaluate pathology of the anterior-inferior glenoid rim. Ectopic calcification, indicative of labral detachments, or a glenoid rim fracture in the anterior-inferior quadrant is visualized on this view when often missed on the standard axillary view. This view is obtained with the patient in supine position, the arm abducted at 90 degrees on an arm board and internally rotated. The x-ray tube is placed at the hip, abducted 25 degrees, and directed downward 25 degrees from behind and above the shoulder, to pass through the coracoid.

An alternative way to visualize the anterior-inferior glenoid rim is the Ciullo supine axillary view, obtained with the arm abducted and externally rotated when the tube is placed at the hip.[119]

Additional views to evaluate the degree of tearing in the rotator cuff include the Fukuda pushup views.[55] Both arms are pushed upward as the patient bears his or her weight on the hand down at his or her side. If the acromial-humeral interval is less than 4 mm, it is considered diagnostic of a rotator cuff tear. Cuff tears do not produce fixed superior migration early, but when the acromial humeral interval is 6 mm or less on standard non–weight-bearing views, a cuff tear is anticipated.[166]

The AC joints are best visualized when they do not overlie the spine of the scapula. A 15-degree cephalad tilt view that is shot at approximately one-third normal exposure will allow demonstration of the joint and any early osteolytic or arthritic changes.[141]

CT arthrotomography has been the most reliable technique to assess the integrity of the glenoid labrum[136] (Fig. 3-45). Anterior detachments are best seen when the arm is scanned in internal rotation, and posterior detachments when the arm is in external rotation. These positioning maneuvers relax the capsule and allow for better detail when tears are present.

Additional tests to evaluate for shoulder impingement lesions include imaging of the rotator cuff with ultrasound,[43,96] the gold standard of shoulder arthrography,[11] and, more recently, MRI.[86] For lesions with a full-thickness rotator cuff tear less than 1 cm in diameter, the ultrasound and MRI are more difficult to interpret. All three examinations have an accuracy approaching 95%. Double-contrast shoulder arthrotomography in a large series had an accuracy of 99%, with additional information as to the size of the tear.[109]

Eccentric glenoid wear and fractures are best evaluated by the CT scan. Stiffness, size, or pain often precludes adequate plain axillary views beyond establishing the lack of a dislocation. Anterior rim fractures of the glenoid (see Fig. 3-3) with dislocations and eccentric posterior glenoid wear in arthritis (Fig. 3-46, *A*) are the two most frequently encountered conditons.

Three-dimensional plastic models, reconstructed from the uncompressed CT tape, further elucidate the amount of glenoid and humeral head distortion (Fig. 4-46, *B*). These reconstructions have been valuable in surgical planning, in shortening operative proce-

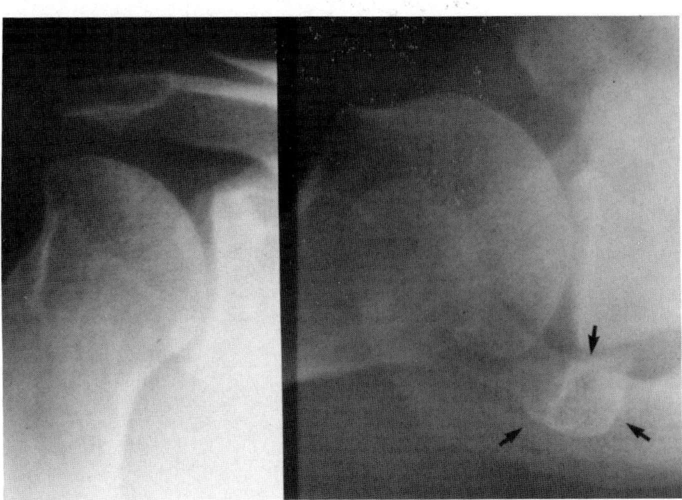

FIG. 3-44. External rotation and axillary view of a patient with a missed tuberosity avulsion. In the external rotation view, deficiency of the top portion of the humeral head is seen. In the axillary lateral view the retracted tuberosity is seen adjacent to the glenoid and no longer attached to the glenoid.

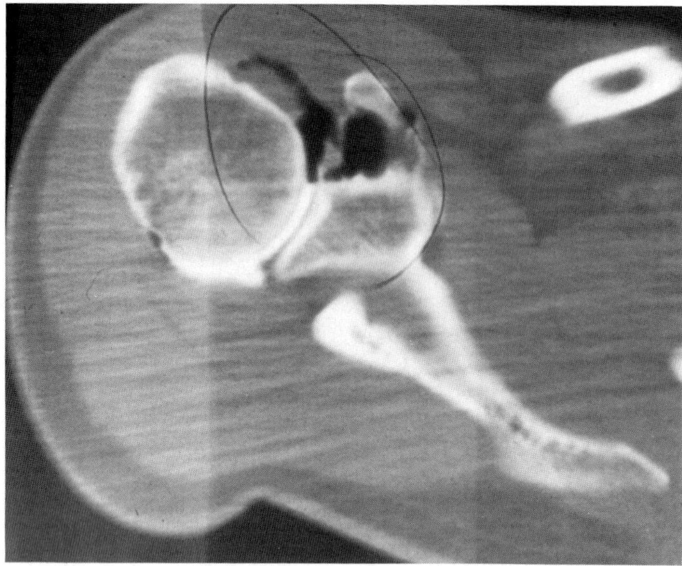

FIG. 3-45. CT arthrotomography showing partial erosion of the anterior glenoid with disruption of the anterior glenoid labrum. Positive contrast outlines the area of disruption where the anterior inferior labrum is no longer attached.

A

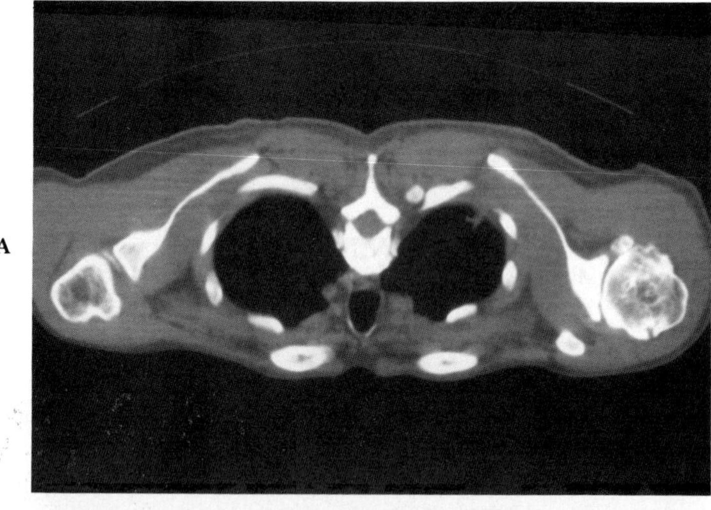

B

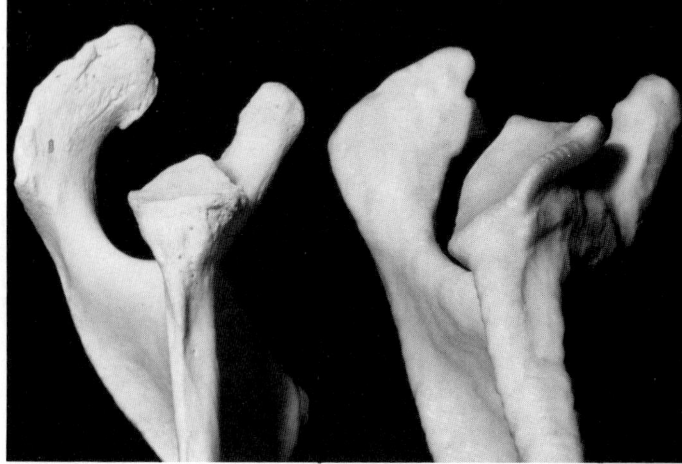

FIG. 3-46. A, CT arthrotomography demonstrates eccentric wear of the glenoid in this athlete with posterior erosion. **B,** Three-dimensional reconstructions of the glenoid allow the surgeon to compare a normal scapula to the amount of erosion to determine whether or not bone grafting is necessary at the time of surgical reconstruction.

dures, and for better visualization of the bony anatomy without widespread muscle detachment in shoulder arthroplasty.[120,121]

The conventional CT scan is also a valuable adjunct to roentgenographs in athletes with infection, osteomyelitis, foreign bodies, and soft tissue abscesses. Increased uptake on skeletal scintography may indicate neoplastic, infectious, posttraumatic, degenerative, and arthritic lesions.[151]

Early signs of asceptic necrosis of the proximal humerus are most easily seen on the MRI. Later, the crescent sign is visualized on plain roentgenographs.

Additional testing for instability can be done with an evaluation of the shoulder performed while the patient is under anesthesia, with[118,119] or without[41,118] C-arm fluoroscopy. Displacement of the humeral head, greater than 50% beyond the glenoid rim, denotes generalized laxity or pathologic instability. This examination is correlated with the other clinical findings.

Electrophysiologic Testing

EMG and nerve conduction studies are obtained routinely to evaluate cervical radiculopathy, brachial plexus injuries, or distal nerve entrapment lesions and also after fracture-dislocations or their treatment in which nerve deficits are anticipated.

These specialized tests confirm the clinical findings from the history and physical examination of the athlete with a painful shoulder. Only with an accurate diagnosis can meaningful comparisons of nonoperative and operative treatments be undertaken.

SUMMARY

An accurate history and thorough physical examination can yield a provisional diagnosis, subsequently confirmed by adjunctive laboratory or roentgenographic evaluation. The clinician well versed in the complete physical examination of the shoulder can facilitate the diagnostic work-up, avoid unnecessary tests, and provide direct, clear avenues of treatment to the athlete with a shoulder problem.

REFERENCES

1. Adelsberg A: The tennis stroke: an EMG analysis of selected muscles with rackets of increasing grip size, Am J Sports Med 14(2):139, 1986.
2. Albright JA et al: Clinical study of baseball pitchers: correlation of injury to the throwing arm with method of delivery, Am J Sports Med 6(1):15, 1978.
3. Allman FL: Fractures and ligamentous injuries of the clavicle and its articulations, J Bone Joint Surg 49A:774, 1967.
4. Andrews JR and Carson WG: The arthroscopic treatment of glenoid labrum tears in the throwing athlete, Orthop Trans 8(1):44, 1984.
5. Andrews JR and Gillogly S: Physical examination of the shoulder in throwing athletes. In Zarins B et al, editors: Injuries to the throwing arm. Philadelphia, 1985, WB Saunders Co.
6. Arendt EA: Multidirectional shoulder instability, Orthopedics 11(1):113, 1988.
7. Ariel G: Body mechanics. In Zarins B et al, editors: Injuries to the throwing arm. Philadelphia, 1985, WB Saunders Co.
8. Arntz CT and Matsen FR III: Disabling scapulothoracic snapping. Abstract submitted to American Shoulder and Elbow Surgeons Annual Meeting, Las Vegas, Nevada, February 1989.
9. Aronoff GM and Evans WO: Evaluation and treatment of chronic pain at the Boston Pain Center, J Clin Psychiatry 43(8):4, 1982.
10. Atwater AE: Biomechanics of overarm throwing movements and throwing injuries, Exerc Sport Sci Rev 7:43, 1979.
11. Bangert BA, Pathria MN, and Resnick D: Advanced imaging of the shoulder, Surg Rounds Orthop (June):48, 1989.
12. Barnes DA and Tullos HS: An analysis of 100 symptomatic baseball players, Am J Sports Med 6(2):62, 1978.
13. Bateman JE: Nerve injuries about the shoulder in sports, J Bone Joint Surg 49(4):785, 1967.
14. Becker G: Diagnosis: the cornerstone of treatment in chronic pain. Paper presented at meeting of Yale Orthopaedic Association, Turtle Bay, Oahu, Hawaii, November 1986.
15. Becker G: Personal communication, June 1989.
16. Bennett GE: Shoulder and elbow lesions distinctive of baseball players, Ann Surg 126 (July): 107, 1947.
17. Bennett GE: Elbow and shoulder lesions of baseball players, Am J Surg 98:484, 1959.
18. Benton J and Nelson C: Avulsion of the coracoid process in an athlete, J Bone Joint Surg 53A(2):356, 1971.
19. Bergfeld JA, Andrish JT, and Clancy WG: Evaluation of the acromioclavicular joint following first- and second-degree sprains, J Sports Med 6(4):153, 1978.
20. Bigliani LU et al: The relationship between the unfused acromial epiphysis and subacromial impingement lesions, Orthop Trans 7(1):138, 1983.
21. Bigliani LU and Wolfe IN: Biceps tendon rupture in the athlete. In Current therapy in sports medicine, St Louis, 1985, The CV Mosby Co.
22. Biondi J and Bear TF: Isolated rupture of the subscapularis tendon in an arm wrestler, Orthopaedics 11(4):647, 1988.
23. Bland JH, Merritt JA, and Boushey DR: The painful shoulder, Semin Arthritis Rheum 7:21, 1977.
24. Blazina ME and Satzman JS: Recurrent anterior subluxation of the shoulder in athletics—a distinct entity, J Bone Joint Surg 51A(5):1037, 1969.
25. Blom S and Dahlback CO: Nerve injuries in dislocations of the shoulder joint and fractures of the neck of the humerus, ACTA Chir Scand 136:461, 1970.
26. Bonnin JG: Spontaneous subluxation of the sternoclavicular joint, Br Med J 2:274, 1960.
27. Booth RE and Marvel JP: Differential diagnosis of shoulder pain, Orthop Clin North Am 6(2):353, 1975.
28. Bosworth DM: The supraspinatus syndrome: symptomatology, pathology, and repair, J Am Med Assoc 116:2477, 1941.

29. Boyer DW: Trapshooter's shoulder: stress fracture of the coracoid process, J Bone Joint Surg 57A(6):862, 1975.
30. Bremner RA: Nonarticular, noninfective subacute arthritis of the sternoclavicular joint, J Bone Joint Surg 41B:749, 1959.
31. Brewer BJ: Athletic injuries: musculotendinous unit, Clin Orthop 23:30, 1962.
32. Brown JT: Early assessment of supraspinatus tears: procaine infiltration as a guise to treatment, J Bone Joint Surg 31B(3):423, 1949.
33. Brunet ME et al: Atraumatic osteolysis of the distal clavicle: histologic evidence of synovial pathogenesis, Orthopedics 9(4):557, 1986.
34. Bryan WJ, Schauder K, and Tullos HS: The axillary nerve and its relationship to common sports medicine shoulder procedures, Am J Sports Med 14(2):113, 1986.
35. Cahill BR: Osteolysis of the distal part of the clavicle in male athletes, J Bone Joint Surg 64A(7):1053, 1982.
36. Cahill BR, Tullos HS, and Fain RH: Little League shoulder, J Sports Med 2:150, 1974.
37. Clancy WG: Shoulder problems in overhead-overuse sports, Am J Sports Med 7(2):138, 1979.
38. Codman EA: The shoulder. Malabar, Fl, 1984, Robert E. Kreiger Publishing Company. (Reprint of Private Press 1934 Publication, Thomas Todd.)
39. Coene LN: Axillary nerve lesions and associated injuries, thesis, de Kempenaer, Oegstgeest, Holland, 1985.
40. Coene LN and Narakas AO: Surgical management of axillary nerve lesions, isolated or combined with other infraclavicular nerve lesions, Peripheral Nerve Repair and Regeneration 3:47, 1986.
41. Cofield RH and Irving JF: Evaluation and classification of shoulder instability, Clin Orthop 223:32, 1987.
42. Cofield RG and Simonet WT: The shoulder in sports, Mayo Clin Proc 59:157, 1984.
43. Crass JR and Craig EV: Noninvasive imaging of the rotator cuff, Orthopedics 11(1):57, 1988.
44. Danielsson L: Ruptur av. m. pectoralis major, en brottningsskada, Nordisk Med 72:1089, 1964.
45. Deltoff MN and Bressler HB: Atypical scapula fracture—a case report, Am J Sports Med 17(2):292, 1989.
46. Derebery UJ and Tullos WH: Low back pain exacerbated by psychological factors, West J Med 144:574, 1986.
47. Drez D: Suprascapular neuropathy in the differential diagnosis of rotator cuff injuries, Am J Sports Med 4(2):43, 1976.
48. Ebel R: Uber die Ursachen der Axillaris Parese bei Schulterluxation, Mschr Unfallheilk 76:445, 1973.
49. Engle G: Psychogenic pain and the pain-prone patient, Am J Med 26 (June):899, 1959.
50. Faure G and Daculsi G: Calcific tendinitis: a review, Ann Rheum Dis 42 (suppl):49, 1983.
51. Ferretti A, Cerullo A, and Russo G: Suprascapular neuropathy in volleyball players, J Bone Joint Surg 69A(2):260, 1987.
52. Ford CV: The somatizing disorders, Psychosomatics 27(5):327, 1986.
53. Fronek J, Warren RF, and Bowen M: Posterior subluxation of the glenohumeral joint, J Bone Joint Surg 71A(2):205, 1989.
54. Fukuda H, Hamada K, and Kobayashi Y: "Push-up views" for the massive rotator cuff tears—a new roentgenographic projection. Paper presented at the American Shoulder and Elbow Surgeons, Fifth Open Meeting, Las Vegas, Nev, February 12, 1989.
55. Fukuda H and Neer CS II: Archer's shoulder—recurrent posterior subluxation and dislocation of the shoulder in two archers, Orthopedics 11(1):171, 1988.
56. Gainor BJ et al: The throw: biomechanics and acute injury, Am J Sports Med 8(2):114, 1980.
57. Garth WP, Leberte MA, and Cool TA: Recurrent fractures of the humerus in a baseball pitcher, J Bone Joint Surg 70A(2):305, 1988.
58. Gerber C and Granz R: Clinical assessment of the shoulder, J Bone Joint Surg 66B:551, 1984.
59. Glick JM et al: Dislocated acromioclavicular joint: follow-up study of 35 unreduced acromioclavicular dislocations, Am J Sports Med 5(6): 264, 1977.
60. Glousman R et al: Dynamic EMG analysis of the throwing shoulder with glenohumeral instability, Orthop Trans 11(2):247, 1987.
61. Goldstein R: Psychological evaluation of low back pain, SPINE: State of the Art Reviews 1(1):103, 1986.
62. Goldstein R: Personal communication, June 1989.
63. Gregg JR et al: Serratus anterior paralysis in the young athlete, J Bone Joint Surg 61A(6):825, 1979.
64. Hansen NM: Epiphyseal changes in the proximal humerus of an adolescent baseball pitcher, Am J Sports Med 10(6):380, 1982.
65. Hawkins RJ and Kennedy MD: Impingement syndrome in athletes, J Sports Med 8(3):151, 1980.
66. Hawkins RJ and Hobeika PE: Impingement syndrome in the athletic shoulder, Clin Sports Med 2(2):391, 1983.
67. Hawkins RJ and Neer CS II: Missed posterior dislocations of the shoulder. In Bateman JE and Welsh RP, editors: Surgery of the shoulder, Philadelphia, 1984, BD Decker.
68. Hawkins RJ and McCormack RG: Posterior shoulder instability, Orthopedics 7(1):101, 1988.
69. Henry JH and Genung JA: Natural history of glenohumeral dislocation revisited, Am J Sports Med 10:135, 1982.
70. Hill HA and Sachs MD: The grooved defect of the humeral head: a frequently unrecognized complication of dislocations of the shoulder joint, Radiol 35:690, 1940.
71. Hirasawa Y and Sakakida K: Sports and peripheral nerve injury, Am J Sports Med 11:420, 1983.
72. Hopkinson WJ, Ryan JB, and Wheeler JH: Glenoid rim fracture and recurrent shoulder instability, Complic Orthop (March/April):36, 1989.
73. Howell SM et al: Normal and abnormal mechanics of the glenohumeral joint in the horizontal plane, J Bone Joint Surg 70A(2):227, 1988.
74. Hoyt WA: Etiology of shoulder injuries in athletes, J Bone Joint Surg 49:755, 1967.
75. Ishikawa H et al: Osteochondritis dissecans of the shoulder in a tennis player, Am J Sports Med 16(5):547, 1988.
76. Jobe FW: Shoulder problems in overhead-overuse sports, Am J Sports Med 7(2):139, 1979.
77. Jobe FW: Treating problem elbows in baseball pitchers, Orthop Today, 1986.
78. Jobe FW: Impingement problems in the athlete. In Barr JS, editor. Instructional Course Lectures 38. Park Ridge, Ill, 1989, American Academy of Orthopaedic Surgeons.
79. Jobe FW et al: The relationship of anterior instability and rotator cuff impingement in the throwing athlete. Presented at the American Shoulder and Elbow Surgeons Annual Open Meeting, Las Vegas, Nev, February 12, 1989.

80. Jobe FW and Jobe CM: Painful athletic injuries of the shoulder, Clin Orthop 173:117, 1983.
81. Kaplan PE and Kernahan WT Jr: Rotator cuff rupture: management with suprascapular neuropathy, Arch Phys Med Rehab 65:273, 1984.
82. Kennedy JC, Hawkins R, and Krissoff WB: Orthopaedic manifestations of swimming, Am J Sports Med 6(6):309, 1978.
83. King JW, Brelsford HJ, and Tullos HS: Analysis of the pitching arm of the professional baseball player, Clin Ortho Rel Res 67:116, 1969.
84. Kiviluoto O et al: Immobilization after primary dislocation of the shoulder, Acta Orthop Scand 51:915, 1980.
85. Kline DG and Lusk MD: Management of athletic brachial plexus injuries. In Schneider RC et al, editors: Sports injuries, Baltimore, 1984, Williams & Wilkins.
86. Kneeland JB et al: Rotator cuff tears: preliminary application of high resolution MRI with counter-rotating loop gap resonators, Radiology 160:695, 1986.
87. Kretzler HH and Richardson AB: Rupture of the pectoralis major muscle, Orthop Trans 11(1):76, 1987.
88. Leach RE and Schepsis AA: Shoulder pain, Clin Sports Med 2(1):123, 1983.
89. Leffert RD: Thoracic outlet syndrome. A correspondence newsletter to the American Society for Surgery of the Hand, December 12, 1988.
90. Leffert RD: Lesions of the brachial plexus revisited. Barr JS, editor: Instructional Course Lectures 38. Park Ridge, Ill, 1989, American Academy of Orthopaedic Surgeons.
91. Leffert RD and Gumley G: The relationship between dead arm syndrome and thoracic outlet syndrome, Clin Orthop 223:20, 1987.
92. Lipscomb AB: Baseball pitching injuries in growing athletes, J Sports Med 3(1):25, 1975.
93. Lipscomb AB, Thomas ED, and Johnston RK: Treatment of myositis ossificans traumatica in athletes, Am J Sports Med 4(3):111, 1976.
94. Lombardo SJ et al: Posterior shoulder lesions in throwing athletes, J Sports Med 5(3):106, 1977.
95. Lundberg BJ: The frozen shoulder, ACTA Orthop Scand Suppl 19, 1969.
96. Mack LA et al: US evaluation of the rotator cuff, Radiology 157:205, 1985.
97. Magni G and deBertolini C: Chronic pain as a depressive equivalent, Postgrad Med 73(3):79, 1983.
98. Maki NJ: Cineradiographic studies with shoulder instabilities, Am J Sports Med 16(4):362, 1988.
99. Mariani PP: Isolated fracture of the coracoid process in an athlete, Am J Sports Med 8(2):129, 1980.
100. Matsen FA: TUBS-AMBRI—pneumonics to differentiate traumatic instability from multidirectional instability, American Academy of Orthopaedic Surgeons, Summer Institute, San Diego, September 7-11, 1988.
101. McCue FC, Gieck JH, and West JO: Throwing injuries to the shoulder. In Zarins B et al, editors: Injuries to the throwing arm, Philadelphia, 1985, WB Saunders Co.
102. McEntire JE, Hess WE, and Coleman SS: Rupture of the pectoralis major muscle, J Bone Joint Surg 54A(5):1040, 1972.
103. McGlynn FJ, El-Khoury G, and Albright JP: Arthrotomography of the glenoid labrum in shoulder instability, J Bone Joint Surg 64A:506, 1982.
104. McLaughlin HL: Rupture of the rotator cuff, J Bone Joint Surg 44A(5):979, 1962.
105. McLeod WD: The pitching mechanism. In Zarins B et al, editors: Injuries to the throwing arm: Philadelphia, 1985, WB Saunders Co.
106. McLeod WD and Andrews JR: Mechanisms of shoulder injuries, Phys Ther 66(12):1901, 1986.
107. McMaster WC: Anterior glenoid labrum damage: a painful lesion in swimmers, Am J Sports Med 14(5):383, 1986.
108. Mestdagh H, Drizenko A, and Ghestem P: Anatomical bases of suprascapular nerve syndrome, Anatomia Clinica 3:67, 1981.
109. Mink JH, Harris E, and Rappaport M: Rotator cuff tears: evaluation using double-contrast shoulder arthrography, Radiol 157:621, 1985.
110. Moynes DR et al: Electromyography and motion analysis of the upper extremity in sports, Phys Ther 66(12):1905, 1986.
111. Neer CS II: Anterior acromioplasty for chronic impingement syndrome in the shoulder, J Bone Joint Surg 54A:41, 1972.
112. Neer CS II, Craig EV, and Fukuda H: Cuff tear anthropathy, J Bone Joint Surg 65A:1232, 1983.
113. Neer CS II and Foster CR: Inferior capsular shift for involuntary inferior and multidirectional instability of the shoulder, J Bone Joint Surg 62A:897, 1980.
114. Neer CS II, Watson KC, and Stanton FS: Recent experience in total shoulder replacement, J Bone Joint Surg 64A:319, 1982.
115. Neer CS II and Welsh RP: The shoulder in sports, Orthop Clin North Am 8(3):583, 1977.
116. Neviaser JS: Adhesive capsulitis of the shoulder, Med Times 90:783, 1962.
117. Nicholas JA, Grossman RB, and Hershman EB: The importance of a simplified classification of motion in sports in relation to performance, Orthop Clin North Am 8(3):499, 1977.
118. Norris TR: C-arm fluoroscopic evaluation under anaesthesia for glenohumeral subluxations. In Bateman J and Welsh P, editors: Surgery of the shoulder, Philadelphia, 1984, BC Decker Co.
119. Norris TR: Diagnostic technique for shoulder instability. In Stauffer ED, editor: American Academy of Orthopaedic Surgeons, Instructional Course Lectures 34, St Louis, 1985, The CV Mosby Co.
120. Norris TR: Bone grafts for glenoid deficiency in total shoulder replacements. The shoulder. Proceedings of the Third International Conference on Surgery of the Shoulder. Tokyo, 1987, Professional Postgraduate Services.
121. Norris TR: Unconstrained prosthetic shoulder replacement. In Watson M, editor: The shoulder. London, 1989, Churchill Livingstone.
122. Norris TR: Recurrent posterior subluxations: hospital medicine, New York, 1989, Cahners Publishing Co.
123. Norris TR and Bigliani LU: Analysis of failed repair for shoulder instability—a preliminary report. In Bateman J and Welsh P, editors: Surgery of the shoulder, Philadelphia, 1984, BC Decker, Inc.
124. Norris TR and Bigliani LU: Complications following the modified Bristow procedure for shoulder instability, J Bone Joint Surg Ortho Trans 11:232, 1987.
125. Norris TR et al: The unfused acromial epiphysis and its relationship to impingement syndrome, Orthop Trans 7(3):505, 1983.
126. Nuber GW et al: Fine wire electromyography analysis of muscles of the shoulder during swimming, Am J Sports Med 14(1):7, 1986.
127. O'Brien SJ et al: Capsular restraints to anterior posterior motion of the shoulder, Orthop Trans 12(1):143, 1988.

128. Pappas AM, Goss TP, and Kleinman PK: Symptomatic shoulder instability due to lesions of the glenoid labrum, Am J Sports Med 11(5):279, 1983.
129. Pasila M et al: Early complication of primary shoulder dislocations, Acta Orthop Scand 49:260, 1978.
130. Perry J: Anatomy and biomechanics of the shoulder in throwing, swimming, gymnastics, and tennis, Clin Sports Med 2(2):247, 1983.
131. Pettrone FA: Shoulder problems in swimmers. In Zarins B et al,editors: Injuries to the throwing arm, Philadelphia, 1985, WB Saunders Co.
132. Poindexter DP and Johnson EW: Football shoulder and neck injury: a study of the "stinger," Arch Phys Med Rehabil 65:601, 1984.
133. Poppen NK and Walker PS: Normal and abnormal motion of the shoulder, J Bone Joint Surg 58A:195, 1976.
134. Poppen NK and Walker PS: Forces at the glenohumeral joint in abduction, Clin Orthop 135:165, 1978.
135. Quigley TB: Injuries to the acromioclavicular and sternoclavicular joints sustained in athletes, Surg Clin North Am 43(6):1551, 1963.
136. Rafii M et al: Athlete shoulder injuries: CT arthrographic findings, Radiology 162(2):559, 1987.
137. Resnick D: Shoulder pain, Orthop Clin North Am 14:81, 1983.
138. Richardson AB: Overuse syndrome in baseball, tennis, gymnastics, and swimming, Clin Sports Med 2(2):379, 1983.
139. Richardson AB, Jobe FE, and Collins HR: The shoulder in competitive swimming, J Sports Med 8(3):159, 1980.
140. Robertson WC, Eichman PL, and Clancy WG: Upper trunk brachial plexopathy in football players, J Am Med Assoc 241(14):1480, 1979.
141. Rockwood CA Jr: Posterior dislocation of the shoulder. In Rockwood CA Jr. and Green DP, editors: Fractures in adults, Philadelphia, 1984, JB Lippincott Co.
142. Rokous JR, Feagin JA, and Abbott HG: Modified axillary roentgenogram, Clin Orthop 82:84, 1972.
143. Rome HP and Harness DM: Psychological and behavioral aspects of chronic facial pain, Otolaryngol Clin North Am 22:6, 1989.
144. Rowe CR: Shoulder subluxation in the athlete. In: Current therapy in sports medicine, St Louis, 1985, The CV Mosby Co.
145. Rowe CF: Recurrent transient anterior subluxation of the shoulder, the "dead arm" syndrome. Clin Orthop 223:11, 1987.
146. Rowe CR, Pierce DS, and Clark JG: Voluntary dislocation of the shoulder: A preliminary report on a clinical electromyographic and psychiatric study of 25 patients, J Bone Joint Surg 55A:445, 1973.
147. Rowe CR and Zarins B: Recurrent transient subluxation of the shoulder, J Bone Joint Surg 63A:863, 1981.
148. Ryu RKN et al: An electromyographic analysis of shoulder function in tennis players, Am J Sports Med 6:481, 1988.
149. Sain J and Andrews JR: Proper pitching techniques. In Zarins B et al, editors: Injuries to the throwing arm, Philadelphia, 1985, WB Saunders Co.
150. Santavirta S and Kiviluoto O: Transverse fracture of the humerus in a shotputter: a case report, Am J Sports Med 5(3):122, 1977.
151. Sartoris DJ and Resnick D: Imaging the painful shoulder: what studies to order, J Musculoskel Med 5(7):21, 1988.
152. Schwartz PA, Torzilli PA, and Warren RF: Capsular restraints to anterior-posterior motion of the shoulder. Presented at the 33rd Annual Meeting, Orthopaedic Research Society, San Francisco, January 19-22, 1987.
153. Shuman WP et al: Double-contrast computed tomography of the glenoid labrum, Am J Roentgenol 141:581, 1983.
154. Simonet WT and Cofield RH: Prognosis in anterior dislocation. Presented at American Orthopaedic Society for Sports Medicine, Anaheim, Calif, March 9-10, 1983.
155. Sisto D et al: An EMG analysis of the elbow in pitching, Am J Sports Med 15:260, 1987.
156. Stanish WD and Lamb H: Isolated paralysis of the serratus anterior muscle: a weight training injury, Am J Sports Med 6(6):385, 1978.
157. Stewart MJ: The acromioclavicular joint in the throwing arm. In Zarins B et al, editors: Injuries to the throwing arm, Philadelphia, 1985, WB Saunders Co.
158. Tibone JE et al: Surgical treatment of tears of the rotator cuff in athletes, J Bone Joint Surg 68A(6):887, 1986.
159. Tullos HS and King JW: Lesions of the pitching arm in adolescents, J Am Med Assoc 220(2):264, 1972.
160. Tullos HS and King JW: Throwing mechanism in sports, Orthop Clin North Am 4(3):709, 1973.
161. Tullos HS et al: Unusual lesions of the pitching arm, Clin Orthop 88:169, 1972.
162. Turkel SJ et al: Stabilizing mechanism in preventing anterior dislocation of the glenohumeral joint, J Bone Joint Surg 63A:1208, 1981.
163. Uhthoff HK, Sakar K, and Maynard JA: Calcifying tendinitis—a new concept of the pathogenesis, Cline Orthop 118:164, 1978.
164. Van Nes CP and Van Nes JF: Serratus paralysis, Arch Chir Neerly 21(1):85, 1969.
165. Warren RF: Instability of shoulder in throwing sports. In Stauffer ED, editor: American Academy of Orthopaedic Surgeons, Instructional Course Lecture 34: St Louis, 1985, The CV Mosby Co.
166. Weiner DS and McNab I: Superior migration of the humeral head: a radiological aid in the diagnosis of tears of the rotator cuff, J Bone Joint Surg 52B:524, 1970.
167. Weiss J: The painful shoulder. In Kelly WN et al, editors: Textbook of rheumatology, Philadelphia, 1981, WB Saunders Co.
168. Welsh RP: Dislocations of the shoulder: acromioclavicular and sternoclavicular joints. In Welsh, RP and Shephard RJ, editors: Current therapy in sports medicine 1985-1986, Philadelphia, 1985, BC Decker, Inc.
169. Whitaker JH: Arm wrestling fractures—a humerus twist, Am J Sports Med 5(2):67, 1977.
170. Zuckerman JC and Matsen FA III: Complications about the glenohumeral joint related to the use of screws and staples, J Bone Joint Surg 66A(2):175, 1984.

CHAPTER 4 Diagnostic Imaging of the Shoulder

Mahvash Rafii ***Jeffrey Minkoff***
Vincent DeStefano

There is no simple flow sheet by which diagnostic tests and treatments for the athlete with a disabled shoulder may be ordained to the satisfaction of all treating physicians. Only a few decades ago the primary weapon in the diagnostic armamentarium was the physician's examination. Third-party carriers and doubtful patients were not available in any numbers to undermine the physician's diagnosis. While the physical examination became more sophisticated throughout the

ACKNOWLEDGMENT: Grateful acknowledgment is made for the services of Mrs. Barbara O'Hara for the preparation of the ultrasonography discussion, pp. 142-155.

1970s and 1980s, with the common recognition of such entities as impingement and multidirectional instability, the sophistication of roentgenographic diagnostics has grown to a much greater extent, and arthroscopy has developed as well. Today, documentation of pathologic conditions has become a critical factor in American medicine. It satisfies the patient, the carrier, and the physician that the treatment direction is appropriate; perhaps more importantly, objective testing reveals whether anything serious is being overlooked, such as a tumor.

Many factors are involved in determining the extent and nature of the documentary evidence to be secured. They include the severity of manifested symptoms, the activity for which the disabled limb is to be used, expediency requirements (as with professional athletes), the expertise of the physician for the limb segment being treated, the availability and effectiveness of special diagnostic tests within the community, and the variance in treatment approaches by different physicians for a given pathologic entity. These factors constitute the essence of a needed resolve between the radiologist and the sports medicine physician. The radiologist is charged with a descriptive interpretation of roentgenographic studies performed. The sports medicine physician, on the other hand, is charged with the ordering of such studies, and most importantly, the translation of their descriptive interpretations into a practical treatment plan.

The sports clinician ordinarily encounters a variety of shoulder afflications in his or her practice. Some are sport specific and must be kept in mind. Cofield and Simonet[15] provide a partial list:

1. Weight lifters—inflammatory acromioclavicular arthritis with resorption of the distal end of the clavicle
2. Baseball pitchers—ossification of the posterior glenoid region[71]
3. Tennis serve and baseball pitching acceleration phase—impingements
4. Gymnastics—strains, impingements, and instabilities, especially attributable to the use of rings
5. Trap-shooters—fractures of the coracoid
6. Swimmers—impingement, especially on the breathing side (The parameters of "swimmer's shoulder" were defined by Kennedy and Hawkins [1974] and are associated with internal rotation and adduction and CT arthrographic findings of anterior labral detachment.[74])

This list is only a small sample of the wide array of athletically related disorders that may or may not be sport specific. Most of these conditions fall within several categories of pathology: glenohumeral instability, capsulolabral disorders, rotator cuff disease and impingement, acromioclavicular disorders, and a miscellaneous category, which includes pathologic states ranging from calcareous diseases to tumors simulating injuries. Few sports physicians would attempt to diagnose and/or treat any of these prospective disorders without the benefit of a roentgenographic assessment. Before 1970, other than for the intermittent use of arthrography, roentgenography consisted primarily of plain roentgenograms. However, there have since appeared a progression of sophisticated and "high-tech" roentgenographic techniques that have substantially enhanced the accuracy (sensitivity and specificity) of diagnosis of the above-indicated abnormalities. These techniques have included the development of "specialized" views, glenohumeral and bursal arthrography, arthrotomography, computed tomographic (CT) arthrography, sonography, and magnetic resonance imaging (MRI).

There is a great variance among clinicians in their capacities and confidence in the physical diagnosis of the symptomatic shoulder. No matter how confident the physician, nor how certain the apparent diagnosis, there remains an ultimate doubt, even if only with respect to the specificity or quantity of the suspected pathologic condition; certainly, there is little or no disadvantage in performing one or more of the corroborative roentgenographic procedures currently available. Deterrents to this pursuit might include:

1. An over-confident physician and/or undemanding patient
2. Mutual selection of an empirical or arbitrary program of conservative management—a conscious deferment of surgical considerations
3. A decision to bypass the less invasive diagnostics for an arthroscopic evaluation with the potential added benefit of a therapeutic response
4. A special expediency reasonably precluding testing delays
5. Failure of insurance to cover one or more of the proposed roentgenographic tests
6. Absence of facilities for the performance of these tests or expertise in their interpretation

Regardless of any possible deterrents, there are many advantages to the performance of the specialized tests. For the patient who potentially has a surgically treatable problem, the tests may indicate in advance whether there is any reasonable benefit to be gained from surgery. Their ability to detail the pathologic condition may also help in surgical planning: open versus closed, period of expected disability (how long out of work or school), and inpatient versus outpatient treatment. For the patient without intention of surgery or with a diagnosis of a nonsurgical condition, the tests might reveal an intractable problem, treatable only by surgery (such as a bucket handle tear of the glenoid labrum). These tests rarely produce a false-positive result. More often, they produce a false-negative or under-reading of the pathologic state. The potential consequence is that in some instances an appropriate treatment course is not pursued. In most cases, however, these tests corroborate the presence of the pathologic condition and enhance the surgeon's and patient's confidence in the treatment protocol. Objective documentation also better satisfies third-party carriers with respect to approvals, provides a mobile exhibit to facilitate second opinions, and reduces the chances of certain litigious allegations.

This chapter presents the techniques and indications for each of the roentgenographic techniques currently available for the diagnosis of the more common sports-related afflications of the shoulder. The selection of tests and their relative reliability for each condition are outlined within reason at the present level of knowledge.

CONVENTIONAL (PLAIN) ROENTGENOGRAPHY

Trauma and Instability

Most orthopedic surgeons include conventional or plain roentgenography as a part of their evaluation of a shoulder disability. There is some variance, however, in defining those projections that constitute the so-called routine views of the shoulder. Is the objective to demonstrate the most evident pathologic state with the fewest number of roentgenograms, or is it to attempt to discover even more subtle abnormalities by ordering an expanded group of views as a routine? Thoroughness, cost, time efficiency, and the suspected disorder may each be a factor shaping the routine. The suspected disorder is vital in considering the selection of one or more of the "special" or "sports" views to better delineate a particular portion of the glenoid or humeral head. In describing an approach to painful athletic injuries of the shoulder, Jobe and Jobe[55] indicate that the initial evaluation should include three views of the shoulder: anteroposterior views in internal and external rotation and a transaxillary lateral view; a West Point view may be helpful to demonstrate the anteroinferior portion of the glenoid. DeSmet[26] described an anterior oblique (Y-view) projection (see Fig. 4-6) by which he was able to detect scapular and humeral head fractures undetected by the routine views outlined above. This scapular "Y-view" was cited by Rubin et al[111] as an important diagnostic aid in shoulder trauma. Pavlov and Freiberger[96] reenforce the adage that two films at right angles are important in the evaluation of all fractures. They maintain that the evaluation of the traumatized shoulder joint requires the taking of a transscapular view (Y-view) in conjunction with either a frontal or tangential view of the joint.

In any case, the routine views most commonly obtained for evaluating shoulder disorders always include **anteroposterior (AP) views** with internal and external rotation of the humerus (Fig. 4-1). These views provide a profile of the acromioclavicular (AC) and glenohumeral joints, the humeral head, and the tuberosities. They provide information about alignment, arthritic changes, and calcific deposits about the joint. Routine examination often also includes one of the **axillary projections** for tangential visualization of the glenohumeral joint and glenoid margins in order to assess alignment of the former and infractions and irregularities of the latter (Fig. 4-2). The commonly employed axillary view requires meticulous positioning with the arm in abduction (Fig. 4-3). DeSmet[27] has demonstrated its value in the nontraumatized shoulder. However, it is often poorly tolerated by patients with an acute shoulder injury. Hence the routine examination of patients following acute trauma, especially when fractures or dislocations are suspected, requires that the patient be positioned with minimal or no movement of the arm. The roentgenographic projections most often employed include an anteroposterior view without rotating the arm, and a **transthoracic lateral projection** (Fig. 4-4). These projections are usu-

Routine views

- AP (internal and external rotation)
- Axillary view
- Lateral in scapular plane (Y-view)

A

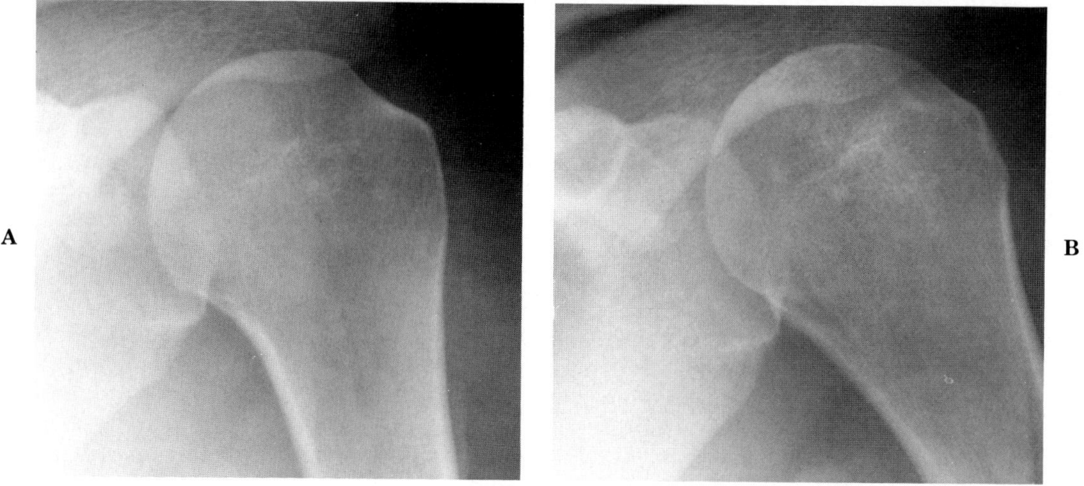

B

FIG. 4-1. Normal anteroposterior views of the left shoulder in external rotation **(A)** and internal rotation **(B).**

A

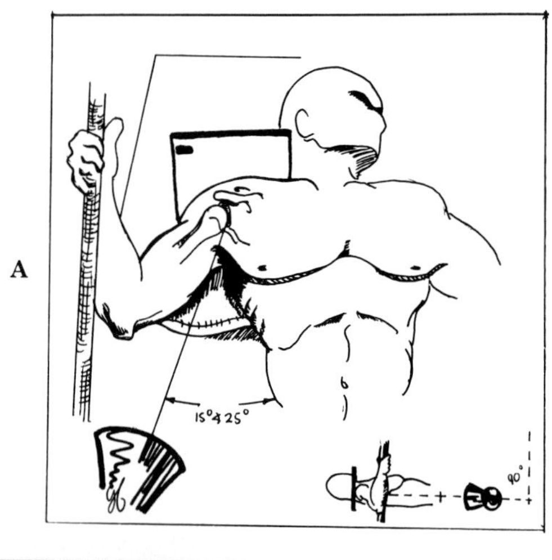

B

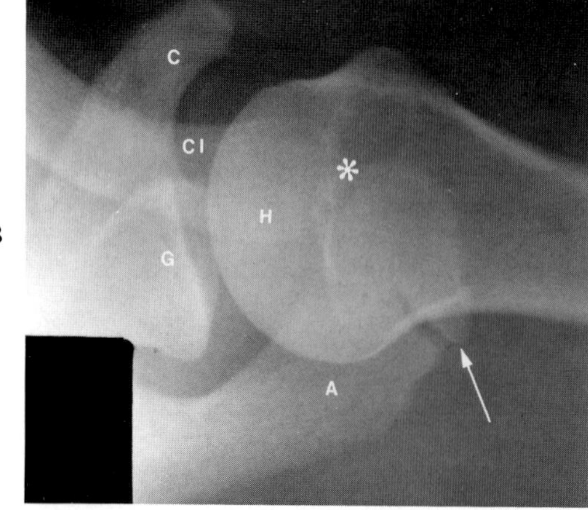

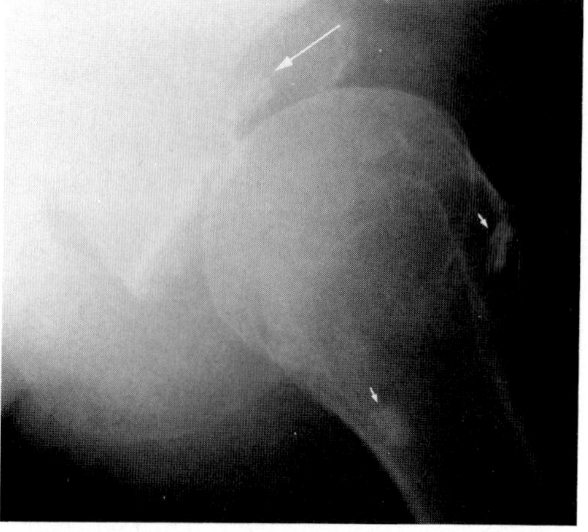

C

FIG. 4-2. Routine supine axillary view. Demonstrates the glenohumeral joint in craniocaudad orientation. Useful for evaluation of the glenohumeral joint alignment, the glenoid margins, and the acromion process. **A,** The patient is supine with the arm in neutral rotation and 45 degrees abduction. The film cassette is placed perpendicular to the table against the top of the shoulder. The x-ray beam is horizontal to the axilla at an angle of 15 to 25 degrees from the sagittal plane. **B,** *Normal. A,* Acromion; *C,* coracoid; *Cl,* clavicle; *G,* glenoid; *H,* humeral head. NOTE: Anterior acromion is formed by a secondary ossification center and is nonunited *(arrow)*. *AC joint. **C,** Anterior instability. The humeral head is subluxed anteriorly. Ossification of an existing Bankart lesion is visualized *(large arrow)*. Osteocartilaginous loose bodies are present *(small arrows)*. (**A** redrawn from Norris TR: Diagnostic techniques for shoulder instability. In: AAOS Instructional Course Lecture, vol 34, St. Louis, 1985, The CV Mosby Co.)

A

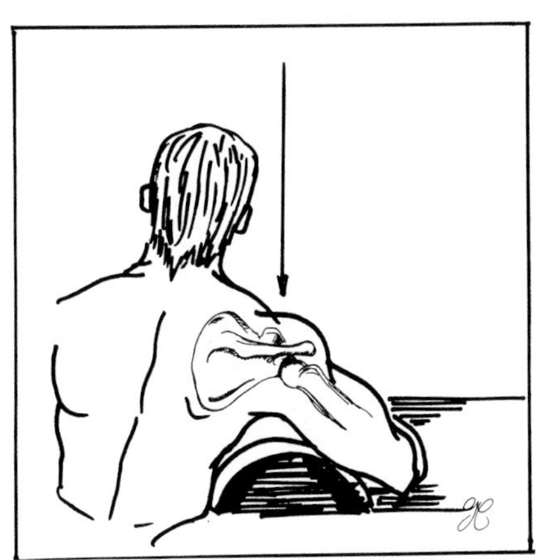

B

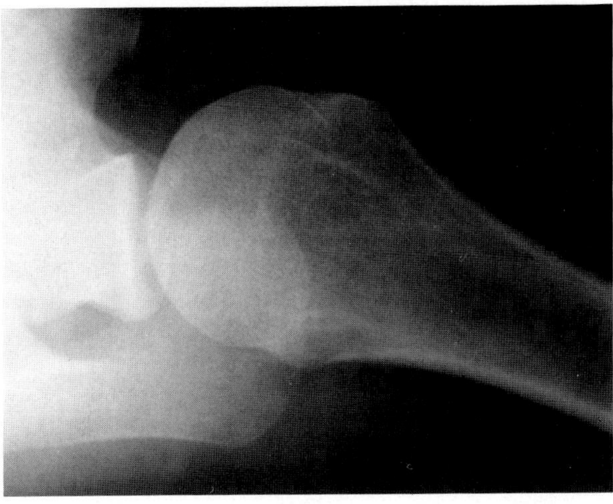

FIG. 4-3. Axillary view. Superoinferior projection. Similar to routine supine axillary view in its demonstration of the anatomic constituents of the shoulder joint. **A,** The patient is sitting with his side against the table. The arm is abducted over the curved cassette. The x-ray beam is directed in a superoinferior direction. This view may also be obtained using a regular cassette. The use of a curved cassette eliminates the excess magnification of the image because of decreased subject-film distance. **B,** Normal.

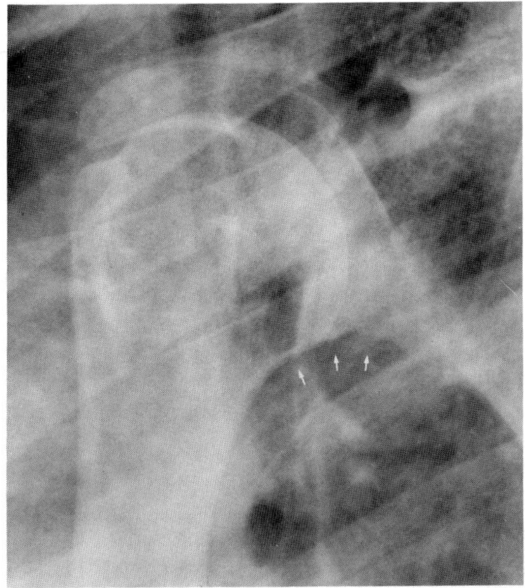

FIG. 4-4. Normal transthoracic lateral view of the shoulder. On this view the humeral shaft, the greater tuberosity, and the humeral head are clearly visualized in a true lateral projection. The coracoid process is visualized arching over the humeral head, which in turn partially ovelaps the glenoid fossa. Line continuity of the lateral scapular margin and the surgical neck of the humerus, forming the scapulohumeral arch *(arrows)*, is an indicator of normal glenohumeral alignment.

ally sufficient for detecting anterior dislocations (best seen on the AP view) and for evaluating displaced fractures of the proximal end of the humerus (Fig. 4-5). They may fail to demonstrate small fractures about the joint. Contrary to common belief, the transthoracic lateral view is not particularly good for the detection of dislocations and requires painstaking scrutiny for the detection of subtle changes in scapulohumeral alignment. A **Y-view** (anterior oblique projection) should be performed because of its ability to detect dislocations and fractures of the proximal end of the humerus (Fig. 4-6). Finally, a **posterior oblique view** (tangential anteroposterior) should be added for additional capability in the detection of dislocations (Fig. 4-7).

Posterior dislocations are notoriously diffi-

A

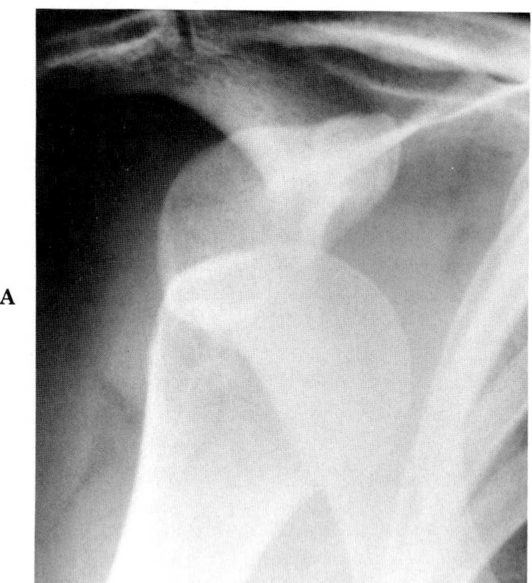

B

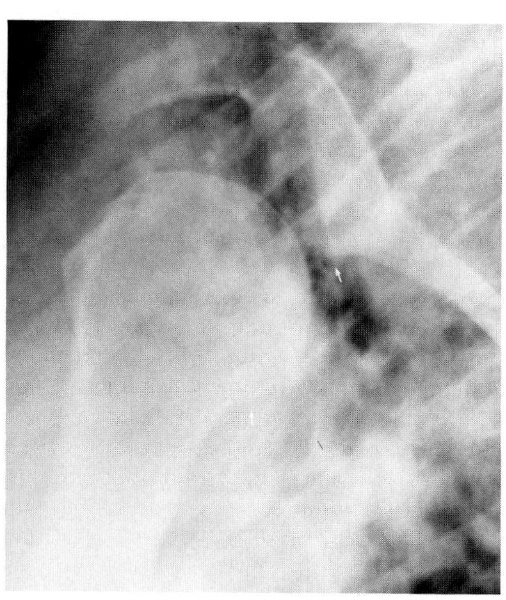

FIG. 4-5. Anterior dislocation of right shoulder. **A,** Anteroposterior view. Anterior dislocation of the humeral head is readily recognized by its marked medial displacement under the coracoid process. **B,** Transthoracic lateral view. Disruption of the scapulohumeral arch *(arrows)* is an indication of glenohumeral malalignment.

A

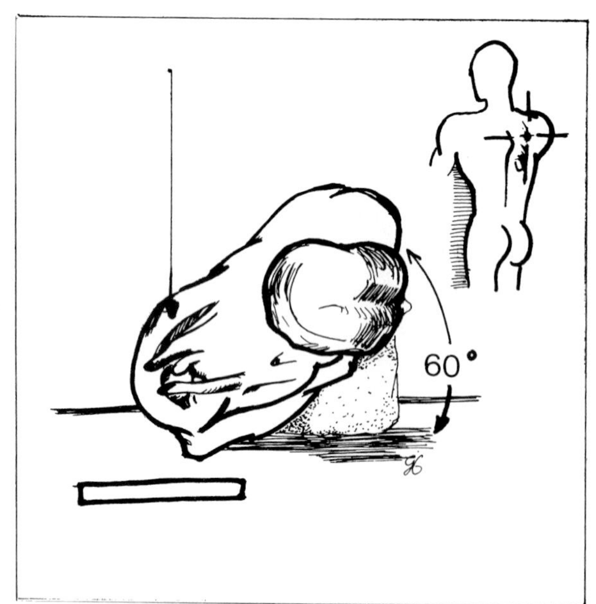

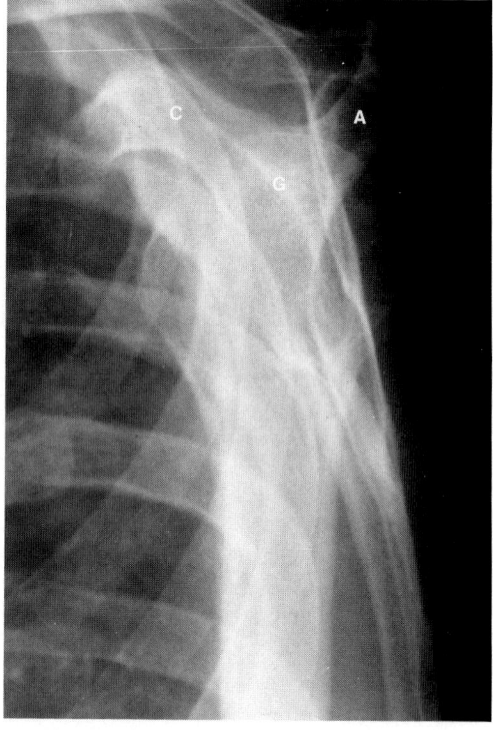

FIG. 4-6. Anterior oblique (Y-view). Proximal humerus and scapula are projected in the lateral position. Useful for evaluation of fractures and dislocations. **A,** Patient is in upright position and the shoulder being studied is anteriorly rotated 60 degrees. The x-ray beam is in posteroanterior direction and is perpendicular to the cassette. **B,** The coracoid *(C)* and the acromion *(A)* processes and the lateral border of the scapula form the figure of Y, in the center of which the glenoid fossa *(G)* is projected enface. The humerus is in the true lateral projection and the humeral head overlaps the center of the figure Y.

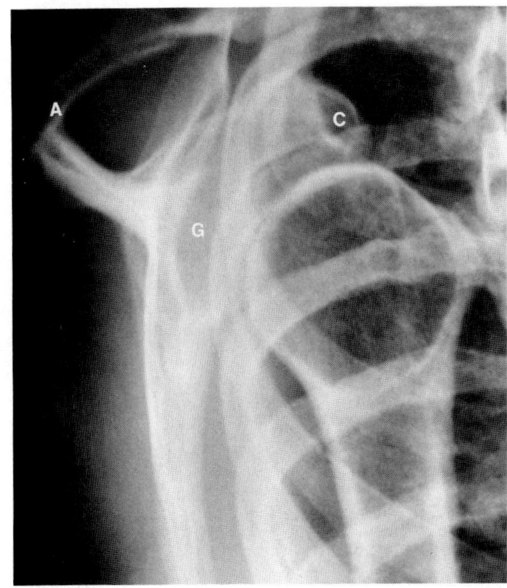

C

FIG. 4-6, cont'd. C, Anterior dislocation. The anteriorly displaced humeral head is demonstrated below the coracoid process in this projection. The glenoid fossa is "empty," signifying the presence of a dislocation. (**A** redrawn from Norris TR: Diagnostic techniques for shoulder instability. In AAOS: Instructional Course Lectures, vol 34, St. Louis, 1985, The CV Mosby Co.)

A

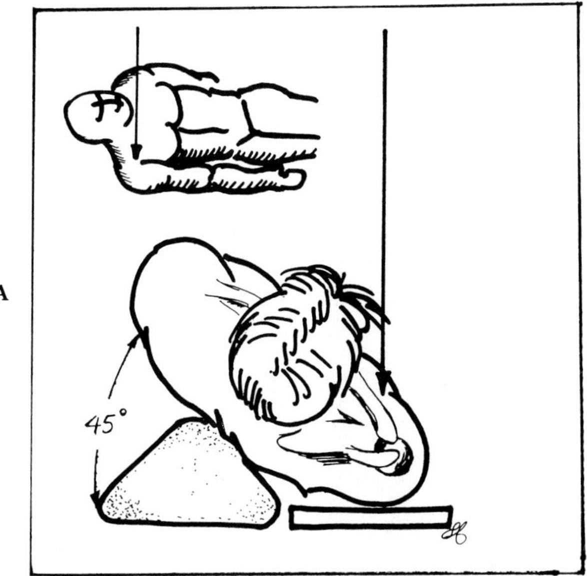

FIG. 4-7. Posterior oblique or true (tangential) anteroposterior view. The glenohumeral joint is visualized in anteroposterior orientation. Useful for evaluation humeral fractures and suspected posterior dislocation. **A,** The patient is supine or upright and the shoulder being studied is posteriorly rotated 45 degrees. The x-ray beam is directed anteroposteriorly and perpendicular to the cassette.

Continued.

cult to detect and may go unrecognized without employing specific views (Fig. 4-8). Vastamaki and Solonen[121] report that the diagnosis of posterior dislocation or fracture-dislocation is often delayed and that an axillary view is essential in suspected cases. Bloom and Obata[7] reenforce the diagnostic dilemma of the posterior dislocation and cite the report of Arndt and Sears,[2] which indicates that in 50% of such cases the diagnosis is tardy. Bloom and Obata sought to reconcile this dilemma of tardy diagnosis with that of attempting to position an acutely injured shoulder, and with the wisdom of Vastamaki and Solonen, by creating "Velpeau axillary" and "angle-up" views. These axillary projections can demonstrate a posterior displacement of the humeral head without a need to position the patient in a painfully compromising manner (Fig. 4-9). Horsefield and Jones[53] describe the "Stripp axial" view designed to evaluate the shoulder of the acutely injured

B

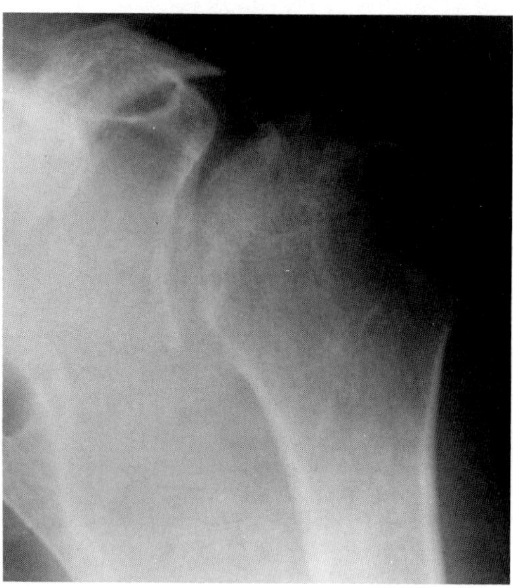

C

FIG. 4-7, cont'd. B, Normal. The glenohumeral joint space is clearly visualized. **C,** Posterior dislocation. The glenohumeral joint space is obliterated because of posterior dislocation of the humeral head, which is hinged and locked against the posterior glenoid margin. (**A** redrawn from Norris TR: Diagnostic techniques for shoulder instability. In: AAOS: Instructional Course Lecture, vol 34, St. Louis, 1985, The CV Mosby Co.)

A

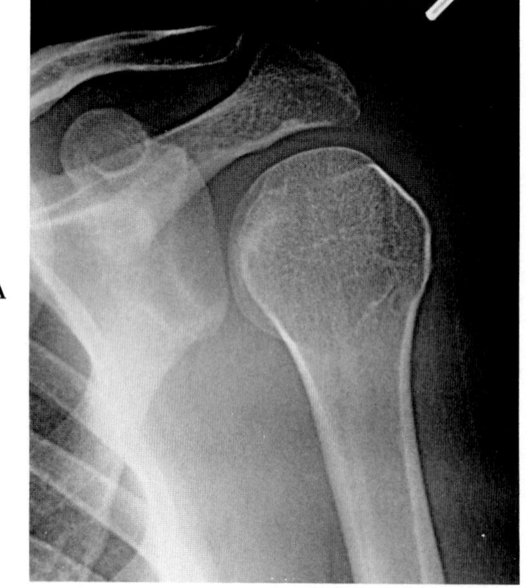

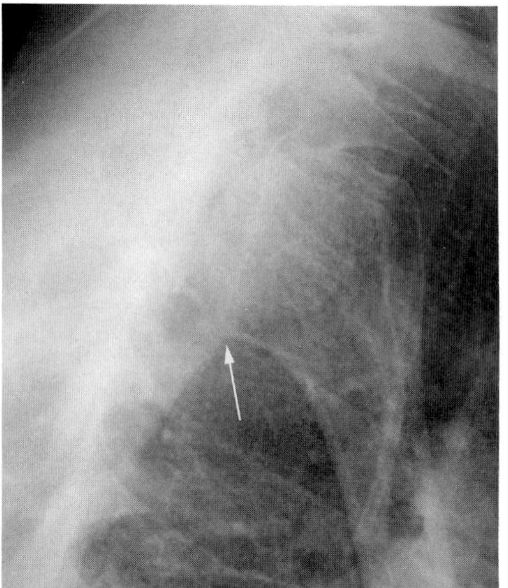

B

FIG. 4-8. Posterior dislocation. Initial roentgenographic examination of left shoulder in anteroposterior **(A)** and transthoracic lateral view **(B)**. **A,** There is widening of the glenohumeral joint space. The humeral head is lateral to the posterior glenoid margin instead of the overlap that is normally seen in this position (see Fig. 4-1). **B,** There is distortion of the glenohumeral arch with a sharp angle between the lateral scapular margin and the humeral neck *(arrow)*. Above findings are both suggestive of an abnormal glenohumeral alignment. A Y-view is obtained to confirm presence of a dislocation.

C

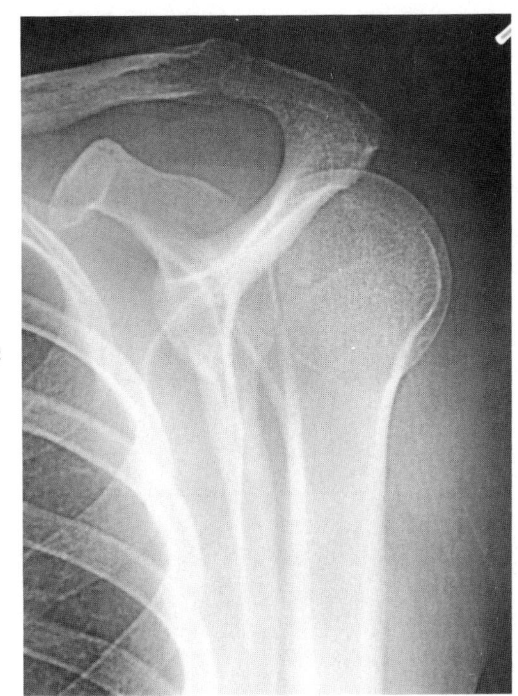

FIG. 4-8, cont'd. C, Tangential scapular *(Y)* view. The humeral head is posteriorly dislocated.

A

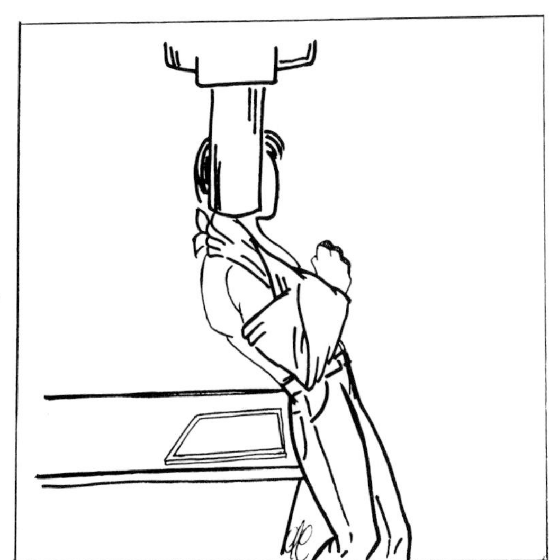

B

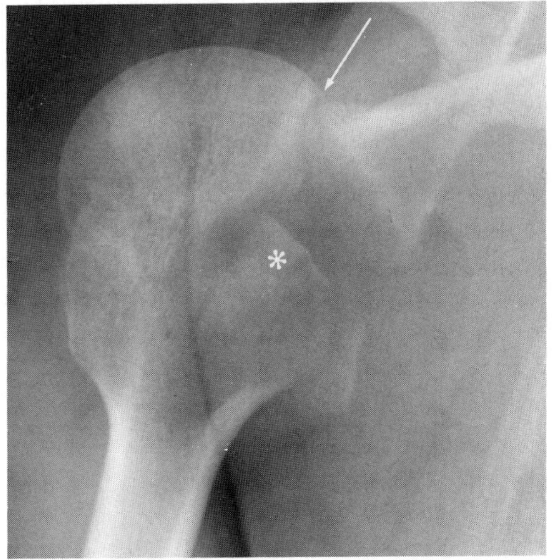

FIG. 4-9. Velpeau axillary view. A craniocaudad view of the glenohumeral joint is obtained. Useful for evaluation of the glenohumeral alignment in suspected posterior dislocation. **A,** Patient stands with back against the x-ray table. The patient arches backward over the table until the shoulder is above the cassette, which is lying on the table. The superoinferior x-ray beam is then directed through the shoulder and perpendicular to the cassette. **B,** Posterior fracture dislocation. In addition to a comminuted fracture of the humeral neck and tuberosities, the major portion of the humeral head is posteriorly dislocated and is hinged against the posterior glenoid margin. A smaller segment of the head (*) is impacted. (**A** redrawn from Bloom MH and Obata WG: J Bone Joint Surg 49A(5):943, 1987.)

45°
40″
45°
A

B
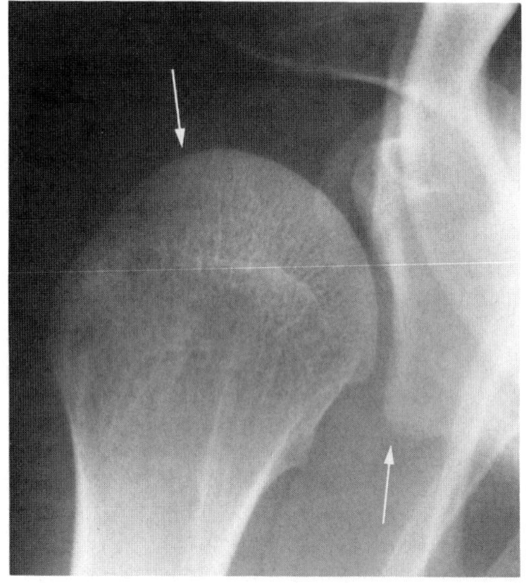

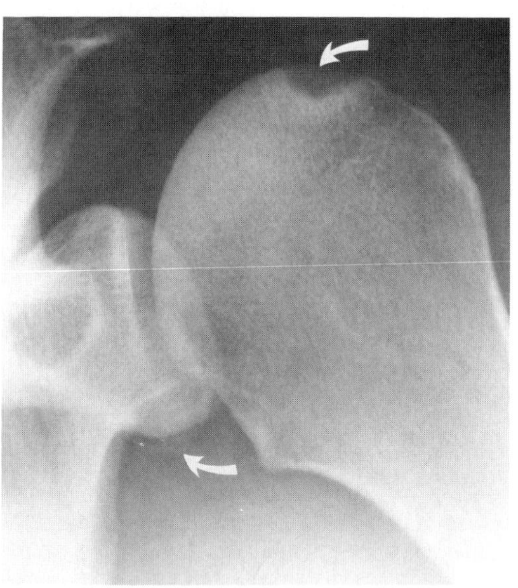
C

FIG. 4-10. Apical oblique or craniocaudad view. The glenohumeral joint is projected in a craniocaudad orientation. Useful for evaluation of fracture dislocations. Specifically good for demonstration of Hill-Sachs and Bankart lesions. **A,** Patient is in upright position and the shoulder being studied is 45 degrees posteriorly rotated. The roentgenographic beam is in an anteroposterior and 45 degrees caudad direction. A variation of this view may be obtained with the patient supine. **B,** The glenohumeral joint is tangentially visualized. Craniocaudad angulation of the x-ray beam provides a tangential view of the posterosuperior aspect of the humeral head and the anteroinferior aspect of the glenoid margins *(arrows)*. **C,** Anterior instability. Hill-Sachs defect of the humeral head and ectopic ossification along the anterior glenoid margin are visualized *(arrows)*. (**A** redrawn from Garth WP, Slappey CE, and Ochs CW: J Bone Joint Surg 66A(9):1450-1453, 1984.)

patient who is unable to abduct because of pain. Another view that is useful in demonstrating glenohumeral instability and that requires no movement of the painful shoulder is the apical oblique projection (Fig. 4-10). Garth et al[37] stated that this view, which provides a coronal profile of the glenohumeral joint, is an excellent detector of the hallmark criteria of instabilities of all ages: glenohumeral displacements, Hill-Sachs lesions, and Bankart fractures or ossifications. Nevertheless, they admitted that the West Point view of Rokous et al[108] was much more likely to detect Bankart lesions (Fig. 4-11).

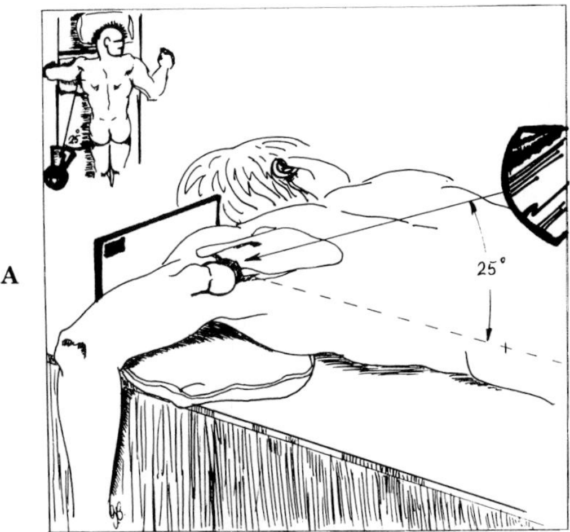

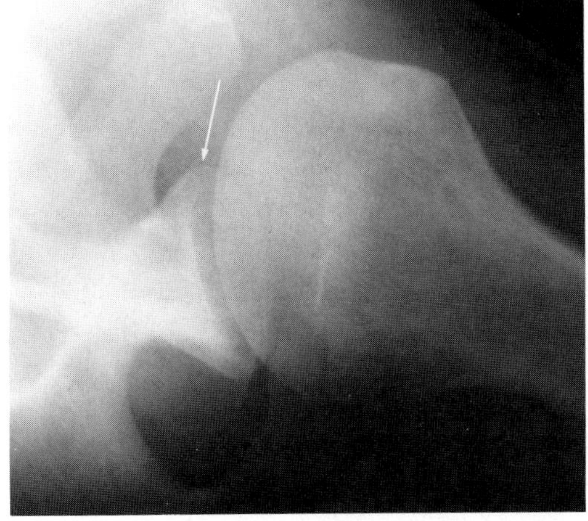

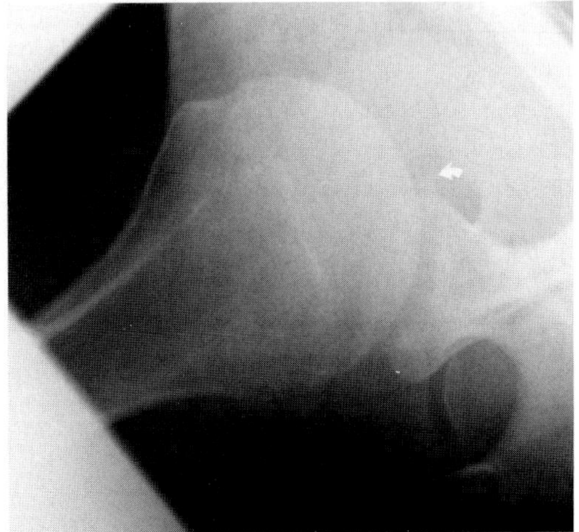

FIG. 4-11. Westpoint axillary view. The anteroinferior glenoid margin is visualized without structure superimposition. Specifically used for detecting osseous Bankart lesion. **A,** Patient is in prone position with shoulder propped up over a pillow. The arm is in internal rotation and hanging down from the edge of the table. The x-ray beam is angled downward 25 degrees from the horizontal plane and 25 degrees from the sagittal plane of the body. **B,** The anteroinferior glenoid margin is visualized without obstruction *(arrow)*. **C,** Anterior instability. Ectopic bone formation (osseous Bankart lesion) of anterior glenoid margin is visualized *(arrow)*. (**A** redrawn from Norris TR: Diagnostic techniques for shoulder instability. In: AAOS, Instructional Course Lecture, vol 34, St. Louis, 1985, The CV Mosby Co.)

Roentgenographic Signs of Instability

Hill-Sachs lesion. It is evident that the lesions of chronic or recurrent glenohumeral dislocations and subluxations are often not optimally visualized on the standard roentgenographic views alluded to above. The compression fracture of the posterolateral portion of the humeral head was first reported by Flower[34] in 1861, then subsequently by Eve[33] in 1880. However, it was Hill and Sachs[52] who ultimately immortalized this lesion as an accompaniment of recurrent anterior dislocation of the shoulder in a classic article in 1940. The article credits Pilz (1925) with having demonstrated that the detection of this posterolateral defect of the head is dependent on the roentgenographic technique employed. While the lesion is frequently visualized on an anteroposterior internal rotation view (Fig. 4-12), it is most likely to be seen to good advantage by a Stryker notch view (Fig. 4-13). Pavlov et al[96] studied 83 patients with combinations of anterior shoulder subluxations

Hill-Sachs lesion

- Compression fracture of the posterolateral humeral head
- Results from anterior dislocation
- Best seen on AP in internal rotation or Stryker notch view

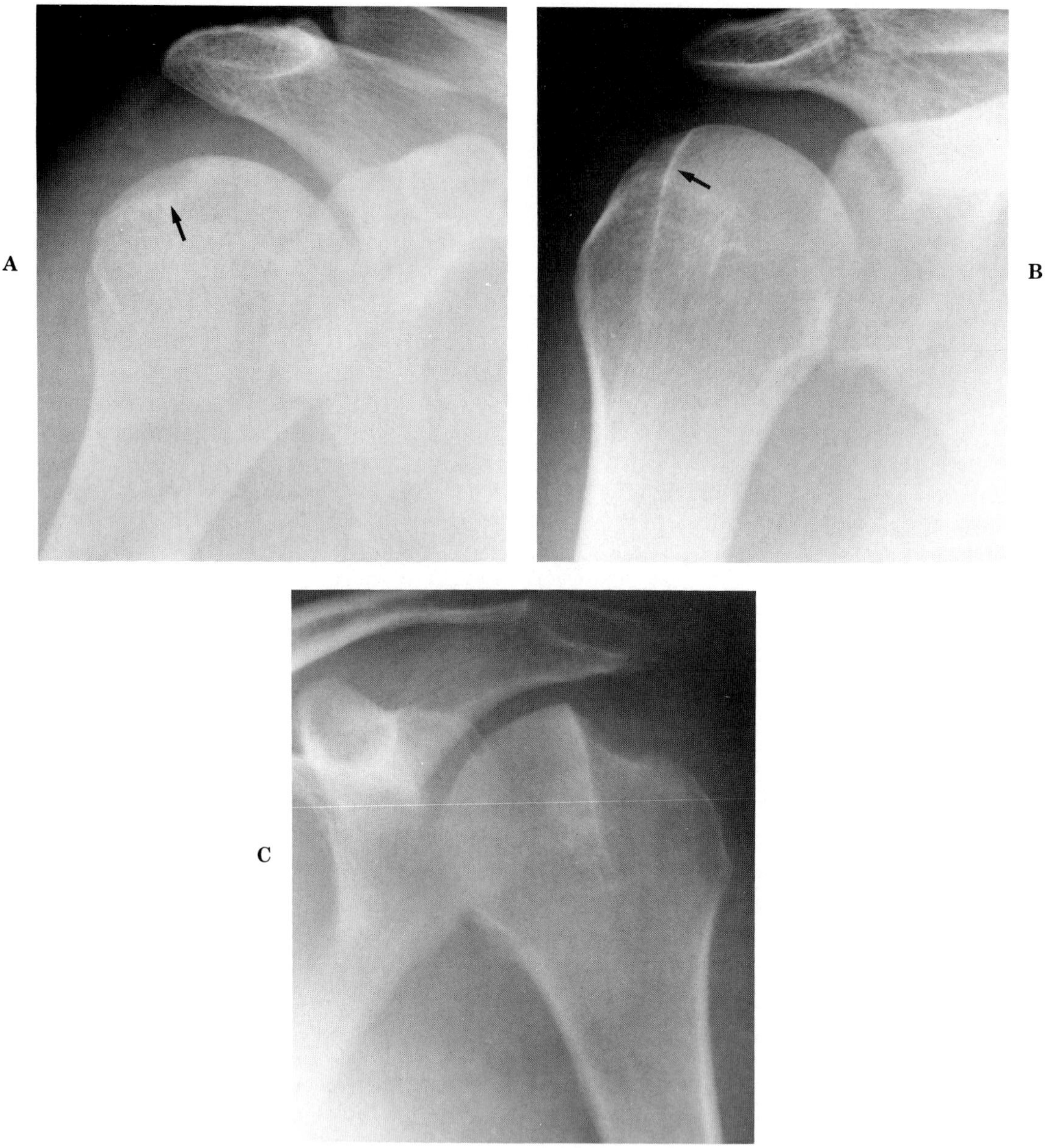

A

B

C

FIG. 4-12. Hill-Sachs lesion: **A, B,** and **C.** Anterioposterior views of right shoulder **(A** and **B)** and left shoulder **(C)** in three different patients. **A,** This small Hill-Sachs defect is projected as a dense band, parallel to the posterosuperior aspect of the humeral head *(arrow)*. **B,** The posterosuperior articular surface of the humeral head is irregular and is outlined by a dense vertical band medially. This sclerotic band shows the extent of this Hill-Sachs lesion *(arrow)*. **C,** A large defect of the humeral head is visualized.

and dislocations and reached the same conclusion. Danzig et al[23] performed cadaveric studies and clinical evaluations on a series of dislocations and concluded that the optimal means for detecting the Hill-Sachs lesion was a combination of three views: an anteroposterior view with 45 degrees of internal rotation of the humerus, a Stryker notch view, and a modified Didiee view[30] (Fig. 4-14).

In 1934 Hermodsson[51] described an axillary view performed with the patient supine (Fig. 4-15). This view was conceived to demonstrate the "Hermodsson fracture" (Hill-Sachs lesion) of the humeral head. In a study of 27 shoulders with recurrent anterior shoulder dislocations, Rozing et al[110] could demonstrate the lesion in only 12 shoulders using the Hermodsson view, whereas the Stryker notch

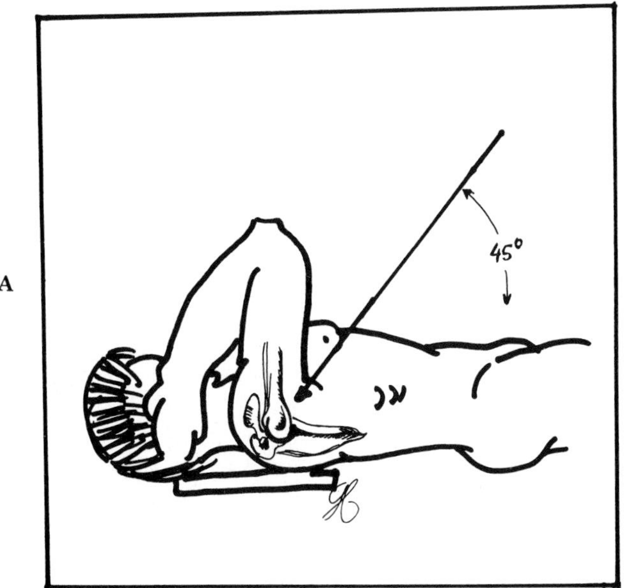

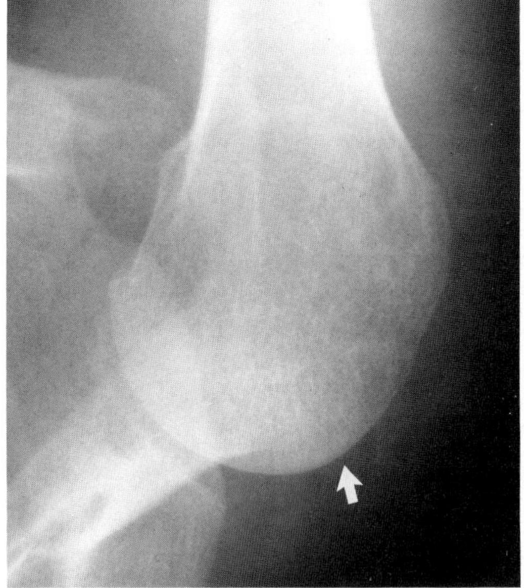

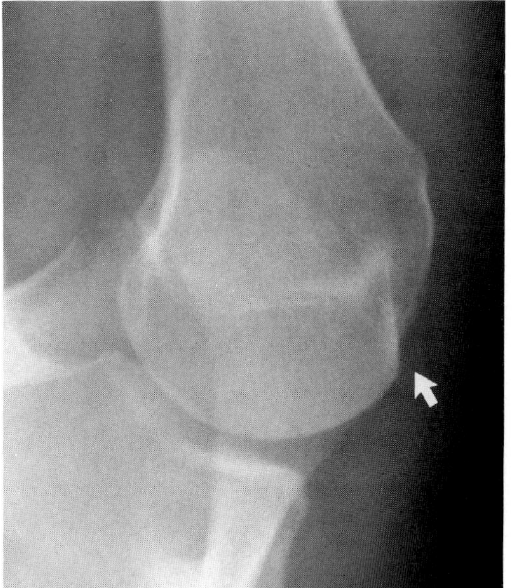

FIG. 4-13. Stryker notch view. Posterosuperior aspect of the humeral head is tangentially projected. Specifically useful for demonstrating Hills-Sachs defect. **A,** The patient is supine. The arm is elevated 90 degrees and the elbow is flexed so that the palm of the hand is on the ear or resting on the side of the head. The humerus is parallel to the sagittal plane of the body. The roentgenographic beam is directed to the axilla 45 degrees from the horizontal plane. A variation of the view may be obtained with a 10-degree cephalad angulation of the beam. **B,** The posterosuperior aspect of the humeral head seen in profile *(arrow)*. **C,** Anterior instability. Hill-Sachs defect is visualized *(arrow)*. (**A** redrawn from Rozing PM, deBakker HM, and Obermann WR: Acta Orthop Scand 68:479, 1967.)

view identified the lesion in 25 of the shoulders. Warren[123] distinguishes between dislocators and subluxators and cites Pavlov et al,[96] who discovered the Hill-Sachs lesion in 80% of the former and in only 25% of the latter.

Bankart lesion. In 1923 Bankart[4] contended that detachment of the glenoid labrum is the essential lesion in recurrent anterior dislocations of the glenohumeral joint. Regardless of any controversy centering about this contention, the radiologist has come to regard the presence of an "osseous" Bankart lesion (fracture or ectopic bone formation about the anterior glenoid rim) as pathognomic evidence of anterior instability.[5,8,96] In 1972 Rokous et al[108] reported a new axillary view, now re-

A

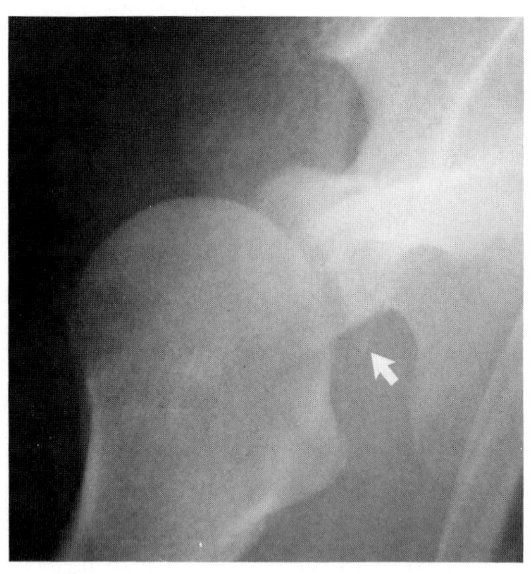

B

FIG. 4-14. Didiee view. Posterosuperior aspect of the humeral head and anterior glenoid margin are projected. Useful for demonstration of Hill-Sachs and Bankart lesions. **A,** Patient is in prone position. The arm is internally rotated and the dorsum of the hand rests on the iliac crest. The roentgenographic beam is directed to the humeral head in the plane of the humeral shaft and 45 degrees to the horizontal plane. **B,** Anterior instability. Ectopic ossification (osseous Bankart lesion) is visualized *(arrow)*. (**A** redrawn from Rozing PM, deBakker HM, and Oberman WR: Acta Orthop Scand 68:479, 1967.)

A

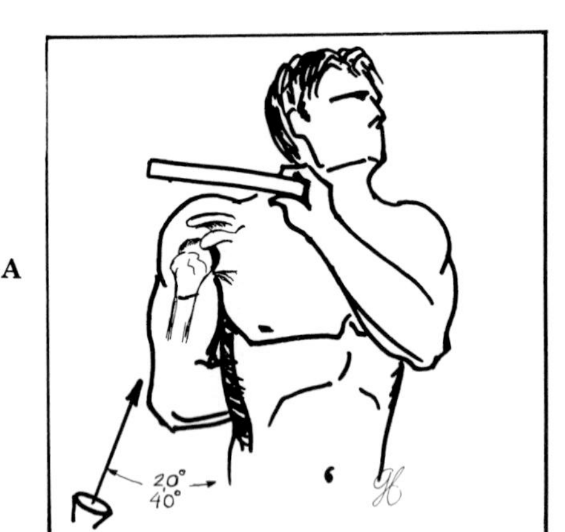

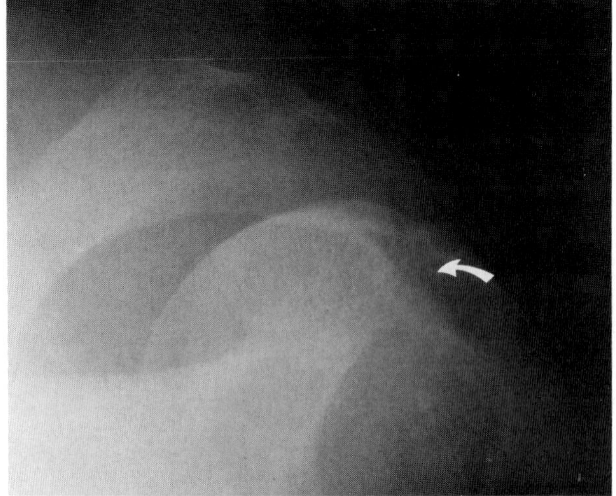

B

FIG. 4-15. Hermodsson view. The posterolateral aspect of the humeral head is visualized without superimpositions for evaluation of Hill-Sachs defect. **A,** The patient is upright and holds the cassette with the opposite hand against the top of shoulder. The arm is internally rotated and the hand rests against the back. The x-ray beam is directed to the back of the humeral head at an angle of approximately 30 degrees from the sagittal plane or the humeral axis. **B,** Hill-Sachs defect *(arrow)*.

ferred to as the **West Point view** (see Fig. 4-11), which was conceived for the specific purpose of demonstrating the Bankart lesion.

Norris recommends assessment of the anteroinferior glenoid findings of instability by either the West Point prone axillary view or the supine external rotation axillary view of Ciullo[91] (Fig. 4-16). He indicates that while the West Point view gives better detail, the Ciullo view is less difficult to obtain for the uninitiated technician.

Pavlov et al report that the osseous Bankart lesion is best documented on the West Point and Didiee views.[96] The latter view was de-

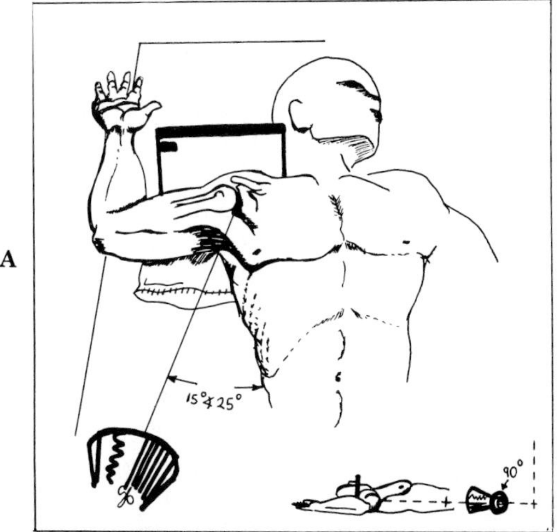

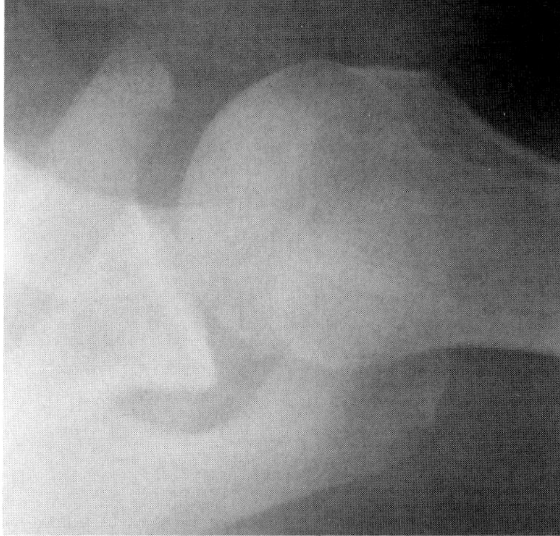

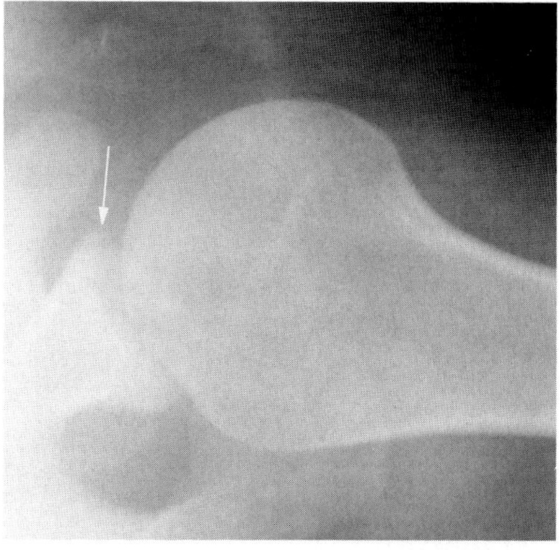

FIG. 4-16. Supine external rotation axillary view of Ciullo. For improved visualization of anteroinferior glenoid margin. Useful for Bankart lesion. **A,** The patient position is similar to that for a routine axillary view. However, the arm is abducted 90 degrees and externally rotated. **B,** Normal. **C,** Small osseous Bankart lesion is visualized *(arrow)*. (**A** redrawn from Norris TR: Diagnostic techniques for shoulder instability. In: AAOS Instructional Course Lectures, vol 34, St. Louis, 1985, The CV Mosby Co.)

scribed by Didiee in 1938[30] and has value as well in the detection of the Hill-Sachs lesion, as already indicated (see Fig. 4-14). The apical oblique or craniocaudad oblique view also has an advantage in that it can reveal both pathognomic lesions of instability, the Hill-Sachs lesion, and the Bankart lesion (see Fig. 4-10). Furthermore, it is simpler to obtain than either the West Point or the Stryker notch view. Mizuno and Hirohata,[83] using a modified West Point view, found anterior displacement of the humeral head in 11% of traumatic anterior subluxations and in 89% of involuntary multidirectional subluxations.

Posterior instability. Consideration to chronic posterior instability must not be forsaken amidst the more voluminous information regarding anterior instabilities. The main contribution made by conventional roentgenology for the diagnosis of posterior instability, according to Gambrioli et al,[35] is the special Y-view projection demonstrating the classic anterolateral lesion of the humeral head; this is the counterpart of the Hill-Sachs lesion described by McLaughlin.[73] Posterior instability counterparts of the Bankart fracture and fracture of the greater tuberosity are fractures of the posterior glenoid rim and of the lesser tuberosity. Routine supine axillary views may reveal the McLaughlin fracture as well as deformities of the glenoid margin in patients with posterior instability (Fig. 4-17). Warren[123] admonishes that both the Stryker notch and the West Point views must be care-

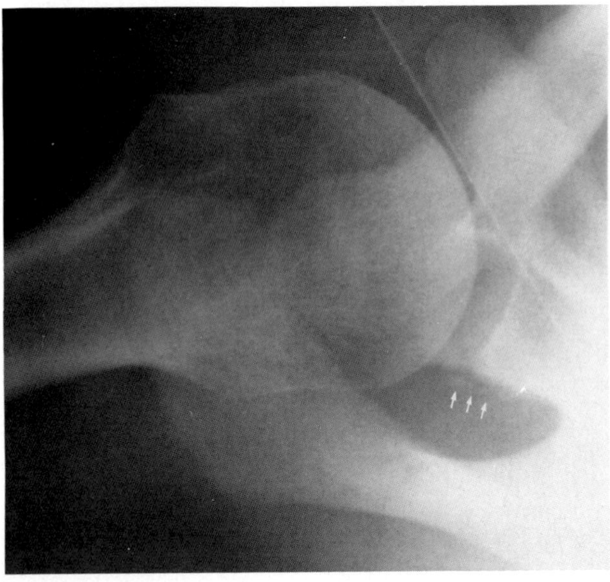

FIG. 4-17. Posterior instability, axillary view. Same patient as in Fig. 4-19. The posterior glenoid margin is irregular and ectopic ossification is present *(arrows)*.

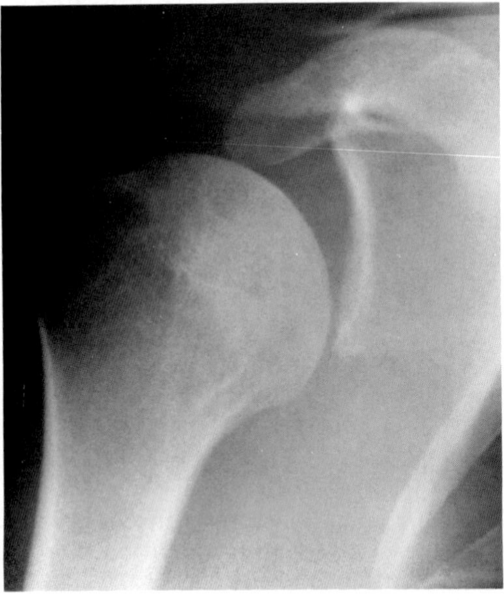

FIG. 4-18. Inferior instability. True anteroposterior view of the right shoulder with addition of 10-pound weight to the forearm. Inferior displacement of the humerus and glenohumeral malalignment is demonstrated.

fully evaluated for posterior glenoid lesions indicative of posterior subluxation. In a study of 50 shoulders with recurrent (involuntary) posterior subluxation, Hawkins et al[50] found no abnormalities on routine roentgenograms. Seventeen of these shoulders were subjected to stress roentgenograms and cineroentgenography, which demonstrated posterior instability.

Dynamic roentgenography. According to Norris,[91] the conventional roentgenographic evaluation of inferior glenohumeral instability may be enhanced by the addition of well-padded 20-pound gauntlet forearm weights, which reveal an increased acromiohumeral interval (Fig. 4-18).

Anterior and posterior drawer tests such as those described by Gerber[38] and recorded by roentgenographs may be performed with the patient awake or anesthetized to corroborate the presence of an instability, its direction, and its magnitude (Fig. 4-19). Confirmation and documentation of the findings in such instances is best accomplished with C-arm fluoroscopy.[91] It must be appreciated that posterior displacement of the humeral head up to 50% of its width may be within normal limits.[91]

Discussion. In reviewing the morass of available views designed to evaluate traumatic lesions and/or instabilities of the glenohumeral joint, one finds that certain trends are evident. Anteroposterior views with both internal and external rotation of the humeri are definite standards. The externally rotated view is not very valuable for instability evaluation but reveals tuberosity fractures and calcifications about the rotator cuff. In acutely traumatized patients, motion of the arm may be too painful or inhibited by a dislocation. In such instances an anteroposterior view may

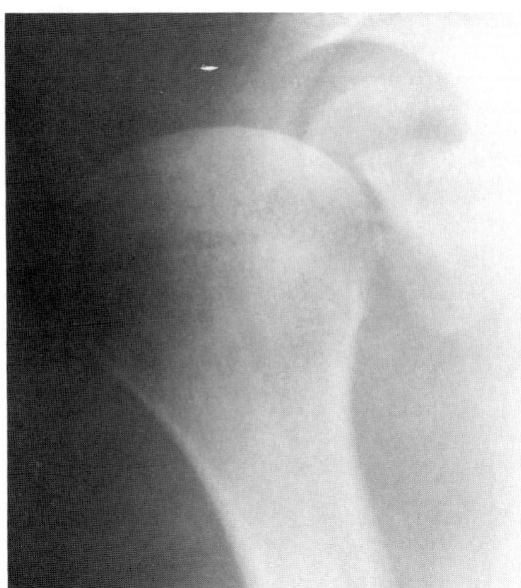

FIG. 4-19. Posterior instability. Craniocaudad (apical oblique) view of the right shoulder (same patient as in Fig. 4-17) was obtained while posterior stress was being applied. Marked posterior displacement of the humeral head is demonstrated. (Courtesy of Dr. Ramesh Gidumal, NYU Medical Center.)

be performed without rotation of the arm. The AP view may be further complemented by the addition of a "true" anteroposterior view (in the posterior oblique position), which permits the joint to be visualized tangentially. The transthoracic lateral view is also used in this circumstance, but as pointed out by Kornguth and Salazar[67] in their evaluation of 161 abnormal shoulders after trauma, the view has relatively poor success in detecting glenoid rim fractures, Hill-Sachs lesions, and scapular body fractures. Supine axillary views fail to reveal a number of lesions with consistency, and since positioning for these views may be too painful for many patients, other views must be considered with regularity. The "Velpeau axillary," "angle up," "Stripp" axial, and anterior oblique views are helpful for patients whose arms cannot be manipulated because of pain.

The format and severity of instability (e.g., subluxation versus dislocation) may bear upon the yield of roentgenographic evidence for its existence on one or more of the axillary or oblique views selected for diagnosis. Garth et al[37] suggested that the size of a Hill-Sachs lesion had no apparent relationship to the chronicity or recurrence rate of instability. Though views such as the Didiee and apical oblique are capable of revealing both Hill-Sachs and Bankart lesions, other views may be more proficient in the detection of one or the other of these lesions. Table 4-1 is a collation of studies by various authors who have attempted to compare the efficacies of different views for the detection of a variety of traumatic and instability lesions.

Acromioclavicular Joint

The acromioclavicular joint is ordinarily well visualized on all anteroposterior views of the shoulder. There is, however, a technical difficulty in the roentgenographic examination of the acromial arch region on the anteroposterior projection. The thickness of the proximolateral aspect of the shoulder is considerably less than that of the glenohumeral and axillary regions. Therefore optimal visualization of the latter regions is often achieved at the expense of the acromioclavicular joint and subacromial regions. The use of the appropriately designed filters can overcome this problem. These filters may be in the form of a graduated aluminum plate attached to the x-ray tube with its thicker end up against the top of the shoulder. They may also come in the form of a silicone rubber pad placed on the shoulder. Vezina[122] has employed a silicone absorption filter to enhance clarity of the acromioclavicular window even when performing such studies as arthrotomography in evaluating a ruptured rotator cuff. In any case, when a filter is used the beam is more attenuated by the filter's proximal end, preventing overpenetration of the proximal portion of the shoulder.

Visualization of the acromioclavicular joint is also enhanced by a 15-degree cranial angulation of the x-ray beam (Fig. 4-20). This joint, however, has a variable orientation. Neviaser[87] indicates that the plane of the acromioclavicular joint varies from vertical to nearly horizontal. When acromioclavicular joint separation is suspected, it is common practice to examine the joint with 5 to 15 pounds of weight attached to the patient's wrists. This examination most often includes both shoulders for purposes of comparison. The apposition of the acromion to the articular end of the clavicle is evaluated, as is the coracoclavicular interval.[124] The usual coracoid to clavicle distance is 1.1 to 1.3 cm; an increase in this interval is indicative of a coracoclavicular ligamentous disruption (Fig. 4-21). With increasing severity of the grade of sprain and elevation of the lateral portion of the clavicle, there is a progressive widening of the acromioclavicular joint.[95] Horizontal instability of the clavicle is not appreciated by standard roentgenographic techniques. Oc-

TABLE 4-1 The efficiency of various roentgenographic views in evaluation of shoulder abnormalities

A. Instability

1. Adapted from Rozing PM, deBakker HM, and Obermann WR: Acta Orthop Scand 68:479, 1967.
Twenty-seven shoulders, with recurrent anterior dislocation Hill-Sachs defect seen in 26; Bankart defect seen in 10.

View	*Hill-Sachs*	*Bankart*
45-degree craniocaudal	22/27	10/10
Stryker notch	25/27	1/10
Didiee	7/27	Not reported
Frontal (AP)	7/27	Not reported
Hermodsson	12/27	0/10
Axial	0/27	2/10

COMMENTARY: 45-degree craniocaudal view has high yield for both lesions. Stryker notch view excellent for Hill-Sachs.

RECOMMENDATION: Do craniocaudal view first, and if defect is not seen, do Stryker notch view. West Point and Didiee views may be added to see Bankart lesion.

2. Adapted from Danzig LA, Greenway G, and Resnick D: Am J Sports Med 8(5):328, 1980.
The Hill-Sachs Lesion in 15 patients with anterior shoulder dislocation.

View	*Result*
AP external rotation	1/15
AP internal rotation 45 degrees	*15/15
Axillary	7/15
AP internal rotation 20 degrees	4/15
PA external rotation 45 degrees	10/15
PA internal rotation 45 degrees	*12/15
Stryker notch	*14/15
Modified Didiee	*12/15

RECOMMENDATION: Take three views to show Hill-Sachs: AP (or PA) in 45-degree internal rotation, Stryker notch, and Didiee.
*Views that are particularly efficacious.

3. Adapted from Pavlov H et al: Clin Orthop 194: 153, 1985.
a. A study of 83 patients with unilateral anterior shoulder instability.

View	*Hill-Sachs*	*Bankart*
Internal rotation	92%	15%
External rotation	32%	65%
Axillary	44%	66%
West Point	51%	70%
Stryker Notch	92%	11%
Didiee	35%	71%

COMMENTARY: Maximal yield in diagnosing the lesions of anterior instability are achieved with three combined views: AP internal rotation, Stryker notch, and either West Point or Didiee.

b. (1)

Lesion	Bankart or Hill-Sachs	Hill-Sachs and Bankart	Isolated Hill-Sachs	Isolated Bankart	Normal
%	82%	16%	61%	5%	18%

(2)

	Hill-Sachs (with or without each other)	Bankart
Subluxations	66%	40%
Dislocations	77%	15%
Combined	87%	20%

COMMENTARY: Isolated Hill-Sachs occurs much more often than isolated Bankart. One or the other is often present, but they occur together infrequently. The type of instability bears upon defect incidence.

B. General Trauma

1. Adapted from DeSmet AA: Am J Radiol 134:515, 1980.

Acute Trauma	*AP External Rotation*	*AP External and Internal Rotation*	*Anterior Oblique*	*AP Internal Rotation and Anterior Oblique*
Anterior dislocation	0	0	0	8
Humeral head fracture	2	0	*1	4
AC separation	0	0	0	5
Clavicle fracture	0	0	0	3
Scapular fracture	0	1	3	2

NOTE: 60-degree anterior oblique = Y view.

COMMENTARY: In this series four fractures (*) would have been missed without an anterior oblique projection. It may be obtained at 45 degrees or 60 degrees and requires no movement of the humerus.

TABLE 4-1—cont'd. The efficiency of various roentgenographic views in evaluation of shoulder abnormalities

B. General Trauma—cont'd.

2. Adapted from Kornguth PJ, and Salazar AM: Am J Radiol 149(1):113, 1987.

Abnormality	*n.*	*AP Percent*	*Lateral Percent*	*Y-View Percent*	*Apical Oblique Percent*
Humerus fracture	56	100	70	68	93
GH dislocation	34	100	94	91	100*
Clavicle fracture	22	100	9	68	73
Glenoid rim fracture	7	39	0	11	94†
AC Separation	14	100	14	21	14
Hill-Sachs lesion	5	42	8	8	100‡
Scapular fracture	9	90	30	50	50

COMMENTARY: Twenty of 161 abnormalities would have been missed in a study of 511 traumatized shoulders if an apical oblique (45-degree posterior oblique with 45-degree caudal angulation) view was not performed. It is a good view to show posterior glenohumeral dislocation (*), glenoid rim fractures (†), and Hill-Sachs lesions (‡).

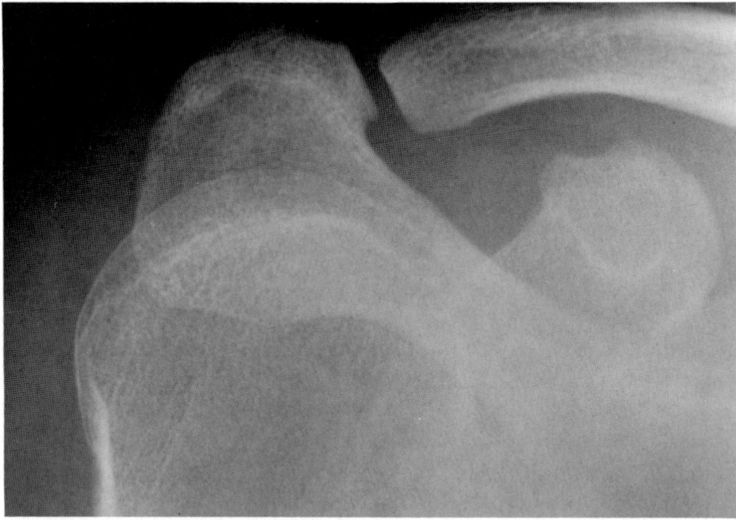

FIG. 4-20. Normal right acromioclavicular (AC) joint. Cranial angulation of the roentgenographic beam projects the AC joint above and clear of the acromion process.

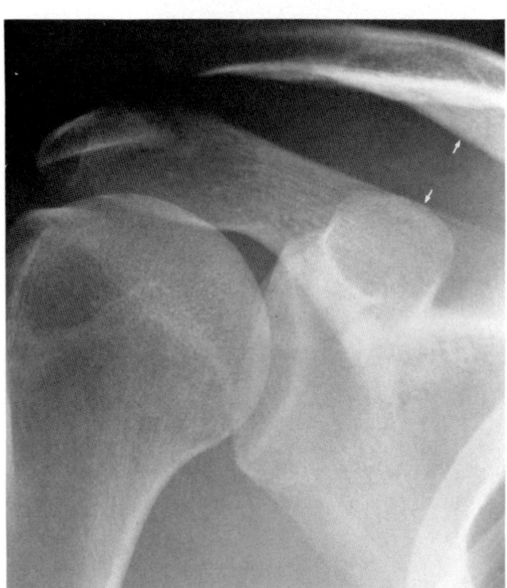

FIG. 4-21. Coracoclavicular ligament disruption. Anteroposterior view of right shoulder following acute trauma. AC joint separation is evident. The coracoclavicular distance *(arrows)* of 1.7 cm indicated ligamentous disruption.

casionally, intraarticular fractures may mimic a separation on physical inspection and/or accompany a separation (Figs. 4-22 and 4-23). Realistically, the search for fractures is perhaps more important than the evaluation for separation, since the latter is most readily discerned by physical examination. Except for the most flagrant separations, such as the subcutaneous variety of the Rockwood classification,[107] which requires a reattachment of the large extrinsic muscles, sports physicians are moving away from early operative fixations of the joint or even protracted immobilizations[18] in favor of early mobilization and strengthening.

Examination of the chronically separated joint may reveal a displaced, enlarged, and arthritic clavicular head and/or ossifications where the coracoclavicular ligaments had existed (Fig. 4-23).

Conventional Roentgenography in Search of the "Supraspinatus Syndrome"

According to Jobe and Jobe,[55] "the most common shoulder problem in sports medicine is impingement syndrome associated with bursitis, rotator cuff inflammation and tears, and bicipital tendinitis." The presence of impingement or the "supraspinatus syndrome" implies the existence of symptoms and/or functional disability emanating from one or more of the tissues of which the subacromial region is comprised. Most commonly these manifestations result directly or indirectly from the inflammation or tearing of the rotator cuff and/or the existence of an obstruction to tissue glide within the subacromial space. The role of available diagnostic roentgenography for this entity and its related pathologic conditions is variable, because it is predicated on the patronage of prescribing physicians whose need for quantified proof of diagnosis and prognosis is variable. The diagnosis of rotator cuff tears and impingements is based upon a spectrum of evidence that ranges from circumstantial to pathognomonic. With respect to the rotator cuff, physical examination can provide reasonably strong evidence of disruption in many cases, but pathognomonic demonstrations are accomplished only by roentgenography (arthrography, sonography, and MRI) and surgery. Impingement, on the other hand, is perhaps most confidently diagnosed by physical examination. Roentgenography merely adds credence to a strong circumstantial case. Unfortunately, there is no objective and quantitative measure of impingement. In fact, impingement is not even a single entity but a syndrome that may be multiply derived from a gamut of pathologic states. It is an eponym for a group of painful motion syndromes about the shoulder having some abnormality of glide of the subacromial structures, as a common denominator.

Preoperative roentgenographic evaluation must be pursued for those patients and surgeons concerned with a quantitative assessment of pathologic conditions, a measure of the difficulty of the intended surgery, an an-

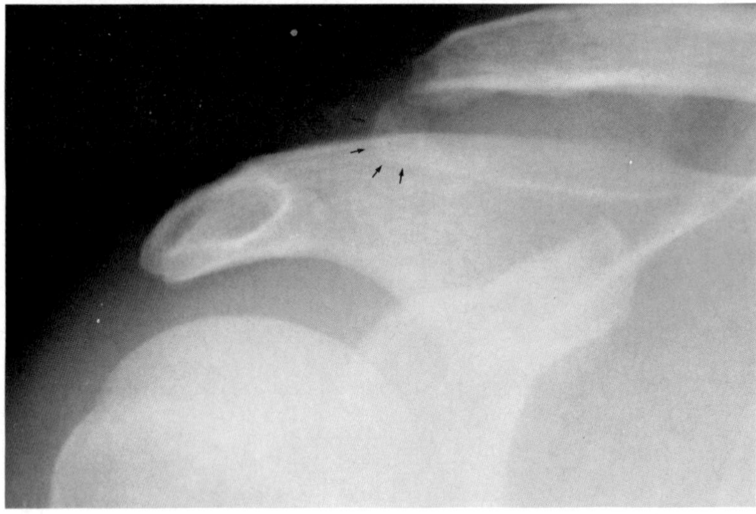

FIG. 4-22. Intraarticular fracture of the distal clavicle with AC separation. A fracture of the distal end of the clavicle with involvement of its articular surface is demonstrated following acute trauma in this major league hockey player. The articular fracture fragment is displaced and rotated inferiorly *(arrows)*.

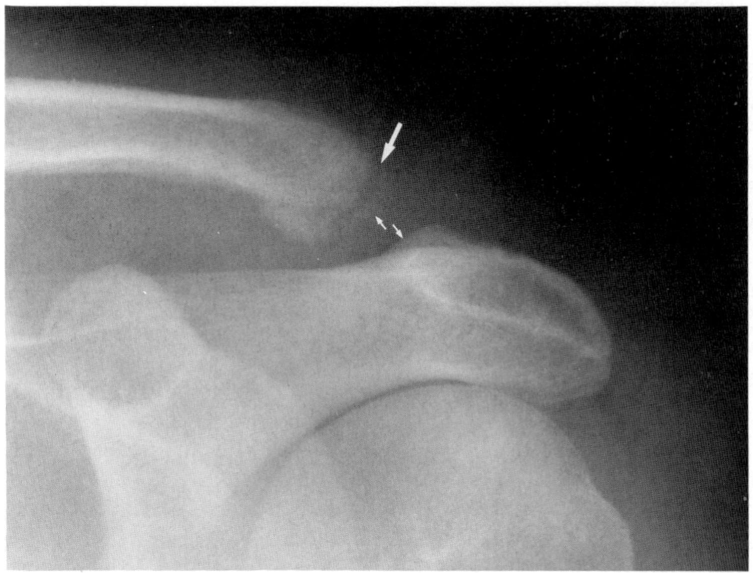

FIG. 4-23. Intraarticular fracture of the distal clavicle. A healing fracture is evident *(long arrow)*. The articular component remains properly aligned with the acromial articular surface *(small arrow)*.

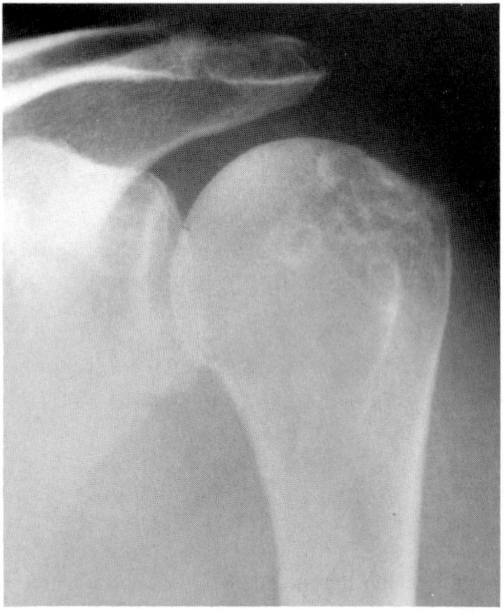

FIG. 4-24. Rotator cuff disease. Anteroposterior view of left shoulder. There are multiple cystic erosions of the anatomic neck and greater tuberosity regions. The tuberosity is flattened and the humeral head is sclerotic.

ticipation of the duration and quantity of postoperative disability, and a foreknowledge of predictive success and prognosis.

Disease of the rotator cuff tendons and dysfunction attributable to alterations of the anatomy and mechanics of the periacromial region are intimately related. These entities are also intimately related with respect to the conventional roentgenographic signs they produce, especially in more chronic cases.

In 1961 Golding[43] reported that cystic erosion of the anatomic neck is pathognomonic of a tear of the rotator cuff. Godsil and Linscheid[42] observed conventional roentgenographic alterations in 100% of patients between 36 and 76 years of age with rotator cuff tears. The duration of cuff disease in the 59 patients studied was difficult to deduce. The degenerative changes observed included the following: (1) subcortical cystic erosion at the angle of cuff insertion into the greater tuberosity and (2) late sclerosis of the acromioclavicular joint and humeral head (implying their mutual articulation) (Fig. 4-24).

Both Golding[43] and Godsil and Linscheid[42] reported their observations before the renaissance of the concept of impingement. The issue is raised as to which of the roentgenologic observations are attributable to rotator cuff disease and which to impingement.

Impingement within or about the coracoacromial arch was an established source of shoulder disability long before Neer[84] reacquainted orthopaedists with it in 1972. According to Ciullo,[13] the athletic impingement syndrome was first described in baseball pitchers (1906) by Codman. Gerber et al[40] refer to the works of Meyer (1922) and Watson Jones (1943) as additional cornerstones in the establishment of impingement as a disabling entity for shoulders.

Conventional roentgenography generally reveals no evidence of impingement in its ear-

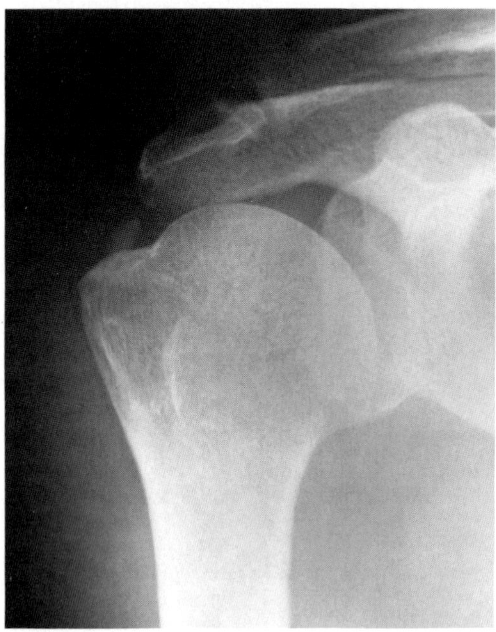

FIG. 4-25. Calcific tendonitis, right shoulder. Amorphous calcium deposition is present in the immediate vicinity of the greater tuberosity and in expected orientation of the supraspinatous tendon. The tuberosity is sclerotic, also a manifestation of impingement syndrome.

lier stages when the soft tissues are the primary source of involvement.[15] Repetitious trauma to these tissues induces a progression of fibrin deposition, edema and inflammation, granulation formation, and tissue calcification or ossification (Fig. 4-25). Only the latter may be detected by conventional roentgenography. Hence, conventional roentgenographic evidence of impingement only becomes evident in stage III[85] (see Chapter 8) cases when tendon degeneration and/or rupture have already occurred.[49] The characteristic roentgenographic findings of impingement thus relate more to the middle-aged groups rather than to the younger groups of patients with the syndrome.

Ellman et al[32] operated on 50 nonathletic patients with shoulder pain, three quarters of whom had clinical manifestations of Neer's impingement stages II or III.[85] Conventional roentgenography revealed greater tuberosity cysts in 60% and rarefaction or sclerosis in 76%. There were acromial cysts in 30% and lateral or inferior sclerosis in 74%. A concave acromial undersurface (from articulation with the humerus) was present in 36%. These findings bear more than a casual similarity to those reported by Godsil and Linscheid[42] in cases of documented rupture of the rotator cuff. Cone et al[17] reported their findings in cases of shoulder impingement. Consistent among their findings were bony proliferation, sclerosis, and cystic changes of the greater tuberosity. These changes are more often seen in association with the presence of subacromial traction spurs, while a flattened, sclerotic appearance is most likely to be seen when there is an associated complete rupture of the rotator cuff. The "cuff arthropathy" referred to by Neer[85] obviously encompasses the changes resulting from impingement. While Neer contends that impingement precedes cuff tears and is responsible for 95% of all cuff tears, it is difficult to determine the chronology of roentgenographic findings attributable to each. It would certainly seem that sclerosis of the greater tuberosity, acromion, and humeral head and the concave undersurface appearance of the acromion are findings largely attributable to an associated complete rupture of the rotator cuff (Fig. 4-26). Since some of these findings imply an articulation of the humeral head with the acromion as a consequence of a reduction of tissues occupying the acromiohumeral interval, it is appropriate to interrupt the discussion of impingement in favor of a discussion of conventional roentgenography of the ruptured rotator cuff.

Beltran et al[6] refer to the work of Bretzke et al (1985) in stating that the thickness of the supraspinatus is approximately 6 mm. Diminution of the interval between the humeral head and the acromion, which is occupied by the supraspinatus and its surrounding soft tissues, implied rupture of the rotator cuff. Petersson and Redlund-Johnell[98] studied almost 200 shoulders of almost 100 patients with neither symptoms nor degenerative changes. They measured the shortest distance between the inferior aspect of the acromion and the top of the humeral head. Remembering that the space is occupied by acromial periosteum, areolar tissue, and bursa, as well as by the supraspinatus, the measured intervals on anteroposterior roentgenographs were as follows:

♂: 9.7 mm (+/− 1.5 mm) to 10.2 mm (+/− 1.7 mm)

♀: 9.2 mm (+/− 1.4 mm)

The interval diminished with age in males only. The authors stated that a space of less than 6 mm is abnormal in a middle-aged person (see Fig. 4-20). Upward subluxation of the humeral head, according to Cofield,[14] is almost always more pronounced on external than on internal rotation views (see Fig. 4-26, *C*).

The acromiohumeral interval may bear

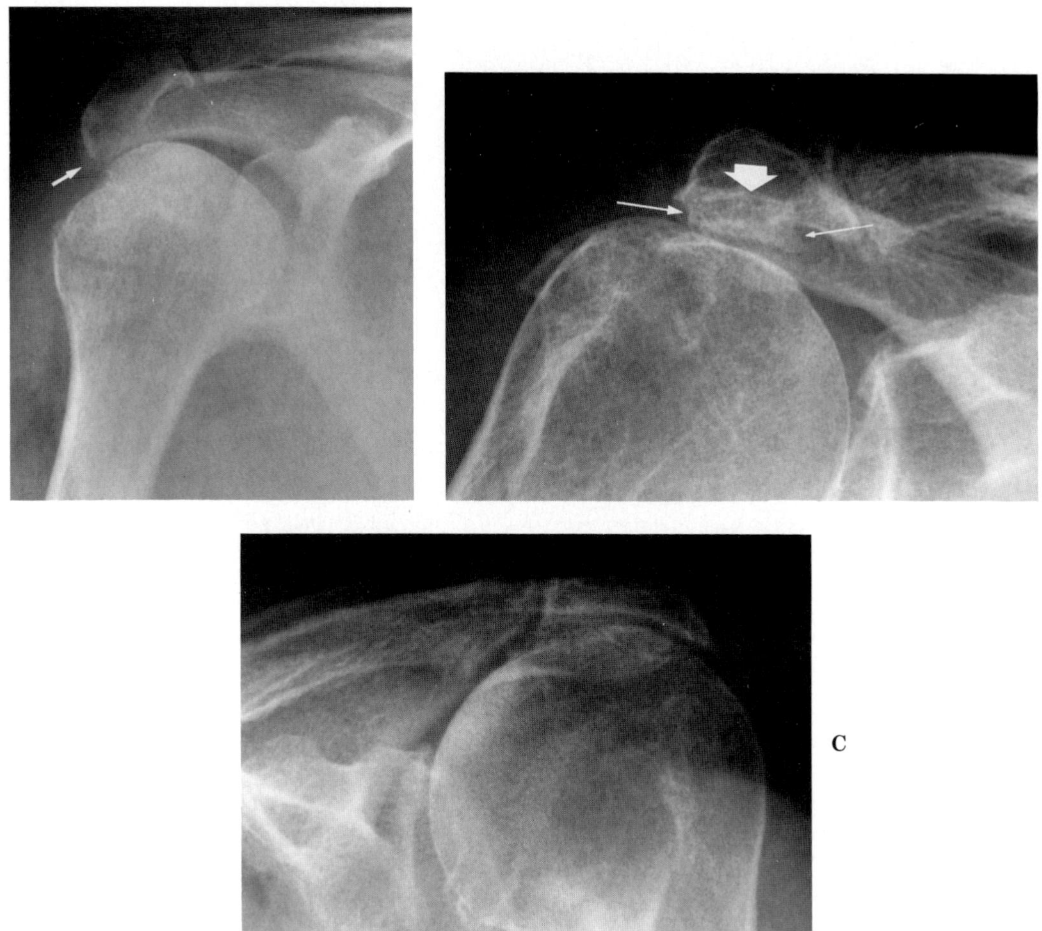

FIG. 4-26. Rotator cuff disease and impingement. **A,** Right shoulder; both the greater tuberosity and the acromion process are sclerotic. Hypertrophic changes of the peripheral margin of the acromion are also evident *(arrow)*. **B,** Right shoulder. There is bone formation *(long arrows)* along the undersurfaces of the acromion process *(large arrow)*. This occupies the subacromial space and is conformed to the humeral head contour. **C,** Left shoulder. Superior migration of the humeral head is evident. The anterior acromion process and the distal clavicle have developed a concave appearance as a result of articulation with the humeral head.

prognostic as well as diagnostic import. In their study, Ellman et al[32] found that patients whose acromiohumeral distance was less than 7 mm had larger tears and less strength and motion than others after cuff repair.

A discussion of impingement may now be resumed with the knowledge that the most flagrant roentgenographic evidence of its presence is observed in association with complete ruptures of the rotator cuff.

Petersson and Gentz[97] studied 47 shoulders of patients with arthrographically proven supraspinatus ruptures, 50 normal shoulders, and 170 cadaveric shoulders, of which 54 had partial or complete supraspinatus rupture. Among the groups studied just over 50% of shoulders with supraspinatus ruptures had distally pointing acromioclavicular osteophytes, while less than 15% of the remaining shoulders had them (Fig. 4-27). In addition, the "ruptured" groups manifested anterior lipping of the acromion in 20% to 25% of shoulders, as described by Neer.[84] The contentions of Petersson and Gentz[97] and of Kessel and Watson,[56] who found the acromioclavicular osteophytes in one third of their supraspinatus ruptures, would point up the importance of scrutinizing the acromioclavicular joint in such cases.

Anterior acromial "spurs" (see Fig. 4-26, *A* and *B*) and distally pointing acromioclavicular spurs have thus been identified as two important additional findings of impingement, the latter being particularly associated with

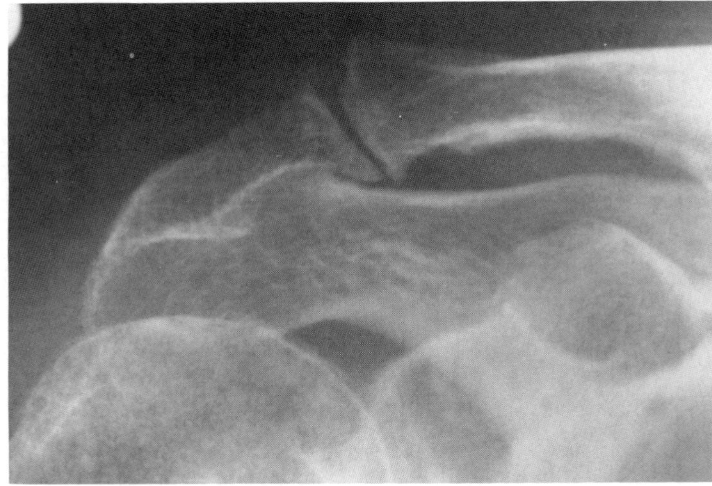

FIG. 4-27. Acromioclavical spur. Anteroposterior view with upward angulation of the beam demonstrates inferiorly pointing osteophytes of the acromioclavicular joint.

ruptures of the supraspinatus. Neer has repeatedly played up the importance of the anterior acromion in the creation of symptomatic impingements[84,85] and contends that the posterior half of the acromion is not involved in the impingement process. He further asserts[85] that individuals with a less sloped acromion and a more prominent anterior edge on its undersurface are predisposed to cuff tears secondary to impingement, and that it is therefore logical to perform acromioplasty at the time of every cuff repair. Cone et al[17] reported some interesting observations about the relationship between subacromial spurs and other findings associated with their presence. One third of their patients evidencing such spurs also had spurs about the intertubercular sulcus, which appeared on bicipital groove views. Nearly half the patients with subacromial spurs had degenerative changes of the acromioclavicular joint as opposed to only 15% of those without subacromial spurs.

Kessel and Watson,[56] who add the eponym of "painful arc syndrome" to those of "impingement" and the "supraspinatus syndrome," discount the portent of the subacromial spur. However, they reassert the importance of the acromioclavicular spurs (rather than the spurs of the anterior acromion). They develop a theme that the varying manifestations (symptoms and roentgenographic signs) of their "painful arc syndrome" are in fact attributable to different subtypes of impingement.

Kessel and Watson[56] studied nearly 100 patients with painful arc syndromes. Using physical examination, local anesthetic injections, and contrast roentgenography to determine the sites and sources of problems, they determined that patients afflicted with the syndrome were divisible into three distinct groups of equal distribution. The third of patients with the posterior type had no visible pathologic condition, no acromioclavicular disease, pain on internal rotation, and an excellent response to conservative management. The third with the anterior type had no visible pathologic condition, no acromioclavicular disease, pain on external rotation, and an occasional need for surgery. The last third, with a superior type, had acromioclavicular disease and rotator cuff degeneration. Decompressive surgery was often needed.

The findings of Cone et al are consistent with the concept of multifocal impingements and the use of impingement tests ascribable to several arcs of shoulder motion.[17] Their fluoroarthrography studies revealed a correlation in some patients between the production of pain with elevation of the arm and the point at which the humeral tuberosities and acromion were in their closest apposition. In these cases pain was maximal during abduction of 70 to 120 degrees and 20 to 30 degrees of external rotation or during 70 to 120 degrees of elevation and more than 30 degrees of internal rotation.

Conventional roentgenography offers little in documenting impingement in its earlier stages. Special roentgenography to be presented in the ensuing sections has more to offer in this regard, particularly with respect to tears of the rotator cuff. In the advanced stages of impingement, the roentgenographic signs discussed in the preceding paragraphs offer testimony in support of operations predicted on the concept that the acromial arch region is responsible for the production of symptoms. Evidence presented in this section has derived largely from studies of nonathletic populations.

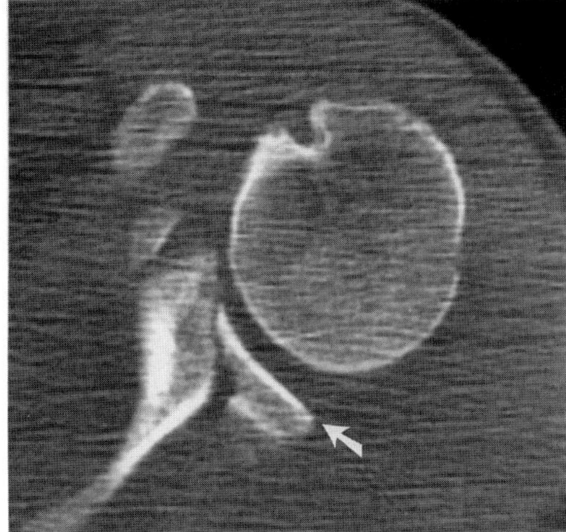

FIG. 4-28. Comminuted fracture of the left glenoid. This single CT section shows that the major articular component of the glenoid as a whole is displaced posteriorly *(arrow)*. The humeral head remains in alignment with this major fragment, while a small fragment is displaced and rotated anteriorly. Superoinferior displacements are determined by viewing all axial sections.

COMPUTED AXIAL TOMOGRAPHY

General Concepts

The modern-generation computed tomography (CT) scanners are capable of producing high-resolution images with excellent detailing of the bony architecture. Software packages are available that can selectively enhance either soft tissue or bony detail; they can enlarge focal segments of images or "regions of interest" as the images are being reconstructed; and they provide capability for image reformation in sagittal, coronal, or oblique planes. Additional computer hardware and software is obtainable for three-dimensional reconstruction and display.

CT of the shoulder without enhancement by contrast media is indicated when plain roentgenography has failed to adequately substantiate a suspected osseous or periarticular abnormality (Fig. 4-28). CT is beneficial for the evaluation of acute intraarticular fractures, such as comminuted fractures of the humeral head, as an aid to surgical planning (Fig. 4-29). It is also of value in the recognition of some ossifications and fractures associated with glenohumeral instability. Obviously, it can document any existing degree of glenohumeral dislocations.[29] Less often CT

Shoulder CT assets

- Intraarticular fractures
- Periarticular ossification or calcification
- Humeral head fractures

A 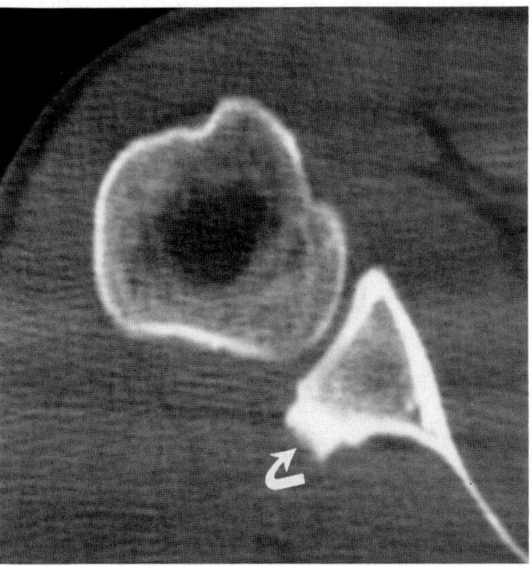

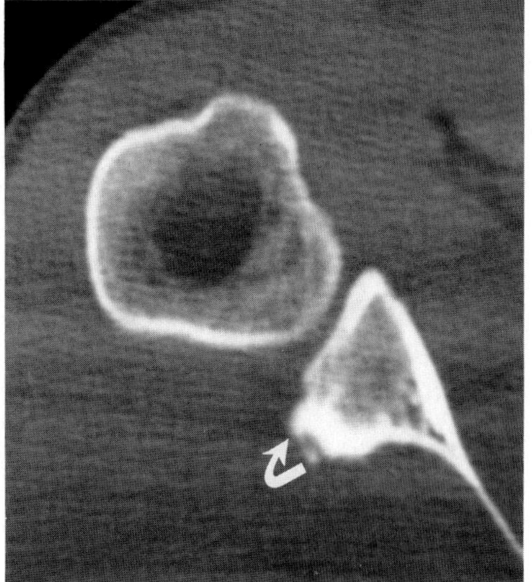 B

FIG. 4-29. Ossification of the posterior glenoid margin in a baseball pitcher. Consecutive CT sections of the right shoulder (A and B) at approximately mid glenoid level. An ossific ridge is formed along the posterior glenoid margin *(arrows)* at the site of insertion of the posterior joint capsule.

is indicated when there is reason to suspect the presence of osseous or soft tissue tumors about the shoulder.

Technique

The imaging technique for the shoulder ordinarily requires patients to be placed in the supine position with the arm at the side. For patients with very wide shoulder girdles, the contralateral arm must be manipulated to a position that allows the hand to cradle the back of the patient's head. In this way the formation of striking artifacts on axial images resulting from a wide shoulder girdle is avoided.

Slice thickness will vary in accordance with the pathologic entity suspected. Ordinarily, 5 mm thick sections provide adequate bony detail and are suitable for the evaluation of traumatic lesions of the shoulder. The slice thickness can be increased to 10 mm when larger lesions of the paraarticular structures are suspected. This is in contradistinction to the thinner, 3 mm sections commonly used in performing CT arthrography.

The hard copies are produced twice, first with wide window settings (2000/200) for bone viewing, and then with narrow window settings (500/50) for the viewing of soft tissue detail.

Scapulometry and Instability

Seltzer and Weissman[117] used CT scapulometry to evaluate certain parameters in normal patients and those with shoulder instability. The only finding of interest was the maintenance of the humeral head in the central third of the glenoid on all cuts in normal shoulders but not necessarily in those with instability. Past investigators such as Saha[112,113] have devised scapulometric techniques for the purpose of determining telltale version and torsion abnormalities of unstable shoulders. Cyprien et al[22] devised their own group of measurements and concluded that angular and torsional values vary little between normal and recurrently dislocating shoulders. While index of contact between the humeral head and glenoid is smaller in patients with recurrent anterior dislocation than in normal patients, Cyprien et al found no consistent deviations of humeral retroversion in the group of dislocators.

Norris[91] claims that lesions and version of the glenoid and humeral head are best revealed with computeruzed axial tomography and may be a particular help in the planning of bony reconstructions.

Gambrioli et al[35] indicate that CT scanning is valuable in the determination of three morphologic factors that Saha[113] determined to be pertinent to anterior instability:

1. *Glenoid tilt*—orientation of the glenoid articular surface in relation to the plane of the shoulder
2. *Angle of retroversion*—proximal end of the humerus
3. *Glenohumeral index*—ratio of maximal diameters (transverse) of the glenoid and humeral head

However, Gambrioli et al[35] studied 50 normal subjects, 24 patients with anterior instability, and 9 patients with posterior instability and found no relevance of these factors to a distinction between the groups studied.

When considering operative approaches for posterior instabilities unresponsive to conservative management, Warren[123] uses CT and axillary roentgenograms to determine the degree of glenoid version. If the version is abnormal and the angle exceeds 20 degrees, Warren considers an osteotomy of the scapular neck. It is an interesting corollary that failing to demonstrate version alteration of the glenoid in cases of anterior instability, Gambrioli et al[35] were able to demonstrate an increase in glenoid cavity retroversion inferiorly in chronic cases of posterior instability. Presumably this is attributable to the erosive changes of the posteroinferior portion of the glenoid over time, indenting its profile on scan cuts at inferior glenoid level.

Obviously there must be a better resolve to the controversy concerning the value of scapulometry in the formulation of surgical indications for instability. Surely the interpretation of CT requires a different and more sophisticated knowledge of anatomy. Deutsch et al[29] point out that the interpretation of shoulder pathology examined by CT is largely predicated upon a knowledge of axial anatomy. For example, the glenoid is mildly retroverted superiorly and undergoes a transition to anteversion as more caudad sections are taken.

Subcoracoid Impingement

Subcoracoid impingement was described in 1909 by Goldthwait; as with other impingement forms, roentgenographic evidence is limited, even on CT.[40] This form of impingement produces dull anterior shoulder pain with distal radiation, aggravated by forward flexion and internal rotation. While the more common varieties of impingement produce pain on full forward flexion, the subcoracoid type produces maximal pain in the forward flexion arc from 80 degrees to 130 degrees and at 90 degrees of abduction with the humerus internally rotated.[39]

Gerber et al performed CT scapulometry to determine its relevance to the diagnosis of this syndrome.[39,40] These studies revealed a narrowed coracoid-to-humeral head distance with the arm abducted and internally rotated in patients with clinically diagnosed impingement. Furthermore, patients with signs of subcoracoid impingement were 1.5 times more likely to produce a reduction of the coracohumeral space with the arm flexed and internally rotated than with the arm at the side. Recommendations for coracoacromial ligament and coracoid tip resection were made on the basis of these studies.

CONVENTIONAL SHOULDER ARTHROGRAPHY

General Concepts

Arthrography of the shoulder was initially described by Oberholzer (1933), who used air as a contrast medium to evaluate capsular distortions that occurred after dislocations. In 1939 Lindblom and Palmer used single contrast arthrography to document ruptures of the rotator cuff.[70] As recently as 1968 Killoran et al[60] indicated that arthrography of the shoulder was not in widespread use despite its ability to demonstrate the character of the glenohumeral capsule and ruptures of the rotator cuff. Ghelman and Goldman[41] were responsible for the popularization of double contrast arthrography (1977). The diagnostic use of arthrography (with and without CT or tomography) has been expanded to include the evaluation of the glenoid labrum. On occasion distention arthrography has been used in the treatment evaluation of the frozen shoulder.

The two popular techniques used today are single and double contrast arthrography.

Technique of Single Contrast Arthrography

Routine roentgenographic examination of the shoulder is performed before the arthrographic procedure. Anteroposterior, internal-external, axillary, and bicipital groove views are obtained and reviewed. The procedure is performed with the patient supine on the fluoroscopic table. While most orthopaedic surgeons prefer to aspirate or inject a shoulder through a posterior approach, most roentgenologists prefer an anterior approach to the joint.

After sterile preparation of the shoulder region and the infiltration of a local anesthetic, a 20-gauge, 3.5 cm long disposable spinal needle is inserted into the glenohumeral joint using fluoroscopic guidance. If the injection of a small amount of positive contrast material confirms an intraarticular position of the needle, 16 ml of contrast medium is injected and the needle is withdrawn. The contrast agent most often used is 60% meglumine diatrizoate.

Four views are obtained after withdrawal of the needle: anteroposterior views in internal and external rotation, an axillary view, and a bicipital groove view. Unless a complete tear of the rotator is immediately evident, the same views are repeated after the joint is exercised.

Technique of Double Contrast Arthrography

This technique has been advocated for enhanced visualization of the rotator cuff, the joint surfaces, and the labrum (Fig. 4-30). The contrast medium used consists of 4 ml of a positive contrast agent admixed with ⅓ ml of 1/1000 epinephrine and 12 ml of room air. After the injection of contrast medium, anteroposterior views are taken with the patient in the upright position with 5-pound weights fastened to the wrists.

To enhance visualization of the rotator cuff, Garcia[36] hangs 6 to 10 pounds of weight from the patient's wrist. On anteroposterior views with 15 degrees caudal angulation of the central beam, the acromiohumeral space is increased an average of 25 to 35 mm, the tendons of the biceps and rotator cuff are well separated, and the shape of the torn segments is well visualized. An axillary view is then taken with the patient in the supine position. As with the single contrast technique, if a complete tear of the cuff is not immediately evident, the joint is exercised and the roentgenographic series is repeated.

Errors and Morbidity

False-negative arthrographic studies are obviously a problem when rotator cuff tears are incomplete, either intratendinous or on the superior surface, or when they have been sealed by encompassing granulations. Full thickness tears are easier to detect. Nevertheless, Killoran et al[60] caution that errors can be made when there is inadequate distribution of contrast; a tardy arrival of contrast within the bursa may be seen on delayed films. This is the rationale for the routine taking of roentgenograms before and after exercise when a tear is not immediately evident. Direct and inadvertent injection into an enlarged bursa can also be misconstrued as a complete tear of the rotator cuff.

A

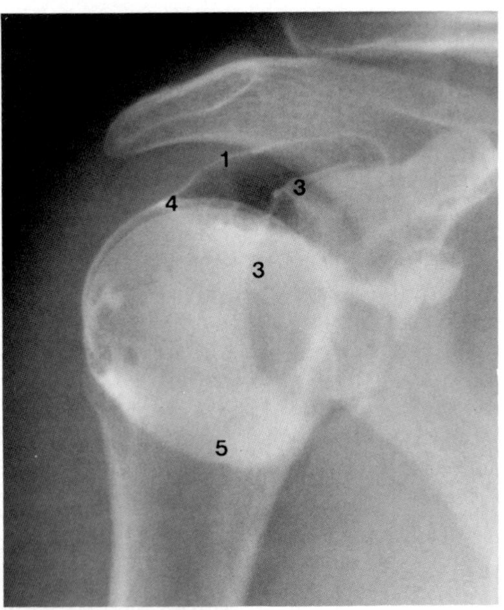

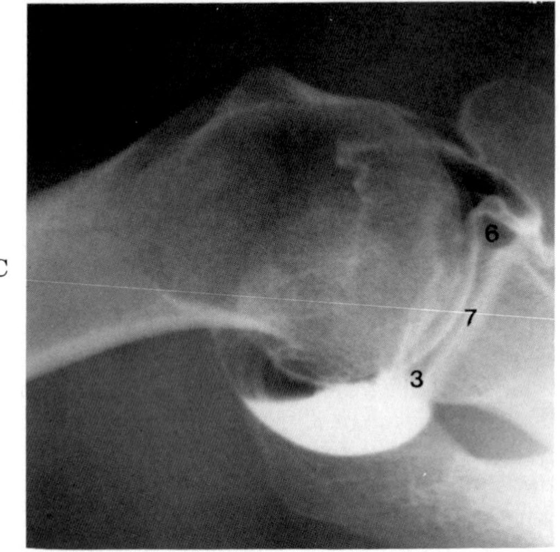

FIG. 4-30. Normal double contrast shoulder arthrogram of right shoulder. Anteroposterior views with patient standing and holding 5-pound weight, in external rotation **(A)** and internal rotation **(B).** The undersurface of the rotator cuff *(1)*, the long head of the biceps tendon, *(2)* the superior and posterior glenoid labrum *(3)*, the humeral articular surface *(4)*, and the joint capsule *(5)* are optimally visualized. **C,** Supine axillary view. The glenohumeral articular components are visualized. The excess positive contrast is pooled in the posterior joint space and therefore the anterior glenoid labrum *(6)* is clearly visualized. A prone axillary view improves visualization of the posterior glenoid labrum *(3)*, which in this view is partially obscured by pooling of contrast material. The glenoid articular cartilage *(7)* is also clearly seen.

Shoulder arthrography (single or double contrast) with or without the use of epinephrine or local anesthetics as a diluting agent has, in general, been a safe procedure. Anaphylactoid reactions, chemically induced synovitis, and even infections have occurred as a consequence of arthrography, especially in its early years. Patients are most apprehensive, however, of the pain associated with the placement of a needle in their shoulder joint and of the painful aftermath reported to them by others who had undergone the procedure. Severe postprocedural pain has not been commonly reported. In the authors' experience such pain occurs most commonly among patients with severe pain before studies are done.

Hall et al[47] could find little morbidity attributable to arthrography in a 30-year review of the English-language literature. Nevertheless, significant shoulder discomfort occurred within 48 hours of the procedure in 74% of

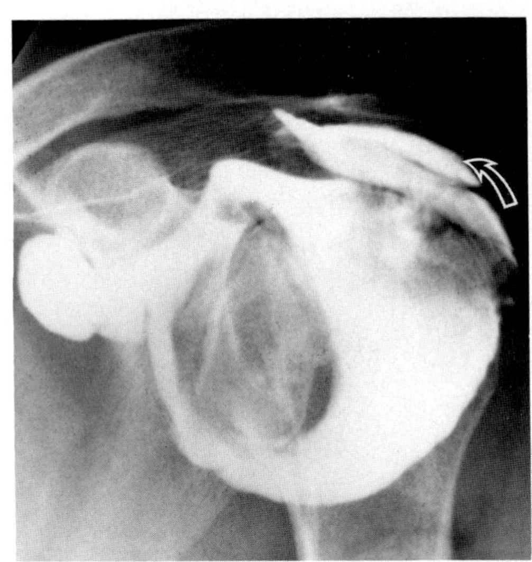

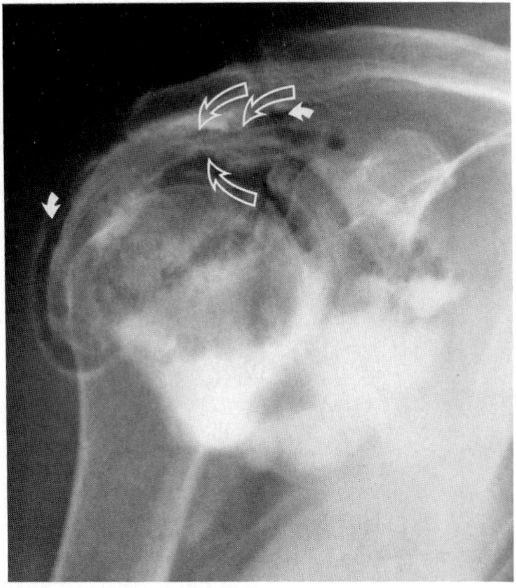

FIG. 4-31. Complete rotator cuff tear. Single and double contrast techniques. **A,** Single contrast arthrogram of left shoulder. There is opacification of the subcromion-subdeltoid bursa *(arrow)* indicating a rotator cuff tear. Although no significant degeneration of the cuff is seen, the site of the tear and the nature of torn tendinous margins cannot be determined because of pooling of contrast material. **B,** Double contrast arthrogram of right shoulder. The subacromion-subdeltoid bursa is mostly opacified by air *(solid arrows)*. The rotator cuff is covered by positive contrast material. The site of tendinous tear and the quality of the tendinous margins are well demonstrated *(hollow arrows)*.

72 patients evaluated. The least discomfort was reported in the group subjected to double contrast arthrography. This was so despite the advocated use of epinephrine with its potentiating effects for the double contrast technique. Its use is unnecessary in single contrast arthrography, and it is rather mandatory for CT arthrography or arthropneumotomography for prolongation of the time during which an optimal tomographic study can be performed.

In a 1985 sequel study to their 1981 study,[47] Hall et al[48] found that moderate or severe delayed exacerbation of baseline discomfort after shoulder arthrography occurred in only 14% of those examined with metrizamide, an anionic medium, and in 45% of those studied with the conventional double contrast technique. Hence, postprocedural pain is related to several factors, including a direct irritant effect of contrast material on the synovium and the hyperosmolar nature of these agents. The latter phenomena result in diffusion of fluids across the synovium, causing further joint distention. These effects are greater with sodium salts, rather than the meglumine salt of the contrast medium most commonly employed in arthrography. In conclusion, the double contrast arthrographic technique using the meglumine salt of the positive contrast agent without the addition of epinephrine is associated with the lowest morbidity rate. However, epinephrine must be used when arthrotomographic techniques are employed for evaluation of the glenoid labrum. Nonionic contrast agents are likely to be safer though their higher cost is a prohibitive factor.

Single Versus Double Contrast Arthrography

There is a consensus that the double contrast arthrography is capable of revealing more information about the character of a cuff tear. Mink et al[81] found double contrast arthrography to have a greater than 99% accuracy in the detection of surgically proven full-thickness tears. Pavlov and Freiberger[95] indicate that while an accurate diagnosis of a torn rotator cuff can be made by single contrast arthrography, double contrast arthrography better delineates the size of the tear and the character of its edges (Fig. 4-31).

Goldman and Ghelman[44] report that while both single and double contrast techniques are accurate in diagnosing full thickness and inferior surface tears of the rotator cuff, only double contrast arthrography can demonstrate the quality of the tendon ends and help delineate the width of a tear. Mink et al,[81] using three grades to distinguish tear size and three grades to distinguish cuff quality, found

A

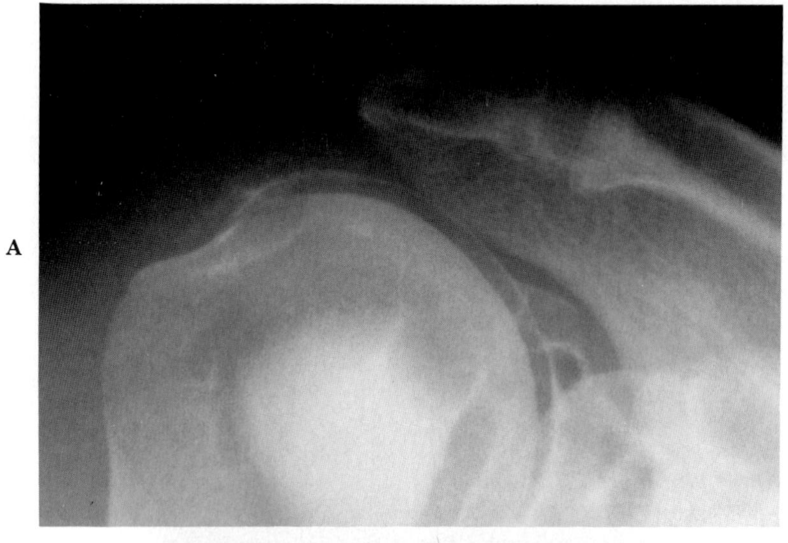

B

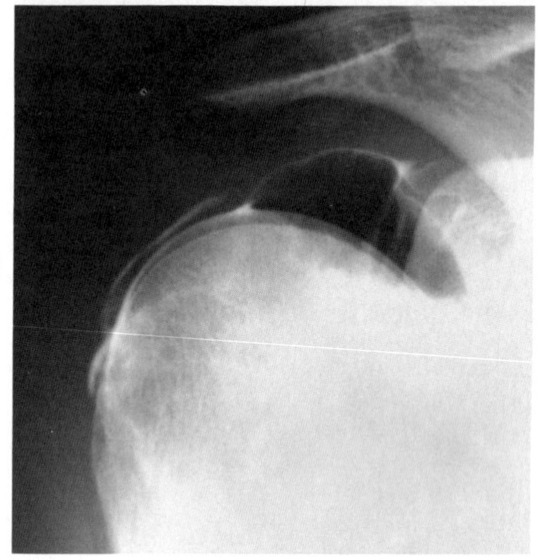

FIG. 4-32. Incomplete rotator cuff tears. **A,** Supraspinatous tear near its tuberosity insertion. A superficial fissurelike tear is visualized communicating with a longitudinal intratendinous tear. **B,** Infraspinatus tear originating at the site of posterior greater tuberosity insertion. Two tears are visualized, one forming a long intratendinous component.

that they did not err by more than a grade as determined by surgical correlation. On the other hand, Ellman et al[32] found that neither single nor double contrast arthrography was of consistent accuracy in quantitating the size of a tear before surgery.

Neer[86] indicates that double contrast arthrography with or without tomography requires special experience in attempting to identify the size of identifiable tears in the rotator cuff. Cofield[14] states that double contrast arthrography reveals more information about the synovium and articular surfaces and, when combined with tomography, may define the size of a tear. However, Cofield indicates that the single contrast arthrogram will usually suffice for the diagnosis of a cuff tear and probably with fewer false-negative results.

Arthrography and the Rotator Cuff

A suspected tear of the rotator cuff is the most common indication for shoulder arthrography.[44]

Incomplete tears of the rotator cuff are either of the intratendinous or deep surface variety and each may heal without surgery[90] (Fig. 4-32). While tears of the undersurface of the cuff may be appreciated as an ulcerlike collection of contrast, intrasubstance tears

A 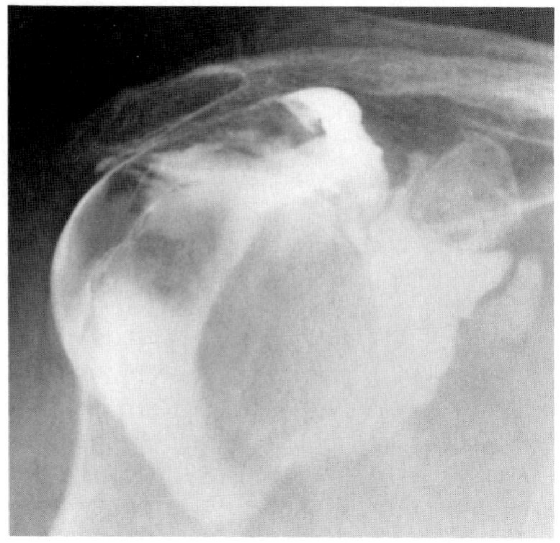 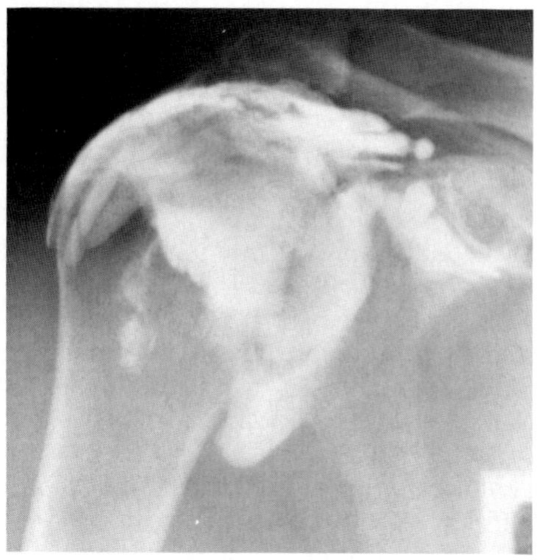 B

FIG. 4-33. Complete rotator cuff tear, single contrast techniques. **A,** There is opacification of the subacromion-subdeltoid bursa, indicating the presence of a rotator cuff tear. **B,** There is opacification of the subacromion-subdeltoid bursa and virtually total communication with the glenohumeral joint space because of disruption and severe degeneration of the rotator cuff tendon.

will most likely escape detection by arthrography. The import of such tears with respect to symptoms or treatment is to some extent speculative and controversial.[60] Thus Neviaser and Neviaser[90] reason that the object of an evaluation for the treatment of a "cuff problem" is the differentiation between complete and incomplete tears. By this hypothesis, the diagnostic pursuits necessary for this distinction are of vital importance, and roentgenography is the most reliable pursuit. By this hypothesis, each patient will a full-thickness cuff tear should undergo surgery.

While the authors vehemently disagree with such dogmatic formulae, and specifically with this one, investigative roentgenography for cuff tears must not be undervalued.

Killoran et al[60] indicate that the easiest diagnosis to make by arthrography is a complete rupture of the cuff, since contrast extrudes blatantly into the subacromial bursa (Fig. 4-33). Neer[85] maintains that arthrography is the most reliable method of detecting a complete tear of the rotator cuff. Arthrograms, in his opinion, are indicated for patients over 40 years of age with an unresponsive impingement syndrome, sudden weakness of the shoulder after trauma, bicipital tendon rupture with persistent shoulder symptoms, and certain glenohumeral instabilities that are chronic or have occurred *de novo* in patients over 40 years of age.

> **Indications for arthrography (Neer)**
>
> - Unresponsive impingement syndrome (>40 years of age)
> - Sudden weakness after trauma
> - Bicipital tendon rupture
> - Glenohumeral instability (>40 years of age)

The Neviasers[88-90] recommend five arthrographic views in the evaluation of musculotendinous pathology, adding an anteroposterior view with the arm abducted to the four views reported in the sections on technique. They claim that the presence of contrast material in the subdeltoid bursa on any of the five views should be considered diagnostic of a tear.

Importance of Discovering a Cuff Tear

Among the critical diagnostic functions of the shoulder arthrogram is the determination of rotator cuff integrity. The discovery of a tear of the rotator cuff, especially a full thickness tear, is of theoretical significance in the understanding and management of patients manifesting pain and/or weakness of the shoulder. Aggressive surgeons such as the Neviasers[90] suggest the repair of all full-thickness tears. Yet many patients with full thickness tears respond well to conservative management. It is always debatable whether the manifestations of weakness and pain are particularly caused by the cuff tear, or by associated impingement, relative overuse, or rehabilitation of inadequate quantity or specificity. In this regard, the study of Calvert et al[11] is of particular interest. This group studied 20 patients with double contrast arthrography after operative repair for a torn rotator cuff. Most of the patients experienced a complete remission of pain and return of shoulder elevation despite the discovery that contrast leaked into the subacromial bursa in 18 of the 20 patients studied. It is not stated, though implied, that a deimpingement was performed concurrently with the cuff repair to account for the remissions. While Calvert et al conclude that arthrography may not be helpful in the evaluation of cuff repair failures, there is another question to ponder. To what extent do leakages of contrast into the bursae of unrepaired tears implicate the cuff as the primary source of pain or motion restriction? If good operative results can be achieved despite the demonstration of leakage subsequent to repair through defects in excess of 2 cm, then the value of arthrography as an indicator for surgery may be inappropriately exaggerated.

It is noteworthy in the study of Calvert et al[11] that the only two patients with no contrast leakage were the only two patients under 50 years of age. The implications are that tear duration or the quality of surrounding tissue are of importance.

Detailing a Cuff Tear—Size and Character

It has already been established that among the alleged advantages of the double contrast technique (conventional or with CT or tomographic enhancement) is its ability to portray the size of a tear and the quality of the remaining tendon in which it is situated (Fig. 4-31, *A*) There is some controversy regarding the efficacy of the technique for the purpose specified.

Calvert et al[11] refer to the work of Post, Silver, and Singh (1983),[99] which failed to demonstrate a correlation between the quantity of collected contrast in the bursa and the size of the defect. Neviaser[87,88] refutes the ability of arthrography to determine the size of the defect, whereas Goldman and Ghelman[44] and Calvert et al[11] maintain that size may be estimated using double contrast arthrography. Kilcoyne and Matsen[59] found good correlations between defect sizes estimated by arthropneumotomography and those observed at surgery.

In the opinion of the authors, there is little doubt that the double contrast techniques are superior in elucidating the tear characteristics with reasonable, though not absolute, accuracy. They are less concerned with this issue than with the more practical issue of whether such information is useful in treatment. The study of Calvert et al might refute the validity of cuff-induced symptoms in many cases. Exposition of cuff tear details is nevertheless of importance to the treatment philosophies of a number of surgeons for purposes of planning an approach or for objective documentation of the nature of existing pathologic conditions for records, research, or insurance carriers.

Timing the Study

If the surgeon accepts the philosophy of Neviaser and Neviaser[90] that an acute full-thickness tear should be repaired expediently if large, then the timing of the arthrogram is of some importance. The Neviasers suggest an outside delay of 2 to 3 weeks, after which time the retraction of the edges will increase the difficulty of reconstruction.

Cuff Tears and Glenohumeral Instability

The entities of glenohumeral instability and rotator cuff tear are not often considered as cohabiting pathologic states within the same shoulder. Reeves[106] has indicated that rupture of the supraspinatus is not an uncommon finding when performing arthrography on patients with acute dislocations. Other authors have been even more definitive on the subject.

In the experience of Neviaser and Neviaser[90] a tear of the rotator cuff is a more common accompaniment of an anterior dislocation than an axillary nerve palsy. Therefore, they maintain, the persistence of an inability to abduct after 1 to 2 weeks calls for an arthrogram when an axillary nerve injury has been ruled out by examination.

While tears of the cuff occurring in conjunction with acute instability episodes may heal, there are instances when cuff pathology may have existed before a dislocation or when newly acquired cuff lesions may fail to heal. In less acute circumstances, Kneisl et al,[65] studying patients with shoulder pain with and without instability, found rotator cuff pathology in 12% of patients with instability.

Arthrography and the Unstable Shoulder

The use of arthrography for the evaluation of glenohumeral instability dates back to Lindblom (1938). Even approaching the early 1970s, when orthopaedists were reluctant to operate upon a patient reporting instability without roentgenographic documentation, the capsular shadows perceived on arthrography were welcome corroborators of the sus-

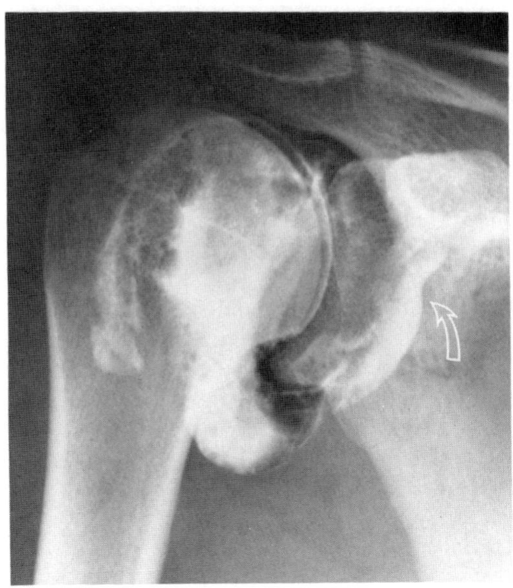

FIG. 4-34. Anterior instability. Double contrast arthrogram in a patient with history of prior dislocations. The anterior capsule is extended more medially than normal. This has resulted in almost complete obliteration of the notch normally seen between the subscapularis bursa and the joint capsule *(arrow)*.

pected diagnosis (Fig. 4-34). Today the capsular patterns of different instabilities are reasonably well defined, and even labral and Bankart lesions are determinable without enhancement by tomography or CT.

In Kummel's study[68] of 10 unstable shoulders subjected to arthrography and surgery, three types of arthrographic defects were noted and confirmed: (1) defect of the anteroinferior capsule, filled with contrast anterior to the glenoid; (2) extravasation beyond the capsule; and (3) enlarged and irregular axillary pouch (Fig. 4-34).

Mizuno and Hirohata[83] specifically studied patients with clinical evidence of traumatic, recurrent subluxation of the shoulder. Using double contrast arthrography, they determined that there is pooling of contrast material (a "cap shadow") over the humeral head in looser-jointed patients with inferior and/or multidirectional instability when traction is applied to a slightly adducted arm.

Mink et al[82] studied 12 shoulders with documented or suspected glenohumeral instability. Their technique included upright internal and external rotation, supine axillary, prone axillary, and bicipital groove views. Nine of 12 arthrograms revealed a torn labrum.

Mizuno and Hirohata[83] have described the special use of arthrography to diagnose labral tears with a relatively high positive predictive value. The presence of a Bankart lesion is demonstrable by a subscapular leakage of contrast and only when the arm is in an externally rotated position. Mizuno and Hirohata[83] observed subscapular leakage in 75% of their anterior subluxations and in only 5% of their involuntary multidirectional subluxations. They found that posterior tangential views are helpful in attempting to assess Bankart lesions. This modified West Point view demonstrates the labrum as a radiolucent shadow on the anterior and posterior portions of the glenoid, a shadow that is not observed when the labrum or glenoid cartilage has been damaged. The demonstration of a detached labrum requires a good superoinferior view. There were no false-positive results among 35 patients who were operated upon. False-negative outcomes could not be determined.

It is of historical and some practical interest to know that conventional arthrographic techniques have capability for detecting multiple components of glenohumeral instability. Still, the specificity and sensitivity of conventional arthrographic techniques do not begin to match those of CT arthrography and arthrotomography, especially with respect to labral and osseous lesions.

Frozen Shoulder and Distention Arthrography

Moderate pressure is required to inject the smaller quantity of contrast material (5 to 10 ml) accepted by the tighter joint with diminutive or absent subscapularis and axillary recesses (Fig. 4-35). On very rare occasions the pressure distention needed for the study results in symptomatic relief and improved motion of the afflicted shoulder. The value of arthrography is not necessarily confined to diagnosis and surgical planning. In 1976 Older et al,[92] referring to Duplay's (1872) initial use of shoulder manipulation for the stiff shoulder, reported on a group of six patients they treated for stiff shoulders with distention arthrography. They distended shoulders with contrast under fluoroscopic control and obtained good results (increased motion and decreased pain) in five of the six patients. Average follow-up was nearly 2 years from the time of distention. Ten years previously (1965) Andren and Lundberg had reported on a much larger series with a short follow-up.[1] Inconsistent results were observed. These efforts are largely of historical interest now that arthroscopy accomplishes distention, fibro-

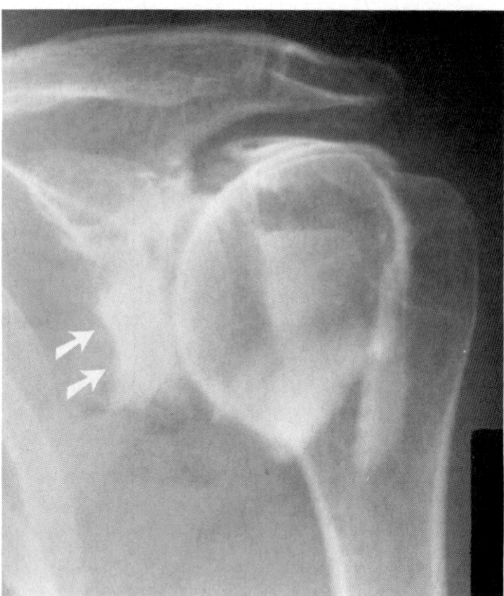

FIG. 4-35. Frozen shoulder. Double contrast arthrogram of left shoulder. Less than half the usual amount of contrast material could be injected. Patient experienced severe pain. The joint capsule and recesses are retracted. There is extravasation of contrast material along the anterior aspect of the capsule over the scapula *(arrows)*. This occurred after forceful injection of contrast material.

lysis, and visual guidance without the dangers of forcible, blind manipulation.

SPECIALIZED ARTHROGRAPHY

Subacromial Bursography

Subacromial bursography is a procedure that has been sporadically performed and studied.[17,68,120] Purposeful bursography was initially performed in the 1930s by Lindblom.[70] As remarked on in the section on conventional roentgenology, subacromial bursography may be accomplished inadvertently while attempting to perform a glenohumeral arthrogram.[68]

When a bursogram is performed in conjunction with an arthrogram, the thickness of the cuff is readily determined.[120] Subacromial bursography may reveal information about the superior surface of the cuff, which is not obtainable by arthrography alone. In addition, bursography can provide knowledge about impingement.[17] Its usefulness, however, may be overshadowed by the skills necessary for its performance and interpretation.

The subacromial bursa is adherent to the greater tuberosity and rotator cuff distally and to the undersurface of the acromion and the coracoacromial ligament proximally. It has a usual volume capacity of 4 to 6 ml.[68] The subacromial and subdeltoid components of the bursa are usually confluent. A subcoracoid component extending more inferiorly is not often present.[120]

In principle, the technique of subacromial bursography is simple. A 20-gauge spinal needle is inserted immediately under the anterior margin of the acromion and 3 to 4 ml of contrast agent is injected. The bursa is usually opacified after slight motion of the arm. The entry of contrast material into the bursa is confirmed with an anteroposterior, internal rotation view of the shoulder.[68] Nonopacification may be seen in severe instances of bursitis.

Lie and Mast[69] were able to image a variety of disorders using bursography: degenerative rotator cuff tear, mechanical impingement, and adhesive bursitis. When a complete tear of a rotator cuff tendon is present, the contrast escapes into the glenohumeral joint. Incomplete tears of the superior cuff surface are less likely to be discovered by finding contrast-filled craters as might be found on the glenohumeral (undersurface) surface of the cuff. The implication is that subacromial bursography adds little, if anything, to the diagnosis of disorders of the rotator cuff when compared to glenohumeral arthrographic techniques.

Lie and Mast[69] express a much more positive attitude with respect to the role of subacromial bursography in the diagnosis of impingement. They go so far as to say that the normal clearance of the humeral tuberosities relative to the coracoacromial arch is demonstrable only by subacromial bursography. In the presence of an intact cuff, mechanical impingement is recognized by progressive distention of the bursa as the arm is elevated into abduction. Supposedly, this distention is a consequence of the failure of the humeral head to freely clear the arch.

In a very limited series of patients subjected to bursography, Cone et al[17] discovered rotator cuff tears and impingement evidenced by the pooling of contrast material in the subdeltoid portion of the bursa. Bursatomography was not found to enhance the observations discernible by simple bursography and fluoroscopy alone.

Strizak et al[120] studied the value of bursography in the evaluation of impingement components in 15 cadavers and 31 symptomatic patients. When the findings of bursography are normal, a diagnosis of subacromial impingement should be regarded as dubious. In fact, Strizak et al maintain that when the bursogram is normal, deimpingement surgery

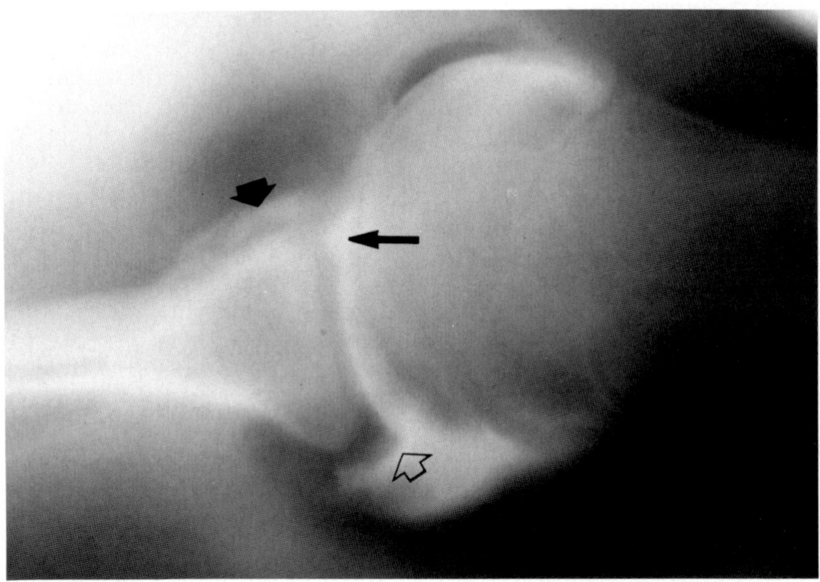

FIG. 4-36. Arthropneumotomography in anterior instability. Tomographic section of the left glenohumeral joint in the axillary position, following double contrast arthrography. The anterior glenoid labrum is torn *(long arrow)*. There is stripping of the joint capsule; this has initiated ectopic bone formation over the scapular neck region *(short arrow)*. The posterior glenoid labrum is normal *(hollow arrow)*. (Courtesy of Dr. Georges El-Khoury, Professor of Radiology and Orthopedics, The University of Iowa Hospitals and Clinics.)

has a poor prognosis in young, healthy athletes failing to respond to conservative management. Abnormal bursograms were those demonstrating an absent, small, or irregularly shaped subacromial bursa, with or without evidence of a cuff tear or thinning.

Arthropneumotomography

This technique is employed essentially for the evaluation of the glenoid labrum. Conventional, thin-section roentgenographic tomography is performed after double contrast arthrography has been done. Two variations of this technique have been described[9,31] based upon the manner in which the patient is positioned and the projection in which tomographic sections are obtained. One technique utilizes an anteroposterior projection with a 45-degree posterior rotation of the shoulder. The images obtained with this format best demonstrate the superior and inferior portions of the labrum.[9] The middle portions of the labrum, anterior and posterior, are less well defined and are best seen by the other method, which employs an axillary projection.[31,62] The patient is positioned so that the scapula is perpendicular to the plane of the film and the arm is extended so that the patient appears to be taking a breath while swimming the crawl. This technique projects the anterior and posterior portions of the labrum in favor of the superior and inferior portions.

Double contrast arthrotomography was apparently introduced to the modern literature in 1979 when El-Khoury et al[31] described the value of the technique in the reading of labral or capsular lesions of eight patients with instability (Fig. 4-36).

Kleinman et al[62] expanded upon the report of El-Khoury et al,[31] who studied 67 arthrotomograms of patients with a variety of shoulder complaints not necessarily derived from instability per se. For the examinations performed with surgical confirmation they claimed to have had a sensitivity of 100% and a specificity of 80% for labrocapsular lesions. Braunstein and O'Connor[9] reported a small series of surgically proven labral tears predicted by arthrotomography.

Pappas et al[93] reported no false-positive or false-negative results in a study of 37 labral tears confirmed by surgery using double contrast arthrotomography. They stress that axillary arthrotomography is especially useful in the detection of subtle labral lesions.

The use of arthropneumotomography for the evaluation of the labrum and capsule may have had diagnostic value in the era preceding the advent of CT arthrography. Mink et al[82] contended that polytomography-augmented arthrography may be at least as accurate as double contrast arthrography in defining labral pathology, but increases the dose of radiation to the patient. CT arthrography is more accurate than either technique and imposes less radiation than tomography.[28]

Contrary to the arguments of such investigators as El-Khoury et al[31] that double contrast arthrotomography is a valuable screener of patients with shoulder pain and/or instability, Kneisl et al[65] feel otherwise. Their studies revealed good reliability of the procedure for the planning of a "lesion-specific" operative procedure among patients with instability. However, its low sensitivity for labral lesions and partial cuff tears leave its value in question for painful but stable shoulders.

Arthropneumotomography has also been used in the evaluation of full-thickness rotator cuff lesions for purposes of surgical planning and prognostication. As already discussed, the premise that surgical planning is aided by a knowledge of the size of a cuff tear and the character of the surrounding tissues has been a stimulus to the "improvement" of arthrographic techniques. Kilcoyne and Matsen[59] comment about the evolution from Lindblom's[70] single contrast method to Goldman and Ghelman's double contrast technique[44] (by which cuff quality and tear size may be estimated) and compare these with their own arthropneumotomographic evaluation. This technique, culminating the 40-plus year evolution, is based on double contrast arthrography but with the addition of complex motion tomography in the upright position to better demonstrate cuff tears. Kilcoyne and Matsen[59] perform upright arthrography first and then proceed with tomography when a tear is identified by conventional radiography. A transscapular view is sometimes helpful in identifying the more elusive tears of the subscapularis, infraspinatus, and teres minor. Employing their technique in 33 shoulders that underwent subsequent surgery, they found a good correlation between predicted and actual pathologic conditions with specific reference to the size of cuff tears and the quality of the adjacent tissues. Nevertheless, the use of tomographic arthrography with its increased radiation exposure seems too heroic a technique to consider when conventional arthrography is relatively revealing, and when the absolute importance of defining the details of cuff lesions is a subject of controversy.

CT Arthrography

Value of CT Arthrography

In this era of arthroscopic labral reattachments and capsular advancements, surgeons of varied skills may hope to determine the planning of an open versus a closed procedure and attempt to predict the duration of postoperative disability on the basis of an accurate, minimally invasive diagnostic test. CT arthrography is not foolproof, but approaches fulfilling the objectives of documentation and planning.

Kleinman et al[62] express many of these thoughts in contemplating the performance of either CT arthrography or arthrotomography of the shoulder. They state that the need for preoperative study in the patient with documented instability "is dictated by the general approach of the orthopedic surgeon." In other words, it is a function of what the surgeon desires to learn or to gain from the procedure: extent of labral disruption, corroboration of the direction of instability, or diagnostic reaffirmation for the patient. Obviously, in the patient without obvious instability, the indications include a search for labral tears or for the discovery of an unsuspected instability. Either procedure may lead to findings that could avert an invasive procedure or help the physician avoid the selection of an inappropriate surgical approach. Despite its described benefits in assessing the glenohumeral joint, CT arthrography falls well short of arthroscopy when possible impingements must be evaluated in addition to localized glenohumeral lesions and when one considers that the arthroscope is not only diagnostic, but is at the same sitting prepared to implement a therapeutic resolve for a number of complex problems in the hands of a sophisticated arthroscopist.

DeHaven et al[24] express the relative advantages and disadvantages of CT arthrography versus arthroscopy in Table 4-2.

Arthrotomography Versus CT Arthrography

Though we have had no experience with arthrotomography, it would appear that the technique is reasonably accurate in delineating pathologic conditions of the labrum.* On the other hand, we have had considerable experience with CT arthrography, and along with other investigators† attest to its accuracy in the discovery of both labral and capsular pathologic conditions.

Rafii et al[102] report that CT arthrography is particularly accurate in the detection of disturbances of the capsular attachments to the scapula that characterize glenohumeral instability. Deutsch et al[28] relate that CT arthrography is more comprehensive and accurate, requires less technical expertise to perform,

*References 9, 28, 31, 62, 65, 72.

†References 24, 75, 100-102, 118, 119.

TABLE 4-2 CT arthrography versus arthroscopy

	Advantages	Disadvantages
CT arthrography	Delineates capsular redundancy, loose bodies, glenoid rim lesions Is less invasive Reveals rotator cuff ruptures	Poorly delineates partial cuff tears and bicipital labial complex Uses ionizing radiation Poorly delineates impingement
Arthroscopy	Delineates most soft tissue abnormalities, including partial cuff tears and the bicipital-labral complex Does not use ionizing radiation Diagnoses and treats impingement	Does not always identify instability or capsular redundancy Is an invasive procedure with general anesthesia

From DeHaven JP et al: A prospective comparison study of double contrast CT arthrography and shoulder arthroscopy. Walter Reed Army Medical Center. Paper presented at the AAOS in San Francisco, January 1987.

requires less difficulty with positioning to gain reliable images, and requires less radiation. Furthermore, in experienced hands, the arthrotomographic procedure requires nearly an hour to perform,[62] almost one half hour more than is needed for CT arthrography. It is the opinion of the authors that the clinicians reporting the use of arthrotomography might have preferred to have used CT arthrography had it been as readily available as it is today.

Technique

Following a conventional double contrast arthrogram, a CT scan of the shoulder is performed. With the newer generation of scanners, this will add approximately 15 minutes to the duration of the examination. The patient is examined in the supine position and the arm is placed at the side with the palm against the thigh (neutral position).[100-102] The neutral position of the arm is the one most commonly employed.

Deutsch et al[28] examined their patients with the arm in neutral or slight internal rotation. Singson et al[119] examined shoulders in neutral and occasionally in internal or external rotation. McNiesh and Callaghan[75] and DeHaven et al[24] performed examinations in neutral or in external rotation. The position of the arm plays a role in the movements of air and contrast, which may enhance or diminish visualization of a given area of study. The neutral position allows fairly uniform dispersement of contrast media. An externally rotated position may adversely prejudice interpretation of the anterior joint structures. At NYU Medical Center, additional sections with the arm in external rotation are obtained specifically to enhance visualization of the posterior portion of the glenoid labrum; otherwise a neutral position of the arm is routinely employed. This is in accord with Deutsch et al[28] who explain that the externally rotated position enhances posterior labral visualization by relaxing the posterior capsule and forcing air to move posteriorly.

In the context of air-contrast dispersements, Randelli et al[104] indicate their experience with false-positive results wherein a localized accumulation of contrast had been misconstrued as labral fragmentation. This can occur with inadvertent positioning of the needle within the labrum, especially early on in the learning curve. Adequate distention and even distribution of contrast is necessary for proper interpretation of the soft tissues. Variation in the quantities of positive contrast material or even the use of air alone has been reported.[28] The joint is scanned with 3 mm thick slices by the authors. Using special software, the computer can generate high-resolution, magnified images of the shoulder region. Wide window settings (3000/300) are used for producing hard copy images that allow various densities (bone, soft tissue, and contrast media) to be adequately resolved. Excellent visualization of the glenoid labrum, the capsular structures, including the glenohumeral ligaments and the joint surfaces, is achieved by this technique.[100] Additionally, the osseous and the periarticular structures are optimally visualized and can be evaluated for possible unexpected lesions (Fig. 4-37).

The evaluation of the extent of rotator cuff tears and degeneration by direct sagittal computerized tomography (DSCT) has also been described.[6] According to Beltran et al,[6] DSCT performed with the patient seated between the gantry and the scanner table reveals greater diagnostic accuracy in the detection of rotator cuff lesions than either axial CT scanning or double contrast arthrography with plain films. Twenty-nine lesions were detected in 24 symptomatic patients: 14 by arthrogram, 19 by axial CT, and 27 by DSCT. Hence, DSCT is better for cuff pathology and axial CT arthrography is better for labral lesions.

A

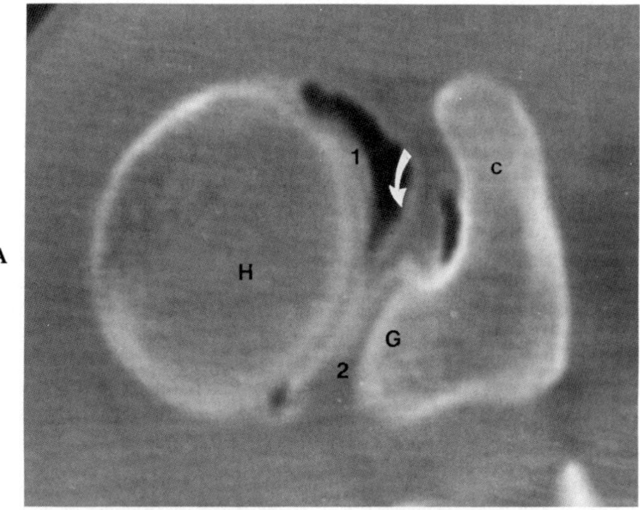

B

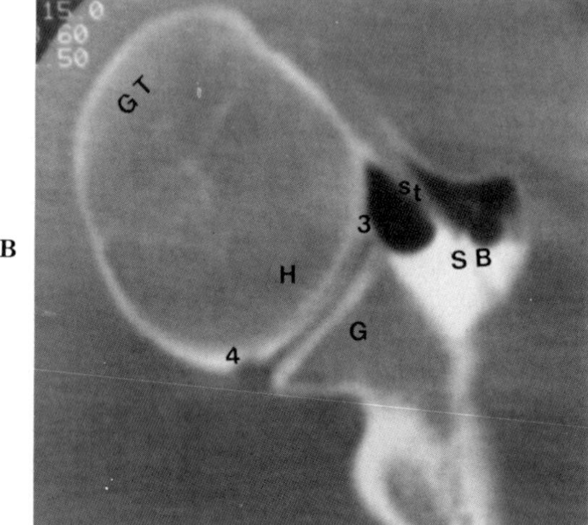

C

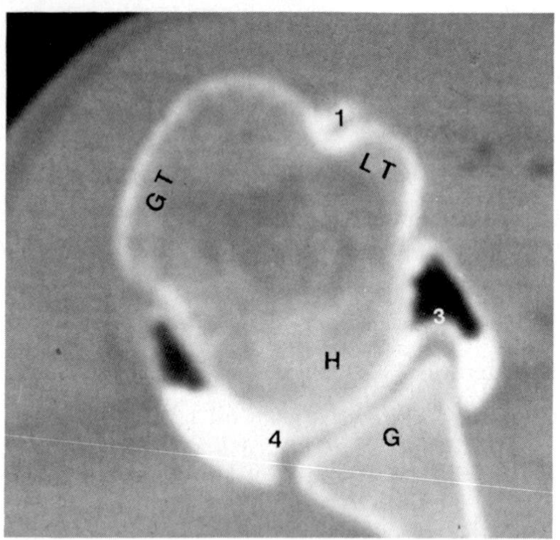

FIG. 4-37. Normal CT arthrogram of right shoulder. Representative images from proximal **(A),** middle **(B),** and distal **(C)** aspects of the glenohumeral joint. *C,* coracoid process; *G,* glenoid; *H,* humeral head; GT, greater tuberosity; *LT,* lesser tuberosity; *SB,* subscapularis bursa; *ST,* subscapularis tendon; *1,* long head of biceps tendon; *2,* superior glenoid labrum; *3,* anterior glenoid labrum; *4,* posterior glenoid labrum. **A,** The long head of biceps tendon and the superior glenoid labrum merge and form a common insertion onto the superior glenoid margin. The anterior aspect of the joint capsule in this vicinity forms the superior glenohumeral ligament *(arrow).* **B,** The subscapularis bursa is formed below the coracoid process as a medial extension of the synovial lining of the joint capsule along the superior free margin of the subscapularis tendon. **C,** Below the subscapularis bursa, the anterior capsule extends for a distance (individually varied) medially, forms a smooth reflexion over the glenoid, and blends with the anterior glenoid labrum. The posterior capsule is intimately related to the posterior glenoid labrum. (**C** reproduced with permission from Rafii M et al: Am J Sports Med 16:352, 1988).

Isolated Labrum Lesion

CT arthrography has its greatest value in the evaluation of "isolated" labral lesions and of labral and capsular lesions associated with glenohumeral instability. Isolated and instability lesions of the labrum are sometimes difficult to distinguish. The isolated varieties are most traditionally associated with throwing type mechanisms. Rafii et al[101,102] observe that athletes with no clinical instability had frequently demonstrable detachments of the superior labrum, the inner margin of which is weakly attached to the glenoid.[8] The second most frequent labral tear in the athlete with a stable shoulder is that of the middle anterior portion of the glenoid. Just as the superior labral detachment has been postulated by Andrews, Carson, and McLeod (1985)[102] to result

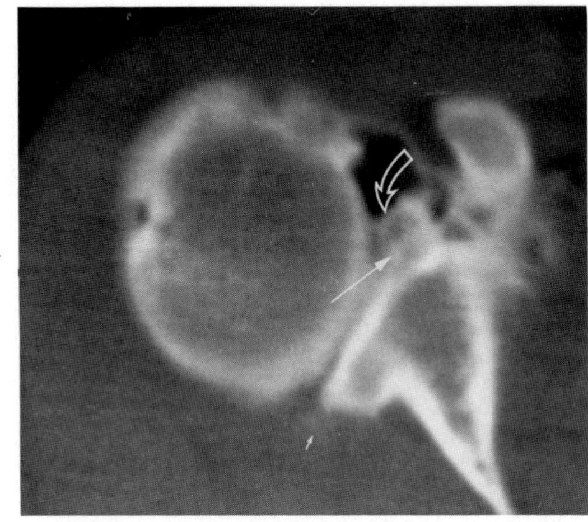

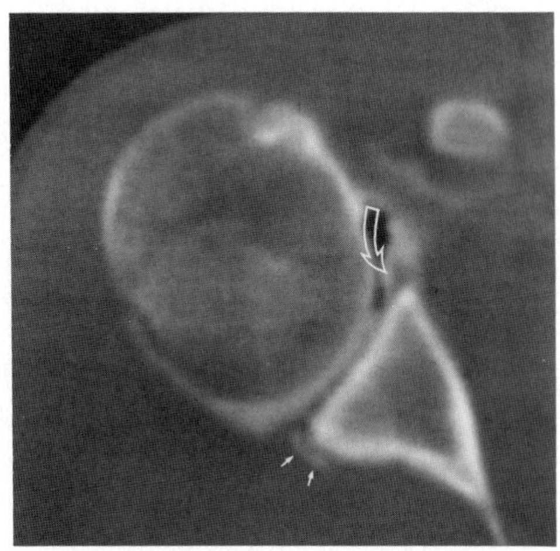

FIG. 4-38. Isolated glenoid labrum tear. Major league pitcher with right shoulder pain. **A** and **B,** CT arthrogram images from the proximal aspect of the glenohumeral joint. The anterior glenoid labrum is irregularly torn *(curved arrow)* and detached from the glenoid margin *(long arrow)*. Inferior to these levels the labrum was normal. Also noted is a calcific ridge formed along the posterior capsular margin within the expected site of capsular attachment *(short arrows)*.

from the pull of the biceps tendon during the throwing act, middle anterior lesions may be a consequence of labral impingement between the humeral head and subscapularis tendon during the act of throwing (Fig. 4-38).

According to Zarins and Matthews,[125] these labral tears occur in the anterosuperior or anterior portions of the glenoid. Vertical longitudinal or circumferential tears are seen with the greatest frequency, followed by flap tears and then complex tears. The labral lesions of instability occur more commonly, though not exclusively, about the lower hemisphere of the glenoid.

In a study of autopsy and patient shoulders, Kohn[66] discovered a high incidence of labral pathology by gross or arthroscopic examination that could not be correlated to symptoms. He concluded that most glenoid labral lesions have little clinical relevance. DePalma's studies of aging in the shoulder joint are worth mentioning at this point.[25] They revealed a progressive degeneration of the labrum after the second decade. These changes are comprised of detachment of superior labrum from the glenoid (which exceeds an incidence of greater than 60% in the fifth decade) and thinning and fraying of the inferior portion of the labrum. It may be the case that many of these degenerative changes are not productive of symptoms. Nevertheless, it is evident, particularly in an athletic population, that many labral tears produce symptoms that are relieved by arthroscopic debridement. In fact, some of these tears produce not only pain and clicking, but also a sense of instability within the joint (functional instability). Pappas et al[93] go to great lengths in creating a distinction between labrum-produced, or "functional," instability treatable by excision and "anatomical," or glenohumeral, instability, which may require labral repair and capsulorrhaphy. Obviously, this distinction is important in surgical planning and in patient counseling, and it is one that can be made with CT arthrography.

Shuman et al[118] studied 11 sequential patients with suspected labral pathology associated with a variety of signs and symptoms, and in each instance in which a labral tear was discovered on CT arthrography, it was confirmed at surgery. All negative studies were confirmed at surgery as well. Deutsch et al,[28] based on surgical correlation to CT arthrography, found a sensitivity for anterior labral lesions of 100%. CT arthrography is currently the most accurate roentgenographic means for the detection of lesions of the labrum. DeHaven et al,[24] using CT arthrography to evaluate a group of patients with symptoms derived from multiple pathologic conditions, found high sensitivities for loose body detection and labral lesions; they found relatively poor sensitivities (less than 70%) in diagnosing lesions of the rotator cuff, the bicipital-labral complex, and the Hill-Sachs lesion. While specificities were 100% for the cuff, loose body, posterior labral lesion, Hill-Sachs lesion, and bicipital-labral complex, there was less than 75% specificity and a less than 90% accuracy for anterior labral lesions. This may, in part, relate to the fact that they studied patients with the arm in an externally rotated position, which, as already indicated, is best for enhancing posterior lesions.

Labral Morphology

As pointed out in the section on the isolated labrum, the labrum can manifest a variety of tears. However, frank tears are not the only morphologic labral alterations that can be appreciated arthroscopically. The labrum can appear atrophic or degenerated, loose or floppy, or even distorted in contour. The significance of each of these findings is not always clear. The morphologic characteristics of the labrum as seen by CT arthrography are often different than those which may be appreciated by direct viewing using arthroscopy, lending more confusion and speculation to their significance.

McNiesh and Callaghan[75] studied 72 shoulders by double contrast CT arthrography between 1984 and 1988. They noted labra which they considered to be unusually small (though nondegenerated), some with cleavages within the normally sharply truncated shadow, and even one that was notched. They considered these to be normal variants, since subsequent arthroscopies demonstrated no apparent abnormalities in any of these labra. The corrugations that frequently develop within labra after the second decade may help to explain some of these variants.[25] They might also result from peripheral detachment or laxity as in the knee, where a normal meniscus will often appear convoluted when there exists a near or distant locus of peripheral separation.

Working with a variety of co-workers, Rafii[100-102] noted numerous morphologic alterations in the evaluation of labra CT arthrography. Labral eversion, attenuation, hypertrophy, and floppiness (loss of truncation) were among the findings noted. While not even a majority of those studied eventually underwent surgery, these labral findings were considered to be abnormal and not always readily appreciated by arthroscopy. It is postulated that configurational alterations of the labrum may be more readily identifiable by the definitive geometry created by air/contrast lines than by direct gross inspection. The meaning of the morphologic variants appreciated by CT arthrography has also been speculated upon by the authors. The floppy labrum probably results from a tear with subsequent degeneration. The everted labrum is also associated with tear or detachment. The hypertrophied labrum may result from tearing with inflammation and/or hydrops (Fig. 4-39). DePalma's work[25] revealed that a natural progression of hypertrophy occurs within the superior portion of the labrum with aging (Fig. 4-40). DePalma ascribed this hypertrophy to the formation of synovial tabs and fringes particularly about the anterior portion of the labrum.

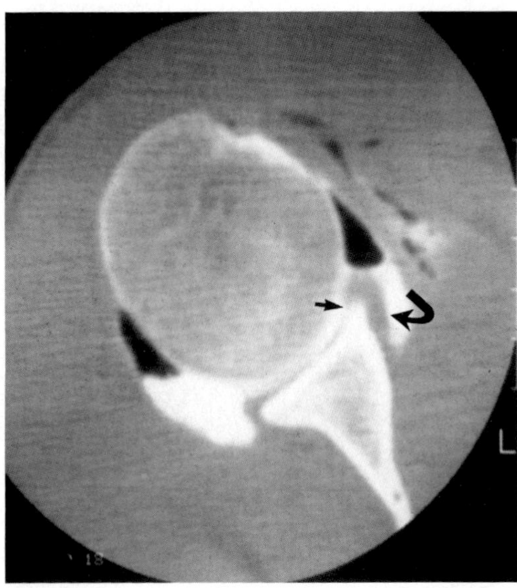

FIG. 4-39. Tear and enlargement of the glenoid labrum. Same patient as in Fig. 4-44, *A*). An anterior labrum tear *(straight arrow)* was detected one week following acute trauma to the right shoulder in this professional hockey player. The torn labrum is rather enlarged and the adjacent soft tissues of the capsulolabral junction are thickened *(curved arrow)*.

Whether the discovery of morphologic variants other than obvious tears relates to the isolated labral problem, to instability, or to neither, is not altogether clear. It is not yet established whether these changes have import and reliability in the planning of lesion-specific surgery.

Unstable Shoulder—Capsule and Labrum

Glenohumeral instability is most often discoverable by history and physical examination and is frequently documented by conventional roentgenography, as discussed on p. 93. However, when no bony lesions are present on conventional roentgenography, even with special views, and when there is a need for more precise evaluation of the suspected pathologic condition, special roentgenography such as computed tomographic arthrography becomes important.[61]

CT arthrography has value in the reaffirmation of a suspected instability, the discovery of subtle or unsuspected instability, the determination of the direction of instability, and

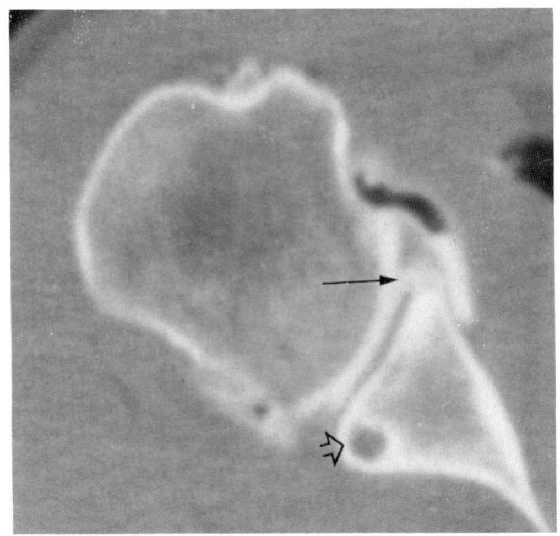

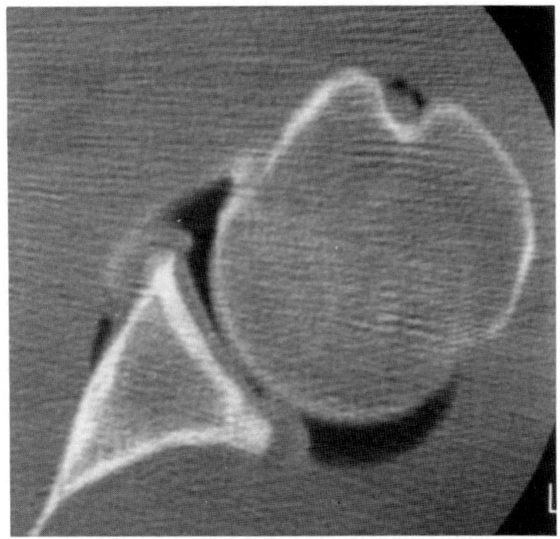

FIG. 4-40. Degenerative disease of the glenohumeral joint. **A,** Right shoulder pain in a middle-aged tennis player. The anterior and posterior glenoid labra are enlarged. The anterior labrum is also partially detached from the glenoid margin, which shows osteophyte formation *(solid arrow)*. A subarticular cyst of the posterior labrum is also present *(hollow arrow)*. **B,** Degenerative disease in a veteran baseball player. The anterior glenoid labrum and the articular cartilage of the humeral head and glenoid are attenuated. There is an osteophyte off the anterior glenoid margin. The posterior glenoid margin is irregular.

the characterization of the type of labral lesion associated with the instability. At times, the diagnosis of the unstable shoulder can be difficult.[61] Many patients are poor at perceiving a sense of sliding and merely experience pain as a manifestation of glenohumeral displacement. Many are too apprehensive to be adequately examined or refuse to submit to surgery or even general anesthesia for purposes of diagnosis. In these instances, the CT arthrogram can be especially helpful in defining soft tissue and bony abnormalities not detectable by conventional roentgenography.

In an early study, Kinnard et al[61] performed CT arthrography upon 10 unstable shoulders of which seven had documented instability. All 10 were noted to have had an increase in the size of the anterior recess, which, by the way, may be of no significance; seven patients had intraarticular septate adhesions; three had labral amputations, and two patients had glenoid rim fractures not discovered by "routine" roentgenography. All of the findings in this rudimentary study were substantiated by subsequent surgery.

Fifty-four shoulders, 40 with involuntary dislocations and 14 with involuntary subluxations, were studied by Singson et al.[119] Eighty-five percent of the shoulders had sustained athletic trauma. Anterior labral abnormalities were present in almost 100% of cases on CT arthrography. Surgical corroboration revealed *no* false-positive findings and only two false-negative findings based on either an inadequate study or an inadequate prospective interpretation of positive evidence.

Randelli[104] cautions that large capsular recesses must not automatically be assumed to represent an instability. The capsular recesses, particularly the axillary and subscapular recesses, vary considerably in size and shape among normal shoulders. Only marked anterior capsular enlargement and/or detachment should be interpreted as a definite sign of instability (Fig. 4-41). This statement is corroborated by Rafii et al.[100]

Capsular recesses

- Large ones may represent normal variation
- Not a sine qua non of instability
- If detached, more likely to represent instability

Singson et al[119] found roentgenographic capsular evidence of instability in almost 80% of cases and consisted of the following: (1) medial scapular insertion; (2) glenoid stripping or detachment; and (3) capsular widening or redundant anterior recess.

The import of the location of the glenohumeral capsular insertion into the scapula is reinforced by Rothman et al.[109] They indicate

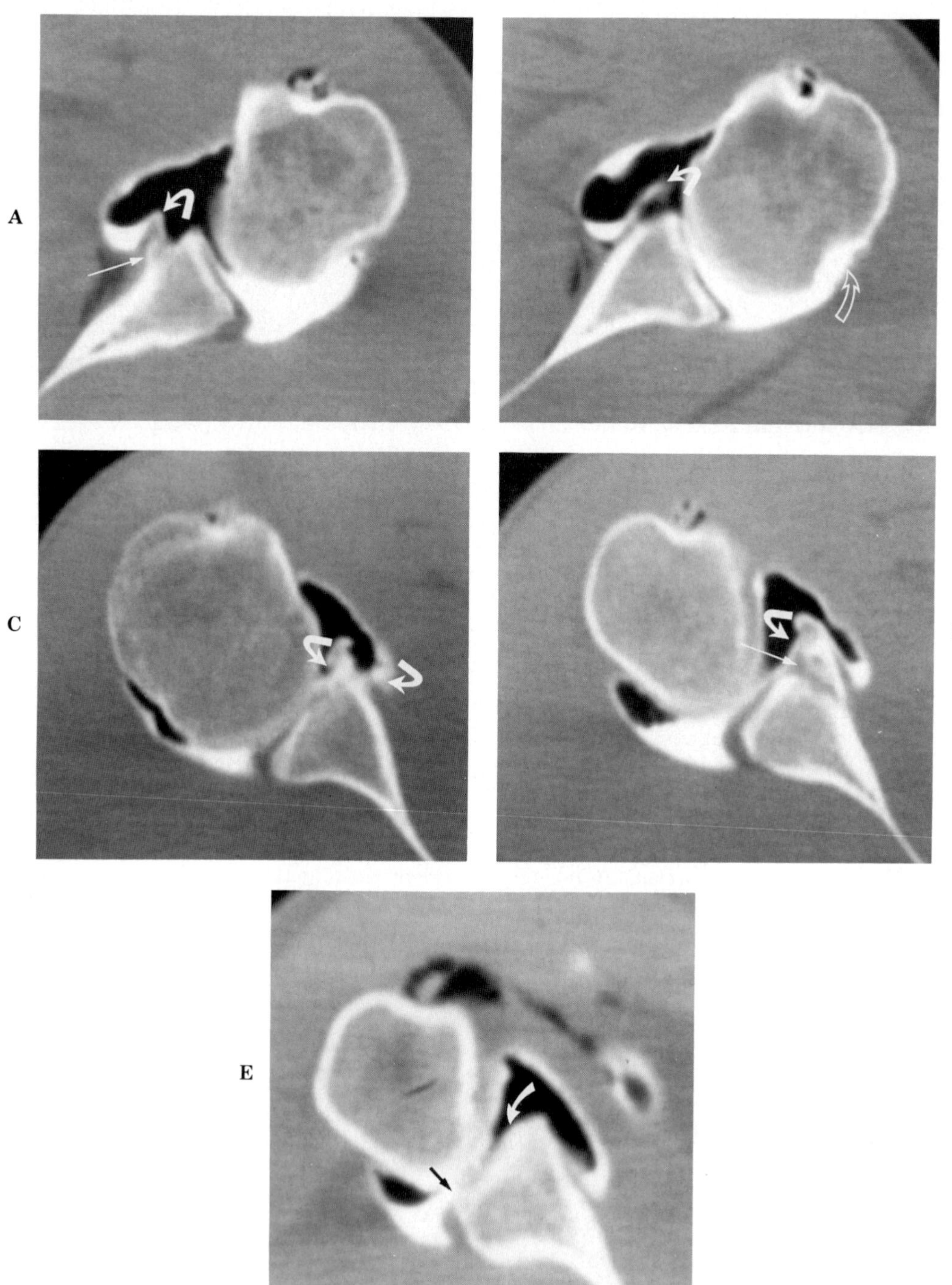

FIG. 4-41. Anterior instability. Recurrent dislocations and subluxations. Various morphologic configurations of capsulolabral lesions. **A** and **B,** Recurrent dislocation of left shoulder. The glenoid labrum *(curved arrow)* is detached and considerably attenuated. The capsulolabral junction is also detached and an enlarged anterior pouch is formed. The anterior glenoid margin is deficient and ectopic calcification is noted *(long arrow)*. A Hill-Sachs defect is also demonstrated *(hollow arrow)*. **C** and **D,** Recurrent subluxation of right shoulder. The anterior capsulolabral complex is irregularly torn in all aspects *(curved arrows)*. A fracture of anterior glenoid margin is demonstrated *(straight arrow)*. **E,** Recurrent dislocation of right shoulder. The anterior glenoid labrum is totally absent and stripping of the anterior capsule is evident. The articular cartilage of the glenoid and the osseous glenoid margin are deficient *(white arrow)*. Also, a tear of the posterior glenoid labrum is visualized *(black arrow)*.

that the more distal capsular insertions (types II and III) onto the neck, rather than onto the glenoid (type I), are more likely to be associated with anterior instability. Rafii et al[101] reported that capsular findings of instability included stripping of the anterior capsule from the scapular neck; thickening and/or irregularity of the capsular and periosteal soft tissues about the anterior portion of the scapula; capsular tears with or without leakage; periosteal bone formation about the scapular neck; and anterior or posterior capsular redundancy. One or more of these findings were present in all cases of glenohumeral instability (see Fig. 4-41).

Capsular findings associated with instability

- Stripping of anterior capsule from scapular neck
- Thickening/irregularity of capsule/periosteum
- Capsular tears
- Periosteal bone formation along scapula neck
- Capsular redundancy

Singson et al[119] found no essential differences in the labral lesions of recurrent subluxation and dislocation. However, capsular abnormalities were more frequent and dramatic in shoulders with recurrent dislocation. They reported that 90% of patients with a widened subscapular bursa had anterior dislocations, while those with only cicatricial responses within the tendon of the subscapularis tended to have only subluxations. However, it must be pointed out that subscapular cicatrix may only be deduced from circumstantial evidence.

Rafii et al[100-102] observed that all anterior instabilities were associated with lesions of the anterior portion of the labrum, which included frank tears, detachments, absences, and attenuations. In occasional cases the labrum remains intact and a frank tear is not seen (Fig. 4-42). Labral lesions on the side of the glenoid opposite the direction of instability were not uncommonly observed (see Fig. 4-41, *E*). Such tears were not necessarily construed to represent a posterior instability. An instability on the side of the glenoid with a tear was most definitely accepted when there was an associated tear of the capsule, glenoid rim fracture, or peculiarity in the scapular insertion of the capsule (Fig. 4-43). This is in keeping with the findings of Singson et al[119] who report that in nearly all cases in which an anterior form of instability existed an anterior labral lesion is present; all patients with posterior instability (uni- and multidirectional) have concomitant anterior as well as posterior labral lesions.

Labral findings associated with instability

- Tears
- Detachment
- Absence
- Alteration

Rafii et al[100-102] stress the dilemma of diagnosing mild uni- or multidirectional instabilities and of distinguishing instabilities from isolated labral lesions, such as those resulting from throwing activities. They further indicate the additional burden of establishing these diagnoses in the wake of a new and acute injury (Figs. 4-44 and 4-45).

While experts in athletic medicine may be embarrassed or reluctant to admit that they are unable to discover or define all cases of instability by physical evaluation of patients in the awake or anesthetized state, the difficulty nonetheless exists in a number of instances. Even when an instability of limited magnitude is discovered, there remains the task of assigning to it a clinical (symptomatic) relevance. The concepts expressed by Pappas et al[93] of "functional instability" and by Rafii et al[102] of "unobtrusive laxity" are not just a source of additional confusion, but are loose ends in the determination of practical treatment designs.

Rafii and her radiologist colleagues at New York University Medical Center have come to appreciate the pressures for both accurate and expedient diagnosis in professional athletes. New York University orthopaedic surgeons have submitted their players for roentgenographic evaluation in an effort to gain a greater specificity of knowledge without first resorting to more invasive techniques that could lead to complications or unnecessary player days missed in this highly visible population. CT arthrography is best suited to this task, at least until magnetic resonance imaging techniques for the shoulder become more reliable. The primary concern, of course, is the incidence of false-positive or false-negative results, both of which are extremely low. A second concern pertains to those acute cases in which CT arthrography defines ex-

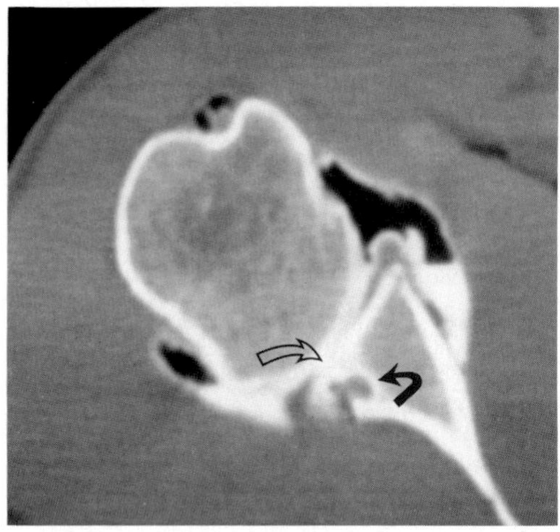

FIG. 4-42. Anterior instability. Recurrent subluxation of right shoulder. There is a small notch at the junction of the glenoid labrum and the glenoid articular cartilage *(white arrow)*. The labrum is rounded in contour, but does not otherwise show a tear. Also there is small ectopic calcification adjacent to the glenoid margin *(black arrow)*. A frank tear was not seen at arthroscopy.

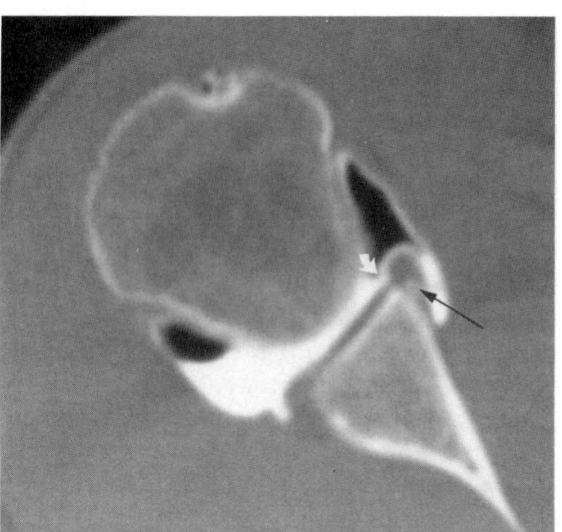

FIG. 4-43. Posterior instability, right shoulder. The posterior glenoid labrum is torn, and there is detachment and displacement of the torn glenolabral complex *(hollow arrow)*. The osseous glenoid margin is deficient and shows a cystic type defect *(solid arrow)*. This configuration is the result of glenoid margin fracture. There is an enlarged anterior capsule with medial attachment near the scapular neck. This results from presence of large inferior subscapularis bursa in this patient. One should be alerted to the possible presence of anterior instability in this instance.

A

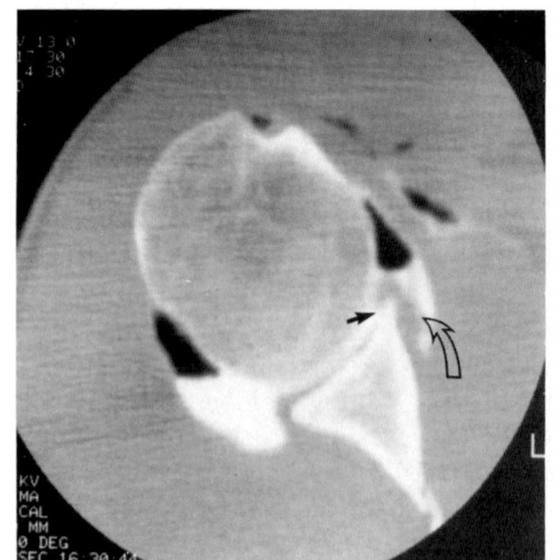

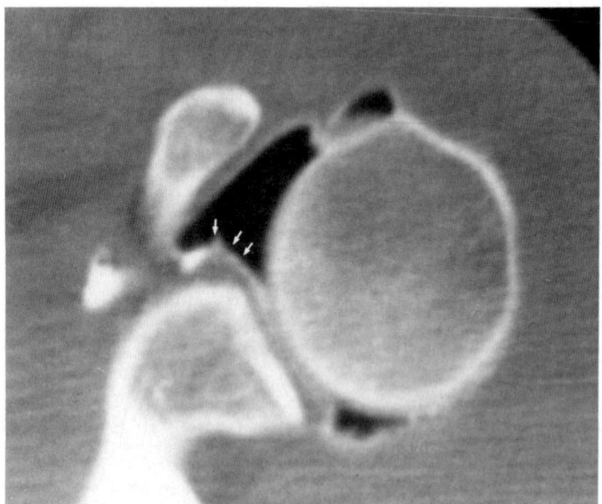

B

FIG. 4-44. Glenoid labrum tear resulting from acute trauma. **A,** CT arthrogram of right shoulder in a professional hockey player 3 days after acute trauma (same patient as in Fig. 4-39). The anterior labrum is shown to be torn and partially detached *(solid arrow)*. There is no stripping of the capsule. However, the capsulolabral junction is swollen *(hollow arrow)*. This finding was not considered to be a solid evidence for persistent joint instability and none was demonstrated at arthroscopy. Anterior instability became apparent at subsequent clinical examination. **B,** Professional hockey player following acute trauma to left shoulder. Representative image from proximal aspect of the joint. The anterior glenoid labrum is deformed and shows many surface of irregularities. The entire anterior labrum showed similar abnormality. No capsular abnormality was detected. Subsequently, laxity was clinically documented. No follow-up CT arthrogram was done to evaluate any interval change. (**B** reproduced with permission from Rafii M et al: Am J Sports Med 16:352, 1988.)

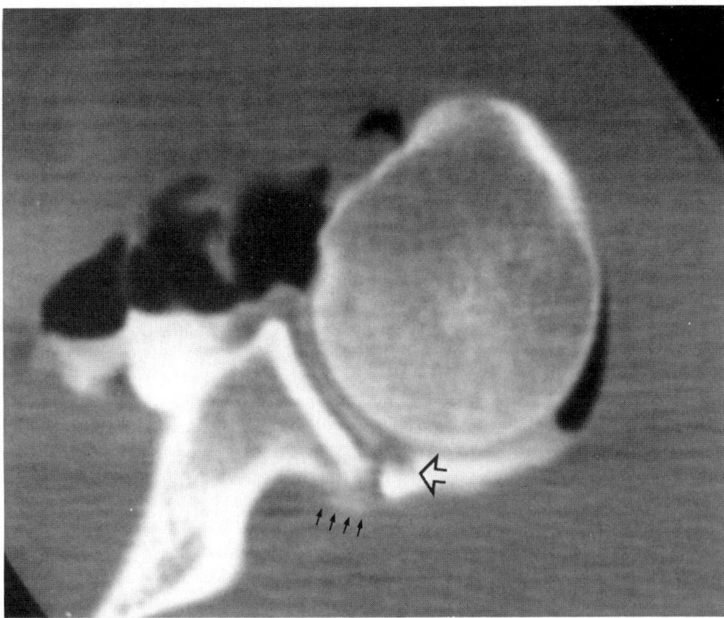

FIG. 4-45. Posterior shoulder instability. Professional hockey player following acute trauma to left shoulder. Representative CT arthrogram image at the upper aspect of the joint, with a rather prominent subscapularis bursa visualized anteriorly. The posterior glenoid labrum is torn and detached, floating within the posterior aspect of the joint *(hollow arrow)*. There is extravasation of the contrast material beyond the capsulolabral junction, indicative of capsular tear *(small arrows)*. This finding was considered to be a manifestation of persistent instability.

isting pathologic conditions but fails to predict the role of the condition in the natural history of the problem. For example, between 1984 and 1987, three professional hockey players sustained acute shoulder trauma evaluated by CT arthrography. In two of the three, isolated anterior labral pathology (detachment) was evident by CT arthrography or arthroscopy, without detectable glenohumeral instability under anesthesia (see Fig. 4-44). Both players subsequently manifested anterior subluxation on examination within 24 months (by J.M.) and without a second acute traumatic episode. The third player was not arthroscoped after CT arthrography revealed evidence of posterior instability (see Fig. 4-45). His symptoms were of pain and not instability until nearly 8 months after the injury, when he began to experience recurrent episodes of posterior subluxation (which have been well tolerated). It is interesting that Hawkins et al,[50] reporting in a large series of patients with recurrent posterior subluxation, indicated that most were unable to recall an initial episode of trauma in which the shoulder came out. Instability appeared and progressed insidiously with time.

Rafii et al[102] specifically studied 61 shoulders with symptoms deriving from athletic trauma or performance in patients between 15 and 40 years of age. They observe that high level athletes with glenohumeral instability had fewer dramatic labral lesions and less capsular stretching than the population at large, which may relate to their youth and/or their resilience in achieving an elite status.[101,102]

Hill-Sachs Lesion

Among the alleged disadvantages of CT arthrography and arthrotomography is a diminished ability to detect the Hill-Sachs lesion.[24] In the series reported by Rafii et al[101] only two Hill-Sachs lesions were identified among 14 competitive athletic patients with a known anterior instability. Using CT arthrography, a Hill-Sachs lesion was identified in less than 40% of the 54 unstable shoulders studied by Singson et al.[119] Other reports, however, are more positive. Deutsch et al[28] state that computerized arthrotomography is highly sensitive in the detection of Hill-Sachs lesions and may detect these lesions when conventional roentgenography or arthrography fail to do so. Gambrioli et al[35] determined that CT revealed the Hill-Sachs lesion with a similar accuracy to that of conventional roentgenographic views such as the Didiee, but with better definition of the extent of the lesion.

In any case, if the only Hill-Sachs lesions missed by CT arthrography are those which are too small to require a specific treatment for the bony defect, then the only potential loss in diagnostic confirmation of instability is the failure to detect the Hill-Sachs lesion. This is a small loss, since in virtually all but some newer cases of instability, the accurate delineations of Bankart lesions of the glenoid-labrum complex and the character of the capsular insertion onto the scapula by CT arthrography are sufficiently diagnostic of instability.

MAGNETIC RESONANCE IMAGING

This newest imaging modality without the use of ionizing radiation has brought what amounts to a revolution to the field of diagnostic imaging. The impact of musculoskeletal imaging is significant because of the exquisite resolution of various soft tissue structures. Also, magnetic resonance imaging (MRI) has the capability for multiplanar imaging (including oblique planes by several commercially available units), which allows for imaging in anatomically suitable planes for gathering information most helpful for recognition of pathologic conditions.

Advantages of MRI

- High soft tissue contrast
- Multiplanar imaging capability
- Absence of bone artifacts
- Absence of ionizing radiation
- Noninvasive

The principal advantages of MRI are summarized by Huber et al[54]: high soft-tissue contrast, multiplanar imaging capability, absence of bone artifacts, and an absence of ionizing radiation or other invasive elements. This imaging modality, which is still in the developing stages, has particularly affected the imaging of the peripheral joints and has already proved its efficacy in the imaging of the hip, knee, and ankle joints. Noninvasive, and with a much greater capacity for the depiction of the ligamentous structures and the periarticular soft tissues, MRI has already eliminated the need in many cases for the more invasive technique of knee arthrography and even diagnostic arthroscopy. MRI is more effective than CT in the demonstration of shoulder joint anatomy because of its capability for multiplanar imaging and its superior resolution of soft tissue structures.[54]

Signal Generation

The MR images are formed on the basis of signals that are received from the various tissues. The MR signal is based on the presence and the density of mobile protons in various tissues. The cortical bone, fibrocartilage, fibrous tissue, tendons, and ligaments produce no signal and are depicted as black regions on MR images. Fat produces the highest signal, appearing as bright or white areas. Water and water-containing tissue elements such as muscles induce various ranges of medium signal intensity. The MR signals are produced by magnetized protons, which are then excited by a radiofrequency. The signals, or "echos," are detected and transmitted with the same or a different coil system from that which generated the original radiofrequency. The varied characteristics of signals obtained in short or long ranges of "listening" can help in determining the nature of some tissue elements and may therefore help in detecting pathologic processes. For example, fluids such as joint effusion produce a medium signal intensity and may blend with periarticular tissue when short-range intervals of signal gathering are used. In long ranges of pulse sequence, the intensity of signal from fluids is greatly increased. For example, effusion is depicted as bright, providing an arthrogram effect that is easily distinguished from adjacent structures.

The developiment of MR technique for imaging of the shoulder joint has proved to be a challenging task. The shoulder is difficult to image because of the space limitations within the housing of the MR magnet and because the shoulder cannot be positioned in the center of the magnet where the highest ranges of signal-to-noise (S/N) ratios are achieved. Seeger et al[114] explain that these problems can be overcome by combining high resolution scanning with the use of a surface coil for the shoulder.

MR imaging of the peripheral joints became a clinical reality mostly after the development of high resolution imaging techniques and the development of surface coils intended for gathering MR signals from small regions of the body. The peripheral location of the shoulder, however, necessitated further changes in imaging techniques. Ordinarily the center of the field of view is in the vicinity of the center of the magnet, where the highest S/N ratio is obtained. While peripheral images are possible to obtain, they have poor resolution. The development of an off-center zoom technique has eliminated this problem by shifting the center of the field of view to the periphery as much as needed to produce high resolution magnified images of the shoulder region.

Technique

The MR examination of the shoulder is obtained with the patient supine and with the arms extended along the sides. With the palm against the thigh, the humerus will be in a position midway between internal and external rotation, which is most suitable for imaging of this joint. The rotator cuff muscles also are in a relaxed state. Seeger et al[116] perform MR scanning with the arm in internal rotation, a position that they consider more

A

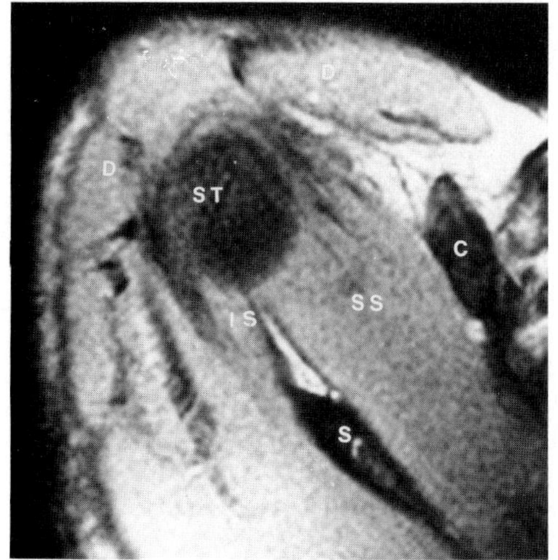

B

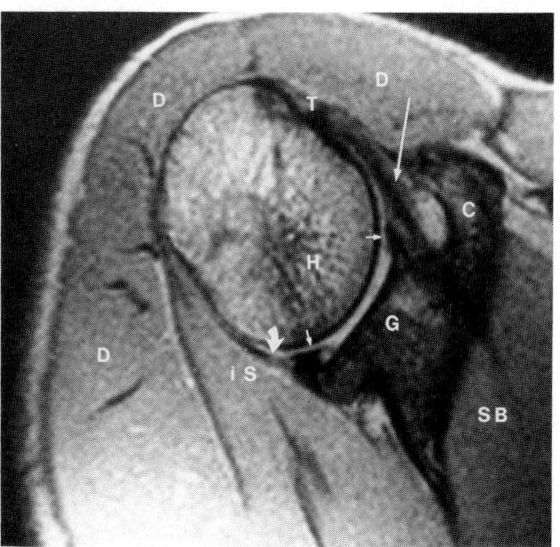

C

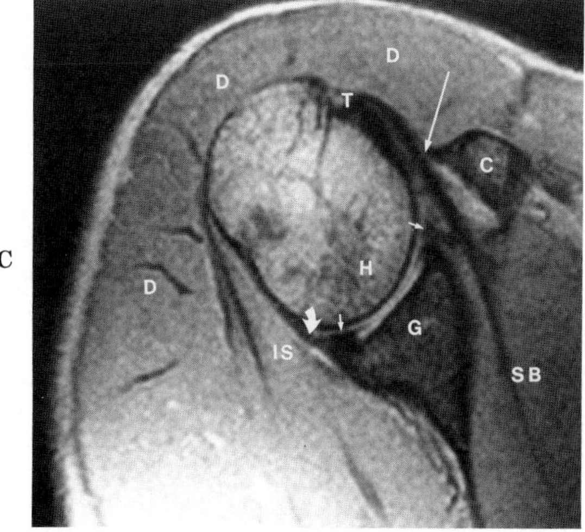

FIG. 4-46. Magnetic resonance imaging of right shoulder. Normal anatomy in axial **(A,B,C)** and anatomic coronal plane **(D,E). A,** Axial image at the level of supraspinatus fossa of the scapula. At this level the supraspinatus muscle and tendon are visualized. The plane of the coronal images is based on the orientation of this muscle in each individual. A small portion of the infraspinatus muscle is also visualized with its tendon overlapping the supraspinatus tendon. **B** and **C,** Axial images at the level of the base of the coracoid process **(B).** At this level and below the coracoid process **(C),** the glenohumeral articulation and the glenoid labrum (anterior and posterior segments) *(short arrows)* and the subscapularis, the infraspinatus, and the deltoid muscles are visualized. The anterior joint capsule and the subscapularis tendon *(long arrow),* which emerges from medioinferior margin of the coracoid process, extend laterally to the lesser tuberosity. A cross-section of the long head of the biceps tendon is seen at the top of the bicipital groove. The posterior capsule *(curved arrow)* extends from the posterior labrum along with the infraspinatus muscle and tendon to the greater tuberosity. **C,** Axial MR image below the coracoid process. The subscapularis muscle and tendon are visualized in continuity.

Continued.

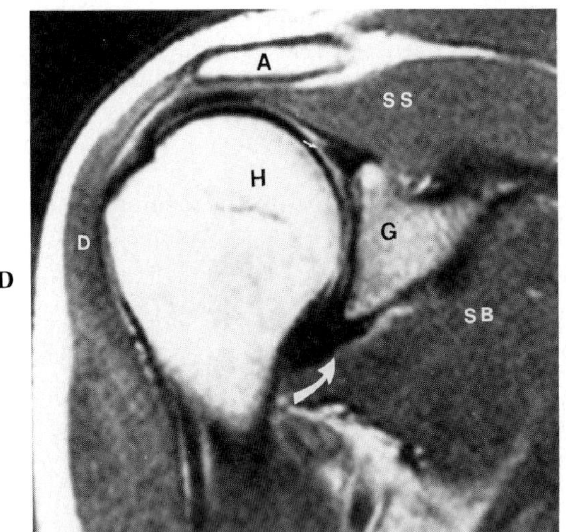

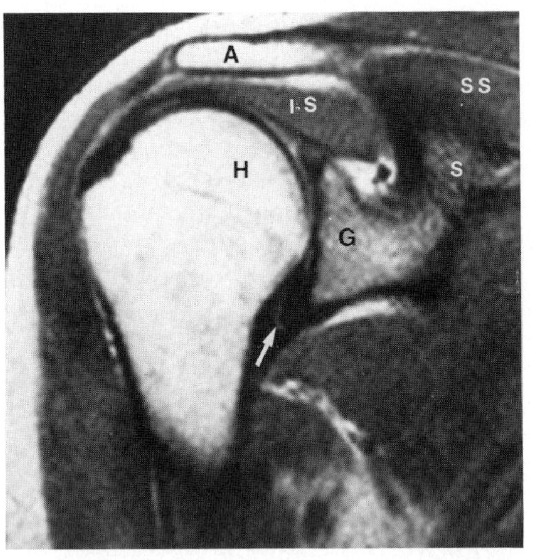

FIG. 4-46, cont'd. D, Anatomic coronal plane MR image of right shoulder oriented along the longitudinal axis of the supraspinatus muscle and tendon. The supraspinatus, the subscapularis, and the deltoid muscles are visualized extending within the subacromial space and inserting onto the greater tuberosity. The superior glenoid labrum is visualized *(short arrow)*. The inferior labrum blends with the axillary pouch of the joint capsule from which it can not be differentiated because of the normal lack of signal from both structures *(curved arrow)*. **E,** Anatomic coronal plane MR image slightly posterior (lateral) to **D.** At this level, the infraspinatus muscle is visualized (lateral to the scapular spine) emerging from behind the scapular spine. A portion of the supraspinatus muscle is also visualized medial (anterior) to the scapular spine. The musculotendinous junction and the tendon of the infraspinatus are visualized within the subacromial space extending toward the greater tuberosity. The inferior glenoid labrum is partially outlined on this image, probably as a result signal arising from a small amount of joint fluid *(arrow)*. *A*, acromion; *C*, coracoid process; *D*, deltoid; *G*, glenoid; *H*, humeral head; *IS*, infraspinatus; *SB*, subscapularis; *SS*, supraspinatus; *T*, long head of biceps tendon.

convenient to the patient and more revealing of the pathologic state related to subacromial impingement. The imaging of the rotator cuff, the subacromial space, the acromioclavicular, and the glenohumeral joints are best achieved by imaging in at least two planes (Fig. 4-46): (1) the oblique coronal (anatomic coronal) and (2) the axial planes. The anatomic coronal plane of the shoulder is individually varied and is best determined in each patient by obtaining a series of axial or "scout" images. The oblique plane images are best made parallel to the course of the supraspinatus tendon. These images are most suitable for evaluation of the supraspinatus tendon and the subacromial space, the AC joint, the glenohumeral joint, and the superior and inferior glenoid labrum. The axial images are centered on the glenohumeral joint and are most helpful for evaluation of the anterior and posterior rotator cuff, the capsule, and the labral elements. The superficial rotators and the neurovascular bundle are also well demonstrated. Oblique sagittal plane images (parallel to the glenoid) could also be obtained. These images provide a cross-section of the cuff tendons in the lateral to medial direction.

The use of MR contrast material has been reported in evaluation of various joints. While this is an interesting concept, several drawbacks exist. The contrast agent most commonly employed, Gadolinium DTPA, is rather costly. The procedure requires insertion of a needle into the joint under fluoroscopy before transferring the patient to the MR room. This eliminates one advantage of MR imaging of the joint, that is, its noninvasive nature. If injection is intended one may continue to employ CT arthrography of the shoulder.

An historical review of pilot reports on MR imaging of the shoulder that addresses the structures visualized by imaging in various planes may be summarized as follows.

Huber et al,[54] in an early report on MRI of the shoulder, suggested that the rotator cuff is most usefully imaged on coronal and sagittal views.

Middleton et al[80] studied normal MR anatomy of the shoulders of six volunteers. They found that the deltoid was the most prominent structure, could be identified in all planes, and was easily distinguishable from the rotator cuff because of an interspace of fat in which the subdeltoid bursa and the coracoacromial ligament are identified. They detected the rotator cuff tendons most easily in the coronal and sagittal planes, as did Huber.[54]

Seeger et al[115] report that the coracoclavicular ligaments, acromioclavicular joint, and superior humeral head articular cartilage are well seen in the coronal plane. They indicate that the sagittal plane reveals the horizontal axis of the acromion and its relationship to the supraspinatus tendon, while the oblique plane shows the supraspinatus muscle and tendon in continuity and their relationship to the acromion and acromioclavicular joint.

According to Seeger et al[114] the low signal glenoid labrum is well depicted with axial scanning, and with internal rotation the anterior labrum is larger at all levels than the posterior labrum. It is demarcated from the adjacent capsule and cuff by a thin rim of medium to high intensity produced by synovial folds within the cavity.

Kieft et al[57] devised an "anatomically shaped surface coil." They indicate the most advantageous planes for viewing the various structures of the shoulder are as follows:

1. *Axial plane*—best for the biceps tendon, glenohumeral joint, articular surfaces, glenoid labrum, and neurovascularbundle
2. *Oblique plane*—(perpendicular to the glenoid) best for the rotator cuff, glenohumeral joint, and acromioclavicular joint
3. *Sagittal plane*—best for the neurovascular bundle and for staging bone tumors

With the technique presently employed in MR examination of the shoulder, the normal anatomy may be seen in one, two, or three planes with an excellent resolution. The rotator cuff tendons and the glenoid labrum are well visualized (see Fig. 4-46). The central aspect of the cuff tendons are entirely devoid of signal, while the intervening regions show medium signal intensity. Also these tendons may each have several components separated by septae and adding to the complexities of generated signals.[80] However, the distal aspect of the supraspinatus tendon that is most susceptible to pathologic conditions is more uniform. The pathologic changes of the rotator cuff tendons are depicted as areas of inhomogeneous signals derived from the inflammatory reaction or obvious interruption of the tendon, in cases of tendon tear[63] (Figs. 4-47 and 4-48). Seeger et al[116] studied 107 symptomatic shoulders and diagnosed impingement in 53. Three types of impingement signs were recognized: type I—subacromial bursitis; type IIa—supraspinatus tendinitis; and type IIb—tendonitis with areas of tendon disruption. While complete tears of the rotator cuff were all accurately diagnosed (18/18), partial tears were missed by MRI. The glenoid labrum is similarly visualized as a signal void outlined by signal derived from surrounding elements (hyaline articular cartilage of the glenoid and humeral head and the small amounts of joint fluid covering the joint surfaces). The pathologic changes of the labrum are determined mostly on the basis of abnormal contours, relations to the glenoid margin, and areas of abnormal signal intensity (Figs. 4-49 and 4-50).

Kieft et al[58] studied 13 patients with recurrent anterior dislocation with both MRI and CT arthrography. MRI accurately identified all Hill-Sachs lesions and glenoid rim fractures. Only one labral pathology was not accurately identified. Capsular alterations and insertional stripping were poorly visualized on MRI unless large joint effusions were present. Seeger et al[115] also studied 35 shoulders with recurrent anterior dislocations and subluxations. In the 20 cases with surgical documentation, all labral abnormalities and humeral head defects found had been accurately depicted by MRI.

Current Status

The authors must emphasize to the reader that MRI of the shoulder is merely in its infancy. Furthermore, the greater technical demands of imaging this joint, which is eccentrically placed within the magnet, and which has so many diverse structures within a small area, curtail the accuracy of pathology depiction in comparison to other peripheral joints. Similarly, while there is already a plethora of articles about MRI of the knee, there is virtually only a handful of articles pertaining to imaging of the shoulder.

So far, at least, there has been adequate documentation about the normal MR anatomy of the shoulder.[115] Pathologic changes defining characteristics of the capsulotendinous elements have also been published, and reports regarding impingement, cuff arthropathy, and labral pathology have recently appeared in the literature.* Despite the availability of other well-established and reasonably accurate imaging modalities, such as conventional and CT arthrography, it would appear that MRI has much to offer, even in its formative stages of development. However, its true diagnostic impact must await refinements in technique and more extensive and comparative clinical studies.

---

*References 46, 58, 64, 114-116.

A

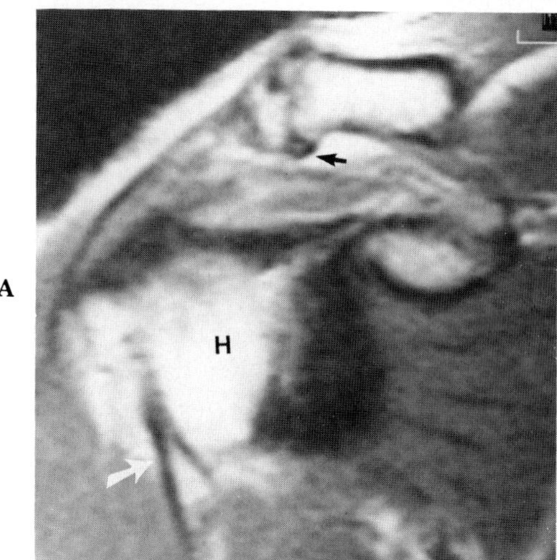

B

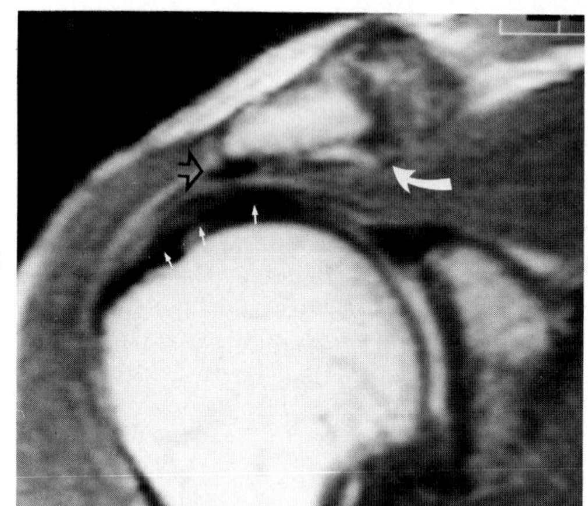

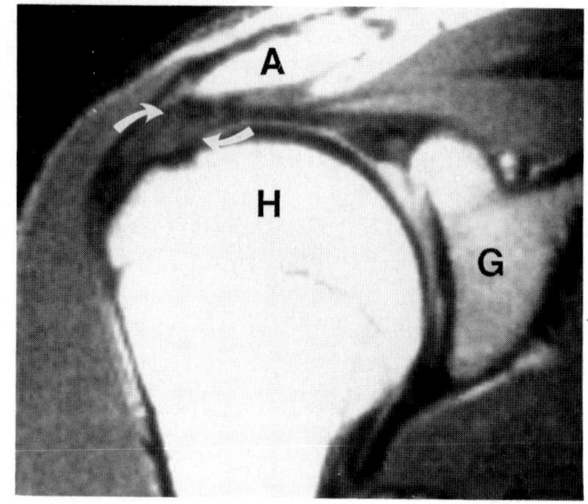

C

FIG. 4-47. Impingement syndrome and rotator cuff tendonitis. **A** and **B,** MR images of the right shoulder in anatomic coronal plane; **A** is anterior (medial) to **B. A,** This coronal image is at the most anterior aspect of the joint, with the humeral head *(H)* and the long-head of the biceps tendon *(white arrow)* visualized. There is an inferiorly pointing osteophyte of the AC joint *(black arrow).* **B,** This section through the supraspinatus muscle and tendon again demonstrates degenerative manifestations of the AC joint with hypertrophic changes *(curved arrow)* impinging upon the musculotendinous junction. Also an area of hypertrophic change is present at the periphery of the acromion process *(hollow arrow).* The supraspinatus tendon has an inhomogeneous appearance with a linear area of increased signal along its length *(small arrows).* This is indicative of tendonitis and may also indicate interstitial tendon tear. There is no complete tendon tear demonstrated. **C,** MR image of the right shoulder in the anatomic coronal plane. There is marked swelling of the distal aspect of the supraspinatus tendon (distance between *curved arrows*). Also the peribursal fat is obliterated indicating subacromial-subdeltoid bursitis. *A,* Acromion. *G,* Glenoid, *H,* Humeral head.

Certainly, on the basis of the clinical studies thus far available and our experience, it is evident that the most osseous, bursal, and tendinous manifestations of mechanical impingement can be detected. Our experience with MR scanning at 1.5 Tesla has shown a sensitivity of greater than 92% in detection of partial or complete cuff tears. At this time some partial or small complete tears of the rotator cuff may not be accurately differentiated from one another or from tendonitis. However, MR has the capability of detecting certain lesions that are usually not detectable by shoulder arthrography such as intratendinous or bursal surface partial tears or full-thickness tears that are sealed by the synovial lining of the joint.

Thus far, clinical experience suggests that lesions of the glenoid labrum are detectable by MRI, but sometimes without the clarity with which they are seen by CT arthrography. The capsular lesions associated with instability are less well visualized. It is not likely that the sensitivity and accuracy of MRI in detecting labral lesions will approach that of CT arthrography in the very near future, unless the joint is distended by fluid or an MRI contrast agent.

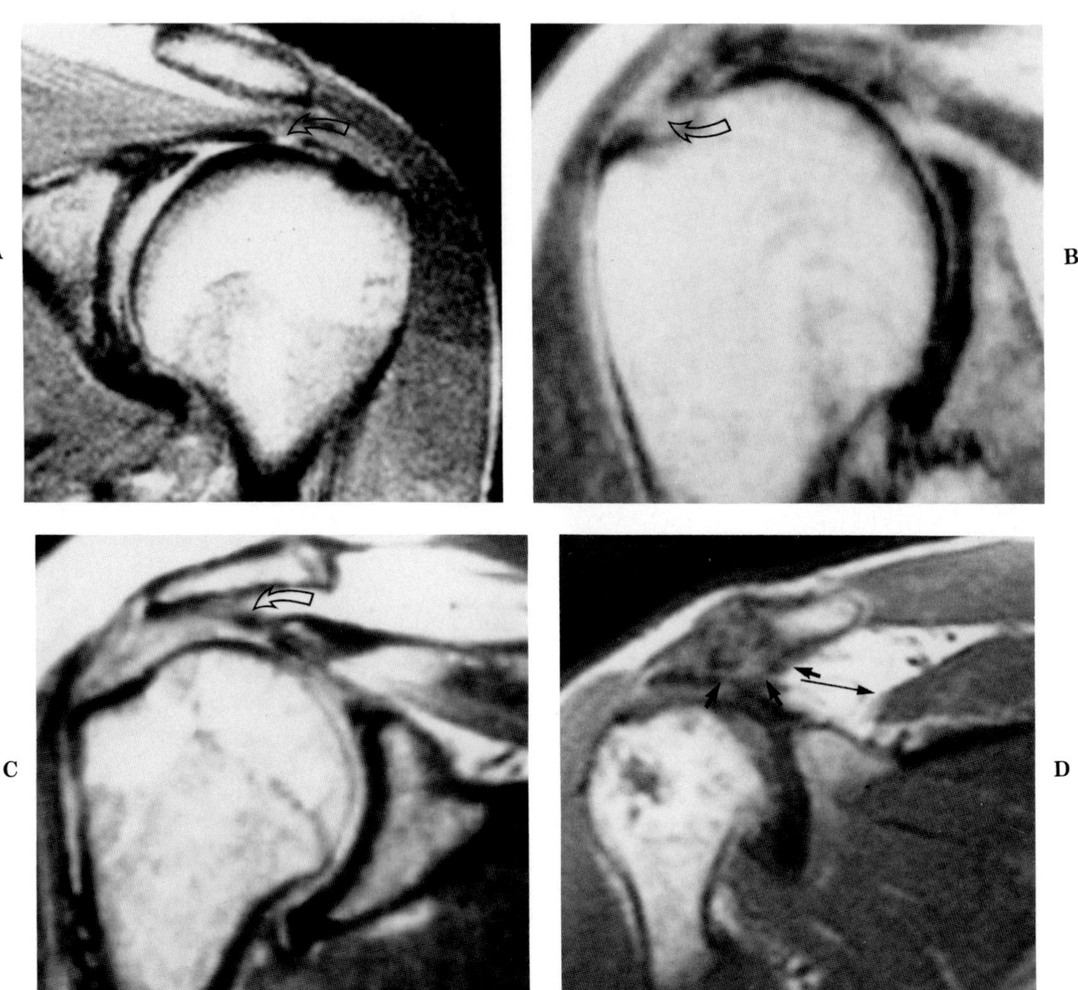

FIG. 4-48. Advanced impingement and various rotator cuff tears. **A,** Partial cuff tear. MR image of the left shoulder in the anatomic coronal plane in a 20-year-old football player. A small defect of the inferior surface of the supraspinatus tendon is demonstrated (*arrow*). **B,** Small full-thickness tear. MR image of the right shoulder in anatomic coronal plane. A small defect at the tuberosity insertion of the supraspinatus tendon is visualized extending from the bursal to the synovial surfaces (*arrow*). **C,** Large cuff tear. MR image of the right shoulder in anatomic coronal plane. There is a large defect of the supraspinatus tendon, which shows marked degeneration of its torn and retracted margin (*arrow*). **D,** Massive chronic rotator cuff tear. There is superior migration of the humeral head with no recognizable tendinous structures seen within the markedly diminished subacromial space. The retracted and atrophic supraspinatus muscle is seen in the supraspinatus fossa (*long arrow*). The articular aspects of the AC joint are irregular and prominent because of degenerative disease (*short arrows*).

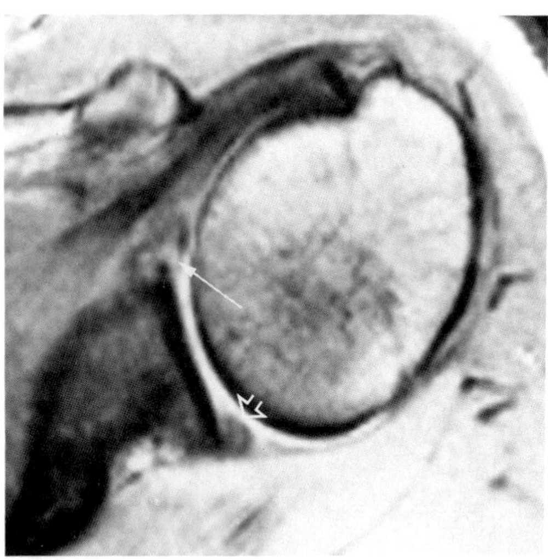

FIG. 4-49. Glenoid labrum tear. Axial MR images of the left shoulder at the proximal aspect of the glenohumeral joint. There is an abnormal configuration of the anterior glenoid labrum, which is separated from the glenoid margin with an area of increased signal intensity *(solid arrow)*. This indicates tear and detachment. The posterior labrum has a normal configuration, but demonstrates normal signal intensity *(hollow arrow)*. This is indicative of partial tear.

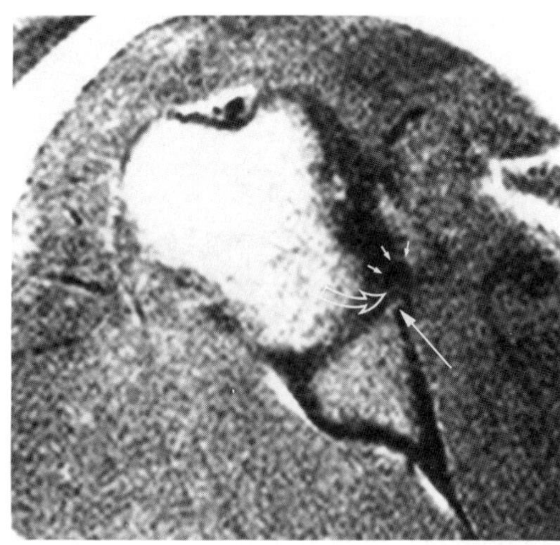

FIG. 4-50. Anterior shoulder instability. Recurrent subluxation in an 18-year-old tennis player. MR image of the right shoulder at the inferior aspect of the glenoid. The anterior glenoid margin is flattened, and there is outgrowth of bone along the plane of the glenoid articular survace *(long arrow)*. The glenoid labrum, which is relatively normal in contour *(short arrows)*, is totally detached from the deformed glenoid margin *(curved arrow)*.

The basic advantages offered by MRI for the shoulder at this time are that it is noninvasive and provides a comprehensive, multiplanar evaluation of the joint, which can detect a moderate quantity of pathologic changes. Its most promising diagnostic advantage over other roentgenographic techniques is its ability to demonstrate, at once, the collective components of impingement. Its principal disadvantage is its high cost.

ULTRASONOGRAPHY

Ultrasonography is another technique that is noninvasive to patients. It is most valuable in the evaluation of the rotator cuff. The difficult learning curve needed for reliable interpretation has undoubtedly been a deterrent to the popularity of shoulder ultrasonography. As pointed out by Balogh et al[3] ultrasonography, like MRI, may be studied in all planes, and the use of a "real-time" probe permits almost a cine-evaluation of evolving echogenicity in the study of tendon damage. Studies such as those of Pattee and Snyder[94] attest to the efficacy of ultrasonography as an excellent screener for suspected cuff tears of both full and partial thickness. In their study of patients by ultrasonography, arthrography, and arthroscopy, they found that nearly 80% of cuff tears discovered arthroscopically were detected by ultrasonography. While the arthrogram detected full-thickness tears with an 80% sensitivity, its sensitivity for partial tears was only 50%. Only 12 of 20 patients with negative arthrograms had negative sonograms.

Physics of Ultrasound

Sound waves are vibrations of gases, liquids, or solids that are quantitated in terms of Hertz(Hz), the international unit of frequency, equal to one cycle per second. Those in the range of 20 to 20,000 Hz are audible to the human ear. Sound vibrations below 20 Hz are termed "subsonic" and those above 20,000 Hz are termed "ultrasonic." Frequencies 1 to 15 million Hz or megaHertz(MHz) are used for medical diagnostic ultrasonography.

Since acoustic waves of sufficiently high frequency can be made to travel in a beam with little spreading, such a beam can explore a physical medium and detect inhomogeneities by reflection (echo). Ultrasonography is the technical procedure in which the transmitted and reflected properties of an ultrasound beam are imaged and recorded after passage through a particular area of the body. An ultrasound beam travels through tissue at a fixed rate, and thus the distance traveled by the beam and echo, when imaged, indicates

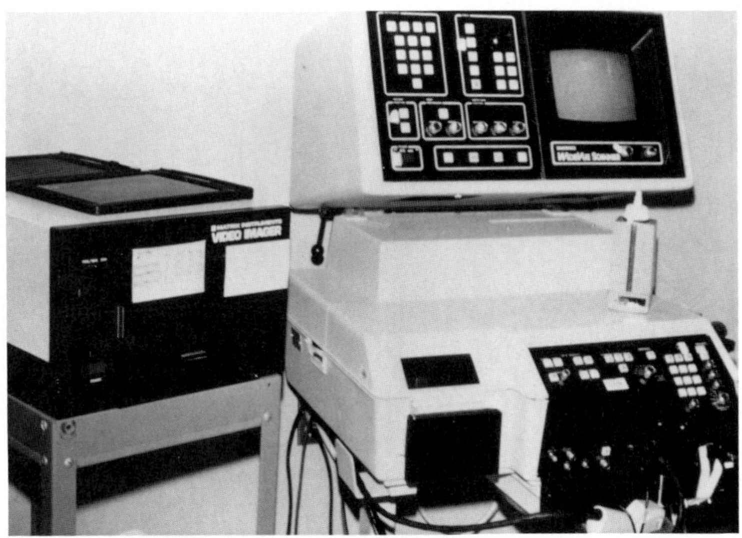

FIG. 4-51. Real-time small parts mechanical sector scanner with 10 MHz transducer

the proportional distances between the structures traversed.

When an ultrasound beam is transmitted through a medium and strikes a second medium of altered density, a portion of the energy is reflected at the tissue boundary (interface) while the remaining energy penetrates the second medium. Diagnostic data are obtained by imaging the echoes at tissue boundaries. The interfaces relevant to the study of the rotator cuff are those between the differing soft tissue media of the deltoid muscle, rotator cuff, and bony humerus.

Technique

A real-time mechanic sector scanner employing a 7.5 or 10 MHz transducer is most often used (Fig. 4-51). A patient is scanned while seated with the humerus resting against the patient's side or slightly extended and in neutral or slight external rotation.

In this position, the region of insertion of the supraspinatus tendon into the greater tuberosity of the humerus lies uncovered anterior and lateral to the shadowing effect of the acromion process, exposing to the transducer the "critical zone" of vascularity where most rotator cuff ruptures occur.[105] The more proximal portion of the rotator cuff beneath the acromion process may be exposed by shrugging the shoulder and occasionally by simultaneously extending the humerus at the glenohumeral joint. The more lateral and posterior portions are uncovered by internal rotation of the humerus.

The bicipital groove and greater tuberosity are used as landmarks for localizing the supraspinatus tendon, which is scanned in the longitudinal (sagittal) and transverse planes (Figs. 4-52 and 4-53). Emphasis is placed on the anterior or supraspinatus portion of the cuff since most tears occur in this area, but the more posterior portions containing the tendinous insertions of the infraspinatus and teres minor should also be routinely scanned. Most investigators image the subscapularis only when clinical suspicion points to this area. The intraarticular and extraarticular portions of the tendon of the long head of the biceps, including the bicipital groove of the humerus, are scanned in the transverse plane (Fig. 4-54). The tendon is also imaged in the longitudinal plane along its long axis.[20,75,78-80] (Fig. 4-55).

Normal Ultrasonographic Anatomy

Rotator Cuff

The relevant anatomy of the shoulder region is easily imaged and compared with the opposite member for diagnostic purposes. The rotator cuff appears as a well-marginated band of homogenous echogenicity between the humeral head below and the deltoid muscle above. Acoustic shadowing from the acromion establishes the limit of visualization medially, while distally the aponeurosis of the rotator cuff tapers in two directions, laterally into its bony insertion as well as posteriorly.

The rotator cuff band is bordered superiorly and inferiorly by echogenic lines of higher amplitude. The superficial line marks the interface of the deltoid muscle and rotator cuff and identifies the location of the subdeltoid bursa, which in its normal nondistended state

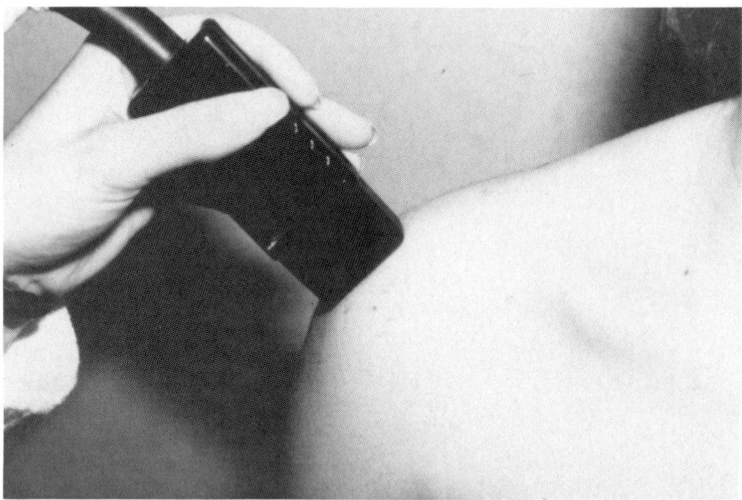

FIG. 4-52. Transducer aligned in the longitudinal (sagittal) plane of the supraspinatus tendon

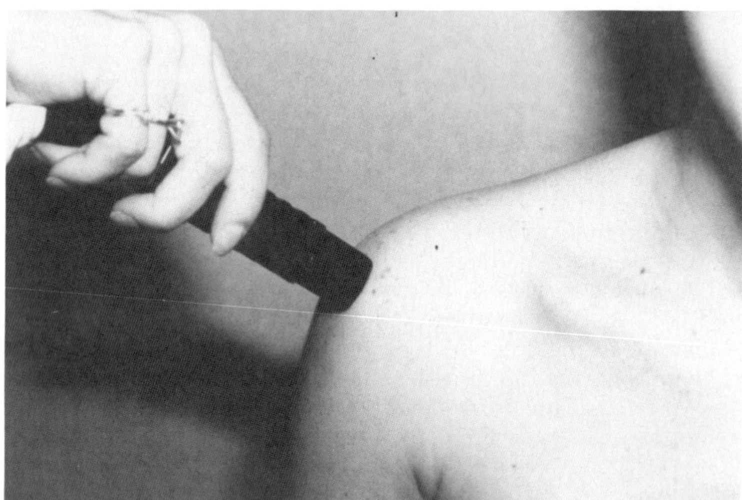

FIG. 4-53. Transducer aligned in the transverse plane of the supraspinatus tendon

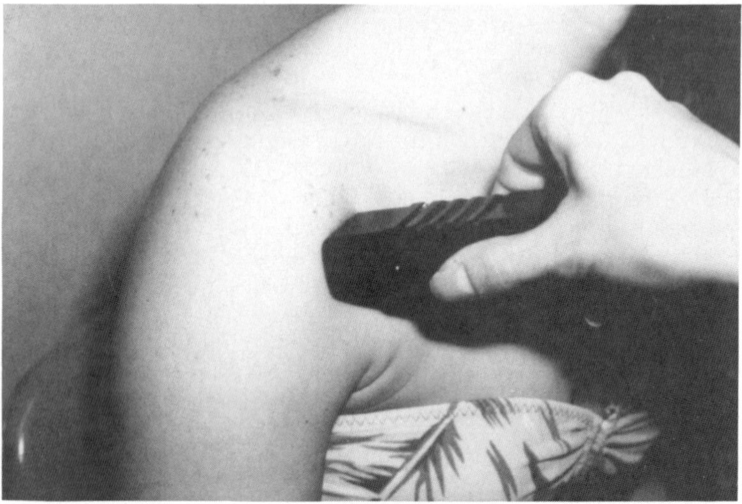

FIG. 4-54. Transducer aligned in the transverse plane of the tendon of the long head of the biceps

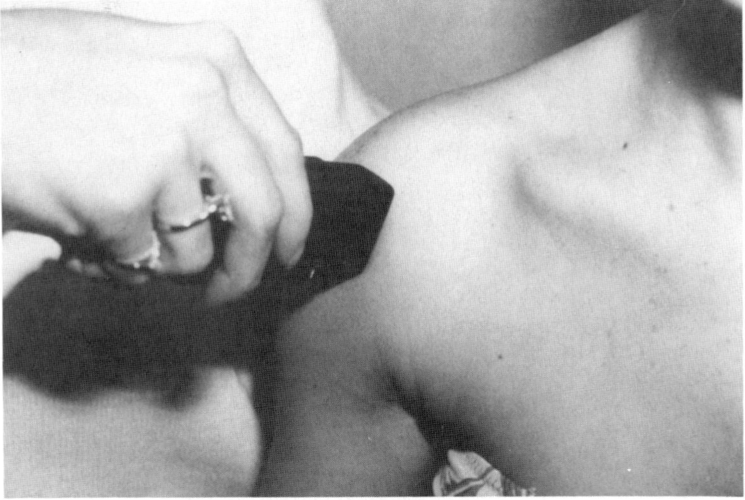

FIG. 4-55. Transducer aligned in the longitudinal (sagittal) plane of the tendon of the long head of the biceps

is not resolved as a separate structure. The deep echogenic line results from reflections at the proximal humerus.

The average thickness of the anterior cuff is 6 mm and the posterior cuff 3.6 mm.[20] In most instances, the rotator cuff band is thicker than the deltoid, which tends to diminish somewhat beyond the sixth decade of life. Physiologic age-related cuff thinning is represented sonographically as a homogenous although hypoechoic band, which is symmetrical with the opposite side. Increased gain settings may be used to evaluate its internal characteristics. While focal inhomogeneities can occur in normal subjects, the echogenicity of the rotator cuff is relatively homogenous and equal to or brighter than that of the suprajacent deltoid (Figs. 4-56 to 4-60). Comparison with the opposite side allows abnormalities to be differentiated from the physiologic reduced echogenicity seen in the elderly.

Biceps Tendon

On transverse scan the tendon of the long head of the biceps appears as an echogenic ellipse within the bicipital groove of the humerus. More proximally the tendon is found adjacent to the humeral head delineated superiorly and posteriorly by the supraspinatus and inferiorly and anteriorly by the subscapularis (see Fig. 4-59). On longitudinal scans the tendon appears as a narrow band of tissue between the humerus and deep surface of the deltoid. Its echogenicity is greater than that of the deltoid muscle (see Fig. 4-60).[77-79]

Abnormal Ultrasonographic Anatomy

Rotator Cuff

When the ultrasonic evaluation of the symptomatic shoulder is considered equivocal, the imaged asymptomatic side acts as a control providing a comparison with normal. Major diagnostic criteria for rotator cuff rupture have been established; they include the following.*

Focal thinning. Focal thinning of the rotator cuff is considered a very reliable sign of rupture with a reported 100% predictive value.[79] While isolated tears in the posterior aspect of the rotator cuff are uncommon, suspected pathologic posterior thinning can be differentiated from normal posterior thinning by the presence of an abrupt transition between the normal and abnormal portions of the cuff. Pathologic thinning is almost always more pronounced than physiologic tapering and symmetry is lost with the normal opposite side. Further, normal-appearing cuff tissue is not seen in an area of pathologic thinning (Figs. 4-61 and 4-62).

The intact portions of the tendons maintain the thickness of the tendon plane in smaller or incomplete tears, but the low-level echogenicity of normal tendon is replaced by high level echoes, resulting from the many fibrous interfaces in the bursal proliferations.

An uncommon pattern of sonographic abnormality is represented as a factitious irregular thickening of the cuff with foci of in-

*References 10, 19-21, 75, 76-79.

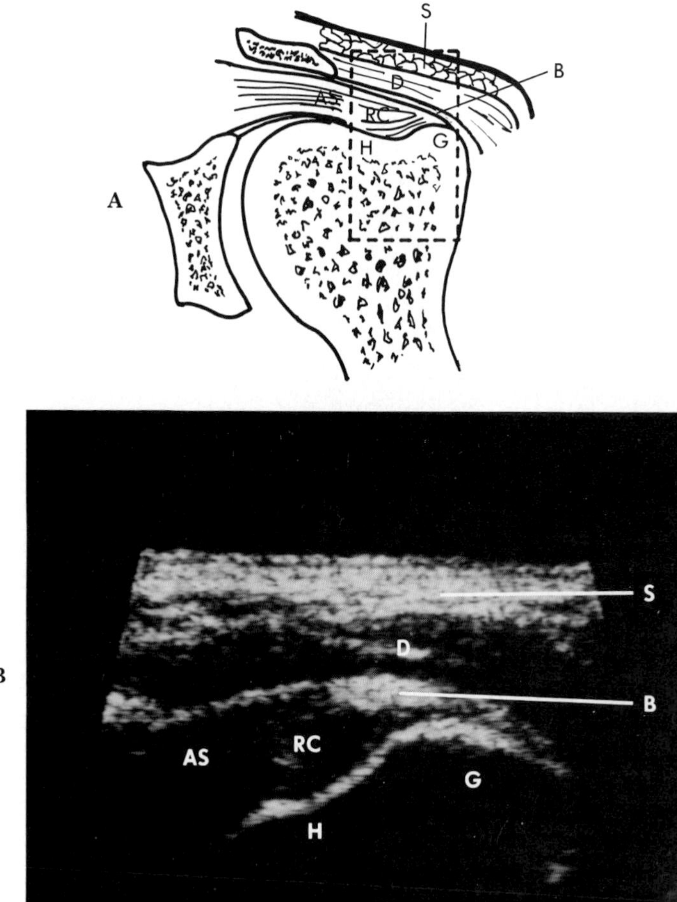

FIG. 4-56. Schematic **(A)** and sonographic **(B)** representations of the normal shoulder as seen in the longitudinal (sagittal) plane. *S*, subcutaneous fat; *D*, deltoid muscle; *B*, echogenic line marking deltoid and rotator cuff interface and the location of the subdeltoid bursa (normally not imaged as a distinct structure); *AS*, area of acromion shadowing; *RC*, rotator cuff tendon; *H*, humerus; *G*, greater tuberosity. Note relative thickness and echogenicity of deltoid and rotator cuff images.

creased and decreased echogenicity. The thickened appearance is caused by hypertrophied bursal elements, which are sonographically inseparable from the tendon undergoing degenerative change in the region of the tear (Fig. 4-63).

Nonvisualization. In large tears in which the torn edge of the rotator cuff retracts under the acromion, ultrasonography demonstrates close apposition of the deep surface of the deltoid muscle to the entire humeral head (Fig. 4-64). Complete nonvisualization has also been reported to carry a 100% predictive value for diagnosing rotator cuff tears.[80]

Focal discontinuity. Small areas of discontinuity are more difficult to interpret and provide a source of false-positive sonograms because of the presence of echogenic inhomogeneities seen in normal subjects (Fig. 4-65). This finding is more reliable when the discontinuity is large, well defined, and clearly asymmetric when compared with the opposite side. When the edge of the tendon is visible it may appear as a simple termination of the normal tendon or a hyperechoic and thickened border; at times it tapers toward the torn edge (Fig. 4-66).

A normal area of discontinuity is present on transverse scans between the intraarticular portion of the tendon of the long head of the biceps and the adjacent supraspinatus. This can be differentiated from a tear by first imaging the biceps tendon extraarticularly in the intertubercular groove of the humerus and following it proximally over the humeral head. This strict delineation of the biceps tendon

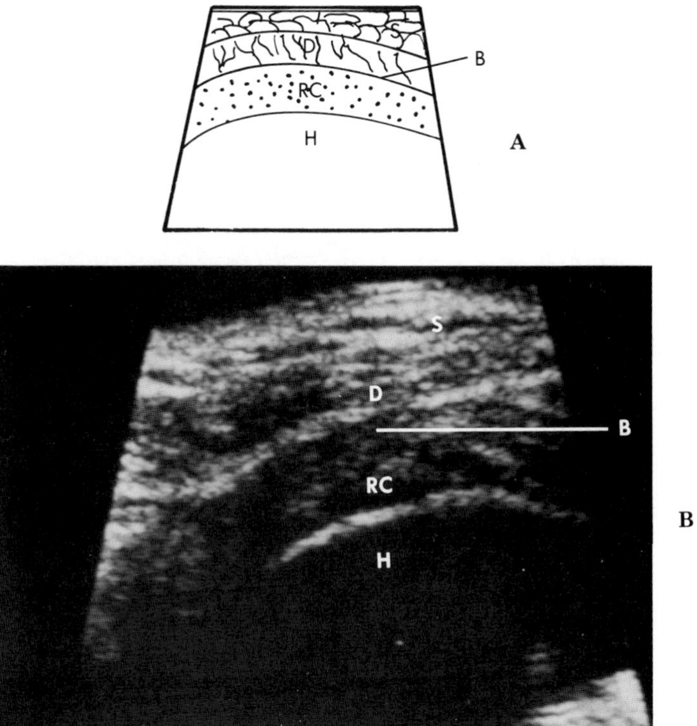

FIG. 4-57. Schematic **(A)** and sonographic **(B)** representations of the normal shoulder as seen in the transverse plane. Same keys as Fig. 5-56.

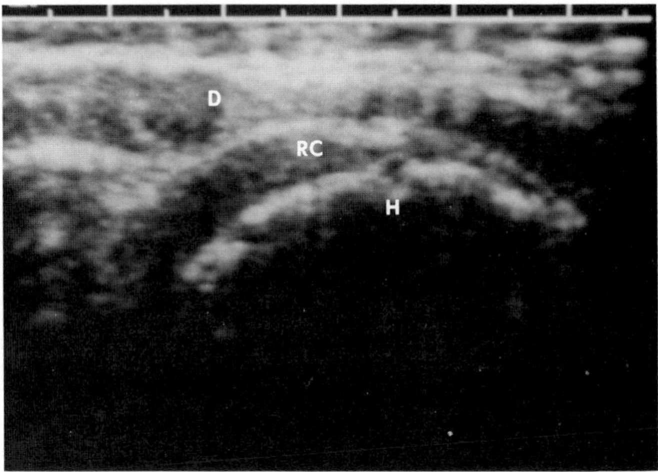

FIG. 4-58. Transverse scan in an asymptomatic subject demonstrating normal posterior thinning of rotator cuff. **D,** deltoid; *RC*, rotator cuff; *H*, humerus.

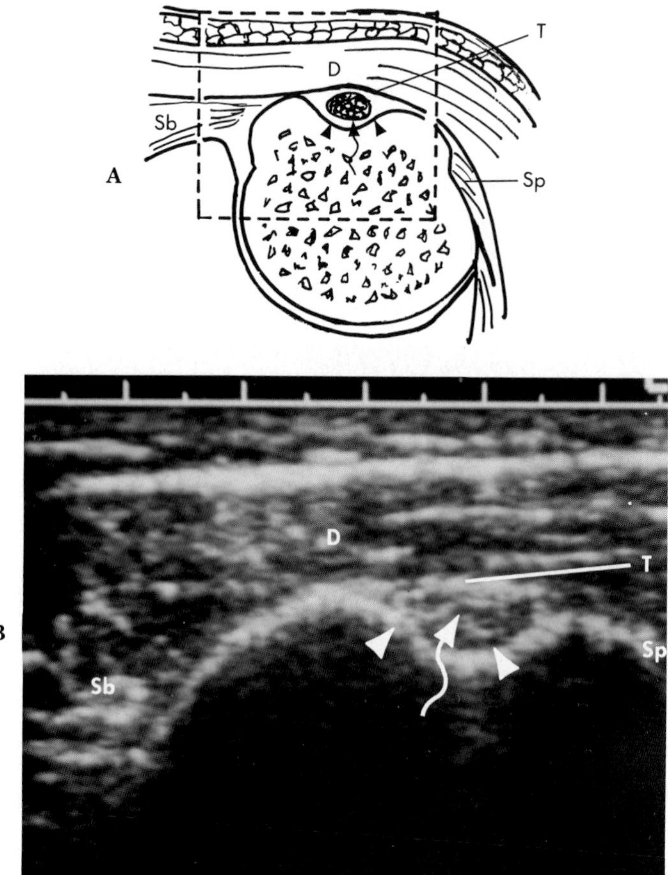

FIG. 4-59. Schematic **(A)** and transverse sonographic **(B)** representations of the normal tendon of the long head of the biceps in the bicipital groove of the humerus. *D*, deltoid; *T*, transverse humeral ligament; *Sb*, subscapularis; *Sp*, supraspinatus. *Arrowheads*, bicipital groove; *Curved arrow*, bicipital tendon; *H*, humerus.

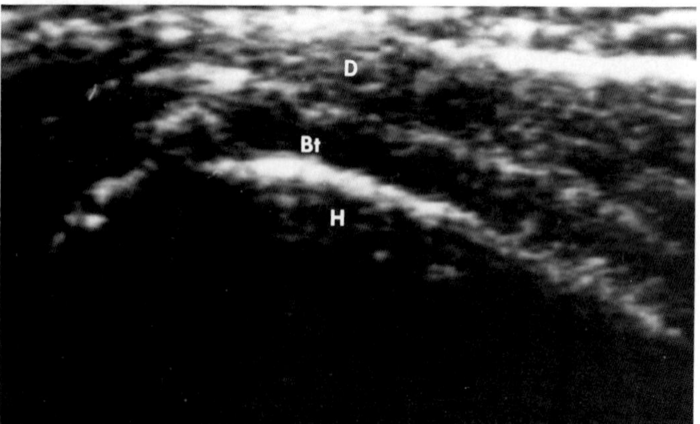

FIG. 4-60. Longitudinal scan showing tendon of the long head of the biceps between the humerus and deep surface of the deltoid. *D*, deltoid; *RC*, rotator cuff; *H*, humerus.

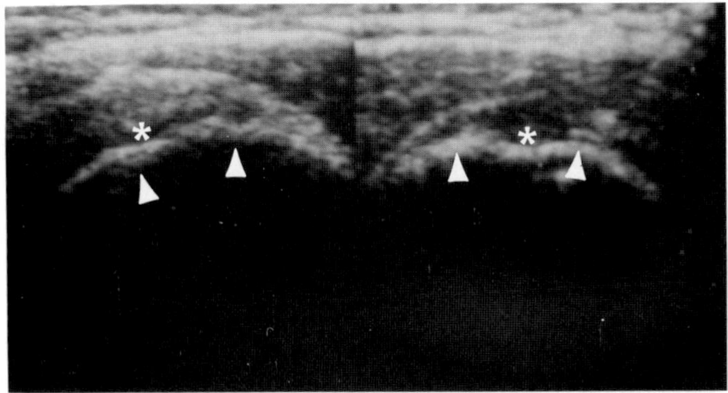

FIG. 4-61. Bilateral transverse sonograms in patient with right rotator cuff tear. Note marked thinning and absence of normal appearing cuff tissue on right. *Star* (*), rotator cuff; *Arrowheads*, humerus.

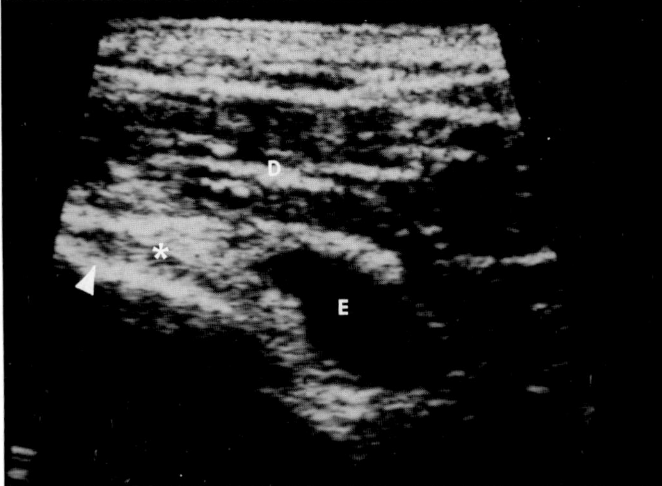

FIG. 4-62. Tranverse sonogram in a patient with complete rupture of the rotator cuff demonstrating markedly thinned and hyperechoic cuff tissue and effusion. *Star* (*), thinned hyperechoic cuff tissue; *E*, effusion; *Arrowheads*, humerus; *D*, deltoid.

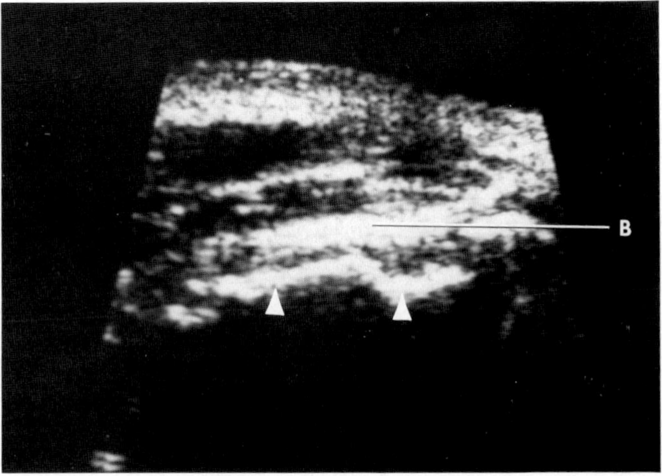

FIG. 4-63. Longitudinal scan in patient with complete rotator cuff rupture demonstrating bursal hypertrophy and marked thinning of rotator cuff. **B,** bursal hypertrophy; *Arrowheads*, humerus.

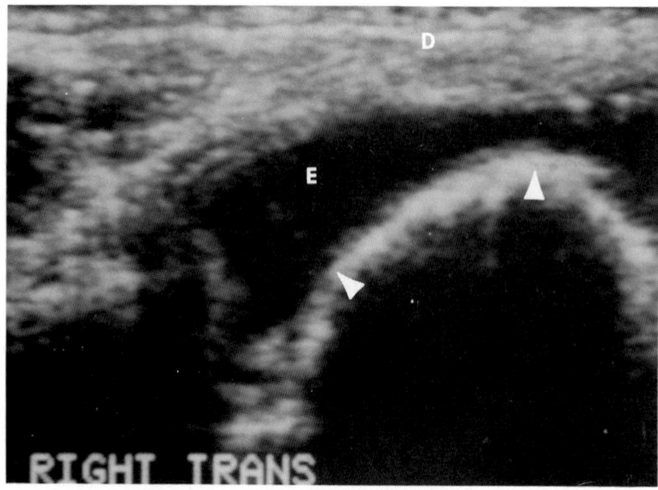

FIG. 4-64. Transverse sonogram demonstrating complete nonvisualization of rotator cuff in a patient with a large rupture that has retracted proximally. The deltoid is separated from the humeral head by a large effusion. *Arrowheads,* humerus; *E,* effusion; *D,* deltoid.

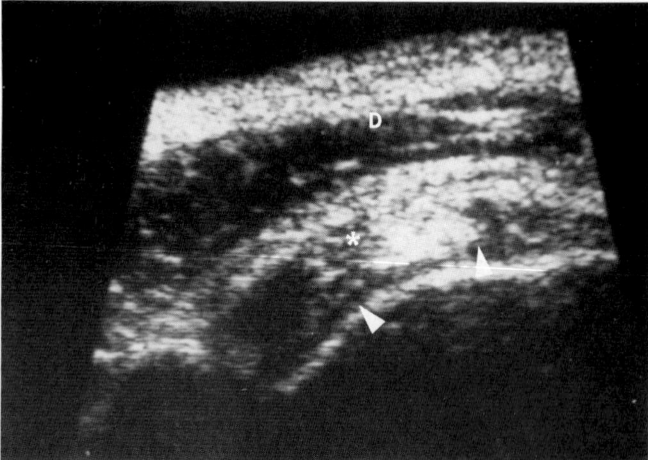

FIG. 4-65. Transverse sonogram in an asymptomatic shoulder revealing areas of echogenic inhomogeneity in the rotator cuff band. *D,* deltoid; *Star (*),* rotator cuff; *Arrowheads,* deltoid.

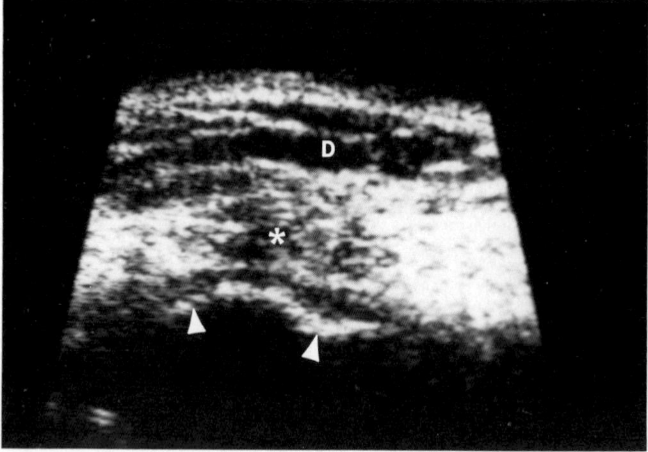

FIG. 4-66. Longitudinal sonogram demonstrating area of focal discontinuity in a patient with a moderate-sized cuff tear. *D,* deltoid; *Star (*),* area of focal discontinuity in rotator cuff band; *Arrowheads,* humerus.

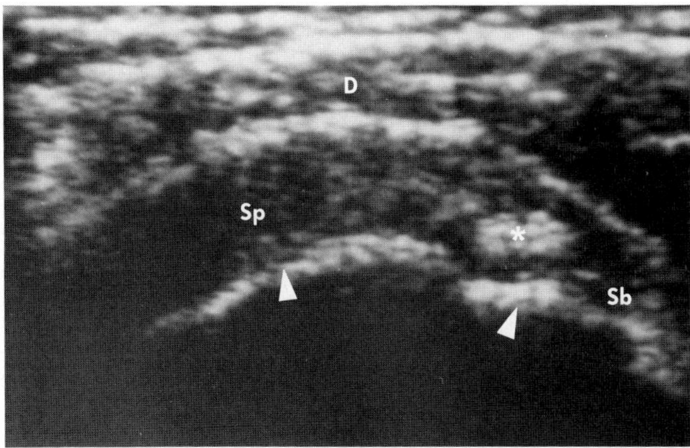

FIG. 4-67. Transverse sonogram demonstrating physiologic discontinuity surrounding intraarticular portion of biceps tendon. *D*, deltoid; *Sp*, supraspinatus; *X*, biceps tendon; *Sb*, subscapularis; *Arrowheads*, humerus.

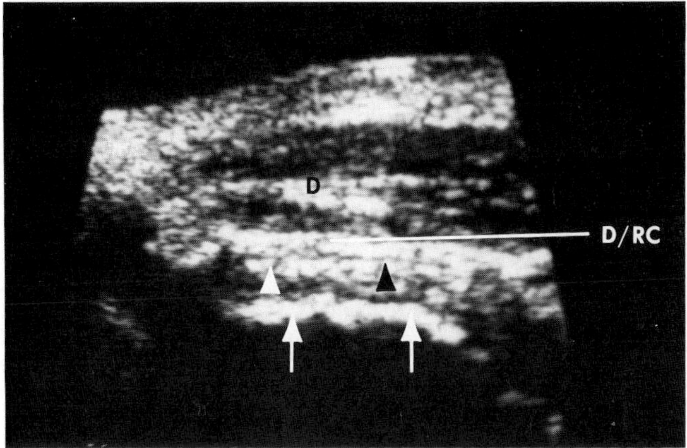

FIG. 4-68. Longitudinal sonogram in a patient with rotator cuff rupture demonstrating a central echogenic band that was not present on the opposite control. *D*, deltoid; *Arrowheads*, central echogenic band; *D/RC*, deltoid-rotator cuff interface; *Arrows*, humerus.

also serves to differentiate this portion of the normal shoulder anatomy from a hyperechogenic focus resulting from a cuff tear (Fig. 4-67).

Central echogenic bands. Granulation tissue and hypertrophied synovium filling the tear defect can result in the presence of a hyperechogenic band replacing the normal homogenous echogenicity of the rotator cuff. Close comparison with the opposite side is mandatory since echogenic bands may occur in normal shoulders (Fig. 4-68).

The presence of calcareous lesions in the rotator cuff must be determined by study of routine roentgenograms, since such deposits will produce hyperechogenic foci (Fig. 4-69).

Nonspecific changes. Abnormal findings such as joint or bursal fluid, atrophy of the deltoid, and bursal hypertrophy, while not bearing a consistent association with rotator cuff tears or other shoulder lesions, do nonetheless bolster one's confidence that the shoulder has pathologic changes.

Biceps Tendon

Effusion. Effusions of the sheath of the tendon of the long head of the biceps appear on transverse scans as a penumbral area of decreased echogenicity (Fig. 4-70) and are often associated with other pathologic entities afflicting the glenohumeral joint, the most common being tears of the rotator cuff. Other lesions reported in association with effusions of the tendon sheath include adhesive capsulitis, fractures of the glenoid, osteochondral loose bodies, and subacromial fibrosis.[79]

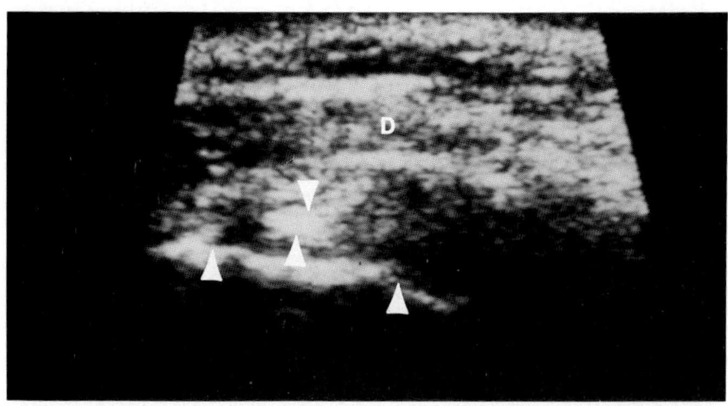

FIG. 4-69. Longitudinal scan in a patient demonsrating a hyperechogenic focus in the rotator cuff band caused by an area of calcific tendonitis. *D*, deltoid; Arrowheads, hyperechogenic focus (calcific deposit); *Arrows*, humerus.

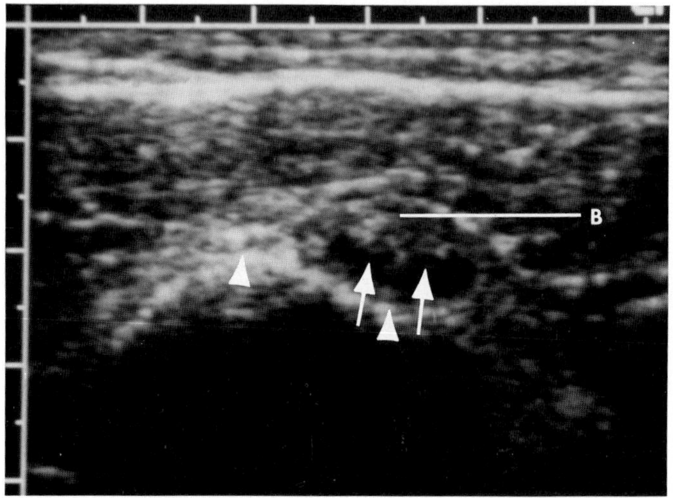

FIG. 4-70. Tranverse scan of the bicipital groove demonstrating an effusion of the bicipital sheath appearing as an area of hypogenicity situated between the floor of the bicipital groove and the biceps tendon. The patient had a complete rotator cuff rupture. *B*, biceps tendon; *Wavy arrows*, effusion; *Arrowheads*, humerus.

Nonvisualization. Nonvisualization of the biceps tendon from its humeral groove suggests dislocation or rupture; tendon sheath effusion and asymmetric hyperechoic foci within the tendon are indicative of chronic degenerative change.

Hyperechoic foci. Sonography can help delineate the site of biceps tendon rupture: visualization of the tendon within the groove places the rupture intraarticularly and allows for proper preoperative planning when surgery is anticipated (Fig. 4-71).

Loose bodies. Osteochondral loose bodies in the tendon sheath are likely to present as echogenic foci casting an acoustical shadow within a sheath effusion.

Advantages

Ultrasonography is quick, noninvasive, and painless and carries no risk of infection or allergic reaction. In most institutions its cost is only 75% or 80% that of an arthrogram and includes the routine investigation of the opposite shoulder with no morbidity.

Examination of the normal and abnormal biceps tendon is more readily and accurately accomplished with ultrasound than with contrast. Middleton et al[79] have reported considerably higher sensitivity, specificity, and accuracy values with ultrasonography when the two studies are compared.

Ultrasonography may be of greatest value in the detection of partial intersubstance ro-

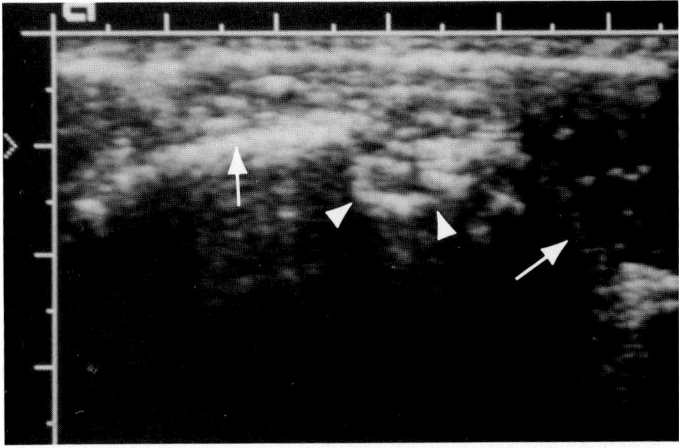

FIG. 4-71. Transverse scan of the bicipital groove in a patient with a proximal rupture of the tendon of the long head of the biceps. Scan reveals absence of the tendon from the groove, which contains echogenic fibrous tissue. *Arrowheads*, bicipital groove; *Arrows*, humerus.

tator cuff tears, which are often not visualized by standard arthrography.

Dynamic ultrasonographic imaging may add a new dimension to the motion study of normal and abnormal rotator cuff mechanics. These studies have shown the normal rotator cuff to glide smoothly beneath the coracoacromial arch during its excursion and suggest that the coracoacromial ligament functions as a pulley, guiding the superior rotator cuff and changing the direction and degree of the cuff indentation in abduction. Abnormal cuff mechanics have been demonstrated as a buckling or hesitancy of the cuff beneath the coracoacromial arch during motion, which corresponds with the patient's complaints of impingement pain.[16,45]

Limitations

Ultrasonographic interpretation may be confused by altered anatomy secondary to large calcific deposits, bony deformity, or inferior subluxation of the glenohumeral joint.

In the presence of morbid obesity the transducer may not be capable of adequately penetrating to the level of the rotator cuff.

Ultrasonography of the postoperative rotator cuff is often confusing, since abnormal echogenicity resembling a tear in a patient who has not undergone surgery and distortion or absence of soft tissue planes about the tendon persist indefinitely. As rotator cuff tears enlarge, the appearance changes from that of an echogenic area to a gap or defect. The finding of an unequivocal defect in the rotator cuff tendon is the only reliable sign of a recurrent rotator cuff tear (Fig. 4-72).

When exaggerated anatomic variations render ultrasonographic interpretation difficult, arthrography is a more appropriate diagnostic tool.

Current Status

A review of available literature uncovers a paucity of original authors and lends mute testimony to the reality that ultrasonography of the rotator cuff and biceps tendon is a new technique not presently in widespread use. While ultrasonography appears to offer accurate data in the hands of an experienced few, it remains for many an investigational procedure of unproved merit.

Diagnostic accuracy and constancy are dependent on the clinician and rely in good measure on the correct anatomic placement of the transducer, underscoring the importance of an initial interdisciplinary collaboration to include cadaveric and intraoperative study of the rotator cuff and its environs.

Notwithstanding current limitations, recent developments in the application of ultrasonography to the study of the shoulder have fostered cautious optimism that it may replace arthrography as the primary screening test for the diagnosis of abnormalities of the rotator cuff and biceps tendon.

SUMMARY

The standard roentgenographic evaluation of the shoulder invariably includes anteroposterior views in internal and external rotation, and usually includes an axillary view. While these views will detect the preponderance of traumatic and nontraumtic osseous lesions,

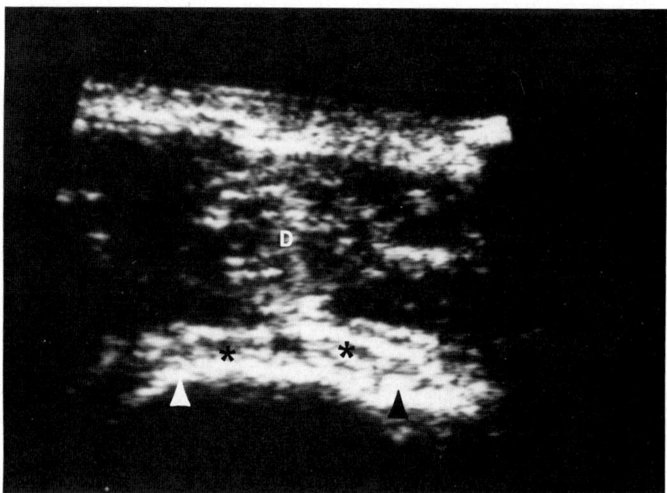

FIG. 4-72. Longitudinal scan in a patient with a recurrent rotator cuff tear. Rotator cuff band is absent and bursal elements lie opposed to the humeral head. *D*, deltoid; *Star* (*), bursal elements and granulation tissue; *Arrowheads*, humerus.

they often fail to detect posterior dislocations, certain scapular fractures, Hill-Sachs lesions, and the glenoid rim lesions of throwing and/or instability. Specialized views for the detection of these abnormalities have been reported. They include anterior (Y) and posterior oblique views, West Point and Ciullo axillary views, the Stryker notch, Hermodsson, and Didiee views. Some specialized views are of particular value for the assessment of the painful shoulder because they require no manipulation of the arm. Included among these views are the apical (craniocaudad) oblique, Velpeau, angle-up, and Stripp axial views. The anterior oblique and Didiee views each have a capability for the detection of both the Bankart and Hill-Sachs lesions of anterior instability. Conventional roentgenography is able to demonstrate evidence of only the intermediate or more advanced stages of subacromial impingement. To a large extent, this evidence is indistinguishable from that which is ascribable to cuff arthropathy.

Simple CT has a limited role in studying the shoulder. It has value in defining some bone tumors and in the clarification of certain fractures, such as those of the humeral head with multiple parts. It can be of value in the assessment of subluxations and fractures of the clavicular articulations, especially those with the sternum. On rare occasion, CT scapulometry is used to analyze version of the scapular neck. The analysis may be useful in the planning of surgical osteotomies for posterior glenohumeral instability. Anecdotally, it should be indicated that CT scapulometry appears to have some reliability in the confirmation of subcoracoid impingement.

Simple arthrography of the shoulder remains a standard for the evaluation of full-thickness and inferior surface tears of the rotator cuff. Its use has been reported for the evaluation of capsular and even labral abnormalities of instability. However, its capacities in this regard are not comparable to those of CT arthrography. Double contrast arthrography provides more information about cuff tear morphology than does the single contrast technique. It also tends to produce less post-procedural pain. The use of subacromial bursography has been sparsely reported to have value in the diagnosis of impingement and superior surface cuff tears. The benefits of the technique for these purposes are too limited, and technical demands are too exacting to ever allow bursography to become a popular procedure.

Arthropneumotomography can effectively demonstrate lesions of the labrum, but it is a less reliable, more time-consuming procedure than CT arthrography, and it imposes a greater quantity of radiation upon the patient. CT arthrography is presently the best roentgenographic procedure for demonstrating pathology of the capsulo-labral-osseous complexes. It demonstrates labral tears, Bankart lesions, abnormal capsular distensions and insertions, and even the directions of an instability. Yet it is relatively inefficacious in demonstrating pathologic changes of impingement other than cuff tears or degeneration. Cuff disease is probably better seen using direct sagittal rather than axial forms of CT arthrography.

While arthrography is the most commonly used procedure in the search for rotator cuff tears, the value of arthrography is largely limited to the demonstration of full-thickness types. It is invasive by virtue of the injection of contrast media and the need for radiation. Ultrasonogrphy, on the other hand, is a noninvasive, reliable screener of the rotator cuff. In expert hands, it offers the advantages of diagnosing partial as well as full-thickness tears without radiation or needles. The use of ultrasonography in the shoulder, however, has not become widespread; this procedure can only reveal pathologic conditions relative to the cuff; in addition, expertise in ultrasonographic interpretation of the shoulder is not rapidly developed.

Magnetic resonance imaging is the newest of the radiographic techniques. It is noninvasive and it provides images in multiple planes with equally good resolution. It can image virtually every structure and every tissue about the shoulder. In its present, formative stage of development, it is the diagnostic tool "most likely to succeed." It can demonstrate the labrum and the capsule, portraying abnormalities with less clarity of detail than CT arthrography. It can demonstrate most tears of the rotator cuff with good reliability. MRI can show subacromial bursitis and is a fairly reliable diagnostic study for impingement. In fact, there is no roentgenographic modality that is definitively diagnostic of this entity during its earlier stages. It is expected that the MRI will surpass all other roentgenographic methods for the accurate diagnosis of any shoulder pathology. Today, MRI stands as a noninvasive screener of shoulder lesions. Its inordinate expense has been a deterrent to its use. Extensive studies of accuracy, sensitivity, and specificity of shoulder MRI are conspicuously lacking in the literature.

In the early 1980s, arthroscopy of the shoulder was an infant procedure. Major pathologic states of the shoulder were treated by arthrotomy when surgery was indicated. By the middle 1980s, excisional arthroscopy (e.g., labral tear) and deimpingement were well established, and arthroscopically directed capsulorrhaphy for instability had been intiated. In the late 1980s arthroscopy has advanced to include acute capsulolabral repair and/or reconstruction, even before an instability is necessarily evident and the repair of some discrete cuff tears within the avascular zone. CT arthrography, with its detailing of cuff tears, labral disruptions, and directions of instability, has been a valued predictor and prognosticator of surgical needs. However, the sophistication of arthroscopic surgery may presently be progressing more rapidly than that of shoulder roentgenography. To determine whether to perform an arthroscopic procedure or to open a shoulder, whether a labrum is completely torn or simply detached, or whether an impingement is of sufficiently confined geography to be treated arthroscopically, the arthroscopist must use a roentgenographic procedure that is capable of spelling out the pathologic process in consummate detail. CT arthrography combined with MRI can offer sufficient detail in many cases, but not reliably in nearly all.

REFERENCES

1. Andren L, and Lundberg BJ: Treatment of rigid shoulders by joint distension during arthrography, Acta Orthop Scand 36(1):45, 1965.
2. Arndt JH, and Sears AD: Posterior dislocation of the shoulder, Am J Roentgenol 94:639, 1965.
3. Balogh, B et al: Sonoanatomy of the shoulder, Acta Anat 126:132, 1986.
4. Bankart ASB: Recurrent or habitual dislocation of the shoulder joint, Br Med J 2:1132-1133, 1923.
5. Bankart ASB: The pathology and treatment of recurrent dislocation of the shoulder joint, Br J Surg 26:23, 1938.
6. Beltran J et al: Rotator cuff lesions of the shoulder: evaluation by direct sagittal CT arthrography, Radiology 160(1):161, 1986.
7. Bloom MH, and Obata WG: Diagnosis of posterior dislocation of the shoulder with use of the Velpeau axillary and angle-up roentgenographic views, J Bone Joint Surg 49A(5):943, 1967.
8. Bost FC, and Inman VT: The pathological changes in recurrent dislocation of the shoulder: a report of Bankart's operative procedure, J Bone Joint Surg 24:595, 1942.
9. Braunstein EM, and O'Connor G: Double contrast arthrotomography of the shoulder, J Bone Joint Surg 64A(2):192, 1982.
10. Bretzke CA et al: Ultrasonography of the rotator cuff: normal and pathologic anatomy, Invest Radiol 20:311, 1985.
11. Calvert PT et al: Arthrography of the shoulder after operative repair of the torn rotator cuff, J Bone Joint Surg 68B:147, 1986.
12. Ciullo JV: Swimmer's shoulder, Clin Sports Med 5(1):115, 1986.
13. Ciullo JV, Koniuch MP, and Teitge RA: Axillary roentgenography in clinical orthopedic practice, Orthop Trans 6(3):451, 1982.
14. Cofield RH: Tears of rotator cuff, Mayo Clin Proc 258, 1980.
15. Cofield RH, and Simonet WT: Symposium on sports medicine. II. The shoulder in sports, Mayo Clin Proc 59(3):157, 1984.
16. Collins RA, Gristina AG, Carter RE: Ultrasonography of the shoulder: static and dynamic imaging, Orthop Clin North Am 18:351, 1987.

17. Cone RO III, Resnick D, and Danzig L: Shoulder impingement syndrome: radiographic evaluation, Radiology 150(1):29, 1984.
18. Cox J: Personal communication, 1989.
19. Crass JR et al: Ultrasonography of the rotator cuff: surgical correlation, J Clin Ultrasound 12:487, 1984.
20. Crass JR et al: Ultrasonography of the rotator cuff, Radiographics 5:941, 1985.
21. Crass JR, Craig EV, and Feinberg SB: Sonography of the postoperative rotator cuff, Am J Radiol 146:561, 1986.
22. Cyprien JM et al: Humeral retroversion and glenohumeral relationship in the normal shoulder and in recurrent anterior dislocation (scapulommetry), CORR 175 p. 8, May 1983.
23. Danzig L, Greenway G, and Resnick, D: The Hill-Sachs lesion, Am J Sports Med 8(5):328, 1980.
24. DeHaven JP et al: A prospective comparison study of double contrast CT arthrography and shoulder arthroscopy. Walter Reed Army Medical Center. Paper presented at the AOSS in San Francisco, January 1987.
25. DePalma AF: Surgery of the shoulder, ed 3, Philadelphia, 1983, JB Lippincott Co, p. 100.
26. DeSmet AA: Anterior oblique projection in radiogaphy of the traumatized shoulder, Am J Radiol 134:515, March 1980.
27. DeSmet AA: Axillary projection in radiography of the non-traumatized shoulder, Am J Radiol 134:511, March 1980.
28. Deutsch AL et al: Computed and conventional arthrotomography of the glenohumeral joint: normal anatomy and clinical experience, Radiology 153:603, 1984.
29. Deutsch AL, Resnick D, and Mink JH: Computed tomography of the glenohumeral and sternoclavicular joints, Orthop Clin N Am 16(3):497, 1985.
30. Didiee J: Le radiodiagnostic dans la luxation recidivante de l'epaule, J Radiol Electrol 14:209, 1930.
31. El-Khoury GY et al: Arthrotomography of the glenoid labrum, Radiology 131:333, May 1979.
32. Ellman H, Hanker G, and Bayer M: Repair of the rotator cuff, J Bone Joint Surg 68A(8):1136, 1986.
33. Eve FS: A case of subcoracoid dislocation of the humerus with formation of an indentation on the posterior surface of the head, Medico-Chir Trans Soc (London) 63:317, 1880.
34. Flower WN: On the pathological changes produced in the shoulder joint by traumatic dislocation, as derived from an examination of all the specimens illustrating this injury in the museums of London, Trans Path Soc (London) 12:179, 1861.
35. Gambrioli PL, Maggi F, and Randelli M: Computerized tomography in the investigation of scapulo-humeral instability, Ital J Orthopaed Traumatol 11(2):223, 1985.
36. Garcia JF: Arthrographic visualization of rotator cuff tears , Radiology 150(2):595, 1984.
37. Garth WP, Slappey CE, and Ochs CW: Roentgenographic demonstration of instability of the shoulder: the apical oblique projection, J Bone Joint Surg 66A(9):1450, 1984.
38. Gerber C: Clinical assessment of instability of the shoulder, J Bone Joint Surg 66B(4):551, 1984.
39. Gerber C et al: The subcoracoid space, CORR 215 p. 132, February 1987.
40. Gerber C, Terrier F, and Ganz R: The role of the coracoid process in the chronic impingement syndrome, J Bone Joint Surg 67B(5):703, 1985.
41. Ghelman B, and Goldman A: The double-contrast shoulder arthrogram: evaluation of rotary cuff tears, Radiology 124:251, 1977.
42. Godsil RD, and Linscheid RL: Intratendinous defects of the rotator cuff, CORR 69 p. 181, 1970.
43. Golding RC: The shoulder—the forgotten joint, Br J Radiol 35(411):149, 1962.
44. Goldman AB, and Ghelman B: The double-contrast shoulder arthrogram, Radiology 127:655-663, June 1978.
45. Gristina AG, Collins RA, and Carter RE: Diagnostic ultrasound of the shoulder, Abst Orthop Trans 10:214, 1986.
46. Hajek PC et al: MR arthropathy: pathologic investigation, Radiology 163:141, 1987.
47. Hall FM et al: Morbidity from shoulder arthrography: etiology, incidence, and prevention, Am J Radiol 136:59, 1981.
48. Hall FM et al: Shoulder arthrography: comparison of morbidity after use of various contrast media, Radiology 154:339, 1985.
49. Hawkins RJ, and Kennedy JC: Impingement syndrome in athletes, Am J Sports Med 8:151, 1980.
50. Hawkins RJ, Koppert G, and Johnston G: Recurrent posterior instability (subluxation) of the shoulder, J Bone Joint Surg 66A(2):169, 1984.
51. Hermodsson I: Rontgenologische studien uber die traumatische und habituellen schultergelenk-verrenkungen nach vorn und nach unten, Acta Radiol Suppl 20:1, 1934.
52. Hill HA, and Sachs MD: The grooved defect of the humeral head: a frequently unrecognized complication of dislocation of the shoulder joint, Radiology 35:690, 1940.
53. Horsefield D, and Jones SM: A useful projection in radiography of the shoulder, J Bone Joint Surg 69B(2):338, 1987.
54. Huber DJ et al: MR imaging of the normal shoulder, Radiology 158:405, 1986.
55. Jobe FW, and Jobe CM: Painful atheltic injuries of the shoulder, Clin Orthop Rel Res 173:117, 1983.
56. Kessel L, and Watson M: The painful arc syndrome, J Bone Joint Surg 59B:166, 1977.
57. Keift GJ et al: Normal shoulder: MR imaging, Radiology 159(3):741, 1986.
58. Kieft GJ et al: MR imaging of anterior dislocation of the shoulder: comparison with CT arthrography, Am J Radiol 150:1083, 1988.
59. Kilcoyne RF, and Matsen FA: Rotator cuff tear measurement by arthropneumotomography, Am J Radiol 140:315, 1983.
60. Killoran PJ, Marcove RC, and Freiberger RH: Shoulder arthrography, Am J Radiol 103(3):658, 1968.
61. Kinnard P et al: Assessment of the unstable shoulder by computed arthrography, Am J Sports Med 11(3):157, 1983.
62. Kleinman PK et al: Axillary arthrotomography of the glenoid labrum, Am J Radiol 141:993, May 1984.
63. Kneeland JB et al: Rotator cuff tears: preliminary application of high-resolution MR imaging with counter rotating current loop-gap resonators, Radiology 160(3):695, 1986.

64. Kneeland JB et al: MR imaging of the shoulder: diagnosis of rotator cuff tears, Am J Radiol 149:333, August 1987.
65. Kneisl JS, Sweeney HJ, and Paige ML: Correlation of pathology observed in double contrast arthrotomography and arthroscopy of the shoulder, Arthroscopy 4(1):21, 1988.
66. Kohn D: The clinical relevance of glenoid labrum lesions, Arthroscopy 3(4):223, 1987.
67. Kornguth PJ, and Salazar AM: The apical oblique view of the shoulder, Am J Radiol 149(1):113, 1987.
68. Kummel BM: Arthrography in anterior capsular derangements of the shoulder, CORR 83 p. 170, March-April 1972.
69. Lie S, and Mast WA: Subacromial bursography, Radiology 144:626, 1982.
70. Lindblom K: Arthrography and roentgenography in ruptures of tendons of the shoulder joint, Acta Radiol 20:548, 1939.
71. Lombardo SJ et al: Posterior shoulder lesions in throwing athletes, Am J Sports Med 5(3):106, 1977.
72. McGlynn FJ, El-Khoury G, and Albright JP: Arthrotomography of the glenoid labrum in shoulder instability, J Bone Joint Surg 64A(4):506, 1982.
73. McLaughlin H: Posterior dislocation of the shoulder, J Bone Joint Surg 34A(3):584, 1952.
74. McMaster WC: Anterior glenoid labrum damage: a painful lesion in swimmers, Am J Sports Med 14(5):383, 1986.
75. McNiesh LM, and Callaghan JJ: CT arthrography of the shoulder: variations of the glenoid labrum, Am J Radiol 149:963, 1987.
76. Middleton WD et al: Ultrasonography of the rotator cuff: technique and normal anatomy, J Ultrasound Med 3:549, 1984.
77. Middleton WD et al: Ultrasonography of the biceps tendon apparatus, Radiology 157:211, 1985.
78. Middleton WD et al: Pitfalls of rotator cuff sonography, Am J Radiol 146:555, 1986.
79. Middleton WD et al: Ultrasonographic evaluation of the rotator cuff and biceps tendon, J Bone Joint Surg 68A:440, 1986.
80. Middleton WD et al: High resolution MR imagining of the normal rotator cuff, Am J Radiol 148:59, March 1987.
81. Mink JH, Harris E, and Rappaport M: Rotator cuff tears: evaluation using double-contrast shoulder arthrography, Radiology 157:621, 1985.
82. Mink JH, Richardson A, and Grant TT: Evaluation of glenoid labrum by double-contrast shoulder arthrography, Am J Radiol 133:893, November 1979.
83. Mizuno K, and Hirohata K: Diagnosis of recurrent traumatic anterior subluxation of the shoulder, CORR 179 p. 160, October 1983.
84. Neer CS: Anterior acromioplasty for the chronic impingement syndrome in the shoulder: a preliminary report, J Bone Joint Surg 54A:41, 1972.
85. Neer CS: Impingement lesions, CORR 173 p. 70, 1983.
86. Neer CS, and Welsh RP: The shoulder in sports, Orthop Clin N Am 8(3):583, 1977.
87. Neviaser RJ: Anatomic consideratons and examination of the shoulder, Orthop Clin N Am 11(2):187, 1980.
88. Neviaser TJ: Arthrography of the shoulder, Orthop Clin N Am 11(2):205, 1980.
89. Neviaser RJ: Tears of the rotator cuff, Orthop Clin N Am 11(2):295, 1980.
90. Neviaser RJ and Neviaser TJ: Lesions of musculotendinous cuff of shoulder: diagnosis and management. Chapter 11, pp. 239-57.
91. Norris TR: Diagnostic techniques for shoulder instability. In AAOS: Instructional course lecture, vol 34, 1985, p. 239.
92. Older MWJ, McIntyre JL, and Lloyd GJ: Distension arthrography of the shoulder joint, Can J Surg 19:203, 1976.
93. Pappas AP, Gross TP, and Kleinman PK: Symptomatic shoulder instability due to lesions of the glenoid labrum, Am J Sports Med 11:279, 1983.
94. Pattee GA, and Snyder SJ: Sonographic evaluation of the rotator cuff: correlation with arthroscopy, Arthroscopy 4(1):15, 1988.
95. Pavlov H et al: The roentgenographic evaluation of anterior shoulder instability, Clin Orthop 194:153, 1985.
96. Pavlov H, and Freiberger RH: Fractures and dislocations about the shoulder, Semin Roentgenol 13(2): 1978.
97. Petersson CJ, and Gentz CF: Ruptures of the supraspinatus tendon, CORR 175 p. 143, April 1983.
98. Petersson CJ, and Redlund-Johnell I: The subacromial space in normal shoulder radiographs, Acta Orthop Scand 55:57, 1984.
99. Post M, Silver R, and Singh M: Rotator cuff tear, CORR 173 p. 78, March 1983.
100. Rafii M et al: CT arthrography of capsular structures of the shoulder, Am J Radiol 146:361, 1986.
101. Rafii M et al: Athlete shoulder injuries: CT arthrographic findings, Radiology 162(2):559, 1987.
102. Rafii M et al: CT arthrography of shoulder instabilities in athletes, Am J Sports Med (in press).
103. Randelli M, and Gambrioli PL: Glenohumeral osteometry by computed tomography in normal and unstable shoulders, CORR 208 p. 151, July 1986.
104. Randellil M, Odella F, and Gambrioli PL: Clinical experience with double-contrast medium computerized tomography (arthro-CT) in instability of the shoulder, Ital J Orthopaed Traumatol 12(2):151, 1986.
105. Rathbun JB, and McNab I: The microvascular pattern of the rotator cuff, J Bone Joint Surg 52B:540, 1970.
106. Reeves B: Arthrography of the shoulder, J Bone Joint Surg 48B(3):424, August 1966.
107. Rockwood CA: Fractures and dislocations about the shoulder. II. Subluxations and dislocations about the shoulder. In Rockwood CA, and Green DP, editors: Fractures, ed 2, Philadelphia, 1975, JB Lippincott Co, p. 722.
108. Rokous JR, Feagin JA, and Abbott HG: Modified axillary roentgenogram: a useful adjunct in the diagnosis of recurrent instability of the shoulder, Clin Orthop 82:84, 1972.
109. Rothman RH, Marvel JP, Jr, and Hepenstall RB: Anatomic considerations in the glenohumeral joint, Orthop Clin N Am 6:341, 1975.
110. Rozing PM, deBakker HM, and Obermann WR: Radiographic views in recurrent anterior shoulder dislocation, Acta Orthop Scand 57:328, 1986.
111. Rubin SA, Gray RL, Green WR: The scapular "Y" view—a diagnostic aid in shoulder trauma, Radiology 110:725, 1974.
112. Saha AK: Anterior recurrent dislocation of the shoulder, Acta Orthop Scand 68:479, 1967.

113. Saha AK: Dynamic stability of the glenohumeral joint, Acta Orthop Scand 42:491, 1971.
114. Seeger LL et al: MR imaging of the normal shoulder: anatomic correlation, Am J Radiol 148:83, January 1987.
115. Seeger LL et al: Shoulder MR. Paper presented at the annual meeting of the Radiological Society of North America, Chicago, November 1987.
116. Seeger LL et al: Shoulder impingement syndrome: MR findings in 53 shoulders, Am J Radiol 150:343, 1988.
117. Seltzer SE, and Weissman BN: CT findings in normal and dislocating shoulders, J Can Assoc Radiol 36(1):41, 1985.
118. Shuman WP et al: Double-contrast computed tomography of the glenoid labrum, Am J Radiol 141:581, September 1983.
119. Singson RD, Feldman F, and Bigliani L: CT arthrographic patterns in recurrent glenohumeral instability, Am J Radiol 149:749, October 1987.
120. Strizak AM et al: Subacromial bursography, J Bone Joint Surg 64A(2):196, 1982.
121. Vastamaki M, and Solonen KA: Posterior dislocation and fracture-dislocation of the shoulder, Acta Orthop Scand 51:479, 1980.
122. Vezina JA: Compensation filter for shoulder radiography, Radiology 155(3):823, 1985.
123. Warren RF; Instability of shoulder in throwing sports. In: Staufer ES editor: AAOS: Instructional course lectures, vol. 34, St. Louis, 1985, The CV Mosby Co.
124. Zanca P: Shoulder pain-involvement of the acromioclavicular joint, Am J Radiol 112:493, 1971.
125. Zarins B, and Matthews LS: Evaluation and treatment of glenoid labrum tears. In Jackson DW editor: Shoulder surgery in the athlete, Rockville, MD 1985, Aspen Publications, p. 31.

CHAPTER 5 Shoulder Arthroscopy

Francis X. Mendoza
C. Alexander Moskwa, Jr.

The concept of using a small telescope to visualize a joint directly was introduced by Takagi in Japan in 1918. Employing a 7.3 mm cytoscope, he inspected a cadaveric knee and thereby inaugurated the field of arthroscopy.[39] In 1930 Burman reported on the arthroscopic examination of various cadaveric joints, including 25 shoulders. Using both anterior and posterior portals, he concluded that the shoulder is the easiest of all joints to visualize.[5] Although many contemporary orthopaedic surgeons would disagree with Burman's conclusion, there is no doubt that shoulder arthroscopy has significantly increased in popularity and use.

Shoulder arthroscopy has followed a development parallel to that of knee arthroscopy. Although at present it is not as universally established as knee arthroscopy, shoulder arthroscopy has grown to be the second most performed arthroscopic procedure.[20] It is beyond the stage of being predominantly an investigative or diagnostic tool, and it currently can be used for surgical treatment of certain conditions.

Shoulder arthroscopy

Advantages
- Less invasive than open surgery
- Permits direct visualization
- Allows earlier rehabilitation

Disadvantages
- Skill dependent on case volume

The advantages of shoulder arthroscopy are that it is less invasive than open surgery, permits direct visualization of intra- and extraarticular pathologic conditions, and allows earlier rehabilitation, with return to activities of daily living. A major disadvantage is that the physician's skill with shoulder arthroscopy is generally correlated to his or her experience. It is no surprise that those orthopaedic surgeons well trained in knee arthroscopy have found an easier transition to the art of shoulder arthroscopy than those without such previous experience.

HISTORY AND PHYSICAL EXAMINATION

A diligent history and physical examination, supplemented with plain roentgenograms, form the cornerstone of the appropriate diagnosis in the overwhelming majority of shoulder conditions. If necessary, additional studies, such as plain roentgenograms of cervical spine, electrodiagnostic studies, arthrograms, computerized tomograms and, most recently, magnetic resonance imaging, can be helpful after a review of the initial plain shoulder roentgenograms to substantiate the diagnosis further. In our experience, shoulder arthroscopy cannot be depended upon to reveal the diagnosis in most situations.

Shoulder position (lateral decubitus)

Intraarticular visualization
60 degrees abduction
5 to 10 degrees forward flexion

Subacromial visualization
5 to 15 degrees abduction
Zero to 10 degrees forward flexion

SURGICAL SETUP

The patient usually receives a general anesthetic to assure good relaxation. It is critical to perform a gentle examination of the shoulder during anesthesia on all patients undergoing arthroscopy, since it will afford an opportunity to assess shoulder motion and instability, if appropriate, with complete joint relaxation.

A lateral decubitus position (Fig. 5-1) is commonly used for most patients, with the involved shoulder up. The patient rests with anterior and posterior pelvic posts stabilizing the pelvis, an axillary pad under the uninvolved arm, and careful padding and positioning of all bony prominences. To enhance distention of the joint, longitudinal traction of 10 to 15 pounds is applied, with Buck's traction on the forearm directed through a commercially available shoulder suspensory device. This traction apparatus must permit changes in the degree of shoulder abduction and forward flexion (Fig. 5-2). Various authors have offered a wide range of recommendations of shoulder abduction and forward flexion to obtain maximal visualization of the joint while avoiding the neurovascular structures. Our experience indicates that approximately 60 degrees of abduction, with 5 to 10 degrees of forward flexion, allows best glenohumeral (intraarticular) visualization, while 5 to 15 degrees of abduction, with zero to 10 degrees of forward flexion, maximizes visualization of the subacromial space.

Other methods of positioning the patient exist, such as the semirecumbent or beach-chair position.[37] Here, shoulder joint distraction is accomplished via gravity—the weight of the arm—assisted by gentle manual downward traction by the surgical assistant. Although this position is more comfortable for the surgeon, our experience reveals that it does not provide the same degree of visualization as one obtained in the lateral decubitis position, especially in muscular athletes.

EQUIPMENT

In virtually all cases, the standard 30-degree angle, 4.0 or 4.5 mm arthroscope can be used in the shoulder, as in the knee. Other pieces of equipment common to knee and shoulder arthroscopy include a high-intensity fiberoptic light source; a camera; a video monitor and recorder; cannulae with sharp and semiblunt trocars; an 18-gauge spinal needle; a gravity-based irrigation system; and an as-

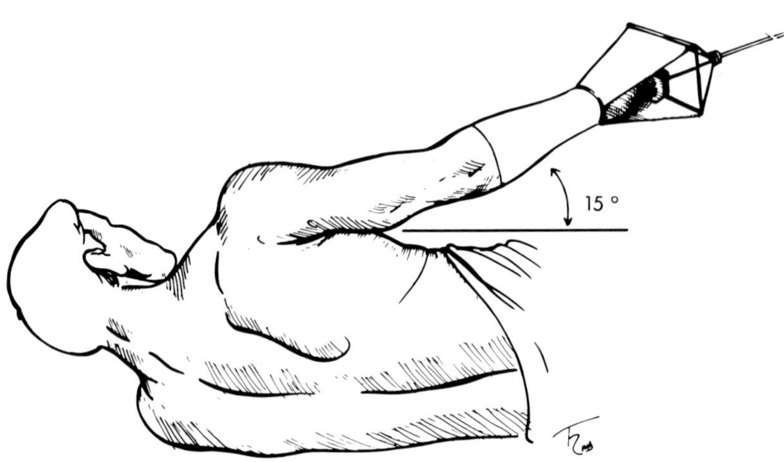

FIG. 5-1. Lateral decubitus position with longitudinal traction in 5 degrees, 15 degrees abduction, and 0 to 10 degrees of forward flexion maximizes visualization of the subacromial space.

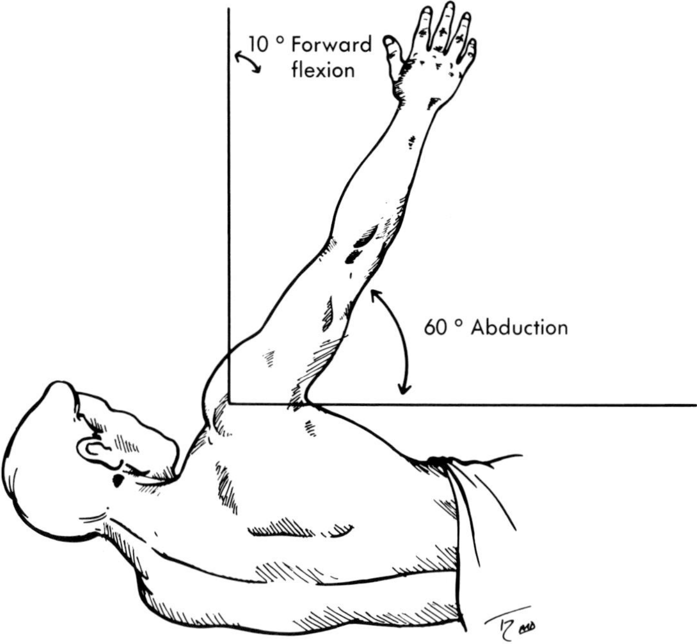

FIG. 5-2. Lateral decubitus position with longitudinal traction in 60 degrees of abduction with 5 to 10 degrees of forward flexion enhances glenohumeral intraarticular visualization.

sortment of arthroscopic instruments, such as probes, scissors, punches, and graspers. A power-driven rotary shaver with variable speed, suction capability, and interchangeable blades and burrs is also necessary for debridement purposes. Instruments specific for shoulder arthroscopy include a cannula system with a diaphragm to prevent leakage of fluid when instruments are passed through it, a Wissinger rod to assist in creation of an anterior intraarticular portal, and an electrocautery generally used during subacromial procedures.

Equipment

- Routine arthroscopy setup
- Cannula system for instrument interchange
- Wissinger rod
- Intraarticular electrocautery

PORTAL SELECTION

With the patient sterilely prepared and draped, the following bony landmarks are palpated and outlined with a sterile pen: the distal clavicle, the tip of the coracoid process, and the anterolateral and posterolateral borders of the acromion. The ideal portal for joint inspection and instrumentation should meet the following criteria:

1. A relatively avascular tissue plane should be entered.
2. Adjacent neurovascular structures should be protected.
3. Tissue bulk should be minimized to assure maximal visualization of the joint and instrument maneuverability.
4. The technique of creating the portal should be reproducible.

Portal site selection

- Through relatively avascular plane
- Avoid or protect adjacent neurovascular structure
- Minimize tissue bulk
- Technique reproducible

Many portals have been successfully used for shoulder arthroscopy. Nonetheless, procedures involving the glenohumeral joint (intraarticular) (Fig. 5-3) necessitate different portals than those procedures performed in the subacromial space (extraarticular) (Fig. 5-4).

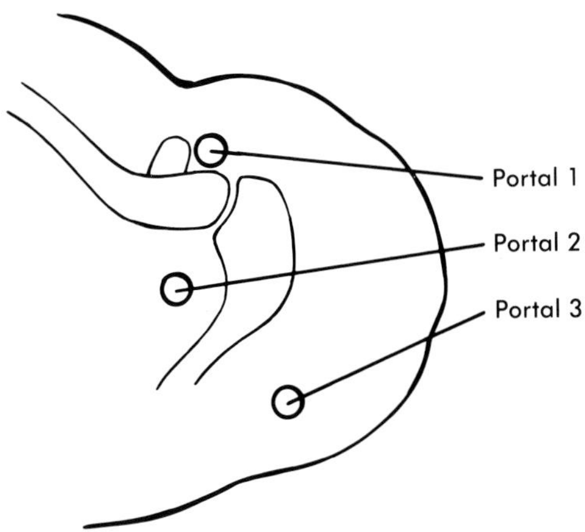

FIG. 5-3. Intraarticular portals. *Port 1,* The anterior portal remains lateral and in line with or just superior to the tip of the coracoid process. *Port 2,* The accessory portal for additional instrumentation or improved inflow is located superiorly just posterior to the acromioclavicular joint. *Port 3,* The posterior portal is located in the "soft spot" 1 cm medial and 2 cm inferior to the posterior lateral corner of the acromion.

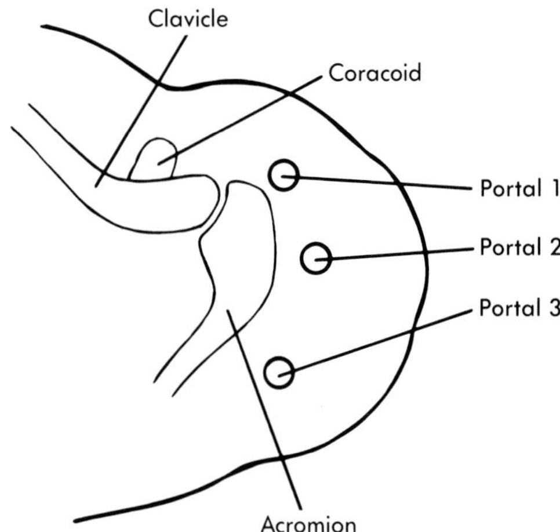

FIG. 5-4. Extraarticular subacromial portals. *Port 1,* The instrument portal is in line with and 3 cm distal to the anterolateral acromial edge. *Port 2,* The arthroscopic portal is located 1.5 cm to 2 cm anterior and 1.5 cm inferior to the posterior lateral of the acromion. *Port 3,* The posterior inflow portal is located 2 cm below the posterior acromial edge and lateral to the acromiolclavicular joint.

Intraarticular Portals

The **posterior portal** has been accepted as the standard for the initial entry into the shoulder joint. In a cadaveric study using 51 shoulders, Rojvanit[36] found that the posterior approach had a wider field of view as compared to the anterior and superior approaches, and better anatomic orientation was obtained.

The posterior intraarticular portal is located approximately 1 cm medially and 2 cm inferiorly to the posterolateral corner of the acromion. The location corresponds to the palpable posterior "soft spot" of the shoulder, which represents the interval between the infraspinatus and teres minor muscles. With the middle finger palpating the coracoid process and the thumb on the posterior soft spot, the surgeon inserts an 18-gauge spinal needle through the soft spot directed at the coracoid process. Approximately 30 centiliters of sterile saline are injected through the spinal needle to distend the shoulder joint and to demonstrate free backflow, thereby confirming joint entry. The spinal needle is then withdrawn, and a small incision is made through the skin. The arthroscopic sheath with its semisharp trocar is used to penetrate the soft tissues into the shoulder. A blunt trocar should be inserted before any further manipulation within the shoulder joint. Adequate joint distention is maintained with a continuous gravity inflow of saline from elevated saline fluid bags.

An **anterior intraarticular portal** is then made by advancing the arthroscope to the anterior capsule, where the "intraarticular triangle," consisting of the humeral head, glenoid, and biceps tendon, is visualized, as described by Matthews et al[21] (see Plate 1). The authors confirm through anatomic studies that instruments passing through the area cause little risk to adjacent neurovascular structures. Further safety is ensured if the anterior portal remains in the area lateral and adjacent or just superior to the coracoid process.

Two common techniques exist for the safe and reproducible method used to create an anterior intraarticular portal. The arthroscopic sheath may be advanced anteriorly to abut against the anterior capsule within the intraarticular triangle between the superior and middle anterior glenohumeral ligaments (see Plate 2). The arthroscope is then exchanged for a Wissinger rod, which is advanced through the arthroscopic sheath to rest at the previously determined point on the anterior capsule and just lateral or adjacent to the coracoid process. An anterior skin incision is made over the tip of the Wissinger rod, and a cannula is placed over the anteriorly existing rod and advanced in a retrograde fashion into the joint. The rod is then removed, and the accessory anterior portal is ready to accept instruments or an arthroscope.

An alternate method for the creation of an anterior intraarticular portal is described by Matthews et al,[21] who employed a 22-gauge spinal needle entering through the intraarticular triangle under arthroscopic visualization. The needle is placed superior to the middle glenohumeral ligament but inferior to the biceps tendon. After satisfactory placement is confirmed, a small skin incision is made, and a semisharp trochar and cannula are inserted following the previously defined angle to create the anterior portal (see Plate 3).

A third **accessory intraarticular portal** may at times be necessary for improved fluid inflow or additional instruments. This portal may be created adjacent to the initial anterior portal, using the previously described techniques. Care must be taken to remain somewhat more superior and lateral to the coracoid process to avoid jeopardizing the musculocutaneous nerve. An alternative site for this accessory portal is located superiorly on the shoulder just posterior to the acromioclavicular joint (see Plate 4). From that point, an 18-gauge spinal needle is aimed toward the center of the axilla and monitored arthroscopically as it enters the joint through the superior posterior capsule just posterior to the posterior glenoid rim. The needle is then withdrawn, and a cannula with a semisharp trocar is inserted through the previously defined track establishing the **superior portal**.[31] Only the muscular portions of the trapezius and supraspinatus are traversed in creating this portal. However, rigorous technique must be employed to avoid violating the tendinous portion of the supraspinatus.

Extraarticular Portals (Fig. 5-4)

The technique for performing subacromial endoscopic procedures demands that different portals be used.[31] The arthroscope is inserted into the subacromial space through a posterolateral subacromial portal located approximately 1.5 to 2.0 cm anterior and 1.5 cm inferior to the posterolateral edge of the acromion. A posterior subacromial portal used for inflow is placed 2 cm below the posterior acromion and angled toward the anterior edge of the acromion. An instrument portal is generally selected in line with the anterior edge of the acromion and lies approximately 3 cm distal to the anterolateral edge.

ARTHROSCOPIC ANATOMY

A detailed knowledge of normal anatomy and its variants is absolutely essential for arthroscopic surgery. All anatomic structures and viewing orientation can be related to four anatomic landmarks (see Plate I): (1) articular surface of the humeral head; (2) articular surface of the glenoid; (3) tendon of the long head of the biceps; and (4) tendon of the subscapularis.

Consistent anatomic landmarks

- Humeral head articular surface
- Glenoid articular surface
- Long head of biceps tendon
- Tendon of the subscapularis

The humeral head and glenoid face opposite one another and contain smooth articular cartilage covering their surfaces. A normal sulcus exists circumferentially on the humeral head, which represents an area of bare bone between the insertion of the capsule and the edge of the humeral articular cartilage.[8] An increase in size of this bare area posteriorly should not be considered pathologic, since it is thought to be part of the normal aging process. Clinically, one must be careful not to confuse this normal bare area of posterior humeral head with a Hill-Sachs lesion, which represents a pathologic denuding of the posterior humeral cartilage secondary to anterior glenohumeral instability (see Plate 5).

The glenoid is surrounded by a wedge-shaped labrum and is intimately related to the capsule and ligaments. It is important to note that not all detachments of the labrum are pathologic. DePalma[8] noted that superior labral detachments frequently occur with advancing age. Our experience suggests that symptoms from anterior superior labral tears do occur but are uncommon.

The tendons of the long head of the biceps and of the subscapularis are both prominent structures within the glenohumeral joint. The biceps tendon can be followed arthroscopically from its insertion at the supraglenoid tubercle and superior labrum (see Plates 6 and 7) to its exit at the opening of the bicipital groove. Two rare variants of the biceps tendon should be noted: double-headed biceps and intracapsular biceps,[8] which may lead to initial confusion during arthroscopy. Located at approximately 90 degrees to the glenoid, the biceps tendon forms the anterior border of the insertion of the supraspinatus before entering the bicipital groove (see Plate 7). Thus the biceps tendon is helpful in locating the rotator cuff, where the supraspinatus tendon will be seen just superior to it. The infraspinatus and teres minor tendons can also be seen by directing the arthroscope farther posteriorly and superiorly.

Biceps tendon variants

- Double-headed tendon
- Intracapsular

The superior edge of the subscapularis tendon is also an intraarticular structure and can be seen against the anterior capsule (see Plate 8). It, too, courses at approximately 90 degrees to the glenoid, and it is roughly parallel in orientation to the biceps tendon. The subscapularis tendon is helpful in locating the capsular ligaments. Of the three capsular ligaments, the inferior glenohumeral ligament is usually the largest, and its superior band can be seen crossing the superior edge of the subscapularis tendon at about 90 degrees near its attachment to the glenoid (see Plate 9). The middle glenohumeral ligament crosses the superior edge of the subscapularis at approximately 60 degrees (see Plate 9), and it is slightly anterior to the superior band of the inferior glenohumeral ligament. The smallest capsular ligament, the superior glenohumeral ligament, is usually obscured from view by the biceps tendon. It can, however, be seen by switching to an anterior or superior portal.

With an intimate familiarity with the four anatomic landmarks of the articular surfaces of the humerus and glenoid, the long head of the biceps tendon, and the subscapularis tendon, one can view nearly the entire glenohumeral joint in an orderly fashion. A standardized viewing sequence is important, so that no accessible area is overlooked. Many different regimens for systematically viewing the glenohumeral joint have been proposed, and the selection of a particular regimen is at the discretion of the arthroscopist.

Our approach is to access the aforementioned orienting landmarks completely at the start. We then proceed anteriorly to view the anterior capsule, glenohumeral ligaments, and subscapularis recess and its opening. The examination then goes to the superior portion of the glenohumeral joint, followed by the inferior and posterior portions, where the rotator cuff and capsule are inspected. With this approach, the entire joint has been inspected, and all critical structures are noted.

INDICATIONS

The indications for shoulder arthroscopy have yet to be definitely outlined and substantiated by long-term prospective studies. Diagnostic shoulder arthroscopy should be limited to the occasional patient in which the history, physical examination, plain roentgenograms, and other less invasive diagnostic tests failed to reveal the diagnosis.

Subacromial Impingement and Rotator Cuff Tears

The use of arthroscopic surgery in the subacromial space has been shown to be quite effective in the appropriate patient. As defined by Neer,[29,30] the impingement syndrome is a mechanical compression of the rotator cuff by the subacromial arch. The diagnosis continues to be a clinical one, and the treatment is dependent upon the stage of impingement. Stage 1 impingement consists of a mechanical bursitis and inflammation of the rotator cuff tendons, which is reversible and thus responsive to conservative treatment. State 2 impingement consists of a bursitis, tendonitis, and fibrosis within the soft tissues, which compromise the subacromial space. Nonoperative treatment is generally successful, with avoidance of overhead activities, the use of oral inflammatory medication, the prudent use of one or two cortisone injections, and strengthening exercises for the rotator cuff musculature. If symptoms persist for a year or more, these patients may be candidates for a decompressive procedure.

An arthroscopic subacromial decompression is recommended by many physicians for those stage 2 patients without acromioclavicular joint involvement. This technique was introduced by Ellman in 1985.[11] In a 1-to 3-year follow-up of the initial 50 cases, Ellman[12] found that 88% had good-to-excellent results. Similar favorable results have been reported by others.[15,25,28]

An open surgical procedure continues to be the most efficient method of decompressing stage 2 shoulders with concomitant acromioclavicular joint involvement.

Stage 3 subacromial impingement consists of advanced stage 2 pathologic findings, with an additional rotator cuff tear. The use of surgical arthroscopy is limited with respect to treatment of stage 3 disease. There is little

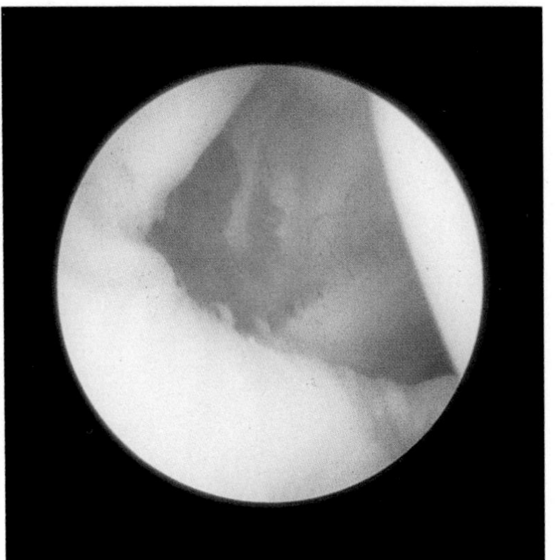

PLATE 1. Four intraarticular landmarks are visualized. Inferiorly—glenoid articular surface. Extreme right—humeral head articular surface. Extreme left—long head of biceps tendon. Subscapularis tendon coursing obliquely from behind humeral head toward glenoid surface.

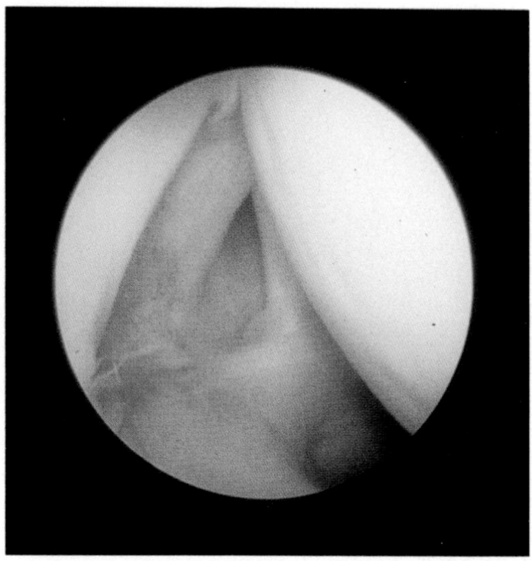

PLATE 2. Anterior capsule visualized within borders created by superior glenohumeral ligament on left, superior edge of subscapularis tendon on right, and middle glenohumeral ligament along base.

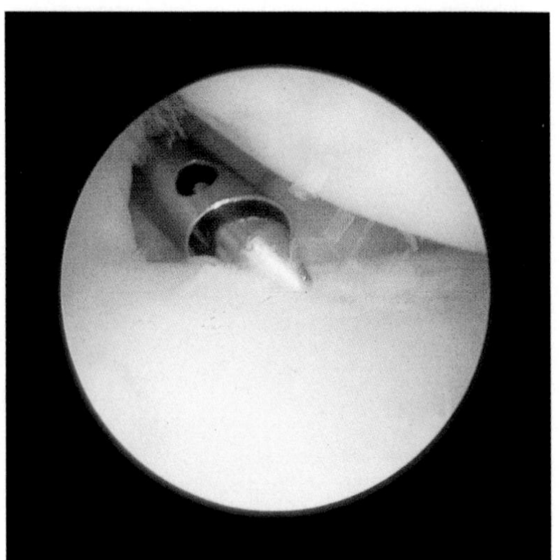

PLATE 3. Trochar and cannula enter joint anteriorly through intraarticular triangle.

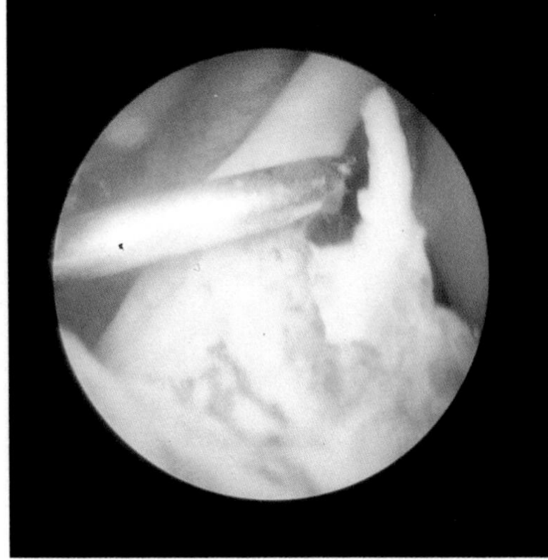

PLATE 4. Spinal needle enters joint through accessory portal, providing a posterior superior view of long head of biceps tendon origin and anterior superior lateral tear.

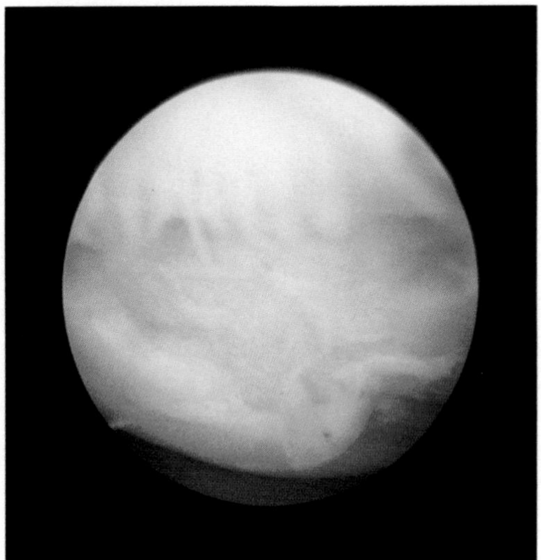

PLATE 5. Hill-Sachs lesion. A pathologic denuding of the posterior humeral head cartilage secondary to anterior glenohumeral instability.

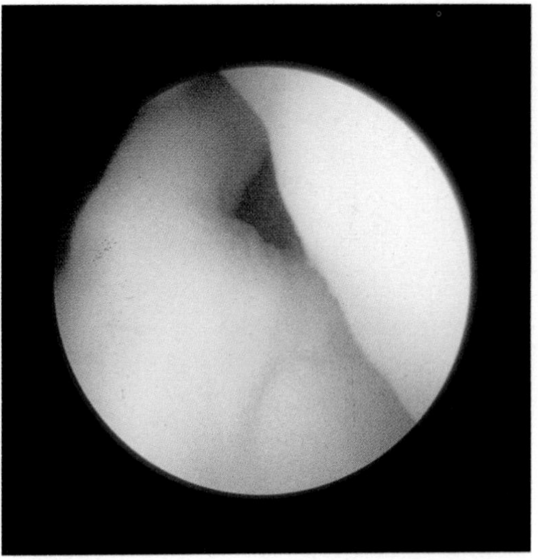

PLATE 6. The origin of the long head of biceps tendon from the supraglenoid tubercle and anterior labrum.

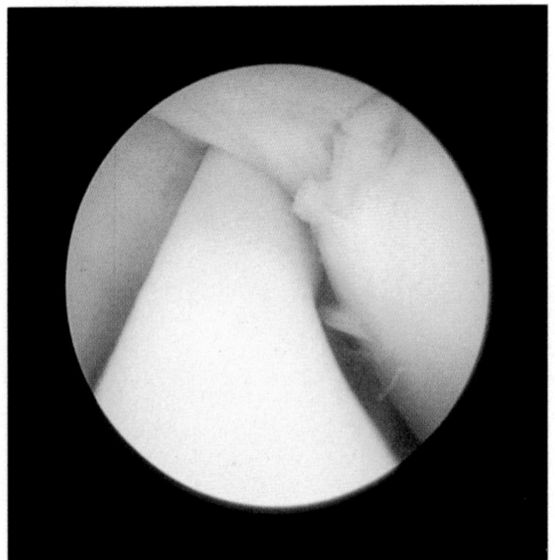

PLATE 7. The long head of biceps tendon is seen existing just before the entrance to the bicipital groove. The humeral head is identified on the right. The tendon traversing the exit of the biceps tendon is the supraspinatus.

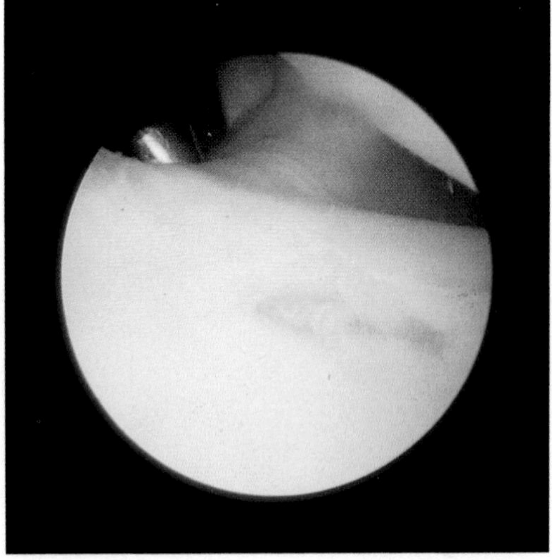

PLATE 8. The insertion of the oblique broad band of ligamentous tissue consisting of the middle and inferior glenohumeral ligaments is identified with a spinal needle. The more vertically oriented superior edge of the subscapularis tendon is visualized in the background.

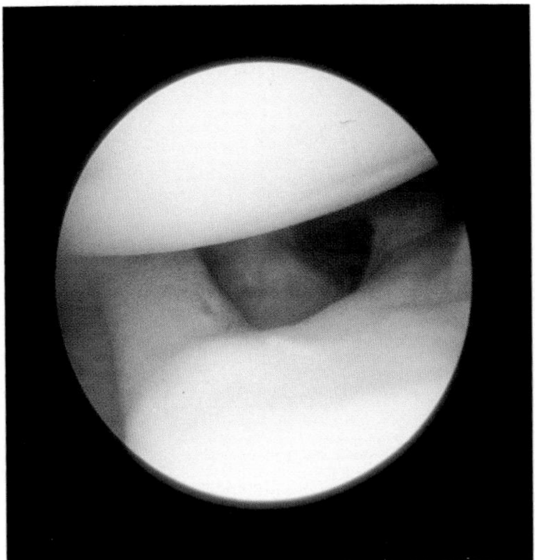

PLATE 9. Identified from left to right are the long head of biceps tendon, the superior ligament, and the superior and middle glenohumeral ligaments. The subscapularis tendon edge is not visualized in the background.

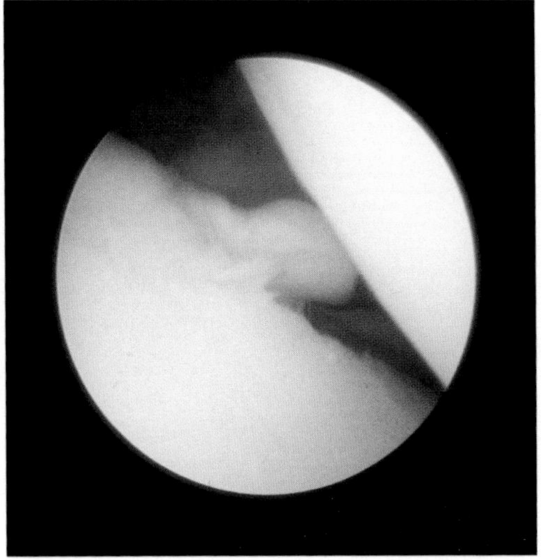

PLATE 10. A detached anterior labrum consistent with recurrent anterior glenohumeral subluxations.

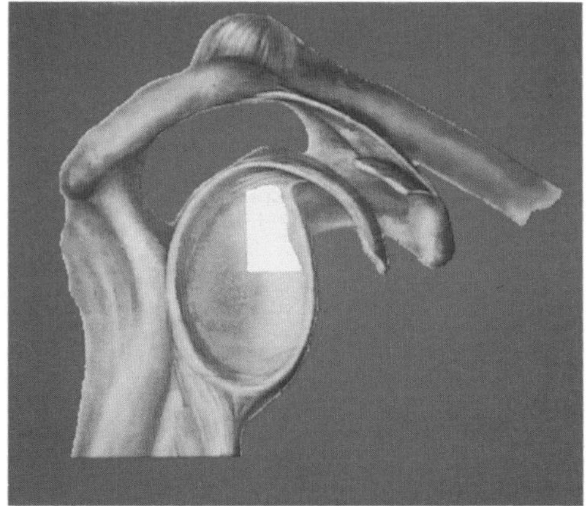

PLATE 11. Although anterosuperior quadrant (yellow) labral tears without time detachments are commonly identified, they are not necessarily symptomatic.

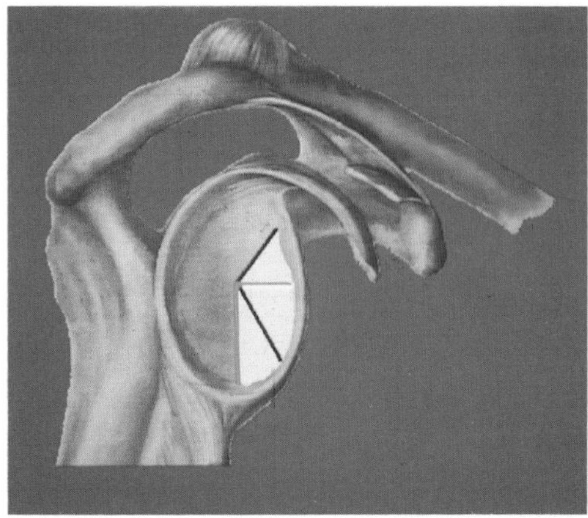

PLATE 12. Anterior lateral tears associated with instability extend from the anterosuperior quadrant into the inferior quadrant (black) or are confined to the inferior quadrant (red).

scientific evidence that debridement of a partial rotator cuff tear leads to an increased healing response, although clinical improvements have been noted. In the largest retrospective series to date, Ogilvie-Harris[33] found that arthroscopic debridement of partial rotator cuff tears led to clinical improvement in only 50% of patients. Poor results were obtained in debriding complete or previously repaired tears of the rotator cuff. Andrews,[1] on the other hand, reported that 85% of competitive athletes with partial tears of the supraspinatus portion of the rotator cuff had good-to-excellent results after an arthroscopic debridement. Ellman[13] recommended that an arthroscopic decompression follow the debridement of a partial tear in hopes of minimizing its progression to a complete tear. Again, further scientific study is necessary in order to support these findings and better define the role of arthroscopy in treating rotator cuff tears.

Our experience is that arthroscopy is helpful in identifying small-to-incomplete tears of the rotator cuff that are not identified by an arthrogram, and that judicious debridement may be of some value at the time of an arthroscopic subacromial decompression. In complete tears, however, arthroscopic debridement in the athlete, despite decompression, is of little value, since symptoms attributable to weakness and discomfort commensurate with the size of the tear will manifest themselves during attempts at high-performance use of the shoulder. Furthermore, this may worsen the athlete's condition, with possible extension of the tear and an exacerbation of the overall condition. Some of the more demanding open rotator cuff repairs that we have encountered have been failures after an arthroscopic debridement, where loss of tendon substance has been thought to compromise the open repair directly.

Instability

The term "shoulder instability" encompasses the entire spectrum, from uni- to multidirectional and from subluxation to frank dislocation. Current thinking reflects that glenohumeral instability is dependent upon an interrelationship between the capsule, labrum, glenohumeral ligaments, and rotator cuff tendons, as well as the humeral head and bony glenoid.

Use of shoulder arthroscopy to treat instability is still in its developmental stages. In recent years Johnson has popularized a technique of an arthroscopic staple capsulorrhaphy. After scarification of the anterior scapular neck, the glenohumeral ligaments were grasped with a tine of a staple and advanced and fixed into the newly created bony bed. Nottage[32] reported that double-contrast computed arthrotomography is useful in helping to select patients for staple capsulorrhaphy by identifying large labral lesions with sufficient tissue suitable for the procedure.

Other arthroscopic procedures include screw fixation[40] of the advanced capsule or placing sutures[27] through the anterior scapular neck, tying them posteriorly to obtain fixation of the anterior capsulorrhaphy. Although early results with all of these techniques have been encouraging, Johnson[17,35a] reports a 21% recurrence rate of instability after the arthroscopic staple capsulorrhaphy in 106 shoulders with a minimal 2-year follow-up. This does not compare favorably with currently accepted open surgical repair failure rates of 3%.[35] Furthermore, the placement of metallic devices into the scapular neck has been replete with problems in open surgical procedures,[42] and their use arthroscopically must be weighed accordingly.

The diagnosis of shoulder instability is still primarily based on the history and clinical findings. It is uncommon when shoulder arthroscopy is needed for the diagnosis. Cofield[7] found that approximately 90% of arthroscopy was either optional or unnecessary in diagnosing or altering the treatment of cases of shoulder instability. In difficult cases of recurrent subluxations, a careful evaluation of the shoulder with the patient under anesthesia, supplemented with image intensification and perhaps an arthroscopic evaluation, may be effective in yielding the diagnosis.[9]

Zarins[41] has found that the direction of abnormal subluxations can be inferred by the location of the labral pathology present at the time of arthroscopy. Other arthroscopic findings that may be supportive of recurrent glenohumeral subluxations include attenuation of the inferior glenohumeral ligament, glenoid changes of fraying, tearing, or true detachments (see Plate 10), a peripheral erosion of the glenoid cartilage, loose bodies, or a humeral head Hill-Sachs lesion (see Plate 5).[6,14,23,26]

Arthroscopic findings in subluxation

- Labral tears
- Inferior glenohumeral ligament attentuation
- Glenoid fraying, tearing, or erosion
- Loose bodies
- Humeral Hill-Sachs lesion

Labral Tears

Labral pathology is currently an area of much interest. Labral fraying and tears are known to occur with instability, as well as degenerative conditions.[8] Mechanical symptoms arising from labral tears unassociated with clinical glenohumeral instability (functional tears) have been described. More recently, we have identified tears of a nonfunctional nature associated with chronic subacromial impingement.

Pappas[34] divided labral lesions into those occurring with instability and those that are functional and cause painful clicking in the stable shoulder. Treatment in the former group must be directed primarily at the clinical instability. On the other hand, open debridement of functional tears leads to improvement.

Andrews[2] found that functional anterosuperior labral tears are also seen in throwing athletes complaining of pain or popping during the throwing motion, and that, after an arthroscopic debridement of these tears, many athletes had excellent or good results and returned to pitching.

We[24] have found that anterosuperior glenoid labral tears without true detachments occur more commonly than previously believed but are not necessarily symptomatic. These tears generally extend from the long head of the biceps tendon distally, but they are confined to the anterosuperior quadrant of the glenoid and do not cross the equator into the inferior quadrant (see Plate 11). This configuration of tear is frequently found in shoulders of athletes suffering from stage 2 subacromial impingement, and successful results continue to be obtained by a subacromial decompression without debridement of the labral tear, further supporting the nonfunctional nature of this type of tear. Much more uncommon is the throwing shoulder with symptoms suggestive of recurrent anteroinferior subluxations, which cannot be shown to be clinically unstable. This latter group of shoulders with an additional concomitant anterosuperior labral tear has improved, with return to throwing, after an arthroscopic debridement of the labral tear. This supports the functional nature of the tear. Labral tears associated with anteroinferior glenohumeral instability have been shown to extend from the anterosuperior quadrant of the glenoid to the inferior quadrant, or they remain confined in the inferior quadrant[24] (see Plate 12). Arthroscopic debridement of these lesions as a sole treatment is contraindicated, and a repair against the stability continues to be the most effective treatment.

Bicipital Tendonitis

Intraarticular fraying and synovitis of the biceps tendon are often seen in overhead throwers, as well as in older individuals in conjunction with degenerative arthritis.[8] These pathologic implications remain unclear. Nonetheless, some authors arthroscopically debride the tendon and enlarge the entrance into the bicipital groove.[33] Partial and complete tears of the biceps tendon are more often noted as part of the impingement syndrome, and therapeutic intervention should be directed there. Mechanical symptoms resulting from a ruptured intraarticular biceps tendon stump are uncommon but may be eliminated by an arthroscopic debridement of the stump.

Glenohumeral Arthritis

The role of arthroscopy in this entity depends on the severity of the disease.[33] In mild osteoarthritis, Ogilvie-Harris obtained successful results with debridement of chondral debris and synovium in about two thirds of cases. In severe osteoarthritis only one third of patients had favorable results. Early rheumatoid arthritis without roentgenographic evidence of disease had improvement after arthroscopic synovectomy with approximately 1-year follow-up. Long-term results are still pending.

Adhesive Capsulitis

After arthroscopy of 24 patients with adhesive capsulitis, Ha'eri[16] found no significant intraarticular abnormality, except a decreased glenohumeral joint volume in 16% of patients. Although a more rapid recovery from this condition has been reported after arthroscopy, presumably by stretching soft tissue contractures,[33] we have found that improvement is short-term, and an intensive course of physical therapy is overall a more effective and predictable method of treatment without the attendant risk of surgery.

Loose Bodies

Loose bodies of the glenohumeral joint are a telltale sign and can occur in association with conditions such as instability, arthritis, chondromatosis, or an osteochondral fracture. Although retrieval of loose bodies can be accomplished arthroscopically in the shoulder without resorting to open techniques,[22] emphasis should be placed on treatment of the primary condition rather than only on the loose bodies.

Calcific Tendonitis

A large single calcific deposit may be amenable to arthroscopic needling and curettage after failure of conservative methods.[12] However, if multiple or small deposits exist, the technical difficulties encountered in locating the tendinous deposits and their boundaries within the surrounding chemical bursitis may be such that an open procedure is necessary for proper treatment.

Other Conditions

Shoulder arthroscopy has been successfully used for irrigation and debridement or septic shoulders, biopsy of tissue in polymyalgia rheumatica,[10] and other conditions, including synovectomy and treatment of pigmented villonodular synovitis.

COMPLICATIONS

In his reported series of 439 surgical shoulder arthroscopies, Ogilvie-Harris[33] reported a complication rate of 3%, all of which were without residual sequelae. These complications included massive leakage of fluid from the shoulder, abrasion of the articular cartilage, sepsis, and musculocutaneous nerve palsy.

Fluid leakage into the surrounding soft tissues poses a theoretical complication of neurovascular compromise, but the fluid usually begins to resorb within the first 12 hours.[19]

Neurologic injury is a potential serious complication that can be minimized with careful arthroscopic technique. In anatomic studies Bryan[4] demonstrated the potential for direct nerve injury because the standard posterior portal of entry passes only from 0.5 cm to 2.5 cm superior to the main trunk of the axillary nerve. Transient neurologic compromise ranging from paresthesias to palsies has been reported, with an incidence of 10% to 30%.[18] The commonly affected nerves are the musculocutaneous and ulnar.[3] Positioning of the upper extremity and the degree of applied traction have been found to be contributing factors. The positions of least strain on the brachial plexus that allow maximal visualization are 45 degrees of forward flexion and 90 degrees of abduction, or 45 degrees of forward flexion and 0 degrees of abduction.[18]

In a recent survey on arthroscopy of the knee and other joints, the Arthroscopic Association of North America reported that anterior staple capsulorrhaphy for shoulder instability had a complication rate of 5.3%—the highest rate of any joint arthroscopic procedure. Subacromial decompression had a rate of only 0.76%[38] Surgical failures were not included in these statistics. Thus anterior staple capsulorrhaphy must be regarded as a technique necessitating further refinement.

SUMMARY

Shoulder arthroscopy has, without a doubt, increased our knowledge of anatomy, as well as of pathology. Although its role as a diagnostic tool in the shoulder is currently minimal, its effectiveness as a surgical tool is ever increasing. Its continued success can only be further enhanced by a sound understanding of the appropriate preoperative diagnosis. Long-term results of surgical arthroscopy are still pending in many areas, but the future of this minimally invasive alternative to open surgery is encouraging.

REFERENCES

1. Andrews JR, Broussard TS, and Carson WG: Arthroscopy of the shoulder in the management of partial tears of the rotator cuff: a preliminary report, J Arthroscopy 1:117, 1985.
2. Andrews JR, Carson WG, and McLeod WD: Glenoid labrum tears related to the long head of the biceps, Am J Sports Med 13:337, 1985.
3. Andrews JR, Carson WG, and Ortega K: Arthroscopy of the shoulder: technique and normal anatomy, Am J Sports Med 12:1, 1984.
4. Bryan WJ, Schauder K, and Tullos H: The axillary nerve and its relationship to common sports medicine shoulder procedures, Am J Sports Med 14:113, 1986.
5. Burman MS: Arthroscopy or the direct visualization of joints: an experimental cadaver study, J Bone Joint Surg 13:669, 1931.
6. Caspari RB: Shoulder arthroscopy: a review of the present state of the art, Contemp Orthop 4:523, 1982.
7. Cofield RH: Arthroscopy of the shoulder, Mayo Clin Proc 58:501, 1983.
8. De Palma AF: Surgery of the shoulder, ed 3, Philadelphia, 1983, JB Lippincott Co.
9. Dolk T, and Gremark O: Arthroscopy and stability testing of the shoulder joint, Arthroscopy 2:35, 1986.
10. Douglas WAC, Martin EA, and Morris JH: Polymyalgia rheumatica: an arthroscopic study of the shoulder joint, Ann Rheum Dis 42:311, 1983.
11. Ellman H: Arthroscopic subacromial decompression, Orthop Trans 9:48, 1985.
12. Ellman H: Arthroscopic subacromial decompression: analysis of one to three year results, Arthroscopy 3:173, 1987.
13. Ellman H: Shoulder arthroscopy: current indications and techniques, Orthopaedics 11:45, 1988.
14. Garth WP, Allman FL, and Armstrong WS: Occult anterior subluxations of the shoulder in noncontact sports, Am J Sports Med 15:579, 1987.
15. Gartsman GM: Arthroscopic treatment of stage II

subacromial impingement, Orthop Trans 12:731, 1988.
16. Ha'eri GB, and Maitland A: Arthroscopic findings in the frozen shoulder, J Rheumatol 8:149, 1981.
17. Deleted in proofs.
18. Klein AH, et al: Measurement of brachial plexus strain in arthroscopy of the shoulder, Arthroscopy 3:45, 1987.
19. Lilleby H: Shoulder arthroscopy, Acta Orthop Scand 55:561, 1984.
20. Lombardo SJ: Arthroscopy of the shoulder, Clin Sports Med 2:309, 1983.
21. Matthews LS, et al: Anterior portal selection for shoulder arthroscopy, J Arthroscopy 1:33, 1985.
22. McGinty JB: Arthroscopic removal of loose bodies, Orthop Clin N Am 13:313, 1982.
23. McGlynn FJ, and Caspari RB: Arthroscopic findings in the subluxating shoulder, Corr 183:173, 1984.
24. Mendoza FX, Nicholas JA, and Reilly J: Anatomic patterns of anterior glenoid labrum tears, Orthop Trans 11:246, 1987.
25. Mendoza FX, Nicholas JA, and Rubinstein MP: The arthroscopic treatment of subacromial impingement, Clin Sports Med 6:573, 1987.
26. Mizuno K, and Hirohata K: Diagnosis of recurrent traumatic anterior subluxation of the shoulder, Corr 179:160, 1983.
27. Morgan CD, and Bodenstab AB: Arthroscopic Bankart suture repair: technique and early results, Arthroscopy 3:111, 1987.
28. Morrison DS: Correlation of acromial morphology and the results of arthroscopic subacromial decompression, Orthop Trans 12:731, 1988.
29. Neer CS II: Anterior acromioplasty for the chronic impingement syndrome in the shoulder: a preliminary report, J Bone Joint Surg 54A:41, 1972.
30. Neer CS II: Impingement lesions, Clin Orthop 173:70, 1983.
31. Nottage WM: Shoulder arthroscopy: portals and surgical techniques, Tech Orthop 3:23, 1988.
32. Nottage WM, Duge WD and Fields WA: Computed arthrotomography of the glenohumeral joint to evaluate anterior instability: correlation with arthroscopic findings, Arthroscopy 3:273, 1987.
33. Ogilvie-Harris DJ, and Wiley AM: Arthroscopic Surgery of the shoulder: a general appraisal, J Bone Joint Surg 68B:201, 1986.
34. Pappas AM, Goss TP, and Kleinman PK: Symptomatic shoulder instability due to lesions of the glenoid labrum, Am J Sports Med 11:279, 1983.
35. Rockwood CA, Jr, and Green DP: Fractures in adults, ed 2, Philadelphia, 1984, JB Lippincott Co.
35a. Rockwood, CA, Jr. Shoulder arthroscopy, editorial, J Bone Joint Surg 70A:639, 1988.
36. Rojvanit F: Arthroscopy of the shoulder joint—a cadaver and clinical study. I. Cadaver study, J Jpn Orthop Assoc 58:1035, 1984.
37. Skyhar MJ, Altcheck DW, and Warren RF: Shoulder arthroscopy in the seated position, Orthop Rev 10:1033, 1988.
38. Small NC: Complications in arthroscopy: the knee and other joints, Arthroscopy 2:253, 1986.
39. Takagi K: Practical experiences using Takagi's arthroscope, J Jpn Orthop Assoc 8:132, 1933.
40. Wolf EM: Arthroscopic anterior shoulder capsulorrhaphy, Tech Orthop 3:67, 1988.
41. Zarins B: Current concepts in the diagnosis and treatment of shoulder instability in athletes, Med Sci Sports Exerc 16:444, 1984.
42. Zuckerman JD, and Masten FA: Complications about the glenohumeral joint related to the use of screws and staples, J Bone Joint Surg 66A:175, 1984.

CHAPTER 6 Acromioclavicular Complex

John A. Bergfeld

Injuries to the acromiocoracoclavicular ligament complex are a common problem in athletics.

MECHANISMS OF INJURY

A knowledge of the pertinent anatomy is important in understanding the rationales for intervention (Fig. 6-1). The box below summarizes the AC complex components.

The acromioclavicular (AC), coracoclavicular (CC) complex is usually injured by a fall in which the athlete lands on the tip of his acromion, forcing the scapula caudally[2,18] (Fig. 6-2). If the clavicle does not break, then the acromioclavicular and coracoclavicular ligaments may be sprained. Other mechanisms of injury include a direct lateral blow on the shoulder (crushed in a pile-up) or a posterior blow to the scapula. An indirect injury may result from a fall on the outstretched arm or elbow. These are rare mechanisms by far. The fall in which the outer edge of the shoulder (tip of the acromion) is landed on is the most common mechanism. Injury to the acromiocoracoclavicular complex is common in football, rugby, ice hockey, skiing, wrestling, horseback riding, and, to a lesser extent, basketball, tumbling, and soccer.

AC-CC complex

- Acromioclavicular joint—Acromioclavicular ligaments
- Coracoclavicular interval—Coracoclavicular ligament (conoid and trapezoid)

CLASSIFICATION OF INJURIES

Prioritization of injuries developed by Rockwood allows us to effectively group the injuries for diagnosis, treatment, and prognosis[18] (Fig. 6-3). Grade I injuries represent a mild sprain of the acromioclavicular coracoclavicular ligaments, with no anatomic disruption of either the AC joint or the coracoclavicular ligaments.[2] Grade II represents a partial displacement of the AC joint, less than the width of the clavicle, representing a second degree sprain of both the AC and CC ligaments. Grade III represents complete loss of the integrity of the AC ligaments and coracoclavicular ligaments. Grade IV is a posterior dislocation of the clavicle on the acromium, with complete disruption of the AC joint and ligaments, although the coracoclavicular ligaments may remain intact. Grade V represents complete loss of the acromioclavicular joint, ligaments, and coracoclavicular ligaments, as well as the trapezius and deltoid muscle attachment to the clavicle and acromion. Often the acromion buttonholes through the mus-

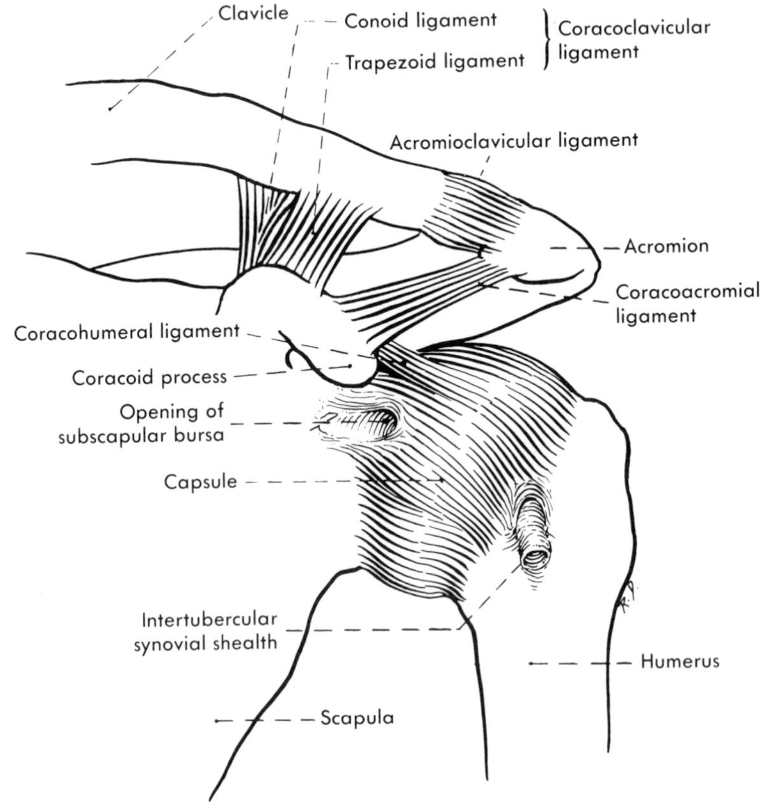

FIG. 6-1. Ligaments of the acromial end of the clavicle and the anterior aspect of the shoulder joint.

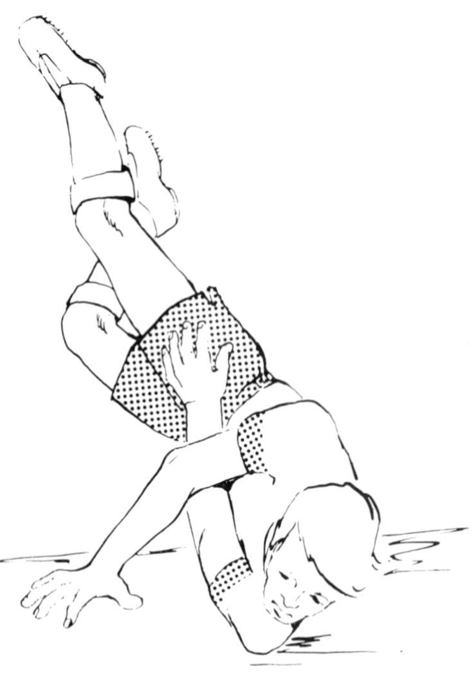

FIG. 6-2. The most common mechanism of injury is a direct force that occurs from a fall on the point of the shoulder.

-cle. Grade VI represents the clavicle being displaced inferiorly to the coracoid. This is a very rare injury in athletics, and usually occurs only with massive trauma, such as that sustained in a motorcycle or motor vehicle accident.

ACUTE INJURIES

Grade I

The Grade I injury is the most common injury, but often goes unnoticed until the day after the injury, and sometimes until the late sequela of posttraumatic arthritis causes discomfort in the shoulder. Physical examination is characterized by point tenderness directly over the acromioclavicular joint, a good diagnostic point to differentiate this injury from

Grade I injury

- Point tenderness on acromioclavicular joint
- No instability of joint
- Minimal or no loss of shoulder motion
- Normal roentgenogram

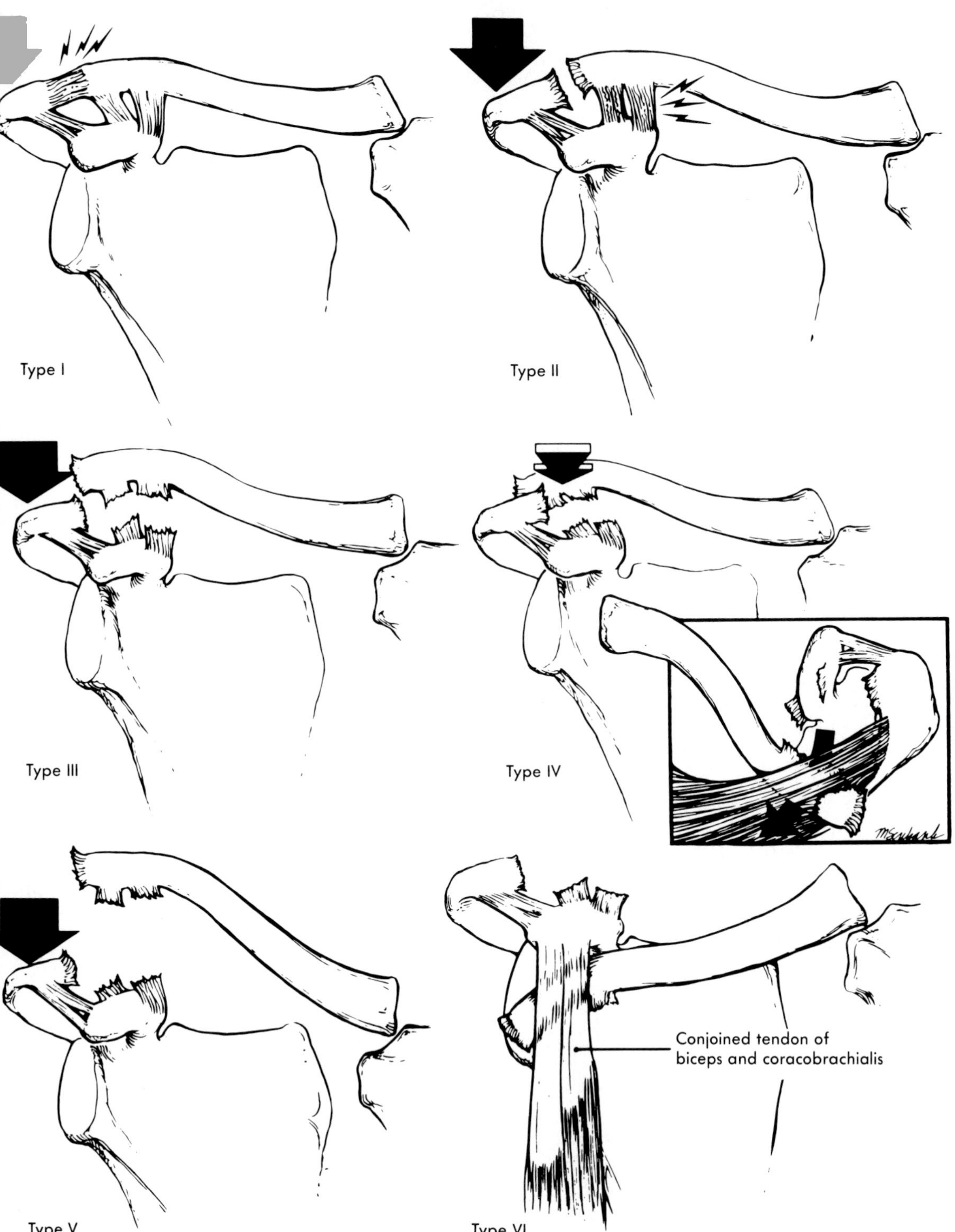

FIG. 6-3. Rockwood's classification of injuries to the acromioclavicular, coracoclavicular complex. (From Neer CS, and Rockwood CA: Fractures and dislocations of the shoulder. In Rockwood CA, and Green DP, editors: Fractures in adults, Philadelphia, 1984, JB Lippincott Co.)

the shoulder pointer (contusion on the acromion), or strain of the rotator cuff. The joint will be stable, and often there is no loss of motion of the shoulder joint; the athlete reports only mild discomfort at the extremes of motion, especially abduction. Roentgenograms will be negative. A good physical examination should preclude the need for stress roentgenograms to rule out further injury.

Treatment

Treatment of the acute grade I injury is symptomatic. These measures include ice, antiinflammatory medication, and padding of the shoulder to prevent direct pressure over the joint (Fig. 6-4). Often the athlete is able to return to competition immediately, and certainly within 2 days to 2 weeks, depending upon the sport.

Grade II

With this injury the athlete is usually aware of the injury because of the pain and functional disability. Physical examination reveals mild laxity of the AC joint, and a step-off that may be felt between the clavicle and the acromion. There will be limitation of abduction and adduction of the shoulder. Roentgenograms without stress will show the classic appearance of the acromion being depressed less than the width of the clavicle. Occasionally the roentgenograms will be normal, and stress roentgenograms will be necessary (Fig. 6-5). We find the need for stress a rare situation. After some experience, one should be able to tell if there is instability of the AC-CC complex on a physical examination.

Grade II injury

- Moderate discomfort
- Palpable (mild) AC joint step off
- Limitation of abduction and adduction

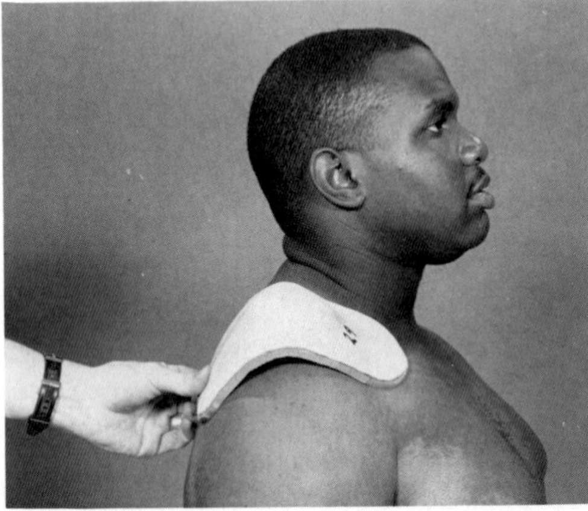

FIG. 6-4. Following grade I injury, the shoulder is padded to allow return to competition.

Stress views

- Specific views must be taken of the AC joint
- Proper exposure and angulation of the beam is essential
- Stress roentgenograms require passive stretching of the joint, with weights suspended from both the injured arm and the contralateral arm
- Often the patient is mistakenly asked to hold the weights in the hands, with the resulting muscle contraction negating the displacement of the joint

Treatment

Treatment of this injury is again symptomatic, but now one must be more aggressive in supporting the joint. Usually a sling is sufficient, but I often use a modified Kinney-Howard sling to get proper support of the joint (Fig. 6-6). The length of treatment depends upon the symptoms, and competition in all but a few sports that produce unusual stress across the AC joint (i.e., parallel bar). The athlete may return to sports usually as soon as he or she is free of pain; this requires anywhere from 1 to 4 weeks. The deformity that is initally present with the joint will remain a permanent deformity. Before going on to Grade III, IV, and V injuries, further discussion of the Grade I and II injuries is warranted.

LONG-TERM SEQUELAE

Grade I and II Injuries

Often little concern is given to the sequela of Grade I and II injuries in the textbooks for general orthopaedics. These injuries may cause significant problems for the athlete in the future. A follow-up study of midshipmen carried out at the U.S. Naval Academy by Andrish and Bergfeld in 1973,[4] and a similar study repeated, by Cox at the U.S. Naval Academy,[11] revealed a surprisingly large number of persistent positive physical findings and roentgenographic changes, and significant symptoms (Table 6-1).

The positive physical findings consist of

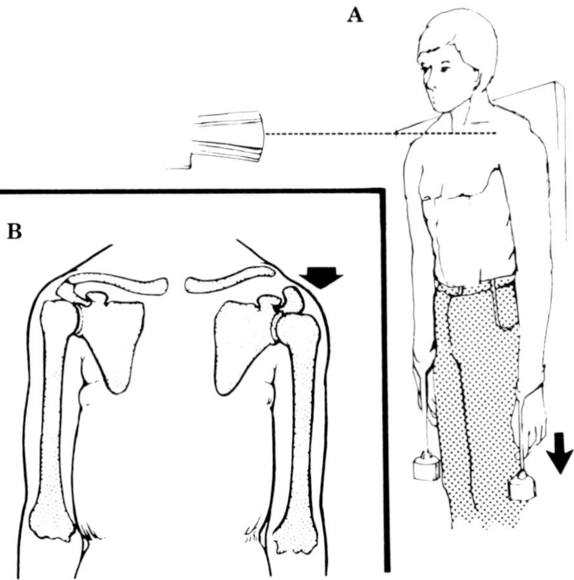

FIG. 6-5. Technique of obtaining stress roentgenographs of the acromioclavicular joint. **A,** Anterior posterior roentgenographs are made of both acromioclavicular joints with 10 to 15 pounds of weight hanging from the wrists. **B,** The distance between the superior aspect of the coracoid and the undersurface of the clavicle is measured to determine whether or not the coracoclavicular ligaments have been disrupted. One large horizontal-positioned 14 × 17-inch roentgenograph cassette can be used in small patients to visualize both shoulders on the same film. In large patients it is better to use two horizontal-placed smaller cassettes and take two separate roentgenographs for the measurements.

TABLE 6-1 Long-term findings in grade I and II AC injuries

	Grade I	Grade II
Positive physical examination	43%	71%
Abnormal roentgenogram	29%	48%
Support system	3.5%* 9%†	13%* 23%†

*Data from Cox JS: Am J Sports Med 5:258, 1977.
†Data from Bergfeld JA et al: A J Sports Med 6:153, 1978.

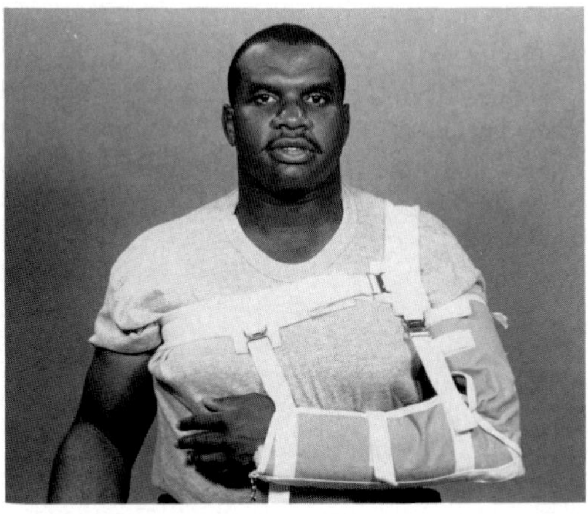

FIG. 6-6. Modified Kinney-Howard sling for proper support of AC joint.

thickening and prominence of the acromioclavicular joint. Abnormal roentgenographic findings include post-traumatic changes about the AC joint, loss of the joint space, bony spurring, and soft tissue calcification. A minor roentgenographic finding commonly linked to the first degree AC separation is **osteolysis of the lateral clavicle.** This was an identical finding in these studies, and did not correlate with symptoms. Many authors postulate that this osteolysis is caused by avascular necrosis of the lateral clavicle secondary to undecompressed pressure from intraarticular hematoma in a first degree injury.[9,14] I have seen an osteolytic clavicle recalcify, and I have also noted avascular necrosis in a resected lateral clavicle that had been symptomatic after grade I AC injuries.

The significant after symptoms in athletes with osteolysis grade I injuries include pain with heavy activity, such as dips between parallel bars, bench pressing heavy weights, and overhand serving in tennis, as well as throwing a ball. The cause of these symptoms is usually the incongruity of the AC joint as the result of tearing of the meniscus between the clavicle and the acromion, or simply posttraumatic arthritis with loss of the articular surface and spur formation.

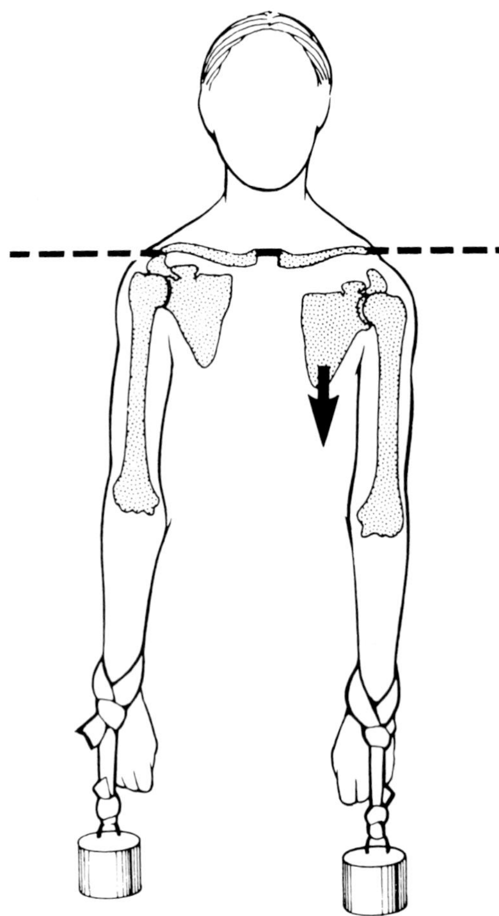

FIG. 6-7. Schematic drawing of a patient with a complete grade III acromioclavicular dislocation. The major deformity seen in this injury is a downward displacement of the scapula and upper extremity and *not* an upward elevation of the clavicle.

Treatment of Chronic Symptoms

Treatment of the chronically symptomatic grade I and grade II injury is to first assure that there is full strength of the joint. Consideration can be given to a corticosteroid injection, which will often resolve the inflammatory response. Injections can be repeated 1 or 2 times if there is persistent discomfort. Surgical resection of the lateral clavicle will yield good results. The lateral 1½ cm of the clavicle should be resected to achieve satisfactory improvement in the athlete's symptoms.

The grade I and II injury to the AC joint in the athlete should not be taken lightly, because he or she may have problems in the future. Fortunately, the steroid injection or, if needed, the resection of the lateral clavicle, gives generally satisfactory results.

ACUTE INJURIES

Grade III

Grade III injury is more severe, and the injured athlete will experience immediate pain, limitation of motion, and possible disability. Often the athlete comes out of the participation supporting his or her shoulder with the opposite arm. Inspection of the shoulder will reveal the downward displacement of the acromion and often one hears that the clavicle is riding high (Fig. 6-7). This is an illusion because the clavicle remains at the same level as it's counterpart; it is the scapula that is driven caudally. The clavicle is freely movable and there is complete loss of integrity of the AC joint and coracoclavicular ligaments. An occasional patient may have a posterior subluxation or dislocation of the clavicle in relation to the acromion (Rockwood's grade IV).

Grade III injury

- Severe pain
- Marked limitation of motion
- Downward acromion displacement

In the mild Grade IV, the coracoclavicular ligaments will remain intact. In the Grade III injury, although there is complete loss of the ligamentous stability, the trapezius and deltoid muscles are only partially torn from the clavicle. As with any injury, especially involving the shoulder, careful neurologic examination should be carried out. It is interesting to note that it is rare to see a brachial plexus injury associated with a Grade III acromioclavicular sprain in the athlete. I believe the dissipation of the energy through rupturing of the AC and CC ligaments relieves the abnormal stress on the brachial plexus. It may also be that the blow to the shoulder that causes the brachial plexus injury is more toward the top of the shoulder and closer to the spine, such as might occur in making a tackle in American football (see injuries to brachial plexus).

Treatment

Treatment of the grade III injury has changed in the past 15 years. In 1974, a poll of Chairmen of the Teaching Programs revealed the 95% responded that this injury required surgery to restore the normal anatomy, although a similar recent survey by Cox[11] found only 40% of the respondents believed surgery was necessary. An informal poll of orthopaedists who treat athletes exclusively raises the percentage of those advocating nonoperative treatment to approximately 90%. This is not to say that nonoperative treatment may return the anatomy to normal, but, as Hippocrates said, "No impediment, small or great, will result from such an injury (grade III AC separation), however there would be [malposition] or deformity, for the bone cannot be properly restored to its rational situation."[1]

Before proceeding further, let me say that grade V injury (complete loss of the attachment of the trapezius and deltoid muscles) should be repaired surgically, as this is a severe loss of muscle and ligamentous integrity of the AC joint. Resultant deformity is such that functional use of the shoulder is severely compromised. Fortunately, this is a rare injury in all sports, except motorcycling.

Several considerations must go into the treatment of the very common grade III injury. There are problems and complications in both open and closed methods (Table 6-2).

Overall, a 5% to 10% incidence of significant problems can be anticipated with a grade III AC injury, no matter whether it is treated by closed or open means.

A review of the literature reveals a multiplicity of surgical procedures designed for acromioclavicular separations.* At present, there appear to be three basic procedures commonly performed: (1) AC joint fixation with wires,[6] (2) circumferential dacron or wire immobilization of the coracoid and clavicle,[16,19] and (3) screw fixation of the clavicle to the coracoid.[7] After personally treating many of these injuries, using all of the above methods at one time or another, I have elected to now treat these injuries by closed method. The closed method falls into two categories—symptomatic and aggressive[5,13,22,23] (Table 6-3).

TABLE 6-2 Complications or problems in treating Grade III injury

Closed Method	Open Method
Deformity	Anesthesia
Patient intolerance	Infection
Failure to obtain reduction	Cosmetic scar
Failure to maintain reduction	Fixation device failure a. breaks become loose b. migrate c. erode through bone d. second operation to remove
Postimmobilization joint stiffness	Expense
Compression neuropathy	Time loss from competition
	Longer than nonoperative treatment
Common Problems (Open and Closed Treatment)	
Posttraumatic arthritis	
Deformity versus scar	
Calcification of soft tissues	
Pain and disability with sports activity	

Closed symptomatic treatment. Closed, symptomatic treatment might be called, by some, skillful neglect. This term is because any method will require attention to the details of splint adjustment and rehabilitation. The closed symptomatic treatment has many advantages, including earlier return to competition.[5,15] One hundred percent will have some residual deformity of the AC joint. Approximately 5% to 10% of the individuals will find the cosmetic appearance disturbing. However, little correlation is found between

*References 3, 8, 10, 17, 20, 21.

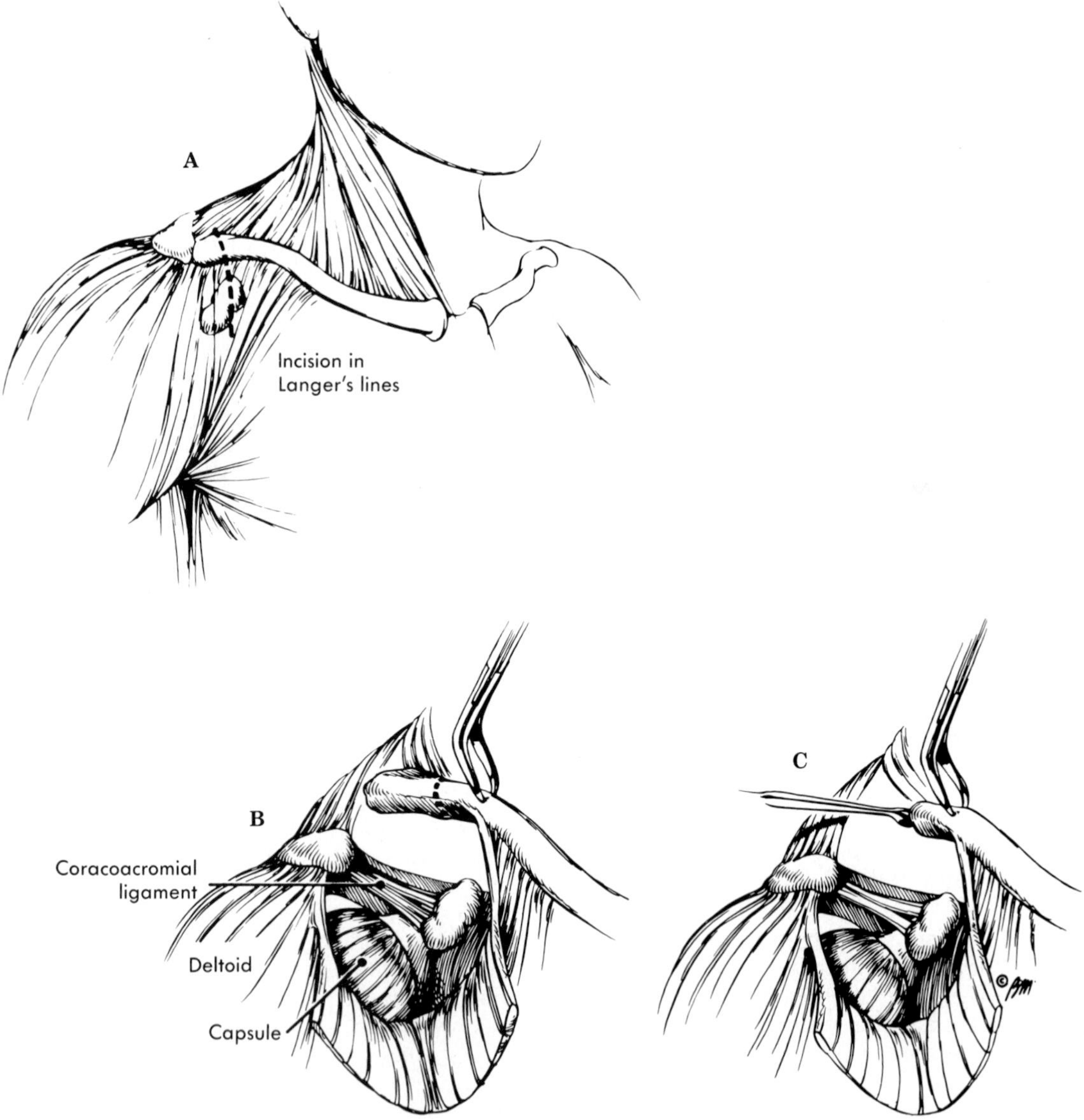

FIG. 6-8. A through **H,** Author's method to reconstruct a type III acromioclavicular dislocation. See text for description. Preoperative *(left)* and postoperative *(right)* x-rays of a chronic type III A/C dislocation treated with an acromioclavicular reconstruction. There are degenerative changes in the acromioclavicular joint that were causing pain in this laboring man. The coracoacromial ligament will be used to reconstruct the coracoclavicular ligaments. Following removal of the distal 1¼ inches of the clavicle the coracoacromial ligament, which was detached from the acromion, was transferred into the medullary canal of the distal clavicle. The coracoclavicular lag screw will hold the clavicle in position for 8 to 12 weeks until there is secure fixation of the ligament to the clavicle.

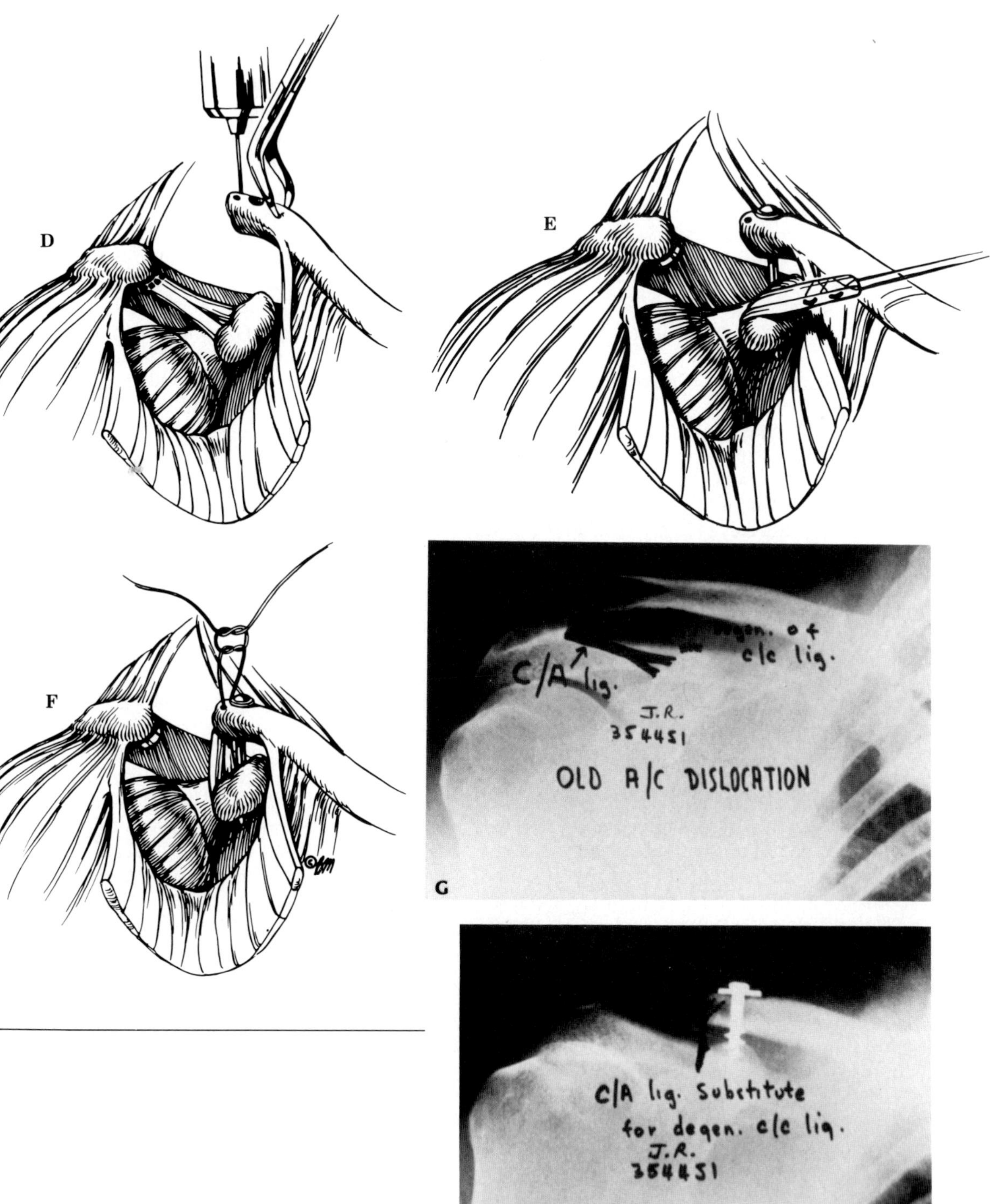
D
E
F
degen. of
c/c lig.
C/A lig.
J.R.
354451
OLD A/C DISLOCATION
G
C/A lig. Substitute
for degen. c/c lig.
J.R.
354451
H

TABLE 6-3 Closed treatment

Symptomatic	Aggressive
Immobilization for comfort	Reduce with a splint
Begin rehabilitation when tolerated	Attempt to maintain reduction
	Begin rehabilitation when tolerated

the final roentgenogram, the clinical appearance,[12] and the incidence of significant pain and disability. Like other methods the closed symptomatic treatment yields a 5% to 10% incidence of later problems requiring medical attention.

Closed aggressive treatment. The closed aggressive treatment has other advantages for certain situations. An attempt is made to restore normal anatomy, therefore the resultant deformity will not be as severe as with the closed symptomatic treatment. These techniques are difficult to carry out, however, if patient's compliance is poor, and particularly after 3 weeks from the initial injury. The closed aggressive treatment has the same incidence of persistent significant pain and disability as other methods.

Techniques of treatment. If seen at the site of injury, a grade III acromioclavicular joint sprain can often be easily reduced and held with a modified "Kinney-Howard sling." Once the acromioclavicular joint is reduced, the athlete is given pain medication and instructions to keep the shoulder quiet, not to remove the sling unless there is severe pain, and report for daily adjustment of the sling. If symptomatic treatment is elected, the acromioclavicular sling is discontinued when the symptoms allow, usually after 7 to 10 days. While the patient is in the sling, isometric exercises are begun; the sling is loosened for range of motion exercises and these are performed through the range of motion with the athlete or the therapist supporting the acromioclavicular joint. Progressive resistance exercises are begun as soon as they can be tolerated by the athlete.

If agressive treatment is elected, then an attempt is made to keep the joint reduced for 6 full weeks, during which time isometric exercises are instituted and periodic checks of sling position are made. Experience shows that patent compliance drops off after approximately 3 weeks, and one finds the sling on only in the doctor's office or the training room.

More commonly, the athlete is seen several hours after the injury and moderate to severe swelling as well as pain is present. An attempt to reduce the joint and support it with the AC sling is a difficult, uncomfortable experience for the athlete, and frustrating for the physician, therapist, or trainer. If one applies a sling, and only tightens it for pain reduction, this is also often unsuccessful. An injection into the area with local anesthetic can assist in obtaining a good reduction, essentially a hematoma block, much like treatment of a Colles fracture. The joint is fixed in the sling. This often requires admission to the hospital, where pain medication and attention to the sling at frequent intervals can be carried out. With both symptomatic and aggressive treatment, once the sling is discontinued, the athlete is allowed to return to competition when he or she can demonstrate a full range of motion and reasonable strength in the shoulder. A recent report by Walsh[24] showed that there was no decrease in strength compared to the normal shoulder in the third degree AC separations treated by nonoperative means, as opposed to a 19.8% deficit in those shoulders treated surgically. This report tends to give support to nonsurgical treatment of this problem, especially in the athlete or worker who requires good strength in his or her shoulder.

In certain grade III injuries, closed treatment may not be satisfactory. This might be a body builder or fashion model who, for cosmetic reasons, absolutely needs to restore normal anatomy. In the question of a throwing athlete, the need to restore anatomy also may arise, although a majority of the team orthopaedic surgeons treating throwing athletes often resort to closed method of treatment. A preferable technique is the method described by Bosworth[7] and popularized by Rockwood.[18] The AC joint is debrided and the coracoclavicular ligaments are repaired as best as possible. The AC joint, now reduced, is held with a lag screw (or, in some instances, a Dacron tape is used).

Braided PDS suture can be used in place of a Dacron tape. This material loses its strength and dissolves within the body after 8 to 10 weeks, thereby negating the need to go back and cut the tape or remove the lag screw. At the time of surgery, all muscles are repaired.

LONG-TERM SEQUELAE

Grade III Injuries

For the athlete who has the residuum of a third-degree AC separation with significant pain and disability, I prefer a modification of the procedure described by Weaver and Dunn.[25] This consists of resection of the lateral clavicle, reconstruction of the coracoclavicular ligaments using the coracoacromial ligament, and stabilization of the coracoid to the clavicle using a lag screw or Dacron tape (Fig. 6-8). With this technique, the screw must be removed and or the tape cut at 8 to 10 weeks postoperatively.

Often there is a severe calcification and scarring in the area of the coracoclavicular ligaments, making any reduction of the space between the clavicle and the coracoid very difficult. In this situation, a simple resection of the lateral clavicle is appropriate.

POSTERIOR DISLOCATION

The clinician should look closely for the third-degree posterior dislocated clavicle because this injury tends to have an increased incidence of chronic functional disability. Acutely, there may be difficulty reducing this separation with a sling, necessitating an open reduction. Most often, the examiner can determine by physical examination that the clavicle is posterior to the acromion. If the examiner is unable to determine this, a hint that there is a posterior subluxation of the clavicle on the acromion is indicated by the clavicle and acromion being at the same level, although there is a widened space between the acromion and the clavicle. If there is any question that there is a posterior dislocation of the clavicle, a CT scan with comparison to the opposite shoulder is often helpful.

In our clinic, we have treated one young patient who sustained an interesting posterior subluxation of the clavicle, having split through its periosteum. The athlete then began to regenerate a second clavicle in its final position, necessitating resection of the distal portion of the initial clavicle, which was ruptured posteriorly. Posterior subluxation of the clavicle tends to occur, in our experience, in the younger athlete, and most commonly in wrestlers. It is not a common injury in the person who is fully skeletally mature.

REHABILITATION

As with all athletic injuries, rehabilitation should begin as soon as possible to avoid the deleterious effects of immobilization. As soon as the shoulder is stabilized, by sling or surgically, isometric contraction of the shoulder musculature should be instituted. After surgical treatment, a gentle, full range of motion of the joint can be started when shoulders are pain free. Light resistive exercises can be begun at 3 weeks and weight lifting at 8 to 10 weeks.

With closed treatment, range of motion can be started after 2 weeks, with an assistant stabilizing the acromioclavicular joint. Eventually, the athlete will be able to stabilize his or her own AC joint with the opposite hand. Modified resistive exercise can be started immediately, progressing to full progressive resistance exercise at 8 to 10 weeks after injury. Returning to sports activity must be individualized, depending on the athlete and his or her sport.

REFERENCES

1. Adams FL: The genuine work of Hippocrates, vol 1, 2, New York, 1986, William Wood.
2. Allman FL Jr: Fractures and ligamentous injuries of the clavicle and its articulation, J Bone Joint Surg 9A:774, 1967.
3. Bailey RW: A dynamic repair for complete acromioclavicular joint dislocation, J Bone Joint Surg 47A:858, 1985.
4. Bergfeld JA et al: Evaluation of the acromioclavicular joint following first and second degree sprains, Am J Sports Med 6:153, 1978.
5. Bjerneld H et al: Acromioclavicular separations treated conservatively, Acta Orthop Scan 54:743, 1983.
6. Bloom FA: Wire fixation in acromioclavicular dislocation, J Bone Joint Surg 27:273, 1945.
7. Bosworth BM: Acromioclavicular separation—a new method of repair, Surg Gynecol Obstet 73: 866, 1941.
8. Browne J et al: Acromioclavicular joint dislocations—comparative results following operative treatment with and without primary distal clavisectomy, Am J Sports Med 5:258, 1977.
9. Cahill BR: Osteolysis of the distal part of the clavicle in male athletes, J Bone Joint Surg 64A:1053, 1982.
10. Cook FF et al: The Mumford procedure in athletes: an objective analysis of function, Am J Sports Med 16(2):97, 1988.
11. Cox JS: The fate of the acromioclavicular joint in athletic injuries, Am J Sports Med 5:258, 1977.
12. Glick JM et al: Dislocated acromioclavicular joint follow-up study of 35 unreduced acromioclavicular dislocations, Am J Sports Med 5:264, 1977.
13. Imatani RJ et al: Acute complete acromioclavicular separations, J Bone Joint Surg 57A:328, 1975.
14. Jacobs P: Post-traumatic osteolysis of the outer end of the clavicle, J Bone Joint Surg 46B:705, 1964.
15. McDonald PB et al: Comprehensive functional analysis of shoulders following complete acromioclavicular separation, Am J Sports Med 16(5):475, 1988.
16. Monem MS and Balduini FC: Coracoid fractures as a complication of surgical treatment by coracoclavicular tap fixation, Clin Orthop 168:133, 1982.
17. Mumford EB: Acromioclavicular dislocation, J Bone Joint Surg 23:799, 1941.
18. Neer CS and Rockwood CA: Fractures and dislocations of the shoulder. In Rockwood CA and Green DP, editors: Fractures in adults, vol 1, Philadelphia, 1984, JB Lippincott Co.

19. Nelson CL: Repair of acromioclavicular separations with knitted dacron graft, Clin Orthop 143: 289, 1979.
20. Park JP et al: Treatment of acromioclavicular separation, Am J Sports Med 7:65, 1979.
21. Powers JA and Bach PJ: Acromioclavicular separation—closed or open treatment, Clin Orthop 104:213, 1974.
22. Smith MJ and Stewart MJ: Acute acromioclavicular separation, Am J Sports Med 7:65, 1979.
23. Stewart MJ: The acromioclavicular joint in the throwing arm. In Zarins B et al, editors: Injuries to the throwing arm, Philadelphia, 1985, WB Saunders Co.
24. Walsh WM et al: Shoulder strength following acromioclavicular injury, Am J Sports Med 13:153, 1985.
25. Weaver JK and Dunn HK: Treatment of acromioclavicular injuries, especially complete acromioclavicular separation, J Bone Joint Surg 54A:1187, 1972.

Figs. 6-2, 6-3, 6-5 and 6-8 reproduced from Neer CS and Rockwood CA: Fractures and dislocations of the shoulder. In Rockwood CA and Green DP, editors: Fractures in adults, vol 1, Philadelphia, 1984, JB Lippincott Co.

CHAPTER 7 Instability of the Shoulder

Michael J. Skyhar
Russell F. Warren
David W. Altchek

CLASSIFICATION OF INSTABILITY

The following classification of shoulder instability is used at the Hospital for Special Surgery in New York (HSS) (see outline below). The essential components of the classification system include frequency of occurrence, etiology, direction, and degree of instability.

Shoulder Instability Classification

A. Frequency
   1. Acute
   2. Recurrent
   3. Fixed (chronic)
B. Etiology
   1. Trauamtic (Macrotrauma)
   2. Atraumatic
      i) Voluntary
      ii) Involuntary
   3. Microtrauma (Repetitive use)
   4. Congenital
   5. Neuromuscular (Erb's palsy, cerebral palsy (CP), seizures)
C. Degrees
   1. Dislocation
   2. Subluxation
   3. Micro—(Transient)
D. Direction
   1. Anterior
   2. Posterior
   3. Inferior
   4. Multidirectional

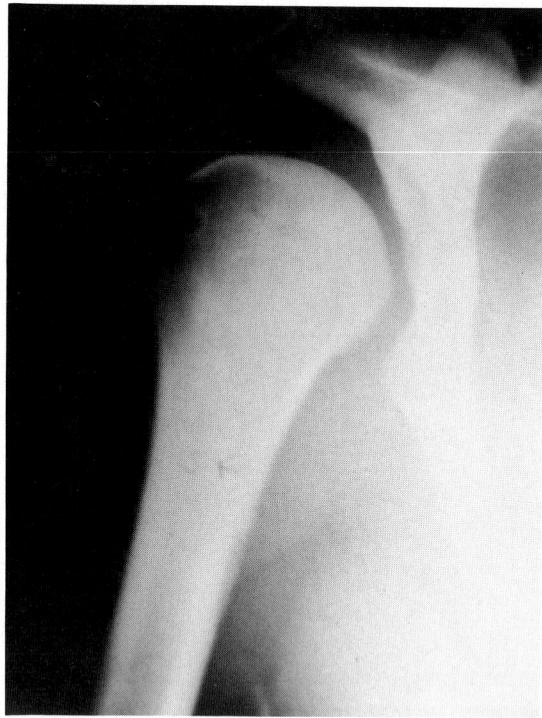

FIG. 7-1. Roentgenogram showing congenital dysplasia of the glenoid.

The classification system allows specific categorization for all types of shoulder instability. Classification systems improve diagnostic forethought, streamline treatment protocols, and facilitate comparative follow-up studies.

Frequency

The initial event, either subluxation or dislocation, is termed "acute," whereas those with repeated episodes are called "recurrent." The term **"fixed dislocation"** refers to the missed episode of a dislocation in which the humeral head is not reduced. This will occur in either a posterior or an anterior direction, resulting in restricted external or internal rotation, respectively.

Etiology

We have found it useful to include the etiology as a descriptive term in dealing with shoulder instability. As part of the classification system, this is based on the degree of trauma involved in the initial episode. The main terms are therefore traumatic versus atraumatic. In addition, a third group consisting of repetitive microtrauma should be considered (swimming, throwing). **Traumatic** episodes occur as specific isolated events in which the patient can describe a specific mechanism of injury. The **atraumatic** group of patients may have an involuntary episode that becomes voluntary over time, or the converse may occur. The atraumatic group includes patients with inherited ligamentous laxity in which the onset may be voluntary or involuntary. Other causes included **congenital,** with glenoid dysplasia (Fig. 7-1), and **neuromuscular** problems. In those situations glenoid shape and abnormal humeral version angles may be altered. Version angles may be altered in Erb's palsy or cerebral palsy, in which muscle contraction results in increased humeral head retroversion.

Rowe[31] has noted that those with a voluntary type of instability may have an underlying psychologic problem. In our experience voluntary instability has been more commonly associated with a prior involutary episode in an emotionally stable patient. In this setting exercise and cessation of the voluntary component are often helpful, but if the involuntary instability persists then operative treatment may be considered and a good result anticipated.

Degree

It is generally accepted that dislocation is more common at the glenohumeral joint than in other joints. Subluxation has been recognized more frequently as a distint clinical entity across the shoulder and may progress to recurrent dislocation. Essentially, subluxation represents increased humeral head translation in the glenoid to a point at which symptoms occur. It implies a degree of laxity of the soft tissues that is greater than "normal." More recently, with the use of the arthroscope, it has been noted that injury to the labrum may exist without obvious subluxation. We suspect that these labral injuries are the result of repetitive translation of the humeral head on the glenoid without obvious subluxation being present. This is frequent in throwing athletes in which humeral head translation (anterior and posterior) would develop high loads on the labrum, resulting in vertical tears or degeneration. With repeated injury this may progress to clinical subluxation if the labral injury affects the inferior glenohumeral ligament.

Direction

Generally it has been noted that anterior instability represents approximately 95% of shoulder instability.[42] More recently posterior shoulder instability has been observed commonly in athletes or loose-jointed individuals. In contrast to anterior shoulder instability, which often is initially seen as dislocation rather than subluxation, posterior instability of a recurrent type is nearly always a subluxation, with dislocation generally being an isolated and uncommon traumatic episode.

Shoulder instability

- **Anterior instability**
  95% of all instability
  Often present with dislocation
- **Posterior instability**
  Usually subluxation
  Dislocation less common

Shoulders with anterior or posterior instability may in addition subluxate or dislocate inferiorly. Termed "multidirectional instability," this may be present in two or three directions, but most will have significant inferior component combined with anterior, posterior, or both. A shoulder may sustain a complete inferior dislocation (luxatio erecta), but this is relatively uncommon in contrast to inferior subluxation. The shoulder may dislocate in one direction and sublux in a second or third. In a small percentage of patients we have seen anterior dislocation with marked posterior subluxation without inferior subluxation noted clinically. From a biomechanical point of view this is difficult to understand, since the inferior glenohumeral ligament should be injured. Possibly sufficient healing has occurred to prevent inferior subluxation but still allows abnormal anteroposterior translation.

PATHOPHYSIOLOGY OF SHOULDER INSTABILITY

A variety of factors may play a role in the development of clinical instability. These may occur as isolated factors or in association with other factors. They include (a) bone configuration, (b) capsule and ligament, and (c) muscle tendon unit. Forces applied to the shoulder have magnitude and direction and therefore can be subjected to vector analysis. Analysis of the resultant force reveals how the glenohumeral joint shares the load among the anatomic structure to create a stable situation. Three situations illustrate this point.

1. If a force is applied directly to the humeral head such that the vector (R) falls within the confines of the glenoid, the bony structure will contain the humeral head and the soft tissues will be lax.
2. If the resultant forces fall outside the confines of the glenoid, the resisting load will be shared by the glenoid and subsequently the ligaments. The soft tissue posteriorly as well as anteriorly would be expected to play a role in shoulder stabilization. The muscle tendon unit may act to create joint compression, also stabilizing this situation.
3. In the third example, the resultant force is directed away from the glenoid. This represents a distraction force as seen with throwing or reaching out suddenly. The bony anatomy is unable to play any role in resisting this type of instability. In this situation the anterior and posterior capsule will tighten to resist the forces and the muscle tendon unit will fire to compress the joint resisting distraction. In this analysis the subscapularis and infraspinatus would be expected to fire, attempting to decelerate the humeral head. If overloaded, strain might occur to the tendon, resulting in injury.

Contributing factors in shoulder instability

- Bone configuration
- Capsule and ligament integrity
- Motor unit function

Glenoid

The glenoid may be the only structure required to resist a direct force. Unfortunately its dimensions limit this ability. It is an ellipse measuring about 25 by 15 mm, with a radius of curvature less than that of the humeral head. However, the labrum increases the curvature making the glenoid/labral/capsule complex concentric with the humeral head. It may be congenitally dysplastic and result in recurrent subluxation, leading to instability, which presents clinically in an active teenager.

Fortunately, this condition is quite uncommon. Glenoid version angles have been noted by Saha[35] and our own studies to reveal no consistent abnormalities in patients with anterior or posterior dislocation. Humeral head version is usually about 30 degrees of retroversion. This may increase secondary to a muscle imbalance as in Erb's palsy, but in general it has not been implicated in shoulder instability. We have studied the interplay between glenoid version and humeral head version and have found a more parallel surface associated with anterior instability of the atraumatic type only.

Fractures of the glenoid may potentially result in shoulder instability. Generally the new bone seen at the margin of the joint represents ectopic bone formation, but acute fractures do occur. If the head is well positioned following reduction and no fracture fragments are displaced within the joint seen on computed tomography (CT) scan, our tendency initially is to treat these patients nonoperatively. However, if the head is seen to be subluxed or if significant fragments are in the joint, then early surgery and fracture reduction is recommended.

Capsule and Ligaments

The ligaments of the shoulder joint have a variable configuration dependent on the position of the arm. The superior glenohumeral ligament is often absent but the middle and inferior ligaments (anterior and posterior) are consistent structures (Fig. 7-2). Their appearance and function will vary with arm elevation and rotation, making examination in multiple positions important to detect instability. The posterior capsule is attenuated in many patients but inferiorly there is a thickening we have termed the "posterior inferior glenohumeral ligament."[36] Anteriorly the inferior glenohumeral ligament has a well-recognized band ascending superiorly to attach to the labrum. The inferior glenohumeral ligament complex with its anterior and posterior bands acts as a sling under the humeral head, preventing abnormal anterior and posterior translations as well as inferior instability. The middle ligament is a consistent structure that passes across the subscapularis tendon attaching anteriorly on the glenoid. Studies have shown that it acts as a secondary restraint to anterior instability. Previously Turkel et al noted that for a dislocation to occur anteriorly, they had to cut the anterior ligaments from the glenoid, including the superior middle and anterior half of the inferior glenohumeral ligament, as well as the posterior half of the inferior glenohumeral ligament.[40]

In a study performed at HSS, we have similarly evaluated posterior dislocation and found that in a right shoulder, cutting all of the posterior structures from the 6- to 12-o'clock positions did not cause dislocation but did result in some increased posterior translation. Dislocation did not occur until the anterior superior capsule and ligaments from the 12- to 3-o'clock positions were incised (Fig. 7-3).[17]

More recently, studies at our institution with instrumented testing have demonstrated that incising ligaments on one side of the shoulder resulted in increased translation on both sides.[36] When testing a shoulder at 90 degrees of elevation in three planes of horizontal abduction (−30, 0, +30 degrees relative to the scapula), three basic facts became clear. Normal humeral head translation was evenly divided between anterior and posterior. Maximal laxity was seen in the normal shoulder with the arm in the plane of the scapula and averaged 23 mm. The smallest excursion was seen with the arm position at 30 degrees anterior to the scapula, 13 mm. Cutting of the ligaments demonstrated that the superior ligament had little function while the middle ligament acted as a secondary restraint. The inferior glenohumeral ligament with its anterior and posterior bands was the prime stabilizer of the shoulder, resisting anterior, posterior, and inferior translation. The anterior and posterior limbs acted in concert to limit anterior and posterior translation. Only by cutting the posterior limb of the inferior ligament in conjunction with the anterior structures would dislocation routinely occur.[36]

From these experiments we have concluded that the shoulder acts as a circle in that for a dislocation to occur both sides of the circle must be interrupted (Fig. 7-4). Thus in examining shoulders with anterior dislocation one should not be surprised to note increased posterior translation. In addition, surgery on one side of the joint will affect the opposite side. If the anterior structures are over-tightened, as in a Putti-Platt procedure, the humeral head may then slide posteriorly,

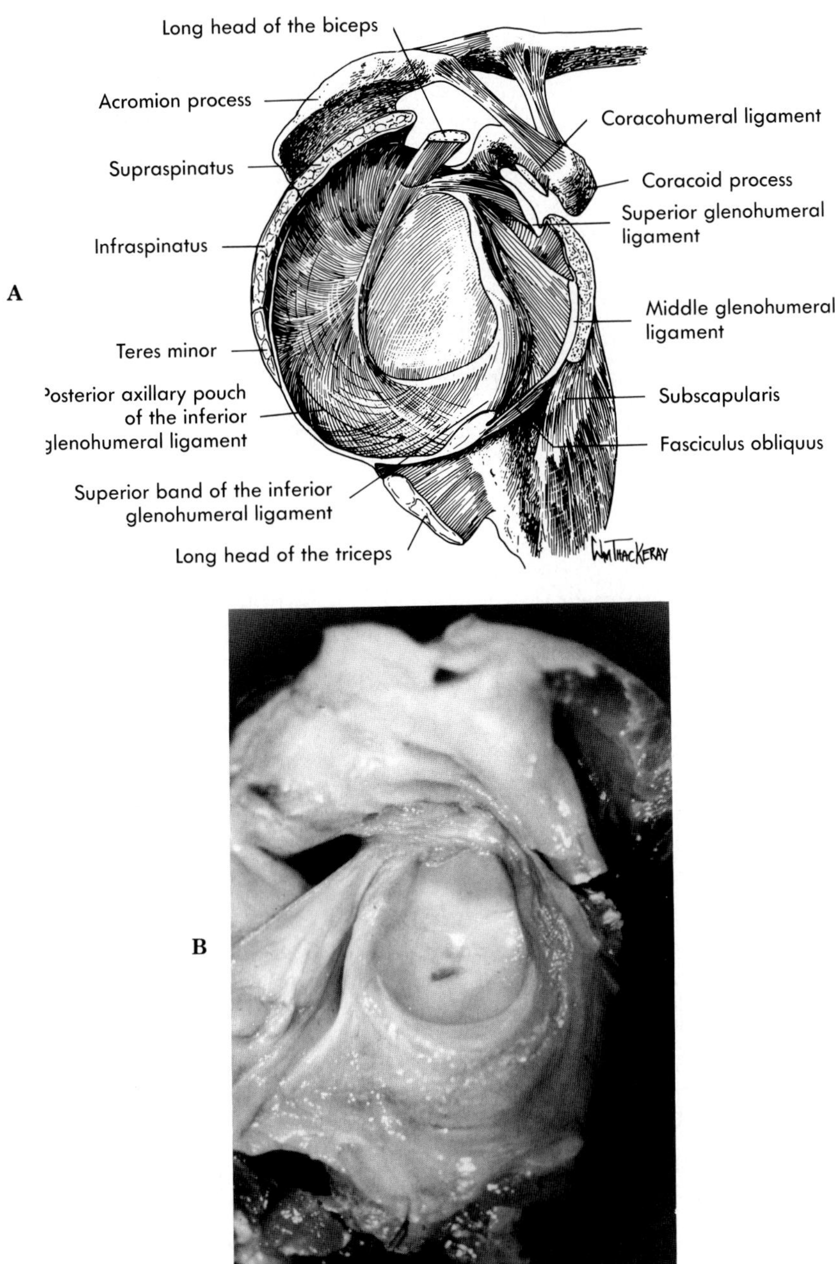

FIG. 7-2. A, Schematic drawing of right glenohumeral capsuloligamentous complex. Note superior, middle, and inferior glenohumeral ligaments. The superior ligament is variable in its presence. **B**, Cadaveric specimen of left glenohumeral capsuloligamentous complex. Compare with schematic drawing.

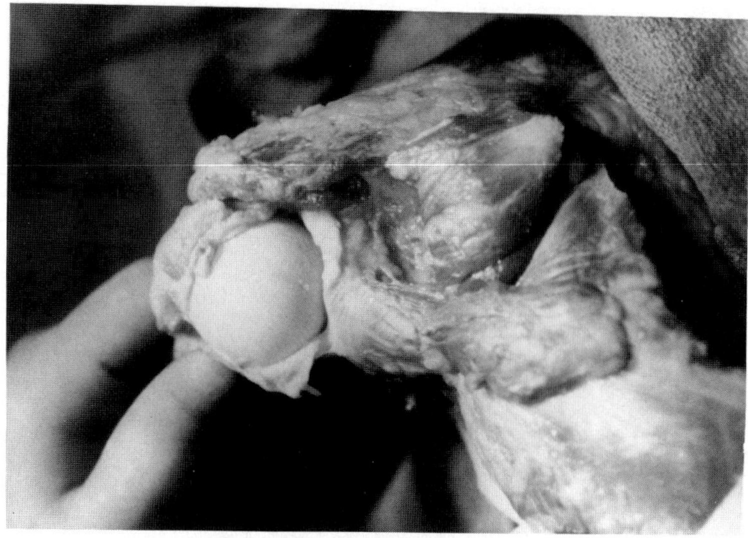

FIG. 7-3. A view of the posterior shoulder. The capsule is cut from the 12- to 6-o'clock position allowing only posterior subluxation. For dislocation to occur, an additional cut in the anterior capsule from the 1- to 3-o'clock position is necessary.

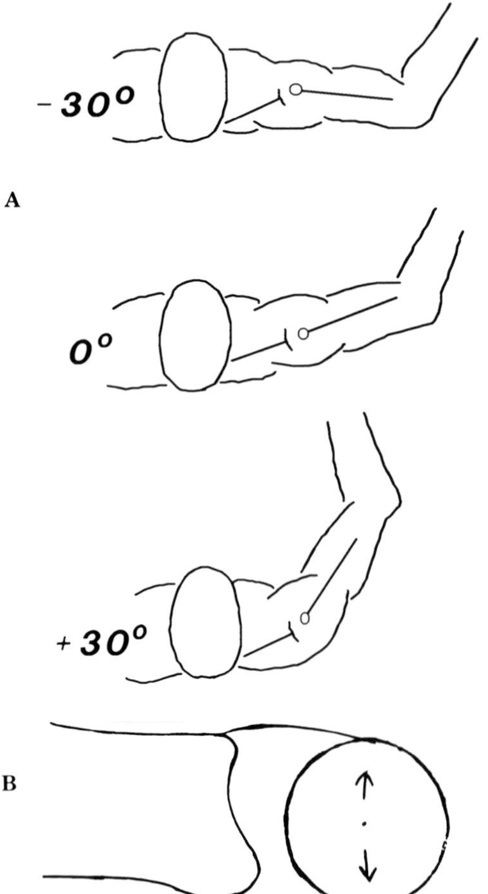

FIG. 7-4. A, With the arm in three planes of horizontal abduction (−30, 0, +30 degrees relative to the scapula) instrumented laxity testing was performed on the glenohumeral joint following selective glenohumeral ligament cutting. **B**, Shoulder as a circle.

resulting in increased stress on the articular cartilage and posterior capsule. These patients may present later with symptomatic posterior instability or, as Hawkins has reported, degenerative arthritis following overtightening in Putti-Platt procedures.[13]

Muscle Tendon Unit

Few objective data concerning the dynamic function of these tissues have been reported. Some static effects are possible in certain positions, with tightening occurring in the tendon raphe of the subscapularis or infraspinatus as the arm is elevated and rotated. Injury to these muscles alone will not allow dislocation to occur. However, with fatigue or certain activities, such as throwing, they may allow abnormally high forces to be generated on the ligament and/or labrum, resulting in injury. Soft tissue injury within the subscapularis is often noted at surgery but may be secondary rather than primary. Muscles passing across joints are able to decrease translations and increase stiffness by creating compression. In addition in the shoulder they may resist distraction forces.

Muscle forces across the shoulder

- Decrease translation
- Increase stiffness
- Create compressive forces
- Resist distraction forces

A

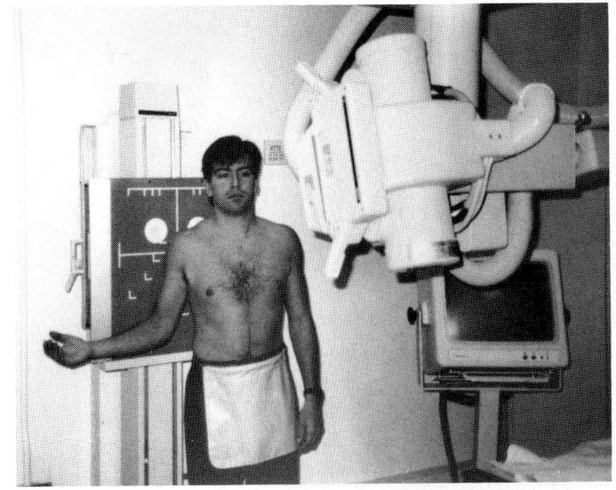

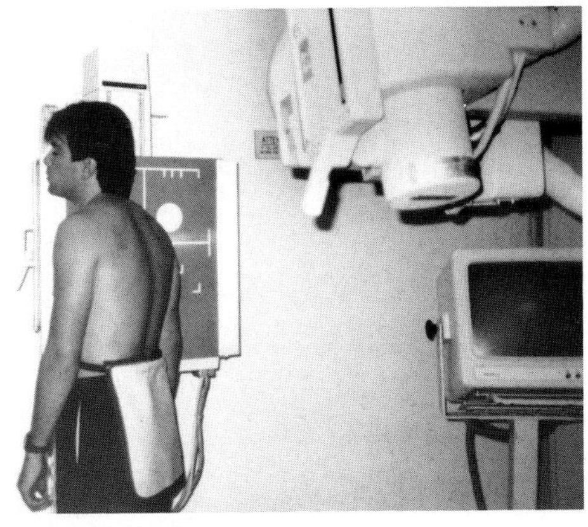

B

C

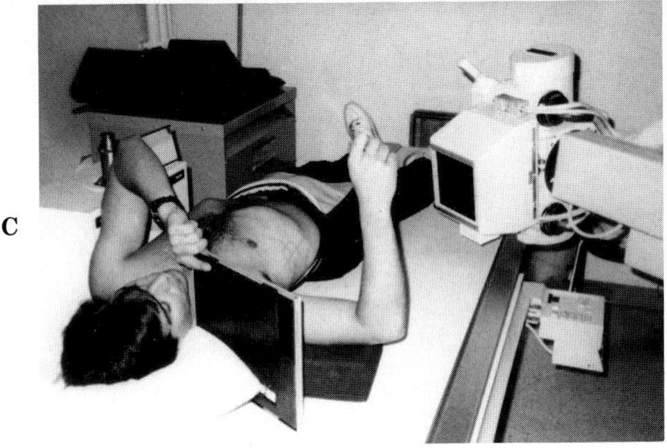

FIG. 7-5. The roentgenographic series for shoulder trauma includes **A**, true AP of the scapula; **B**, true lateral in the scapular plane; **C**, physician assisted axillary.

In Erb's palsy and cerebral palsy, contractures of these tissues will result in altered development of the proximal humerus, resulting in increased stress on the capsule and ligaments, which may in time become symptomatic.

ROENTGENOGRAPHIC EVALUATION

The roentgenographic evaluation of acute shoulder instability should include three views of the glenohumeral joint. These are the true anteroposterior (AP), transscapular or Y views, and a physician-assisted axillary or seated axillary view (Fig. 7-5). These views are useful screening studies for fractures, glenohumeral dislocation, and acromioclavicular (AC) joint pathology. It is very helpful for the physician to assist in positioning the patient's arm for the roentgenographic series.

The roentgenographic evaluation of recurrent shoulder instability was recently reviewed at our institution.[25] A bony pathologic condition of the glenohumeral joint is most completely evaluated with an "instability series." This consists of four roentgenographic views, including an AP view in internal rotation, weighted AP internal rotation view, Stryker notch view, and a West Point modified axillary view.[28] **Bankart lesions** are documented best on the West Point view. A combination of a Stryker notch and AP internal rotation views will define most **Hill-Sachs lesions** in the posterolateral aspect of the humeral head (Fig. 7-6). These two bony lesions are pathognomonic for glenohumeral instability. Other roentgenographic studies that are useful include arthrography, computerized tomography, CT arthrography, arthrotomograms, ultrasound, and magnetic resonance imaging (MRI) (see Chapter 4). Arthrography is most useful for evaluation of the rotator cuff integrity. Computerized tomography is useful for a more detailed evaluation of bony defects of both the glenoid and humeral head. CT scan with contrast will aid evaluation of the labrum anteriorly and posteriorly (Fig. 7-7). It is especially useful for cases of recurrent posterior instability because posterior glenoid defects are not well

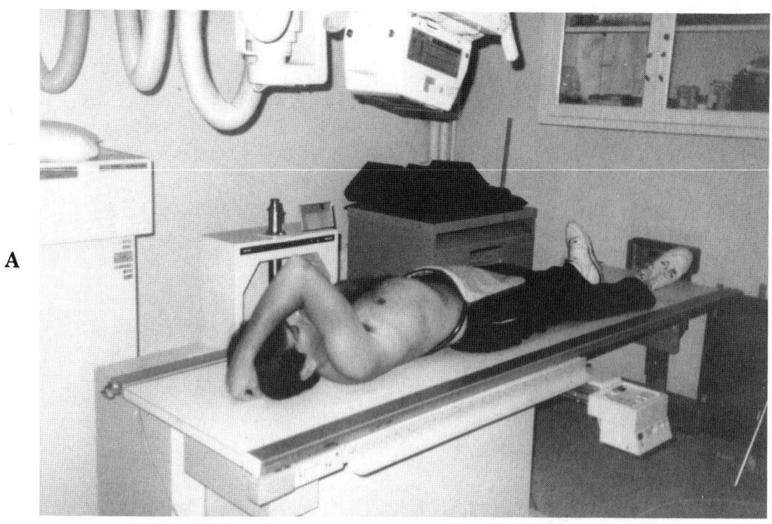

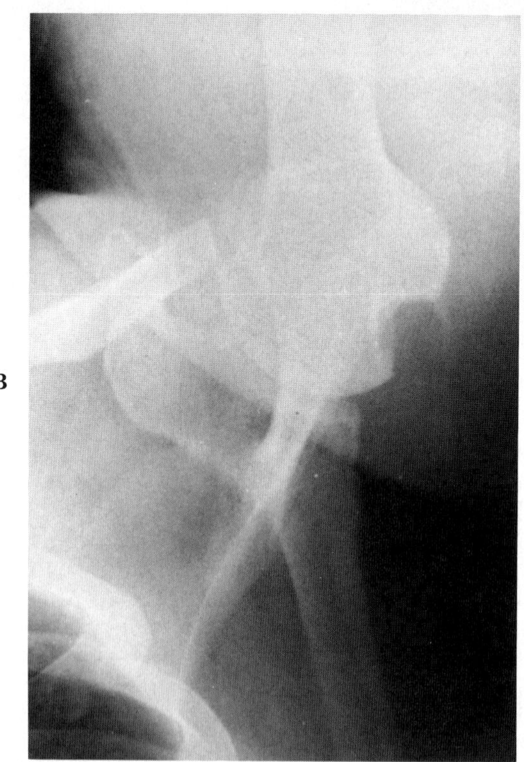

FIG. 7-6. **A**, Method for obtaining Stryker notch roentgenogram of the shoulder. **B**, Stryker notch roentgenogram with a large Hill-Sachs lesion on the posterolateral humeral head.

visualized on standard roentgenograms. MRI is an exciting evolving technique that may become the standard method for imaging the soft tissues about the shoulder.

ANTERIOR SHOULDER INSTABILITY

Acute Traumatic Anterior Dislocation

Dislocation of the glenohumeral joint is defined by complete separation of the articular surfaces, secondary to either direct or indirect forces. A direct force causing shoulder dislocation is uncommon.[27] Indirect force is the most frequent etiology of anterior glenohumeral dislocation. The arm is usually forced into excessive abduction, external rotation, and extension. These forces cause attenuation and disruption of the static and dynamic anterior stabilizers of the joint. The humeral head most commonly dislocates into a subcoracoid position and rarely a subclavicular or intrathoracic position. The dislocated arm is

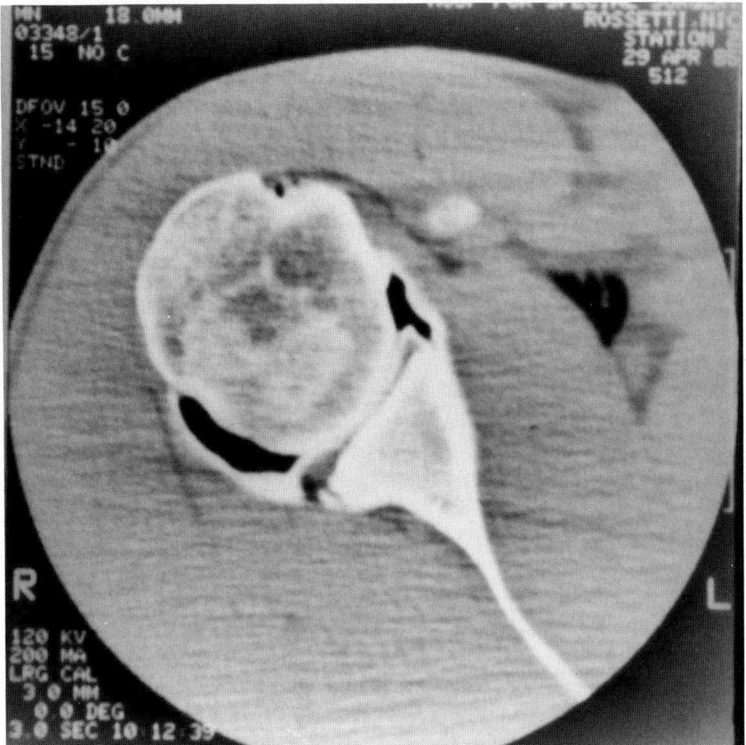

FIG. 7-7. CT arthrogram of shoulder. Note how contrast outlines the entire labrum.

usually very painful, associated with muscle spasm, and causes the patient to become extremely apprehensive.

> **Forces associated with anterior dislocation**
>
> - Abduction
> - External rotation
> - Extension

Unless the traumatic incident is witnessed by the treating physician, a thorough history of the injury mechanism must be obtained. Specific questions about neurologic involvement at the time of the injury must be asked. Physical examination must include a detailed neurologic examination of the upper extremity, including sensory testing in the distribution of the axillary and musculocutaneous nerves.

Ideally, roentgenograms should be obtained before one attempts to reduce a suspected shoulder dislocation. Techniques of reduction and anesthesia vary with the stage of presentation and the physician's expertise. When a young athlete sustains an acute, witnessed dislocation on the playing field, immediate relocation should be attempted. Initially, this would consist of elevation and internal "derotation" of the arm with minimal traction. If this was unsuccessful the patient would be transported to the locker room so a scapular rotation maneuver could be performed.[1] With the patient lying prone on the table, the injured side is allowed to hang in a dependent position off the edge of the table. The scapula is then manipulated to open the front aspect of the joint so that congruence of the head and the glenoid is restored, allowing the joint to relocate. If this is not successful, an intravenous line is started for administration of muscle relaxants and pain medications as needed. At this point, roentgenograms should be obtained to assess the injury more completely. The incidence of fractures increases with age, so in older patients, roentgenograms should always be obtained before manipulation. Simple arm elevation may reduce the dislocation.

The next relocation maneuver we would try is Stimson's.[41] With the affected shoulder hanging free off the edge of the table, weights are used to apply traction to the arm. Five pounds is usually sufficient, although the amount of weight will vary with the size of the patient. After satisfactory muscle relaxation is achieved, traction is applied to the arm in a straight anterior direction with compression of the humeral head.

Another reduction technique uses the double sheet method. The patient is placed in the supine position with the arm and shoulder off the edge of the table. One sheet is placed around the patient's chest and held by an assistant. A second sheet is placed around the patient's upper arm for gentle lateral traction. The physician applies gradual gentle traction to the arm by grasping at the wrist and pulling in an axial direction. The arm is positioned in a comfortable amount of abduction and then slowly traction is increased in the axis of the arm until reduction occurs. Often, gentle traction over a period of up to 5 minutes is required to overcome muscle spasm. With this maneuver, the physician must be fully aware of the fact that undue traction forces may result in damage to the neurovascular and other soft tissues about the shoulder.[6] Iatrogenic fractures as well as displacement of existing fractures may also occur as a result of excessive traction. If this method fails, reduction with the patient under anesthesia should be considered, especially in older people, those with osteopenia, or patients taking steroids.

Roentgenographic confirmation should always be obtained after reduction. The younger athlete is immobilized in a sling for 6 weeks, followed by a rehabilitative program consisting of shoulder strengthening exercises emphasizing internal rotation. Abduction is limited to 90 degrees during the first 2 weeks after sling removal. Although there are conflicting reports in the literature, Yoneda[43] and Simonet[38] in two separate series reported improved results using this method. The rationale is based on studies showing ligament and capsular healing requiring 6 weeks[8,20] and the subsequent risk to the shoulder of immediate return to activity without adequate muscle rehabilitation. At the U.S. Naval Academy, Cox has demonstrated that a prescribed exercise program will lower the recurrence rate.[9]

Care after reduction (initial dislocation)

- 6 weeks in a sling
- Limit abduction (<90°) weeks 7 and 8
- Begin progressive resistance exercise program week 6 (stress internal rotation)

In patients over 40 years of age, there is an increased incidence of cuff tears and adhesive capsulitis after dislocation. These patients are immobilized for only 7 to 10 days, followed by early range of motion and strengthening exercises. If pain persists, an arthrogram is obtained to assess the rotator cuff. Undoubtedly the subsequent level of activity as well as the type of damage sustained at the injury are important contributing factors.

The risk of recurrent dislocation will depend mainly on the study patient's age at the time of the index dislocation. In Rowe's[32] classic study of 324 anterior dislocations, the redislocation rate in patients under 20 was greater than 90%, while after the age of 40 the rate falls below 25%. In patients over the age of 50 recurrences, while uncommon, can occur. In a previous study by Kinnet[16] this was associated with excessive generalized ligamentous laxity.

Recurrent Anterior Instability

Classification

Recurrent anterior shoulder instability can be classified into the following subgroups: traumatic or atraumatic, voluntary or involuntary, subluxation or dislocation. Factors that influence placement within the recurrent subgroups include the magnitude of force the joint experiences, extent of previous injuries, and ligamentous laxity (Fig. 7-8).

Recurrent anterior shoulder dislocation from repetitive macro- or microtrauma can be quite disabling. The extent of disability will vary significantly among patients. The clinical spectrum ranges from traumatic redislocations without interval instability or pain to daily painful dislocations while performing activities of daily living.

Recurrent anterior instability classification

- Traumatic versus atraumatic
- Voluntary versus involuntary
- Subluxation versus dislocation

Atraumatic shoulder dislocation can be either voluntary or involuntary. Voluntary dislocators usually have a long history of being able to dislocate the shoulder with minimal apprehension or discomfort. Although commonly associated with generalized ligamentous laxity or connective tissue disorders, this can also occur in patients with normal muscular development and no apparent increase in joint laxity.[31] Unfortunately, some patients use this trick to control their environment. It is important to sort out these patients when considering treatment options. Some patients

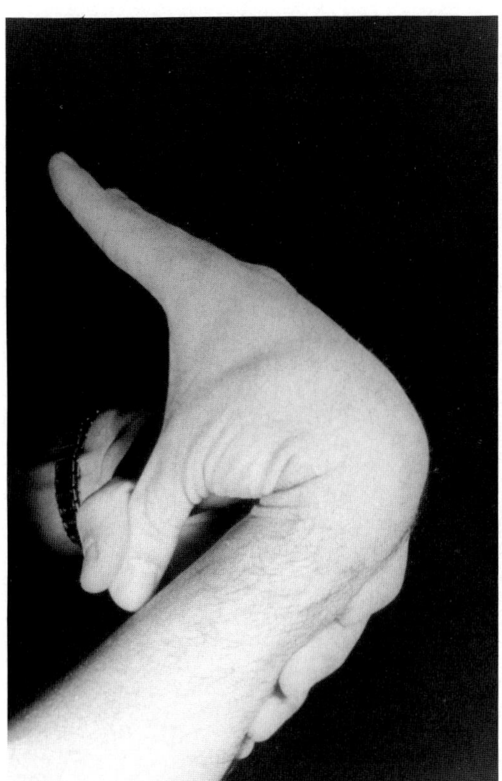

FIG. 7-8. All patients with shoulder instability should be evaluated for generalized ligamentous laxity. It is more commonly found in patients with multidirectional instability.

eventually lose control of the situation and begin to dislocate involuntarily and cannot participate in normal activities without having the shoulder dislocate. Although patients with voluntary instability are often psychologically normal, psychiatric evaluation should be considered before surgical intervention if a program of rotator cuff exercises is unsuccessful.

Shoulder subluxation may be defined as increased humeral head translation on the glenoid. We have defined subluxation, based on our anatomic studies, as head translation greater than one half the width of the glenoid but less than the sum of one half the glenoid and one half the humeral head.[36] It has been stated that participation in certain sports activities such as throwing and swimming will often lead to increases in AP translation of the involved shoulder when tested for stability. Although most patients may be asymptomatic, others, including high performance athletes, become symptomatic because of the capsule and particularly the labrum undergoing repeated stress at the extremes of motion. This can lead to labral damage that will vary from small tears to complete detachment.

Clinical Findings

The clinical presentation is usually one of pain. If a thrower complains of painful clicking or the so-called dead arm syndrome[34] while in phase I of throwing (cock-up phase), the diagnosis may not be difficult. However, the pain is often posterior, or the patient may present with a classic impingement syndrome from repetitive traction and compression of the rotator cuff during subluxation. It is not uncommon to see clinical overlap between subluxation and the impingement syndrome in which symptoms of both conditions may occur, often resulting in inappropriate or incomplete surgical treatment.

Physical Examination

Evaluation of patients with painful anterior subluxation must be carried out with a thorough understanding of the mechanisms that produce the patients' complaints. Pain in phase I of throwing often indicates anterior instability. However, pain with follow-through (phase III), while usually associated with posterior subluxation, can also be seen in patients with anterior instability secondary to traction. Range of motion should be assessed with arms both at the side and abducted to 90 degrees, paying particular attention to internal and external rotation. Frequently, patients with anterior instability will have some loss of external rotation with the arms at the 90-degree position secondary to apprehension. With the arm at the side, where apprehension will not play a role, losses of 15 to 20 degrees of external rotation with respect to the opposite normal arm are common. Stress testing with the patient supine at the edge of the table should be performed anteriorly, inferiorly and posteriorly to evaluate the type of instability (Fig. 7-9). Crepitance should be noted, especially if it produces pain. A clinical test that is useful to indicate the presence of inferior instability we have termed the "sulcus sign."[41] A sulcus sign is defined as the presence of a prominent depression noted inferiorly below the acromion while traction is applied on the wrist in an inferior direction.[41] The arms must be completely relaxed and hanging at the patient's side to elicit this sign (Fig. 7-10). This finding is commonly present in multidirectional instability. A complete motor examination should also be performed, especially noting any axillary nerve dysfunction.

Treatment

Considerations for deciding which treatment options are viable include the patient's age, occupation, activity level, dominant side,

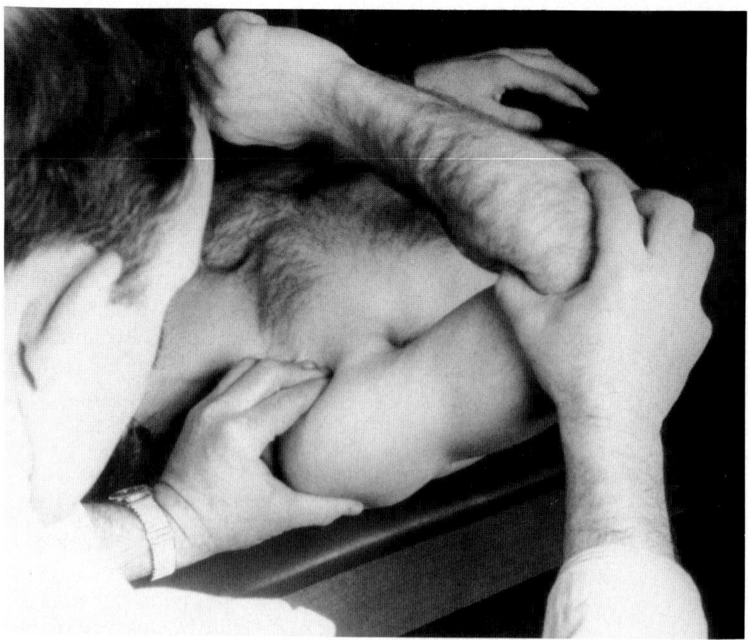

FIG. 7-9. Stress testing is an integral part of examining a shoulder for instability. Stress should be applied in each of the anterior, posterior, and inferior directions, with the arm in many different positions.

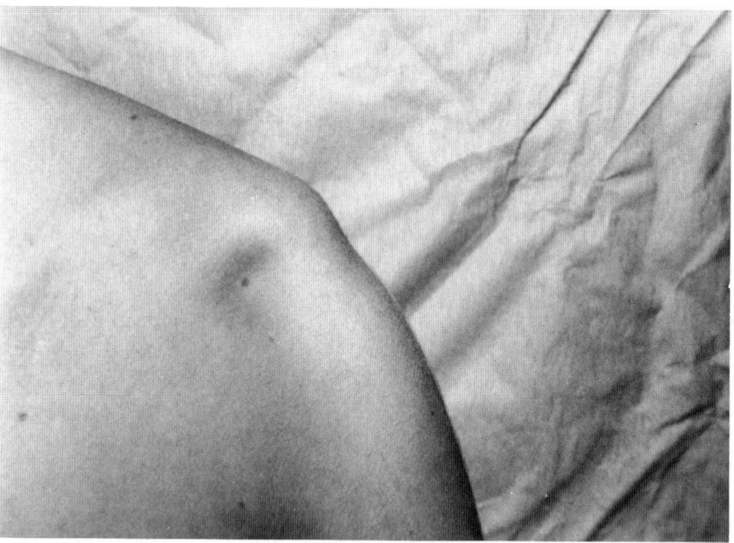

FIG. 7-10. The sulcus sign manifests as a hollowing inferior to the acromion when downward traction is applied to the dependent arm.

general health, ligamentous laxity, and reliability.

Conservative management. The goals of conservative management should include restoration of strength and range of motion. In the athletic population, one is frequently faced with treating tendonitis secondary to instability-induced traction on the rotator cuff structures. Patients who develop acute traumatic anterior shoulder subluxation should initially be placed at complete rest. For an individual with acute traumatic subluxation, a period of immobilization with the arm internally rotated at the side for 5 weeks is recommended to potentially decrease the recurrence rate. In those patients with more gradual onset, a shorter period of rest to decrease the local inflammation may be allowed. In both cases, however, a flexibility and strengthening program is mandatory and any loss of external rotation must be regained before returning to any overhead sporting activities. With loss of motion of the shoulder, abnormal glenohumeral stresses may be generated as a result of asynchronous muscle activity attempting to compensate to regain full power. This may contribute to rotator cuff inflammation. Rotation exercises are carried out with the arm at the side as well as with the arm abducted 90 degrees. This can be performed on Cybex equipment (Lumex Corporation, Lake Ronkonkoma, NY), simple spring exerciser, pulley systems, or Theraband. In addition, exercises are performed to develop trapezius and deltoid as well as the periscapular musculature. These include the rhomboids, latissimus dorsi, and serratus anterior, which are often ignored in exercise programs. These muscles help the scapula to act as a moving platform from which the arm functions. As strength and flexibility return, the patient may gradually increase his or her activity. It usually requires 6 weeks to regain strength and motion and 6 weeks to graduate to full activity.

Treatment considerations

- Age
- Occupation
- Activity level
- Dominant side
- General health
- Ligamentous laxity
- Reliability

In patients who are refractory to conservative treatment, operative treatment should be considered. The use of arthroscopic versus the open techniques depends upon the pathologic condition and the patient's needs. For instance, open treatment will often fail to return a thrower back to his preinjury status; thus arthroscopy may be considered first for these patients. However, for a patient whose instability only manifests itself in certain activities, the possibility of giving up these activities and avoiding surgery should be discussed. Surgery becomes the treatment of choice when, despite an adequate trial of conservative therapy, a patient's instability precludes normal activities of daily living or sports from the standpoint of either pain, apprehension, or limited shoulder motion.

Surgical treatment. A specific clinical diagnosis and accurate evaluation of the pathologic state at surgery are critical when choosing a surgical procedure to treat anterior shoulder instability. Particular attention should be paid in determining whether the instability is a unidirectional anterior laxity or associated with a concomitant inferior laxity. An accurate examination of both shoulders under anesthesia should be performed before any skin incisions. The patient's history and physical examination of the shoulder in the office usually will provide the correct diagnosis. In some patients apprehension may preclude an adequate examination of the shoulder; however, the position producing the apprehension is helpful diagnostically. The examination under anesthesia (EUA) is performed in a similar fashion to that in the office, noting especially the directions and magnitude of instability. Some experience is helpful when performing an examination with the patient under anesthesia, because the degree of nonpathologic humeral head translation may be greater than expected, particularly posteriorly. Norris has observed that approximately 50% of the humeral head may be uncovered posteriorly during a normal examination (see Chapter 3). Our studies have demonstrated that the head will translate anteriorly and posteriorly with equal distance if the arm is placed in the plane of the scapula at 0° of rotation. If it is posterior the excursion anteriorly will decrease, while if it is anterior (i.e., follow-through position in throwing) the posterior excursion will decrease.[36]

To stress the right shoulder, the examiner, while kneeling next to the patient, holds the patient's elbow with his right hand, gently applying an axial load (see Fig. 7-9). The left hand palpates the humeral head and acts as a fulcrum to lever the head anteriorly or posteriorly. The degree of humeral head translation is noted with the arm abducted 90 degrees and in neutral rotation. Flexion or extension of the arm while in this position can be used to amplify instability (see Fig. 7-9). Increasing external rotation will tighten the anterior capsule, thus preventing the examiner from noting the translation. Similary, internal rotation will tighten the posterior capsule, decreasing perceived posterior laxity. By altering the degree of rotation and axial load, the optimal arm position for provoking maximal glenohumeral instability can be found.

At HSS, shoulder instability is graded. Grade I, or subluxation, implies greater than 50% humeral head translation on the glenoid without dislocation. The presence of grinding on the labrum should be noted. Grade II is frank dislocation without locking. Grade III is dislocation associated with the ability to lock the humeral head over the edge of the glenoid. Generalized ligamentous laxity should be factored in when assessing the outcome of any examination performed with the patient under anesthesia.

HSS shoulder instability grading scale

- Grade I—subluxation
  Greater than 50% humeral head translation on the glenoid without islocation
- Grade II—dislocation
- Grade III—locked dislocation

Before surgical procedures are described in detail, a few general principles regarding shoulder surgery need to be discussed. If the diagnosis based on clinical examination and EUA is still in doubt, arthroscopy of both the glenohumeral joint and subacromial space is indicated before any open procedures. When an open anterior procedure is performed, the adequacy of the anterior capsule and its attachment to the glenoid are noted. Some detachment of the labrum from the glenoid is seen in about 80% of our patients. If no labral detachment is noted, the lateral capsular attachments must be inspected for patency.[5] The presence of a rotator interval must be evaluated, because this lesion can precipitate and potentiate anterior shoulder instability.[24] If none of these lesions is present, generalized ligamentous laxity should be considered and evaluated before surgery. Examining the shoulder after releasing the subscapularis is also advisable, because the stability of the humeral head within the capsule can be directly observed. If a Bankart lesion is present, the lesion should be anatomically reattached to the glenoid. The T-plasty[41] or inferior capsular shift[23] may be used when the inferior capsule and glenohumeral ligament are lax, allowing abnormal inferior humeral head translation. By shifting the capsule superiorly and medially, the axillary recess will be reduced, eliminating inferior and anterior translation of the head. If the labrum is detached, it is reattached to the bony glenoid when the T-plasty is closed. If the labrum and capsule are intact, then the limbs of the capsular T-plasty are sutured to the labrum. (See section on multidirectional instability.)

The quality of the bone stock of the glenoid and humeral head should be carefully evaluated both preoperatively with roentgenograms and during the operation. Bone loss anteriorly on the glenoid is usually in the 10% to 20% range. If excessive bony loss is present (>30% of the glenoid) a bone block procedure in addition to capsular reattachment is considered. *Procedures involving routine use of coracoid transplantation to the anterior glenoid have no sound physiologic basis and probably are not indicated unless there is severe anterior bone loss.* Hill-Sachs lesions are present in over 80% of recurrent dislocations but in only 25% of patients with subluxation.[25] There is occasional concern over the size of the Hill-Sachs lesion. Several operations have been suggested, such as filling in the defect with a bone graft, performing rotational osteotomy of the humeral head, or transplanting the infraspinatus tendon into the defect. These types of procedures are not necessary if the anterior soft tissue repair is performed adequately. The repaired capsule will decrease the anterior translation of the humeral head, preventing the defect from catching on the anterior edge of the glenoid. Operations that are designed to limit external rotation of the arm, such as the Putti-Platt or Magnuson-Stack, are also not indicated if proper anterior capsular repair is performed. Limitation of external rotation, if excessive, (i.e., less than neutral) may result in forcing the humeral head posteriorly. This has been noted particularly after a Putti-Platt procedure.[13] This occurs as a result of the increased posterior translation that accompanies a shoulder which dislocates anteriorly. The injury to the inferior ligament (anterior and posterior) allows increased posterior translation and thus a tight anterior structure will force the head posteriorly across the joint, resulting in force concentration and shear on the articular cartilage.

Open procedure. Our basic operation is a modified Bankart type of procedure in which the capsule and labrum, if present, are reattached to the glenoid, assuming it is detached. If inferior laxity is also present, a capsular T-plasty procedure is indicated. Most of our patients are anesthetized with an interscalene block, but some still receive general anesthesia. The patient is placed supine with the arm abducted 45 degrees on an arm board. The head of the bed is elevated 30 degrees (Fig. 7-11). A folded sheet is placed behind the interscapular area to lift the chest forward. If the pad is placed behind the scapula, it will close down the glenohumeral joint anteriorly, making the exposure more difficult.

The skin incision is placed in the anterior

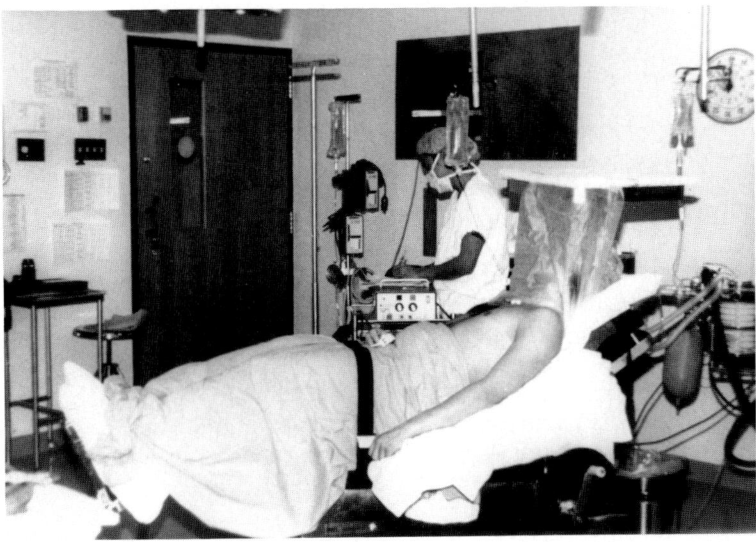

FIG. 7-11. Patient position for open shoulder surgery. A folded sheet is placed behind the interscapular area.

skinfold to help minimize postoperative scar widening. The incision starts just lateral to the coracoid and extends distally approximately 6 cm toward the anterior axillary fold. If desired, it may be placed low in the axilla as Leslie described.[19] The Leslie incision provides for improved cosmesis but requires considerable subcutaneous dissection to create a normal pathway through the deltopectoral interval. For those patients with multidirectional instability, the Leslie incision is not recommended. The cephalic vein is identified and retracted laterally with the deltoid, since fewer branches enter medially. In the proximal incision, care must be taken not to cut the vein because it crosses the wound just distal to the coracoid. Occasionally, the vein is absent or arborized, making dissection of the interval more difficult. The coracoid is a good landmark for identification of the deltopectoral interval. Once the interval has been separated, the clavipectoral fascia will be encountered. The fascia is incised just lateral to the muscle belly of the short biceps. The coracoacromial ligament is then isolated and partially excised near the coracoid. Downward traction on the arm facilitates this maneuver. The conjoined tendon is partially incised just distal to the coracoid, leaving a small edge of the tendon laterally for reattachment. We have not found it necessary to perform osteotomy on the coracoid, because simple partial tenotomy will allow adequate exposure. It is important, however, to cut the tendon close to the coracoid because of the musculocutaneous nerve. The nerve enters the muscle belly approximately 49 mm from the tip of the coracoid, but 5% of 61 specimens recently reviewed had a branch 1.0 to 2.5 cm from the coracoid.[4]

The inferior border of the subscapularis muscle and the anterior humeral circumflex vessels should be easily seen. If not, the superior 1 to 2 cm of the pectoralis major insertion may be obliquely incised for exposure. The arm is then externally rotated and a roll of towels placed under the elbow. The anterior humeral circumflex vessels are then suture-ligated near the subscapularis tendon insertion. A curved Kelly clamp is then used to bluntly dissect the subscapularis tendon off the capsule, starting inferiorly from approximately 2 to 3 cm medial to the lesser tuberosity. By separating the tendon from the capsule medially, the surgeon can avoid inadvertent entry into the capsule. The tendon is then incised obliquely in the coronal plane to gain length. The capsule is exposed medially and laterally as far as possible. Also, the inferior capsule should be exposed to at least the 6-o'clock position on the glenoid, avoiding the axillary nerve. Once the capsule is cut, further inferior exposure is very difficult. If a rotator interval is found, it should be closed at this time, or if there is inferior translation and a T-plasty is planned, the interval may be used as part of the T. The capsule is incised at the edge of the glenoid in a vertical fashion, avoiding lateral deviation of the cut inferiorly. If inferior laxity is present, and a T-plasty is anticipated, a transverse capsular incision at about the 3- to 4-o'clock position on the glenoid is performed first. The labrum is then inspected. If no labral detachment is seen, a vertical incision is made either medially along the glenoid, or laterally along the humeral head to complete the T-plasty incision. If there is marked inferior laxity, both medial and lateral incisions can be made to perform an H-plasty (Fig. 7-12). (See section on multidirectional shoulder instability, p. 207.) In approximately 85% of our athletic patients, some degree of labral detachment is noted. However, this is significantly less in the atraumatic type of instability.

The area of capsular detachment off the glenoid is extended medially and proximally to allow placement of a retractor along the medial glenoid neck. A ring retractor (Fakuda) is then inserted into the joint to provide exposure of the entire glenoid (Fig. 7-13). The joint is then irrigated to remove loose bodies, which are present in 10% of our traumatic dislocations. The glenoid is then prepared by using an osteotome to create a groove vertically oriented 3 to 4 mm medial to the bony edge. This provides a bleeding bony surface for enhanced capsular healing and facilitates passage of sutures. Using a dental drill, three to four drill holes are made in the edge of the glenoid, from the 3- to 6-o'clock positions. Nonabsorbable sutures are then passed through the drill holes. With the arm in external rotation, the sutures are passed through the lateral capsular edge to advance the capsule superiorly and also approximate the tissue to bone. The joint must be held in a reduced position while the capsular repair is performed. The goal is to maximize external rotation, setting the arm at 40 to 50 degrees while tightening the capsule in the superior direction. Following the repair, the external rotation of the arm needs to be checked for excessive tightness, and if present, the capsular repair is repeated (i.e., less than neutral rotation). The subscapularis is reattached to the tendon stump with nonabsorbable sutures without tightening the musculotendinous unit. The conjoined tendon is sutured back either to the remaining tendon stump or to the coracoid directly. The wound is drained and the skin closed. The specific steps for performing the T-plasty capsular repair are explained in the section on multidirectional instability.

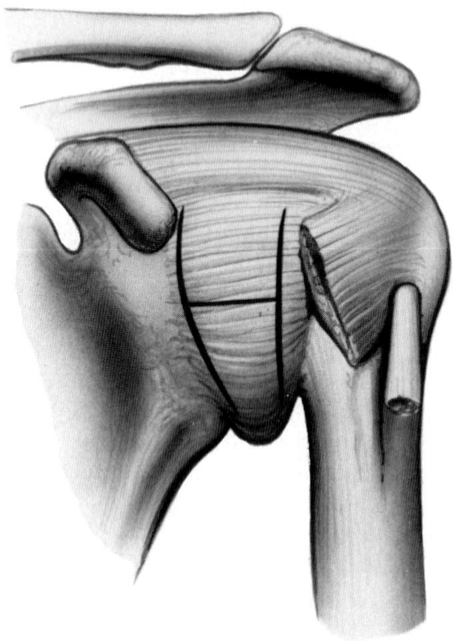

FIG. 7-12. In a T-plasty, a transverse capsular incision is performed first. The labral complex is inspected and then the vertical, medial, and, if needed, lateral incisions of the T-plasty are then performed.

Arthroscopic techniques. Arthroscopy of the shoulder is an extremely valuable and established tool for diagnosing difficult shoulder problems. Technologic advances have allowed this modality to be applied to treating the shoulder for instability. Random arthroscopic excision of loose labral tissue should be avoided. Some labral flap lesions may be debrided, resulting in improvement lasting for a

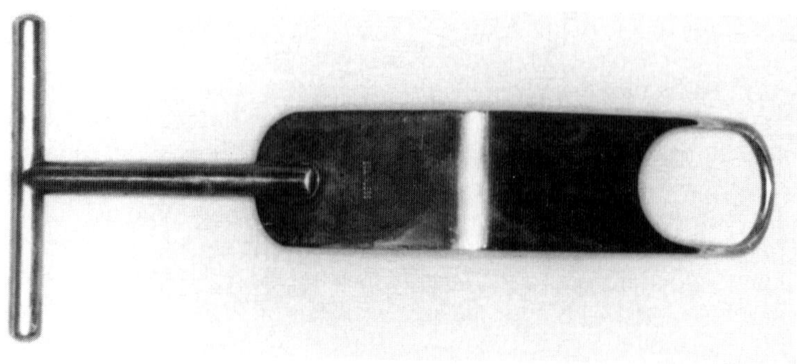

FIG. 7-13. Ring, or Fakuda, retractor.

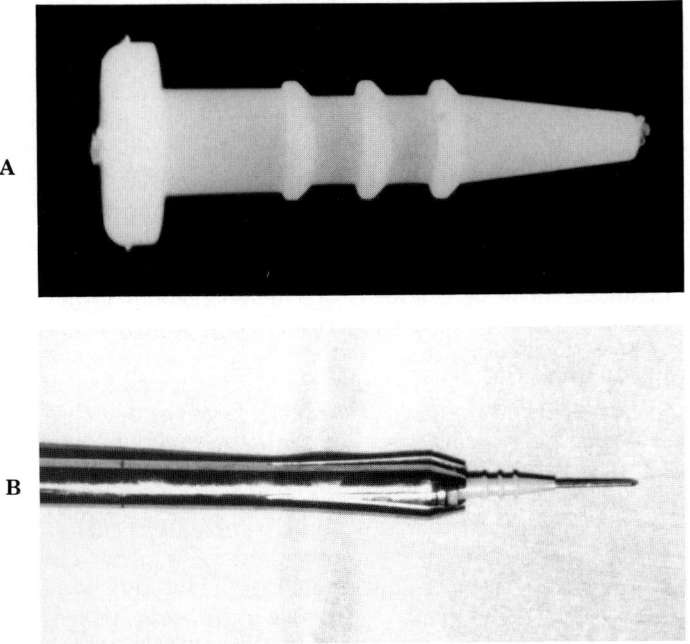

FIG. 7-14. A, Absorbable staple (Acufex) stabilizing the labrum to the glenoid. **B**, The staple is inserted over a guide wire (B).

variable period.[2] If the labral detachment is below the equator of the glenoid, there is usually associated glenohumeral instability. Simple labral debridement could worsen the patient's instability if the attachment of the inferior glenohumeral ligament is compromised. We have used arthroscopic stabilization techniques for treating patients with traumatic unidirectional anterior instability. Technique aside, the basic idea is to reattach the anterior inferior glenohumeral ligament and labrum complex back to bone. Before reattachment, nonfunctional labral tissue should be debrided and the anterior inferior glenoid bone freshened to facilitate soft tissue healing to bone. We have used two different arthroscopic techniques that avoid the use of metallic implants. The first technique involves passing absorbable sutures through the soft tissue complex and then through drill holes in the glenoid.[41,42] The sutures are passed with modified Beath needles drilled from anterior to posterior, through the glenoid. The sutures are tied over fascia and beneath the skin posteriorly.

The second technique involves using an absorbable staple (Acufex Corp.) to reattach the soft tissue to the anterior glenoid. The staple is cannulated and passed into a predrilled hole over a guide wire (Fig. 7-14).[42]

It is conceivable that inferior capsular shifts can be performed using these techniques to treat multidirectional instability. At present we recommend open surgery for multidirectional instability. Unless a surgeon is extremely competent with arthroscopic techniques and fully understands shoulder instability, arthroscopic shoulder stabilizations should not be attempted. We do not recommend the use of metallic implants for open or arthroscopic shoulder stabilizations, because inappropriate positioning, loosening, and subsequent articular injury have occurred all too frequently.

Postoperative rehabilitation. The postoperative rehabilitation is tailored to the individual patient's needs. In the throwing athlete, we are aggressive with early restoration of motion. However, for the nondominant arm or the person with generalized ligamentous laxity, range of motion exercises are delayed. After surgery, the patient's arm is held in a universal shoulder immobilizer. Pendulum exercises are started at 2 weeks and active exercises are added in the third week with progressive increases in external rotation and elevation. The immobilizer is discontinued at about the fourth or fifth week. The degree of external rotation obtained on the operating table should be factored into the rehabilitation, so that the capsular repair will not be stretched or avulsed early on. In throwing athletes, the pendulum exercises are started during the first week with the rehabilitation course following accordingly. The rehabilitation is less aggressive for a nondominant arm than for a dominant arm, and for patients treated for multidirectional instability, the rehabilitation is delayed for 6 weeks.

At 6 weeks aggressive therapy to increase range of motion is undertaken. At 8 weeks strengthening exercises using Theraband are instituted, and exercise to tolerance is permitted. Patients are prevented from carrying heavy loads with the arm in a dependent position for 6 months; this is particularly important if there was an inferior component to the instability, since this will stress the capsular repair. If the patient is involved in throwing sports, 6 months should elapse before resumption of throwing activities to help prevent capsular stretching and possible recurrence. Noncontact sports are resumed at 4 months, while we prefer 6 months' rest from contact sports. Following arthroscopic stabilization we have restricted motion except for pendulum exercises for 4 weeks and then have instituted a slowly progressive motion program similar to that for open techniques.

POSTERIOR SHOULDER INSTABILITY

Posterior instability of the shoulder is less common than anterior instability and often presents more of a diagnostic and therapeutic dilemma. Reasons for this include both a relative lack of understanding of the basic pathophysiologic condition involved and its tendency to present with rather vague symptomatology, which often mimics other clinical disorders, including anterior shoulder instability.

The incidence of posterior shoulder instability varies but has been reported to represent approximately 2% to 4% of patients presenting with an unstable shoulder.[7,29] The exact incidence is hard to determine, because the literature on posterior dislocation and subluxation is relatively small in volume, and many studies discuss subluxation and dislocation interchangeably.[7,10,22,37] Only recently has there been a heightened awareness of posterior instability, with the advances in treatment of sports-related injuries to the shoulder. Symptomatic posterior subluxation is increasingly recognized in the athlete, while posterior dislocation is uncommon.

In this discussion we focus on the more common types of posterior instability using the classification system outlined on p. 181.

Anatomic Considerations

The anatomic structures responsible for posterior shoulder instability and their relative contributions are not well defined in the literature at this time. We have completed a series of cadaver studies at our institution to evaluate the static constraints to posterior translation of the humeral head.[17]

Incising the infraspinatus and teres minor resulted in no significant posterior instability with the shoulder at 90 degrees of abduction and 90 degrees of external rotation. Selective cutting of the intact posterior capsule from the 9-o'clock to 12-o'clock position also caused no increase in posterior shoulder instability. When the capsule was incised to the 6-o'clock position, the shoulder started to sublux posteriorly (see Fig. 7-3), but no dislocation occurred until the anterior, superior capsule was incised, from the 1- to 3-o'clock position, including the superior glenohumeral ligament. Posterior subluxation also occurred when the entire inferior capsule was cut from the anterior border of the inferior glenohumeral ligament to the superior edge of the posterior pouch of the inferior glenohumeral ligament.

When the arm is flexed, adducted, and internally rotated, the capsule posteriorly makes a sling, unfolding like a sail about the humeral head, with the amount of tension depending on the degree of internal rotation applied and the degree of retroversion of the humeral head. At the same time, the anterior capsule is noted to "wind up" like a cord, acting as a tether preventing posterior subluxation or dislocation. Again, the shoulder can be compared to a circle, with stretching or damage to the anterior portion of the capsule, or circle, being an essential component in allowing the head to sublux or dislocate posteriorly.

Factors contributing to posterior instability

- Capsular laxity
- Glenoid retroversion (>10°)
- Humeral head retroversion (>40°)
- Hypoplastic glenoid
- Muscle imbalance
- Generalized ligamentous laxity

Other anatomic factors that may contribute to posterior shoulder instability include glenoid retroversion greater than 10 degrees[35]; retroversion of the humeral head beyond 40 degrees[35]; a hypoplastic glenoid; muscle imbalance; and generalized ligamentous laxity. However, recent studies by Galinat have failed to note any increase in glenoid retroversion in patients with posterior instability.[12]

Acute Traumatic Posterior Dislocation

Although few accurate statistics are available, approximately 98% of all posterior dis-

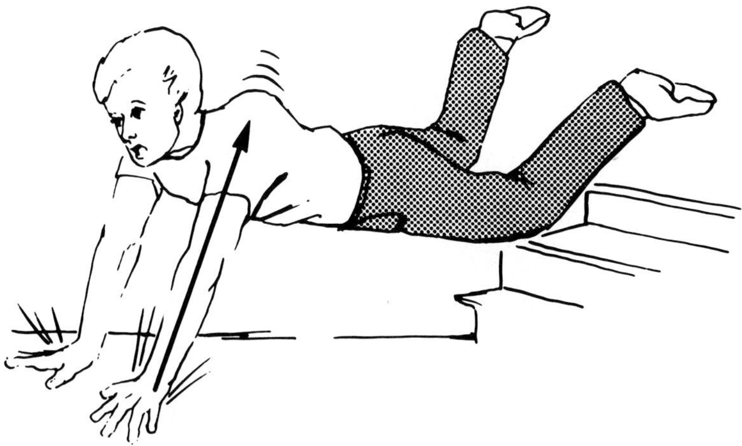

FIG. 7-15. A fall onto an outstretched hand is an example of how indirect forces can cause posterior shoulder dislocation.

locations of the shoulder are subacromial. However, subglenoid and subspinous posterior dislocations have been discussed in the literature.[27]

Mechanism of Injury

The mechanism of injury for posterior dislocation is usually either a direct blow to the anterior shoulder or, more commonly, indirect forces applied to the shoulder that combine flexion, adduction, and internal rotation. The most common causes of posterior dislocation are accidental electric shock and convulsive seizures, in which the stronger internal rotators, including latissimus dorsi, pectoralis major, and subcapularis overcome the weaker external rotators. Another example of an indirect force that can cause posterior dislocation is a fall on an outstretched hand (Fig. 7-15).

Forces leading to posterior dislocation

- Flexion
- Adduction
- Internal rotation

Clinical Findings

Clinical signs and symptoms of posterior dislocation are often overlooked. The repeated incidence of missed diagnosis at first examination is between 60% and 80%.[27] The most likely reason for this is reliance on AP roentgenograms of the shoulder without appropriate lateral or axillary views and, more importantly, an incomplete physical examination.

The patient usually presents with the arm adducted and internally rotated. The coracoid process appears prominent (Fig. 7-16), with the glenoid fossa empty anteriorly and a corresponding bulge posteriorly. Any attempt at abduction and external rotation is quite painful. Another easily recognized sign, if looked for, is the inability of the patient to fully supinate his forearm with the arm forward flexed[33] (Fig. 7-17). A careful neurovascular examination of the involved extremity should be carried out before any attempt at reduction.

Roentgenograms

Roentgenographic evaluation should be obtained to evaluate any associated fractures. The standard trauma series should be obtained, including a true AP view of the shoulder (35 to 45 degrees oblique to the body); a transcapular view at right angles to the true AP film; and a physician-assisted axillary view (see Fig. 7-5). Some classic roentgenographic findings to be aware of are the vacant glenoid sign; the 6 mm rim sign[3]; and the cystic sign. The vacant glenoid sign refers to the void seen in the anterior half of the glenoid fossa in posterior dislocations on a standard AP film of the shoulder. Normally, there is a superimposition of the head of the humerus on the posterior glenoid fossa with the humerus almost filling the glenoid fossa, producing a smooth elliptical shadow resembling the teardrop effect seen in the acetabulum on AP views of the pelvis. The 6 mm rim sign is an extension of

Classic roentgenographic signs of posterior dislocation

- Vacant glenoid sign
- 6-mm rim sign
- Cystic sign

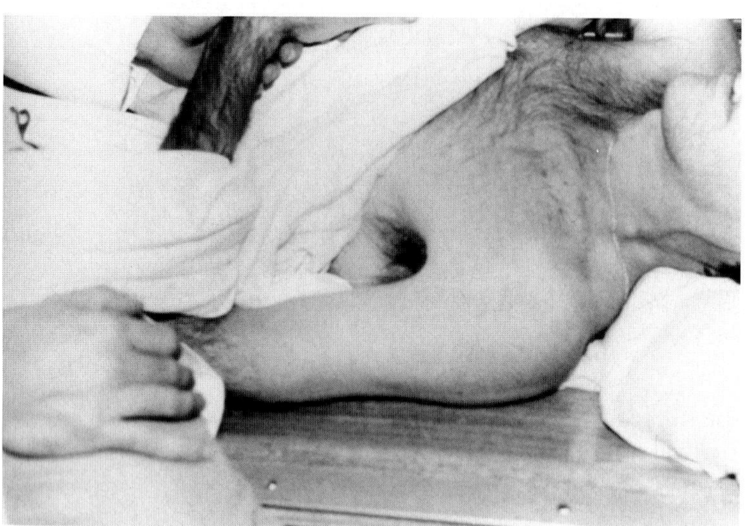

FIG. 7-16. Clinical example of acute posterior shoulder dislocation. Note prominent coracoid and hollowing over glenoid fossa.

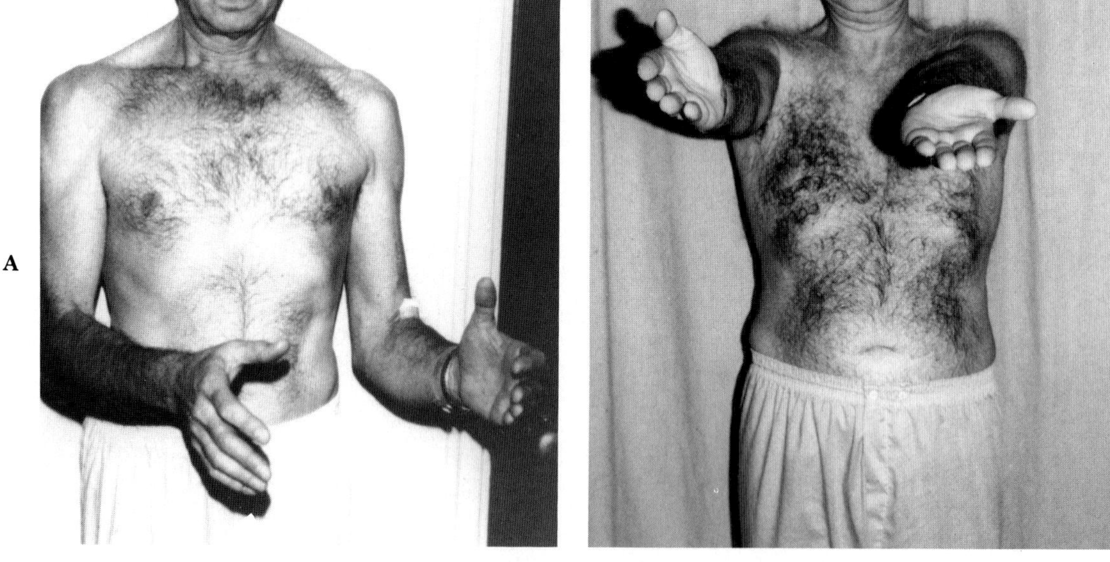

FIG. 7-17. Posterior shoulder dislocation. **A**, Note inability to externally rotate arm. **B**, The patient cannot fully supinate the forearm.

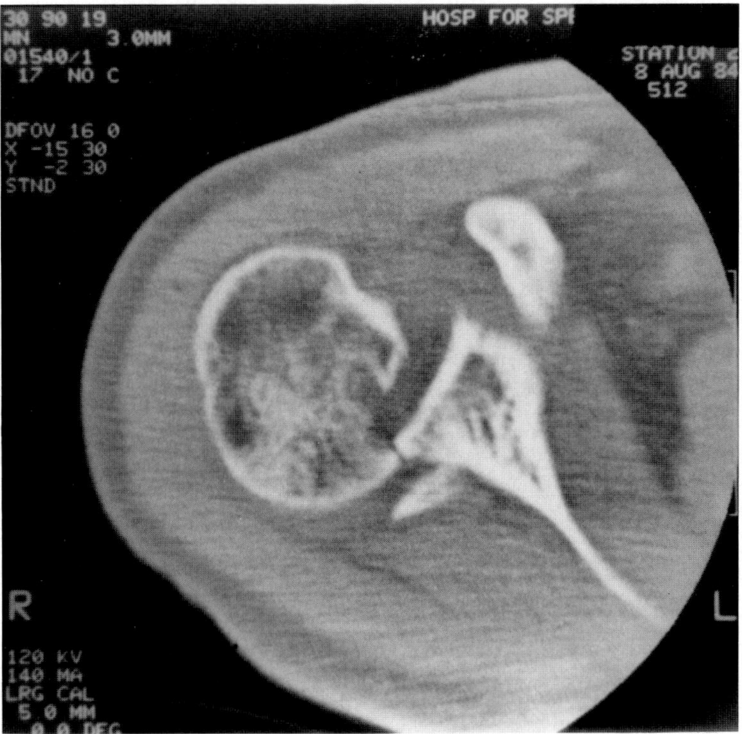

FIG. 7-18. CT scans of the glenohumeral joint are often necessary to fully define bony pathologic conditions associated with posterior dislocation.

the vacant glenoid sign, stating that a space between the anterior rim of the glenoid and the humeral head greater than 6 mm is highly suggestive of a posterior dislocation. It is important to note that these two signs are obliterated on a true AP of the shoulder (45 degrees to the central axis) in which the glenoid fossa is not visualized. The cystic sign refers to the marked lucency in the humeral head present on an internal rotation view of the shoulder. However, this hollow appearance may be seen in normal shoulders in full internal rotation. Axillary views are of critical importance for evaluating the displacement and the degree of notching or fracture of the humeral head. This notch may indicate whether a closed reduction is feasible, since the trauma of a difficult reduction may displace a component of the humeral head. When there is difficulty in getting an adequate evaluation on plain roentgenograms, we have found the CT scan to be quite valuable in defining the pertinent anatomy (Fig. 7-18).

Treatment

Reduction is affected by first obtaining satisfactory patient and muscular relaxation through the use of either diazepam (Valium) or pain medication. With the patient in the supine position, lateral traction is applied with internal rotation to remove the notch from the glenoid, followed by external rotation to relax the posterior capsule. Posterior pressure is then placed on the humeral head to facilitate reduction. As reduction is achieved, the arm is then gently adducted in external rotation and placed at the side.

If the reduction is stable the arm is immobilized in a stockinette, as described by Rowe, with the shoulder in mild extension at the side.[33] If there is a significant defect in the humeral head or if the shoulder is unstable, the arm is best immobilized in a slightly externally rotated position. In younger patients (less than 40 years old) immobilization should be continued for 4 to 6 weeks, followed by an aggressive physical therapy program emphasizing strengthening of the external rotators of the shoulder. In the older patient, the period of immobilization is shorter, lasting approximately 2 to 3 weeks.

The literature regarding recurrence rates is again not firmly established, but recurrences have generally been regarded as being less frequent than is seen with anterior dislocations. One series, reported by Robert and Wickstrom,[26] had recurrences in 38% of the patients (9/24). Patients under the age of 20

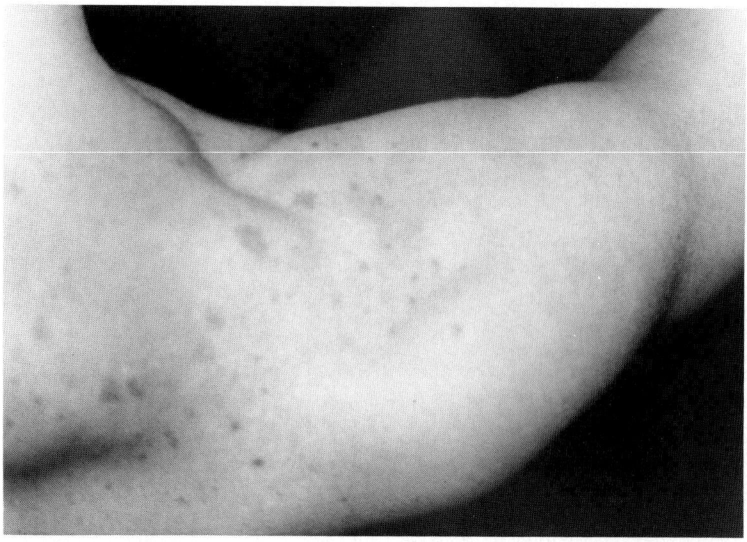

FIG. 7-19. Voluntary posterior shoulder subluxation induced by arm positioning. Note prominence posteriorly.

appear to be at more risk for recurrence than older patients, which is also the case in anterior shoulder dislocation.

Recurrent Posterior Subluxation

Many of the same arguments for recurrent anterior shoulder instability apply to recurrent posterior instability. The etiology may be either traumatic or atraumatic; instability may be voluntary or involuntary; ligamentous laxity plays an important role; combined instability patterns may be present; the extent of disability will vary significantly from patient to patient; and high performance athletes may be more susceptible to instability patterns because of repeated edge loading at the extremes of motion.

Recurrent posterior subluxation, however, differs in other ways from anterior instability patterns. For instance, we have not seen patients with posterior subluxation progress to a recurrent dislocation pattern. In addition, the majority of patients with posterior subluxation present initially with the complaint of pain, with instability as a secondary concern. Apprehension as a subjective complaint or observation during examination is uncommon with posterior subluxation and, if present, should raise the concern that the shoulder may in fact be subluxing anteriorly.

Voluntary Posterior Instability

Two types of voluntary posterior subluxation have been observed. Some patients induce subluxation by appropriate positioning of their arm into flexion, adduction, and internal rotation (Fig. 7-19), whereas others use selective muscle group activation and suppression to create the displacement of the humeral head (Fig. 7-20). The latter group of patients will frequently have a significant in-

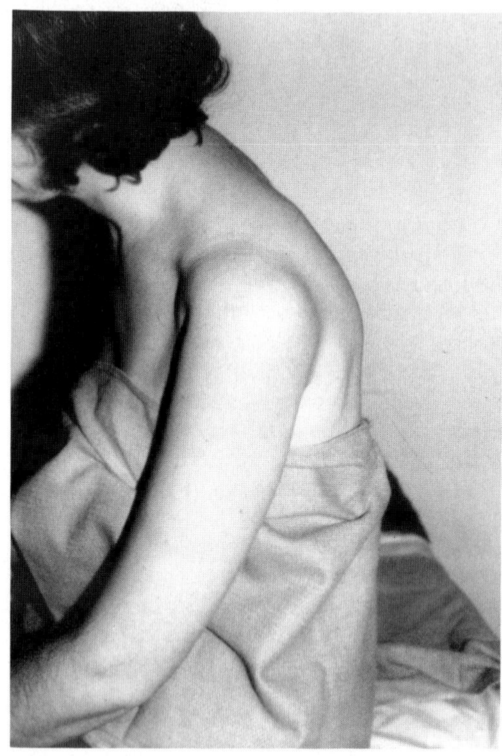

FIG. 7-20. Voluntary posterior shoulder subluxation induced by selective muscle activation. Note prominence of humeral head posteriorly.

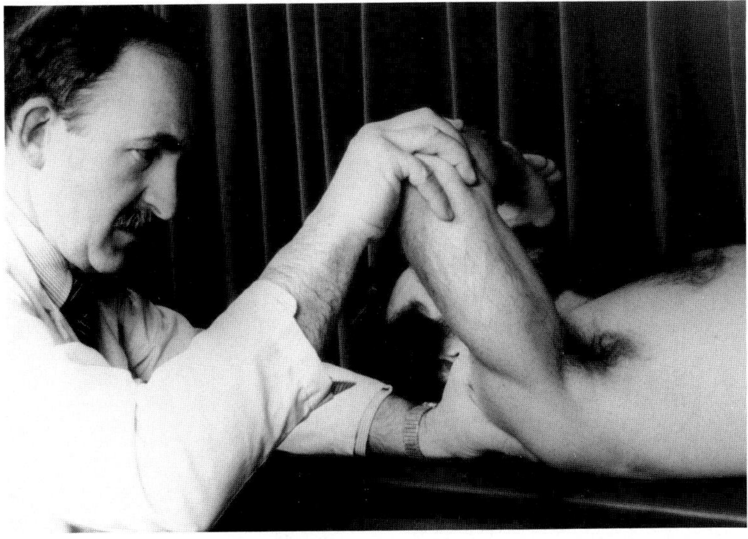

FIG. 7-21. Method for posterior stress testing of the shoulder. Note the examiner's hand position. Complete relaxation is necessary on the part of the patient.

crease in generalized ligamentous laxity. For patients in the former group it is voluntary by position but not muscle control, in contrast to those in the latter group. In both groups the subluxation appears to be a learned maneuver, a result of the patient's awareness of the specific action contributing to the subluxation. Some patients may use this trick to control their environment. These patients may require psychiatric evaluation, particularly those who produce subluxation by contracting the internal rotators. However, the majority of patients with voluntary posterior subluxation do not fall into this category.

Involuntary Posterior Instability

Involuntary recurrent posterior subluxation is often associated with the high forces generated in the follow-through phase of various sports activities. This develops as the humerus is in adduction, flexion, and internal rotation, and maximal contraction is present in the subscapularis, infraspinatus, and deltoid muscle groups.[15] This may be seen in pitchers, in swimmers during the pull-through phase of freestyle, and also occasionally in tennis players while serving or during the initiation of the backhand stroke.

Clinical Findings

The pain with posterior instability may be posterior or anterior or both, because recurrent posterior subluxation can cause reverse Bankart lesions and/or cause pain in the anterior capsule from traction. The abnormal joint biomechanics resulting from persistent instability may also lead to stress-related inflammation in the rotator cuff. The resulting impingement syndrome may become more disabling than the subluxation itself.

The patient with posterior instability will describe the sensation of crepitation and/or clicking in the involved shoulder when in the appropriate position for posterior translation. In a recent review at our institution[11] crepitation or clicking was noted in 90% of the patients with symptomatic posterior subluxation (18/20).

Physical Examination

On physical examination, patients with recurrent posterior subluxation frequently have loss of internal rotation, particularly with the arm at 90 degrees of abduction. Posterior stress testing should be performed with the patient supine, in both 90 degrees of abduction and 90 degrees of forward flexion with adduction and internal rotation (Fig. 7-21). As with anterior instability, we assign a grade to the amount of posterior humeral head translation on physical examination. Instability is graded as 1+ if there is increased motion without a "clunking" sensation of the humeral head "dropping off" the posterior glenoid, 2+ if a jump is noted without locking in the subluxated position, and 3+ if there is actual locking in a dislocated position. Careful examination for multidirectional instability should be performed in addition to examination of the contralateral shoulder. Finally, careful assessment should be made for generalized ligamentous laxity. Four parameters

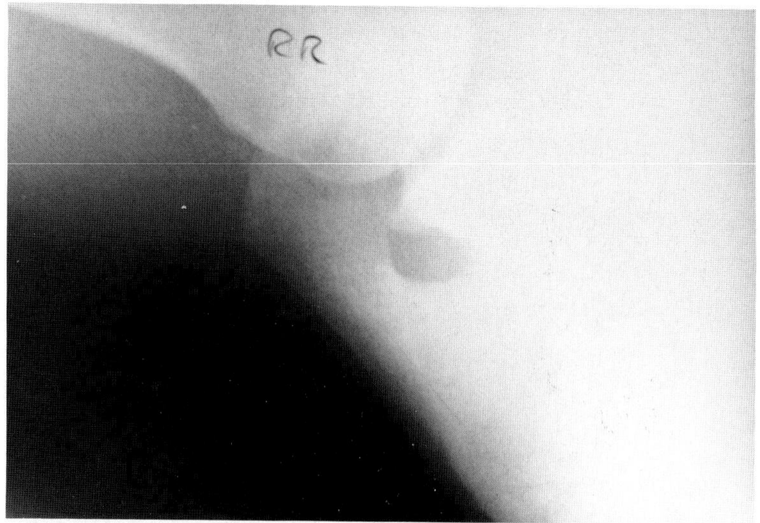

FIG. 7-22. West Point roentgenogram of shoulder. Note capsular calcification along the posterior glenoid labrum. This is present in 20% of patients with posterior instability.

frequently used are the degree of thumb hyperabduction in wrist palmar flexion, the degree of index finger metacarpophalangeal (MCP) joint hyperextension, the degree of elbow hyperextension, and the degree of knee hyperextension.[18]

Roentgenograms

Roentgenographic evaluation of posterior instability should include the instability series described by Pavlov et al[25] for anterior instability, that is, an AP view in internal rotation, a Stryker notch view, and a West Point view. In addition, an AP view in external rotation may be helpful to identify any reverse Hill-Sachs lesions. Of the patients we reviewed recently,[11] 20% demonstrated capsular calcification along the posterior aspect of the capsule and glenoid labrum (Fig. 7-22). An additional 20% were noted to have 2 to 4 mm of bony erosion of the posterior glenoid rim. In general, arthrography and arthrotomography are less useful, because visualization of the labral and capsular pathologic condition does not appear to be as reliable as arthroscopy.

Assessment of ligamentous laxity

- Thumb hyperabduction with wrist palmar flexion
- Index MCP hyperextension
- Elbow hyperextension
- Knee recurvatum

Treatment

Treatment considerations are the same as for anterior instability. Patients with voluntary posterior instability may need psychiatric evaluation, especially if there is consideration being given to any surgical procedure.

Conservative care. The goals for conservative management include (1) avoiding any voluntary episodes of instability or positions that are likely to result in subluxation and (2) restoring normal shoulder motion and strengthening the internal and external rotators, with the emphasis on the external rotators in positions that would not aggravate any preexisting tendonitis. Painful episodes of acute instability are managed initially with sling immobilization and antiinflammatory medications before an aggresive rehabilitation program. Concomitant rotator cuff tendonitis is treated in the standard fashion with a brief period of rest for the acute inflammation (1 to 2 weeks), nonsteroidal antiinflammatory medication, and then a physical therapy program including range of motion and strengthening exercises for the shoulder. In a refractory case, subacromial injection of steroids may be needed. If this is done, the patient must be cautioned that this may temporarily weaken the rotator cuff, and strenuous activity should be avoided for approximately 4 weeks.

Rotator cuff exercises can be performed in many ways, although a simple spring exerciser used initially with the arm at the side and subsequently in 90 degrees of abduction

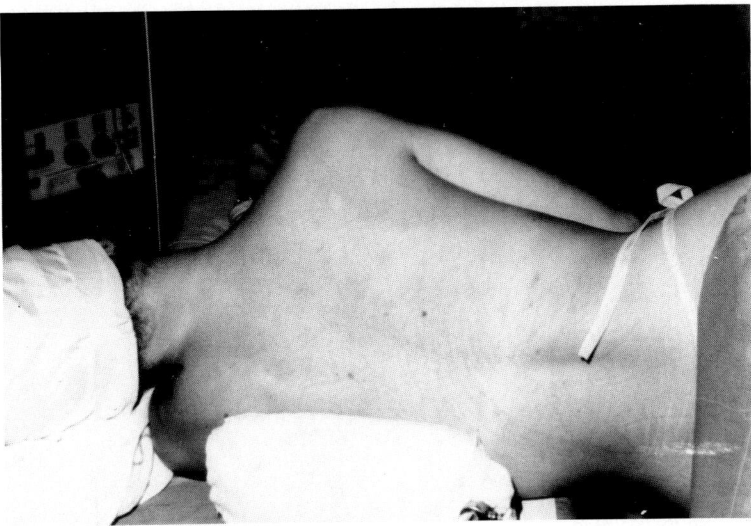

FIG. 7-23. Patient positioning for posterior shoulder surgery. This illustrates the lateral decubitus position. The arm must be draped free to check rotation once the capsular repair is completed.

can be sufficient. An emphasis should also be placed on developing the deltoid and periscapular musculature.

Most patients with posterior instability will respond to an aggressive exercise program, particularly in patients with generalized ligamentous laxity and instability occurring secondary to repetitive microtrauma. Patients whose onset was associated with macrotrauma are less likely to be aided by an exercise program.[11]

Operative care. Operative treatment should be considered in patients who fail an adequate trial of conservative therapy and whose pain and/or instability precludes adequate function of the involved shoulder. A thorough examination under anesthesia is mandatory to confirm or refute preoperative findings. This may or may not include arthroscopy. In addition, the opposite shoulder should be evaluated.

Arthroscopy. Arthroscopy may be of considerable value in treating posterior shoulder subluxation as well as diagnosing it. This appears to be the case in a number of throwers. Arthroscopic debridement of labral lesions, although not affecting their instability, may decrease their pain sufficiently to resume throwing. Subsequent stabilization procedures may be required; however, some of these patients will become asymptomatic when they are no longer placing the shoulder under such high loads. In the athlete in whom posterior subluxation is seemingly caused by repetitive overload, reconstructive surgery will not necessarily allow him to return to a high level of throwing. As such we are more inclined to persist with exercises and possibly labral debridement in that setting. Arthroscopic debridement, while helpful initially, tends to be temporary because symptoms recur in 2 to 3 years if activity is resumed.

Open surgical procedures. As with surgery for anterior instability, surgical procedures for posterior shoulder instability must be designed to treat the pathologic abnormalities present. In patients with no bony glenoid defects and a substantial posterior capsule and infraspinatous tendon, soft tissue repair by itself is usually adequate. When there is deficient glenoid or for patients with generalized ligament laxity and inadequate posterior tissues, we think it is indicated to augment the posterior capsulorrhaphy with a bone block.

The patient is positioned either prone with two chest rolls longitudinally, or in the lateral decubitus position with the involved side up. In either position the arm is draped free to allow accurate determination of external rotation (Fig. 7-23).

We have increasingly used a vertical incision that allows a better scar to form. The horizontal incision has a tendency to widen with time. In using a vertical incision, the incision is oriented vertically over the soft spot of the posterior shoulder from the acromion distally toward the axillary crease. The deltoid fibers are split distally, avoiding the inferior portion where the axillary nerve passes distal to the teres minor. If the exposure is inade-

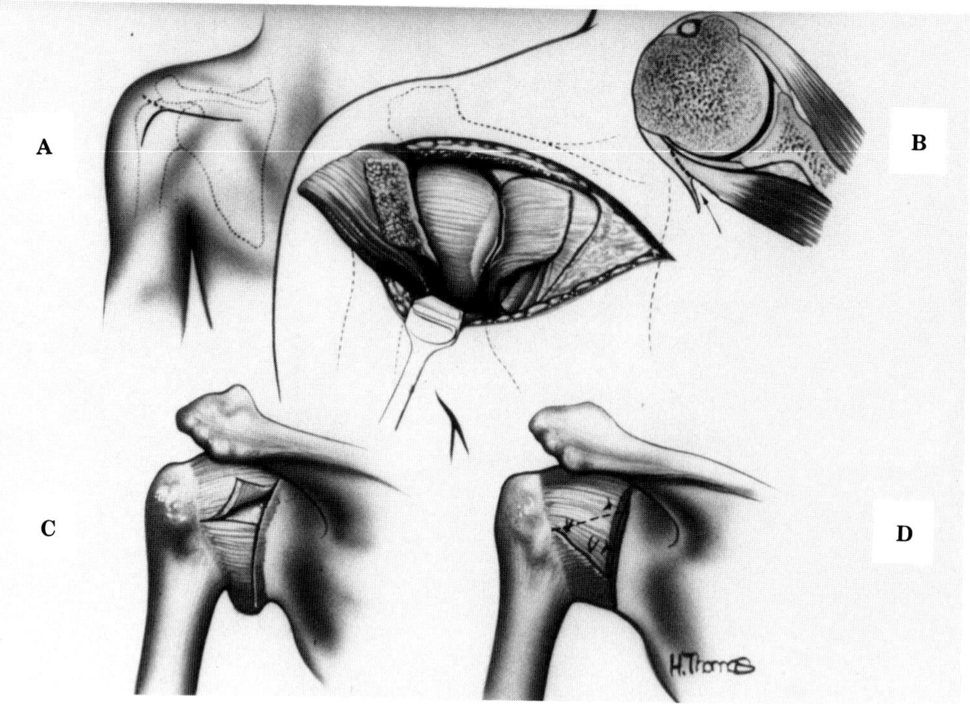

FIG. 7-24. A, The incision for posterior shoulder surgery. **B**, The infraspinatus tendon is incised obliquely to gain length. The lateral flap of tendon, which is still attached to the humeral head, may be used to reinforce the posterior capsular repair. **C**, T-shaped capsular incision. **D**, Completed T-plasty capsulorrhaphy. Note superior advancement of inferior capsular limb and inferior advancement of superior capsular limb. This decreases inferior capsular redundancy.

quate, it may be lengthened medially or laterally to form a Y. If a horizontal incision is used it must be positioned 2 cm distal to the scapular spine. The subcutaneous tissues are dissected and undermined in order to retract the skin and to visualize the fibers of the deltoid. The deltoid muscle is split to reveal the infraspinatus and teres minor (Fig. 7-24).

The infraspinatus tendon is split vertically, leaving a large portion of the tendon laterally. Unfortunately this tendon is often thin and insufficient, but it can be used to thicken the posterior capsule as a rule even if it is not long enough to reach the glenoid.

After dissecting the tendon and muscle off the capsule, one can identify the capsule. Frequently it is thin and translucent with no obvious ligament fibers. It is incised in a T shape at the margin of the glenoid. The labrum and joint are inspected. The labrum often has vertical clefts from subluxation and may be partially detached, but rarely is an extensive Bankart lesion noted as seen anteriorly. All loose bodies and flap tears of the articular cartilage are debrided.

Posterior capsulorrhaphy is performed, and the lateral flap of the capsule is reattached to the glenoid. the repair is accomplished with drill holes through the bone if the labrum is detached or by direct suture if the labrum is intact. In essence, the capsule is advanced superiorly and medially, dependent on the degree of laxity posteriorly and inferiorly. In marked inferior laxity it may be necessary to make an H-shaped capsular incision to allow adequate obliteration of the inferior pouch, as with anterior H-plasty. The arm is held at the side in neutral rotation during suturing of the capsule. The infraspinatus tendon may be used for reinforcement, with reefing of the tendon or direct advancement into the capsule (Fig. 7-24).

In the presence of bony deficiency, marked capsular laxity, or insufficient capsule and infraspinatus tendon, the posterior bone block is used. The graft placement is critical since the primary goal is to increase the size and depth of the glenoid without contacting the humeral head. The technical considerations in adding the bone block are important to the success of the procedure. Generally the graft is obtained from the spine of the scapula and is 3 cm long and about 15 mm wide. The cortex of the glenoid neck is prepared and a

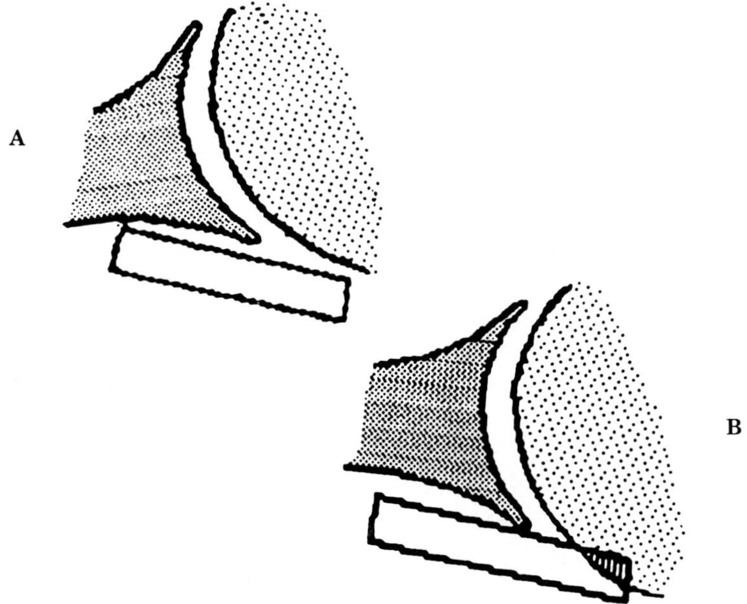

FIG. 7-25. **A**, Correct position of posterior bone block. **B**, Incorrect position of posterior bone block. The bone should not function as a mechanical block to the humeral head.

hole is drilled to ensure the placement of the screw across both cortices while avoiding the joint surface. The capsule repair is then performed, followed by placement of the bone graft. The graft is placed into the posterior inferior quadrant at the margin of the joint. It is our concept that the graft should function to extend the joint so that the soft tissues both anteriorly and posteriorly will prevent subluxation. The graft should not function as a mechanical block to the humeral head (Fig. 7-25).

Postoperatively, the patient is placed in an Orthoplast orthosis made preoperatively with the arm held in neutral rotation and slight extension, in order to minimize any posterior subluxation forces (Fig. 7-26). At 6 weeks a range of motion and strengthening program is begun with the primary emphasis placed on strengthening the internal and external rotator muscle groups. Sports activities involving the shoulder are begun 9 to 12 months after surgery if good strength and a full range of motion have been achieved.

Summary

In summary, the assessment of the posterior subluxation patients should include evaluation of ligamentous laxity, the degree of trauma prior to the onset of symptoms, and voluntary subluxation. While essentially all microtrauma patients are good candidates for the physical therapy program, only some macrotrauma patients with mild to moderate disability may benefit significantly from this program. Patients' compliance and presence of significant emotional problems should be observed at this time. The majority of the macrotrauma patients present with more severe disability and are candidates for posterior capsulorrhaphy. If the posterior capsule and infraspinatus tendon appear incompetent, then augmentation of the reconstruction with a bone block is recommended.

MULTIDIRECTIONAL SHOULDER INSTABILITY

Multidirectional shoulder instability (MDI) is defined as shoulder instability occurring in more than one plane of motion. The combinations of directions of laxity in order of frequency are anteroinferior, posteroinferior, all three directions, and, rarely, anteroposterior without an inferior component. Patients display a spectrum of MDI, ranging from the individual with excessive ligamentous laxity (see Fig. 7-8) (atraumatic type) to one who performs repetitive activities at the extremes of motion, (microtraumatic type), to the person without increased laxity who sustains a violent insult to the shoulder (traumatic type). The concept of the separation of true unidirectional instability from MDI is probably simplistic. A continuum between these two diagnoses exists. Acutely, most if not all anterior

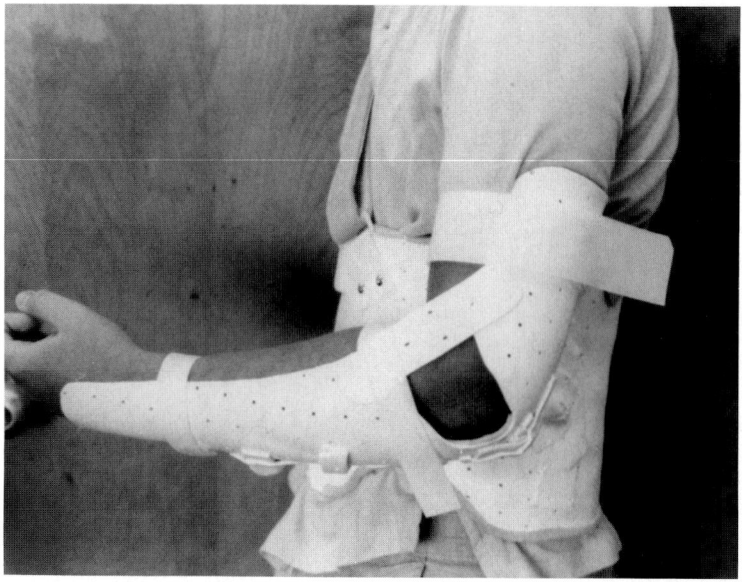

FIG. 7-26. Orthoplast orthosis for arm immobilization following posterior shoulder stabilizaiton.

and posterior shoulder dislocations are associated with some mild inferior laxity or laxity in the opposite direction. The quality of soft tissue healing during conservative treatment as well as the degree of inferior laxity before the injury will determine the subsequent diagnosis of MDI.

Patterns of multidirectional instability

- Anteroinferior
- Posteroinferior
- Anteroposteroinferior
- Anteroposterior

For patients without generalized laxity, a history of multiple violent injuries to the shoulder is usually obtained. Athletes with increased laxity will generally relate repetitive activities such as throwing, swimming, or weight lifting as the cause of instability. This repetitive microtrauma has a cumulative effect on increasing the magnitude of multidirectional instability.

Clinical Findings

The presenting symptoms of MDI will vary according to the predominant directions of instability. Most patients will have a component of inferior laxity. Inferior laxity will manifest as pain and/or clicking with the arm in the dependent position. When lifting objects such as suitcases, the person may experience subluxation or dislocation. Most of these patients will exhibit a sulcus sign, as we have previously described (see Fig. 7-10). The addition of anterior or posterior laxity will then determine which activities cause symptoms. The key point is that patients with MDI are relatively more continuously disabled for any given activity than those with simpler instability patterns.

Roentgenograms

All patients should have an instability roentgenographic series performed. If there is a concern regarding the quality of bone stock in the glenoid or humerus, a CT scan or CT arthrogram may be performed.

Treatment

Conservative Care

Treatment for MDI is initially nonsurgical. Patients with ligamentous laxity are more likely to respond to conservative rehabilitation than those whose MDI is of traumatic origin. Approximately 50% to 70% of patients with MDI and ligamentous laxity will have a favorable response to rehabilitation, especially if they are willing to modify their activities.

Surgical Care

For those patients who fail conservative treatment and for patients with MDI of traumatic origin, open capsular plication is recommended. First, the patient's primary direction of instability must be determined. Most MDI can be rectified using a standard anterior approach to the shoulder. However, if the primary clinical direction of instability is posterior, a posterior approach is used. An extra effort must be made to strip the capsule free of cuff tissue at least to the 6-o'clock position on the glenoid before any capsular incisions are made. The axillary nerve is dangerously close to the inferior capsule during this dissection and the surgeon must be constantly aware of its position to avoid transsection or excessive traction.

Technique. A transverse incision in the capsule is performed first at about the midglenoid level. If a large rotator interval is present, this may be substituted for the transverse limb of the capsular incision to inspect the joint. The quality of the labral tissue and its attachment to the glenoid are then assessed. If the labrum is well attached to the glenoid, then the labral complex is not dissected off the glenoid neck but rather a vertical capsular incision is then made lateral to the labrum. If labral detachment has occurred, a medial vertical capsular incision is made parallel to the glenoid, extending to the 6- or 7-o'clock position inferiorly. If no labral detachment is noted, the vertical incision may be made laterally or medially, with reattachment to soft tissues rather than bone. The inferior limb of the T-capsular incision is shifted superiorly to decrease the inferior capsular redundancy. If after reattachment, inferior redundance and laxity still appear, a second vertical capsular incision is made opposite the first to create an H configuration. Again, the inferior limb is advanced superiorly as needed to eliminate the inferior capsular redundancy. Advancement of the capsule in a mediolateral direction may also be performed if needed at the same time. The superior limb of the capsular T- or H-plasty is then advanced inferiorly and sutured over the inferior limb (Fig. 7-27). The goal is not to limit external rotation of the arm but to restore normal volume and tension to the glenohumeral capsule. If a rotator interval is present, it should be repaired as part of the capsular plication.

Postoperative care. Postoperatively, the patient is immobilized in a sling-and-swathe type of orthosis, which helps to prevent inferior sag of the arm. At times with severe inferior laxity and a poor quality tissue the orthoplast splint is used as previously described. The shoulder is kept immobilized for a full 6 weeks prior to starting any motion. Passive and active assisted motion are performed from 6 to 12 weeks after surgery. Progressive resistive exercises are then added slowly. Full sporting activities are not allowed for 9 to 12 months, until muscle strength and range of motion are symmetric.

Although the operation for MDI is technically demanding, it directly deals with the pathologic state in the capsule. Other procedures that try to indirectly rectify the capsular laxity are not recommended.

COMPLICATIONS OF SURGICAL TREATMENT

Several complications can occur with surgical repair for shoulder instability. Postoperative infection and hematoma formation can occur as in all operations. Meticulous surgical technique, achievement of hemostasis, and use of suction drains and prophylactic antibiotics can decrease the incidence of these problems. If an extensive hematoma occurs, then early evacuation to prevent scarring and restricted motion is suggested.

Complications of surgical treatment

- Infection
- Hematoma
- Neurologic injury
  - Musculocutaneous nerve
  - Axillary nerve
- Recurrent dislocation
- Loss of motion

Neurovascular injuries secondary to surgery are the next group of complications. The musculocutaneous nerve is susceptible to traction neuropraxia as it enters the coracobrachialis. The axillary nerve and posterior humeral circumflex artery are at risk with inferior capsular dissection and repair. If a nerve injury occurs, initial conduction studies may be used to determine if conduction is still present before wallerian degeneration sets in at 48 hours. If conduction occurs it suggests the nerve is still intact. Electromyographic (EMG) studies are obtained at 3 weeks and the patient is followed. There is a tendency to wait too long with these patients in the hope that recovery will occur. If no recovery is occurring and there is no voluntary potential in EMGs, then exploration at 3 months is indicated. Urbaniak has noted that these lesions are frequently complete requiring operative repair.

Failure of the surgical procedure is also a potential complication. This can vary from persistent instability in the shoulder to severe limitation of motion. The reported incidence

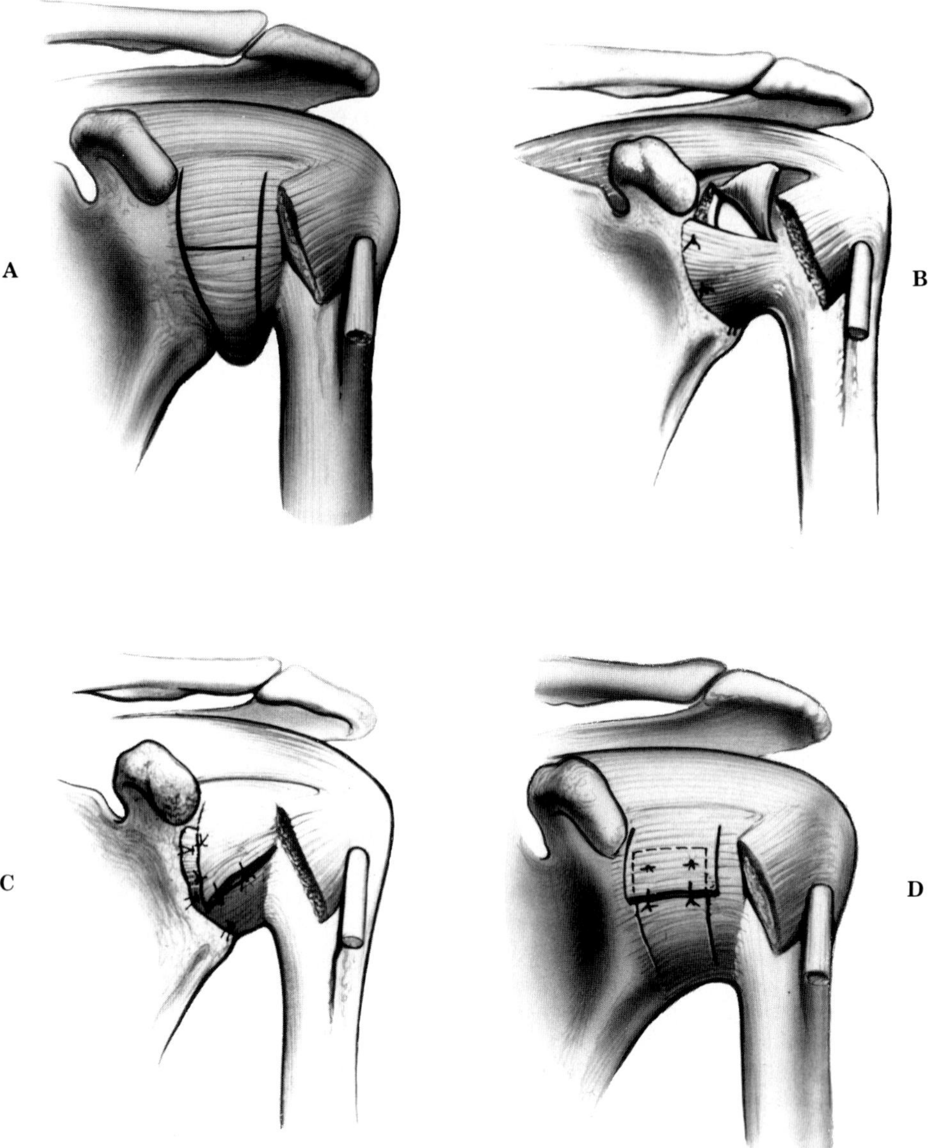

FIG. 7-27. A, Capsular incisions for perfoming a T-plasty or H-plasty. The transverse incision is performed first followed by inspection of the labral complex. **B**, The inferior limb of the T-plasty is advanced superiorly and medially to decrease inferior redundancy. The capsule is sutured to the glenoid or the intact labrum. **C**, The superior limb of the T-plasty is advanced inferiorly to reinforce the repair. **D**, The completed H-plasty. This would be performed for marked inferior laxity.

of recurrent dislocation after surgical repair of anterior instability ranges from 0% to 11%.[14,21,27,30] Provided that pathologic capsular abnormalities have been corrected at surgery, recurrent instability has been very uncommon at our institution. Range of motion losses are a function of surgical technique, tissue contracture, and rehabilitation programs. The capsular tension should be set at 30 to 50 degrees of external rotation on the table and the subscapularis muscle repaired anatomically. Another type of complication concerns the use of hardware about the shoulder. We have advised against the use of any metal implants in or about the shoulder joint in treating shoulder instability because they may loosen with activity.

REFERENCES

1. Anderson D, Zvirbulis R, and Ciullo J: Scapular manipulation for reduction of anterior shoulder dislocation, Clin Orthop 164:181, 1982.
2. Andrews JR, and Carson WG: The arthroscopic treatment of glenoid labrum tears in the throwing athlete, Orthop Trans 8:44, 1984.
3. Arndt JH, and Sears AD: Posterior dislocation of the shoulder, Am J Roentgenol 94:639, 1965.
4. Bach BR et al: An unusual neurological complication of the Bristow Procedure: a case report, J Bone Joint Surg 70A(3):458, 1988.
5. Bach BR, Warren RF, and Fronek J: Disruption of the lateral capsule of the shoulder: a cause of recurrent dislocation, J Bone Joint Surg 70B:274, 1988.
6. Blom S, and Dahlback L: Nerve injuries in dislocations of the shoulder joint and fractures of the neck of the humerus, Acta Chir Scand 136:461, 1970.
7. Boyd HB, and Sisk TD: Recurrent posterior dislocation of the shoulder, J Bone Joint Surg 54A:779, 1972.
8. Clayton ML, and Weir GJ, Jr: Experimental investigations of ligamentous healing, Am J Surg 98:373, 1959.
9. Cox JS: Personal communication.
10. English E, and MacNab I: Recurrent posterior dislocation of the shoulder, Can J Surg 17:147, 1974.
11. Fronek J, Warren RF, and Bowen M: Posterior subluxation of the glenohumeral joint, J Bone Joint Surg 71A:205, 1989.
12. Galinat BJ et al: The glenoid-posterior acromion angle: an accurate method of evaluating glenoid version, Orthop Trans 12(3):727, 1988.
13. Hawkins RJ: Osteoarthritis following an excessively tight Putti-Platt repair, Orthop Trans 12(3):728, 1988.
14. Hovelius L, Thorling J, and Fredin H: Recurrent anterior dislocation of the shoulder: results after the Bankart and Putti-Plat operations, J Bone Joint Surg 61A:566, 1979.
15. Jobe FW et al: An EMG analysis of the shoulder in pitching, Am J Sports Med 12:218, 1984.
16. Kinnet JG, Warren RF, and Jacobs B: Recurrent dislocation of the shoulder after age fifty, Clin Orthop 149:164, 1980.
17. Kornblatt I, Warren RF, and Marchand R: An analysis of the effects of capsular and tendon releases on posterior glenohumeral translation, Orthop Trans 8:89, 1984.
18. Koslin BL, Zeno S, and Meyers A: Joint looseness: a function of the person and the joint, Med Sci Sports Exerc 12:189, 1980.
19. Leslie JT, and Ryan TJ: Anterior axillary incision to approach the shoulder joint, J Bone Joint Surg 44A:1193, 1962.
20. Mason ML, and Allen HS: The rate of healing of tendinitis: an experimental study of the tensile strength, Am J Surg 113:424, 1941.
21. Morrey BF, and James JM: Recurrent anterior dislocation of the shoulder: long-term follow-up of the Putti-Platt and Bankart procedures, J Bone Joint Surg 58A:252, 1976.
22. Mowery CA et al: Recurrent posterior dislocation of the shoulder: treatment using a bone block, J Bone Joint Surg 67A:777, 1985.
23. Neer CS, and Foster CR: Inferior capsular shift for involuntary inferior and multidirectional instability of the shoulder, J Bone Joint Surg 62A:897, 1980.
24. Nobuhara K, and Hitoshi I: Rotator interval lesion, Clin Orthop 223:44, 1987.
25. Pavlov H et al: The roentgenographic evaluation of anterior shoulder instability, Clin Orthop 184:153, 1985.
26. Robert A, and Wickstrom J: Prognosis of posterior dislocations of the shoulder Acta Orthop Scand 42:328, 1971.
27. Rockwood CA: Subluxations and dislocations about the shoulder. In Rockwood CA, and Green DP editors: Fractures in adults, Philadelphia, 1984, JB Lippincott Co., pp 722-860.
28. Rokous JR, Faegin JA, and Abbott HG: Modified axillary roentgenograms: a useful adjunct in the diagnosis of recurrent instability of the shoulder, Clin Orthop 82:84, 1972.
29. Rowe CR: Prognosis in dislocations of the shoulder, J Bone Joint Surg 38A:957, 1956.
30. Rowe CR, Patel D, and Southmayd WW: The Bankart procedure: a long-term end-result study, J Bone Joint Surg 60A:1, 1978.
31. Rowe CR, Pierce DS, and Clark JG: Voluntary dislocation of the shoulder: a preliminary report on a clinical electromyographic and psychiatric study of twenty-six patients, J Bone Joint Surg 55A:445, 1973.
32. Rowe CR, and Sakellarides HT: Factors related to recurrences of anterior dislocation of the shoulder, Clin Orthop 20:40, 1961.
33. Rowe CR, and Zarins B: Chronic unreduced dislocations of the shoulder, J Bone Joint Surg 64A:494, 1982.
34. Rowe CR and Zarins B: Recurrent transient subluxation of the shoulder, J Bone Joint Surg 63A:863, 1981.
35. Saha AK: Recurrent dislocations of the shoulder, ed 2, New York, 1981, Thieme-Stratton.
36. Schwartz RE et al: Capsular restraints to anterior-posterior motion of the shoulder, Orthop Trans 12(3):727, 1988.
37. Scott DJ, Jr: Treatment of recurrent posterior dislocations of the shoulder by glenoidplasty, J Bone Joint Surg 49A:471, 1967.
38. Simonet WT, and Cofield RH: Prognosis in anterior shoulder dislocation, Am J Sports Med 12:19, 1984.

39. Stimson LA: An easy method of reducing dislocation of the shoulder and hip, Med Rec 57:356, 1900.
40. Turkel SJ et al: Stabilizing mechanisms preventing anterior dislocation of the glenohumeral joint, J Bone Surg 61A:1208-1217, 1981.
41. Warren RF: Subluxation of the shoulder in athletes Clin Sports Med 2(2):339, 1983.
42. Warren RF: Personal communication, 1988.
43. Yoneda B, Welsh RP, and MacIntosh DL: Conservative treatment of shoulder dislocation, J Bone Joint Surg 64B:254, 1982.

CHAPTER 8 Impingement and Rotator Cuff Lesions

Keith Watson

The impingement syndrome is one, if not the most common, cause of pain and dysfunction in the athletes shoulder.[2,3,10] The pathomechanics of this syndrome implicate activities that repetitively place the arm in overhead positions. The majority of athletes who manifest this condition participate in baseball, swimming, and tennis, but it is by no means confined to these sports. The importance of its recognition is that impingement is often a progressive condition that, if recognized and treated early, can have a more favorable outcome. Delay in recognition and treatment can allow secondary changes to occur, with resultant limitations in treatment options and expectations.

PATHOPHYSIOLOGY

In response to the demands placed on it, the shoulder has evolved from a massive appendage supporting the weight of the trunk to a light-weight, fully suspended structure that allows the greatest range of motion of any joint in the body. To accomplish this, nature has developed an anatomic arrangement that demands a precise balance among the bony and soft tissues. As in a finely tuned machine, the tolerances are quite precise. Specifically, the rotator cuff functions essentially to maintain a force-couple with the deltoid that secures the humeral head in the glenoid. When this arrangement is compromised, the pull of the deltoid will force the humeral head proximally and the rotator cuff can be compressed (impinged) beneath the unyielding coracoacromial arch.[9] Neer[7] has proposed a progressive staging of this condition that helps to define treatment options as well. According to this scheme, an initial injury will produce acute changes in the rotator cuff, such as edema and hemorrhage. These changes, which are transient and fully reversible, are considered stage 1. In response to repeated irritation over time, fibrosis and chronic tendonitis may develop—a subacute condition considered stage 2. Finally, in response to persistent impingement over time, there are both adaptive and degenerative structural changes in the rotator cuff, bursa, acromial arch, and even the greater tuberosity. Once irreversible structural alterations have occurred, the process is then considered stage 3.

Because the demands an athlete places on the shoulder may exceed those of the average person, the degree and progression of the impingement process is accelerated. Because bone reacts and adapts more slowly than soft tissues, there may be an accelerated rate of wear to the soft tissues that will not be reflected by changes in the bony structures. Therefore, when dealing with the athlete, some have found it convenient to modify these stages. Stage 3 would represent relatively small rotator cuff defects, whereas an addi-

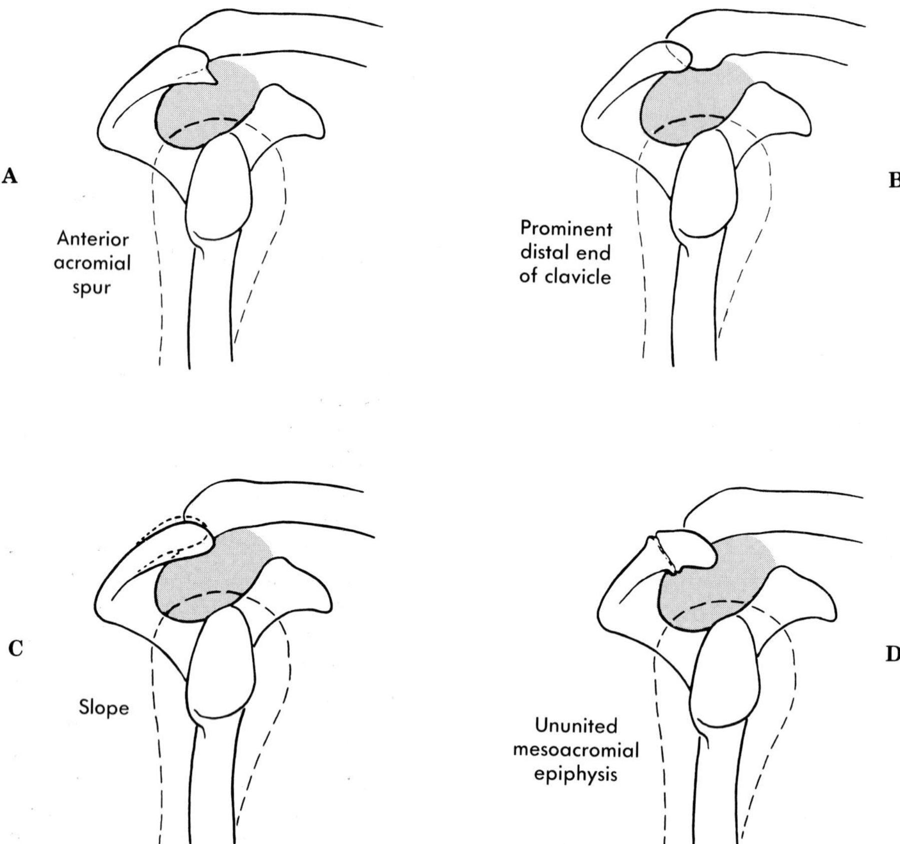

FIG. 8-1. The usual cause of subacromial impingement is narrowing of the supraspinatus outlet or variation in the shape or slope of the acromion. **A,** Anterior acromial spur formation. **B,** Prominence of the distal end of the clavicle or the inferior edge of the acromioclavicular joint. **C,** Flattening of the slope of the acromion. **D,** Nonunion or malunion of the acromion is a less common cause. (Reproduced from Poppen NK: Soft-tissue lesions of the shoulder. In Chapman MW editor: Operative orthopaedics, Philadelphia, 1988, JB Lippincott.)

tional stage 4 subclassification would represent tears larger than 1 cm.[4] In essence, the condition is not necessarily different in athletes, but the body's response is more limited.

What is not clear is who will develop progressive impingement and why? Certainly not everyone who experiences injury to the shoulder or participates in activities that require overhead arm movement will acquire impingement, just as nerve root compression will not develop in everyone who experiences a ruptured disk. Current work suggests there are predisposing anatomic variations that will affect the response of the body to injury or activity.[1]

Variations in the shape and slope of the acromion have been implicated. The concept of the supraspinatus outlet has been proposed to describe this confined space through which the supraspinatus is exposed to impingement.[6] The presence of bony intrusions (e.g., subacromial spurs, inferior acromioclavicular osteophytes, even the presence of an unfused acromial epiphysis) into a supraspinatus outlet is associated with a high probability of impingement (Fig. 8-1). Therefore it can be postulated that an injury (either microtraumatic or macrotraumatic) may occur with resultant reaction in the rotator cuff. However, in individuals who are predisposed by a compromised supraspinatus outlet, the condition does not resolve but becomes one of a viscious cycle, with further use causing further irritation. This concept can explain the predilection for supraspinatus involvement, as well as the variations in presentation with regard to acute injury versus overuse. The concept of impingement can also explain the relationships among bursitis, tendonitis, and rotator cuff tears.

CLINICAL EVALUATION

Diagnosing the cause of shoulder pain in the athlete is difficult because it is almost exclusively a clinical diagnosis. This is especially true for impingement and instability, which are the two most common pathologic conditions.

History

A history of recurrent episodes of pain associated with a particular activity is usually what causes the athlete to seek the treatment of a physician. Often the athlete has been told by the trainer that it is strained or it is bursitis. The usual local remedies—heat, ice, salves, and rest—have not been effective. Quite likely there is no pain unless the athlete is involved in play. Sometimes there is a dull background ache when the athlete is at rest. Most athletes will have a history of some earlier injury, but often are not sure which shoulder was involved. Specific questions regarding fatigue and feelings of looseness may help in directing the examination to rule out instability. It is not unusual for patients with impingement to notice easy fatigability rather than sensations of slipping.

Inspection

Initial examination of the patient should include a visual scan from behind. Specific attention should be paid to identify atrophy of muscle groups, prominence of the acromioclavicular joint, and symmetry of posture. Active elevation and abduction of both arms should reveal any disturbance of the normal scapulohumeral rhythm and the presence of any winging. Palpation can then elicit any areas of sensitivity. Tenderness is not specific for impingement, but would be consistent at the anterior acromion, along the coracoacromial ligament, and at the greater tuberosity. It is particularly important to assess the acromioclavicular joint in this way. The coracoid process is generally tender whenever there is any shoulder problem and is therefore not necessarily a helpful sign. Tenderness at the biceps groove is also consistent with suspected impingement because most episodes of bicipital tendonitis are thought to be secondary to impingement.

Factors contributing to impingement syndrome

- Shape and slope of acromion
- Subacromial spurs
- Inferior acromioclavicular osteophytes
- Unfused acromial epiphysis

Arc of Motion Evaluation

The presence of a painful arc of motion is a significant finding. As the arm is lowered from 120 degrees to 70 degrees, maximum tension is developed in the rotator cuff. If this produces pain, it is suggestive of tendonitis. Jobe and Jobe[4] have further defined this part of the examination to better isolate the supraspinatus. With the shoulder at 90 degrees of abduction, the arm is then brought forward 30 degrees, in line with the spine of the scap-

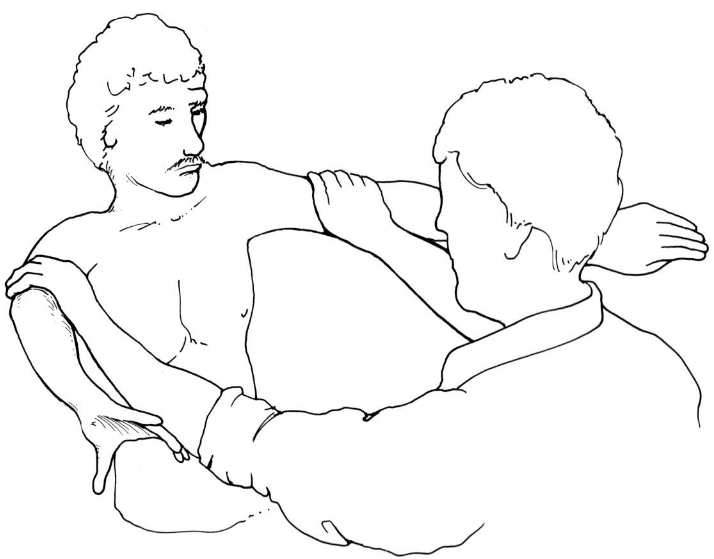

FIG. 8-2. Supraspinatus test. Patient upright, shoulder 90 degrees of abduction, 30 degrees of horizontal adduction, and full internal rotation. Patient maintains position against downward resistance. (Reproduced from Jobe FW, and Jobe CM: Painful athletic injuries of the shoulder, Clin Orthop 173:117, 1983.)

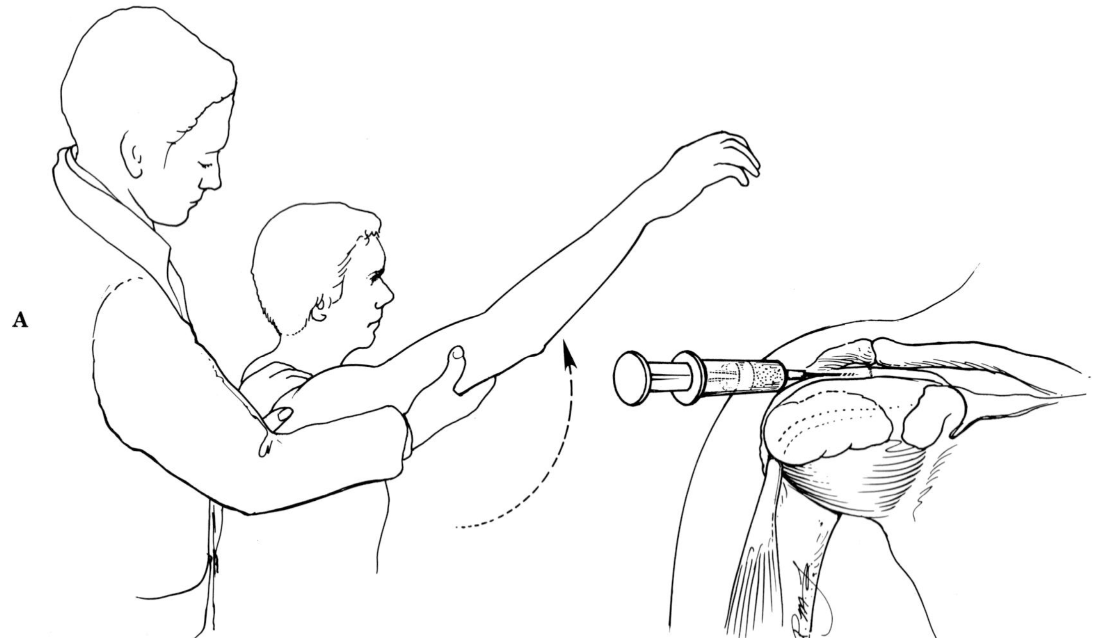

FIG. 8-3. A, The impingement sign is elicited with the patient seated and the examiner standing. Scapular rotation is prevented with one hand while the other hand raises the arm in forced forward elevation. This maneuver produces pain in patients with impingement lesions. **B,** The impingement injection test is useful in separating impingement lesions of all stages from other causes. (Reproduced from Neer CS II: Impingement lesions, Clin Orthop 173:70, 1983.)

ula (i.e., the scapular plane), and then internally rotated so the thumb then points to the floor (Fig. 8-2). Muscle testing against resistance will be more likely to elicit discomfort in patients whose symptoms occur only with strenuous effort.

Impingement Sign

An impingement sign should also be sought (i.e., the production of pain when the arm is forcibly elevated in the forward plane while the scapula is stabilized) (Fig. 8-3, *A*). This will actually compress the irritated tissues and is frequently positive in impingement. If this sign is absent, the diagnosis of impingement should be suspect. A full passive range of motion is necessary for the accuracy of the clinical examination. If stiffness is present, it should be addressed vigorously with stretching exercises and the patient reevaluated. Stiffness can occur as a result of impingement, but also from other causes.

Strength Evaluation

Muscle testing should be undertaken with close attention to the external rotators. The majority of external rotation power comes from the infraspinatus and teres minor. Involvement of the rotator cuff can cause dysfunction either through direct injury or pain. The identification of external rotation weakness indicates a more involved condition.

Injection Test

Finally, if a painful arc, a positive impingement sign, weakness of external rotation—any or all—is identified, then a subacromial injection with a local anesthetic agent—the injection test—is recommended to support the diagnosis. (Fig. 8-3, *B*). In the absence of any additional contributing factors (e.g., acromioclavicular joint stiffness, radiculitis, etc.), the injection should significantly reduce the sensitivity of the subacromial space, usually eliminating painful arc and the impingement sign and restoring external rotation power.

DIAGNOSTIC STUDIES

Roentgenograms

Although subacromial impingement is basically a clinical diagnosis in the later stages of the condition, there can be some diagnostic findings that are corroborative. Bony changes are necessarily slow to develop and are less likely to be of help in the athlete. Changes that are typically seen in the more advanced impingement stages include the development of an anterior acromial spur (an actual morphologic change in the origin of the coracoacromial ligament in response to increased tension in the ligament, much as the heel spur develops in the plantar fascia). Reciprocal changes are seen on the greater tuberosity with the cortical fragmentation and irregularity. Finally, with large defects in the rotator cuff, there may be a decrease of the acromiohumeral interval as the humeral head buttonholes through the defect.

For most athletes, however, these changes will not be found because the dysfunction represented by such changes would have prevented participation much earlier.[10] However, there are some abnormalities detectable on plain roentgenograms that would support a predisposition to the development of impingement in an athlete. These areas should be closely examined and should require three different roentgenographic projections, in addition to "routine" views. A good examination of the acromioclavicular joint is important. It is one of the joints to demonstrate earliest degenerative change, and identification of osteophytic proliferation is important because it can compromise the supraspinatus outlet. Routine views of the shoulder, however, are often overpenetrated, and frequently there is overlapping of bone that prevents a fair assessment of this joint. It is recommended that a 10- to 15-degree cephalad projection be obtained with less penetration. Second, evaluation of the supraspinatus outlet and the profile of the acromion can be of benefit. The identification of a type III acromion would support a clincal diagnosis of impingement. The outlet view is obtained by shooting along the spine of the scapula (as is done in the lateral scapular view of the trauma series) and angling the tube caudad 0 to 10 degrees, depending on the contour of the patient. Third, an axillary view is recommended to rule out the presence of an unfused acromial epiphysis with an increased incidence of impingement.

Roentgenographic signs of impingement

- Anterior acromial spur
- Subchondral sclerosis/cysts of greater tuberosity

Ancillary Tests

Additional diagnostic studies may be of benefit to pin down the diagnosis or better assess the condition of the soft tissues. **Ultrasound** has been recently popularized as an inexpensive and noninvasive technique to evaluate the rotator cuff. For full-thickness tears more than 1 cm in size, it has achieved some success. There is disagreement, however, about its usefulness and accuracy with small tears (less than 1 cm) and partial or incomplete tears of the rotator cuff. In addition, there is some degree of operator dependency with a significant learning curve, which may preclude its usefulness in the general setting. Similarly **MRI scanning** has been viewed as a promising noninvasive technique, but it also has shortcomings, similar to those of ultrasound, in addition to requiring unusual and sophisticated equipment and being relatively expensive.

The importance of **arthrography** in evaluating the condition of the rotator cuff is well recognized, but, unless there is a full-thickness tear, arthrography is not likely to be helpful. In the athletic population, arthrography should be reserved for situations in which there is significant weakness, a major acute injury, or a failure to respond to conservative treatment. Other invasive testing, such as **CT arthrography** and **bursography**, have not produced refinements in the diagnosis of subacromial impingement.

Once again, the diagnosis of subacromial impingement may be made solely on clinical grounds and, especially in the athletic population, diagnostic tests may be negative.

TREATMENT

Once the diagnosis of subacromial impingement has been made, treatment decisions must be undertaken. The desire of the athlete to remain competitive makes this process more difficult. Although this desire is beneficial when it comes to applying oneself to a rehabilitative regimen, it can conflict with the dictates of physiology regarding healing and recovery times. Whether athletic or not, almost all patients want to consider themselves "quick healers" and the athlete, more than anyone, must confront this "time barrier."

Initial treatment must be directed at resting the irritated shoulder. This does not necessarily mean complete inactivity, and certainly not bracing or immobilization, but rather discontinuance of the activity that precipitated the condition. At the same time, it is important to maintain mobility with stretching techniques and muscle tone with isometric and isokinetic exercises that are below the range of sensitivity. In addition, a short course of a nonsteroidal antiinflammatory medication may be helpful in decreasing sensitivity and promoting rapid recovery.

A subacromial injection performed to clarify the diagnosis (injection test) can often be combined with a cortisone derivative to decrease the irritation in the subacromial bursa. (Such injections are made into the bursal space only and never within the tendon tissues). Such injections, although they can provide significant alleviation in symptoms, must be used quite sparingly and only in the acute phase of the condition. Once the acute phase has subsided and the athlete is pain free with full mobility, then the activity may be pursued, but with attention to correcting poor mechanics or techniques that may have initiated the process. It is helpful for the athlete (as well as coaches and trainers) to understand the possible causes of the condition to help identify any easily correctable component. It is important to detect this condition in the early stages, when treatment can be most effective, and to stress the importance of gradual resumption of play, with proper conditioning ahead of time.

Once stiffness and sensitivity have been overcome, then attention should be directed toward recovering tone and strength (see Chapter 11) This is accomplished with a series of exercises performed within the comfort range and not in the impingement arc. Allowance of sufficient time for tissue recovery is essential before the athlete returns to the sport. One of the most common mistakes made is the athlete's attempt to return to the sport too early. The only contraindication to at least 9 months of conservative treatment is the presence of a full-thickness defect in the rotator cuff. (Operative treatment may then be indicated to prevent further progression).

Conservative treatment must be pursued for an extended period because it is the best chance the athlete has to return to his or her sport. The result of operative decompression for high-level athletes has not been adequate to present this as a reliable option.

If conservative measures are inadequate, the athlete faces a difficult choice. He or she must be counseled that more aggressive treatment has proved effective for decreasing pain, but return to preinjury level of competition is not as predictable. The goal of further treatment is, of course, to remove the impingement. Unfortunately, this requires resection of the anterior acromion and coracoacromial ligament.[8] The anatomic sites of impingement have been well identified over the last 2 decades and the importance of the anterior acromion and coracoacromial ligament have been emphasized.

Since the work of Neer in the early 1970s[7], the anterior acromioplasty has taken the forefront in the treatment of advanced subacromial impingement. Attempts to treat early stages of the condition with coracracromial ligament division alone have not withstood the test of time. Certainly, in this younger population it would be attractive to accomplish adequate results using a soft tissue procedure that would necessarily have a shorter period of rehabilitation. Arthroscopy has been shown to be able to remove adequate amounts of the anterior acromion and, although early reports are encouraging, the long term results are unknown. The open procedure described by Neer[7] results in a significant surface of exposed bone, which necessitates a vigorous and prolonged period of rehabilitation. This, along with the unpredictability of the functional outcome, means this procedure should be approached as a final option in the high-level athlete. Obviously this is not as serious a concern to the recreational athlete.

The presence of a full-thickness tear of the rotator cuff as diagnosed by arthrography or arthroscopy dictates decompression and repair or discontinuance. The pathophysiology of the condition precludes healing, and continued participation in the sport would exacerbate the situation. In this situation the athlete is usually caught between the proverbial rock and a hard place.

DISCUSSION

The majority of the work regarding subacromial impingement has been developed working with the older patient (over 40 years of age) in whom this entity is much more likely to occur. Extrapolation of the theories and treatment options into the younger population may not be valid. Certainly, younger individuals do develop rotator cuff tears, and excessive demands placed on an athlete's shoulder may accelerate the pathologic process so that these advanced changes are seen at a younger age. However, a complicated spectrum of shoulder pathology has been implicated in the development of rotator cuff lesions in some young high-level athletes (18 to 35 years of age).[5] This concept identifies a select group of very high-performance throwing athletes who are at risk for developing anterior instability secondary to repetitive microtrauma. The inefficiency of the rotator cuff allowed excessive migration of the humeral head, producing subacromial impingement and (secondarily) damage to the rotator cuff, which from all outward appearances seems to be typical of impingement. The problem, however, is not adequately addressed by treatment for impingement (either conservative or surgical). Treatment of these unique individuals must be directed toward improving the stability of the shoulder and efficiency of the rotator cuff. If conservative measures are inadequate, then it is recommended that stabilization be carried out surgically, but not decompression (see Chapters 7 and 33.) It must be pointed out, though, that this is a special subset of athletes involved at a very high intensity and most athletes with signs and symptoms of impingement will have the classic form.

SUMMARY

The athlete's shoulder is a challenging problem for the sports medicine physician. Many of these patients will manifest problems of attrition and degeneration not expected or anticipated at their age. Because they must often function at the limits of their capabilities, the chance of a "successful" result is markedly diminished. The range of shoulder problems attributable to subacromial impingement (bursitis, tendonitis, rotator cuff tears, frozen shoulder, bicipital tendonitis) makes the shoulder a likely candidate for many athlete's difficulties.

By far, the majority of impingement problems, if identified and treated early, can be resolved with conservative measures. The key is awareness. There is a recognized difference in the impact of the impingement syndrome on the high-level athlete as opposed to the recreational athlete. There is necessarily a greater flexibility in the treatment of the recreational athlete with regard to time and expectations. Unfortunately, the high-level athlete who has the greatest need for a gradual and prolonged recovery period is not in a position to accept this approach.

The emphasis must be on rehabilitation and conservative treatment for the high-level athlete. Operative decompression should be considered when there is a full-thickness defect of unsuccessful conservative treatment for 9 to 12 months. The athlete must understand that operative decompression is effective in the reduction of pain, but not predictable in regard to return of function.

REFERENCES

1. Bigliani LU et al: Morphology of the acromion and its relationship to rotator cuff tears. Orthop Trans 10:228, 1986.
2. Hawkins RJ and Kennedy JC: Impingement syndrome in athletes, Am J Sports Med 8:151, 1980.

3. Jackson PW: Chronic rotator cuff impingement in the throwing athlete, Am J Sports Med 4:231, 1976.
4. Jobe FW and Jobe CM: Painful athletic injuries of the shoulder, Clin Orthop 173:117, 1983.
5. Jobe FW: Impingement problems in the athlete, AAOS Instructional Course Lectures, vol 35, St Louis, 1989, The CV Mosby Co.
6. Neer CS II and Poppen NK: The supraspinatus outlet, Orthop Trans 11:234, 1982.
7. Neer CS II: Impingement lesions, Clin Orthop 173:70, 1983.
8. Penny JW and Welsh RP: Sholder impingement syndrome in athletes and their surgical management, Am J Sports Med 9:11, 1981.
9. Post M and Cohen J: Impingement syndrome: a review of late stage II and early stage III lesions, Clin Orthop 207:126, 1986.
10. Tibone JE et al: Surgical treatment of tears of the rotator cuff in athletes J Bone Joint Surg 68A:887, 1986.

CHAPTER 9 Overview of Soft Tissue Injuries of the Shoulder

Allen B. Richardson

Except for the rare bony fracture of the upper extremity, almost all injuries of the upper extremity in athletes involve the soft tissues, including muscles, tendons, ligaments, bursae, and fibrous (capsular) structures. The diagnosis and treatment of injuries to athletes deal primarily with soft tissue problems, and the shoulder is no exception. This chapter discusses problems in treating the athlete with a soft tissue injury to the shoulder and gives the basic differential diagnosis for dealing with an athlete with shoulder pain.

IMPINGEMENT SYNDROME

Commonly known as "bursitis," "cuffitis," or "supraspinatus syndrome,"[16,17] impingement syndrome is by far the most common soft tissue injury of the shoulder for which an athlete seeks treatment. The work of Neer in 1972[41] has provided great enlightenment to all surgeons in this area.

Anatomy

Anatomically, the rotator cuff (made up of the subscapularis, the supraspinatus, the infraspinatus, and the teres minor muscles) inserts like a cowl onto the humeral head. The overlying acromion serves as the bony attachment for the deltoid muscle; it also acts to protect the rotator cuff from direct blows. The coracoacromial ligament is simply an extension of the acromion anteriorly. As a vestigial connection of the acromion to the coracoid, it really has no currently known function in humans.

The origins of all these muscles on the scapula are slightly caudad to their insertions on the humerus, and all tend to depress (as well as rotate) the humeral head in relation to the glenoid (Fig. 9-1). This is important, since *this depressive function normally helps to prevent the humeral head from migrating upward and impinging the overlying acromion.* Indeed, in older patients one of the roentgenographic signs of a torn rotator cuff is elevation of the humeral head[64] (Fig. 9-2). Rathbun and MacNab[49] have demonstrated a tenuous vascular supply to the anterior rotator cuff, specifically the area of insertion of the supraspinatus and the long biceps tendon.

Biomechanics

In nearly all sports involving the shoulder (all throwing and racquet sports, as well as competitive swimming) emphasis is placed on the power (pull-through) phase, or that phase requiring forced rapid internal rotation and adduction of the shoulder.[50] Most weight-

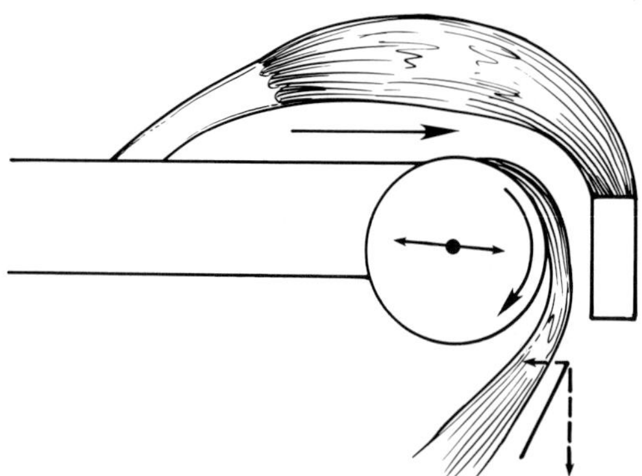

FIG. 9-1 Mechanics of humeral head motion. With the arm fully abducted, contraction of the deltoid muscle leads to superior migration of the humeral head.

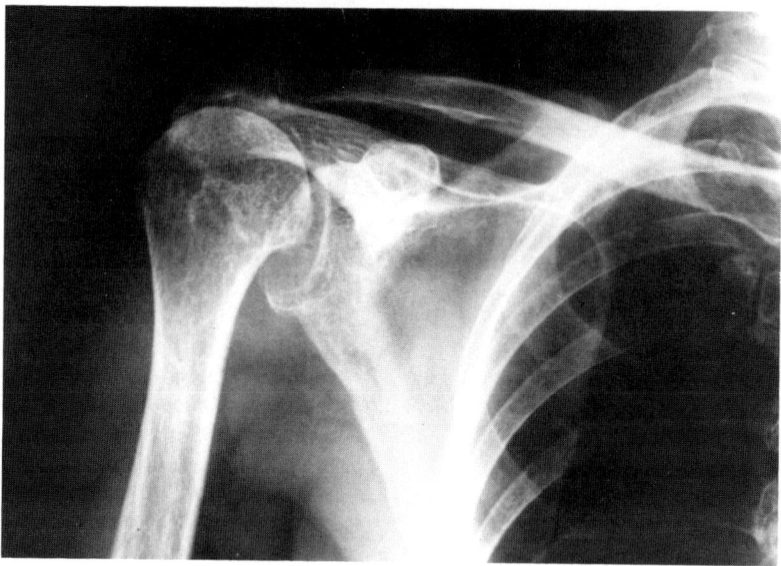

FIG. 9-2 Elevation of the humeral head occurs with large tears of the rotator cuff.

training programs and apparati designed for athletic muscle-strengthening programs concentrate on strengthening the internal rotators of the shoulder. Emphasis is commonly placed on development of the pectoralis major and latissimus dorsi muscles. Relatively few programs emphasize the external rotator muscle groups, which are the muscles of cocking and recovery. External rotation is a function of the posterior cuff musculature—infraspinatus and teres minor.

Because of this relative imbalance between the internal and external rotator muscles of the shoulder, the rotator cuff (the primary external rotator of the shoulder) is unable to prevent the humeral head, and the attachments of the rotator cuff muscles, from migrating proximally and impinging the undersurface of the acromion. Full abduction of the humeral head places the area of attachment of the rotator cuff muscles well under the acromion (Fig. 9-3). With repeated abrasion of this area, the subacromial bursa becomes inflamed, swollen, and scarified, resulting in less effective space between the acromion and the rotator cuff and therefore more impingement.

Most athletes start participating in sports when they are relatively young. By adolescence, many have already experienced symptoms.[60] The average competitive swimmer puts each arm through some 1.5 million strokes per year over a career that may last 8 to 15 years; baseball pitchers might throw as many as 15,000 pitches per year, most of those at very high speeds. It is little wonder that these shoulders eventually wear out and become painful!

Diagnosis

The diagnosis of impingement syndrome is not usually difficult. The patient complains of pain about the acromion, often described as "deep" within the shoulder under the acro-

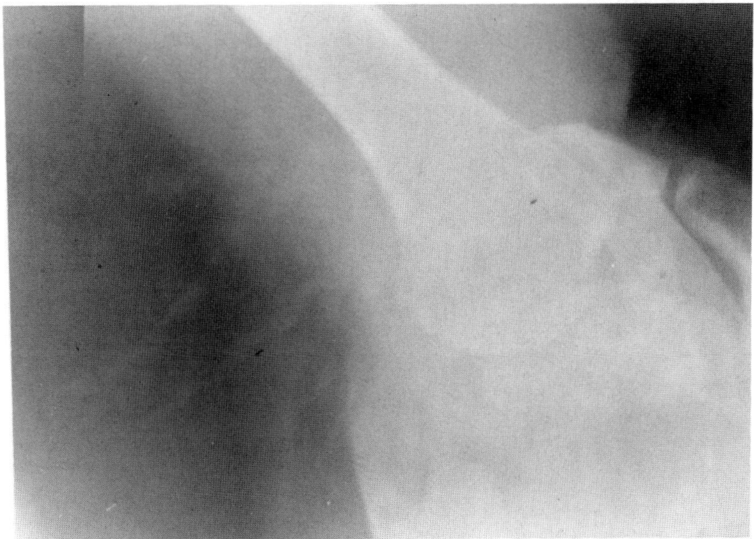

FIG. 9-3 Abduction of the humeral head places the greater tuberosity well under the acromion.

mion. The pain is always diffuse in nature and, depending on which part of the cuff is inflamed, can occur anteriorly about the coracoacromial ligaments, laterally at the insertion of the infraspinatus, or posteriorly at the insertion of the teres minor muscle.

The pain may be aggravated by direct palpation of the insertion of the rotator cuff under the acromion. Hawkins and Kennedy[25] described three stages of clinical symptoms: (1) minimal pain with activity, no weakness, and no restriction of motion; (2) marked reactive tendinitis with significant pain and a diminished range of motion; and (3) pain with significant weakness (rotator cuff tear). The so-called **impingement sign,** which attempts to reproduce the compression of the rotator cuff between the acromion and humeral head, is performed by forcibly forward-flexing the humerus against a fixed acromion.

Neer[41] has also described the "painful arc" of active elevation from 70 to 120 degrees of forward flexion. This is the range of motion during which the area of insertion of the supraspinatus into the greater tuberosity is passing under the anterior acromion and coracoacromial ligament.

Differential Diagnosis

The long biceps tendon is intimately involved with the rotator cuff, interposed between the subscapularis and supraspinatus muscles and attaching to the superior glenoid labrum. As expected, tears of the long biceps tendon can occur in conjunction with subacromial impingement syndrome.[42] Intraarticular ruptures of the biceps tendon may cause pain about the shoulder indistinguishable from impingement syndrome. An arthrogram may yield negative results and, if the tendon does not slide in the bicipital groove, may not produce the familiar deformity of contracture of the biceps muscle of the arm. The only means of diagnosis in this case might be arthroscopic examination (Fig. 9-4).

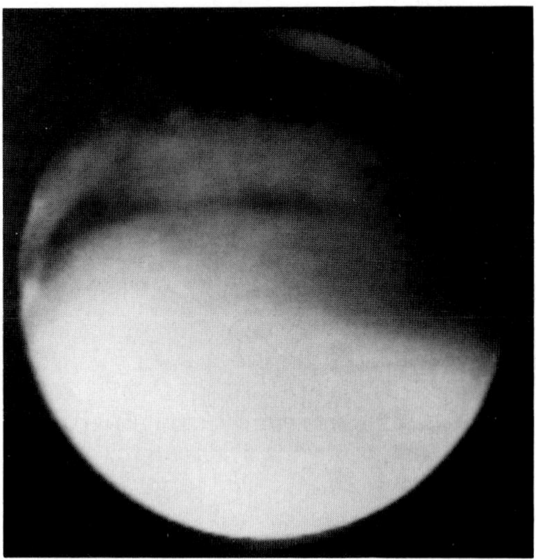

FIG. 9-4 Intraarticular rupture of the biceps tendon. This patient did not demonstrate contracture of the biceps muscle belly.

Extraarticular tears of the long biceps tendon almost always occur in or near the bicipital groove between the tuberosities of the humeral head. The etiology of this rupture is,

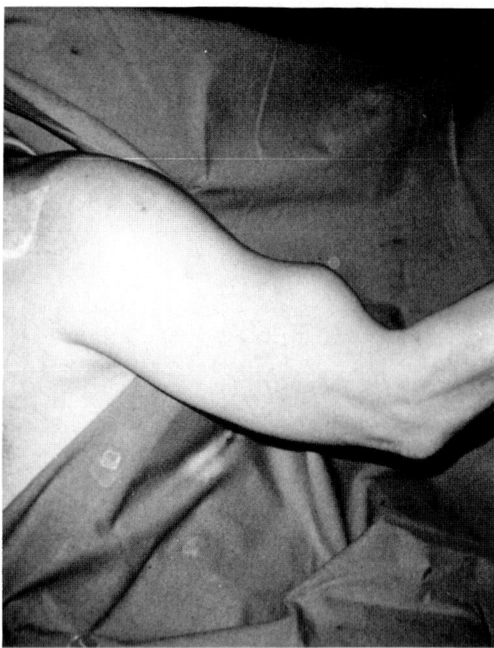

FIG. 9-5 Prominence of the biceps muscle belly following rupture of the long biceps tendon.

once again, impingement of the tendon on the undersurface of the anterior acromion. Contracture of the biceps leads to a very characteristic prominence of the muscle belly (Fig. 9-5). In the great majority of older patients, little disability results from this injury. However, there is some measureable loss of flexion and supination power. In the young active athlete, persistent weakness and pain can result. Treatment in this specific group of patients (young athletes with pain and weakness) is exploration and tenodesis of the ruptured long biceps tendon.* Simultaneous arthroscopic examination of the shoulder will eliminate the missed intraarticular fragment of the tendon and perhaps a tear of the superior glenoid labrum.

McMaster[37] has recently described tears and abrasion of the glenoid labra as a cause of shoulder pain in competitive swimmers. Although the usual pain of "swimmer's shoulder" represents a variation of the impingement syndrome, the physician should always keep in mind that overuse can lead to several distinct but related injuries.

Roentgenographic Findings

Plain roentgenograms are usually unremarkable and show no damage to the bony structures. Particular attention should be directed to inspection of the acromioclavicular joint, since pain resulting from degeneration of this joint can produce symptoms quite similar to subacromial impingement syndrome.

Actual tears of the rotator cuff, except in professional throwers, are rare in athletes under 40 years old unless there is a distinct history of trauma to the shoulder. Suspicion of a rotator cuff tear is certainly increased if the strength of the external rotator muscles of the shoulder is decreased. An anteroposterior roentgenogram of the shoulder does not usually reveal the upward migration of the humeral head seen in larger, global tears.[64] In these cases, a single-contrast arthrogram of the shoulder is helpful in ruling out a tear of the rotator cuff structures. Although the incidence of false-negative results is relatively low, it should be remembered that the area of actual abnormality (abrasion of the upper surface of the rotator cuff against the undersurface of the acromion) is not the undersurface of the rotator cuff; therefore partial tears of the upper surface of the cuff might go unseen on the arthrogram.

Calcific tendonitis, or calcification of the insertion of the rotator cuff, is occasionally seen on plain roentgenograms (Fig. 9-6). Microscopic tears of fibers of the rotator cuff result in inflammation, scarification, and calcification. Although it is conceivable that these calcific crystals are a physical cause of pain, the problem is still one of constant abrasion of the rotator cuff against the acromion, and the calcifications visible on roentgenograms are the result, rather than the cause, of injury.

Treatment

Nonoperative Treatment

The problem of impingement syndrome is clearly one of inflammation of the subacromial bursa and the surrounding structures (the rotator cuff) as a result of a relative lack of sufficient space for movement of the humeral head under the acromion and coracoacromial ligament. The goals of treatment, then, are to

*Editors' note: James Andrew, M.D., has described a relatively simple means of tenodesing the long head of the biceps when replaced extraarticularly. A small incision is made over the medial aspect of the deltoid tuberosity. The tendon is located and looped around the deltoid, finally suturing the tendon to itself. This provides a fixed origin to the biceps, improves the cosmetic appearance, and may help with power return. Intraarticular shoulder symptoms caused by the proximal intraarticular portion of the tendon can be handled arthroscopically.

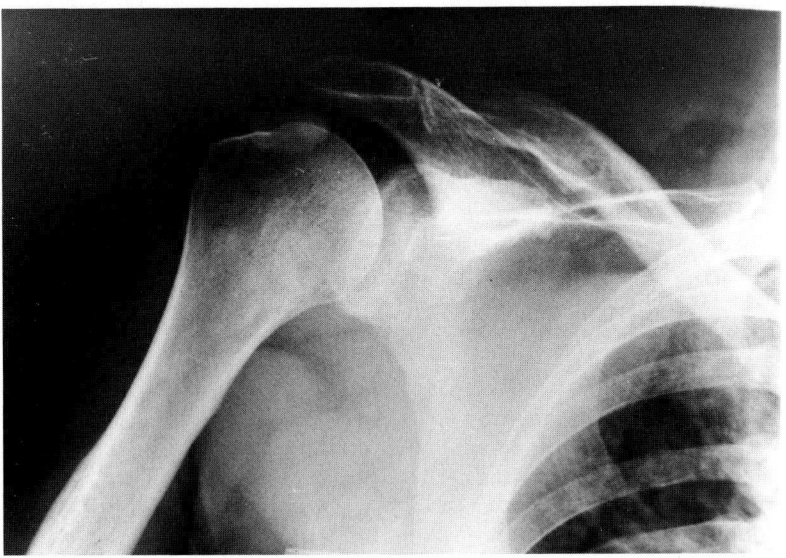

FIG. 9-6 Calcification of the insertion of the rotator cuff.

initially decrease the inflammatory response. This in itself will increase the subacromial space and ultimately increase the space between the acromion and the rotator cuff.

The physician, coach, and athlete should study the athlete's biomechanics and workout schedule. Certain simple changes in the athlete's movements might lead to less pain and better efficiency for the particular sport. For example, the competitive swimmer might increase body roll while swimming freestyle or backstroke, decreasing "swimmer's shoulder" pain and increasing stroke efficiency.[50] Likewise, if a baseball pitcher is "opening up" too soon (turning the body toward home plate well ahead of the throwing shoulder), correction should lead to less shoulder pain and better accuracy and power during the pitching motion.

Certain exercise techniques should be eliminated. For the competitive swimmer, there is little question that the use of hand paddles (which act to increase resistance for the swimmer underwater) produce, increase, and aggravate shoulder pain. There is also some evidence to indicate that excessive overhead weight training, (e.g., bench pressing and military presses) can result in shoulder pain. These should be modified so that stress on the subacromial bursa area is decreased.

Exercises that may increase impingement in swimmers

- Use of hand paddles
- Overhead weight training

Selective rest should be instituted for athletes with shoulder pain. This need not be complete and total rest from their sport. There is usually some type of activity in which the athlete can still participate that can be used to strengthen parts of the athlete's performance. For example, the baseball pitcher who is recovering might work hard on forearm and grip strength, which will certainly help the pitcher's return to throwing.

Ice therapy remains the most practical treatment for impingement syndrome of the shoulder. McMaster et al[38] have demonstrated, in the laboratory, that ice can be effective in decreasing inflammation, producing analgesia, and decreasing muscle spasm. The ice-cup massage is perhaps the easiest and most effective means of applying cold to the inflamed rotator cuff. Commonly available ice-cube packs, ice gels, and packs of frozen vegetables are reasonable alternatives.

If available, physical therapy modalities, such as electrogalvanic stimulation (EGS) and ultrasound, can be helpful. Ultrasound should be used with some caution since it is actually a form of deep heat and can sometimes aggravate the pain of impingement syndrome.

Once the acute pain has resolved, a regular exercise program should be instituted to prevent recurrence of impingement syndrome.

Very simply, all such programs are directed at strengthening the rotator cuff muscles (or the muscles of deceleration, recovery, and cocking). Aronen[7] has described exercises done in the standing position with the arm abducted at 90 degrees to the side; "fly-away" exercises are then done with the thumb upward, neutral, and downward, so that all parts of the rotator cuff are strengthened. The deltoid muscle is also strengthened with this program. Unfortunately, the upward pull of the deltoid may contribute to impingement of the humeral head and the acromion.

A variation of these exercises can be done with the body forward-flexed 90 degrees and supported with the noninvolved arm on a table. The involved arm is then taken through a series of fly-away exercises at three different degrees of abduction (45, 90, 135 degrees), again to strengthen all the muscles of the rotator cuff. In this case, most deltoid function is eliminated. It should be emphasized that these exercises are really more prophylactic than therapeutic.

Injections of corticosteroids remain controversial. Although there is little question that these agents effectively decrease inflammation, there is also ample evidence to indicate that by inhibiting this inflammatory process tissue will not heal as well following injury. At times, however, there is little choice when dealing with chronic and persistent impingement syndrome: the physician either tries a course of no more than four dilute corticosteroid injections or proceeds to a surgical approach to the problem.

Operative Treatment

The goal of any surgical approach to impingement syndrome of the shoulder is direct: to increase the subacromial space. Neer[41] has provided the clearest direction in the approach to subacromial decompression. The undersurface of the acromion is excised along with the coracoacromial ligament, and the subdeltoid bursa is removed. Classically, this was done through a small anterior shoulder incision and, as described, involved detachment of a small part of the deltoid muscle.

The advent of arthroscopy has added an entirely new dimension to decompression of the subacromial space. Visualization with the arthroscope and excision of the undersurface of the acromion and coracoacromial ligament are now the standard of care for decompression and acromioplasty of the subacromial space (see Chapter 5). Not only has this become an outpatient procedure, but also the insult to the overlying deltoid muscle is considerably lower, allowing much faster rehabilitation to overhead (throwing and swimming) activities.

Recuperation following surgical decompression of the subacromial space depends, again, on whether an open or arthroscopic approach was employed. If the approach is arthroscopic, the patient can begin passive range of motion exercises on the day following surgery and continue this through the first 10 days (see Chapter 11). Active range of motion may then start and continue through the next 2 weeks. If progress is good, one may begin easy throwing maneuvers at about 3 weeks after surgery and slowly increase these activities until a full return has been achieved.

Bateman[11] and Jobe[27] have described operative treatment of tears of the rotator cuff in athletes (see Chapter 33). These injuries, as previously mentioned, are unusual in the average recreational athlete. Rehabilitation after surgical repair is prolonged, averaging 13 to 18 months. If a tear of the rotator cuff is confirmed with arthrography or arthroscopy, the athlete must understand that return to full throwing activities might prove extremely difficult.

OVERUSE SYNDROMES

Although the impingement syndrome is fundamentally a problem of friction and abrasion of bony parts (with the rotator cuff being caught between), overuse syndromes imply an overload of activity on a muscle, tendon, ligament, or joint capsule, resulting in inability of that structure to perform its normal duties. The syndrome usually develops in the absence of a specific injury and is an injury of attrition.

Most of these injuries can be categorized depending on whether they occur in the cocking (recovery) phase, the acceleration phase, or the follow-through (deceleration) phase of the throwing motion.

Cocking Phase

The cocking (recovery) phase is that part of the throwing motion in which the arm is brought into a position of preparation for the power (acceleration) phase. The most common problems develop from eccentric muscle loading as a musculotendinous unit is undergoing elongation during contraction. An excellent example[3] occurs when a thrower begins forward shoulder motion too early, resulting in tendinitis of the anterior shoulder muscle tendons. In this case the tendon of the pectoralis major, latissimus dorsi, or anterior shoulder capsule is affected. Barnes and Tullos[10] described anterior shoulder pain in 29 of 56 baseball players, in which five had tendinitis of either the insertion of the pectoralis major or the latissimus dorsi.

Hyperflexibility, which so often leads to improved ability to perform in many sports, may be a liability in some cases, since the joint, tendons, and ligaments will pass well beyond the optimal length of the musculotendinous unit that must control that joint. Repeated stretching of the surrounding capsule can lead to a persistent inflammation of the anterior capsular structures.

Acceleration Phase

The acceleration (power) phase leads most commonly to fatigue injuries about the shoulder. Muscles, bones, ligaments, and tendons will hypertrophy when subjected to a gradually increasing load. If, however, the resistive load is more than the surrounding structures can withstand, a fatigue injury will occur.

A classic example of this has been cited by Fulton et al[21] who interviewed and examined 16 male gymnasts. Eight of these athletes demonstrated a hypertrophic cortical lesion of the upper humerus, at the site of insertion of the pectoralis major and the latissimus dorsi. These muscles, in particular, are important to, and repeatedly stressed by, the male gymnast who must often develop power to hold positions (such as in the ring event) as well as extreme flexibility.

Tullos and King[61] and Tullos et al[62] have described the "spontaneous ball-throwing fracture of the humerus," which has all the characteristics of a stress fracture. After a study of throwing mechanics, Gainor et al[22] noted that the torque developed during the power phase is "considerably larger than the fracture torques of the humerus. . . ." Finally, Adams[1] described osteochondrosis of the proximal humeral epiphysis, in which the force of throwing results in widening, demineralization, and fragmentation of the proximal humeral epiphysis.

Follow-Through Phase

Posterior shoulder pain is characteristic of injuries resulting from the follow-through phase of throwing sports. Most of these injuries are seen in sports requiring a hard forward motion of the upper extremity, such as tennis, baseball pitching, volleyball spiking, and javelin throwing. Jobe et al.,[28,29] in two reports of EMG analysis of the throwing motion, conclude that, immediately after the ball (or javelin) is released, the posterior muscles of the shoulder, and the posterior capsule, must decelerate the arm. As might be expected, most strengthening and exercise programs are directed toward the anterior (power) muscles and little emphasis is given to the muscles that must decelerate the upper extremity following the acceleration phase.

This follow-through phase is characterized by large eccentric loads placed on the posterior structures of the shoulder. Barnes and Tullos[10] described this as "posterior capsule syndrome." Lombardo et al.[32] found posterior shoulder pain in four athletes and related the pain to the cocking and follow-through phases of the throwing arm. Bennett[12-14] describes an exostosis of the posteroinferior glenoid that results from repeated traction of the inferior capsular structures.

The end stage of this repeated stress on the posterior capsular structures is posterior subluxation of the shoulder. Many athletes, in a variety of sports, may develop posterior subluxation of the shoulder. It is not nearly as rare a lesion as reflected in the literature. For most athletes the condition remains asymptomatic; however, if the athlete is very vigorous with overhead, throwing-motion activities, treatment is extremely difficult. Symptoms of posterior shoulder pain and a feeling of instability with throwing are characteristic of the condition (see Chapter 7).

Another injury that usually develops in the follow-through phase is the painful, or **snapping scapula.** Normally there is a small bursa located beneath the medial border of the scapula. It serves to lubricate the motion of the scapula against the thoracic wall. Unfortunately, because of the large amount of motion between the scapula and the chest wall, bursitis can develop, resulting in pain and occasionally a "snapping" sensation as the swollen tissues impinge the underlying rib cage. Diagnosis is straightforward; however, treatment is often difficult and consists of antiinflammatory measures. There is no widely accepted surgical treatment of this condition, although Sisto and Jobe[57] have described excision of the inflamed bursa in professional pitchers.

The diagnosis of injuries of the follow-through phase is almost entirely clinical. Palpation of the tender structures posteriorly will usually allow the physician to identify the pain as emanating from the posterior glenoid and the capsule, or from the teres minor or major

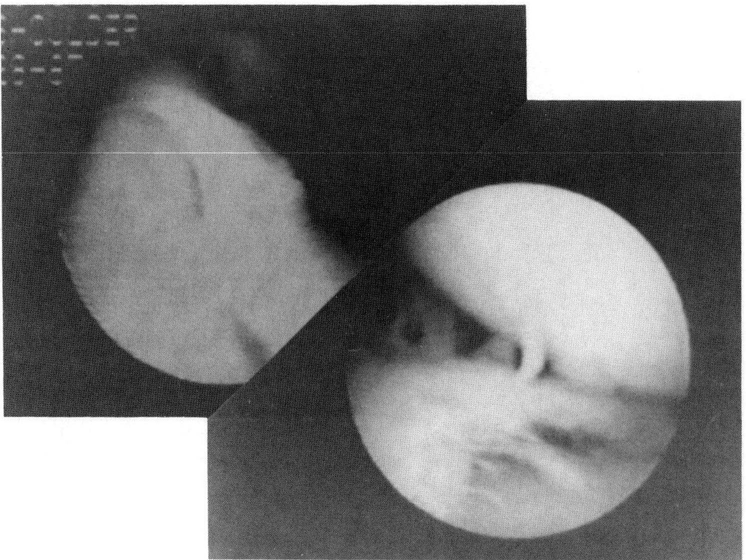

FIG. 9-7 An avulsion of the superior glenoid labrum. Upper left illustration shows the tear extending into the proximal biceps tendon.

muscles. Manual manipulation of the shoulder will usually demonstrate posterior subluxation of the shoulder if it is present. One should be particularly careful to examine the shoulder for all types of instability, since multidirectional instability is always a potential problem and changes the treatment plan drastically. The double-contrast arthrogram[39] is useful in outlining the glenoid labrum, both anteriorly and posteriorly.

The arthroscope is, of course, most accurate in identifying intraarticular pathologic conditions.[18,35] Andrews and Carson[4] and Andrews et al,[6] in describing arthroscopic techniques for the shoulder, advocated simple excision of tears of the glenoid labrum. Although this may eliminate some of the immediate symptoms of shoulder "catching" and "locking," all tears of the labrum indicate some instability of the shoulder and this instability will often become symptomatic at a later date. Therefore, if a labral tear is excised, the surgeon should be aware that this "cure" may only be temporary.

Finally, Andrews et al[5] have described **avulsion of the superior glenoid labrum** by the long biceps tendon (Fig. 9-7). They feel that this develops because of marked contraction of the biceps muscle, which is decelerating the elbow joint, during the follow-through phase. Snyder[58] has termed this the "SLAP (superior labrum anterior-posterior) tear." Surgical treatment presently consists of excision of the torn superior labrum and reattachment of the long biceps tendon as necessary.

TRACTION INJURIES

Avulsion of the Pectoralis Major

Avulsion of the pectoralis major was first described by Patissier[47] in 1822; by 1972, only 44 additional cases had been reported.* The most common site of rupture is at or near the bone-tendon junction. Ruptures occur when the muscle is at full tension and an additional force is added. The most common sources of this additional force are the bench press and breaking a fall by catching one's weight with one arm.

Diagnosis is, again, relatively straightforward. Most patients experience pain and swelling over the anterior aspect of the shoulder joint and relate that "something ripped." Mild to moderate ecchymosis will indicate that bleeding has taken place deep within the shoulder joint. Physical examination may well not demonstrate a defect in the muscle tendon; however, if the patient forcefully claps the hands together, the defect is usually obvious. Although Gudmundsson[23] advocated nonoperative treatment, several authors noted that muscle power is markedly decreased in flexion and internal rotation. Therefore it is

*References 8, 15, 23, 30, 34, 36, 46, 48, 65.

my opinion that operative repair of the ruptured tendon offers the patient the best possible result. This advice applies even to chronic tears of the pectoralis major.

Lateral Acromion Apophysitis

In the adolescent athlete, repeated traction on the lateral acromion by the deltoid muscle can lead to a painful apophysitis of this area. This apophysis usually closes at approximately 16 to 19 years of age, which coincides with the usual age when the athlete is achieving his greatest growth and maturity. Time will usually allow resolution of this problem, and at present I am not aware of an instance in which the lateral acromion required excision with reattachment of the deltoid to the remaining acromion.

PROBLEMS OF INSTABILITY

Anterior Instability

Anterior instability of the glenohumeral joint is perhaps the most common traumatic soft tissue injury about the shoulder in athletes. Its diagnosis and treatment have been described at length in the literature. The "essential" lesion is felt to be the torn anterior glenoid labrum (Fig. 9-8).[9] This labrum is a thick, fibrous expansion of the anterior shoulder capsule.[40] Attached to the labrum are thickened bands of capsule known as the superior, middle, and inferior glenohumeral ligaments, which provide support to the anterior joint during abduction and external rotation (Fig. 9-9). If the humeral head repeatedly subluxes or dislocates from the glenoid, a compression fracture of the posterior humeral head, commonly known as a Hill-Sachs lesion, can develop.

Diagnosis is, again, primarily clinical. The history of the shoulder "coming out" when the arm is in an overhead, externally rotated position is common and classic. Patients will often describe waking with the shoulder either completely or partially dislocated. The "dead arm" syndrome can result from transient anterior subluxations of the shoulder joint.[54] This usually occurs with abduction and extreme external rotation; however, the athlete may not give a clear history of this maneuver. The examiner can usually demonstrate laxity of the shoulder capsule by grasping the scapula in one hand and the humeral head in the other and moving them apart (see Chapter 3).

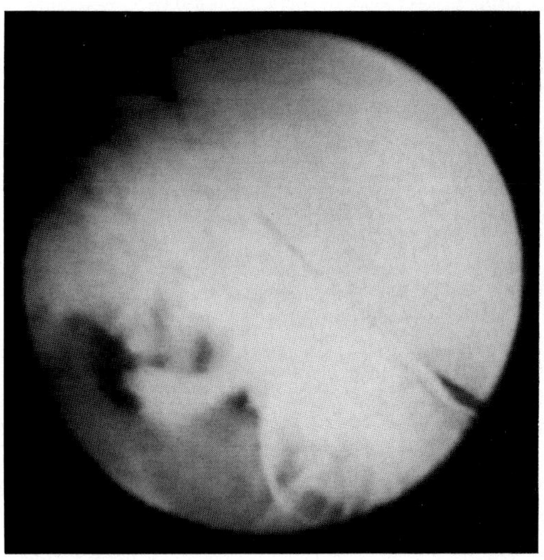

FIG. 9-8 Bankart lesion seen at arthroscopy.

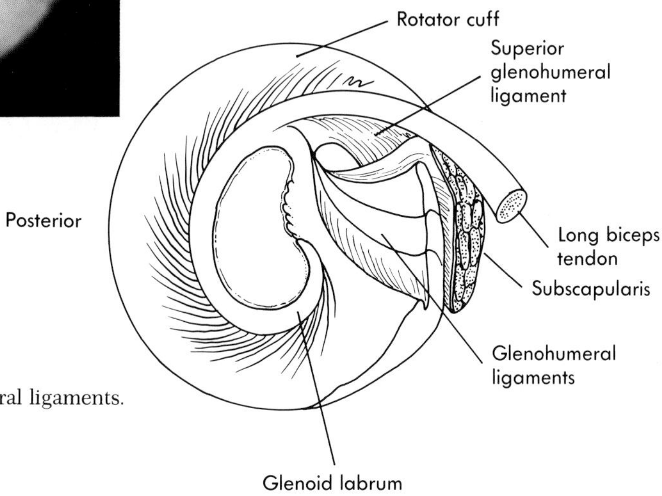

Rotator cuff
Superior glenohumeral ligament
Posterior
Long biceps tendon
Subscapularis
Glenohumeral ligaments
Glenoid labrum

FIG. 9-9 The anterior glenohumeral ligaments.

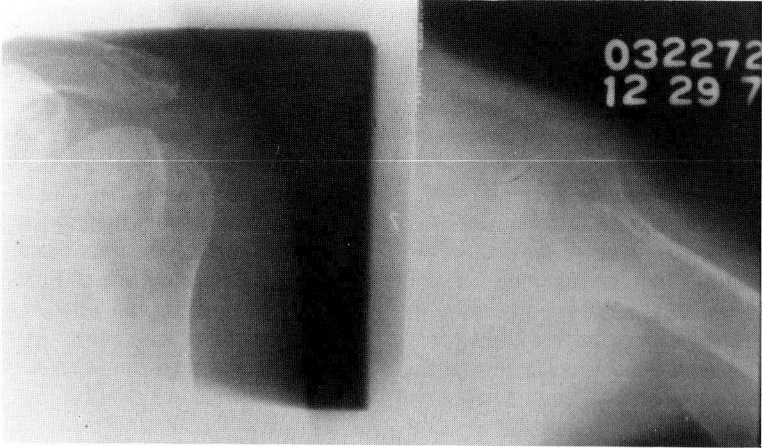

FIG. 9-10 Hill-Sachs lesion.

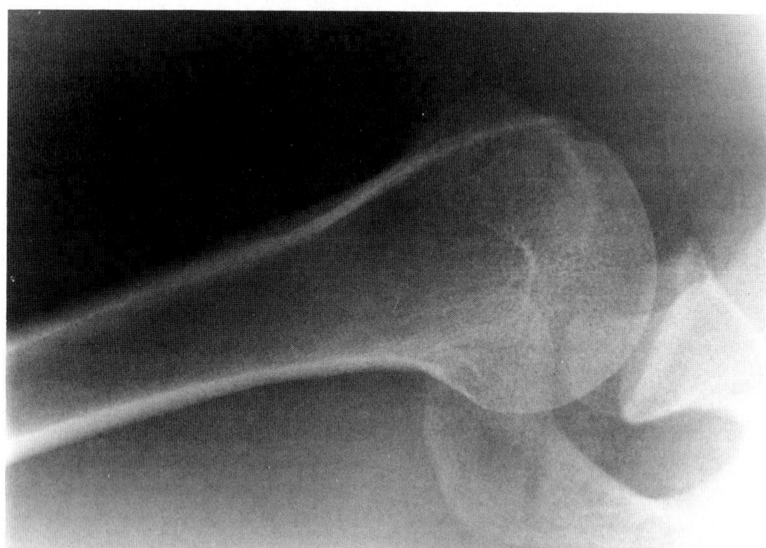

FIG. 9-11 Osteophyte formation of the anterior glenoid neck resulting from recurrent dislocations of the shoulder in a basketball and volleyball athlete.

Roentgenograms, although usually unremarkable, will occasionally reveal two findings:

1. A Hill-Sachs lesion: this is a compression fracture of the posterior humeral head that can often be seen on the anteroposterior roentgenogram with the arm internally rotated (Fig. 9-10).
2. An osteophyte of the anterior glenoid: this represents calcification of the defect in the anterior glenoid labrum (Fig. 9-11). A modified axillary roentgenogram, as described by Rokous et al.,[52] can be helpful in delineating this small osteophyte.

Double-contrast arthrography, as described by Mink et al[39] may also shed light on the diagnosis by showing the torn labrum. Most accurate of all is arthroscopy of the shoulder. Not only can the internal structures of the shoulder be directly visualized, but also the shoulder can be examined with the patient under anesthesia.

Almost all of the recorded procedures to prevent anterior instability of the shoulder are designed to eliminate the laxity of the anterior soft tissue structures that stabilize the shoulder.[63] Therefore a part of their purpose must be to limit abducted external rotation. Early range of motion exercises may allow return to most activities[53]; however, Lombardo and Kerlan[31] have noted that the Bristow procedure does not readily allow the active baseball

TABLE 9-1 Average recurrence rate following surgical repair of the shoulder for anterior dislocation

Procedure	Recurrence
Putti-Platt	3.0%
Magnuson-Stack	4.1%
Bankart	3.3%
Bristow	1.7%

From Rockwood CA and Green DP: Fractures, Philadelphia, 1984, JB Lippincott Co, p. 778.

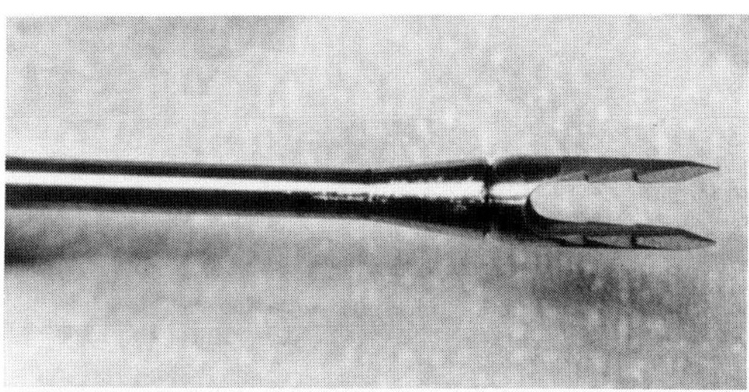

FIG. 9-12 Arthroscopic staple for stabilization of the shoulder. (Made by Instrumaker, Inc.)

pitcher to return to his or her sport. Because flexibility, especially to abducted external rotation, is necessary for very hard throwers, such as pitchers and javelin throwers, the mere presence of anterior instability of the shoulder in these types of athletes may signal the end of their career as a high-speed and power-thrower, regardless of the type of surgery performed.

Of the more common repairs done in the United States, the Bankart repair must remain as that procedure that most tries to recreate the normal anatomy by reattaching a shortened anterior glenoid labrum to the anterior glenoid rim.[9] The Putti-Platt repair[44] attempts to shorten the various anterior structures by sewing the capsule and subscapularis tendon in overlapping fashion in separate layers. The Bristow repair[26] not only places a bone block anteriorly, but also "slings" the conjoined tendon of the short biceps tendon and the coracobrachialis across the humeral head to prevent anterior motion of the head. The Magnuson-Stack procedure[33] reattaches the subscapularis farther laterally on the humeral head in the hope that this will result in a dynamic tightening across the humeral head. The efficacy of all these procedures in preventing future anterior instability of the shoulder is excellent (Table 9-1), and most surgeons determine their choice of procedure by their experience both in training and practice. Where there is recurrence of the instability after surgical repair, a repeat procedure will usually lead to encouraging results.[55] Failure of the initial procedure, however, should prompt the clinician to evaluate the athlete for a multidirectional instability pattern.

Arthroscopic repair of the anterior structures is a new procedure that has the advantages of no hospital stay, a shortened rehabilitation period, and much smaller scars. The most common method available utilizes barbed staples (Fig. 9-12), placed under direct vision, to fix the anterior glenoid labrum and capsule to the glenoid labrum. DuToit[19] described a very similar technique done through an arthrotomy. Cannulated screws and intraarticular suturing through bone are two other methods presently under investigation for application through the arthroscopic incision. Long-term follow-up, comparable to open procedures, is not yet available for these types of procedures, and these techniques should be done by surgeons well versed in shoulder arthroscopy.

Posterior Instability

Posterior instability is a distinctly less common entity than is anterior instability; however, it is not so rare among athletes as it is among the general population.[2,20] Athletes require a certain degree of instability of the shoulder to perform their activities to maximal advantage. I have observed posterior instability (subluxation) in competitive swimmers, volleyball players, throwers, and weight lifters. Voluntary posterior subluxation is probably not treatable; all surgical attempts at repair are probably doomed to failure.

In most cases this condition will remain asymptomatic; unfortunately, in the patient who complains of posterior instability of the shoulder following a documented traumatic episode, surgical stabilization is very difficult. Samilson and Prieto[56] reported good results with tenodesis of the long head of the biceps to the posterior scapular neck. Most authors have realized very equivocal results with stabilization procedures.[24,59]

Multidirectional Instability

In 1980 Neer and Foster[43] reported on the inferior capsular shift procedure as treatment for multidirectional instability of the shoulder. Until that time, the concept of instability of the shoulder occurring simultaneously in several directions was not clearly defined. Since that time, this very difficult entity has been increasingly recognized.

Unfortunately, muscular rehabilitation and exercises are not routinely helpful in preventing instability in the active athlete, and surgical intervention is often necessary. Procedures aimed at stabilization of either the anterior or posterior structures alone are likely to fail. The essential lesion appears to be laxity of the inferior capsule, in particular, the inferior glenohumeral ligament. The inferior capsular shift procedure, described by Neer and Foster, quite simply detaches the lax portion of the inferior capsule from the anterior, inferior, and posterior humeral head and advances it anteriorly and superiorly, thereby eliminating the redundancy of the capsule. The approach is anterior in most cases; however, if the greatest direction of instability is felt to be posteriorly, a symmetric procedure can be done through a posterior approach.

SUMMARY

The approach to the athlete with shoulder pain involves a careful clinical assessment and appropriate roentgenographic or imaging studies to arrive at an exact anatomic diagnosis. The differential diagnosis of most shoulder problems includes impingement syndrome, overuse injuries, traction injuries, and instability. Accurate diagnosis is essential to implementation of appropriate therapy. With proper treatment, most athletes can return to competitive or recreational athletics as they desire.

REFERENCES

1. Adams JE: Little Legaue shoulder: osteochondrosis of the proximal humeral epiphysis in boy baseball pitchers, Calif Med 105:22, 1966.
2. Ahlgren S, Hedlung T, and Nistor L: Idiopathic posterior instability of the shoulder joint, Acta Orthop Scand 49:600, 1978.
3. Albright JA, et al: Clinical study of baseball pitchers: correlation of injury to the throwing arm with method of delivery, Am J Sports Med 6:15, 1978.
4. Andrews JR and Carson WG: The arthroscopic treatment of glenoid labrum tears in the throwing athlete, Orthop Trans 8:44, 1984.
5. Andrews JR, Carson WG, and McLeod WD: Glenoid labrum tears related to the long head of the biceps, Am J Sports Med 13:337, 1985.
6. Andrews JR, Carson WG, and Ortega K: Arthroscopy of the shoulder: technique and normal anatomy, Am J Sports Med 12:1, 1984.
7. Aronen J: Personal communication, 1982.
8. Bakalim G: Rupture of the pectoralis major muscle, Acta Orthop Scand 36:274, 1965.
9. Bankart ASB: Recurrent or habitual dislocation of the shoulder-joint, Br Med J 2:1132, 1923.
10. Barnes DA and Tullos HS: An analysis of 100 symptomatic baseball pitchers, Am J Sports Med 6:62, 1978.
11. Bateman JE: Cuff tears in athletes, Orthop Clin North Am 4:721, 1973.
12. Bennett GE: Shoulder and elbow lesions of professional baseball pitcher, JAMA 117:510, 1941.
13. Bennett GE: Shoulder and elbow lesions distinctive of baseball players, Ann Surg 126:107, 1947.
14. Bennett GE: Elbow and shoulder lesions of baseball players, Am J Surg 98:484, 1959.
15. Berson B: Surgical repair of pectoralis major rupture in an athlete, Am J Sports Med 7:348, 1979.
16. Bosworth DM: An analysis of twenty-eight consecutive cases of incapacitating shoulder lesions, radically explored and repaired, J Bone Joint Surg 22:369, 1940.
17. Bosworth DM: Supraspinatus syndrome: symptomatology, pathology, and repair, JAMA 117:422, 1941.
18. Dolk T and Gremark O: Arthroscopy and stability testing of the shoulder joint, Arthroscopy 2:35, 1986.
19. duToit JG: Recurrent dislocation of the shoulder: a 24-year study of the Johannesburg stapling operation, J Bone Joint Surg 38A:1, 1956.
20. English E and MacNab I: Idiopathic posterior instability of the shoulder, Can J Surg 17:147, 1974.
21. Fulton MN, Albright JP, and El-Khoury GY: Cortical desmoid-like lesion of the proximal humerus and its occurrence in gymnasts (Ringman's shoulder lesion), Am J Sports Med 7:57, 1979.
22. Gainor BM et al.: The throw: biomechanics and acute injury, Am J Sports Med 8:114, 1980.
23. Gudmundsson B: A case of agenesis and a case of rupture of the pectoralis major muscle, Acta Orthop Scand 44:213, 1973.
24. Hawkins RJ: Posterior dislocations of the shoulder, Instructional Course, American Academy of Orthopaedic Surgeons Annual Meeting, New Orleans, January 1972.
25. Hawkins RJ and Kennedy JC: Impingement syndrome in athletes, Am J Sports Med 8:57, 1980.
26. Helfet AJ: Coracoid transplantation for recurring dislocation of the shoulder, J Bone Joint Surg 40B:198, 1958.
27. Jobe FW and Jobe CM: Painful athletic injuries of the shoulder, Clin Orthop 173:117, 1983.
28. Jobe FW et al.: An EMG analysis of the shoulder in throwing and pitching: a preliminary report, Am J Sports Med 11:3, 1983.
29. Jobe FW et al.: An EMG analysis of the shoulder in pitching: a second report, Am J Sports Med 12:218, 1984.
30. Lindenbaum BL: Delayed repair of the ruptured pectoralis muscle, Clin Orthop 109:120, 1975.
31. Lombardo SJ and Kerlan RK: The modified Bristow procedure for recurrent dislocation of the shoulder, J Bone Joint Surg 58A:256, 1976.
32. Lombardo SJ et al.: Posterior shoulder lesions in throwing athletes, Am J Sports Med 5:106, 1977.
33. Magnuson PB and Stack JK: Recurrent dislocation of the shoulder, JAMA 123:889, 1943.
34. Marmor L et al.: Pectoralis major muscle: function of sternal position and mechanism of rupture of normal muscle: case reports, J Bone Joint Surg 43A:81, 1961.
35. Matthews LS, Terry G, and Vetter WL: Shoulder anatomy for the arthroscopist, Arthroscopy 1:83, 1985.
36. McEntire JE et al.: Rupture of the pectoralis major muscle, J Bone Joint Surg 54A:1040, 1972.
37. McMaster WC: Anterior glenoid labrum damage: a painful lesion in swimmers, Am J Sports Med 14:383, 1986.
38. McMaster WC, Liddle S, and Waugh TR: Laboratory evaluation of various cold therapy modalities, Am J Sports Med 6:291, 1978.
39. Mink JH, Richardson AB, and Grant TT: Evalu-

ation of glenoid labrum by double-contrast shoulder arthrography, Am J Roentgenol 133:833, 1979.
40. Moseley HF, and Overgaard B: The anterior capsule mechanism in recurrent anterior dislocation of the shoulder: morphological and clinical studies with special reference to the glenoid labrum and the gleno-humeral ligaments, J Bone Joint Surg 44B:913, 1962.
41. Neer CS: Anterior acromioplasty for the chronic impingement syndrome in the shoulder, J Bone Joint Surg 54A:41, 1972.
42. Neer CS, Bigliani LW, and Hawkins RJ: Rupture of the long head of the biceps tendon related to subacromial impingement syndrome, Orthop Trans 1:111, 1977.
43. Neer CS and Foster CR: Inferior capsular shift for voluntary inferior and multidirectional instability of the shoulder: a preliminary report, J Bone Joint Surg 62A:897, 1980.
44. Osmond-Clarke H: Habitual dislocation of the shoulder: the Putti-Platt operation, J Bone Joint Surg 30B:19, 1948.
45. Pappas AM, Goss TP, and Kleinman PK: Symptomatic shoulder instability due to lesions of the glenoid labrum, Am J Sports Med 11:279, 1983.
46. Park JY and Espinella JL: Rupture of pectoralis major muscle, J Bone Joint Surg 52A:577, 1970.
47. Patissier P: Traite des maladies des artisans (chapter on maladies des bouchers), Paris, 1822, p 162.
48. Pulaski EJ and Chandler BH: Ruptures of the pectoralis major muscle, Surgery 10:309, 1941.
49. Rathbun JB and MacNab I: The microvascular pattern of the rotator cuff, J Bone Joint Surg 52B:540, 1970.
50. Richardson AB, Jobe FW, and Collins HR: The shoulder in competitive swimming, Am J Sports Med 8:151, 1980.
51. Rockwood CA and Green DP: Fractures, Philadelphia, 1984, JB Lippincott Co, p 778.
52. Rokous JR, Feagin JA, and Abbott HG: Modified axillary roentgenogram: a useful adjunct in the diagnosis of recurrent instability of the shoulder, Clin Orthop 82:84, 1972.
53. Rowe CR, Patel D, and Southmayd WW: The Bankart procedure: a long-term end-result study, J Bone Joint Surg 60A:1, 1978.
54. Rowe CR and Zarins B: Recurrent transient subluxation of the shoulder, J Bone Joint Surg 63A:863, 1981.
55. Rowe CR, Zarins B, and Ciullo JV: Recurrent anterior dislocation of the shoulder after surgicare repair, J Bone Joint Surg 66A:159, 1984.
56. Samilson RL and Prieto V: Posterior dislocation of the shoulder in athletes, Clin Sports Med 2:369, 1983.
57. Sisto DJ and Jobe FW: The operative treatment of scapulothoracic bursitis in professional pitchers, Am J Sports Med 14:192, 1986.
58. Snyder S: Personal communication, 1987.
59. Tibone JE et al.: Staple capsulorrhaphy for recurrent posterior shoulder dislocations, Am J Sports Med 9:135, 1981.
60. Tullos HS and King JW: Lesions of the pitching arm in adolescents, JAMA 220:264, 1972.
61. Tullos HS and King JW: Throwing mechanism in sports, Orthop Clin North Am 4:809, 1973.
62. Tullos HS et al.: Unusual lesions of the pitching arm, Clin Orthop 88:169, 1972.
63. Turkel SJ et al.: Stabilizing mechanisms preventing anterior dislocation of the glenohumeral joint, J Bone Joint Surg 63A:1208, 1981.
64. Weiner DS and MacNab I: Superior migration of the humeral head, J Bone Joint Surg 52B:514, 1970.
65. Zeman SC et al.: Tears of the pectoralis major muscle, Am J Sports Med 7:343, 1979.

CHAPTER 10 Degenerative Joint Disease in the Shoulder

John J. Brems

In discussing degenerative joint disease in the athlete, one must first define it as a clinicopathologic condition and second, which is considerably more difficult, one must define an athlete!

In this chapter we will define degenerative joint disease of the shoulder as a pathologic process caused by a mechanical aberration of joint function that results in joint incongruity. This, of course, excludes certain types of degenerative diseases. Rheumatoid arthritis and crystalline and septic processes will purposely be excluded from the following discussion. Further, vascular causes of degenerative disease, such as osteonecrosis, will not be addressed.

Having now defined the condition, I must set about the more difficult task of defining the athlete. Whereas just 10 to 15 years ago one could define an athlete merely by age, now, with an ever-increasing awareness of the benefits of physical activity, the term "athlete" has taken on a wider domain. It is only fair to consider the 7-year-old gymnast as much an athlete as the senior citizen who plays two games of tennis each week.

Perhaps it is too difficult to adequately define our study group from this perspective; nevertheless, in the following discussion we will take a pragmatic approach and discuss degenerative conditions of the shoulder that are commonly associated with competitive and noncompetitive sports activities.

The moving shoulder actually consists of four articulations: the sternoclavicular joint, the scapulothoracic joint, the acromioclavicular (AC) joint, and the glenohumeral joint. Because degenerative joint disease of the sternoclavicular and scapulothoracic joint is exceedingly rare, it will not be considered. However, AC and glenohumeral degenerative joint diseases are very common in the athlete and will be discussed in detail.

ACROMIOCLAVICULAR JOINT

Isolated arthritic conditions of the AC joint have very significant impact on the function of the throwing shoulder. With full elevation of the arm, 20 degrees of axial rotation motion alone occurs at the AC joint. Depalma,[5] in a classic study in 1957, examined 223 sets of human AC and sternoclavicular joints from infant to 94 years of age. Significant changes in the anatomy and composition of the meniscus were directly correlated with degenerative changes. Because the AC joint is so superficial, it is subject to frequent trauma. Further, the joint's small size and incongruence of its mating surfaces lead to high shear stresses and increase the likelihood of degenerative changes.

The treatment of acute injuries is not the subject of this discussion, but the reader is referred to the following synopsis.[7]

History

Patients with degenerative disease of the AC joint may be any age. Most younger patients clearly have a history of trauma within 12 to 24 months of their presentation. At the other extreme are patients who are seen typically over 40 years of age who rarely give a history of any antecedent trauma. Further, in my experience, patients who are seen in middle age with AC arthritis have associated subacromial impingement and rotator cuff pathologic conditions in the majority of circumstances. The most common symptoms are pain with overhead activity and particularly with activities that require use of the arm across the midline. With the arm adducted, compression of the AC joint occurs. Because of this, patients frequently complain of pain at night when they roll over on their affected shoulder.

Physical Examination

The examination of any part of the shoulder begins by inspection. Often, prominence of the AC joints is seen together with significant muscular atrophy about the involved shoulder (Fig. 10-1). One should not mistake the prominence of a remote second- or third-degree AC joint separation with degenerative changes necessarily (Fig. 10-2). True arthritis of the joint has osteophytic changes on both the clavicular and the acromial side of the joint. When the examining physician then palpates the joint, there is tenderness directly over the AC region. There may or may not be observable instability, especially if there is pain, but one should assess superior-inferior and anterior-posterior stability.

Passive and active ranges of motion are then examined. Characteristic changes include pain with elevation, but minimal, if any, pain with external rotation, because this lateral maneuver results in only minimal motion at the AC joint. As noted, passive or active motion with the arm moving in front of the body characteristically produces pain (Fig. 10-3).

In the throwing athlete, it may be difficult to differentiate the pain of subacromial origin from that of AC joint origin. Here, the "injection test" is most valuable. An injection of 10 ml of 1% lidocaine without epinephrine is given in the subacromial bursa (Fig. 10-4), and the shoulder is reexamined. With the sub-

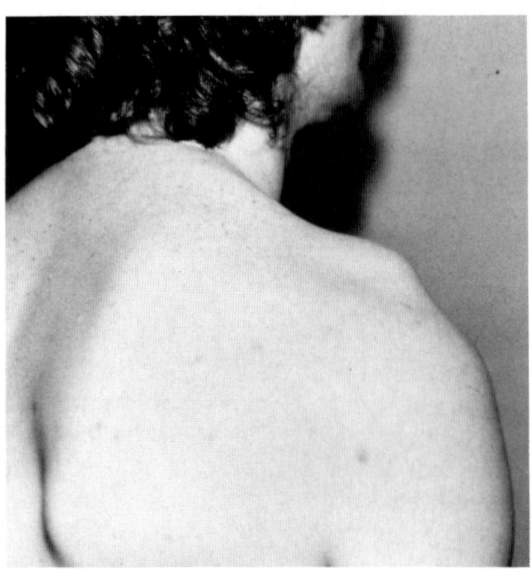

FIG. 10-1 This 40-year-old javelin thrower demonstrates the marked prominence of an arthritic AC joint. There has been no past history of AC joint separation, and the prominence is caused solely by the hypertrophic spurring on both the clavicular and acromial sides of the AC joint. Also note the marked atrophy of the supraspinatus and infraspinatus fossae.

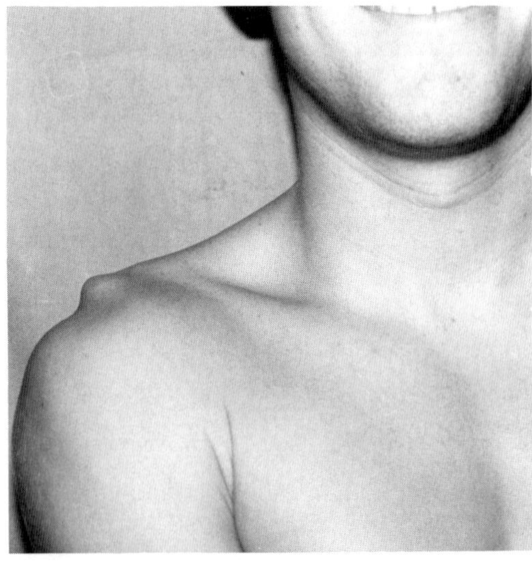

FIG. 10-2 This 30-year-old baseball player sustained an acute trauma by falling on the point of his left shoulder. He demonstrates the clinical findings of an acute third-degree AC joint separation. One would expect no muscular atrophy in an acute situation. Further, palpation of the acromial side of the AC joint would indicate osteophytes if a chronic degenerative process was present.

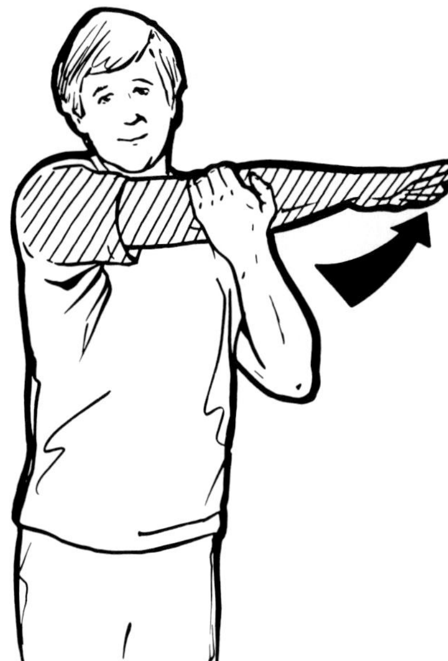

FIG. 10-3 This figure demonstrates the position that most characteristically reproduces the pain of AC joint pathologic conditions. Forcing the arm across the chest in this adducted position compresses the AC joint and is likely to reproduce symptoms.

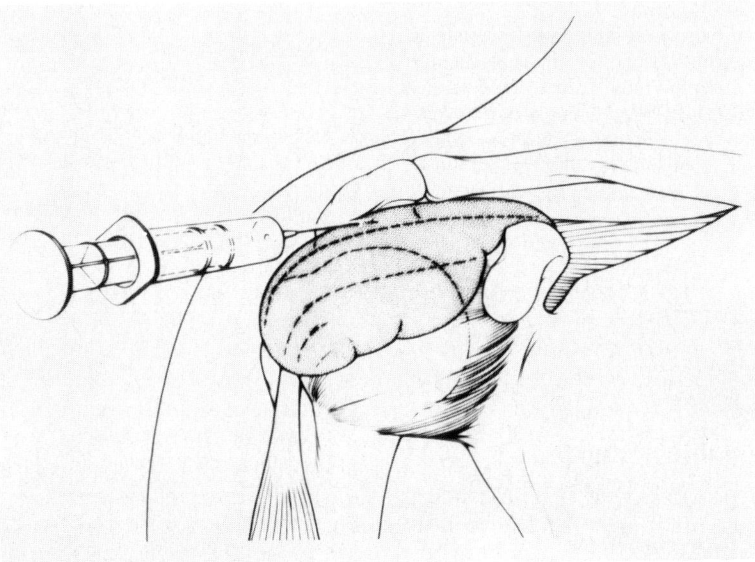

FIG. 10-4 As described, the injection test is performed by placing lidocaine initially in the subacromial bursa. If the pain persists following the subacromial injection, the lidocaine is then brought in from above and placed directly in the AC joint.

acromial mechanism now anesthetized, the pain of impingement and cuff tear should be eliminated. If the patient's symptoms abate following the injection, the pathologic condition is *not* at the AC joint. If the patient's symptoms persist and are still referable to the AC joint, then a further injection of 6 ml of 1% lidocaine is given into the AC joint. The patient is once again examined and the pain associated with AC joint pathologic conditions should now improve. I have found the diagnostic value of this test increased while performing the injections in the order described. If one's clinical suspicion is so directed to the AC joint, the injection could be given initially in that joint. In my experience, an injection into the AC joint can also diminish the pain of subacromial impingement. However, the converse is not true unless there is incompetence of the inferior capsule allowing the lidocaine to enter from the underlying subacromial bursa. In severe degenerative joint

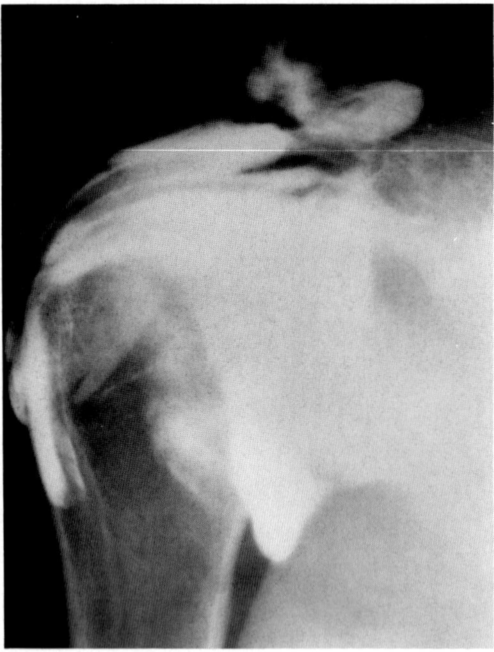

FIG. 10-5 This arthrogram shows an incompetent AC joint capsule. The contrast can readily be seen entering the AC joint from its undersurface. The contrast agent was initially placed in the inferior aspect of the true glenohumeral joint. When there is a large rotator cuff tear as demonstrated here, there frequently is destruction of the AC joint and repair of the rotator cuff requires concomitant excision of the distal clavicle.

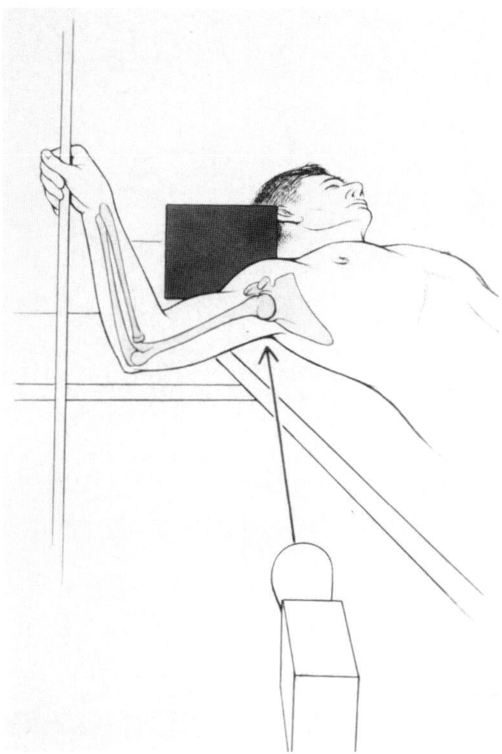

FIG. 10-6 Technique of obtaining the supine modified West Point view. With the patient lying supine and holding an IV pole, the x-ray tube is angled 20 degrees upward from the floor and 20 degrees away from the long axis of the patient's body. This effectively provides the lateral view of the shoulder and AC joint.

disease of the AC joint, the inferior capsule is not present as evidenced by the "geyser sign" seen on arthrography[4] (Fig. 10-5).

Roentgenographic Evaluation

The most appropriate views to obtain when visualizing the AC joint are the true anteroposterior view of the shoulder and the modified West Point view obtained as shown in Figs. 10-6 and 10-7. As in other joint evaluations, one should never accept anything less than two orthogonal views. The roentgenographic findings include irregularity of the joint surfaces, calcification in and about the AC joint capsule, calcification of the coracoclavicular ligaments, and resorption of the lateral end of the clavicle to varying degrees (Figs. 10-8 and 10-9). As mentioned previously, hypertrophic spurring is usually seen on both the acromial and the clavicular side of the joint. Cyst formation in the medial acromion or lateral clavicle is also significant evidence for osteoarthritic degenerative changes.

Roentgenographic findings of AC degenerative joint disease

- Joint surface irregularity
- Calcification of the AC joint capsule
- Calcification of the coracoclavicular ligament
- Hypertrophic spurring
- Cyst formation
- Osteolysis of lateral clavicle (variable)

Treatment

Treatment of any condition must rely on an understanding of the natural history of the pathologic process. However, in the case of the AC joint, the natural history and the rate of progression of the arthritis appear to be activity related. Also, one must remember that, as in most musculoskeletal conditions, the treating physician *never* treats the roentgenograms. Asymptomatic patients with marked degenerative changes roentgenographically need no treatment. Conversely, patients with minimal roentgenographic findings can have

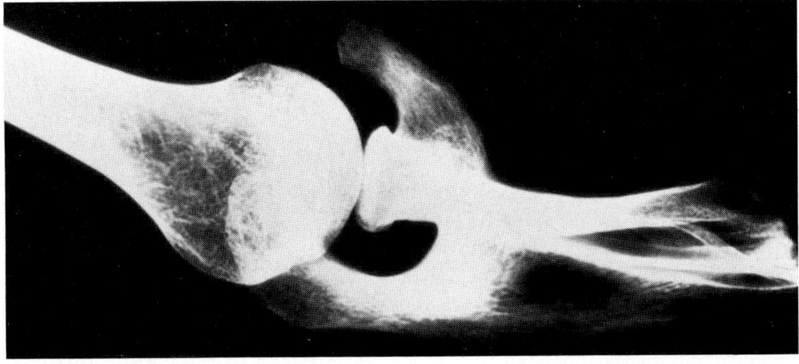

FIG. 10-7 The roentgenographic appearance of this modified West Point view. This provides excellent projection of the glenohumeral joint and AC joint.

A

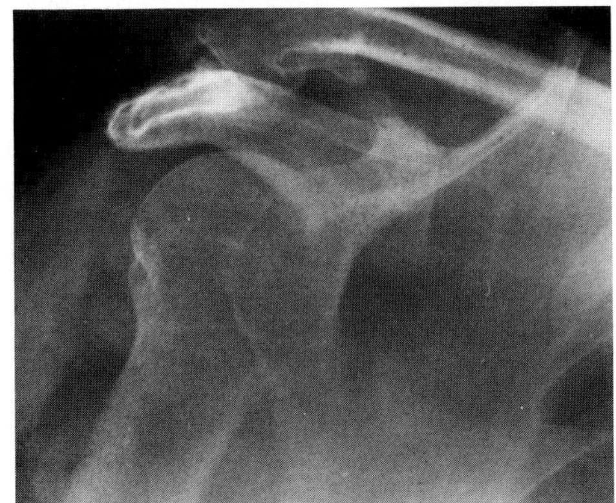

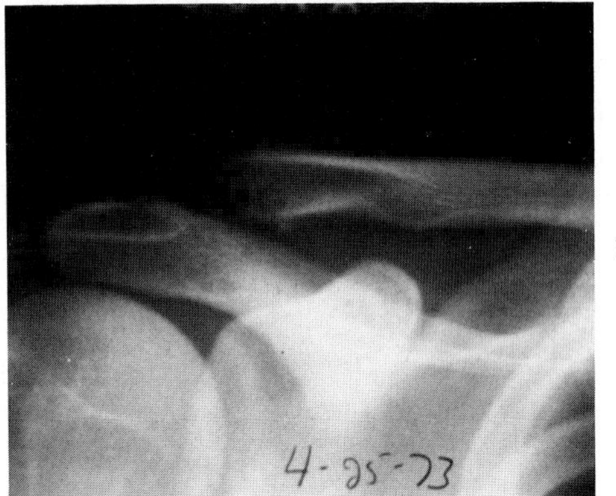

B

C

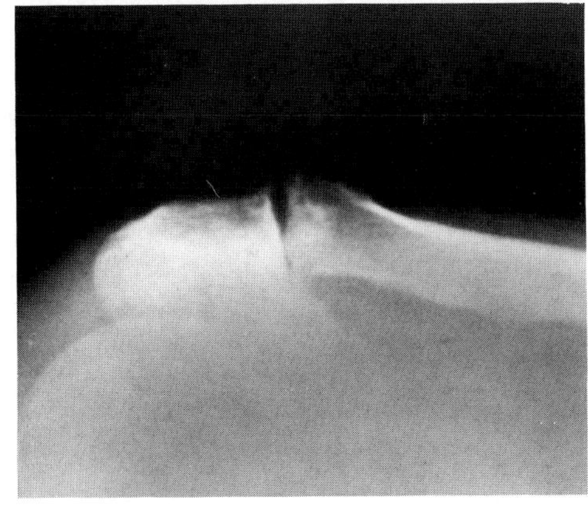

FIG. 10-8 A, Severe arthritis of the AC joint. Note the calcification of the conoid and trapezoid ligament complex, the marked narrowing of the AC joint with irregularity of the joint surfaces, and the osteophyte process involving both the distal clavicle and medial aspect of the acromion. **B,** This roentgenogram of degenerative disease of the AC joint shows significant resorption of the lateral clavicle, cyst formation, and also some early calcification of the conoid and trapezoid ligament complex. **C,** Again, note the AC joint arthritis manifest by joint space narrowing, particularly at the posteroinferior corner of the joint along with cyst formation on both sides of the joint and prominence on the acromial and clavicular portions.

severe disabling pain with recreational and nonrecreational activities.

Nonoperative Management

Nonoperative management of painful degenerative joint disease involving the AC joint begins with modification of activity. Daily stretching and oral nonsteroidal antiinflammatory agents are important adjuncts. Once symptoms abate, a muscle strengthening program involving the trapezius and remainder of the shoulder girdle muscles is initiated. Many nonsteroidal antiinflammatory drugs are available; my preference is one that requires the fewest doses, which (it is hoped) increases patient compliance. The patient must take the medication 2 to 3 weeks before one can evaluate its efficacy. If the initial antiinflammatory medication is not of significant benefit, at least two others of a different chemical class should be tried (Table 10-1). In most patients I reserve intraarticular steroids until two or three oral antiinflammatory agents have been unsuccessful. If a patient is not

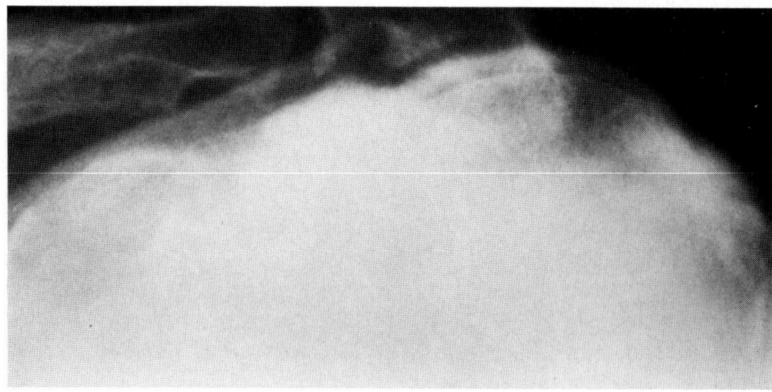

FIG. 10-9 Typical findings of arthritis of the AC joint are seen with significant changes on the acromial side. Taken as part of an arthrogram study, one can see that there is absence of contrast in the AC joint, indicating integrity of the joint capsule.

TABLE 10-1 Chemical classes of nonsteroidal antiinflammatory medications

Chemical Class	Medication
Oxicams	Piroxicam (Feldene)
Salicylates	Aspirin Salsalate (Disalcid) Choline magnesium trisalicylate (Trilisate) Ascriptin
Acetic acids	Indomethacin (Indocin) Sulindac (Clinoril) Tolmetin sodium (Tolectin)
Propionic acids	Ibuprofen (Advil, Motrin) Naproxen (Naprosyn) Fenoprofen calcium (Nalfon) Ketoprofen (Orudis) Flurbiprofen (Ansaid)
Fenamates	Meclofenamate sodium (Meclomen)
Pyrazoles	Phenylbutazone (Butazolidin)
Phenylacetic acids	Diclofenac (Voltaren)

responsive to the oral medications or has other contraindications to them, intraarticular corticosteroids may be given. If the oral agent is beneficial, it should be continued for 8 to 12 weeks after symptoms diminish to minimize the rapid return of symptoms. In addition to medication, it is equally important for the patient to modify activities. As previously mentioned, the use of the arm across the chest compresses the joint and should therefore not be allowed. Repetitive activity with the arm above the shoulder should also be kept to a minimum for the first 4 weeks of treatment. After the first month, patients may be allowed nonrepetitive use of the involved arm. Loss of motion, stiffness and crepitus are common sequelae when treatment consists solely of limiting activity. Therefore daily stretching is also an important component of the nonoperative management of this condition. The patient must stretch in external rotation, internal rotation, and elevation at least once each day and at most twice each day during this recovery period (Fig. 10-10).

Operative Management

If nonoperative management fails to alleviate the patient's symptoms, surgical excision of the lateral clavicle may be indicated. This procedure was first described by Mumford[9] and Gurd[6] in 1941. Details of the technique are readily found in standard texts,[13] but a few points should be emphasized. For this procedure to be successful, the coracoclavicular ligaments must be intact. If these ligaments are incompetent, significant instability of the medial clavicle remnant usually results in pain and marked weakness of elevation and forward throwing motions.

When performing the osteotomy of the clavicle, an osteotome should be used instead of a reciprocating saw. The saw creates bone dust and debris that may result in myositis ossificans of the deltoid muscle. Further, it has much more potential to cause soft tissue injury, involving especially the deltoid and trapezius muscles. Careful consideration must be given to the direction of the osteotomy. The anteroposterior and West Point views of the joint should provide a guide as to the angulation required for the clavicular osteotomy. When the osteotomy is complete, the "new" lateral end of the clavicle should represent a near parallelogram that is parallel to the plane of the medial acromion as seen in the diagram (Fig. 10-11).

In the usual case, one resects slightly more

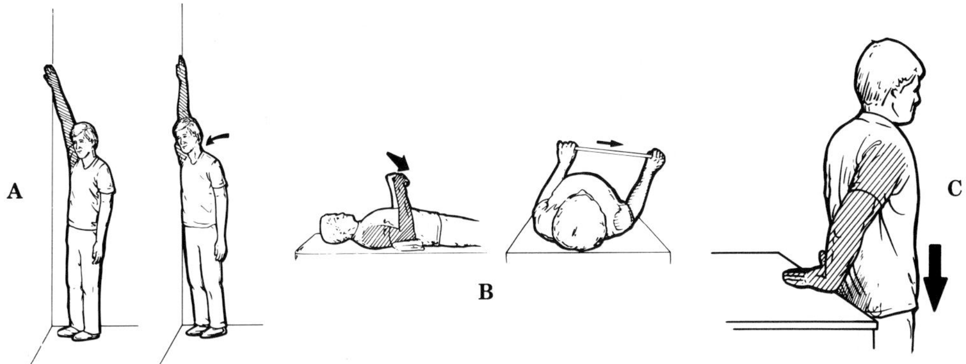

FIG. 10-10 Stretching exercises are an important part in the rehabilitation process of pathologic shoulder conditions. The cardinal motions are demonstrated here. **A,** Passive elevation is performed with the patient standing in the corner and elevating the arm in the plane of the scapula. The patient then leans against the wall, trying to approximate the axilla to the wall itself, as shown. **B,** Supine external rotation is performed using a stick as shown. It is important to keep the elbow off the table so that the humerus remains parallel with the ground. **C,** Internal rotation is performed by having the patient force the thumb along the dorsal area of the spine. This may be done by using the other arm to pull the affected arm up the back, or it may be performed as demonstrated.

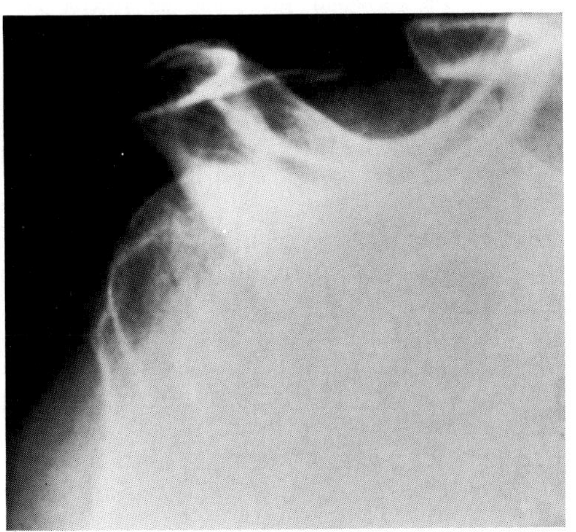

FIG. 10-11 This roentgenogram shows the appearance following resection of the distal clavicle. The angular relationships are important to prevent impingement with motion following the surgery. The lateral aspect of the clavicle is seen with slightly more bone removed inferiorly than superiorly, and the joint remains nearly parallel in appearance when comparing the lateral clavicle and medial acromion in this projection.

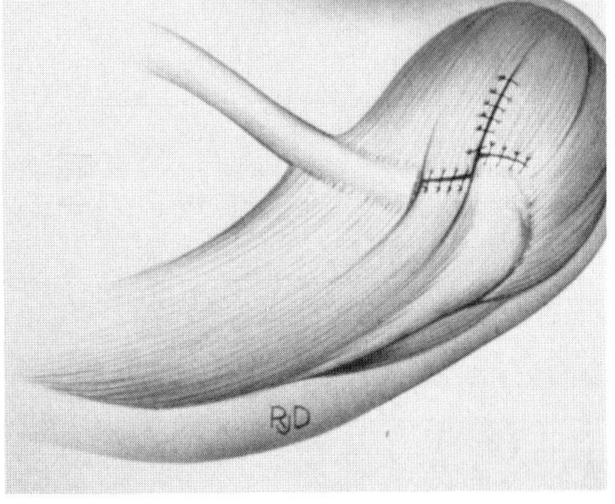

FIG. 10-12 Following clavicular resection, it is imperative to reattach the deltoid muscle to the trapezius muscle directly. The deltoid takes its origin from this lateral clavicle, and failure to reattach this securely results in weakness of elevation; the athlete has difficulty in racquet and throwing sports.

bone posteriorly than anteriorly and slightly more bone inferiorly than superiorly.

The surgeon must also remember the muscle anatomy about the AC joint. The trapezius inserts along the posterior distal clavicle, and the deltoid originates on the anterior distal clavicle. As shown in Fig. 10-12, it is most important to reattach the deltoid origin to the trapezius insertion. Simply repairing the clavicular periosteum is not sufficient, and if this suture line fails the anterior deltoid becomes markedly weak.

Aftercare and Rehabilitation

The aftercare of lateral clavicular resection consists of early passive motion in all planes, but active use of the arm must be restricted for 4 weeks. This permits satisfactory healing of the deltoid to the trapezius muscle. One month after surgery, strengthening programs are begun and the athlete is allowed to return to activity any time thereafter without restriction. Within 3 to 4 months following surgery, the athlete has nearly full range of motion and nearly symmetric strength with the contralateral arm.

GLENOHUMERAL JOINT

This discussion will be of the diagnosis and treatment of glenohumeral joint destruction. Although primary "idiopathic" glenohumeral arthritis is usually not seen until the fifth or sixth decade, a sizable number of patients, usually athletes, have a condition called arthritis of dislocation. This diagnosis was first used by Neer when he reviewed his total shoulder experience.[11] In the cohort of patients who had arthritis of dislocation, the average age at the time of total joint arthroplasty for severe degenerative joint disease was 37 years old. Whether those athletes who use their arms in their chosen sport are at risk for primary glenohumeral arthritis is not known. The association seems dubious outside the spectrum of minor and major instabilities. On the other hand, patients who undergo joint replacement for degenerative disease of the shoulder are not only allowed but also encouraged to return to noncontact sports such as tennis, golf, or swimming.[10]

Arthritis of Recurrent Dislocation

Because instability is a common problem in the athlete, some discussion of this condition seems appropriate. To begin, one again must ask, "What is the natural history of instability?" Untreated, the natural history of the unstable shoulder does not seem to be degenerative joint disease. Clearly, a few patients who come to the orthopaedist in the fifth decade and beyond with severe degenerative disease of the shoulder give a history of untreated instability. Arthritis of dislocation appears to be iatrogenic.

A review of 500 patients who had a degenerative disease of the glenohumeral joint yielded 103 patients who had a history of instability.[1] Ninety-seven of these 103 patients had prior surgery for their instability. Only six patients had a history of untreated instability and developed arthritis in this series. Although this series may not represent a true cross section of the population with instability, it became hard to ignore the findings. In careful studying of these patients, several potential etiologic factors came to light. The most

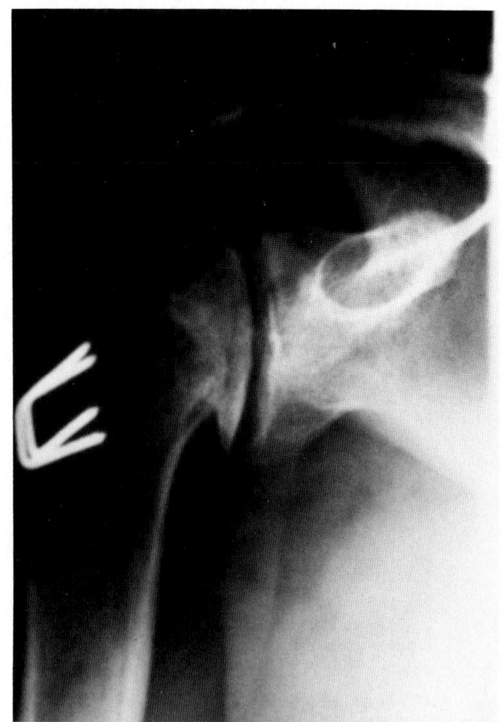

FIG. 10-13 This is the shoulder of a 21-year-old college football player who sustained multiple dislocations. Because he was thought to have anterior instability, repair was with a Magnuson-Stack procedure. However, because of the unrecognized inferior component, he developed the classic arthritis of recurrent dislocation. One can see loss of sphericity of the humeral head with degenerative changes at the glenohumeral joint. The most characteristic findings are inferior glenoid osteophytes along with the osteophyte on the inferior aspect of the humerus. It should be noted that this osteophyte is not only present inferiorly. The more anterior portion of the osteophyte is superimposed on the anatomic neck of the humerus and cannot be visualized in this projection.

common cause identified was the surgeon's failure to recognize the scope of the instability. Anterior instability is thought to be the most common type of instability in the athletic population, hence the popularity of the Bristow, Boyd, Putti-Platt, and Magnuson procedures. Newer concepts of the unstable shoulder include simultaneous components of anterior, inferior, and posterior laxity to varying degrees. When an unrecognized multidirectional instability is repaired with the standard anterior procedures, the humeral head continues to sublux into the areas of untreated laxity (Fig. 10-13). This incongruity becomes exaggerated as the patient returns to activity, and degeneration of the joint then proceeds. In the reported series, 50 of the 103 required either total joint or humeral head replacement

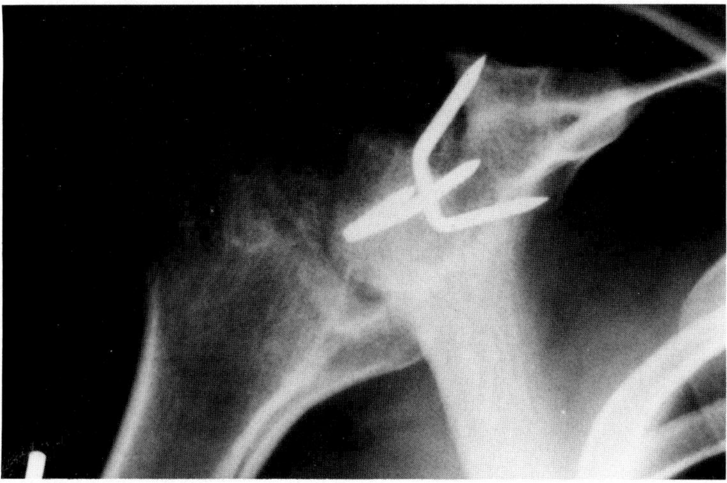

FIG. 10-14 A 19-year-old male following a failed Boyd staple capsulorrhaphy. The staples have become loosened and have migrated, and the shoulder is now in a fixed, subluxed position with severe degenerative changes.

and the average age was only 37 years. The second most common cause of arthritis of dislocation was related to the use of metal around the shoulder. It must be recognized that well-placed screws and staples at the time of surgery may become loose and migrate or they may fracture. If these metallic remnants find their way into the glenohumeral joint, severe destructive arthritis rapidly ensues. The literature has numerous reports on the complications of metal about the shoulder[8,14] (Fig. 10-14).

History

The active athletic patient usually has a chief complaint relating to loss of motion, stiffness, and pain in varying proportions. There is usually no history of acute trauma. If there is a history of instability, it has, more often than not, been surgically treated. Night pain is not as characteristic as with subacromial impingement and rotator cuff pathologic conditions. Pain is usually activity related and relieved by rest. Characteristically, the pain is described as dull, aching, and poorly localizable. Because loss of external rotation is usually seen early in the degenerative process, patients complain of an inability to get their hand behind their head, especially in racquet and throwing sports. Initially, patients get relief from over-the-counter antiinflammatory medications and analgesics.

Physical Examination

In all patients who are being evaluated for shoulder pathologic conditions, a physical examination must begin at the cervical area of the spine (see Chapter 1). The fact that both idiopathic cervical degenerative disease and glenohumeral degenerative disease occur in the same age group makes these conditions difficult, yet mandatory to differentiate. Therefore a well-performed neck examination is critical. The patient is seated, both shoulders simultaneously exposed, and the neck is examined. Range of motion, degree of extension, flexion, rotation, and lateral bend are noted. Especially important is the combined maneuver of extension and lateral bend that may close the neural foramen and reproduce the patient's shoulder symptoms. Any limitation of cervical motion warrants a roentgenographic examination and the anteroposterior, lateral, and oblique planes at the very least.

Clinical findings in glenohumeral degenerative joint disease

- Posterior position of humerus (axis)
- Supraspinatus/intraspinatus atrophy
- External rotation weakness
- Internal rotation contracture
- Loss of elevation

The shoulders are then visually inspected, noting atrophy, symmetry, and "centering" (Fig. 10-15). Degenerative joint disease of the glenohumeral joint characteristically causes posterior glenoid wear (Fig. 10-16). As seen on the clinical photograph, when viewed from a lateral side, the humerus tends to lie more posterior than on the uninvolved side.

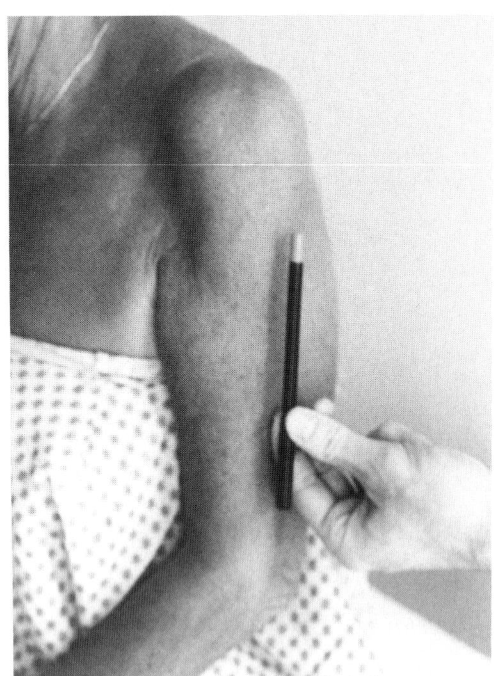

FIG. 10-15 One of the characteristic changes in arthritis of recurrent dislocation and generalized osteoarthritis of the shoulder is posterior migration of the humerus on the glenoid. When observing the patient from the lateral aspect, the more posterior position of the arm with respect to the shoulder becomes evident.

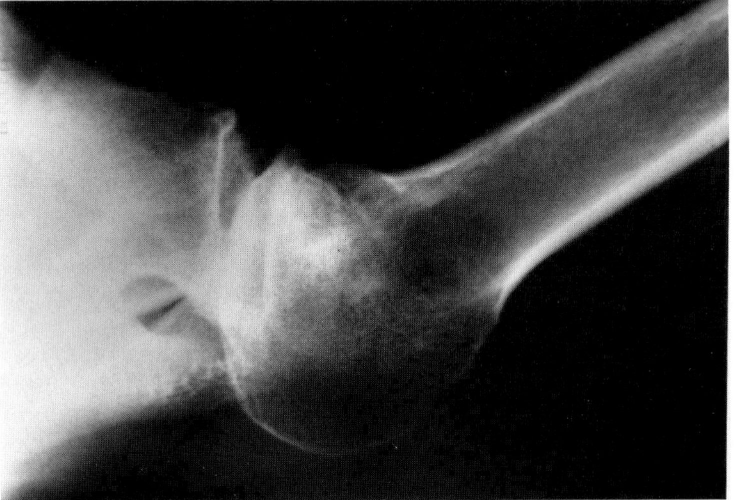

FIG. 10-16 This modified West Point view shows the marked posterior subluxation and migration of this 37-year-old baseball player. This patient had undergone a Putti-Platt procedure because he was thought to have isolated anterior instability. When his anterior capsule was made tight, in the presence of some posterior laxity, the head was forced out the back, causing severe degenerative changes.

There is usually marked atrophy of the supraspinatus and infraspinatus muscles. Because loss of external rotation is so characteristic, the infraspinatus (the only true external rotator of the shoulder) is usually markedly affected. To a lesser degree, clinically, are the supraspinatus and deltoid visibly affected, but a Cybex evaluation will usually demonstrate clear differences between the involved and uninvolved side.

The shoulder is then palpated, and it is imperative to examine the AC joint. Forces that led to the glenohumeral degenerative disease are also present in some magnitude at the AC joint. Concomitant AC arthritis requiring surgical attention at the time of glenohumeral arthroplasty is present nearly 50% of the time in my experience. The sternoclavicular joint should also be examined and palpated at this time.

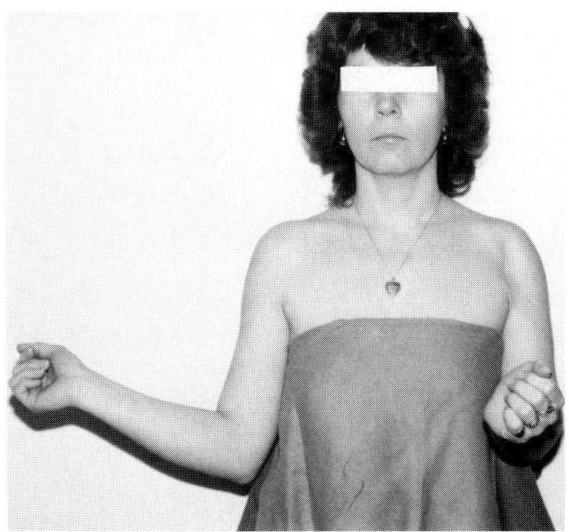

FIG. 10-17 This 27-year-old woman has severe arthritis of recurrent dislocation. She is demonstrating her maximal external rotation of the left shoulder. Careful observation shows several findings of the arthritis of dislocation. There is evidence of previous surgery with an anterior scar and marked atrophy of the anterior deltoid. The loss of external rotation together with the posterior position of the humerus on the shoulder are all clinical signs of this condition.

The patient is then placed supine, and passive range of motion is measured and recorded in both arms. When compared to the normal extremity, there is considerable loss of elevation in the scapular plane. Pain and crepitus are also frequently associated findings during this maneuver. While the patient remains supine, external rotation is measured. This characteristically has the greatest percentage loss when compared to the normal arm (Fig. 10-17). Often, not only is the joint incongruity impeding motion, but also pain in itself limits motion.

The patient is once again placed in the sitting position, and internal rotation and active elevation are measured and recorded. It should be understood that a careful neurologic examination documenting the integrity of the suprascapular and axillary nerve along with the remaining brachial plexus is required.

Roentgenographic Evaluation

As noted previously, the most important roentgenograms to obtain are the true anteroposterior and the modified West Point views (Figs. 10-6 and 10-7). Both of these projections provide an excellent view of a glenohumeral joint. One is able to appreciate the characteristic posterior glenoid wear (Fig. 10-16). The glenoid bone stock available for a glenoid replacement is only seen on the modified West Point view. Further, the AC joint can be roentgenographically evaluated and correlated with the physical examination. The anteroposterior view should include the proximal two thirds of the humeral shaft so one can safely estimate the appropriate humeral component diameter. On the anteroposterior view, only inferior osteophytes are seen, but in fact, these osteophytes are present circumferentially about the anatomic neck of the humerus (Fig. 10-18). Because they are superimposed on the anatomic neck at the periarticular margin (Fig. 10-19), they are seen only in their inferior projection. When clinically indicated, the roentgenographic examination of the shoulder must include a cervical spine series, as previously discussed.

Treatment

Nonoperative Management

Once again, we must consider the natural history of degenerative joint disease involving the glenohumeral joint. Whereas the natural history of untreated arthritis of the shoulder is predictable in the sense of progressive loss of motion and increasing pain, the time course over which it occurs is remarkable for its unpredictability. In that context, treatment of degenerative joint disease of the shoulder by any means is always elective and based on patient symptoms. With both increased activity among patients well into the sixth and seventh decades and the near-normal return of function and strength with shoulder replacement, an increasing role is played in surgical management of the athlete with degenerative joint disease of the shoulder.

Nonoperative management should consist of oral nonsteroidal antiinflammatory agents, a "very occasional" intraarticular corticosteroid, physical therapy primarily for isometric strengthening, and range of motion exercises only to the point of pain. There is little to gain in trying to increase the range of motion in a noncongruent arthritic joint. However, in performing isometric exercises, strength may be maintained in the face of a poorly moving joint. Periods of rest for the joint, along with oral antiinflammatories and isometric strengthening of the infraspinatus muscle, often afford months of subjective relief in the face of clinical and roentgenographic severe shoulder arthritis.

Operative Management

Most surgeons would consider it inappropriate to discuss joint replacements in young active athletic people. Even in 1980 in a standard orthopaedic text, shoulder replacement

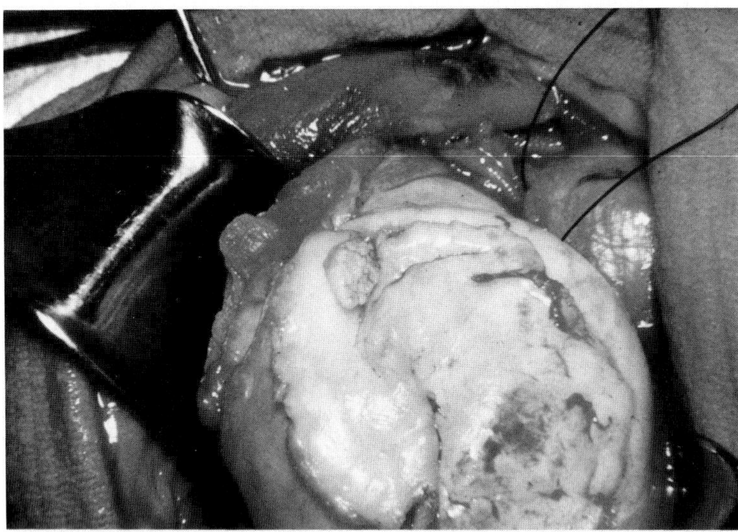

FIG. 10-18 This intraoperative view shows the circumferential nature of the osteophytes on the humeral head. On the anterior projection of this shoulder, only the inferior osteophytes are seen. The more anterior and posterior osteophytes are not seen because they are projected over the anatomic neck of the humerus.

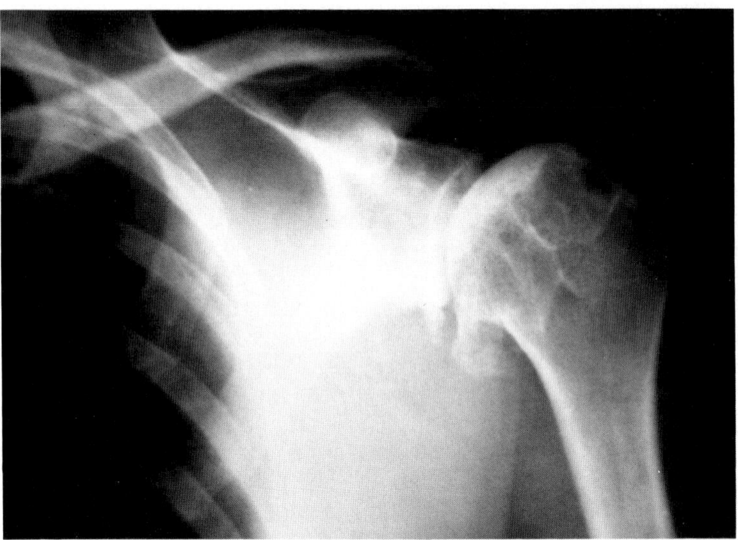

FIG. 10-19 This 40-year-old avid golfer complains of loss of motion. Four years before this roentgenogram, the patient had a Bankart type of repair to correct recurrent anterior instability. Once again, the characteristic inferior glenoid osteophyte is seen along with loss of sphericity of the humeral head. Only the inferior osteophyte is seen, but if one looks carefully at the anatomic neck region of the humerus the anterior and posterior extent of the osteophyte is appreciated.

was considered experimental.[12] Nevertheless, it has been recognized that a large proportion of the indications for surgical management (shoulder replacement) are in young, active, athletic people. Other procedures, including cheilectomy, synovectomy, and joint lavage, should be avoided because those procedures have not been shown to increase motion or alter the natural history of the condition. Those procedures, however, do result in scarring of the muscles, which leads to a poor outcome from subsequent arthroplasty. On the other hand, shoulder replacement, regardless of age, when performed properly, has the potential in these very young active patients to provide near-normal motion and strength. Fusions and resections make it impossible to use muscles effectively, and for

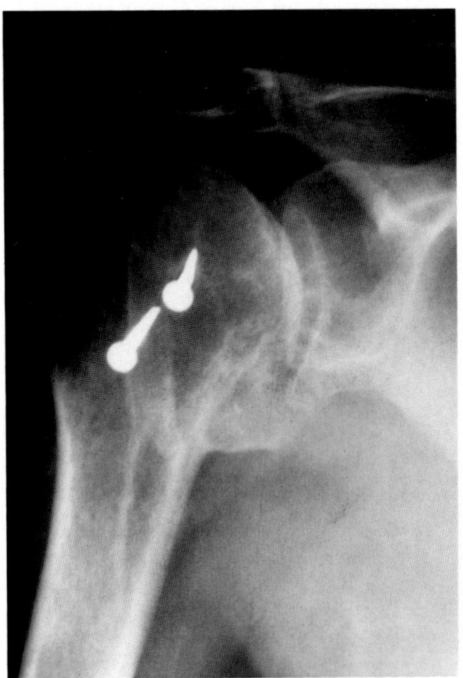

FIG. 10-20 This 27-year-old man has had four previous operations for anterior instability. The roentgenogram shows evidence of a previous Nicola procedure and a Magnuson-Stack type of procedure as evidenced by the nails. Additionally, a Bankart type of procedure was performed with an anterior bone block. Now this patient has severe arthritis of dislocation, markedly limited motion, and severe pain. The only reasonable option in this young patient is shoulder replacement. In the absence of sepsis or paralysis, arthrodesis would not be performed because it would waste potentially good functioning muscle.

this reason those procedures should be considered more radical than shoulder replacement even in the young active age groups.

In Neer's review of 500 shoulder replacements,[11] 95 (19%) had primary idiopathic osteoarthritis. These patients were generally young and actively engaged in activities such as tennis, golf, and swimming. Thirty-two of those 500 had arthritis of recurrent dislocation. This entity is extremely important in a sports medicine patient, as discussed earlier. These patients were very active athletically, and the majority had previous surgery. Most significantly, the patients were young, with the average age of this group being only 37 years. There was no good alternative to shoulder replacement for these patients. Arthrodesis would have laid to waste good, functional muscle. The patient seen in Fig. 10-20 was only 27 years old and had four procedures for instability with resultant severe osteoarthritis. Postoperatively, the patient was engaged in activities including butterfly swimming.

Surgical technique. As with AC joint procedures, the technique of shoulder replacement is available, and in this discussion only additional principles will be given.[2] The principle in all shoulder procedures is to restore normal anatomy. Above all, the surgeon must consider shoulder replacement a soft tissue procedure. One must remove only minimal bone, preserve intact muscles, restore them to their anatomic lengths, and release adhesions.

Principles in shoulder replacement

- Remove minimal bone.
- Preserve intact muscles.
- Restore muscles to anatomic lengths.
- Release adhesions.

My personal preference is to perform shoulder replacements with the patient under regional intrascalene block anesthesia, which offers several advantages over the general anesthetics. There is significantly less blood loss, there is minimal postoperative nausea, and patients are able to ambulate within 2 to 3 hours of their surgical procedure. Analgesia lasts as long as 8 hours and only gradually wears off. The most significant benefit is that the patient is able to observe his or her range of motion following surgery; with the patient sitting on the operating table I place the arm through a range of motion for him or her to see.

The patient is placed in the beach-chair position, and a long deltopectoral incision is made from the clavicle to the deltoid insertion. The deltoid is not removed from its origin on the clavicle and acromion; rather, a portion of its insertion is released when it is necessary for increased exposure. The superior one third of the pectoralis major is released from the humeral shaft, taking care not to injure the tendinous portion of the long head of the biceps muscle. Remembering that 60 to 70 degrees of external rotation is paramount for return to most athletic activities, the surgeon must now assess the external rotation. The subscapularis capsule complex must be lengthened (Fig. 10-21) so that following anterior rotator cuff repair the arm can reach 45 to 50 degrees of external rotation with no tension on the new suture line.

When the humeral osteotomy is performed, great care must be taken to ensure that the axis of the head of the component is above

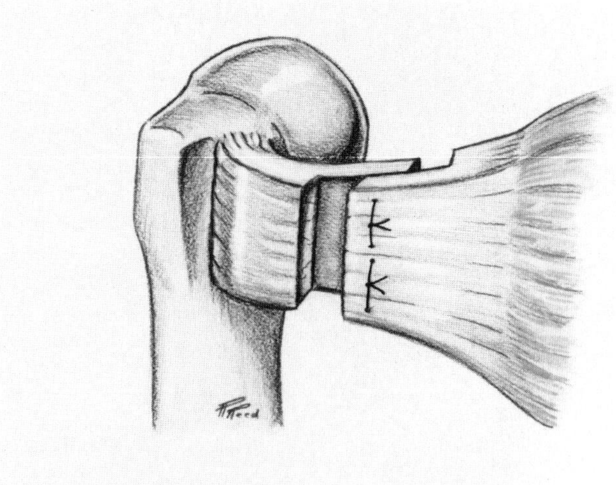

FIG. 10-21 Technique of lengthening the subscapularis capsule complex. The functional success of shoulder replacement depends on adequate external rotation. Because the arthritic process usually results in marked loss of external rotation preoperatively, the surgeon must nearly always lengthen this structure as the shoulder is approached surgically. Despite the previous history of instability, following shoulder replacement for arthritis, the stability of the joint depends on the version of the components and does not depend on a tight anterior subscapularis or capsule complex. When the operative procedure is complete and the shoulder closed, the arm should be able to reach nearly 45 to 50 degrees of external rotation with no tension on the new suture line.

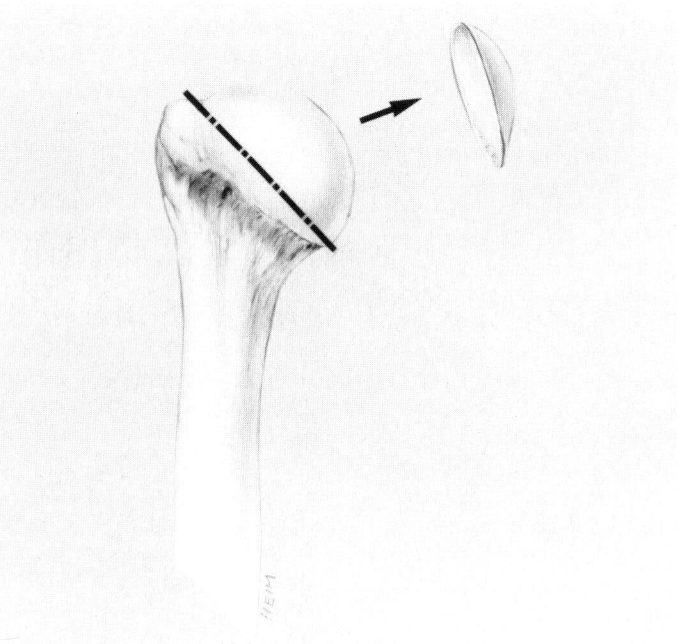

FIG. 10-22 Appropriate location for the humeral osteotomy. The axis of the component must lie above the tip of the greater tuberosity as seen.

the tip of the greater tuberosity (Fig. 10-22). In doing this, the deltoid and rotator cuff muscle lengths are maintained; hence strength recovery is more predictable. The myofascial sleeve of the upper arm must remain taut following replacement to allow full active elevation.

The use of cement in joint arthroplasty has a long, stormy history. However, in shoulder replacements there has never been more than an occasional case report of clinical loosening of either the humeral or glenoid components. In a series presented,[3] glenoid lucency rate was nearly 70% at 5-year follow-up, but none was clinically loose or required revision. More significant was the fact that 68% of the lucent lines were present within 1 week of the operative procedure and less than 7% progressed over the 5-year follow-up period. I believe that cement should be routinely used for the glenoid at present with prior meticulous bone preparation. New glenoid components are becoming available that allow for bone ingrowth. Anatomically, however, there appears to be so little bone available for bio-ingrowth that one should be careful of jumping into a new technology when past methods have offered so few problems. In considering cement for the humeral component, the key is immediate axial and rotational stability. The most important consideration must be early shoulder motion and rehabilitation. If a component cannot be seated firmly, it should be cemented without regard to patient age. With careful technique, however, nearly all humeral components can be placed adequately without the use of methylmethacrylate in the young active athletic patient with primary degenerative joint disease.

Aftercare and Rehabilitation

The physician must be intimately involved in the management of the physical therapy program after replacement. Only the surgeon is aware of the quality of the soft tissues and rotator cuff. Handing the patient a prescription and sending him or her to a physical therapist for rehabilitation is an invitation to failure. All therapy must begin and continue with the surgeon's direction and modification.

Passive range of motion for elevation and external rotation are begun at 48 hours. By the fourth or fifth day, internal rotation stretching is begun. Because the deltoid was not detached, active elevation may begin as soon as 7 to 10 days following surgery if passive motion allows. Patients with osteoarthritis and arthritis of recurrent dislocations should elevate nearly 150 to 160 degrees within 7 days. External rotation should reach at least 45 degrees also within a week's time if appropriate measures were undertaken to lengthen the anterior subscapularis capsule complex at the time of arthroplasty. As the patient's physician, you must encourage and reassure the patient that recovery continues for 9 to 12 months after surgery.

With a properly implanted prosthesis and with proper physician-directed rehabilitation, patients have been allowed to return to nearly all noncontact recreational activities. Football, wrestling, and downhill skiing are not allowed, but most patients engage in activities including tennis, swimming, golf, and basketball. Bowling and other racquet sports are also permitted.

Strengthening exercises below the horizontal are begun with rubber tubing and progress to springs as tolerated; eventually the patients may exercise with free weights to a limit of 50 pounds. Push-ups are allowed, but pull-ups, chin-ups, and overhead Nautilus activity are discouraged.

Athletic activity following shoulder replacement

Permitted (noncontact, recreational)
- Tennis
- Swimming
- Golf
- Basketball
- Bowling

Forbidden
- Football
- Wrestling
- Downhill skiing
- Pull-ups
- Chin-ups

SUMMARY

For the young, active athletic patient who has developed degenerative joint disease of the shoulder, shoulder replacement provides predictable relief of pain and when performed according to previously described surgical principles, patients may return to nearly all activities without restrictions.

REFERENCES

1. Brems JJ: Arthritis of recurrent dislocations, presented at Annual New York Orthopaedic Hospital Alumni Meeting, New York, 1984.
2. Brems JJ and Neer CS: Technique of shoulder replacement. Sound Slide Library, Atlanta, 1985, American Academy of Orthopaedic Surgeons.
3. Brems JJ and Wilde AH: Glenoid lucent lines. In American Academy of Orthopaedic Surgeons: Transactions of Annual Meeting of American Shoulder and Elbow Surgeons, New Orleans, 1986, The Academy.
4. Craig EV: The geyser sign and torn rotator cuff: clinical significance and pathomechanics, Clin Orthop 191:213, 1984.
5. Depalma AF: Surgery of the shoulder, Philadelphia, JB Lippincott Co, 1983, p 232.
6. Gurd FB: The treatment of complete dislocation of the outer end of the clavicle: an hitherto undescribed operation, Ann Surg 113:1041, 1941.
7. Harres TJ and Cox JS: Acromioclavicular injuries and surgical treatment. In Jackson DW, editor: Shoulder surgery in the athlete, Rockville, Md, 1985, Aspen Press, p 119.

8. Lower RF, McNeish LM, and Callaghan JJ: Computed tomographic documentation of intraarticular penetration of a screw after operations on the shoulder, J Bone Joint Surg 67A:1120, 1985.
9. Mumford EB: Acromioclavicular dislocations, J Bone Joint Surg 23:799, 1941.
10. Neer CS and Brems JJ: Shoulder replacement in the active and athletic patient. In Jackson W, editor: Shoulder surgery in the athlete, Rockville, Md, 1985, Aspen Press, p 93.
11. Neer CS, Watson KC, and Stanton FJ: Recent experiences in total shoulder replacement, J Bone Joint Surg 64A:319-337, 1982.
12. Sisk DT: Shoulder arthroplasty. In Edmondson AS and Crenshaw AH, editors: Campbell's operative orthopaedics, ed 6, St Louis, 1980, The CV Mosby Co, p 2415.
13. Wright PE: Dislocations. In Edmondson AS and Crenshaw AH, editors: Campbell's operative orthopaedics, ed 6, St Louis, 1980, The CV Mosby Co, p 452.
14. Zuckerman JD and Matsen FA: Complications about the glenohumeral joint related to the use of screws and staples, J Bone Joint Surg 66A:175, 1984.

CHAPTER 11 Principles of Shoulder Rehabilitation in the Athlete

Francis X. Mendoza
James A. Nicholas
Andrew Sands

The shoulder is the most mobile joint in humans, and, as such, it is frequently injured during athletic activities. This is especially true with modern sports, which tend to overemphasize use of the upper extremity and eye-hand coordination, as well as physical contact.

Shoulder injuries can result from either macrotrauma or microtrauma.[12] Macrotraumatic injuries occur as a result of an explosive force, such as during a tackle in a football game or a fall during a gymnastic maneuver. Microtraumatic injuries, on the other hand, occur from repetitive motions that result in overuse of the shoulder.[10] In this case, the muscle activity and force generated are not necessarily maximal, but the number of times the shoulder is repetitively cycled leads to injury.

All injuries of the athlete's shoulder must be rehabilitated to allow painless range of motion with flexibility and strength. This encourages participation without further injury. The rehabilitation program can be divided into three phases. Phase I emphasizes diminishing the inflammation and discomfort that result from the acute injury or surgical repair. Phase II directs treatment toward achieving and maintaining full, painless range of motion. Phase III concentrates on increasing strength and endurance in all planes of shoulder motion.

The physician and the therapist must communicate during the different phases of rehabilitation, to tailor specific aspects of the treatment to the individual athlete and allow safe and expedient recovery.

It must be remembered that, through the musculoskeletal *linkage system*, the shoulder is intimately related to the cervical spine, as are the elbow and distal arm. To treat the athlete successfully, the shoulder rehabilitation program must incorporate these additional regions.[24] Similarly, it is imperative to continue overall body conditioning during the shoulder rehabilitation program, to facilitate full return of the athlete on completion of treatment.

EVALUATION

Before initiation of treatment after a shoulder injury, a thorough history and physical examination will enable the physician and the therapist to create a treatment program. This allows different aspects within the three phases of rehabilitation to be effectively tailored to the individual athlete.

History

The patient's age, arm dominance, sport and level of competition, as well as any previous injury, should be ascertained.

A detailed description of the current injury, including the position of the shoulder and arm at the time of injury, is necessary to determine whether the injury was predominantly the result of macrotrauma (such as an acute dislocation), or microtrauma (as is often the case with atraumatic subluxations). Knowledge of any previous shoulder injury should include a diagnosis, the type and duration of immobilization, the number of steroid injections, the type of therapy used, the type of surgical repair and findings at the time of surgery, and the athlete's overall response to treatment. Furthermore, a history of injury to the uninvolved shoulder and the treatment for the injury may be useful.

Physical Examination

Examination commenses with observation of the patient's use of the upper extremity while removing outer garments, such as sweaters and coats. Generally, the uninvolved shoulder should be used as a standard of comparison with the injured shoulder. Asymmetry and atrophy are more easily appreciated when both shoulders are observed from behind. The range of motion, both passive and active, should be recorded in degrees for total elevation (Fig. 11-1) and external rotation with the arm at the side and with the arm at 90 degrees of abduction (Fig. 11-2). Internal rotation can be recorded using the spinal vertebrae as landmarks (Fig. 11-3).

The presence of swelling, discrete areas of tenderness, and joint laxity should be noted. Additionally, if appropriate, the presence of an impingement sign and an apprehension sign in the anterior, inferior, or posterior directions should be recorded. Neurologic and vascular examinations of both upper extremities should routinely be performed noting any restrictions of cervical spine motion and discomfort, as well as any differences in the peripheral pulses. Abnormalities in the degree of elbow, wrist, hand motion, and strength should also be recorded.

Manual muscle testing can be accomplished in different functional planes of motion, comparing both shoulders. Quantification of strength can be achieved using a Cybex isokinetic dynamometer or a Nicholas-ISMAT manual tester, although discomfort of the injured shoulder invariably has an adverse effect on the reliability of the results.

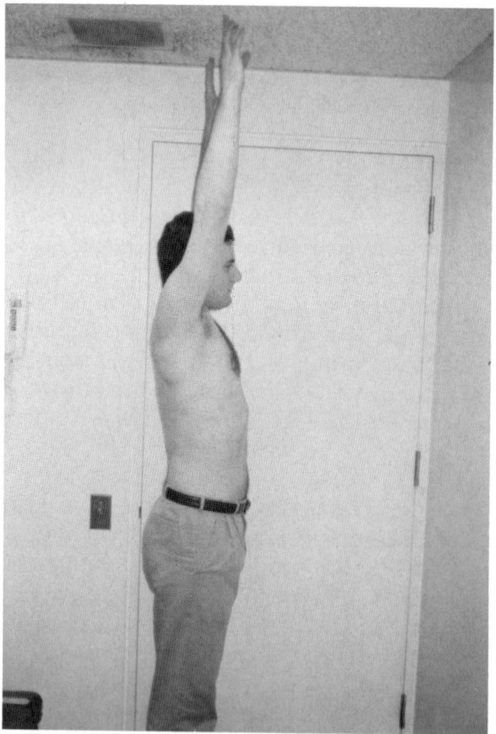

FIG. 11-1. Total elevation is measured from 0 degrees with the arm at the side to 180 degrees.

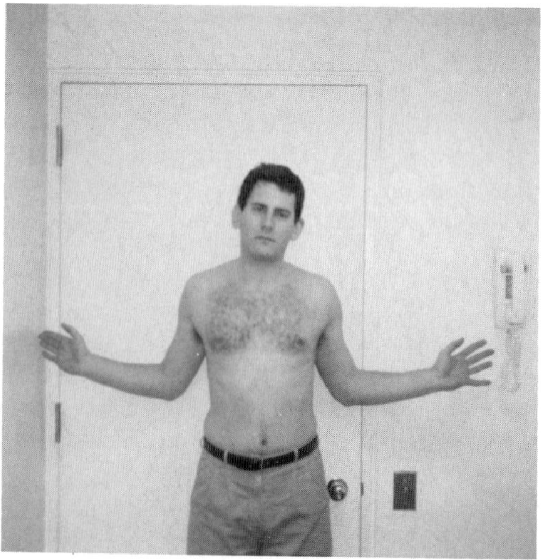

FIG. 11-2. External rotation is measured from 0 degrees with the arm at the side and the elbow flexed to 90 degrees.

BASIC SHOULDER REHABILITATION PROGRAM

The cornerstone to successful shoulder rehabilitation is implementation of a basic three-phase program that will guide the therapist and enable assessment of the athlete's progress as each phase is completed. Although the professional athlete can generally be treated with supervision on a daily basis, the usual frequency of treatment for nonprofessionals is 2 to 3 times a week, with close monitoring of a home exercise program.

General shoulder rehabilitation

- Phase I —Diminish inflammation/discomfort
- Phase II —Achieve full range of motion
- Phase III—Develop strength and endurance

Phase I

The primary goal of phase I treatment is to diminish pain and inflammation during acute and subacute phases of the injury. The type of injury sustained or surgical repair performed will determine the amount of shoulder motion allowed during this period of treatment. For instance, an athletic shoulder injury that results in an acute hemorrhagic bursitis may benefit from 3 to 5 days of sling immobilization. This helps control swelling and discomfort before initiation of range of motion exercises.[23] On the other hand, a shoulder surgically repaired to prevent anterior instability generally requires 2 to 6 weeks of immobilization, depending upon the procedure used, to encourage healing and decrease discomfort before initiation of range of motion exercises. Thus during phase I a variable amount of immobilization is generally necessary.

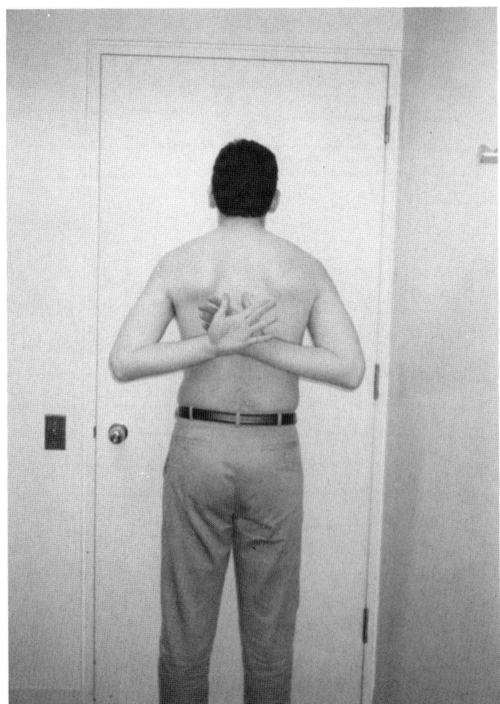

FIG. 11-3. Internal rotation is measured up the back using the spinal vertebrae.

Acutely, during the first 24 to 48 hours after injury, application of ice (cryotherapy) to the area of injury for 10-minute intervals assists in the control of swelling and pain. Discomfort can be further reduced with the use of analgesics, oral nonsteroidal antiinflammatory medication (NSAIDS), and transcutaneous electrical nerve stimulation (TENS).[26] As the athlete progresses into the subacute period, application of heat for 10- to 15-minute intervals, alone or alternated with ice treatments, is beneficial (contrast therapy).[18]

Throughout the phase I period of rehabilitation, isometric contractions of 5-second duration followed by 2- to 3-second relaxations are instituted for the elbow, wrist, and hand. Isometrics can be performed using the uninvolved arm to resist the contraction of the elbow and wrist of the injured extremity while a soft rubber ball or putty is squeezed for hand exercises.

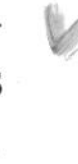

As soon as the acute shoulder discomfort is effectively controlled, overall aerobic and anaerobic fitness of the athlete is maintained. Although immobilization of the injured arm may still be required, use of a stationary bicycle, in conjunction with strengthening and flexibility exercises of both lower extremities, the trunk, and the uninvolved upper extremity, are used.

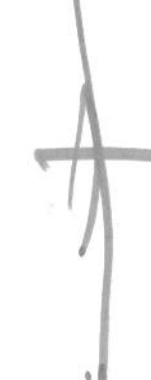

The amount of time necessary to complete phase I is dependent on the degree of swelling

Phase I

- Immobilization
- Cryotherapy
- Analgesics
- NSAIDS
- TENS
- Contrast therapy
- Isometrics
- Maintenance of fitness level

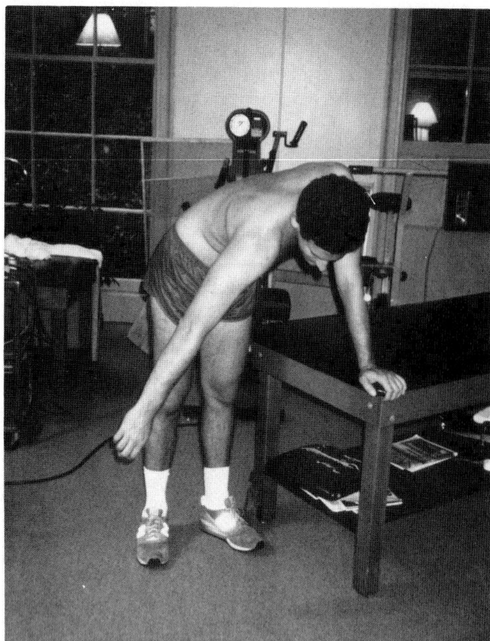

FIG. 11-4. Gentle pendulums can be used as warm-up exercises. They are performed clockwise, counterclockwise, forward and backward, and in an abduction to adduction direction.

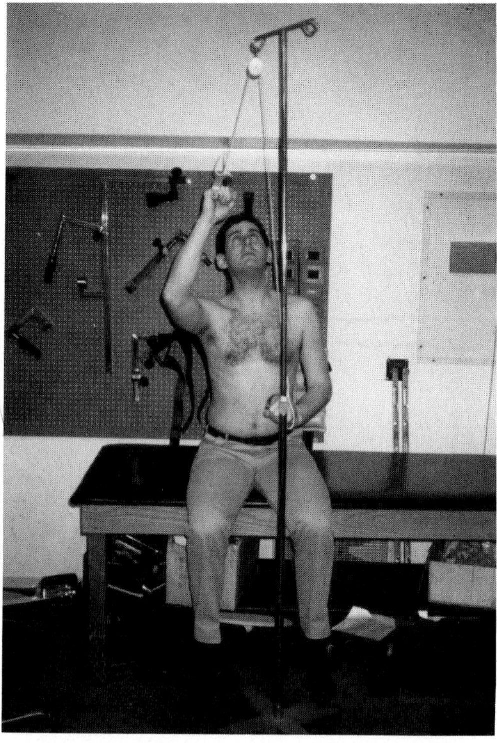

FIG. 11-5. A pulley powered by the uninvolved left arm stretches the right shoulder in total elevation.

and discomfort, as well as the length of time immobilization is needed for healing of soft tissue and/or bone. This phase of rehabilitation generally takes 2 to 3 weeks to complete, but may require up to 6 weeks.

Phase II

Phase II of the shoulder program concentrates on obtaining full, painless range of motion. Any anticipated limitations of motion after a particular injury or surgical procedure should be understood. Aggressive attempts to overcome these limitations may not be appropriate and could cause undue discomfort during rehabilitation.

During this phase of rehabilitation, the therapist works closely with the athlete, using passive-assisted (the therapist or the patient's uninvolved arm passively stretches the injured shoulder) stretching range of motion techniques (Figs. 11-4 to 11-7). This removes any residual shoulder stiffness that resulted from the injury and immobilization. The athlete must be aware that, unlike other aspects of physical therapy, passive-assisted stretching causes some discomfort. Tolerance varies with each individual. To encourage patient participation and minimize discomfort, heat is applied to the shoulder for 10 to 15 minutes before the stretching sessions. Additionally, (TENS) and, more recently, neuromuscular electrical stimulation techniques[2] have been reported to assist in relaxing the patient during maximal soft tissue stretches. Toward the end of a stretching session, heat is applied to the shoulder girdle for 10 minutes; this is followed by the passive stretch being manually sustained during the cooling period to ensure that the motion gained during treatment is not lost.[25] Also, brief, frequent stretching sessions rather than prolonged periods are emphasized.

Since the range of shoulder motion is so extensive, the therapist must regain motion in an orderly manner. Predictably good results continue to be obtained with warm-up pendulum range of motion exercises, followed by passive-assisted stretching in the cardinal planes of total elevation, external rotation with the arm at the side, and internal rotation[22] (Figs. 11-8 to 11-11). Any later stiffness at the extremes of adduction must be eliminated (Fig. 11-12), as well as any residual stiffness that restricts full external rotation at 90 degrees of abduction (Fig. 11-13).

Throughout phase II of the shoulder program, the therapist can use the motion of the uninvolved shoulder as a standard of comparison for the gains achieved after therapy. For optimal function, *the goal of rehabilita-*

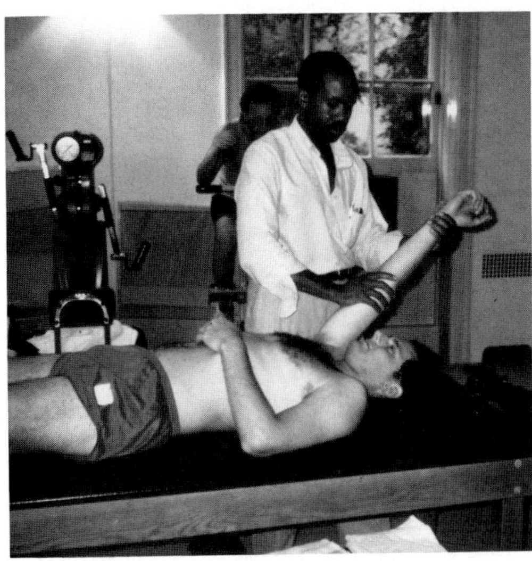

FIG. 11-6. Total elevation stretching assisted by a therapist.

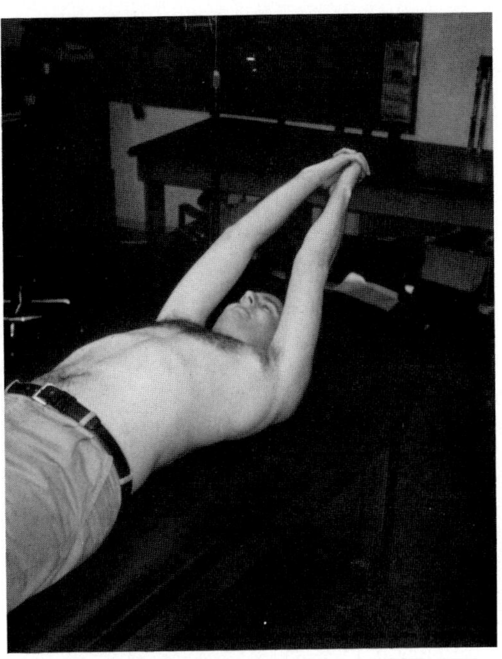

FIG. 11-7. Supine forward elevation stretching of the right shoulder provided by the left, uninvolved, arm.

tion should be to achieve nearly symmetric range of motion in all planes of the shoulder. Nonetheless, with knowledge of the athlete's specific shoulder injury or surgical procedure, it may be desirable to limit a particular shoulder motion. For example, after an anterior dislocation, imposing a mild (10-degree) restriction of motion at the extreme of external rotation may discourage recurrent instability. Similarly, it must be recognized that many athletes involved in sports that require throwing have excessive external rotation of the dominant shoulder with a concomitant loss of internal rotation. This asymmetry may not be pathologic.

On completion of phase II stretching, the athlete enters phase III of the program, which is directed at progressive strengthening.

Phase II

- Passive-assisted range of motion
- Heat
- TENS
- Neuromuscular stimulation

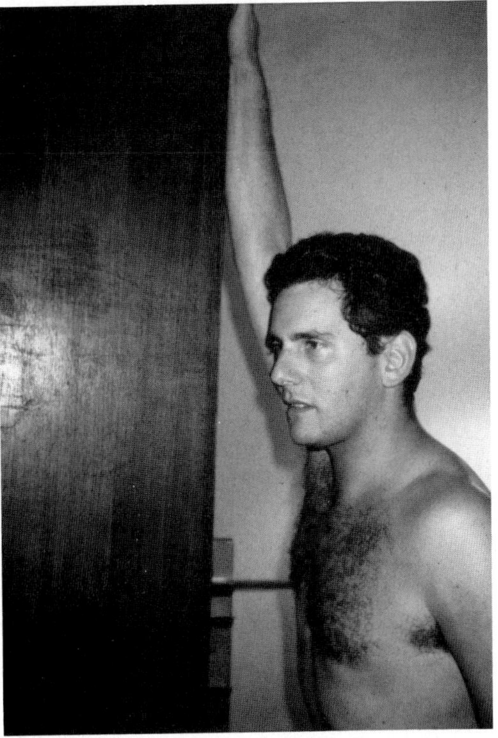

FIG. 11-8. Advanced total elevation stretching by leaning against a door edge.

Phase III

Phase II initially emphasizes strengthening against resistance (isometric), followed by ad-

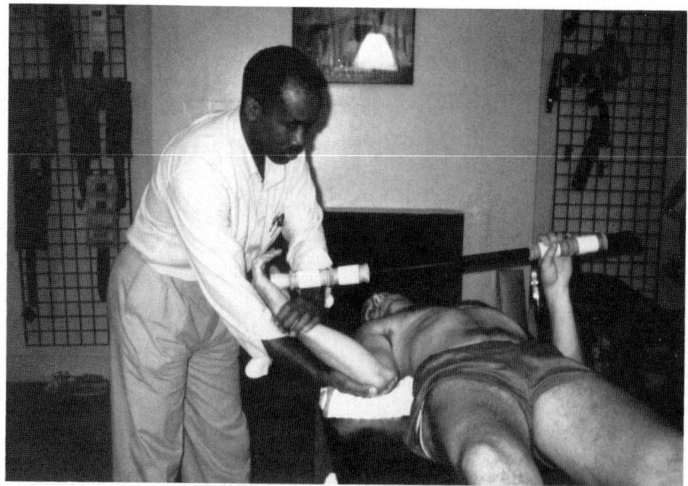

FIG. 11-9. Supine external rotation stretching of the right shoulder with a stick powered by the uninvolved arm or a therapist. A small pillow under the elbow maintains the humerus in the midcoronal plane.

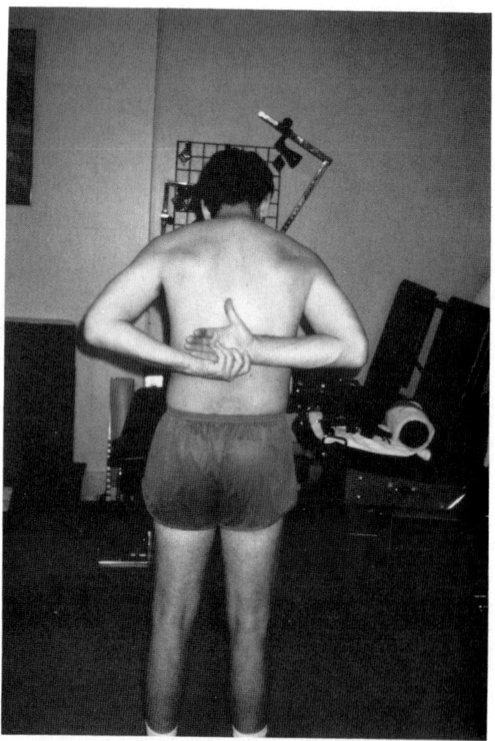

FIG. 11-10. Internal rotation stretching of the right shoulder assisted by the uninvolved left arm.

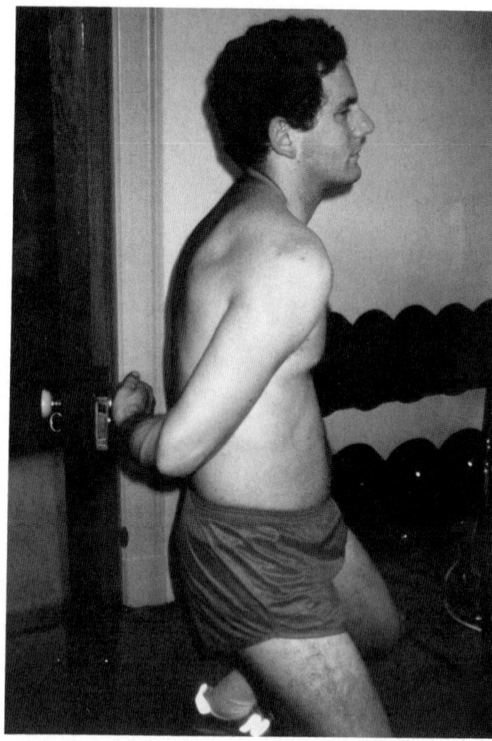

FIG. 11-11. Advanced internal rotation stretching of the shoulder performed by holding a doorknob along the center line of the back and then squatting.

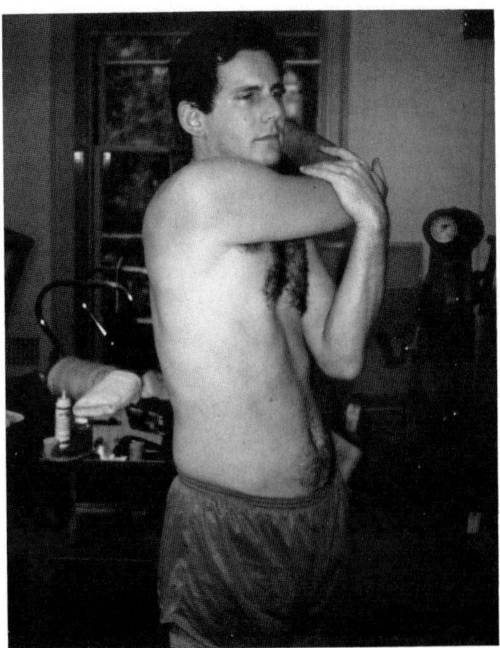

FIG. 11-12. Stretching the posterior right shoulder soft tissues in adduction with a hugging motion powered by the uninvolved left arm.

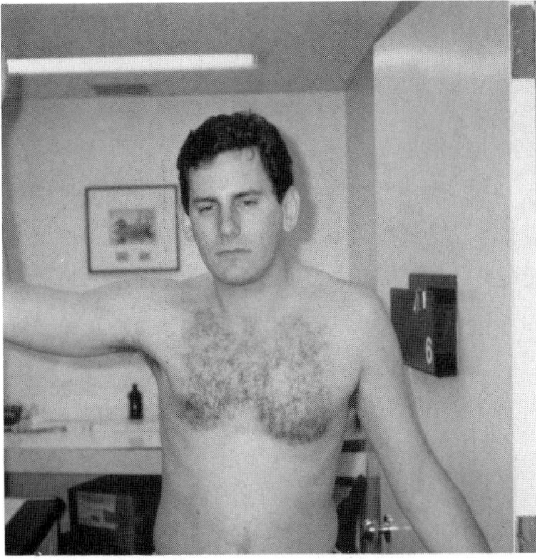

FIG. 11-13. Terminal stretching in 90 degrees of abduction and external rotation can be achieved by leaning in a doorway. This exercise must be used cautiously because it can encourage instability.

vanced (isotonic and isokinetic) strengthening. Each muscle of the rotator cuff should be individually strengthened[13] to facilitate optimal recovery. During phase III, the athlete must perform a gentle daily shoulder stretch in the previously noted cardinal planes of motion to ensure that the range of motion is maintained.

During phase II—as recovery allows—**isometric exercises** are instituted for the internal rotators and adductors, external rotators, abductors, anterior and posterior deltoid muscles, biceps and triceps brachii muscles, and the scapula-stabilizing muscles of the shoulder. This group of exercises is usually performed 10 to 20 times, each with a 5-second contraction and a 2- to 3-second relaxation. The uninvolved extremity and/or a wall is used to resist the contraction. The entire group of shoulder isometrics can generally be performed three times a day.

When the athlete's performance with the isometric contractions improves, the patient then progresses to phase III, with **isotonic strengthening exercises** using surgical tubing or free weights (Figs. 11-14 to 11-19). These exercises are generally most effective if performed slowly and, initially, in the underhorizontal shoulder planes. To promote rhythmic scapula motion and avoid substitution maneuvers, the patient is closely observed during each eccentric and concentric contraction. Short-term discomfort caused by muscle fatigue is acceptable and can be used as a guide to determine the number and frequency of exercise repetitions to be performed. Prolonged discomfort, precipitated by excessive repetitions of exercises or by a particular exercise, should be avoided.

Isometric exercises are performed for all the muscles of the rotator cuff and the surrounding shoulder and scapula muscles. An easy isometric exercise is the "T" exercise, which is performed under the horizontal plane and avoids excessive weight.

As performance increases with isotonic strengthening; the therapist introduces **isokinetic training,** which permits limb exercise at both slow and fast velocities. Slow speeds will focus on residual strength deficits, whereas high-speed training will enhance power and endurance[15,34] (Figs. 11-20 to 11-22). The therapist begins with the underhorizontal planes of motion, then progresses into the cardinal and diagonal planes. The diagonal motions are in functional planes and closely simulate patterns that are necessary for everyday activities[5,32] (Fig. 11-23).

Throughout the isokinetic strengthening period, but on alternate days, the athlete continues more advanced isotonic training in similar planes with free weights or with a Nautilus-type machine. During the advanced strengthening program, continued close supervision is warranted to further encourage

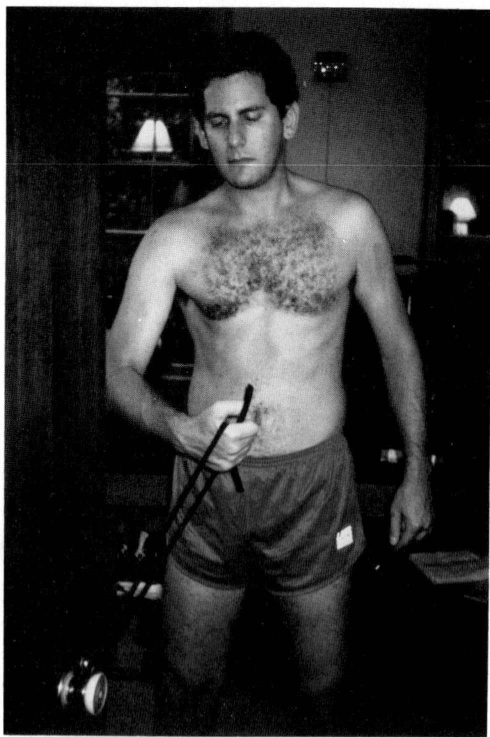

FIG. 11-14. Internal rotators are strengthened using elastic tubing on a doorknob.

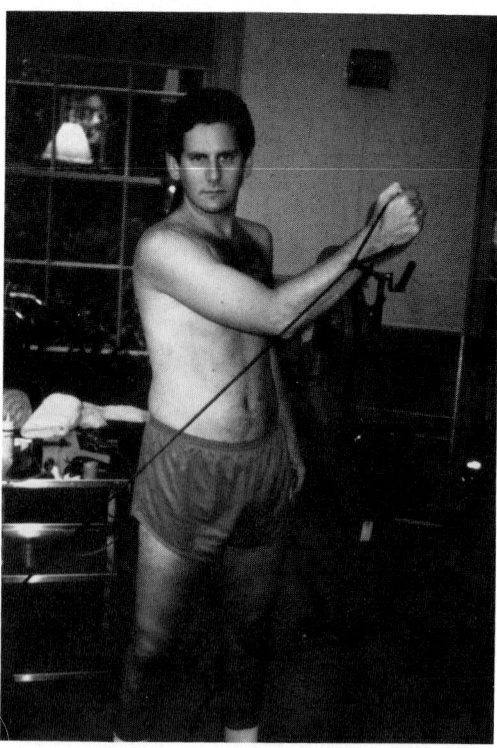

FIG. 11-15. Adductors and internal rotators are strengthened by pulling the elastic tubing across the chest toward the opposite arm.

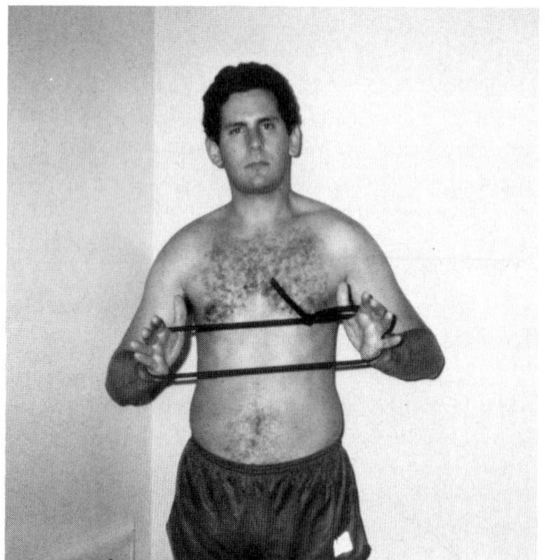

FIG. 11-16. Right shoulder external rotators and abductors are strengthened using the elastic tubing as well as the uninvolved arm.

normal, rhythmic scapular motions.

Generally during this period, the athlete's strength is sufficient to allow limited participation in sports activities. During this period, the athlete's return to sports is monitored and adjusted as progress allows. When clinical examination and strength testing indicate excellent strength has been achieved, the athlete is allowed to return to full activity and continues preinjury conditioning and strength maintenance program.

Phase III

- Maintenance of range of motion with daily stretching
- Isometric exercises
- Isotonic/isokinetic exercises
- Monitoring of progressive return to sports

REHABILITATION OF COMMON SHOULDER INJURIES

Anterior Shoulder Instability

Nonoperative Program

After an anterior/inferior dislocation is reduced or following a traumatic subluxation, assuming no earlier history of instability, rehabilitation should be instituted. Recognizing that the glenohumeral ligaments, capsule, and surrounding musculature have been stretched by the trauma, phase I of the treat-

A 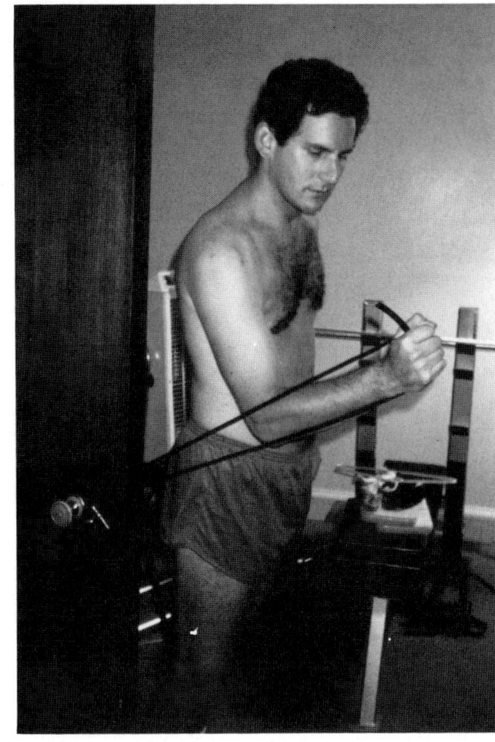

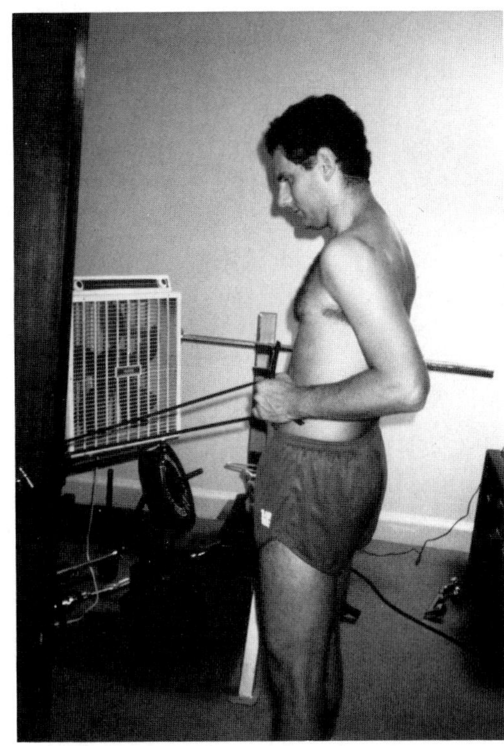 B

FIG. 11-17. Anterior and posterior deltoid muscles are strengthened by **A,** pushing or **B,** pulling the elastic tubing which is anchored on a doorknob.

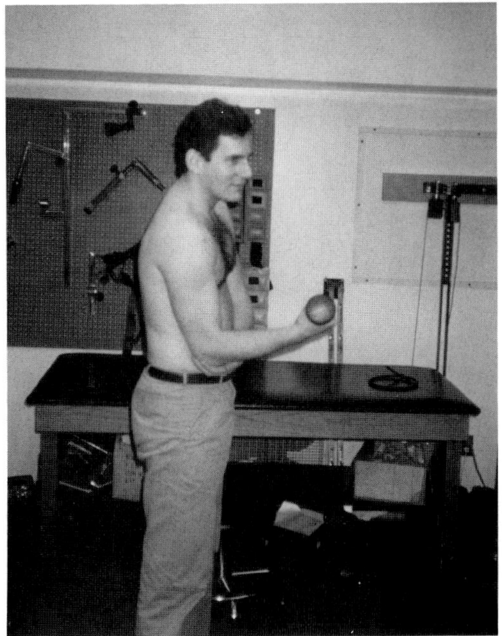

FIG. 11-18. Biceps brachi strengthening can be accomplished with a free weight.

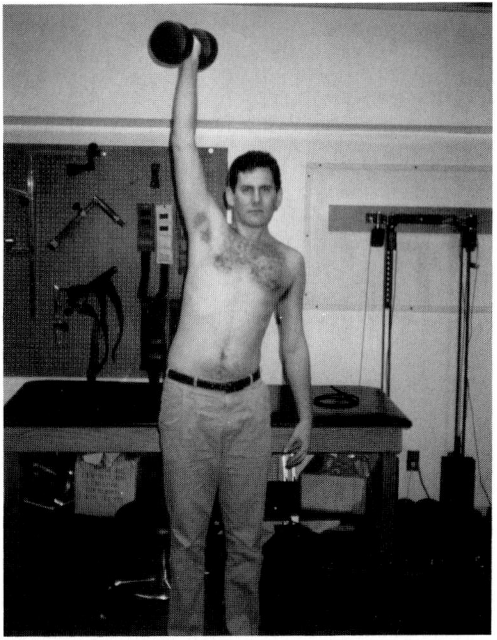

FIG. 11-19. As strength improves, free weights are used in over horizontal planes.

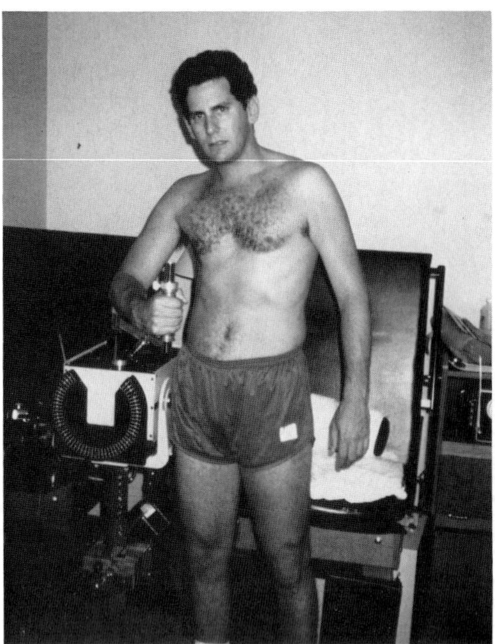

FIG. 11-20. Isokinetic strengthening of the internal rotator muscles.

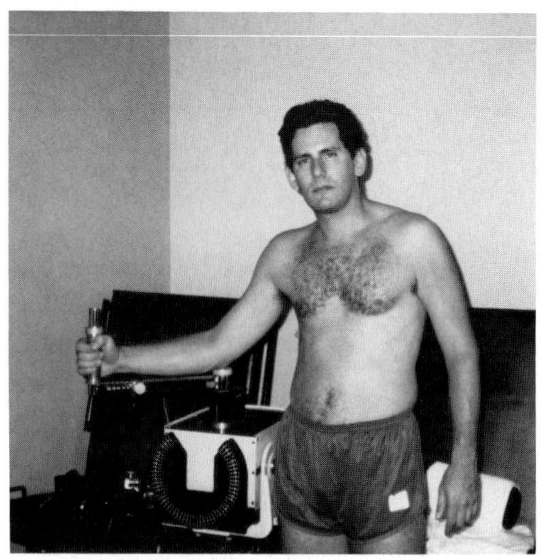

FIG. 11-21. Isokinetic strengthening of the external rotator muscles.

ment emphasizes immobilization with a sling and swathe. Application of ice decreases tissue edema and hemorrhage, and gentle isometric exercises for the elbow, wrist, and hand are initiated while the shoulder is immobilized.

The period of immobilization after glenohumeral dislocations is a topic of considerable debate, and reports range from 0 to 6 weeks.* Additionally, there is evidence that the age of the patient at the time of the first dislocation considerably influences the overall recurrance rate of instability, with rates reported as high as 85% to 90% for patients less than 20 years of age.[29] A well-planned rehabilitation program, however, can decrease the recurrance rate to as low as 25%.[1] In our experience, for best results, the athlete's shoulder should be immobilized from 4 to 6 weeks, depending on his or her age, the sport to which he or she must return, the degree to which the injured shoulder is involved in the sport, and the amount of clinical laxity of the uninvolved shoulder.

During the period of immobilization and when the discomfort allows, isometric contractions of the shoulder musculature are initated within the patient's tolerance. Throughout this period the athlete is instructed to maintain the axis of his or her arm anterior to the midcoronal plane of the body, so as not to encourage anterior instability. On completion of the immobilization period, phase II is initiated, with concentration on gentle, passive, assisted stretching exercises to regain the range of motion.

During phase II, emphasis is placed on the gentle nature of the exercises because these shoulders tend to regain motion rapidly. Progress is enhanced when stretching exercises are supplemented with other soft tissue treatment modalities, such as ice, heat, and TENS. The goals of phase II should be to provide the athlete with painless, full total elevation, full internal rotation, and, ideally, a mild (10-degree) limitation of external rotation with the arm at the side.

The athlete then enters phase III. Strengthening exercises should begin from the underhorizontal position. This encourages stability and diminishes mechanical irritation from the injured capsule and ligaments.[21] The internal rotators are emphasized because

*References 9, 11, 23, 27, 28, 30.

A

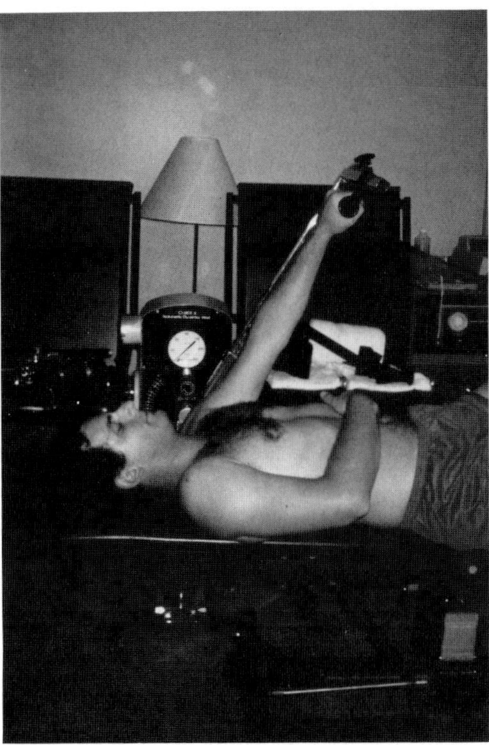

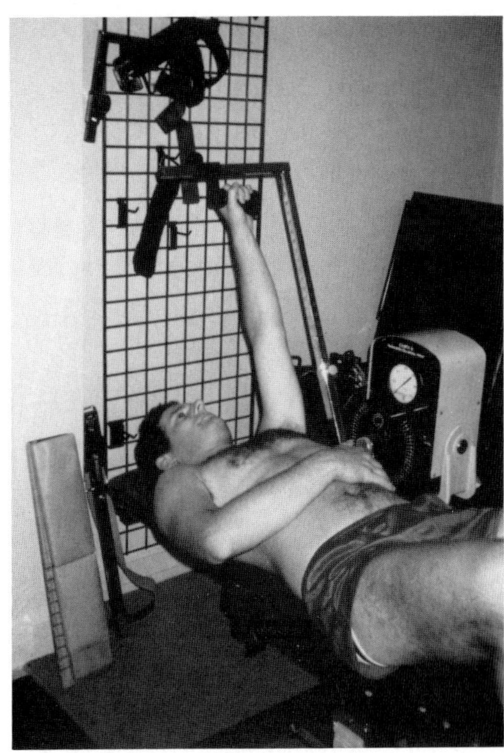

B

FIG. 11-22. Isokinetic strengthening in **A,** forward flexion and **B,** total elevation.

Conservative management after acute anterior dislocation

- Phase I
  - Sling
  - Ice
  - Gentle isometrics for the elbow, wrist, and hand
  - Isometric shoulder work (when comfortable)
  - Aerobic work
- Phase II
  - Gentle range-of-motion
  - Limitation of external rotation
  - Ice
  - TENS
  - Continuation of isometrics
  - Aerobic work
- Phase III
  - *Early*
    - Strength under horizontal plane
    - Emphasis on internal rotators
  - *Mid*
    - Addition of external rotators and shoulder girdle to strength program
    - Initiation of isokinetic work in cardinal planes of motion
  - *Late*
    - Diagonal and sport-specific strength program
    - Endurance work
    - Monitored progressive return to sports

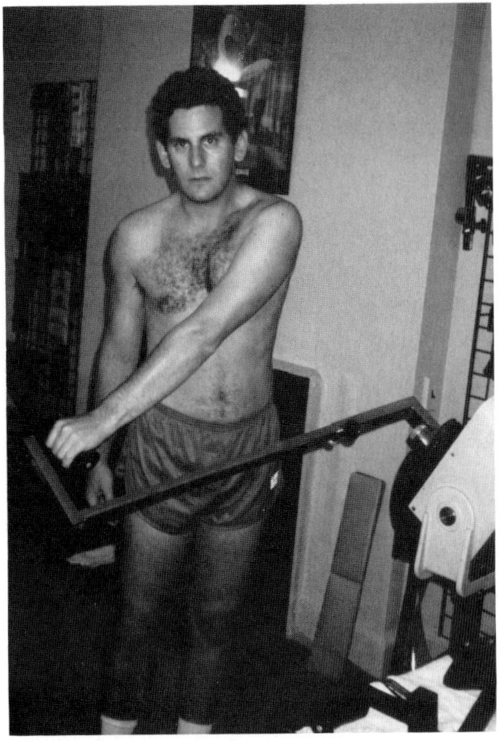

FIG. 11-23. Isokinetic strengthening in diagonal planes of function.

these are the most effective dynamic restraints against anterior instability in the middle to lower ranges of abduction.[4,31] As progress is made, strengthening proceeds to include the external rotators and remaining shoulder musculature. Progressive strengthening is initially used isotonically in the cardinal planes of motion and then advanced isokinetically to the cardinal and diagonal planes of motion.

Before initiation of full, unprotected activity of the arm, the range of motion of the shoulder must be painless, with good strength and endurance as compared to the uninvolved arm. Furthermore, sufficient external rotation at 90 degrees of abduction (the position at which the shoulder is generally most vulnerable to anterior instability) should be obtained without apprehension to allow comfortable participation in the athlete's particular sport. The period of recovery through phases II and III can vary from 6 weeks to 4 months.

Postoperative Program

The principles of rehabilitation of the surgically repaired shoulder against anterior instability are similar to those for the nonsurgically treated shoulder. Modifications depend on the type of procedure used, the time necessary for maturation of the repair, and any imposed motion limitations that are innate to the procedure. As previously noted, progression through all phases can vary and full rehabilitation is generally obtained within 6 months to 1 year.

In our experience,[16] the modified Neer inferior capsular shift repair for anterior instability, supplemented with repair of a detached labrum if present, and bone grafting of a significant glenoid deficiency, has been used in treatment of athletes and yields a high degree of success. The shoulder is generally immobilized in a sling for 6 weeks. Isometric exercises for the elbow, wrist, and hand are used during this period. Thereafter, immobilization by sling is discontinued, and the rehabilitation progresses as previously discussed for the nonsurgically treated athlete after an anterior dislocation. Full, unrestricted use of the arm is generally allowed 9 months after surgery. The average athlete, before resumption of full activity, has regained full total elevation, full internal rotation, and generally lacks 10 degrees of external rotation with the arm at the side. Shoulder strength and endurance are regained without apprehension.

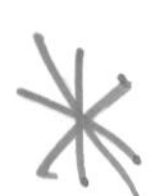

Impingement Syndromes

The impingement syndrome has been characterized as a mechanical compression of the rotator cuff tendons beneath the subacromial arch.[19] In our experience, this syndrome occurs in athletes[3,8,17,23] and can result in a progression of stages, from an acute hemorrhagic, engorged bursitis and tendonitis (stage 1), to a recurrent fibrotic bursitis and tendonitis (stage 2), and finally, to a rotator cuff tear (stage 3).[20] The etiologic cause in most athletes is attributed to microtrauma from activities involving repetitive movement of the arms above the head. Less frequently, macrotraumatic shoulder injuries resulting in recurrent bursitis or in an actual rotator cuff tear have been recognized.

Criteria for return to play

- Painless range of motion
- Strength/endurance parity
- Sufficient external rotation at 90-degree abduction without apprehension

Stages 1 and 2

Nonsurgical treatment of stages 1 and 2 impingement syndromes is generally successful and is based on decreasing rotator cuff inflammation and increasing the strength of the shoulder musculature. As the soft tissue inflammation of the bursa and tendons decreases, their volume effectively decreases, thus encouraging excursion without impingement. Similarly, by strengthening the rotator cuff muscles and the scapula-stabilizing muscles, a dynamic depressor effect on the humeral head is achieved. This maximizes the size of the subacromial space and further enhances function without impingement.

Phase I rehabilitation for either stage 1 (acute) or stage 2 (recurrent) impingement is essentially the same. To discourage reinjury, the athlete is advised to use the involved arm for only light underhorizontal activities. Shoulder isometric exercises are initiated shortly thereafter. In the more extreme case, immobilization by sling may be necessary for a brief period of 3 to 4 days until soft-tissue inflammation diminishes sufficiently to allow light active underhorizontal use of the arm. Nonsteroidal oral antiinflammatories, ice, TENS, and ultrasound treatments have all been used successfully to expedite the diminishment of inflammation of the bursa and rotator cuff tendons.[8]

Within 10 to 14 days, progress usually permits initiation of phase II rehabilitation, primarily aimed at a gentle daily stretch in the cardinal planes of motion. This will prevent shoulder stiffness at the extremes, and the lack of daily repetitive overhorizontal exercises will not encourage the impingement syndrome. On occasion, the prudent use of a steroid injection into the subacromial space may be warranted to enhance progress through phase I or II. Nevertheless, this latter adjunct should be used with extreme discretion; the potential hazards of steroid injections are well known.

When progress through phase II allows, phase III is concomitantly introduced, with isotonic strengthening exercises in the underhorizontal plane for the internal and external rotators, the scapular stabilizers, and the biceps brachii muscle (a humeral head depressor). As strength improves and the phase II daily range of motion stretching exercises become painless, the patient is advanced to isotonic strengthening exercises in the overhorizontal nonpainful planes of motion.

Finally, the therapist begins isokinetic strengthening exercises using a Cybex isokinetic dynameter with progressive advancement into the cardinal and diagonal (overhorizontal) planes. When satisfactory strength and endurance are achieved with full painless range of shoulder motion, and there is no clinical evidence of impingement, rehabilitation is complete.

On occasion, phase II impingement may be refractory to nonsurgical treatment and an operative decompression of the subacromial space is necessary. Traditionally, this type of surgery has been performed in an open manner.[19] In recent years, stage 2 impingement without acromioclavicular joint involvement has been successfully treated by an arthroscopic decompression,[6,7,17] which does not disturb the origin of the deltoid muscle and allows a more rapid return to competitive athletics.

After an arthroscopic decompression, use of immobilization by sling in phase I is brief. The next morning, use of the sling is discontinued and phase II is begun with pendulum range of motion exercises, and passive-assistive stretching in total elevation, external rotation, and internal rotation. Each exercise is performed 20 times, and the entire group is repeated 5 times daily. Light activities of the arm in all planes are encouraged.

Two weeks after arthroscopic surgery, the phase II program is advanced to include stretching in any areas of residual stiffness. Phase III is introduced, with elastic tubing underhorizontal strengthening exercises for the internal and external rotators.

Six weeks after arthroscopy, phase III strengthening is advanced as tolerated. Although complete rehabilitation may require up to 6 months for the higher level athlete, throughout this period, progressive participation in sports that involve repetitive, overhead arm movement is well tolerated.

Stage 3

The conservative treatment of stage 3 subacromial impingement parallels stages 1 and 2. If this approach is unsuccessful, a surgical, open decompression and repair of the rotator cuff tear is recommended.[8,33]

Postoperatively, after sling and swathe immobilization (phase I) for approximately 24 to 48 hours, phase II is begun with pendulum exercises. As patient tolerance allows, passive-assistive total elevation with a pulley, supine external rotation stretching with a stick, and internal rotation stretching exercises are implemented. All four exercises are performed 20 times each, with four to five sessions daily. Throughout this period of phase II, the use of analgesics and the application of heat to the shoulder for 10-minute intervals before and after exercising improve overall patient compliance and performance. The patient is instructed to wear a sling between exercise sessions and while sleeping. Isometrics are used for the elbow, wrist, and hand.

Six weeks postoperatively, phase II passive-assistive stretching exercises are advanced to include supine elevation with and without abduction, and more aggressive internal rotation stretching. The goal of phase II should be to obtain full passive motion in all planes by 3 months. This allows the rotator cuff and deltoid muscle repairs to adequately mature before initiation of active exercises.

Three months after surgery, use of the sling is discontinued and phase III exercises are introduced with shoulder isometrics. The patient is encouraged to use the arm actively in overhead arm movement for natural activities of daily living, without the use of weights. Four and a half months after repair, progress generally allows isotonic strengthening, followed by an isokinetic program as patient tolerance permits.

If the rotator cuff tear was a particularly large one, the rehabilitation program is initially modified by placing the patient in an abduction brace immediately after surgery. Within 48 hours, pulley exercises are begun with the brace in place. Six weeks after repair, the brace is removed and phase II is progressed as previously outlined to include pendulum, external rotation with the stick, and internal rotation stretching exercises. The use of the abduction brace in this manner delays the overall program by 6 weeks. Complete rehabilitation after a stage 3 surgical repair generally takes 9 to 12 months.

SUMMARY

Perhaps because of the emphasis in our society on sports that involve the upper extremities, the shoulder continues to be susceptible to injury. A carefully organized and thorough rehabilitation program can often lead to a more expedient return to athletics and perhaps extend the athlete's career.

The rehabilitation process can be divided into three phases. Phase I deals with the immediate postinjury period, in which immobilization allows for the reduction of inflammation and discomfort, and isometrics are used to maintain muscle tone. The athlete then enters phase II, which focuses primarily on regaining passive range of motion. Finally, phase III emphasizes progressive strengthening by use of isotonic and isokinetic techniques.

Once full range of motion and normal strength have been achieved, the athlete can return to competition without restrictions. A premature return can lead to reinjury or injury of another area as the athlete changes form in an attempt to compensate.

REFERENCES

1. Aronen JG and Regan K: Decreasing the incident of recurrence of first time anterior shoulder dislocations with rehabilitation, Am J Sports Med 12:283, 1984.
2. Baker LL and Parker K: Neuromuscular electrical stimulation of the muscles surrounding the shoulder, Phys Ther 66:1930, 1986.
3. Ciuillo JV: Swimmers shoulder, Clin Sports Med 5:115, 1986.
4. Derscheid G: Rehabilitation of common orthopedic problems, Nurs Clin of North Am 16:709, 1981.
5. Einhorn AR and Jackson DW: Rehabilitation of the shoulder in shoulder surgery in the athlete, Baltimore, 1985, University Park Press.
6. Ellman H: Arthroscopic subacromial decompression: analysis of one to three year results, Arthroscopy 3:173, 1987.
7. Gartsman GM: Arthroscopic subacromial decompression: a clinical study, AAOS Meeting, Atlanta, February 7, 1988.
8. Hawkins RJ and Kennedy JC: Impingement syndrome in athletes, Am J Sports Med 8:151, 1980.
9. Henry JH and Genung JA: Natural history of glenohumeral dislocated—revisited, Am J Sports Med 10:135, 1982.
10. Hill JA: Epidemiologic perspective on shoulder injuries, Clin Sports Med 2:241, 1983.
11. Hovelius L et al: Recurrence after initial dislocation of the shoulder, J Bone Joint Surg 65A:343, 1983.
12. Jobe FW and Jobe CM: Painful athletic injuries of the shoulder, Clin Orthop, 173:117, 1983.
13. Jobe FW and Moynes DR: Delineation of diagnostic criteria and a rehabilitation program for rotation cuff injuries, Am J Sports Med 10:336, 1982.
14. Kennedy JC and Willis RB: The effects of local steroid injections on tendons: a biomechanical and microscopic corrective study, Am J Sports Med 4:11, 1976.
15. Leffert RD and Harris BA: The role of physical therapy in rehabilitation of the shoulder. In Rowe CR editor: The shoulder, New York, 1988, Churchill Livingstone.
16. Mendoza FX, Nicholas JA, and Reilly JP: Neer inferior capsular shift repair for anterior glenohumeral instability, Orthop Trans 10:221, 1986.
17. Mendoza FX et al: The arthroscopic treatment of subacromial impingement, Clin Sports Med 6:573, 1987.
18. Moynes DR: Prevention of injury to the shoulder through exercise and therapy, Clin Sports Med 2:413, 1983.
19. Neer CS: Anterior acromioplasty for the chronic impingement syndrome in the shoulder: a preliminary report, J Bone Joint Surg 54A:41, 1972.
20. Neer CS: Impingement lesions, Clin Orthop 173:70, 1983.
21. Neer CS and Foster CR: Inferior capsular shift for involuntary inferior and multidirectional instability of the shoulder, J Bone Joint Surg 62A:897, 1980.
22. Neer CS and Hugh M: Glenohumeral joint replacement and post-operative rehabilitation, Phys Ther 55:850, 1975.
23. Neer CS and Welsh RP: The shoulder in sports, Orthop Clin North Am 8:583, 1977.
24. Nicholas JA et al: The importance of a simplified classification of motion in sports in relation to performance, Orthop Clin North Am 8:499, 1977.
25. Nitz AJ: Physical therapy management of the shoulder, Phys Ther 66:1912, 1986.
26. Roeser WM et al: The use of transcutaneous nerve stimulation for pain control in athletic medicine: a preliminary report, Am J Sports Med 4:210, 1976.
27. Rowe CR: Prognosis in dislocations of the shoulder, J Bone Joint Surg 380A:957, 1956.
28. Rowe C: Acute and recurrent anterior dislocation of the shoulder, Orthop Clin North Am 11:253, 1980.
29. Rowe CR and Sakellarides HT: Factors related to recurrence of anterior dislocations of the shoulder, Clin Orthop 20:40, 1961.
30. Simonet WT and Cofield RH: Prognosis in anterior shoulder dislocations, Am J Sports Med 12:19, 1984.
31. Turkel SJ et al: Stabilizing mechanisms preventing anterior dislocation of the genohumeral joint, J Bone Joint Surg 63A:1208, 1981.
32. Voss DE et al: Proprioceptive neuromuscular facilitation: patterns and techniques, ed 3, Philadelphia, 1985, Harper & Row.
33. Warren RF: Surgical considerations for rotator cuff tears in athletes, Baltimore, 1985, University Park Press.
34. Wooden MJ: Isokinetic evaluation and treatment of the shoulder. In Donatelli R editor: Physical therapy of the shoulder, New York, 1987, Churchill Livingstone.

CHAPTER 12 Shoulder Equipment

Robert C. Reese, Jr.
T. Pepper Burruss
Joseph Patten

Shoulder pads
Upper arm padding
Shoulder harness

SHOULDER PADS

The shoulder region is often a point of contact in sports. Contact can occur between an athlete's shoulder and another athlete or an object such as a piece of equipment or a playing surface.

Shoulder pads are among the most common pieces of protective equipment used in contact sports. They are designed to protect the shoulder by covering the middle and lateral portions of the clavicle, the acromion, scapular body, and proximal humerus. The area protected will depend greatly on the style and trim of the specific pads used (Fig. 12-1).

There is a great variety of configurations and sizes in shoulder padding. Pads are generally sport specific, but even within sports, shoulder pads can vary by player position and individual requirements. By far the sports that most commonly use shoulder pads are football, hockey, and lacrosse.

In football, the largest pads are often worn by linebackers, who require protection to the shoulder region because of their role as tacklers. They contact opposing players with the shoulder as the point of impact, and the shoulder pads, if appropriate in size and configuration, can protect the region from most contusions and other direct-contact injuries. In contrast, quarterbacks and wide receivers require mobility in the shoulder and arm and often wear shoulder pads with little bulk that allow extensive mobility.

Proper fitting is essential for shoulder protection, while full range of motion of the shoulders, arms, and neck remains unobstructed. Shoulder pads that are too small can allow portions of the region to go unprotected. Conversely, shoulder pads that are too large do not permit normal shoulder mobility, and this restriction can lead to injury. Care must be taken at all times to fit the shoulder pad in relation to the helmet. Interference can occur between the helmet and shoulder pads if the shoulder pads do not allow room for proper helmet fit and head and neck motion.

Additional padding can be used beneath shoulder pads. These are designed to add further impact protection to the region and are generally one of two types: foam or air (Fig. 12-2). These pads are either applied to the shoulder before the shoulder pads are put on or fastened directly to the pads themselves.

Custom padding can also be created for use with shoulder pads. Customizing techniques are most ofen used when an injured area requires additional protection. For example, strips of foam can be secured to the underside of a shoulder pad just anteroposterior to the acromioclavicular (AC) joint (Fig. 12-3). These strips provide relief to the AC joint and can permit the athlete to return to competition with additional protective padding. An alternative to the strips of foam is a high density foam donut. This can be applied directly over the AC joint, either by using adhesive elastic tape or an elastic bandage. Hard shells fabricated from Orthoplast or other thermomoldable plastics can be made for the same purpose and taped directly to the shoulder.

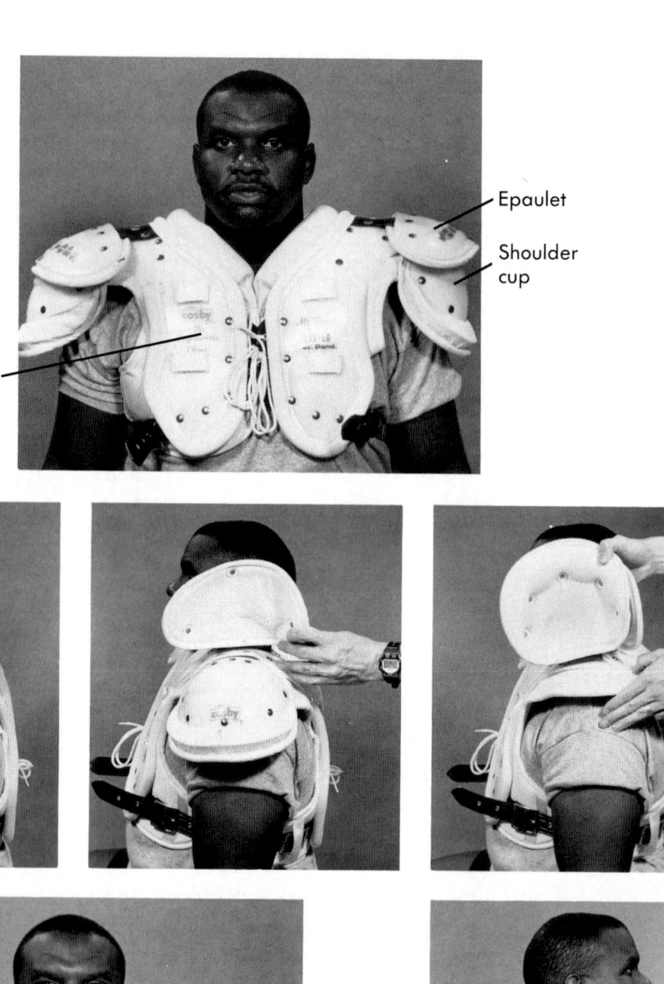

FIG. 12-1. Shoulder pads.

A 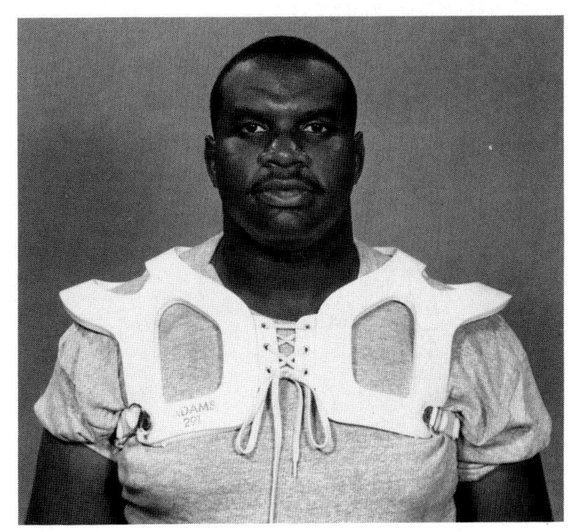

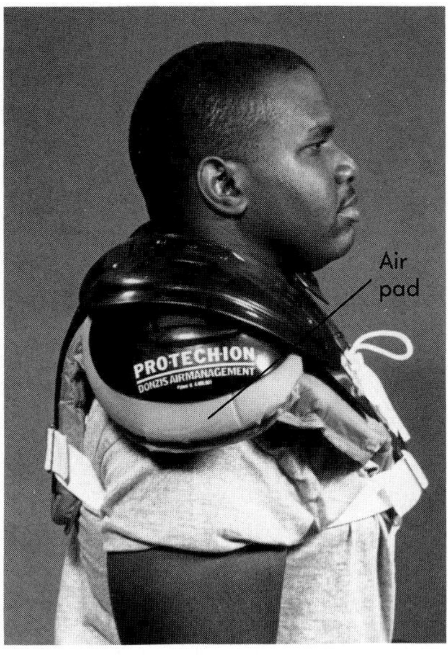

B

FIG. 12-2. Supplemental pads. **A,** Foam. **B,** Air. These go beneath shoulder pads to provide additional protection to the shoulder region.

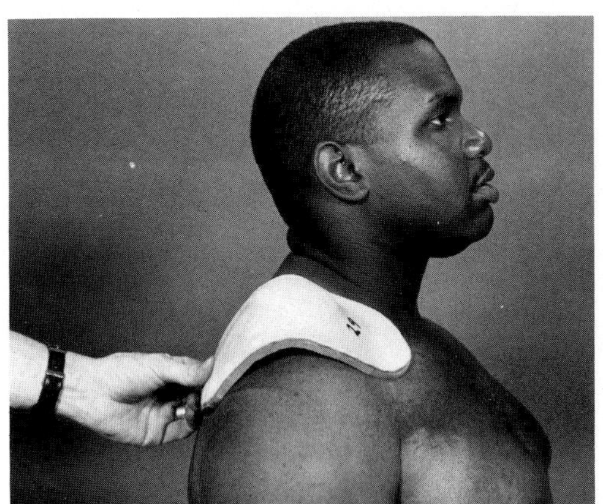

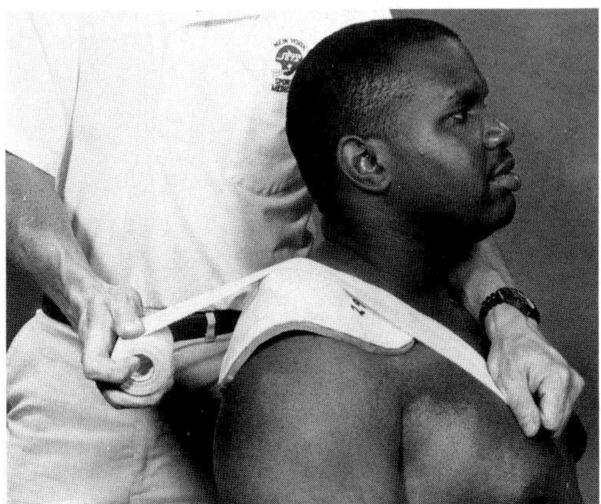

FIG. 12-3. Customized foam is placed on the underside of the shoulder pad to provide additional protection.

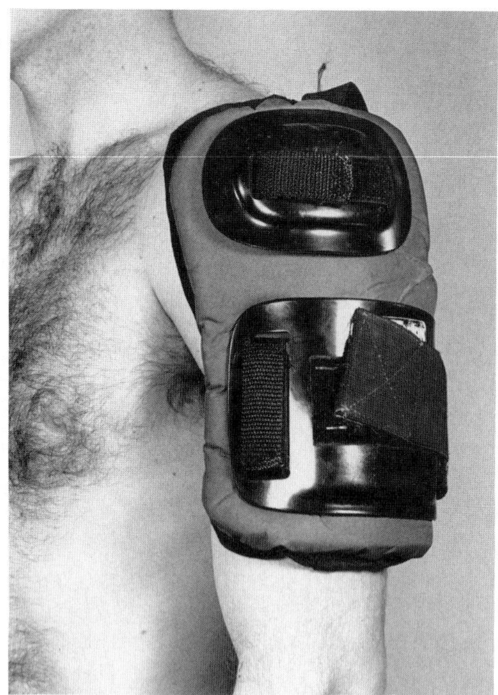

FIG. 12-4. A deltoid pad provides additional protection to the lateral arm.

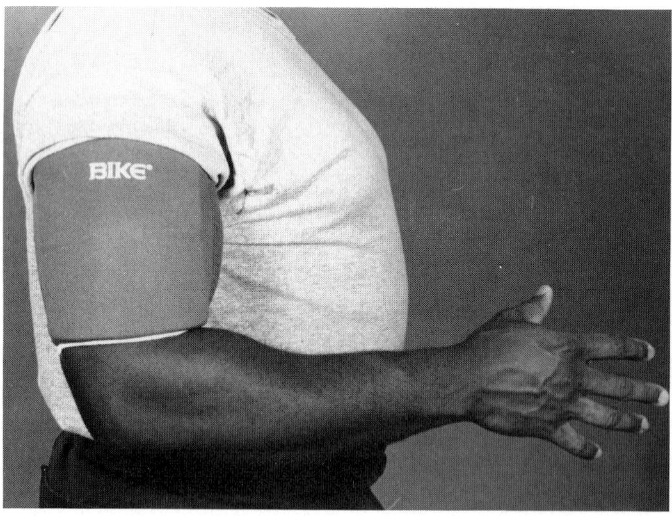

FIG. 12-5. An elastic knee sleeve can provide extra padding to the anterior or posterior arm.

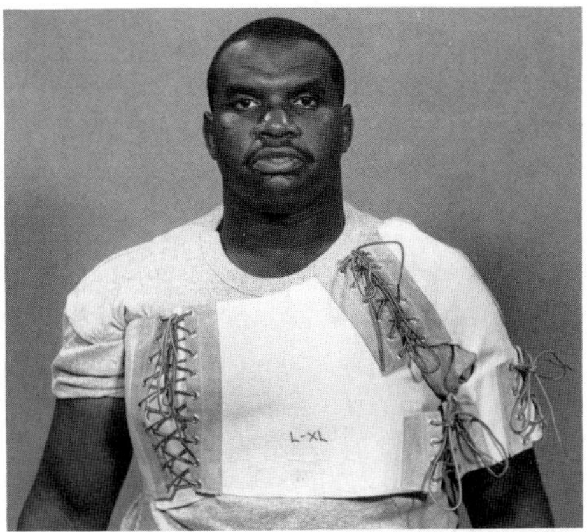

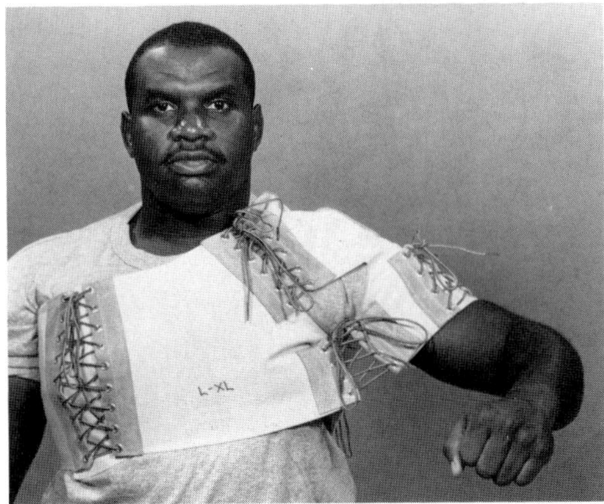

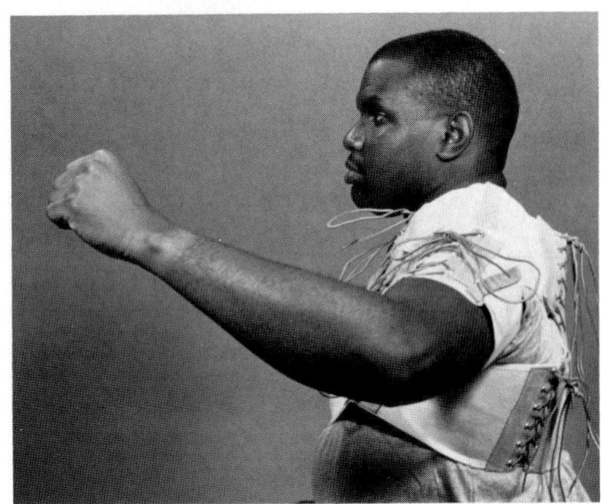

FIG. 12-6. Shoulder harness.

UPPER ARM PADDING

In general, shoulder pads provide sufficient protection for the upper arm. Areas that can sustain injury are the distal deltoid and the proximal and middle thirds of the biceps or triceps. Contusions can occur at the edge of the standard shoulder pads and, if repeated extensive muscle contusion continues, myositis ossificans can result. These areas of ossification can be quite tender and require additional protective padding. Often, firm areas called "blocker's nodes" develop at the site of injury, usually in the lateral aspect of the upper arm.

If additional protection is required at the deltoid insertion, an extension can be added to the standard shoulder pads (Fig. 12-4). It is difficult to protect the anterior or posterior portion of the arm with a hard protective shell. If padding is required in these regions, an elastic knee pad can prove invaluable. These pads can be slipped up the arm and placed over the injured region (Fig. 12-5). Their flexibility permits continued unrestricted motion in the area.

SHOULDER HARNESS

Chronic anterior shoulder instability can, at times, be managed nonoperatively. One of the cornerstones of this treatment is aggressive internal rotator muscle strengthening to assist in maintaining shoulder stability. In contact sports, however, abduction and external rotation forces that exceed the strength of the muscular and capsular restraints can occur at the shoulder. The shoulder harness is a piece of equipment that can be used as an adjunct in the treatment of anterior shoulder instability.

The basic principle of the shoulder harness is that shoulder instability can be controlled by avoiding abduction and external rotation of the shoulder. The design of the harness includes a chest vest, a shoulder cap, and a biceps cuff.

One commercially available harness is the C.D. Denison–Duke Wyre shoulder vest (Fig. 12-6). The brace was developed in the mid-1950s by the late Duke Wyre, former head athletic trainer at the University of Maryland, in conjunction with the late Cedric Denison, former president and chief orthotist of C.D. Denison. At that time, each brace was fabricated to custom-fit the individual athlete. In 1961, standard sizes and designs of the vest were developed and the brace was marketed throughout the United States. The design has remained constant through the years, the only change being the replacement of rawhide laces with nylon nonstretch laces.

The main controlling feature of the harness is the lacing that connects the chest vest to the biceps cuff. This lacing is a direct restraint to shoulder abduction. The degree of limitation can be adjusted by varying the tension of the laces running from the chest to the biceps cuff. In addition, the shoulder cap also is laced to the chest vest, adding additional limitation to abduction and extension range of motion.

These vests come in a variety of standard sizes based on chest and biceps circumference. Right, left, or bilateral models are available. The harness is fitted to the individual; the laces are used to adjust the biceps cuff and the shoulder cap to the chest vest. The degrees of control can be varied by tightening or loosening the various laces. To prevent skin irritation from the vest, the athlete should consider wearing a well-fitted cotton T-shirt beneath the vest.

PART III Elbow

CHAPTER 13 Anatomy and Physical Examination of the Elbow

Thomas E. Anderson

ANATOMY

Surface Anatomy

The superficial anatomy about the elbow is dominated by the bony prominences and the shape of the predominant musculature. The bony prominences include the readily palpable medial and lateral epicondyle as well as the olecranon tip. In the midportion of the arm, the lateral margin and medial margin of the humeral shaft can be palpated. As one nears the elbow, the humerus wings, with the epicondyles being much more distinct. The palpable muscles (Figs. 13-1 and 13-2) include the biceps anteriorly and the biceps tendon and its aponeurosis (lacertus fibrosus) extending medially. The aponeurosis can often be followed distally and medially as it blends with the medial fascia of the forearm. Anteriorly, the brachialis muscle is not readily palpable because of its deep location beneath the biceps muscle and tendon.

Laterally and slightly distal is the extensor muscle group of the forearm. This group, or mobile wad as it is sometimes called,[14] is readily palpable as a group of muscles originating from the lateral distal humerus and epicondyle. The group includes the brachioradialis, extensor carpi radialis longus, and extensor carpi radialis brevis. Just distal to the epicondyle is the tendinous portion of the extensor carpi radialis longus and brevis musculature and the extensor digitorum musculature. The transition between the muscle and tendinous portion is not palpable.

Mobile wad extensors

- Brachioradialis
- Extensor carpi radialis longus
- Extensor carpi radialis brevis

Medially, the flexor pronator muscle group, coming from the medial epicondyle, is also readily palpable. At the proximal portion is a common flexor tendon originating on the medial epicondyle. This group includes the pronator teres, flexor carpi radialis, palmaris longus, and flexor carpi ulnaris. The palmaris longus is absent in 14% of limbs. It may also be present in one forearm and absent in the contralateral forearm.[3]

Flexor pronator muscle group

- Pronator teres
- Flexor carpi radialis
- Palmaris longus
- Flexor carpi ulnaris

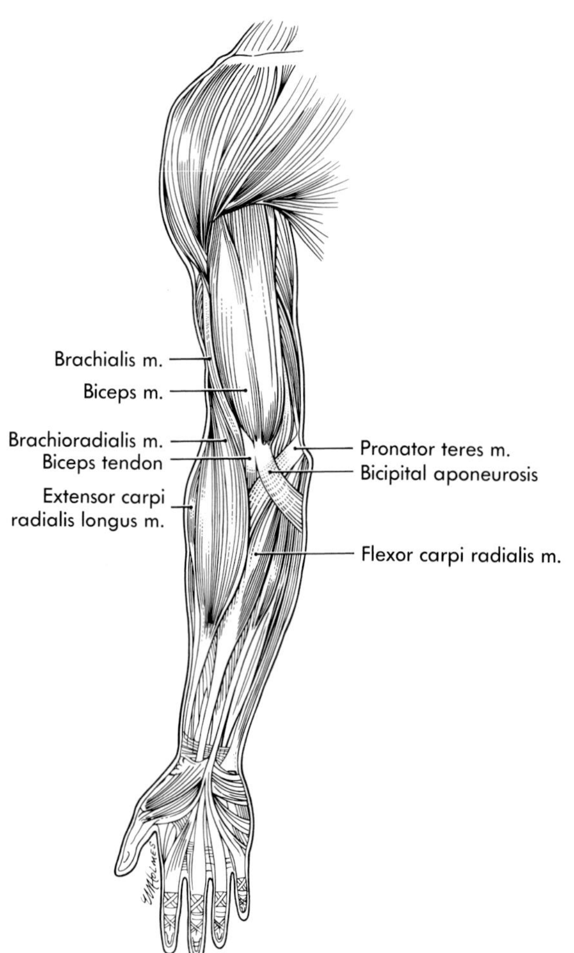

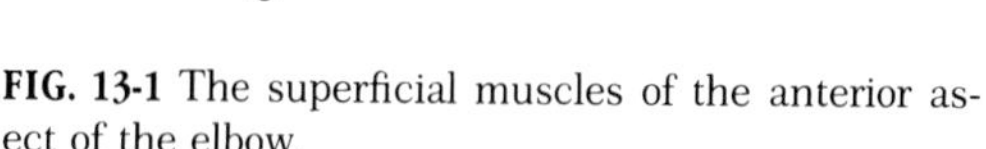
FIG. 13-1 The superficial muscles of the anterior asect of the elbow.

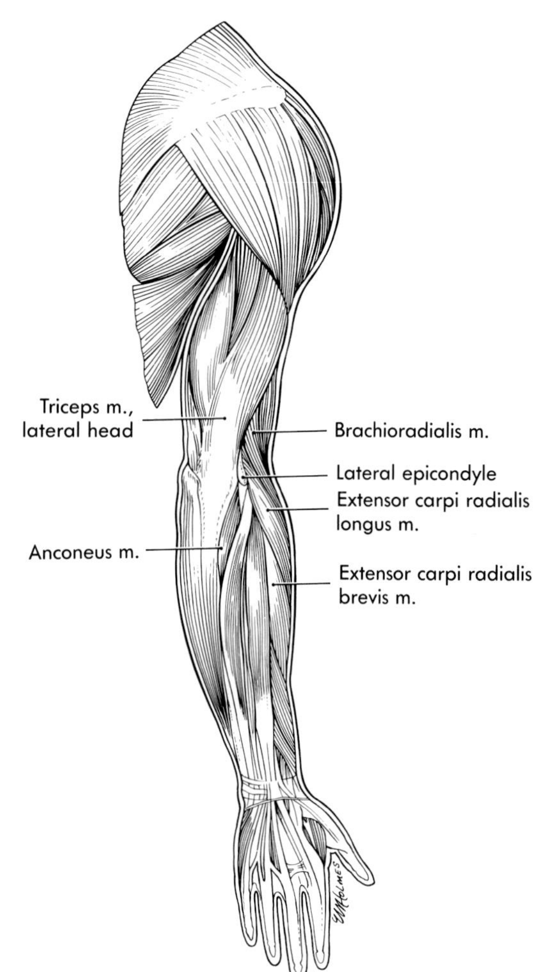

FIG. 13-2 The superficial muscles of the posterior aspect of the elbow.

Posteriorly, the triceps muscle is the dominant structure with its tendinous margins palpable distally as it inserts onto the olecranon. The margin of the triceps tendon can be palpated laterally and can be used in locating portals for elbow arthroscopy. The medial border is also readily palpable, and adjacent to this lies the ulnar nerve. The ulnar nerve is the only nerve about the elbow that is readily palpable in the superficial anatomy. In the distal aspect of the arm it runs along the medial border of the triceps tendon and in the ulnar groove, before disappearing underneath the flexor carpi ulnaris muscle.

Superficial or cutaneous nerves of the forearm are not readily palpable because they are quite small. Along the lateral aspect of the elbow, they run primarily longitudinally and are not a significant problem with lateral surgical approaches to the elbow. Medially, however, they tend to extend from the volar surface to the dorsal surface. These branches of the medial cutaneous nerve of the forearm often cross proposed incisions for exposure of the ulnar nerve or medial epicondyle. Care in avoiding injury to these cutaneous nerves during the exposure will lessen the likelihood of any painful neuroma formation postoperatively. They may, however, be numerous enough and small enough that they are impossible to avoid during the exposure.

At the elbow just medial to the biceps tendon, the brachial artery is palpable. Just distal to the elbow it divides into the radial and ulnar arteries, the division of which is not usually readily palpable. The palpable venous anatomy is the superficial cephalic vein and the basilic vein. The cephalic vein is located laterally, and the basilic vein is located medially in the antecubital area. There are often intercommunication veins between the two primary veins, and these are given various names, such as the median cephalic vein or median basilic vein, depending on the individual pattern.

Deep Soft Tissue Anatomy

Once the skin surface and subcutaneous tissue have been removed, the intervals between the muscles can be visualized. Laterally and anteriorly, the lateral margin of the biceps and brachialis is readily distinguishable from the brachioradialis (Fig. 13-1). In this interval, and just deep to the brachioradialis, lies the radial nerve. Proximal to the elbow joint the radial nerve divides into a deep and a superficial branch. The deep branch of the radial nerve divides the two heads of the supinator muscle. The supinator is the base of this interval and occupies the distal portion. The superficial branch of the radial nerve continues distally along the undersurface of the brachioradialis. Adjacent to the deep branch of the radial nerve lies the recurrent radial artery. It has come off the radial artery, just distal to the biceps tendon, and courses proximally, essentially wrapping around the biceps tendon.[2] This recurrent radial artery needs to be identified when performing an exposure in the area, for example, repair of a ruptured distal biceps tendon, or when exploring the deep radial nerve for entrapment (Figs. 13-3 to 13-6).

An interval is formed medial to the biceps tendon by the tendon and the flexor pronator muscle group. This group is composed from lateral to medial of the pronator teres, the flexor carpi radialis, the variable palmaris longus, and finally the flexor carpi ulnaris. In the interval on the medial side of the biceps tendon lies the brachial artery and median nerve. These course distally, deep to the bicipital aponeurosis. The median nerve sends off several

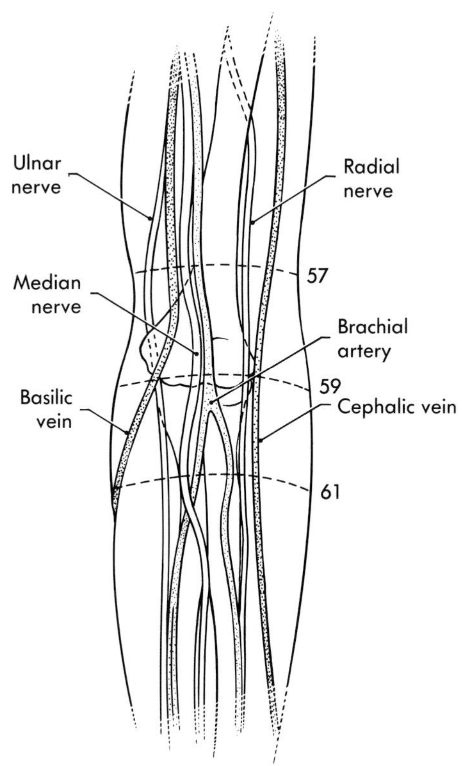

FIG. 13-3 Anterior view of the relationship of the neurovascular structures about the left elbow.

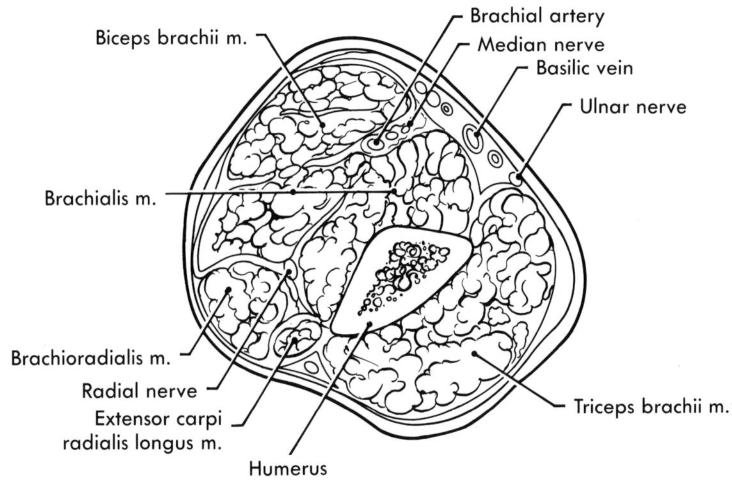

FIG. 13-4 Cross-sectional anatomy correlating with level 57 on Fig. 13-3.

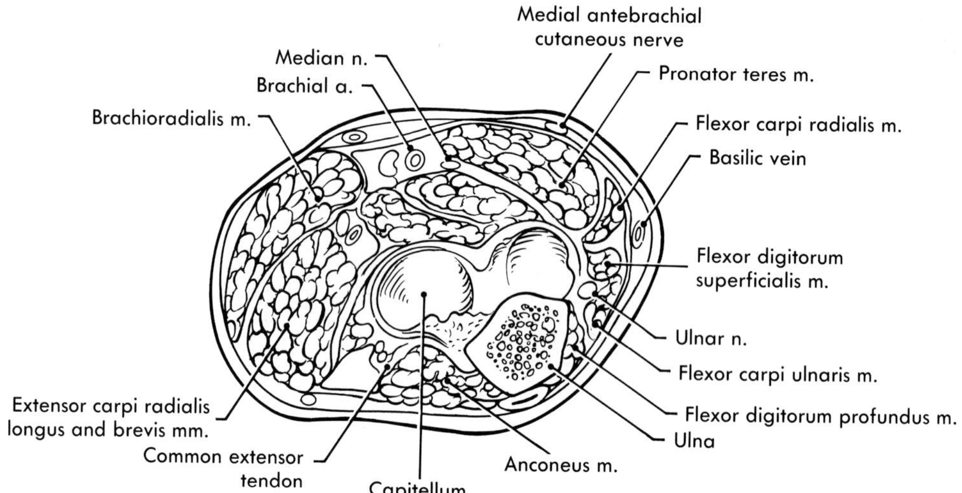

FIG. 13-5 Cross-sectional anatomy correlating with level 59 on Fig. 13-3.

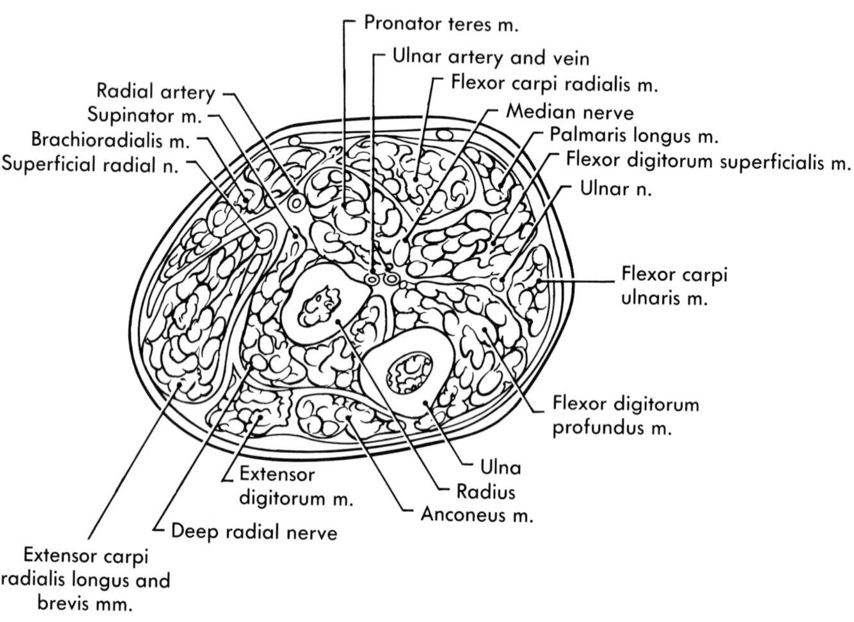

FIG. 13-6 Cross-sectional anatomy correlating with level 61 on Fig. 13-3.

muscular branches before diving deep into pronator teres musculature.

Deep to the pronator teres muscle, the median nerve continues to the flexor digitorum superficialis muscle. The flexor digitorum takes its origin from the medial epicondyle, medial coronoid process of the ulna, and the proximal radius. The brachial artery divides, as it nears the attachment site of the biceps tendon, into the radial and ulnar arteries. The ulnar artery further divides and sends off a recurrent ulnar artery and the common interosseous artery as well. The ulnar artery continues distally, diving deep to the sublimis (or flexor digitorum superficialis) to run between it and the flexor digitorum profundus. It then continues in this plane to the wrist. In approximately 3% of elbows the ulnar artery follows an anomalous course, descending superficial to the flexor muscles.[3]

The deepest layer of muscle in the anterior aspect of the forearm is composed of three muscles. Lateral is the flexor pollicis longus, which comes off the volar shaft of the radius and interosseous membrane. More medially the flexor digitorum profundus comes off the upper volar and medial ulna, as well as the medial coronoid process and interosseous membrane. The third muscle is the pronator quadratus muscle, although this is quite distal in the forearm.

Deep volar musculature

- Flexor pollicis longus
- Flexor digitorum profundus
- Pronator quadratus

The median nerve, after dividing the pronator teres heads, dives deep to the flexor digitorum superficialis and then lies superficial to the flexor digitorum profundus musculature as it courses distally to the wrist. It finally passes through the carpal tunnel, deep to the transverse carpal ligament and ulnar to the palmaris longus tendon (if present). The ulnar nerve, after diving posterior to the medial epicondyle, passes between the two heads of the flexor carpi ulnaris muscle. It then courses distally, lying between the flexor carpi ulnaris and the flexor digitorum profundus muscles. Distal in the forearm the nerve lies adjacent to the ulnar artery, coursing with it toward Guyon's canal at the wrist.

The ulnar artery gives off the common interosseous branch before lying adjacent to the ulnar nerve. The anterior interosseous artery comes off the common interosseous artery and courses distally superficial to the flexor pollicis longus and the profundus muscles. The anterior interosseous artery courses deep to the pronator quadratus just proximal to the wrist. The posterior interosseous artery goes deep to the profundus through the interosseous membrane and is adjacent to the posterior interosseous nerve as the nerve exits the supinator.

The radial artery, after giving off the recurrent radial branch, courses in the interval with a superficial branch of the radial nerve deep to the brachioradialis muscle. As the brachioradialis attaches to the distal radius, the radial artery courses along the superficial palmar aspect of the radius to the level of the wrist. The superficial branch of the radial nerve runs underneath the brachioradialis muscle, coursing distally to the radial and dorsal aspect of the wrist.

Looking at the posterior aspect of the elbow, the most dominant muscle is the triceps, which extends onto the olecranon. Also prominent is the brachioradialis coming off the lateral aspect of the humerus. Just distal to this and lateral is the extensor carpi radialis longus and the extensor carpi radialis brevis musculature. Originating more inferior and somewhat more distal is the extensor digitorum communis musculature and the extensor digiti minimi muscle. Finally, the extensor carpi ulnaris muscle is noted lying on the lateral aspect of the ulna with the flexor carpi ulnaris muscle lying on the medial aspect. Portions of the extensor digitorum communis and extensor carpi ulnaris muscles cover the anconeous, which extends from the lateral epicondyle to the border of the ulna.

Deep to the brachioradialis and extensor carpi radialis longus brevis musculature on the anterior aspect lies the supinator muscle. Portions of the supinator originate from the lateral epicondyle, the radial collateral and annular ligaments, and the ulna shaft below the radial notch. It inserts onto the radius distal to the bicipital tuberosity and along its lateral aspect. Extending down the forearm, the abductor pollicis longus muscle and extensor pollicis brevis muscle originate from the lateral dorsal ulna, the interrosseous membrane, and the dorsal radius.

Just ulnar at this level lie the extensor pollicis longus and extensor indicis proprius, both originating from the dorsal surface of the ulna and the interosseous membrane. These two muscles are felt to have developed later in the pyelogenic history and may be variable in their development at birth.[12] The neural structure in this area is primarily the posterior interosseous (or deep radial) nerve that dives through the supinator. It then courses along to the abductor pollicis longus and extensor pollicis brevis musculature, giving off musculature branches. It finally innervates the extensor pollicis longus and the extensor indicis. These distal nerve branches appear in a fanlike fashion along the area just superficial to the deep muscle group (composed of the abductor pollicis longus, extensor pollicis brevis, extensor pollicis, and extensor indicis proprius).

Osteology

Distal Humerus

The distal humerus is composed of two condyles forming the articular surfaces of the trochlea and capitellum (Figs. 13-7 and 13-8). It develops from a number of separate epiphyses about the distal humerus. These

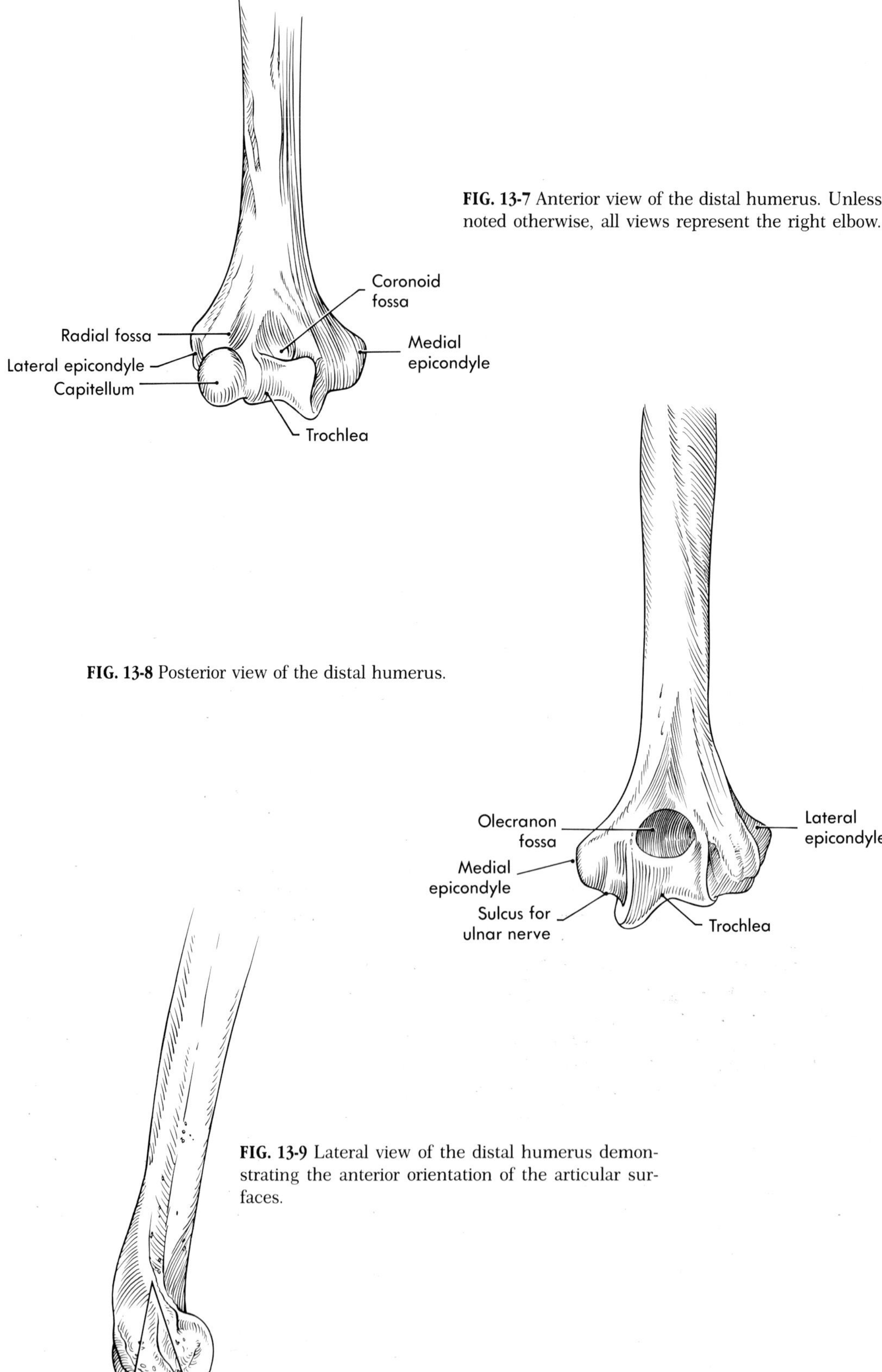

FIG. 13-7 Anterior view of the distal humerus. Unless noted otherwise, all views represent the right elbow.

FIG. 13-8 Posterior view of the distal humerus.

FIG. 13-9 Lateral view of the distal humerus demonstrating the anterior orientation of the articular surfaces.

coalesce at varying ages, and all close at skeletal maturity. Medially (or ulnarly) the epicondyle is quite prominent and serves as a source of attachment for the ulnar collateral ligament and the flexor pronator muscle group. *The size of the prominence of the medial epicondyle provides a mechanical advantage for the ligament and muscle groups that attach there.* Just distal to the epicondyle is the condylar articular surface of the trochlea.

The lateral epicondyle is much less prominent and is located just proximal to the capitellum. This provides less of a mechanical advantage to the attachment of the extensor muscle group as well as the radial collateral ligament. Anterior and proximal to the articular surface are two indentations, or fossa. Laterally, the indentation just proximal to the capitellum accommodates the radial head when the elbow is in full flexion and is referred to as the radial fossa. Just medial to the radial fossa is a deeper fossa that accommodates the coronoid process of the ulna (see Fig. 13-11). The coronoid process gives the fossa its name, the coronoid fossa. The coronoid fossa is just proximal to the trochlea. Posteriorly, the olecranon fits into a deep olecranon fossa in the humerus, allowing full extension of the elbow as well as flexion to approximately 145 to 150 degrees. These bony prominences of the ulna and radius fit quite closely into their respective fossa.

The primary structural integrity of the distal humerus comes from medial and lateral supracondylar columns. The medial column is slightly smaller than the lateral column. The posterior aspect of the epicondyles is relatively flat, and the anterior portions are curved forward. This places the articular surfaces anteriorly and oriented approximately 30 degrees anterior to the long axis of the humerus (Fig. 13-9). The capitellum is spherical in shape over the surface it presents to the radial head. It extends from the radial fossa distally to the distal end of the humerus (Figs. 13-9 and 13-10). It does not continue posteriorly in a circumferential pattern as the trochlea. The axis of the elbow is directed through the trochlea and the capitellum in approximately 6 degrees of valgus as compared to the axis of the epicondyles. Thus the medial trochlea is somewhat longer and projects more distal (see Figs. 13-7 and 13-8).

The trochlea itself is covered with articular cartilage from the coronoid fossa anteriorly to the olecranon fossa posteriorly. This presents a continuous surface of articular cartilage covering the anterior, distal, and posterior aspects of the distal humerus and forms an arc of 300 to 330 degrees.[6] This allows for only a very small area of bone to exist between the coronoid fossa and the olecranon fossa. Indeed, in some individuals only a membrane is present. Occasionally, this area appears to be filled with what roentgenographically looks like a loose body. This, however, is an anatomic variant. The trochlea itself is not symmetric because the medial lip is larger and projects more distal. There is a small groove that appears in the interval between the capitellum and the trochlea that is covered with hyaline cartilage and articulates with the radial head when the elbow is appropriately loaded. This allows for rotation of the radial head without abutting the humerus. In the axial view the distal humerus has approximately 5 degrees of internal rotation of the articular surface in relationship to the epicondylar axis (Fig. 13-10). Medially in the interval between the epicondyle and trochlea is a groove through which the ulnar nerve courses (see Fig. 13-8). More proximally and medially along the area of the intermuscular septum a supracondylar process may be observed in approximately 1% to 3% of the individuals.[3] From this process a fibrous band may attach to the medial epicondyle. This band and bony prominence may form an anomalous insertion of the coracobrachialis muscle and/or origin of the pronator teres. Additionally, it may be involved with aberrant routes of the median and ulnar nerve. The fibrous portion of this complex is termed the ligament of Strothers.

Proximal Radius

The shape of the proximal radius in cross section is almost cylindrical and becomes more elliptical as one goes distal into the forearm. The proximal portion is also termed the radial head, and it articulates with the capitellum.[1] It presents a concave surface to accommodate the capitellum within the cylindric outline of the radial head. Hyaline cartilage covers the proximal radial head as well as the sides of the radial head. This outer surface of the radial head is covered for approximately 240 degrees.[6] The anterior lateral third of the circumference of the radial head is void of cartilage. This area is not involved in articulation. Because it is not normally stressed it is slightly weaker and is prone to fracture when stressed, as in a fall. Distal to the radial head, the bone tapers to the radial neck. Somewhat distal to the radial neck is a prominence of the radial tuberosity on which the biceps tendon attaches (see Fig. 13-7). Often, adjacent to the attachment of the biceps tendon is a small bursa to protect the

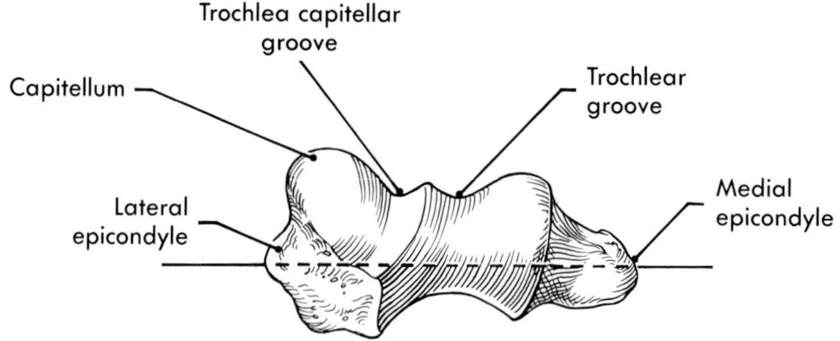

FIG. 13-10 Distal view of the distal humerus. Note medial rotation of the articular surfaces compared to the axis of the epicondyles.

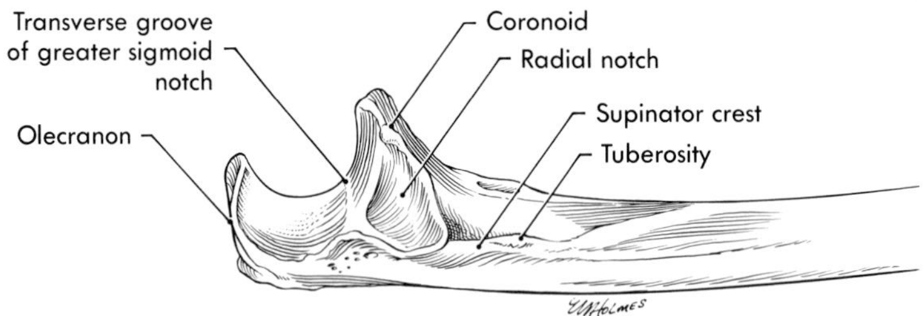

FIG. 13-11 Lateral view of the proximal ulna.

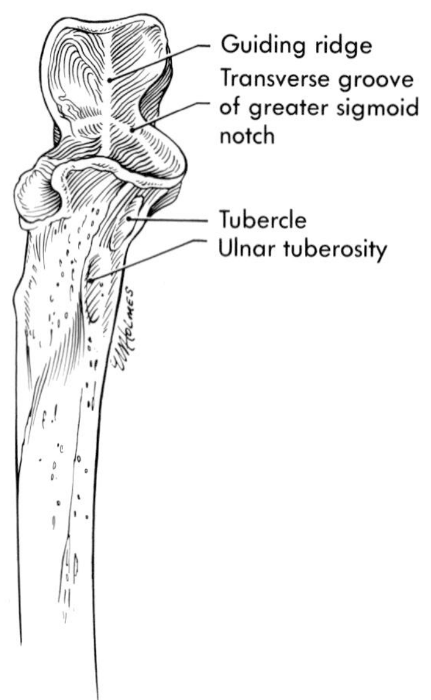

FIG. 13-12 Anterior view of the proximal ulna.

biceps tendon when in full pronation. In addition, the radial head and neck are not colinear with the long axis of the radius. They also form an angle of approximately 15 degrees with the shaft. This is oriented opposite the direction of the radial tuberosity.

Proximal Ulna

The proximal ulna essentially grasps the distal humerus and is responsible for the majority of the bony stability at the elbow. Distal to the elbow the ulna tapers quite rapidly to assume first a triangular shape and then a cylindric shape. Proximally the ulna forms the greater sigmoid notch, which articulates with the trochlea of the humerus. The proximal and distal portions of this notch are composed of the olecranon tip and the coronoid process, respectively. Additionally, the coronoid process serves as an insertion site to the brachialis muscle with the olecranon serving as the attachment of the triceps. Along the lateral aspect of the coronoid process there is a small semilunar notch or radial notch into which the radial head fits that is roughly perpendicular to the long access of the bone. The circular margin of the radial head articulates and is stabilized within the radial notch (Figs. 13-11, 13-12, and 13-17). Just distal to the radial notch is a crest of bone that is the site of the ulnar origin of the supinator muscle. Additionally, on this crest, also called the crista supinatorus, is the insertion of the accessory lateral collateral ligament (see Fig. 13-10). This ligament serves a twofold purpose: to tether the annular ligament and to supplement the radial collateral ligament.

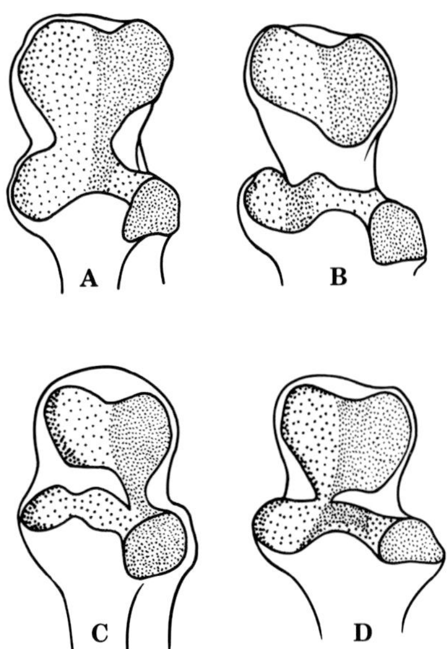

FIG. 13-13 Various configurations of the articular surfaces of the proximal left ulna. Pattern **B** is the most common, representing 63% of cases studied. Pattern **A, C,** and **D** represent 3%, 32%, and 2%, respectively.[6,7]

The medial aspect of the coronoid process serves the site of attachment of the anterior portion of the medial collateral ligament (Figs. 13-12 and 13-16).

The greater sigmoid notch is not covered continuously with hyaline cartilage: indeed, in the majority of cases there is a transverse portion composed of fatty tissue and not hyaline cartilage (Fig. 13-13). With the anterior and posterior portions of the sigmoid notch being composed of articular cartilage, there is normally a depression in the sigmoid notch in the central region. This depression, however, is not apparent on roentgenograms, nor is it apparent on skeletal bone samples, since the area is devoid of articular cartilage and produces a prominence rather than an additional depression of subchondral bone. There is also a longitudinal ridge in the greater sigmoid notch producing a medial and lateral surface (see Figs. 13-12 and 13-13). The sigmoid notch forms an arc of approximately 180 degrees and is angled approximately 30 degrees to the long axis of the ulna. This, coupled with the 300 to 330 degrees of articular surface of the trochlea, allows for between 120 and 150 degrees of flexion of the elbow. Along the lateral aspect of the proximal ulna is a lesser sigmoid notch or radial notch. This depression has an arc of approximately 60 to 70 degrees and articulates with the radial head. This articulation of 60 to 70 degrees, coupled with the radial head surface being covered for 240 degrees of its outside circumference, allows for pronation and supination of 170 to 180 degrees. The greater sigmoid notch is also not completely perpendicular to the longitudinal axis of the ulna. It is in slight valgus angulation with respect to the shaft, representing approximately 4 degrees. This valgus, coupled with the 6 degrees of the distal humerus, creates the **carrying angle**, the angle between the shaft of the humerus and the shaft of the ulna. The carrying angle may normally vary from 10 to 18 degrees with any particular angle being normal only when compared to the contralateral elbow.

The capsule of the elbow joint is covered anteriorly by the brachialis and posteriorly by the triceps. The fibrous portion of the capsule is attached to the humerus anteriorly above the radial and coronoid fossa and posteriorly above the olecranon fossa.[5] Distally, the capsule attaches to the anterior margin of the coronoid medially, as well as to the annular ligament laterally. Posteriorly and distally, the attachment is along the medial and lateral articular margins of the sigmoid notch. Laterally, it attaches along the lateral aspect of the sigmoid notch and blends with the annular ligament.[6] This capsule is normally quite thin and transparent (see Fig. 13-15). Studies by Morrey[6] reveal that the anterior capsule provides a significant portion of varus and valgus stability when the elbow is extended. This appears to be the result of transverse and oblique fiber bands within the capsule itself. The greatest capacity of the capsule is in approximately 60 degrees of flexion and is therefore the most comfortable position when a tense effusion is present.

The synovial membrane courses just deep to the capsule with the exception of the radial and coronoid fossa anteriorly and the olecranon fossa posteriorly. Here the synovial membrane first turns down over pads of fat in the fossa to reach the edges of the articular surfaces; thus the synovium membrane runs over the bone only a short distance to reach the articular cartilage. Most structures within the capsule of the elbow joint either are covered with fat and synovial membrane or are articular cartilage.[5] The fat pads play a significant role in evaluation of effusions of the elbow joint when they are observed in a lateral roentgenographic view of the elbow.

Ligaments

The ligaments about the elbow represent distinct thickening of the capsule of the elbow. These ligaments are located primarily in medial and lateral aspect of the elbow.

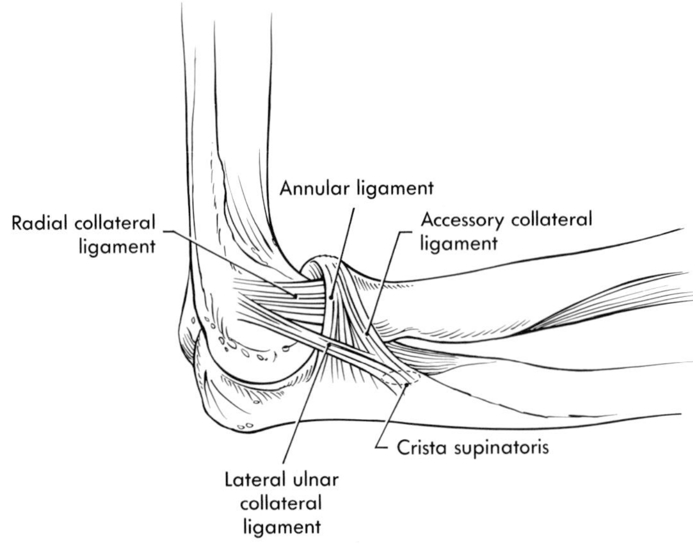

FIG. 13-14 Medial view of the medial collateral ligament bundles.

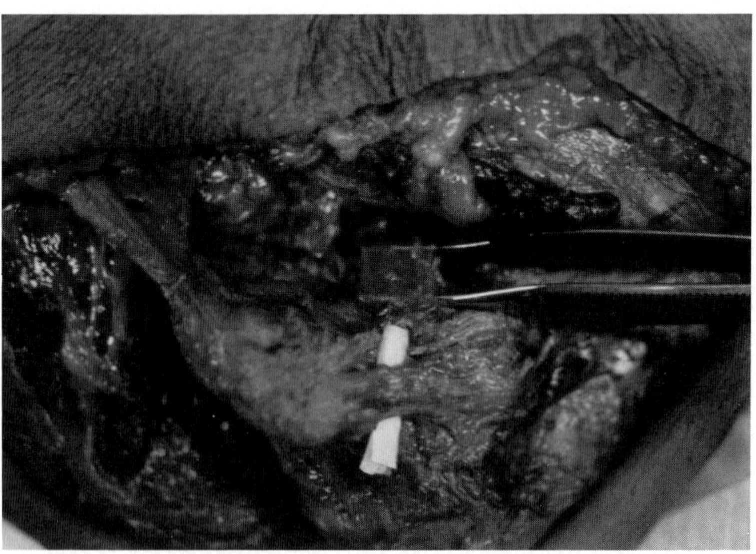

FIG. 13-15 Cadaver dissection of a left elbow. The forceps is beneath the capsule, which can be quite thin. The white marker has been passed deep to the anterior bundle of the ulnar collateral ligament.

Medial Collateral Ligament Complex

The medial collateral ligament of the elbow is the most important ligament for stability of the elbow joint. It is frequently divided into three bundles denoted by their anatomic location—anterior, posterior, and transverse (Fig. 13-14). The posterior bundle appears to provide some support when the elbow is flexed 90 degrees or greater. The transverse ligament has little to do with elbow stability. The origin of the medial collateral ligament is from the medial epicondyle along its distal portion.[6] It inserts along the medial aspect of the coronoid process (Fig. 13-15). The main link to the anterior component of the complex is about 27 mm. The width of the anterior bundles is approximately 4 to 5 mm. There is a slight ridge along the medial side of the olecranon, to which the ligament attaches.

Lateral Collateral Ligament Complex

The lateral ligament complex is formed by the radial collateral ligament, the annular ligament, the lateral ulnar collateral ligament,

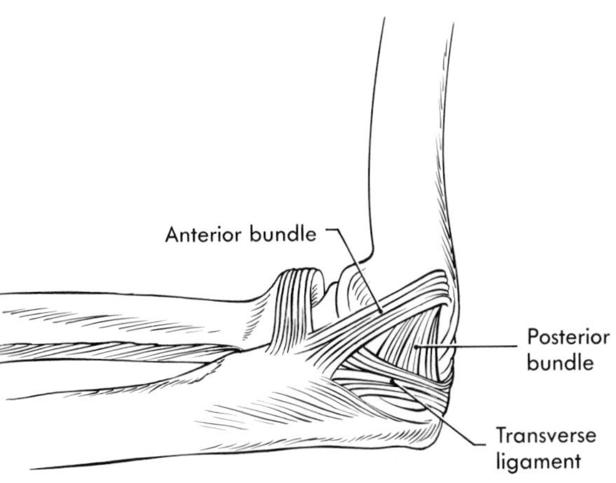

FIG. 13-16 Lateral view of the lateral collateral and annular ligaments.

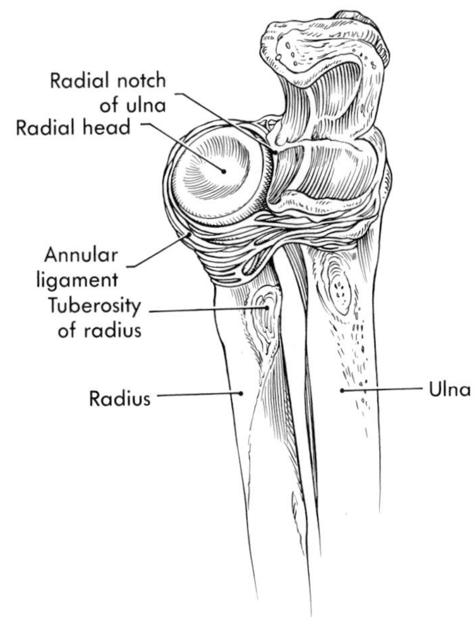

FIG. 13-17 Anterior view of the proximal radioulnar complex. Note the congruency of the radial head, annular ligament, and radial notch of the ulna.

and the accessory collateral ligament.[6] The radial collateral ligament originates from the lateral epicondyle and terminates along the course of the annular ligament (Fig. 13-16). A posterior portion of this ligament extends distally onto the crista supinatorus, which is a small prominence of the lateral ulna just distal to the lesser sigmoid notch. This separate portion is termed the lateral ulnar collateral ligament. Additionally, a band of the annular ligament also joins it at its attachment to the crista supinatorus and is termed the accessory collateral ligament. The annular ligament itself forms the remaining portion of the circle (the initial portion formed by the lesser sigmoid or radial notch) and is attached at the margins of the radial notch of the ulna. This annular ligament fits tightly around the head and upper portion of the neck (Fig. 13-17) and does not allow distal migration of the radius to occur in the adult; however, in the young child or infant this may occur and result in a "pulled elbow." This ligamentous complex combined with the radial notch of the ulna forms a structure with the radial head that is built to very close biomechanical tolerances. Any disruption of this area will often result in a loss of pronation and supination. If any of these structures loses its symmetry, congruous surfaces may no longer be present. This loss of congruity, limiting pronation and supination, is a frequent occurrence following radial head fractures. The origin of the radial collateral ligament appears to be in the anatomic center of rotation.[6]

Bursa

Although there are several bursa noted about the elbow, the most clinically relevant bursa is the olecranon bursa between the olecranon and the skin surface. This is a clinical entity when it has been enlarged because of hematoma, chronic irritation, or rheumatoid synovitis. Occasionally it may need to be surgically excised for relief of symptoms.

PHYSICAL EXAMINATION

An integral part of any evaluation of the elbow is the history and physical examination.[8] The most important question to ask the individual about the elbow is "What bothers you the most about your elbow?" This type of question will elicit the chief complaint and may also aid in getting through some extraneous information as well. Once you have elicited the chief complaint, allow the patient to point to the location where he or she senses the problem is located and ask if there is any radiation of pain or paresthesias from this area. Next, one should ask about the date of onset or reinjury that initiated this problem. Finally, one needs to ask the "how" questions: "How does it bother you now? How have you treated this? How do you make it worse? How do you make it better? How has your training program changed over this time period?"

The actual examination begins initially with **inspection**. One should be able to completely visualize both elbows during the examination. Differences may be noted related to muscle hypertrophy or atrophy, swelling, and also previous surgical incisions.

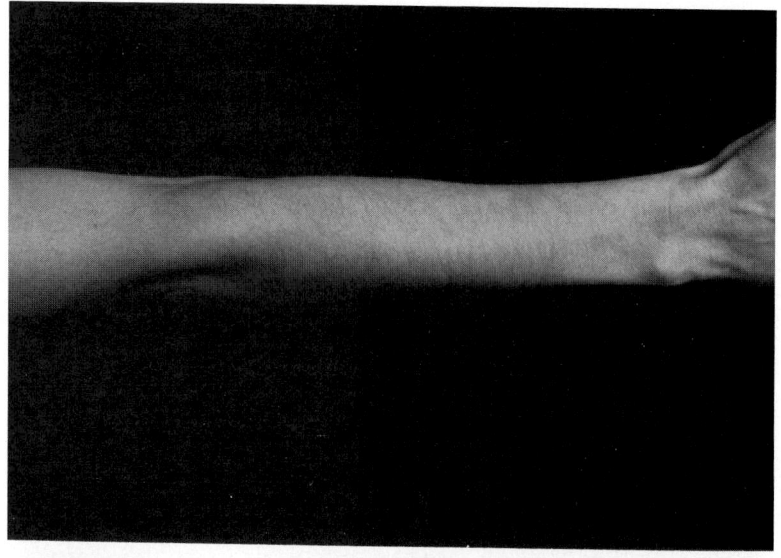

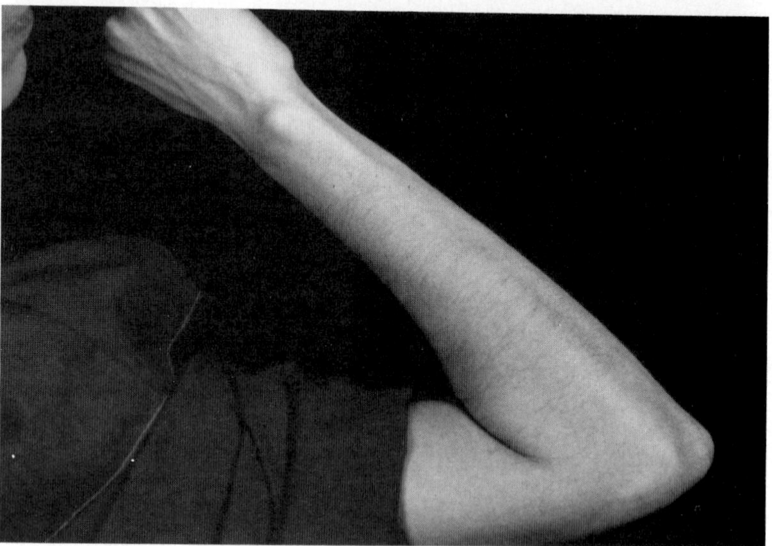

FIG. 13-18 A demonstration of a normal range of motion of the elbow. Symptoms of ulnar nerve entrapment at the elbow may be reproduced when the patient demonstrates range of motion.

Motions should be recorded from full extension, approximately 0 degrees, to full flexion, approximately 150 degrees (Fig. 13-18). Record supination and pronation with the elbow at a right angle. When going through this range of motion, one should note if there is any discomfort noted and have the individual point to the area of this discomfort. A locking or lack of full motion may indicate loose body formation, articular surface defect, or muscle tightness secondary to a muscle strain. Localization of the tenderness by **palpation** is helpful. I will often palpate areas of possible tendonitis or nerve entrapment that do not fit the patient's chief complaint and will utilize these for comparison later when the more painful areas are palpated (Fig. 13-19). The location of the most tender area needs to be noted. The underlying structures that pressure has been applied to in Fig. 13-19, *A*, differ from the structures in Fig. 13-19, *B*. A change in location of the most tender area will change the proposed differential diagnosis.

In an acute injury the pain experienced by the patient may be too great to evaluate the range of motion. A very helpful examination

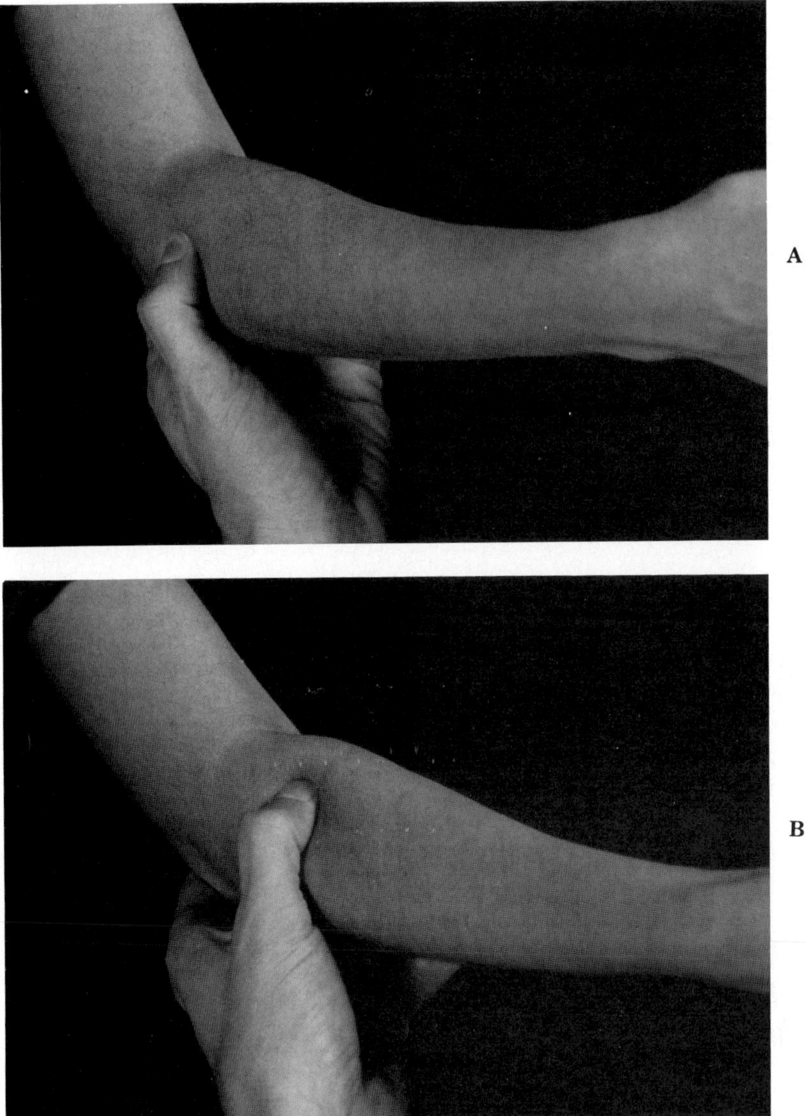

FIG. 13-19 The exact location of the most tender area is important. In **A,** the thumb is over the common extensor tendon and radial head. In **B,** the thumb is over the supinator and radial nerve. This small difference in location is important on the differential diagnosis.

after an acute injury is to palpate the epicondyles and the tip of the olecranon. The line formed by the epicondyles should be perpendicular to the shaft of the humerus. If it is not, a humeral fracture should be suspected. If the position of the elbow is at 0 degrees of flexion the epicondyles and the olecranon should form a straight line. With the elbow flexed to 90 degrees these palpable prominences should form a triangle with the sides adjacent to the olecranon being equal.[11] Should this not be the case either a fracture, a dislocation, or both should be suspected (Fig. 13-20).

Following initial palpation one will then begin the **stress examination** of the elbow. Because of the amount of rotation that occurs at the shoulder and humerus, it is difficult to adequately apply varus or valgus stress to the elbow. This needs to be performed at multiple angles from full extension, approximately 30 to 40 degrees of flexion.[10] The distal humerus should be grasped with one hand while the stress is applied to the distal forearm with the other (Fig. 13-21). Any toggle or play in motion, as well as elucidation of the patient's pain, is significant, especially when compared

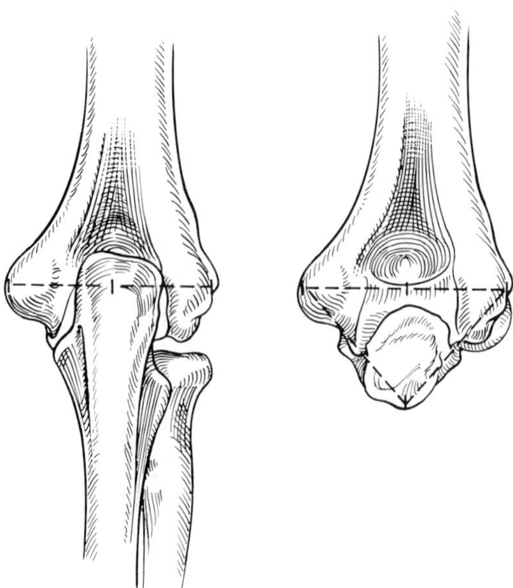

FIG. 13-20 The relationship of the palpable landmarks of the medial and lateral epicondyles of the humerus and the olecranon tip of the ulna. This is demonstrated on full extension and at 90 degrees of flexion of the elbow.

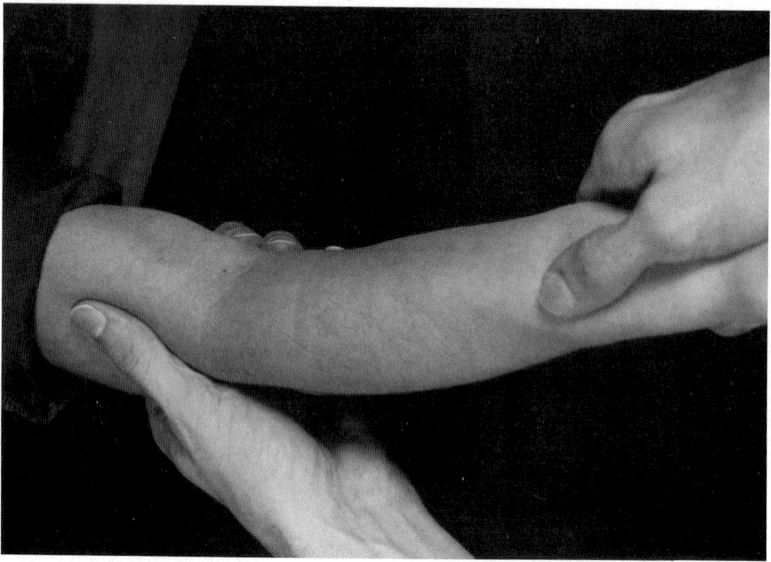

FIG. 13-21 During vagus and valgus stress testing applied to the elbow, one needs to palpate the amount of rotation of the humerus as well. Laxity is best detected at approximately 30 degrees of flexion, which unlocks the olecranon tip from the olecranon fossa.

with the motion of the opposite elbow. The elbow needs to be flexed to 30 degrees to unlock the olecranon from the olecranon fossa when stressing the medial or ulnar collateral ligament.

There are a number of **provocative tests** that can be applied for specific problems. The discomfort of lateral tendonitis can be reproduced if one stresses the extensor carpi radialis longus and brevis muscles or the extensor digitorum communis with the wrist extended (Fig. 13-22). Additionally, discomfort may be reproduced with palmar flexion of the wrist pronation and gradual extension of the elbow, thus stretching the extensor tendon (Fig. 13-22, C). Tightness along the flexor pronator muscle mass or tendonitis may also be elicited with extension of the elbow and dorsiflexion of the wrist (Fig. 13-23).

Palpation of areas that are suspected of being involved by the history obtained should then be performed. The exact location of their

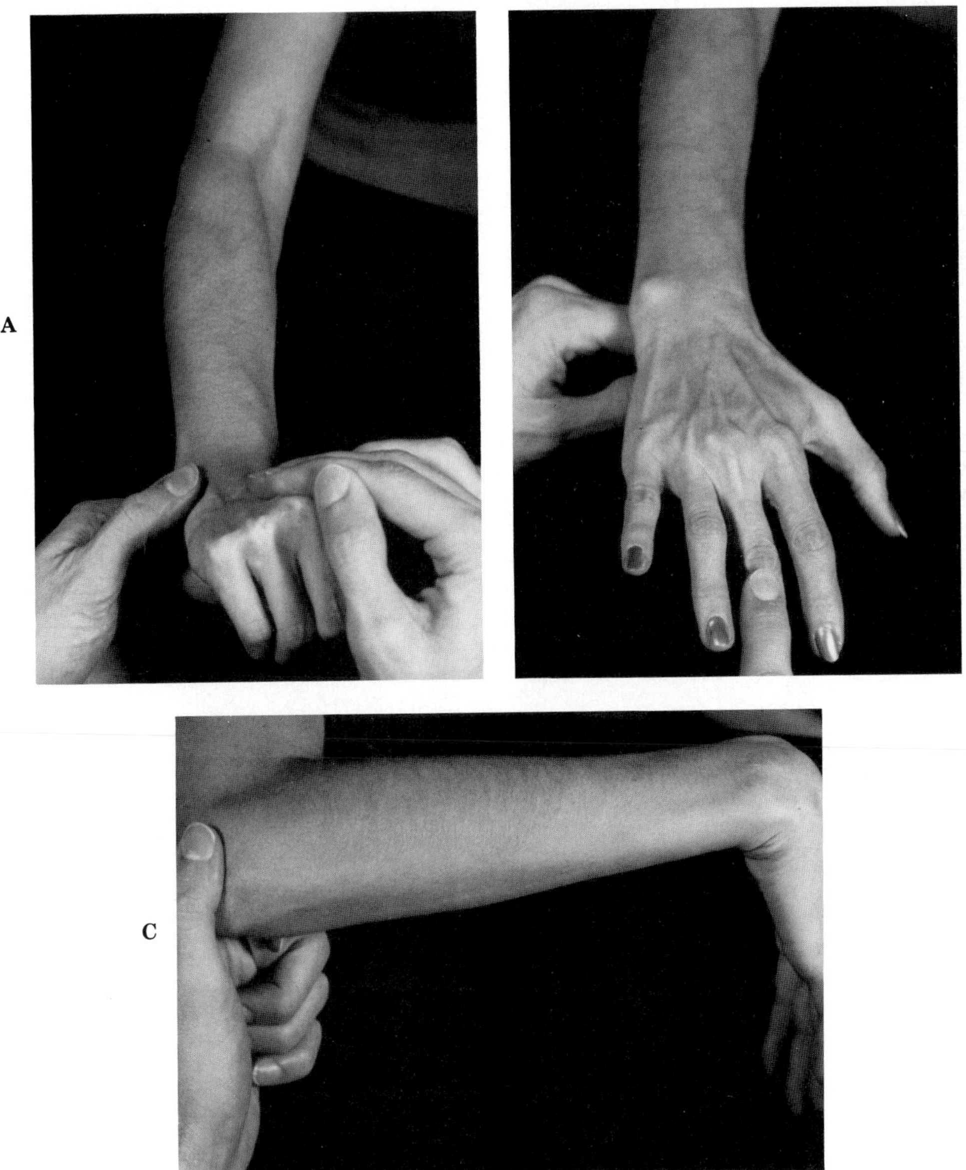

FIG. 13-22 Provocative tests for lateral epicondylitis. **A,** Resisted extension of the wrist. **B,** Resisted extension of the third digit, stressing the extensor digitorum muscle and tendon. **C,** The wrist palmar-flexed and the forearm fully pronated. Extension of the elbow will stretch the common extensor tendon and reproduce symptoms if tendonitis is present.

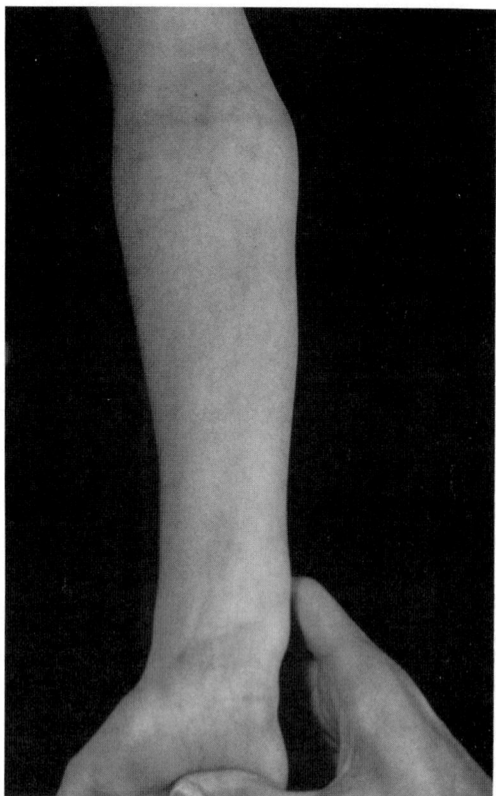

FIG. 13-23 A provocative test for flexor tendonitis is resisted wrist palmar flexion.

tenderness, being in their proximal, middle, or distal portion, is important. At this time, the patient should also be asked to demonstrate any type of motion that re-creates the symptoms most completely. If there is an area of tenderness one must recall the structures beneath this area and try to differentiate the origin of the pain. This may be accomplished by applying stress to these various structures without stressing all of them. At this time one needs to correlate the history with the findings on physical examination and the roentgenographic evaluation. From this, one should have at least a good differential diagnosis of the problem if not the diagnosis. Further diagnostic or therapeutic procedures would then appropriately be planned.

SUMMARY

Diagnosis of specific musculoskeletal problems requires a careful correlation of the patient's symptoms with the physical and roentgenographic examinations. The better the understanding of the underlying anatomy, the more easily the involved structure is identified. Without this understanding one can be led to an incorrect diagnosis when relying on the history or roentgenographic examination alone.

REFERENCES

1. Bogumill GP: Functional anatomy of the shoulder and elbow. In Pettrone FA, editor: Upper extremity injuries in athletes, St Louis, 1987, The CV Mosby Co, pp 67-78.
2. Crenshaw AH: Surgical approaches. In Edmondson AS and Crenshaw AH, editors: Campbell's operative orthopaedics, ed 6, St Louis, 1980, The CV Mosby Co.
3. Grant JC and JCB Boileau: An atlas of anatomy, ed 6, Baltimore, 1972, The Williams & Wilkins Co.
4. Henry AK: Extensile exposure applied to limb surgery, Baltimore, 1945, The Williams & Wilkins Co.
5. Hollinshead WH: Textbook of anatomy, ed 2, New York, 1967, Harper & Row.
6. Morrey BF: Anatomy of the elbow joint. In Morrey BF: The elbow and its disorders, Philadelphia, 1985, WB Saunders Co.
7. Tillman B: A contribution to the functional morphology of articular surfaces, Stuttgart, West Germany, 1978, Georg Thieme, PSG Publishing, (Translated by G Konorza.)
8. Tullos HS and Bryon WJ: Examination of the throwing elbow. In Zarins B, Andrews JR, and Carson WG, Jr, editors: Injuries to the throwing arm, Philadelphia, 1985, WB Saunders Co.
9. Tullos HS and Bryon WJ: Functional anatomy of the elbow. In Zarins B, Andrews JR, and Carson WG, Jr, editors: Injuries to the throwing arm, Philadelphia, 1985, WB Saunders Co.
10. Tullos HS et al: Factors influencing elbow instability. In Murray DG, editor: Instructional course lectures, vol XXX, St Louis, 1981, The CV Mosby Co.
11. Wadsworth TG: Introduction. In Wadsworth TG, editor: The elbow, New York, 1982, Churchill Livingstone.
12. Wood VE: Thumb-clutched hand, congenital hand deformities. In Green DP, editor: Operative hand surgery, New York, 1982, Churchill Livingstone.

CHAPTER 14 Roentgenographic Evaluation of the Elbow

George H. Belhobek

STANDARD ROENTGENOGRAPHIC PROJECTIONS

A standard roentgenographic examination of the elbow joint is the combination of an anteroposterior and a lateral view.

The anteroposterior (AP) projection is produced with the elbow placed on the x-ray cassette in the extended position and the hand positioned in full supination to prevent overlapping of the forearm bones. The anterior surface of the elbow is parallel to the cassette surface. The central x-ray beam is centered perpendicular to the elbow joint. The correct projection has been obtained when the radial head, neck, and biceps tuberosity are slightly superimposed over the proximal ulna. The distal humerus, the proximal radius and ulna, and the elbow joint space are well seen in this projection (Fig. 14-1, *A* and *B*).[1,8]

Lateral Projection

A lateral projection is obtained by placing the 90-degree flexed elbow on the x-ray cassette in the lateral position. The hand is placed in the lateral position and the humeral condyles are perpendicular to the x-ray film. The central x-ray beam is directed perpendicular to the elbow joint. Positioning of the elbow in 90 degrees of flexion is important for proper visualization of the olecranon process and for proper projection of the elbow fat pads. The lateral projection of the elbow provides a lateral view of the distal humerus and the proximal forearm and clearly visualizes the olecranon process (Fig. 14-2).[1,8]

Oblique Projections

Medial and lateral oblique projections are useful in the evaluation of the traumatized elbow. The **lateral oblique view** is made with the elbow extended and the hand rotated laterally to place the posterior surface of the elbow at an angle of 40 degrees to the x-ray cassette. The central x-ray beam is directed vertically to the midpoint of the joint. The correct projection should demonstrate the radial head, neck, and tuberosity free from overlap of the ulna. The external oblique projection optimizes visualization of the radial head and neck area (Fig. 14-3).[1,8]

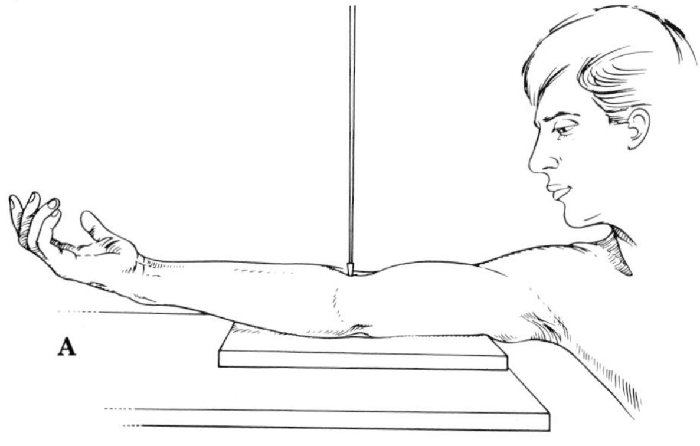

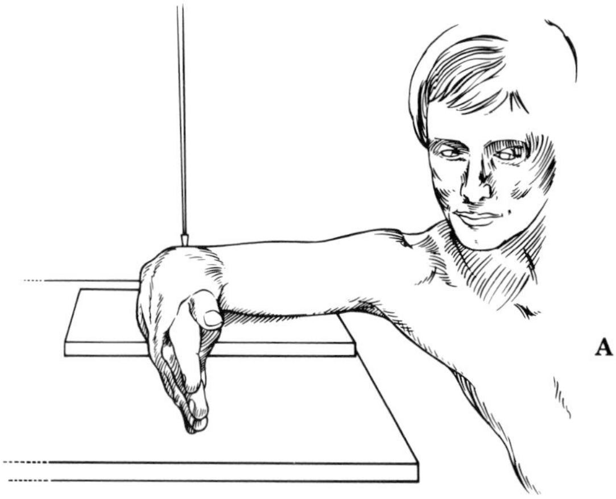

FIG. 14-1. **A,** Anterioposterior projection. **B,** Normal anterioposterior roentgenogram.

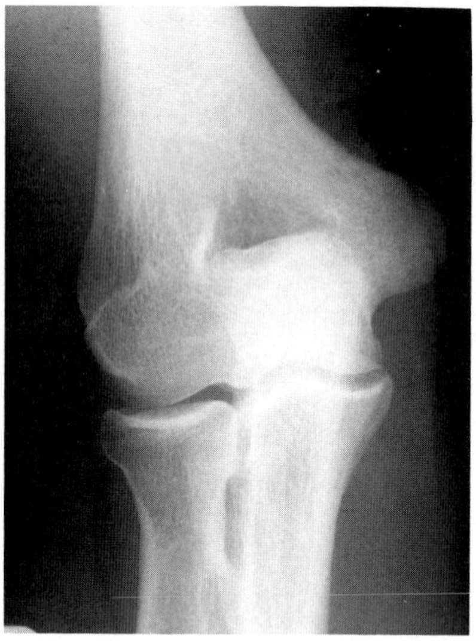

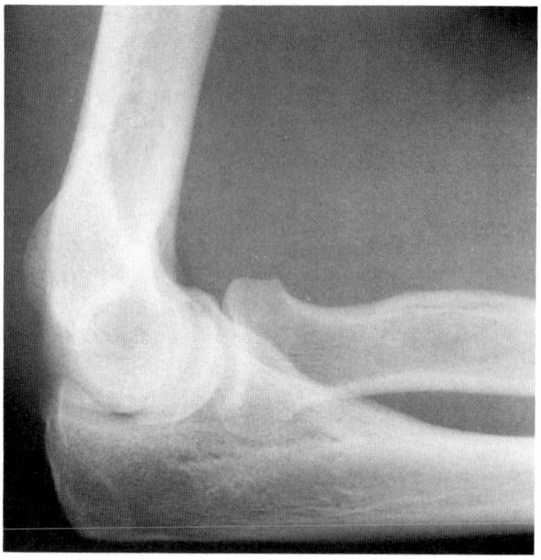

FIG. 14-2. **A,** Routine lateral projection. **B,** Normal lateral roentgenogram.

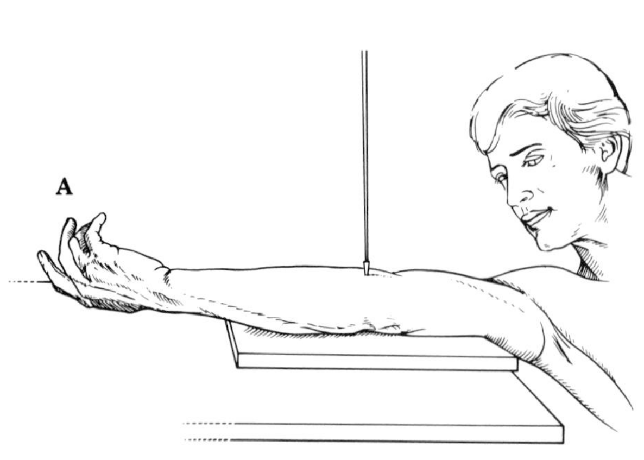

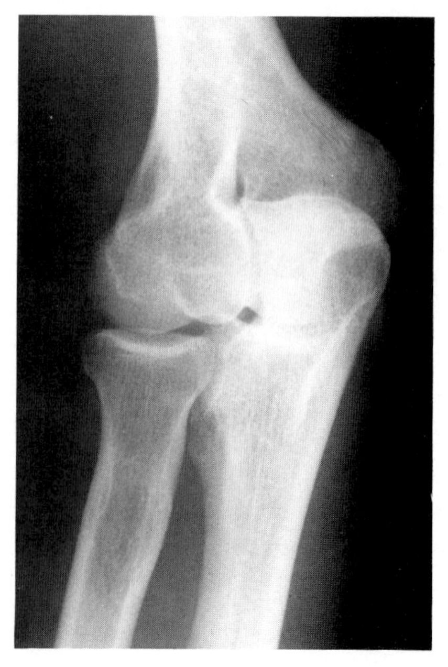

FIG. 14-3. **A,** Lateral oblique projection. **B,** Properly projected lateral oblique roentgenogram.

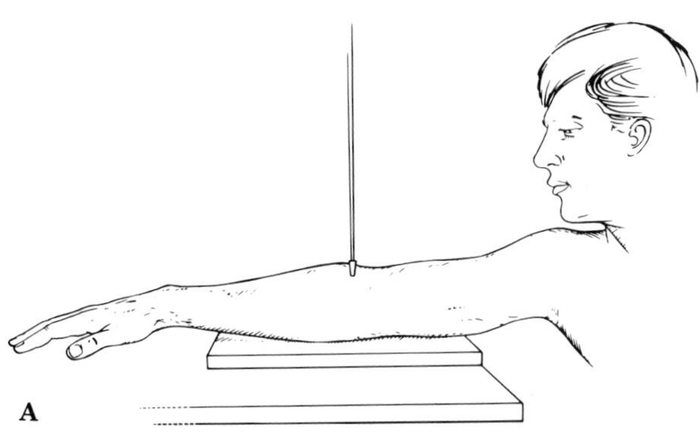

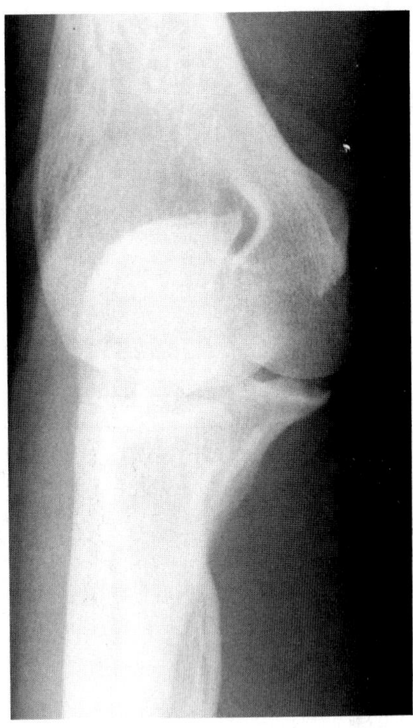

FIG. 14-4. A, Medial oblique projection. **B,** Properly projected medial oblique roentgenogram.

The **medial oblique view** is made with the elbow extended and the hand pronated, with the elbow adjusted so that its anterior surface is at an angle of 40 degrees to 45 degrees to the x-ray cassette. This should project the coronoid process in profile. The radial head and neck are superimposed on the ulna. The internal oblique projection optimizes visualization of the coronoid process of the ulna (Fig. 14-4, *A* and *B*).[1,8]

ADDITIONAL ROENTGENOGRAPHIC PROJECTIONS

The AP, lateral, and external and internal oblique projections are the roentgenograms most commonly ordered to evaluate the elbow joint. These views offer valuable information about the integrity of the bony structures and the elbow joint, the presence of loose bodies, and the periarticular soft tissue calcifications. Subtle bony and soft tissue pathologic conditions, however, may not always be defined by these routine roentgenograms. A number of specialized projections have been described to visualize selected areas of the elbow joint that are not optimally visualized by the standard techniques.

Radial Head Projections

The radial head is a structure that can sustain occult fractures that may be difficult to document on standard roentgenograms of the elbow. In the face of a high clinical suspicion for radial head fracture and nondiagnostic standard roentgenograms, several alternative roentgenographic procedures may be employed to enhance visualization of the radial head.

Roentgenograms of the radial head in various degrees of rotation will improve visualization of this structure. These can be made as spot images obtained under fluoroscopic control or as overhead roentgenograms made during various degrees of rotation of the radius. These procedures project the various surfaces of the radial head in profile, which improves the chances of demonstrating subtle radial head fractures. Optimal fluoroscopic spot images are obtained with fluoroscopic spot film devices employing small focal spot x-ray tubes (0.3 mm or less).

Radial Head–Capitellum View

The radial head–capitellum view is another roentgenographic projection that is useful in evaluating patients with elbow joint injuries. This roentgenogram is made with the elbow placed on the x-ray cassette in the lateral position and in 90 degrees of flexion. The thumb is pointed upward and the humeral condyles are perpendicular to the cassette. The central x-ray beam is angled 45 degrees to the forearm and passes through the radial head dor-

Special elbow roentgenograms

- Radial head projection
- Radial head–capitellum view
- Axial view
- Cubital tunnel view

A

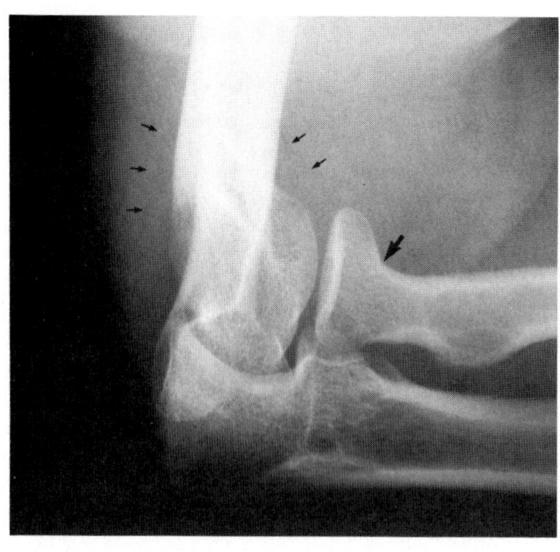

B

FIG. 14-5. A, Radial head–capitellum view. **B,** The radial head–capitellum view may be helpful in demonstrating subtle fractures of the radial head, the capitellum, and the coronoid process of the ulna. This roentgenogram demonstrates a slightly impacted fracture at the base of the radial head *(large arrow)*. Notice the positive fat pad signs indicating the presence of an elbow joint effusion *(small arrows)*.

soventrally.[22] This projection eliminates the overlap at the humeroradial and humeroulnar articulations and projects the radial head anterior to the coronoid process (Fig. 14-5).

The radial head–capitellum view is particularly useful in demonstrating fractures of the posterior aspect of the radial head (those obscured by the overlapping ulna on a conventional lateral view), fractures of the coronoid process, and fractures of the capitellum. Subtle osteochondritis dissecans lesions in the capitellum may be more clearly visualized with the radial head–capitellum view than by standard radiographs.[23,24] The radial head–capitellum view should be employed as an additional roentgenogram when clinical findings strongly suggest an elbow fracture and standard roentgenograms fail to visualize the abnormality.[27]

Axial View

The axial view of the elbow is made by placing the 45-degree flexed elbow on the x-ray cassette and making an x-ray exposure that is perpendicular to the humerus. This view images the olecranon process in an axial projection while the lateral and medial epicondyles are seen in profile (Fig. 14-6).[1,8] The sulcus between the olecranon process and the capitellum, a potential space for small loose bodies, is demonstrated. Osteophytes arising at the medial and lateral aspects of the olecranon–trochlear joint are best seen in this projection (Fig. 14-7). The soft tissues adjacent to the olecranon process and the medial and lateral epicondyles are also demonstrated

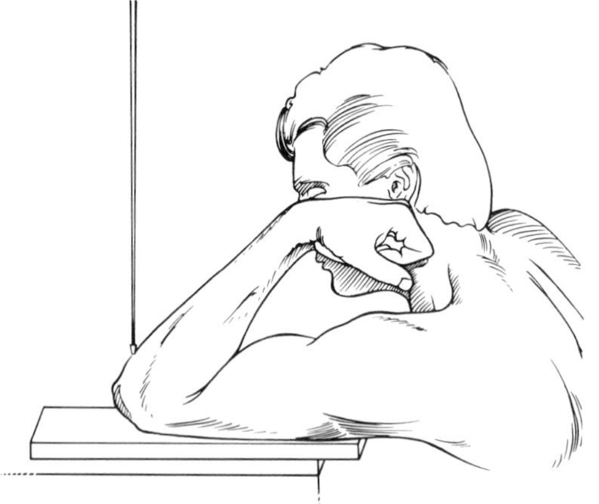

A

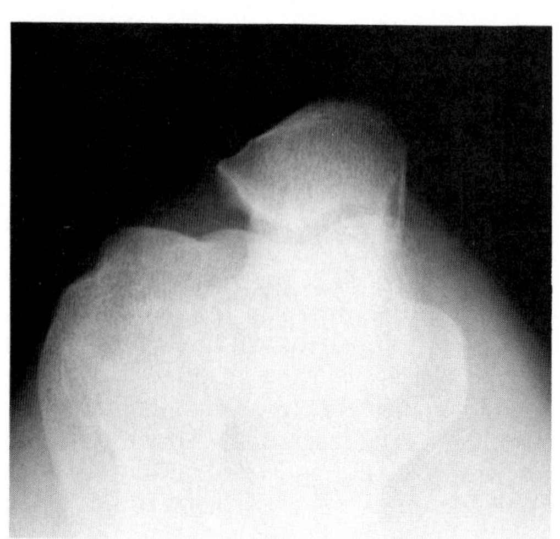

B

FIG. 14-6. A, Axial projection of elbow. **B,** Axial view of normal elbow.

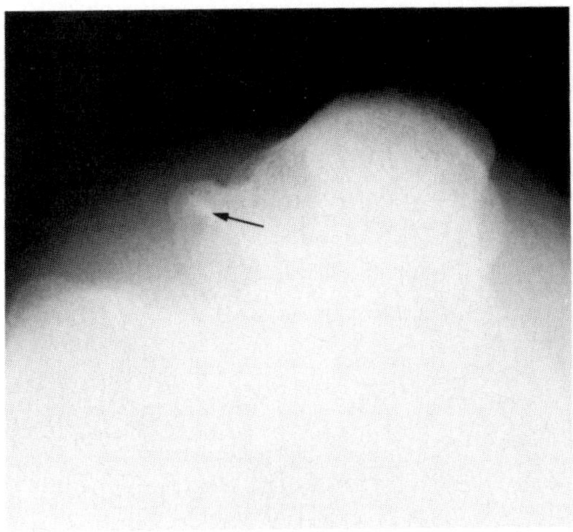

FIG. 14-7. Prominent osteophyte projecting from the lateral aspect of the olecranon process *(arrow)*.

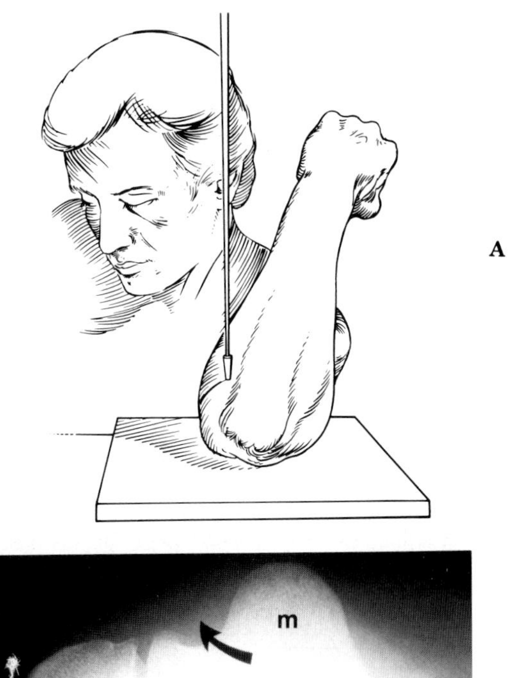

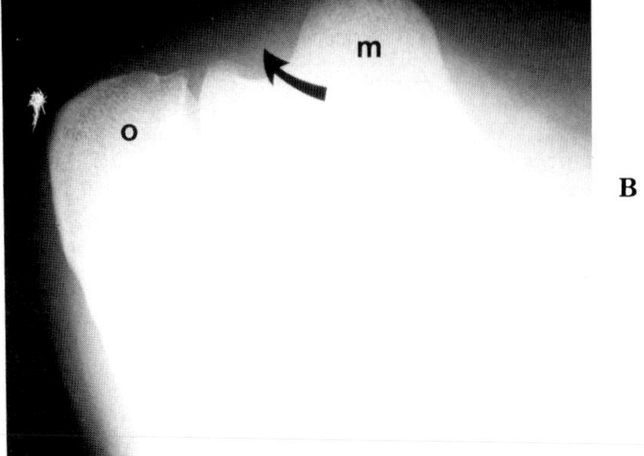

FIG. 14-8. A, Cubital tunnel view. **B,** Cubital tunnel roentgenogram of normal elbow. The curved arrow indicates cubital tunnel. *M*—medial epicondyle, *O*—olecranon process.

for evaluation of postinflammatory or posttraumatic calcification.

Cubital Tunnel View

A roentgenogram to profile the cubital tunnel is made by placing the maximally flexed and 15 degrees externally rotated elbow on the x-ray cassette. This position will cause a vertical x-ray beam to project the cubital tunnel in profile (Fig. 14-8).[55]

The cubital tunnel, the fibroosseous passageway adjacent to the medial aspect of the elbow through which the ulnar nerve courses, was first described by Feindel and Stratford in 1958.[18] The tunnel roof is formed by an aponeurotic arch (the arcuate ligament) that bridges the two heads of the flexor carpi ulnaris muscle. The floor of the tunnel is composed of the medial ligament of the elbow joint. Ulnar entrapment neuropathy, often referred to as cubital tunnel syndrome, can result from medial trochlear osteophytes that elevate the medial ligaments from the floor of the tunnel, resulting in diminished space for the nerve in the tunnel.[55] Lateral shift of the olecranon process during elbow flexion can result in a medial incongruity of the olecranon–trochlear joint space. A medial incongruity of greater than 5 mm is said to be a potential cause of ulnar nerve compression.[55]

ELBOW FAT PADS

Norell[41] in 1954 was the first to suggest that displacement of the posterior fat pad of the elbow was commonly seen in patients with elbow fractures. Bledsoe and Izenstark[7] in 1959 pointed out that displacement of the fat pads anterior to the elbow joint was also seen following elbow trauma.

The roentgenographically visible fat pad anterior to the elbow joint is a summation of the fat collections located in the radial and coronoid fossae. When viewed on the lateral roentgenogram of a normal elbow, these fat collections are superimposed on each other and appear as a radiolucent triangle along the anterior aspect of the distal humerus (Fig. 14-9).

The posterior fat pad at the elbow joint is located in the olecranon fossa. On the lateral view, this posterior fat collection is normally hidden from view by the humeral condyles. The anterior and posterior fat pads are positioned between the flexible joint capsule and the synovium layer of the elbow joint.[40,54]

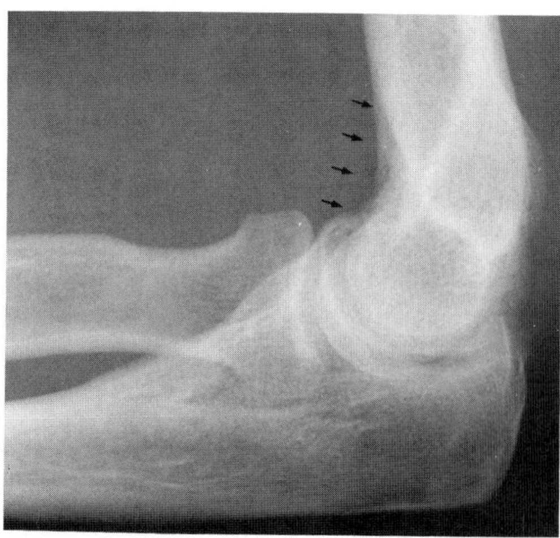

FIG. 14-9. Lateral roentgenogram of the elbow demonstrating the normal appearance of the anterior fat pad *(arrows)*. The posterior fat pad is normally obscured by the humeral condyles.

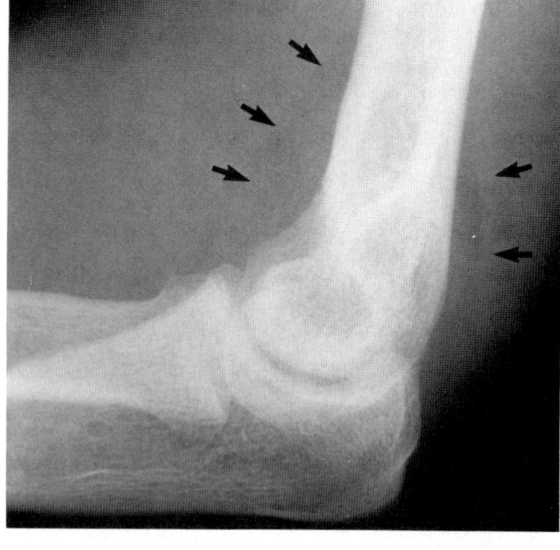

FIG. 14-10. Lateral roentgenogram of the elbow demonstrating positive anterior and posterior fat pad signs *(arrows)*.

Any intracapsular collection of fluid (transudate, exudate, hemorrhage) or tissue leading to capsular distention will cause the anterior fat pad to be displaced anteriorly and the posterior fat pad to be displaced posteriorly. As a result, the anterior fat pad assumes a convex shape on the lateral roentgenogram (ship's sail configuration) while the posterior fat pad will be visualized posterior to the humeral condyles (Fig. 14-10).[40] In acute elbow trauma, positive fat pad signs are the result of intracapsular bleeding secondary to intra-articular fracture.

The roentgenographic projection of the elbow necessary for proper fat pad evaluation is a true lateral view made with 90 degrees of flexion.[25] A slight obliquity of the projection may be enough to obscure the sign.[40] A true-positive fat pad sign following acute elbow trauma is an excellent indicator of an intra-articular fracture. Examinations of the elbow that demonstrate even slight displacement of the fat pads following trauma are likely to reveal fractures if the examiner persists in seeking a positive skeletal finding by using anteroposterior, lateral, oblique, and special roentgenographic views as necessary. Clear roentgenographic evidence of a joint effusion following acute trauma is considered by many as an indication for conservative treatment and radiologic reexamination in 5 to 7 days if initial roentgenograms do not demonstrate a fracture.[9,54]

A false-negative anterior fat pad sign can occur with poor patient positioning, extracapsular fracture, or capsular rupture.[31] According to Murphy and Siegal,[40] a false-positive posterior fat pad sign may occur when the elbow is roentgenographed in extension. A paradoxic positive posterior fat pad sign may occur when the periosteum is stripped from the humerus just proximal to the olecranon fossa, such as with hemorrhage from a supracondylar fracture or subperiosteal neoplasm.[40]

PLAIN ROENTGENOGRAPHIC DIAGNOSIS

Stress Injuries

The elbow is the focus for excessive forces in a number of today's popular sports activities. The elbow is particularly prone to injury in throwing sports such as baseball and javelin and in racquet sports such as tennis and racquetball. The plain roentgenographic examination can demonstrate and document many of these stress-related injuries to the elbow joint.

Slocum[53] was the first to suggest categories of elbow injury based on precipitating stress. A number of authors have elaborated further on this subject.[14,26,32,50,58] Gore et al[21] recently defined five categories of stress-related elbow injuries: diffuse generalized stress, rotational humeral shaft stress, medial tension stress, lateral compression stress, and extension stress. Stresses encountered during the act of pitching are representative of these injury-producing stresses. Effects of these pressures on the elbow joint and the upper extremity are different in the adult and adolescent ath-

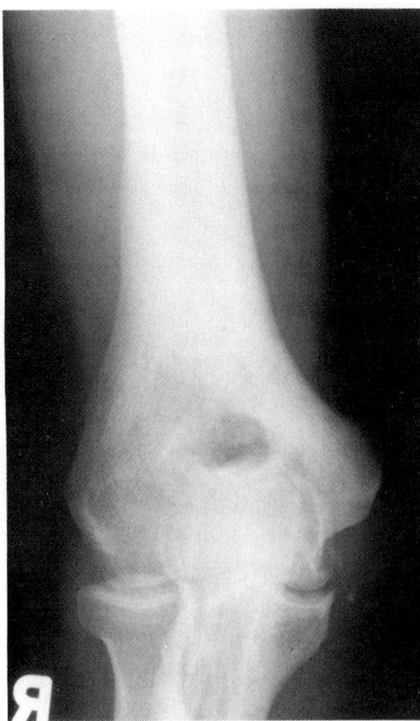

FIG. 14-11. Anterioposterior view of the distal humerus and elbow joint demonstrating cortical and trabecular hypertrophy of the distal humerus in a 28-year-old professional pitcher. This is the result of years of conditioning.

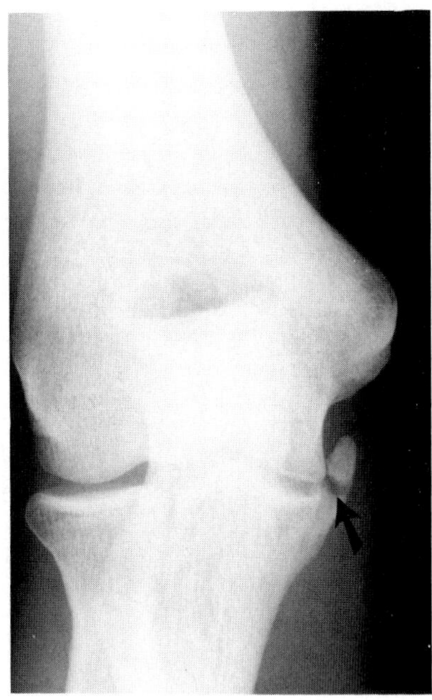

FIG. 14-12. The medial traction spur is a common manifestation of chronic elbow stress in the throwing athlete. In this case, a remote fracture of this spur has healed with a fibrous union *(arrows)*.

lete because of structural differences between the mature and immature skeleton.

Osseous changes about the elbow joint can develop from conditioning of an extremity for the act of throwing or stroking. Conditioning in the mature athlete results in cortical and trabecular hypertrophy and narrowing of the medullary canal of the throwing extremity (Fig. 14-11).[30] The bony hypertrophy is thought to be the result of hyperemia, which leads to accelerated bony remodeling.[21] In the adolescent athlete, diffuse upper extremity stress produces hypertrophy and hypermaturity of the epiphyses and apophyses of the elbow joint.[21,26,32]

The stresses responsible for most elbow injuries from pitching occur during the acceleration phase. The forearm is forced into a valgus attitude with respect to the distal humerus during this phase, which results in distraction forces at the medial aspect of the elbow joint (medial tension stress) and impaction forces at the radial-capitellar articulation (lateral compression stress). In the adult, where the ulnar collateral ligament is the primary medial stabilizer of the elbow, most medial tension injuries result from chronic strain of the ulnar collateral ligament at its attachment on the coronoid tubercle. In the adolescent, the ulnar collateral ligament is relatively lax and the flexor-pronator muscle group becomes the primary medial support for the valgus strain of throwing. Excessive medial tension stresses on the immature skeleton, therefore, result in injury to the medial epicondylar apophysis, the point of attachment of the flexor-pronator muscles.[21,26,32,53]

The most common roentgenographic manifestation of medial tension stress in the throwing adult athlete is a traction spur arising from the medial aspect of the coronoid tubercle (Fig. 14-12). Gore et al[21] reported that 75% of the sixteen professional baseball players they studied for roentgenographic manifestations of elbow stress demonstrated these spurs.

Unusually excessive strain on the ulnar collateral ligament may lead to a cortical avulsion fracture of the medial epicondyle or a rupture of the medial collateral ligament itself. An examination of the elbow under fluoroscopy may be necessary to assess adequately the degree of joint instability following a medial collateral ligament tear. Findings in the injured joint should always be compared with those found during a similar examination of the patient's uninjured elbow.

Posttraumatic changes in the medial epicondylar physis and apophysis may be seen in the juvenile pitcher. This injury has be-

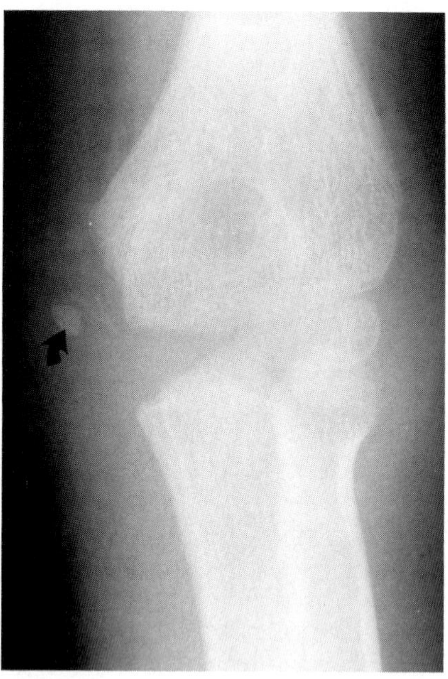

FIG. 14-13. Occasionally a complete avulsion of the medial epicondylar apophysis *(arrows)* can occur from a single stress event. The avulsion fracture illustrated followed a particularly violent throw by this young athlete.

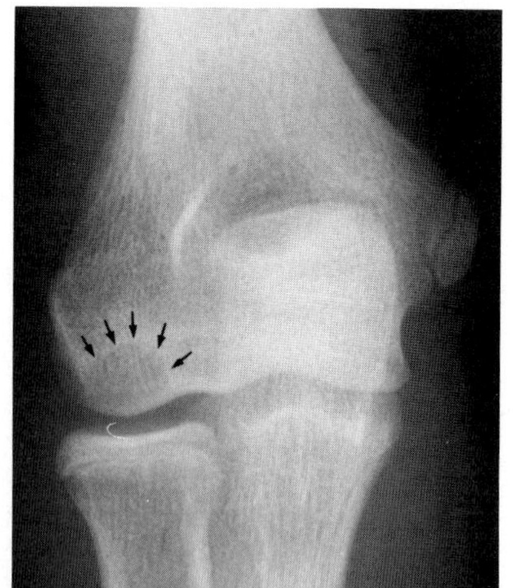

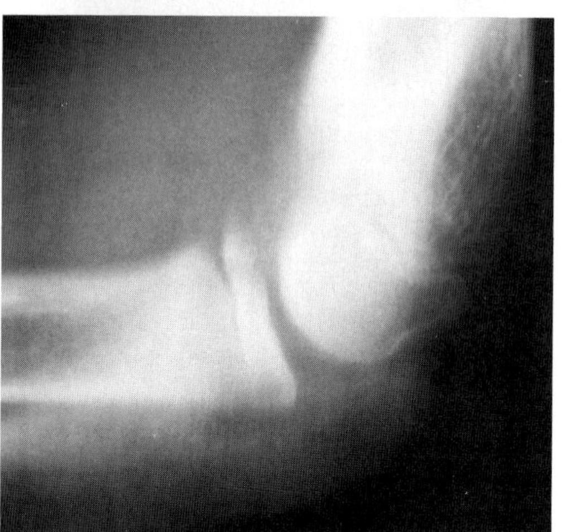

FIG. 14-14. A, The cyst outlined *(arrows)* in the capitellum of this 13-year-old gymnast is compatible with either posttraumatic osteochondrosis or an osteochondral fracture. **B,** The traumatic osteochondrosis of the radial head demonstrated on this lateral tomogram of a 14-year-old pitcher is an unusual manifestation of chronic lateral elbow stress.

come known as little league elbow.[10] The injury is caused by excessive pull of the flexor-pronator muscle group at its insertion on the medial epicondylar apophysis. The radiographic changes seen with little leaguer's-elbow include fragmentation, irregularity, enlargement, and mild separation of the apophysis. These are the result of chronic valgus stress. Occasionally, frank avulsion of the apophysis results from a single traumatic event (Fig. 14-13).[10,32,50] Dr. J. Adams points out, in his review of Larson's Little League Survey published in 1976,[32] that slight widening of the apophyseal plate can result from repeated traction stress and that this finding does not always represent an actual growth plate fracture. The statement is based on his experience that the finding is often seen in asymptomatic patients.

While strong tension forces are applied to the medial aspect of the elbow during the acceleration phase of throwing, equally strong compression forces occur laterally, causing impaction of the radial head on the capitellum. In the adult thrower, Gore et al[21] found that lateral compression forces could occasionally result in an acute osteochondral fracture of the lateral margin of the capitellum. Chronic lateral compartment compression can lead to articular cartilage shaving, which results in degenerative joint disease and loose body formation. Adolescent athletes are more likely to develop lateral compression injuries because they lack the protective cubitus valgus present in adult throwers and because they exhibit a relative laxity of medial joint support.[21] Repeated lateral compression forces in the young thrower can result in osteochondral fractures or traumatic osteochondrosis of the capitellum. Traumatic osteochondrosis of the radial head is an uncommon manifestation of chronic lateral stress.[21,26,32] Subchondral bone deformity, cystic changes, and scattered areas of bone sclerosis are the roentgenographic hallmarks of these injuries (Fig. 14-14, *A* and *B*).

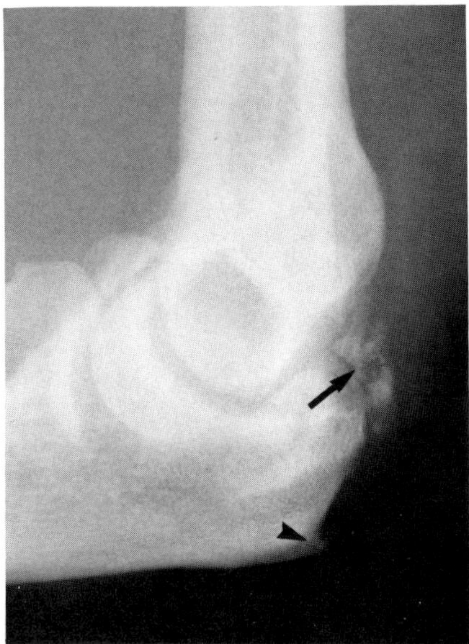

FIG. 14-15. Hypertrophic spurs at the posterior aspect of the olecranon process *(arrowhead)* commonly develop because of violent traction forces that are applied by the triceps tendon during the release and follow-through phase of the pitching motion. Notice the bony excrescences at the posterior tip of the olecranon process *(straight arrow)*.

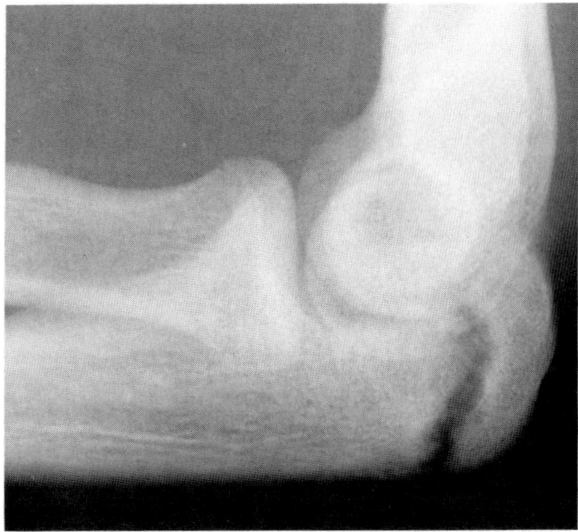

FIG. 14-16. A lateral roentgenogram demonstrates widening of the olecranon apophyseal plate in an adolescent pitcher. The fracture went on to heal with conservative treatment.

During the release and follow-through phases of pitching, the elbow goes from a position of acute flexion to complete extension with the application of a violent force. This force places severe traction on the triceps at its attachment on the olecranon process. In the adult, the repeated pull of the triceps muscle results in formation of traction spurs on the posterior aspect of the olecranon process. Stress or avulsion fractures of the olecranon process may occasionally occur.[21,53,58] Loose body formation is a chronic manifestation of posterior stress (Fig. 14-15). Fractures of the olecranon apophysis have been reported in the adolescent throwing athlete (Fig. 14-16).[44,57]

Loose Body Formation

In the adult, loose body formation may be the result of shaving of the cartilaginous joint surfaces by chronic trauma or the result of fracture of an osteophyte about the elbow joint. Gore et al[21] suggest that the joint incongruity that follows the bony hypertrophy of skeletal conditioning applies pathologic stresses to the synovium, resulting in synovial shredding and metaplasia that leads to loose body exfoliation. In the adolescent, loose bodies may be the result of osteochondral fractures or posttraumatic osteochondroses.[2] The plain roentgenographic projections of the elbow are useful in demonstrating periarticular calcifications and ossifications that are potential loose bodies. Confirmation of a free intra-articular location, however, requires an arthrographic examination.

COMPUTED TOMOGRAPHY

Conventional roentgenographic techniques described in this chapter are an effective means of demonstrating many sports-related injuries of the elbow. However, the axial imaging plane offered by computed tomography (CT) offers an improvement over plain radiography in demonstrating more subtle elbow joint pathologic states. Advances in CT hardware and software allow high-resolution, thin-section axial scans to be obtained with improved contrast resolution.[19] Data obtained from thin-section can be reconstructed in the sagittal and coronal planes. Thin-section studies are particularly helpful in demonstrating subtle fractures, localizing osteophytes and potential loose bodies located out of the plane of conventional roentgenographs, and clarifying joint deformities resulting from significantly displaced fractures of the elbow (Fig. 14-17).

The elbow joint and the upper extremity distal to it can be examined by positioning the arms above the patient's head with the elbows extended and positioned at the level of the scanning gantry. Scans are usually made in a high-resolution algorithm. Patel et al[42] have discussed a modified patient position that may

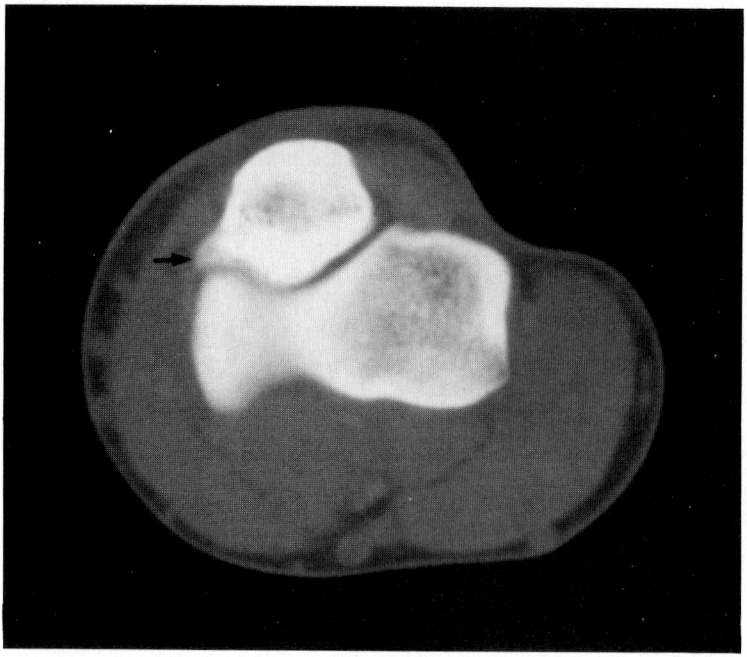

FIG. 14-17. This CT scan made through the condylar region of the distal humerus demonstrates an osteophyte projecting from the lateral aspect of the olecranon process *(arrow)*.

be used when clinical conditions do not allow the patient to be positioned in the scanner in the traditional way. The anatomy and mobility of the proximal radioulnar articulation can also be studied with CT.[12]

RADIONUCLIDE IMAGING

Conventional roentgenographs, particularly in multiple projections, are useful diagnostic tools for demonstrating traumatic injuries of the elbow joint. These examinations are hampered, however, by limited spatial resolution and by the inability of the various roentgenographic projections to visualize all of the complex anatomy of the elbow adequately. While conventional tomography and computed tomography will improve the ability to demonstrate subtle pathologic conditions of the elbow, occult fractures may go undetected unless the appropriate imaging procedure is directed to the location of injury. In addition, several weeks of symptoms will precede any roentgenographic evidence of a stress fracture (e.g., periosteal reaction, endosteal callus, focal bone sclerosis, and ultimately a fracture line).

The radionuclide bone scan, by virtue of its ability to demonstrate physiologic changes in bone, can image the abnormal physiologic changes of a stress injury or an occult fracture considerably earlier than roentgenographic methods can image anatomic evidence of the injury. Early diagnosis of these osseous lesions and their differentiation from soft tissue pathologic states is of primary importance to the competitive athlete who will want to continue training unless significant injury can be documented.[28]

Three-Phase Scanning

Three-phase radionuclide imaging following bolus intravenous injection of 20 mCi (740 MEq) of Tc-99m–labeled methylene diphosphonate (Tc-99m MDP) is the bone-imaging protocol favored by most nuclear orthopaedic specialists.[49]

The three-phase technique consists of: (1) rapid-sequence radionuclide images obtained during the first pass of tracer through the body (vascular phase), (2) blood pool images obtained about 10 minutes after injection (blood pool image), (3) delayed images obtained 2 to 3 hours after injection (delayed image). The three-phase bone scan, therefore, demonstrates the perfusion of a lesion (phase 1), the relative vascularity of a lesion (phase 2), and the relative bone turnover of a lesion (phase 3).[35]

Three-phase bone scan

1. Vascular phase
2. Blood pool images
3. Delayed images

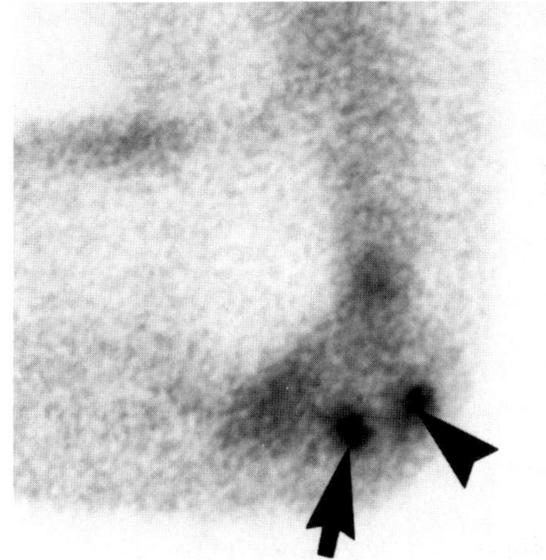

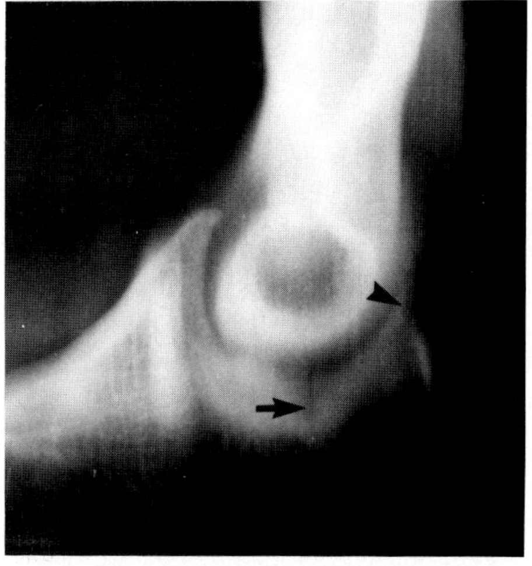

FIG. 14-18. A, This delayed image from a three-phase Tc-99m MDP bone scan was obtained on a 26-year-old professional pitcher with unexplained chronic elbow pain. The scan demonstrates two focal areas of increased radionuclide activity representing foci of abnormal bone metabolism in the olecranon process (*short arrow* and *arrowhead*). **B,** A lateral tomogram of this elbow demonstrates that the more anterior focus of activity corresponds to a stress fracture through the subarticular region of the olecranon process (*short arrow*). The more posterior focus of activity (*arrowhead*) relates to a posttraumatic osteophyte.

Stress Fractures

The radionuclide bone scan has been shown by numerous authors to be highly sensitive in detecting bone stress injuries when conventional roentgenogram are normal.* All three phases of the scan will be positive in the patient with an acute stress fracture. Fractures are imaged as focally intense areas of tracer accumulation involving 50% or more of the bone cortex.[35] A positive bone scan can be expected considerably before the 2 to 3 weeks necessary for documentation of a stress injury with conventional roentgenograms. Conventional tomography or CT scans of the positive area can be helpful in confirming the fracture and in differentiating it from other pathologic conditions that can cause positive three-phase bone scans (e.g., osteoid osteoma or Brodie's abscess [Fig. 14-18]).

Wilcox et al[59] suggest that the pain associated with a stress fracture may not be present before the radionuclide scan becomes positive. The sensitivity of radionuclide scanning in demonstrating active stress injuries is such that when a scan is negative, a stress fracture is quite unlikely.[35,48]

The radionuclide angiogram and blood pool images have been found to be helpful in assessing healing of bone stress injuries. As healing occurs, first the radionuclide angiogram and then the blood pool images will become normal. The intensity of radionuclide uptake on delayed images decreases over 3 to 6 weeks but can still be increased for 8 to 10 months after injury.[49] Simple periosteal reaction is differentiated from a true stress fracture by its superficial and linear scintigraphic appearance compared with the fusiform configuration of a stress fracture.

Occult Fractures

The radionuclide bone scan can also be helpful in documenting and localizing occult posttraumatic fractures when standard roentgenograms are negative. According to Matin,[35] almost all fractures will be detected by bone scintigraphy within 1 day of injury and certainly within 3 days of the trauma. Conventional tomographic or CT images made through the area of the positive scan will help to document the fracture.

ELBOW ARTHROGRAPHY

Roentgenographic techniques, including conventional tomography and CT, have only limited value in evaluating the soft tissues and cartilaginous structures of the elbow joint. Roentgenographic imaging following the intraarticular injection of roentgenographic contrast material provides information about the articular surfaces of the joint, the synovial lining of the joint, and the relationship of peri-

*References 13, 20, 28, 35, 36, 48.

articular calcification to the joint cavity.

Elbow arthrography was first described by Lindblom in 1952.[34] In 1962, Del Buono and Solarino[15] reported the use of double-contrast elbow arthrography in the diagnosis of chondromatosis, osteochondritis dissecans, detached osseous fragments, and posttraumatic calcifications and fibrosis. Since these early reports, the procedure has undergone progressive refinement including the application of conventional tomography[17] and CT.[52]

Techniques

Elbow arthrography can be carried out using either single or double-contrast techniques. Scout roentgenograms of the elbow in at least anteroposterior (AP), lateral, and both oblique projections should precede the arthrographic procedure. Arthrocentesis is generally carried out under fluoroscopic control using a lateral approach to the joint. A 1- or 1½-inch (2.5 or 3.8 cm) hypodermic needle is adequate for this purpose. A posterior approach to the elbow joint has been noted to be helpful in patients who have undergone resection of the radial head.[29]

Standard Arthrography

Single-contrast arthrograms are produced by injecting the volume of water-soluble iodinated contrast material necessary to mildly distend the joint capsule (Fig. 14-19). The contrast material may be diluted with sterile water or saline to decrease its density. This will allow better visualization of intraarticular loose bodies.[6,38] **Double-contrast arthrography** is carried out with 0.5 ml of iodinated contrast material followed by the injection of 6 to 12 cc of room air.

With single-contrast arthrography, standard roentgenograms in the AP, lateral, and both oblique projections are obtained following contrast material injection. Follow-up fluoroscopy of the joint has been noted to be useful.[6,29] Similar roentgenograms are obtained during the double-contrast technique. Pavlov et al[43] suggest that roentgenograms with the elbow in positions that vary the dependent portions of the joint be added to the filming sequence of the double-contrast procedure. The dependent views are said to be helpful in documenting a free intraarticular position of osteocartilaginous bodies.

Arthrotomography

The complexity of the anatomy of the elbow joint makes it difficult to demonstrate all of the articular surfaces in profile on standard roentgenographic projections. The addition of conventional tomography to elbow arthrography is thought by many authors to be the best arthrographic method of evaluating pathologic conditions of the elbow joint.[17,29,38] Arthrotomography provides an improved method of localizing articular cartilage defects and demonstrating small loose bodies com-

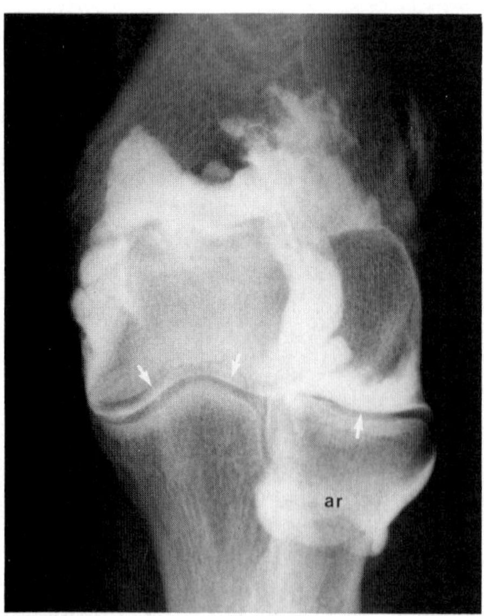

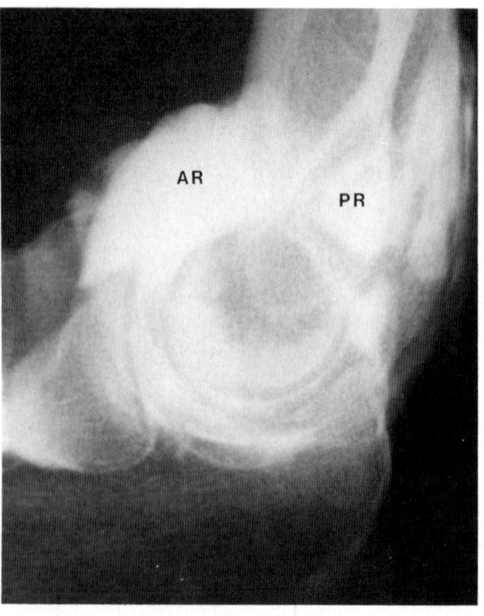

FIG. 14-19. AP **(A)** and lateral **(B)** roentgenograms of the elbow made during a single-contrast elbow arthrogram demonstrate the articular cartilage *(arrows)* with normal filling of the anterior recess *(AR)*, the posterior recess *(PR)*, and the annular recess *(ar)*.

pared with standard elbow arthrography. Arthrotomography is particularly effective when coupled with the double-contrast arthrographic technique. Scout tomograms at about 3 mm intervals in the AP and lateral projections are obtained preceding the arthrogram. Identical sections are then made after the introduction of contrast medium. Tomography is followed by a fluoroscopic examination (Fig. 14-20).

Recently, CT scanning has been suggested as a replacement for conventional tomography in the arthrotomography technique. Thin, high-resolution CT sections (2 to 3 mm thickness) of the elbow's contrast-enhanced anatomy can be reconstructed in multiplanar images following CT scan in a single plane.[52]

Loose Bodies

Elbow arthrography is most commonly employed for the demonstration and localization of intraarticular loose bodies. Arthrography can determine which paraarticular calcific densities seen on plain roentgenograms lie within the joint cavity and which are embedded in the soft tissues. Occasionally, arthrotomography will demonstrate a cartilaginous loose body that has not been suspected on the basis of a plain roentgenographic examination (Fig. 14-21). Intraarticular loose bodies are diagnosed when they are shown to be completely surrounded by air or contrast material and are demonstrated to move freely within the joint during the postarthrography fluoroscopic examination. Calcifications that are fixed in the periarticular soft tissues may move, but less freely than loose bodies. They do not roll over and over and they do not fall into dependent portions of the joint.[29] Decreased joint motion resulting from impingement by thickened synovium or bony prominences can also be documented during arthrotomography and fluoroscopy.

Articular Cartilage

Arthrography may also be helpful in assessing the articular surfaces of patients with osteochondritis dissecans or osteochondral fractures. The plain roentgenographic examination will often suggest subchondral bone irregularity in these patients. Occasionally, however, the only diagnostic information to be obtained will be an articular cartilage defect demonstrated by arthrotomography (Fig. 14-22).

MAGNETIC RESONANCE IMAGING

Magnetic resonance imaging (MRI) is an exciting computerized procedure that has been shown to be useful in demonstrating

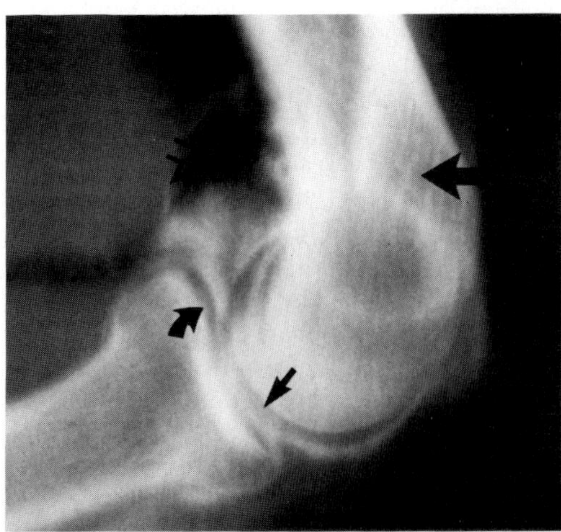

FIG. 14-20. This double-contrast arthrotomogram through the radial capitellum portion of the elbow joint defines the normal articular cartilage of the radius *(curved arrow)* and capitellum *(straight arrow)*. The anterior recess *(open arrowhead)* and posterior recess *(closed arrowhead)* are also demonstrated.

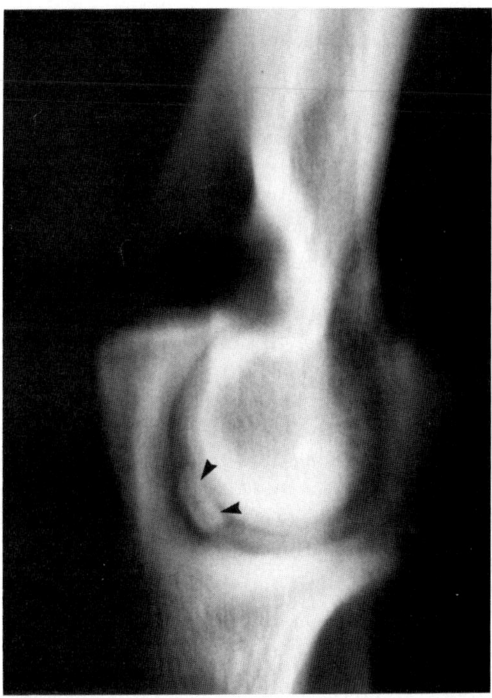

FIG. 14-21. A lateral tomogram made through the ulnar-trochlear portion of the elbow joint during a double-contrast arthrotomogram demonstrates a loose body *(arrowheads)* that was not apparent on routine roentgenograms of the elbow.

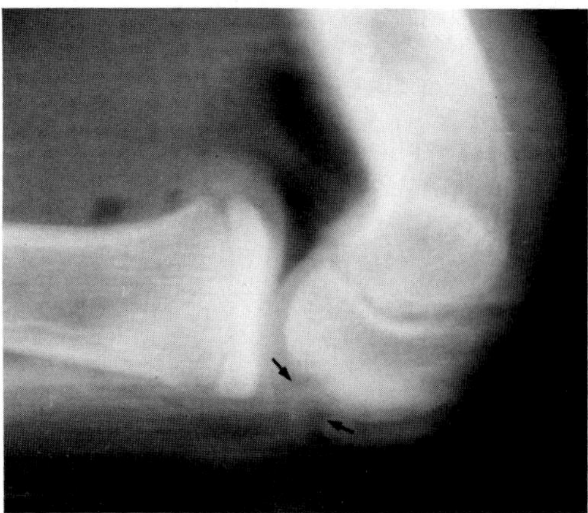

FIG. 14-22. Lateral arthrotomogram through the radial-capitellar portion of the elbow of a 12-year-old pitcher with unexplained elbow symptoms. The arthrotomogram demonstrates an articular cartilage defect that could not be diagnosed on plain roentgenograms and plain tomograms.

traumatic injuries to the musculoskeletal system. This technology, which is based on the principle of nuclear magnetic resonance, produces tomographic images similar to those of x-ray computed tomography but without the use of ionizing radiation.[39]

Technical Considerations

The MR image is created from the interaction between radio waves and hydrogen protons of the body tissues. The MR image is composed of picture elements (pixels) generated by a computer, similar to the mechanism of image production in CT. However, in MR imaging the numeric value of each pixel reflects the intensity of MR signal coming from that volume of tissue rather than the x-ray attenuation of the tissue in that volume element (voxel) as with CT.

The intensity of the MR signal is determined by the density of the resonating nuclei (hydrogen in the present state of development), by proton motion, which is chiefly a function of blood flow, and by two chemical parameters called relaxation times—T_1 and T_2.[47,51] Both normal and abnormal tissues can be characterized by their T_1 and T_2 values, although these values might not be tissue unique. When tissues are altered by disease, their T_1 and T_2 values may change so that pathologic tissues can be distinguished from normal tissues on MR images. Scan techniques (pulse sequences) can be operator selected to enhance either T_1 or T_2 characteristics of tissues, thereby improving the image contrast between normal and abnormal tissues.

TABLE 14-1 Magnetic resonance imaging gray scale: normal anatomy—T_1-weighted spin-echo technique

Anatomic Structure	Signal Intensity	Gray Scale
Areolar tissue	High	White
Yellow bone marrow	High	White
Muscle	Intermediate	Gray
Articular cartilage	Intermediate	Gray
Tendons and ligaments	Low	Gray-black
Flowing blood	Low	Black
Fibrocartilage	Low	Black
Cortical bone	Low	Black

State-of-the-art MR scanners are capable of producing images with excellent spatial and contrast resolution. These images can be obtained primarily in axial, coronal, sagittal, and, with most equipment, oblique planes. Images made with techniques that emphasize T_1 tissue characteristics show excellent spatial resolution and produce the best demonstrations of anatomy; particularly soft tissue anatomy. MR images made with techniques that emphasize T_2 characteristics have a decreased signal-to-noise ratio, which results in images with decreased spatial definition. T_2-weighted images, however, maximize differences in tissue contrast.

The spin-echo imaging technique is currently the most widely employed MR method of imaging musculoskeletal structures. The spectrum of image intensities of normal tissues on T_1-weighted spin-echo pulse sequences is between the very high signal return from fat-containing tissues (fat, yellow bone marrow) and the very low signal return from cortical bone, ligaments, tendons, and fibrocartilage. Fat-containing structures are imaged white on the MR gray scale. Cortical bone is imaged black. The signal intensities of muscle and articular cartilage are intermediate between the intensities of fat and bone and appear gray on the MR gray scale. Vascular structures carrying flowing blood usually demonstrate little signal return and are seen on the black end of the MR gray scale (Fig. 14-23) (Table 14-1).[47] Pathologic processes that cause an increase in the free water of tissue (e.g., tumor, infection, or edema) will cause both the T_1 and T_2 values to be increased. This results in pathologic tissue showing decreased signal (darker) on T_1-weighted scans and increased signal (brighter) on T_2-weighted images compared with

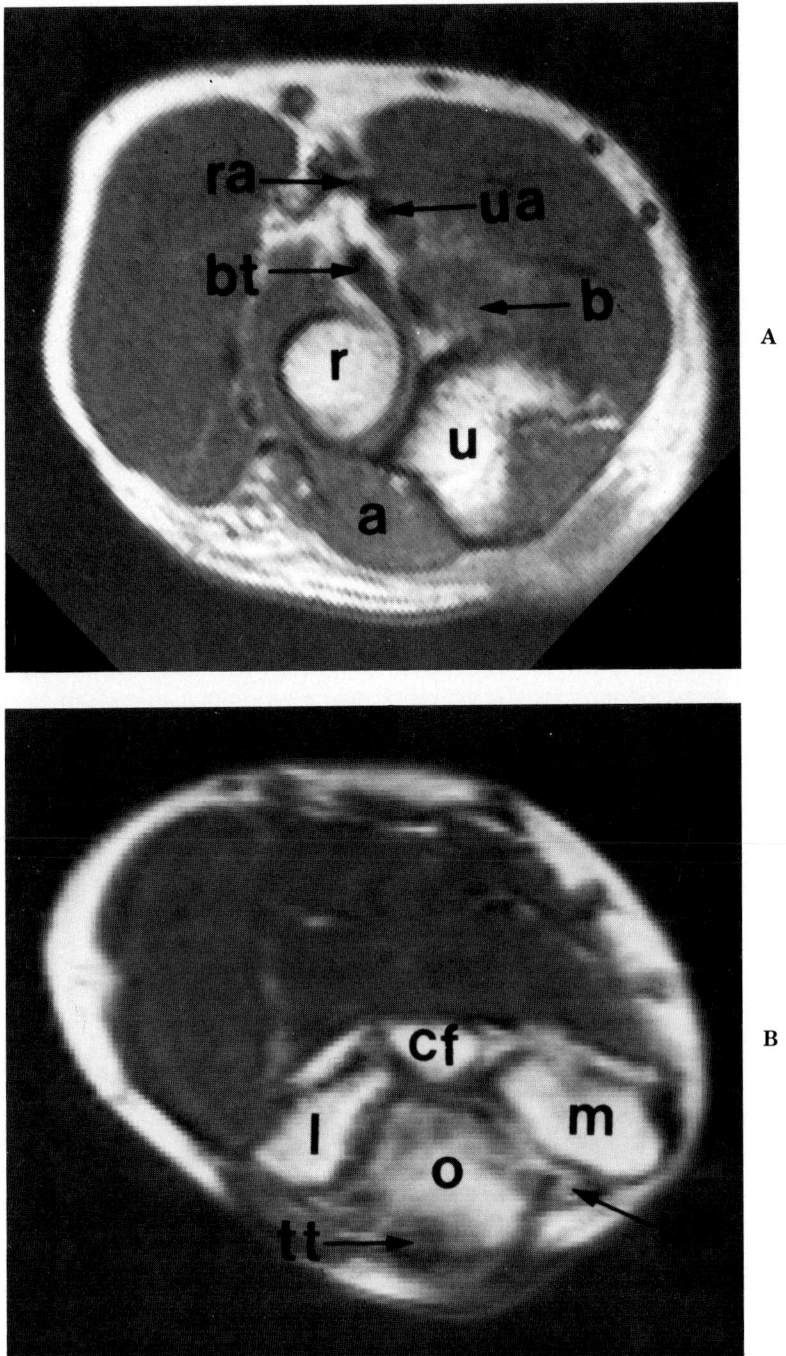

FIG. 14-23. T_1-weighted spin-echo images of a normal elbow (**A**—level of radioulnar articulation; **B**—level of intercondylar region) demonstrate the signal intensities of normal tissues. *r*—radial head, *u*—ulna, *a*—anconeus muscle, *b*—brochialis muscle, *bt*—biceps tendon, *ra*—radial artery, *ua*—ulnar artery, *l*—lateral epicondyle, *m*—medial epicondyle, *cf*—coronoid fossa, *o*—olecranon fossa, *tt*—triceps tendon, *un*—ulnar nerve.

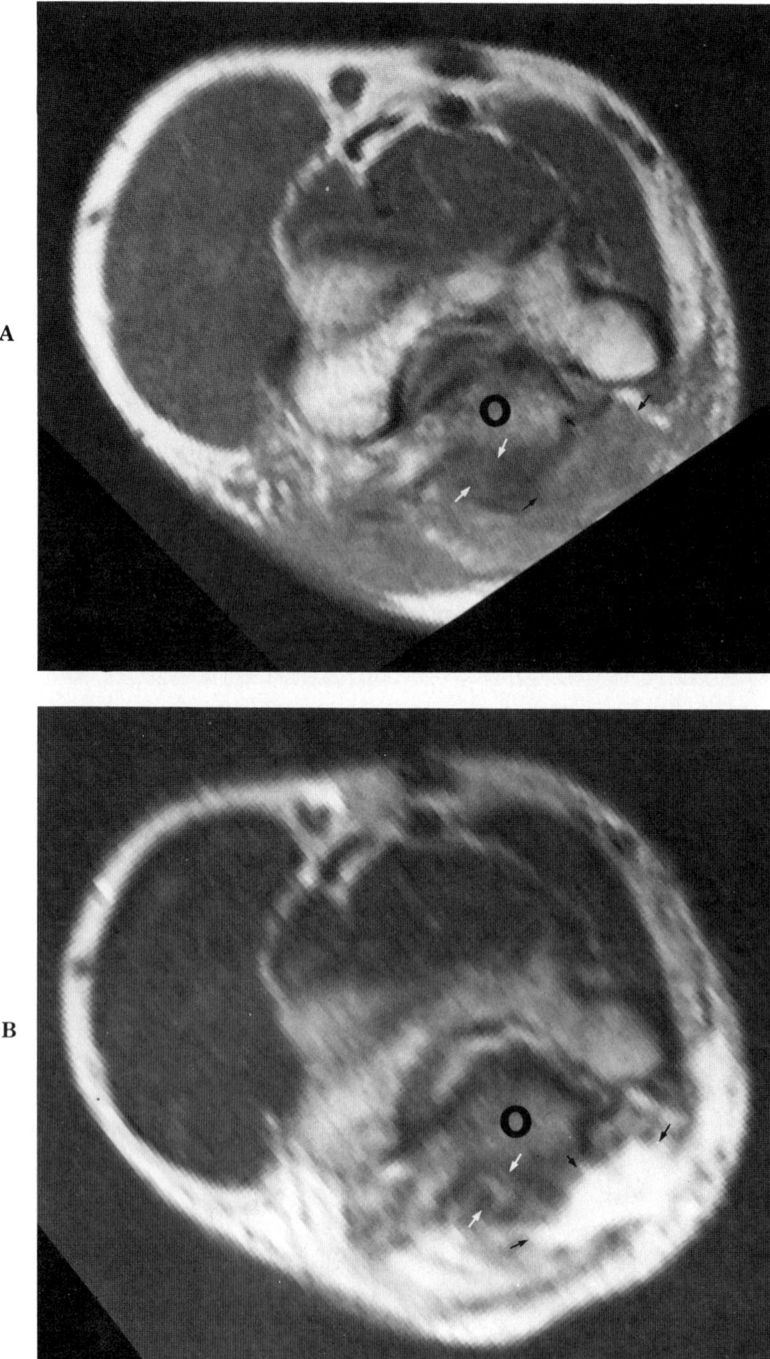

FIG. 14-24. A, The T_1-weighted spin-echo image of a patient with a suspected triceps tendon tear demonstrates decreased definition of the outline of the triceps tendon *(white arrows)* and a soft tissue mass medial to the tendon *(black arrows)*, *o*—olecranon process. Anatomy further defined in Fig. 14-23, *B*. **B,** The corresponding T_2 spin-echo image demonstrates increased signal intensity in the mass, which is consistent with edema or hemorrhage. The findings suggest injury to the triceps tendon and the surrounding soft tissues.

the intensities of corresponding normal tissue. Acute hemorrhage has MR characteristics similar to edema. Subacute hematomas, however, will show relatively bright signal on both T_1- and T_2-weighted pulse sequences.[16,56] Joint effusions produce a bright MR signal on T_2-weighted pulse sequences.[5]

Practical Applications

MRI is a noninvasive method of directly visualizing injuries to such soft tissues as muscle, tendons, and ligaments. Interruptions of the low-signal tendons and ligaments can be seen on T_1-weighted images. The edema and hemorrhage accompanying these injuries have a bright signal on T_2-weighted images (Fig. 14-24).[3,16,51] Muscle tears and associated hemorrhage are easily identified as areas of high-signal intensity on T_2-weighted images.[16]

A volume of information on the use of MR to study pathologic conditions of the knee joint, including ligament injury, meniscus injury, and articular cartilage injury, is now accumulating.[4,33,45,46,60] Advances in MRI technology and the use of local surface coil receivers have led to improved spatial resolution. These improvements will make imaging of smaller joints, such as the elbow, feasible. Recent publications by Middleton et al[37] and Bunnell et al[11] point out that MRI is capable of defining the normal anatomy of the elbow joint. MRI, therefore, has the potential to replace elbow arthrography as the method of diagnosing elbow joint internal derangements.

SUMMARY

A number of procedures that are useful in imaging the elbow joint have been outlined in this chapter. Conventional roentgenograms in standard projections should remain the primary imaging examination for the evaluation of the injured elbow. Specialized roentgenographic projections may provide additional information if they are obtained in appropriate circumstances. Fluoroscopy may provide a cost-effective method of imaging subtle posttraumatic changes.

The use of more sophisticated and costly procedures should be reserved for those cases where appropriate information cannot be obtained with simpler technology. Computed tomography, by virtue of its improved contrast resolution over conventional roentgenographs and its ability to provide images in the axial plane, has proved to be an effective method of documenting injuries in complex anatomical structures, such as the elbow. The three-phase technetium radionuclide bone scan is an efficient method of localizing subtle bone pathologic conditions—providing a "road map" for further analysis with additional imaging techniques.

Arthrography and arthrotomography provide information about the intraarticular and paraarticular structures of the elbow. MRI is proving to be an excellent method of imaging soft tissues such as muscle, tendons, ligaments, and articular cartilage and most certainly will play an important future role in the evaluation of intraarticular and extraarticular injuries to the elbow joint.

The effective use of all of these imaging techniques is predicated on an understanding of their usefulness in providing information about a suspected clinical problem. They should only be ordered after a thorough clinical evaluation has been performed, and the imaging procedure should always be tailored to fit the need of the individual patient.

REFERENCES

1. Ballinger PW: Merrill's atlas of radiographic positions and radiologic procedures, ed 6, St Louis, 1986, The CV Mosby Co, pp 82-93.
2. Bassett LW et al: Post-traumatic osteochondral "loose body" of the olecranon fossa, Radiology 141:635, 1981.
3. Beltran J, Noto AM, and Herman LJ: Tendons: high field strength surface coil MR imaging, Radiology 162:735, 1987.
4. Beltran J, Noto AM, and Mosure JC: The knee: surface coil MR imaging at 1.5 T, Radiology 159:747, 1986.
5. Beltran J et al: Joint effusions: MR imaging, Radiology 158:133, 1986.
6. Blane CE et al: Arthrography in the post-traumatic elbow in children, AJR 143:17, 1984.
7. Bledsoe RC and Izenstark JL: Displacement of fat pads in disease and injury of the elbow: a new radiographic sign, Radiology 73:717, 1959.
8. Bontrager KL and Anthony BT: Textbook of radiographic positioning and related anatomy, ed 2, St Louis, 1987, The CV Mosby Co, pp 112-115.
9. Brodeur AE et al: The basic tenets for appropriate evaluation of the elbow in pediatrics, Curr Probl Diagn Radiol 12(5):1, 1983.
10. Brogdon BG and Crow NE: Little leaguer's elbow, AJR 83:671, 1960.
11. Bunnell DH et al: Elbow joint: normal anatomy on MR images, Radiology 165:527, 1987.
12. Cone RO et al: Computed tomography of the normal radioulnar joints, Invest Radiol 18(6):541, 1983.
13. Dakins DR: Differential diagnosis key to sports injury evaluation, Diagn Imag 9:146, June, 1987.
14. Dehaven KE and Evarts CM: Throwing injuries of the elbow in athletes, Orthop Clin North Am 4(3):801, 1973.
15. Del Buono MS and Solarino GB: Arthrography of the elbow with double contrast media, Ital Clin Orthop 14:223, 1962.
16. Ehman RL and Berquist TH: Magnetic resonance imaging of musculoskeletal trauma, Radiol Clin North Am 24(2):291, 1986.

17. Eto RT, Anderson PW, and Harley JD: Elbow arthrography with the application of tomography, Radiology 115:283, 1975.
18. Feindel W and Stratford J: The role of the cubital tunnel in tardy ulnar palsy, Can J Surg 1:287, 1958.
19. Genant HK: Computed tomography. In Resnick D and Niwayama G, editors: Diagnosis of bone and joint disorders with emphasis on articular abnormalities, Philadelphia, 1981, WB Saunders Co, pp 380-408.
20. Geslien GE et al: Early detection of stress fractures using technetium 99m-polyphosphate, Radiology 121:683-687, 1976.
21. Gore RM et al: Osseous manifestations of elbow stress associated with sports activities, AJR 134:971, 1980.
22. Greenspan A and Norman A: The radial head–capitellum view: useful technique in elbow trauma, AJR 138:1186, 1982.
23. Greenspan A and Norman A: Radial head–capitellum view: an expanded imaging approach to elbow injury, Radiology 164:272, 1987.
24. Greenspan A, Norman A, and Rosen H: Radial head–capitellum view in elbow trauma: clinical application in radiographic-anatomic correlation, AJR 143:355, 1984.
25. Griswold R: Elbow fat pads: a radiography perspective, Radiol Technol 53:303, 1982.
26. Gugenheim JJ et al: Little league survey: the Houston study, Am J Sports Med 4(5):189, 1976.
27. Hall-Craggs MA, Shorvon PJ, and Chapman M: Assessment of the radial head–capitellum view and the dorsal fat pad sign in acute elbow trauma, AJR 145:607, 1985.
28. Holder LE: Radionuclide bone imaging in the evaluation of bone pain, J Bone Joint Surg 64A:1391, 1982.
29. Hudson TM: Elbow arthrography, Radiol Clin North Am 19:227, 1981.
30. Jones HH et al: Humeral hypertrophy in response to exercise, J Bone Joint Surg 59A(2):204, 1977.
31. Kohn AM: Soft tissue alterations in elbow trauma, AJR 82:867, 1959.
32. Larson RL et al: Little league survey: the Eugene study, Am J Sports Med 4(5):201, 1976.
33. Li DKB, Adams ME, and McConkey JP: Magnetic resonance imaging of the ligaments and menisci of the knee, Radiol Clin North Am 24(2):209, 1986.
34. Lindblom K: Arthrography, J Fac Radiol 3:151, 1952.
35. Matin T: Bone scintigraphy in the diagnosis and management of traumatic injury, Semin Nucl Med 13:104, 1983.
36. Maurer AH et al: Three-phase radionuclide scintigraphy of the hand, Radiology 146:761, 1983.
37. Middleton WD et al: MR imaging of the normal elbow: anatomic correlation, AJR 149:543, 1987.
38. Mink JH, Eckardt JJ, and Grant TT: Arthrography in recurrent dislocation of the elbow, AJR 136:1242, 1981.
39. Moon KL, Genant HK, and Davis PL: Nuclear magnetic resonance imaging in orthopedics: principles and applications, J Orthop Res 1(1):101, 1983.
40. Murphy WA and Siegel MJ: Elbow fat pads with new signs and extended differential diagnosis, Radiology 124:659, 1977.
41. Norell HG: Roentgenologic visualization of the extracapsular fat: its importance in the diagnosis of traumatic injuries of the elbow, Acta Radiol 42:205, 1954.
42. Patel RB, Barton P, and Green L: CT of isolated elbow in evaluation of trauma: a modified technique, Comput Radiol 8(1):1, 1984.
43. Pavlov H, Ghelman B, and Warren RF: Double contrast arthrography of the elbow, Radiology 130:87, 1979.
44. Pavlov H, Torg JS, and Jacobs B: Non-union of olecranon epiphysis: two cases in adolescent baseball pitchers, AJR 136:819, 1981.
45. Reicher MA, Hartzman S, and Bassett LW: MR imaging of the knee. Part I—traumatic disorders, Radiology 162:547, 1987.
46. Reicher MA, Hartzman S, and Bassett LW: MR imaging of the knee. Part 2—chronic disorders, Radiology 162:553, 1987.
47. Richardson ML: Optimizing pulse sequences for magnetic resonance imaging of the musculoskeletal system, Radiol Clin North Am 24(2):137, 1986.
48. Roub LW et al: Bone stress: a radionuclide imaging perspective, Radiology 132:431, 1979.
49. Rupani HD et al: Three-phase radionuclide bone imaging in sports medicine, Radiology 156:187, 1985.
50. Schwab GH et al: Biomechanics of elbow instability: the role of the medial collateral ligament, Clin Orthop 146:42, 1980.
51. Sims RE and Genant HK: Magnetic resonance imaging of joint disease, Radiol Clin North Am 24(2):179, 1986.
52. Singson RD, Feldman F, and Rosenberg ZS: Elbow joint: assessment with double contrast CT arthrography, Radiology 160:167, 1986.
53. Slocum DB: Classification of elbow injuries from baseball pitching, Tex Med 64:48, 1968.
54. Smith DN and Lee JR: The radiological diagnosis of post-traumatic effusion of the elbow joint and its clinical significance: the displaced fat pad sign, Injury 10:115, 1978.
55. St. John JN and Palmaz JC: The cubital tunnel in ulnar entrapment neuropathy, Radiology 158:119, 1986.
56. Swensen SJ et al: Magnetic resonance imaging of hemorrhage, AJR 145:921, 1985.
57. Torg JS and Moyer RA: Non-union of a stress fracture through the olecranon epiphyseal plate observed in an adolescent baseball pitcher—a case report, J Bone Joint Surg 59A:264, 1977.
58. Tullos HS et al: Unusual lesions of the pitching arm, Clin Orthop 88:169, 1972.
59. Wilcox JR, Moniot AL, and Green JP: Bone scanning in the evaluation of exercise-related stress injuries, Radiology 123:699, 1977.
60. Wojtys E et al: Magnetic resonance imaging of knee hyaline cartilage and intra-articular pathology, Am J Sports Med 15(5):455, 1987.

CHAPTER 15 Arthroscopy of the Elbow

Howard J. Sweeney

Arthroscopy of the elbow can be a very useful procedure in the armamentarium for therapy of various problems of the elbow joint. The elbow is potentially the most dangerous joint in terms of possible complications experienced in arthroscopic surgery. It is essential that when the elbow is arthroscoped, it be held in a 90-degree flexed position and maximally inflated with liquid before insertion of the arthroscope. These two points will be emphasized a number of times in this chapter because they are key issues in protection against neurovascular damage.

INDICATIONS

The most common indication for arthroscopy of the elbow is the removal of anterior and posterior loose bodies. Synovectomy for rheumatoid arthritis and partial débridement for degenerative joint disease are also valuable procedures. Various bony spurs can be removed from the joint (anteriorly and posteriorly) in an attempt to increase motion. Osteophytes have been removed from the distal humerus, the coronoid process, and the olecranon to reduce pain and to attempt to increase range of motion. Procedures have also been performed to débride osteochondritis dissecans of the capitellum and on occasion to internally fixate the piece in place. It is also to be noted that arthroscopic surgery can be performed on the olecranon bursa, débriding through two of three portals and avoiding a large incision.

Indications for elbow arthroscopy

- Removal of loose bodies
- Synovectomy
- Debridement of osteophytes
- Debridement or fixation of osteochondritis
- Olecranon bursectomy

TECHNIQUE

Initial Setup

Initial setup for arthroscopy of the elbow includes the following steps:

1. The arm is shaved from mid-upper area to mid-forearm and is scrubbed for 10 minutes with soap and water.
2. The patient is given a general anesthesia while lying supine and remains in the supine position.
3. The patient's body is moved to the edge of the table on the side of the affected elbow (Fig. 15-1).
4. A tourniquet is applied to the upper arm and is elevated to 250 mm Hg pressure, subsequent to wrapping the entire arm with an esmark bandage for exsanguination.

5. The forearm is suspended, with the elbow flexed 90 degrees, using Zim Foam material, an ace wrap, a traction spreader, rope, an overhead pulley, and 3 to 4 pounds of weight. The ace bandage should be tight enough around the forearm to stop slippage of the suspension setup (Fig. 15-2).
6. The entire arm is also supported with a standard thigh holder used for knee surgery. This is applied over the arm tourniquet and snugged down loosely. The holder restricts side-to-side motion of the elbow. The superior aspect of the holder is left open, so the surgeon may lift the entire arm superiorly to approach the posterior aspect of the elbow as needed (Fig. 15-3). This same system could be accomplished with two posts, one on either side of the upper arm.
7. The arm is then painted with Betadine,

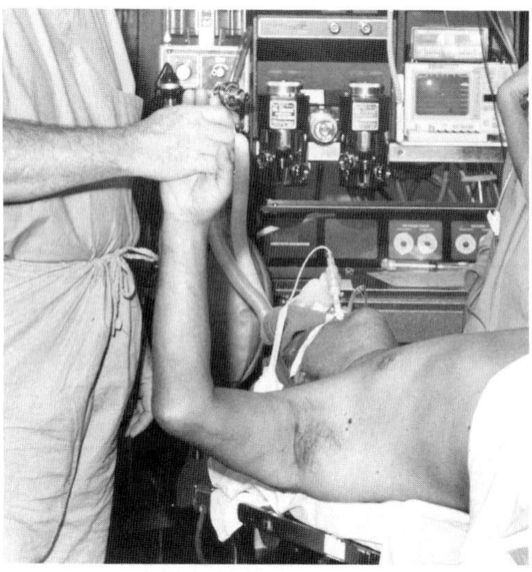

FIG. 15-1. Patient shifted to edge of table, supine position, general endotrocheal anesthesia.

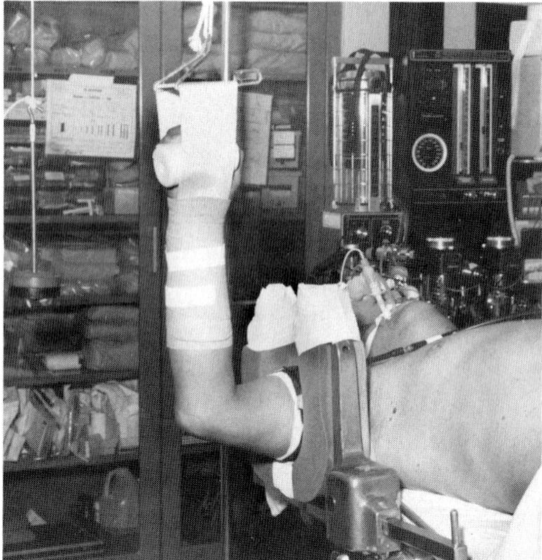

FIG. 15-2. Arm is suspended with elbow at the 90 degree position. Leg holder stabilizes arm. Elbow is easily accessible.

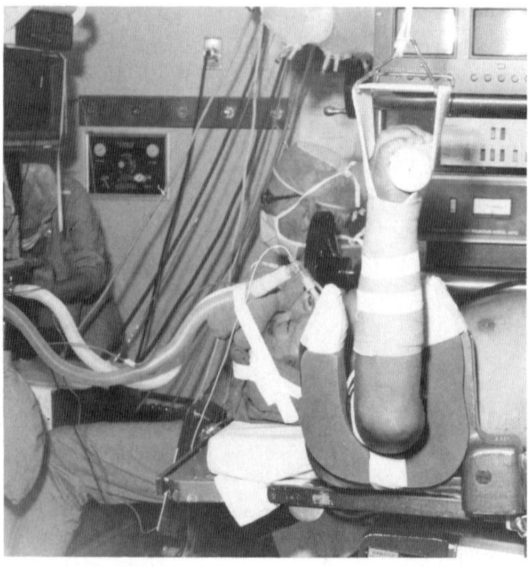

FIG. 15-3. Upper portion of leg holder is kept open to allow elbow extension.

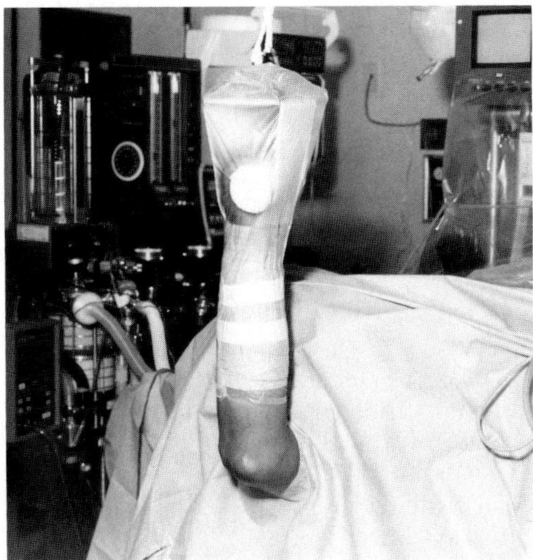

FIG. 15-4. Sterile wrap is applied to suspensory apparatus near operative field.

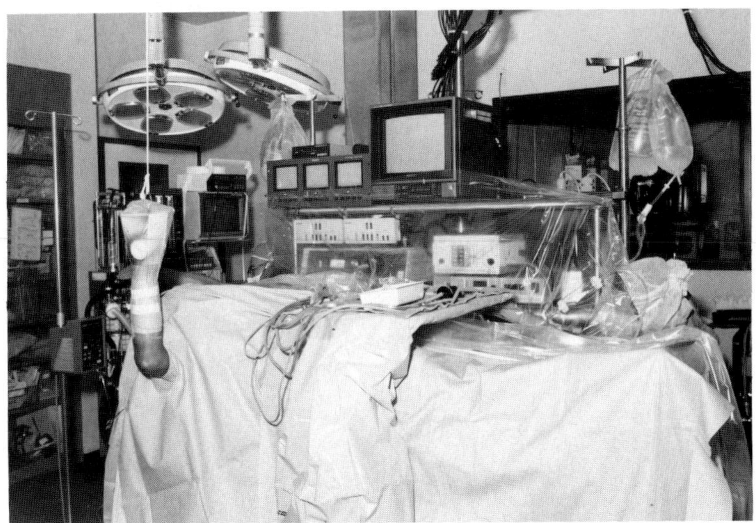

FIG. 15-5. Final preparation and draping.

and sterile draping is carried out.

8. The forearm suspension system is covered with sterile plastic draping material (Fig. 15-4).
9. The television monitor, camera, motorized system, and light source are all placed on the opposite side of the operating table directly across from the surgeon for good, straight-ahead viewing.
10. All the equipment listed in step 9 is covered with a sterile, see-through, plastic drape, for ease of adjustment by the sterile scrub nurse (Fig. 15-5).

Arthroscopic Portals

A variety of portals can be used to visualize the different compartments of the elbow. Portals most commonly used include inferior posterolateral inflow portal, anteromedial, anterolateral, inferior posterolateral, superior posterolateral, and posterior. Establishment of these portals is discussed in the following sections.

Portals

- Inferior posterolateral inflow portal
- Anteromedial
- Anterolateral
- Inferior posterolateral
- Superior posterolateral
- Posterior

Inferior Posterolateral Inflow Portal

The initial approach to the elbow for arthroscopy involves inflation of the joint through a posterolateral approach with either saline or Ringer's lactate solution. An 18-gauge spinal needle is placed posterolaterally in the "soft spot" between the radial head and the olecranon. Forty ml of fluid is passed into the elbow joint using a syringe and extension tubing (Fig. 15-6). One can feel the joint expand anteriorly, and, if the tubing is removed from the needle, there will be adequate flow return from the needle. The initial distention fluid is a combination of Ringer's lactate and epinephrine. Place 1 ampule of epinephrine into 1 L of Ringer's lactate and use 40 ml of this to expand the joint. We never use more than 1 L of this solution.

Initial distention solution

- Ringer's lactate
- Epinephrine

This same location will be used later as a "viewing portal." Also this location is the surgeon's standard approach to aspirate any elbow fluid.

Anteromedial Portal

With the joint well expanded and with the elbow flexed 90 degrees, the initial portal is made anteromedially. This portal is placed 2 cm distal and 2 cm anterior to the medial epicondyle of the humerus (Fig. 15-7). An 18-gauge spinal needle is placed into the joint at that point, and good flow should be obtained before making the definitive arthroscope portal (Fig. 15-8).

The skin is incised with a #11 scalpel blade, taking care not to pass the blade deeply under the skin.

The arthroscopic sheath is then passed into the joint by angling posteriorly toward the joint and aiming at the center of the joint, piercing the joint capsule. One must not pass the scope sheath directly transverse across the elbow because the joint will be missed. Angle directly at the bone and feel your way along the bone. When the trocar is removed, fluid will come forth from the joint. As one tries to puncture the joint capsule, the assistant should maximally inflate the joint through the 18-gauge posterolateral spinal inflow needle (Fig. 15-9).

The arthroscope is placed into the sheath and the joint is inspected. Once again inflate the joint with the needle placed posterolaterally. One can view across the joint in this

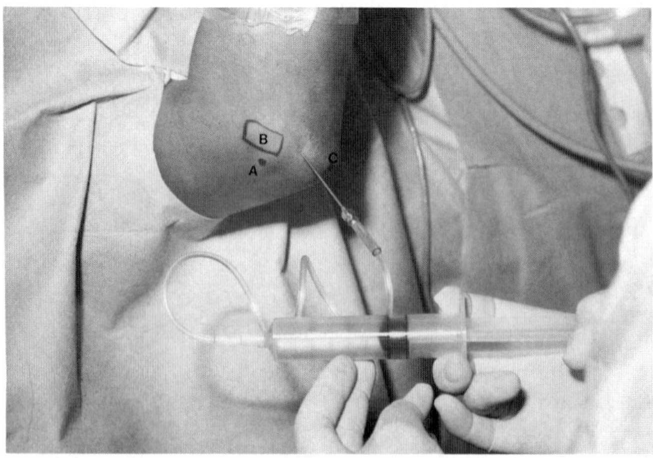

FIG. 15-6. Lateral aspect of right elbow. *A*, Lateral epicondyle. *B*, Radial head. *C*, Tip of olecranon.

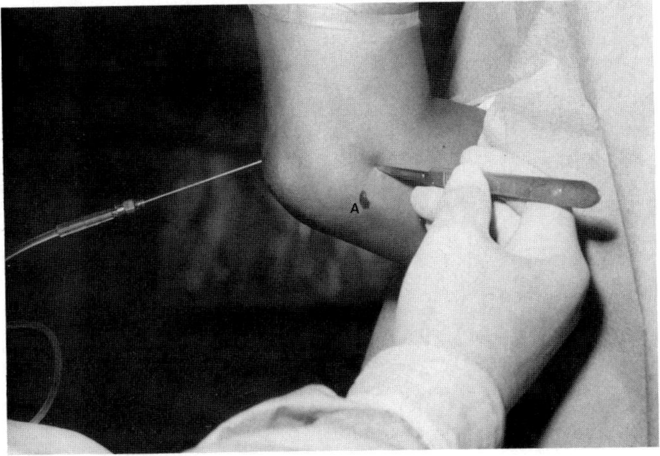

FIG. 15-7. Medial aspect of right elbow. *A*, Medial epicondyle.

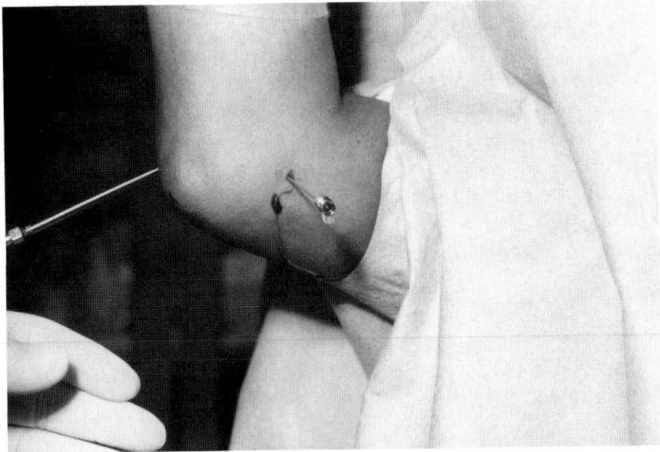

FIG. 15-8. Spinal needle inserted to indentify anteromedial portal site.

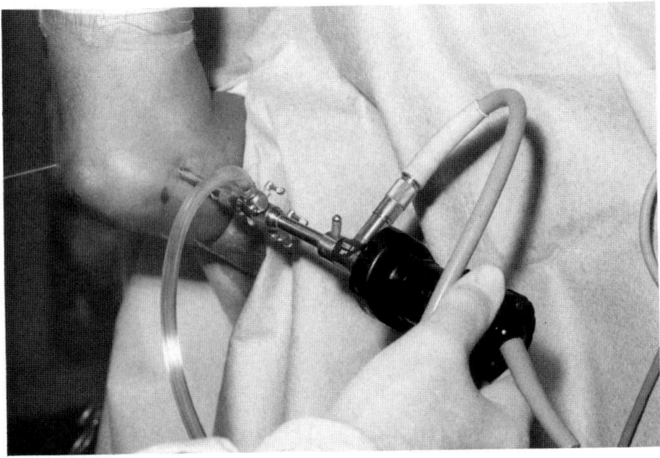

FIG. 15-9. Arthroscope in anteromedial portal.

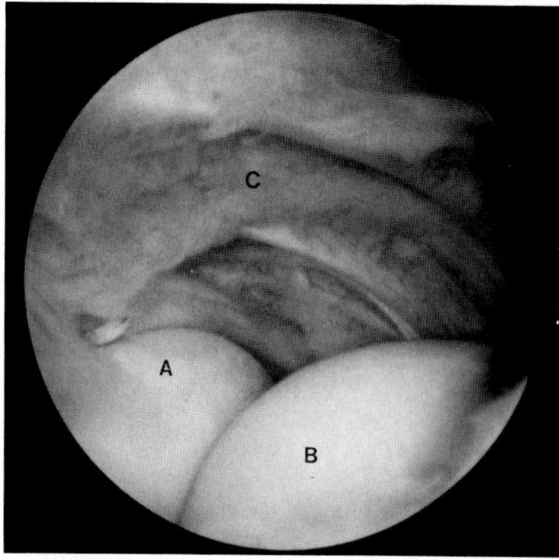

FIG. 15-10. Arthroscopic view from anteromedial portal. *A*, Radial head. *B*, Capitellum. *C*, Synovia anterolaterally.

position and very adequately see the radial head, capitellum, portions of the trochlea, the coronoid process, and the anterior recesses of the joint superiorly. (Fig. 15-10).

One should be sure before making this portal that the patient has not had a previous ulnar nerve transposition.

Anterolateral Portal

To establish an anterolateral portal, the arthroscope is then passed transversely across to the opposite side of the joint, just anterior to the radial head and capitellum. Firmly holding the arthroscope sheath in this position, pass a Wissinger rod through the sheath, puncturing the capsule so it will appear under the skin anterolaterally (Fig. 15-11). Incise skin over the rod and complete passage of rod. In this position one is deep to the radial nerve. This technique adds a great measure of safety to the establishment of this portal (Fig. 15-12).

One now has made anteromedial and anterolateral portals into the joint at this point. With the use of switching sticks, one can move the scope from anteromedial to anterolateral. Either portal can then be used for viewing, probing, or cutting, with inflow through the scope or posterolaterally (Figs. 15-13 to 15-15). These two portals solve most of the problems anteriorly. Dr. Smith, from Seattle, has pointed out the usefulness of 70-degree, 90-degree, and 120-degree scopes in the elbow joint to view either side of the joint.

The anterolateral portal can also be established in very similar fashion to the anteromedial portal, if one wishes to make a direct approach from outside at this point. Locate the lateral epicondyle and establish a point 3 cm distal and 1 cm anterior to the epicondyle. Make a small 5 mm skin incision at this point taking care not to penetrate deeply.

Once again, penetrate with the arthroscope sheath and trocar through the skin portal, angle toward the bone so the joint is entered directly, thus avoiding the radial nerve, which will be anterior to the scope sheath. If this

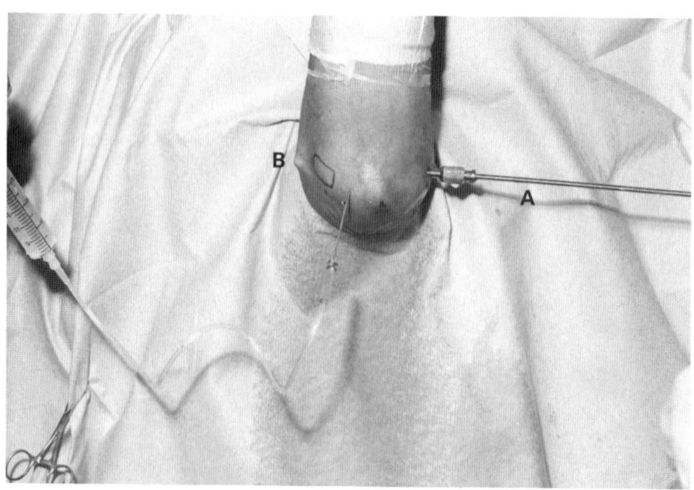

FIG. 15-11. *A*, Wissinger rod. *B*, Rod tenting. Skin anterolaterally deep to radial nerve.

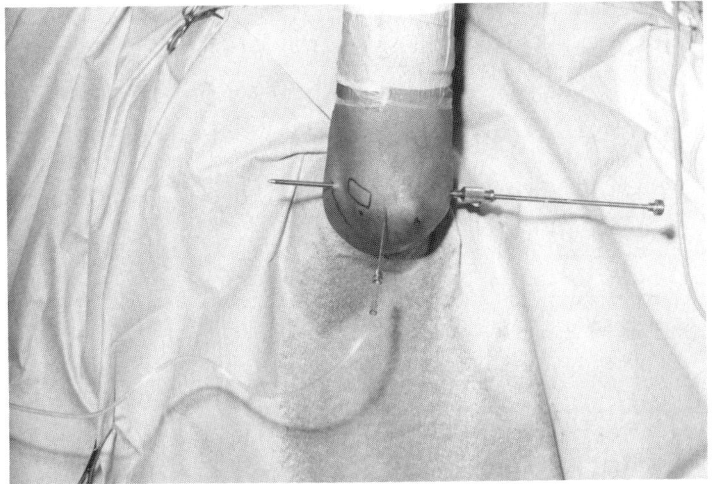

FIG. 15-12. Wissinger rod passed through joint from medial side to lateral side.

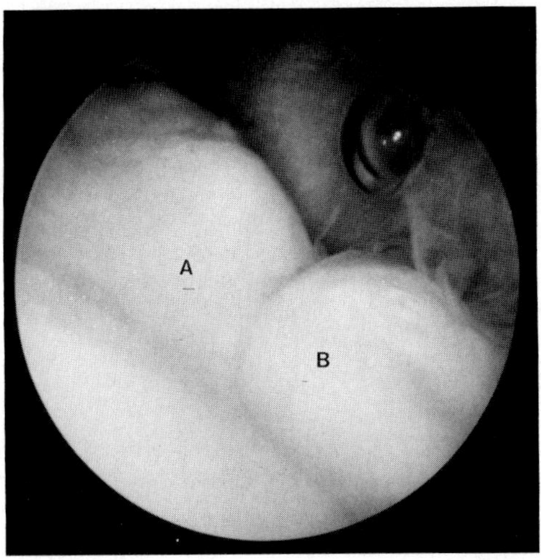

FIG. 15-13. Scope now in anterolateral portal viewing medially. *A*, Trochlea. *B*, Coronoid Process.

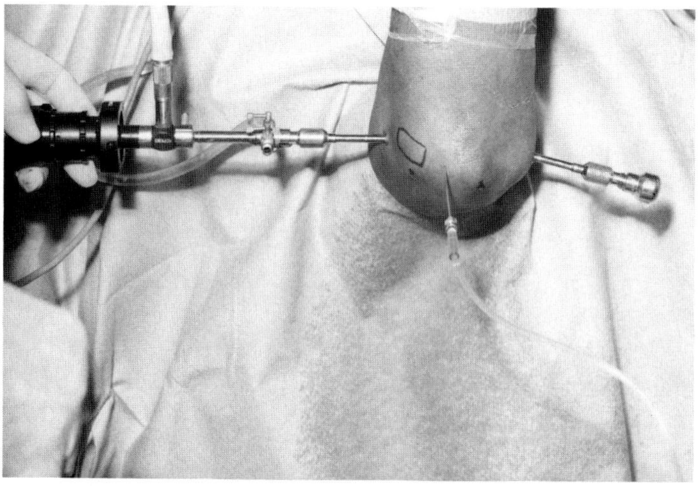

FIG. 15-14. Scope anterolateral with inflow and synovial resector anteromedial. Eighteen-gauge spinal needle lateral—not being used at the moment.

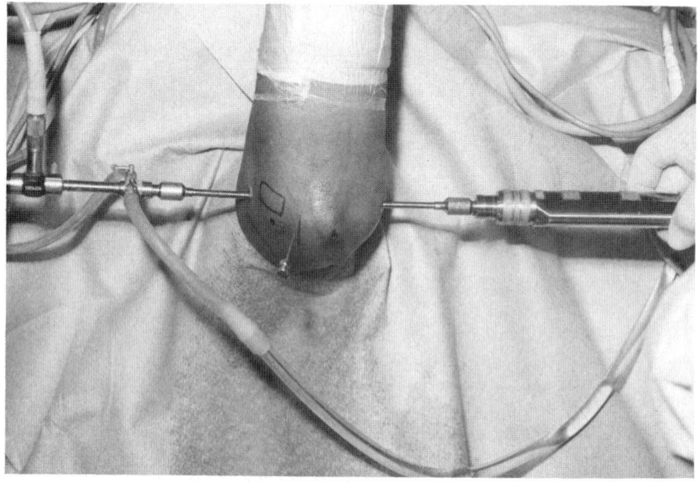

FIG. 15-15. View of joint from anterolateral portal looking medially.

anterolateral portal is used initially, the scope can be passed across to the opposite side of the joint anteromedially and then the Wissinger rod can be used to establish an anteromedial portal.

There is discussion whether it is safer to start anterolateral or anteromedial with the initial portal. It has been our feeling they are of equal danger in terms of the relationship of the brachial artery, median nerve, and radial nerve to the distended joint capsule in the 90-degree flexed position.

Lynch,[9] Meyers, Whipple, and Caspari demonstrated that flexion of the elbow to 90 degrees and distention of the joint greatly increases the distance between the scope sheath and various nerves. They found the mean distance between the scope sheath in the anterolateral portal and the radial nerve was 4 mm before and 11 mm after maximal distention. Using the same technique, they found "the median nerve was a mean distance of 4 mm anterior to the sheath without distention and 14 mm anterior with 35 to 40 cc of distention."

Techniques to avoid nerve injury

- Flex elbow to 90 degrees
- Distend joint maximally

Inferior Posterolateral Portal

The inferior posterolateral portal is placed in the "soft spot" on the lateral side of the elbow between the radial head and the olecranon. The surgeon already has had the inflow needle in this spot; the same portal should be used for putting the scope in posterolaterally. The joint is inflated through one of the anterior portals using a syringe to produce as much distention as possible for posterolateral scope penetration. A 4 mm or 2.7 mm scope can be used (Fig. 15-16). This portal shows the radial head, the lateral side of the olecranon, and a portion of the capitellum. By moving the elbow back and forth these areas can be seen quite well. Then the arthroscope is directed along the lateral side of the olecranon toward the posterior aspect of the elbow, looking for osteophytes along the lateral surface of the olecranon.

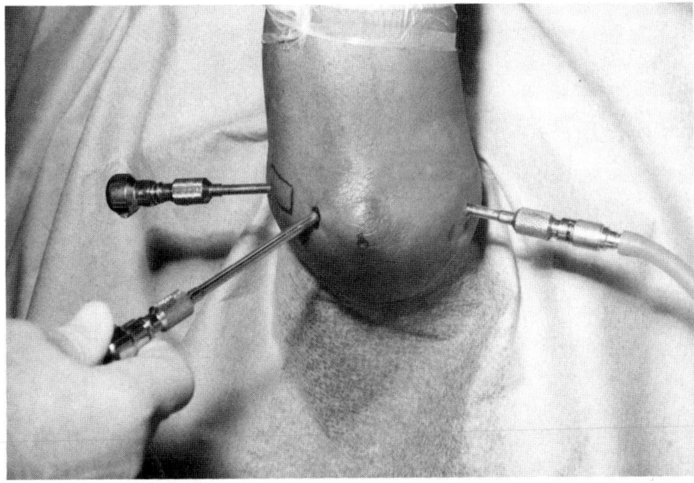

FIG. 15-16. Direct lateral portal into "soft spot." Inflow anteromedially. Cannula with blunt trocar left in place anterolaterally to stop outflow through this portal and help maintain joint distension.

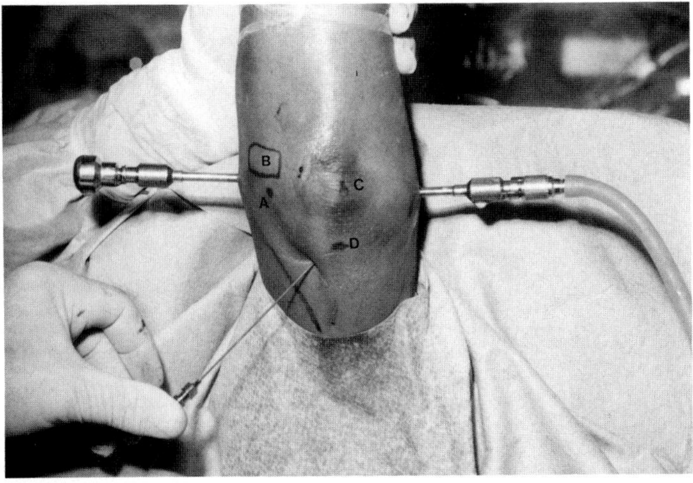

FIG. 15-17. Posterolateral portal. *A*, Lateral epicondyle. *B*, Radial head. *C*, Olecranon. *D*, Proximal tip olecranon—needle being inserted posterolaterally.

Superior Posterolateral Portal

A portal can be placed posterolaterally 3 cm proximal to the olecranon tip and 2 to 3 cm lateral from that point, aiming directly into the olecranon fossa. This portal is located near the lateral edge of the triceps and posterior to the lateral epicondyle of the humerus (Fig. 15-17).

Posterior Portal

A portal can be made directly into the olecranon fossa by measuring 3 cm proximal to the tip of the olecranon, passing through the triceps tendon directly into the olecranon fossa for triangulation purposes (Fig. 15-18).

When establishing posterior portals, distend the elbow fully through an anterior portal to distend the posterior area as much as possible. Reducing the elbow flexion to 20 degrees or 30 degrees will also help for successful posterior capsular entry.

Completion of Procedure

To complete arthroscopy of the elbow, take these steps:

1. Flush joint well with Ringer's lactate solution.
2. Bupivacaine HCL and Marcaine HCL (Marcaine) 0.25% may be instilled into the joint to reduce postoperative pain. I prefer not to use this because of possible dissection of Marcaine into anterior elbow structures, producing confusing neurologic pictures postoperatively.
3. Suture all portals with subcuticular 5-0 Vicryl sutures. I believe this reduces chances of retrograde infection (for knee arthroscopy, no sutures are used).
4. Remove drapes, arm-holding devices, and tourniquet. Check distal circulation for adequacy.
5. Apply sterile 4-inch by 4-inch dressings and wrap from MP joints to mid-upper arm with well-applied Ace bandage and place in a sling with 90-degree elbow flexion.
6. Elevate elbow on two pillows in recovery room.
7. Discharge patient the same day after again checking neurovascular status.
8. Check patient in the office within 2 to 3 days of surgery.

Postoperative Care

Dressings can be replaced with band-aids in 48 hours. Motion is started as soon as possible, and a sling is used only for a day or two postoperatively. Patients are advised to avoid getting the elbow wet for at least 48 hours, and total immersion in water is prohibited for 10 days.

COMPLICATIONS

The 1986 Report from the Arthroscopic Associates of North America Complications Committee was based on 1569 elbow arthroscopies out of a total of 395,566 arthroscopies reported. Small[12] reported the "average responding surgeon doing elbow arthroscopy was doing 0.74 cases per month." One radial nerve injury was reported. Thomas[13] also re-

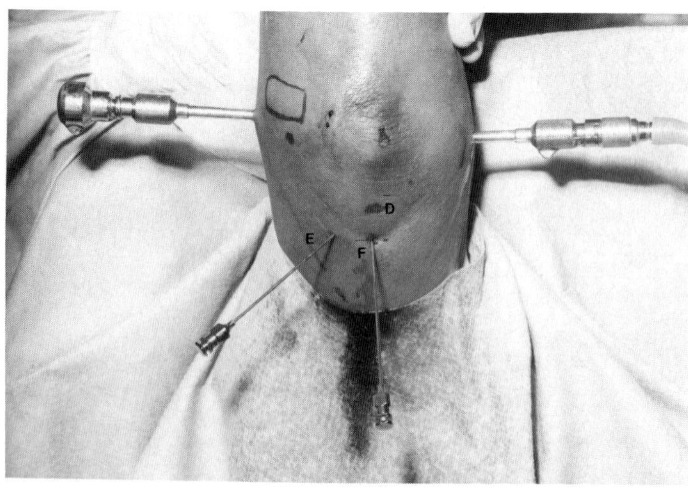

FIG. 15-18. Straight posterior portal through triceps. *D*, Proximal tip of olecranon. *E*, Posterolateral portal. *F*, Straight posterior portal.

ported a case of radial nerve damage in 1987. The potential for serious nerve damage is evident, based on anatomy, and must be guarded against.

SUMMARY

Thus far the indications for elbow arthroscopy are not totally developed. However, the following list represents our present views on the subject:

1. Loose bodies, or suspicion of loose bodies, is the primary indication. Anterior loose bodies are the easiest to remove (Fig. 15-19).
2. Various types of chronic synovitis (e.g., rheumatoid arthritis, pigmented villonodular) may be helped by arthroscopic synovectomy (Fig. 15-20).
3. Bands of scar, located intraarticularly, that restrict motion may be excised.
4. Osteochondritis dissecans of the capitellum can be débrided. Dr. L. Johnson[8] has reported intraarticular fixation of fragment with cannulated screws followd by successful healing.
5. Resection of intraarticular spurs of olecranon, coronoid, and humerus can be done. Results of resection of various spurs still await long-term results.

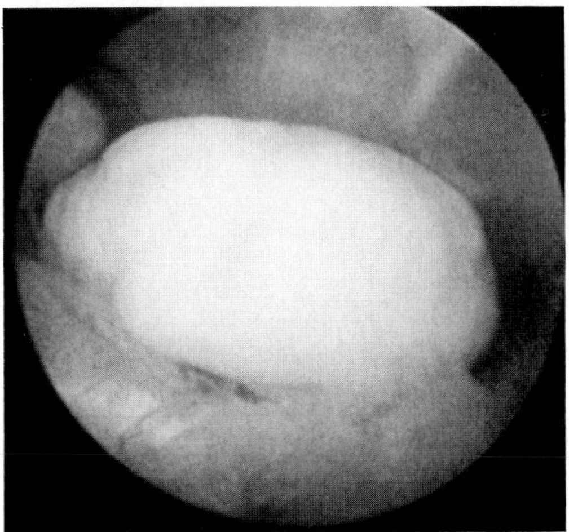

FIG. 15-19. Large loose body lying anterolaterally in elbow joint.

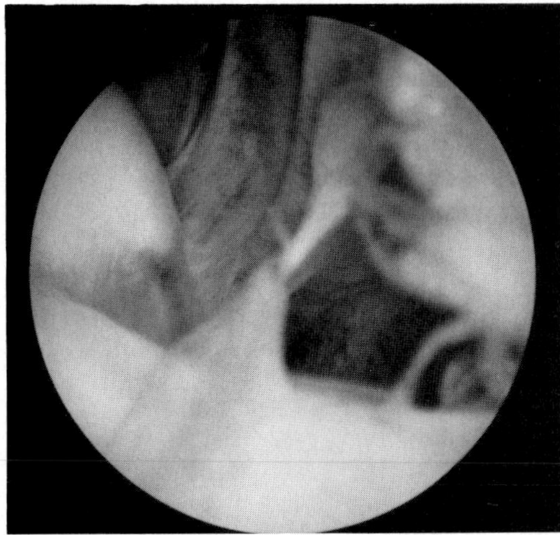

FIG. 15-20. Synovitis, nonspecific—anterior elbow compartment.

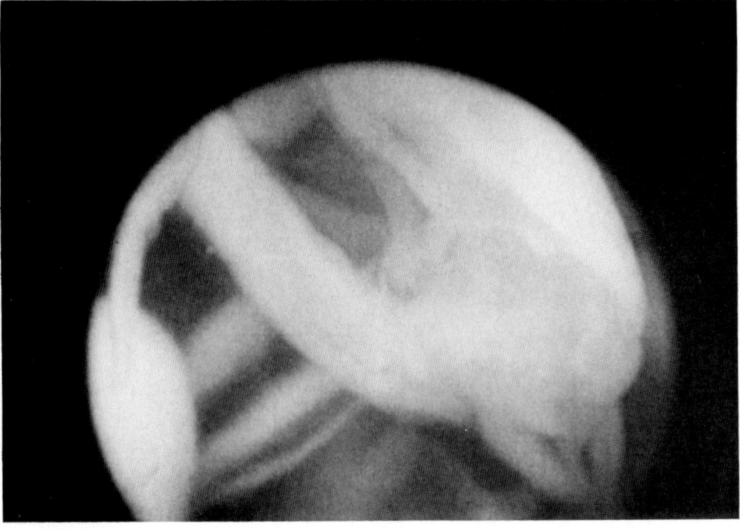

FIG. 15-21. Interior view, olecranon bursa.

6. The "diagnostic problem" can be handled. The patient complains of pain and/or swelling, but no answer has appeared from the work-up. Elbow arthroscopy becomes a very valuable diagnostic tool.
7. Olecranon bursitis can be débrided arthroscopically, avoiding wound sloughs and possible ulnar nerve damage from open bursal resections (Fig. 15-21).

Keeping these indications in mind, the sports medicine physician can now use arthroscopy of the elbow as a potent tool in the diagnosis and treatment of a variety of elbow conditions. Attention to detail is important to avoid potential complications during the procedure.

REFERENCES

1. Andrews JR: Arthroscopy of the elbow, Arthroscopy: The Journal of Arthroscopic and Related Surgery 1(2):97, 1985.
2. Andrews JR: Bony injuries about the elbow in the throwing athlete, Instruct Course Lect-34:323, 1985.
3. Andrews JR: Arthroscopy of the elbow, Clin Sports Med 5(4):653, 1986.
4. Boe S: Arthroscopy of the elbow, Acta Orthop Scand 57:52, 1986.
5. Dutka M: Elbow and wrist arthroscopy: perioperative nursing care, Orthop Nurs 5(4):5, 1986.
6. Eriksson E: Arthroscopy and arthroscopic surgery in a gas versus a fluid medium, Orthop Clin North Am 13(2):293, 1982.
7. Guhl JF: Arthroscopy and arthroscopic surgery of the elbow, Orthopedics 8(10):1290, 1985.
8. Johnson L: Elbow arthroscopy, In Arthroscopic Surgery, Chap 16, 1986, p 1446.
9. Lynch GJ: Neurovascular anatomy and elbow arthroscopy: inherent risks, Arthroscopy: The Journal of Arthroscopic and Related Surgery 2(3):191, 1986.
10. McGinty JB: Arthroscopic removal of loose bodies, Orthop Clin North Am 13(2):313, 1982.
11. Morrey BF: Arthroscopy of the elbow, Instruct Course Lect 35:102, 1986.
12. Small NC: Complications in arthroscopy: the knee and other joints, Arthroscopy: The Journal of Arthroscopic and Related Surgery 2(4):253, 1986.
13. Thomas M: Radial nerve damage as a complication of elbow arthroscopy, Clin Orthop 215:130, 1987.

CHAPTER 16 Acute Injuries to the Elbow

James B. Bennett
Hugh S. Tullos

Acute injuries to the elbow in athletes are common. Diagnosis is not always easy. Factors that can aid accurate diagnosis include the location of pain about the elbow joint, the patient's age, and the sports activity involved. The examining physician must understand both the structural anatomy of the elbow and the biomechanics of the elbow joint as it relates to the specific activity. With this understanding, complaints of pain with activity may be better localized and the specific pathology treated.[3,22]

ANATOMIC CONSIDERATIONS

Osseous Structures

Anatomically the elbow is a hinge joint composed of the distal humerus, which is divided into the capitellum and trochlear articulation. The proximal ulna, which articulates with the trochlea, is composed of a coronoid process and an olecranon process, forming the greater sigmoid notch. The proximal radius articulates with the capitellum as well as with the proximal ulna, which is constrained by the annular ligament. Bone stability of the elbow joint is confined to the coronoid trochlear articulation and the radiocapitellar joint. The olecranon process offers little varus-valgus stability, assuming ligamentous competency is maintained, and then only in complete extension[17] (Fig. 16-1).

Cadaver studies as well as clinical studies have demonstrated that the olecranon can be surgically removed without violating elbow stability up to the insertion of the anterior oblique ligament of the medial collateral ligament complex.[1,21] The joint capsule with the brachialis anterior and the triceps posterior is normally thin and offers little stability.

Capsular thickness, however, can change markedly in pathologic injury states, producing an elbow flexion contracture.

The primary ligament support of the elbow is the **medial collateral ligament** complex. The origin of the medial collateral ligament is medial and inferior to the medial epicondyle with a fanned insertion from the coronoid through the olecranon process. The medial collateral ligament is composed of the thickened parallel fibers of the anterior oblique portion of the ligament. They are organized so that some fibers remain taut throughout the

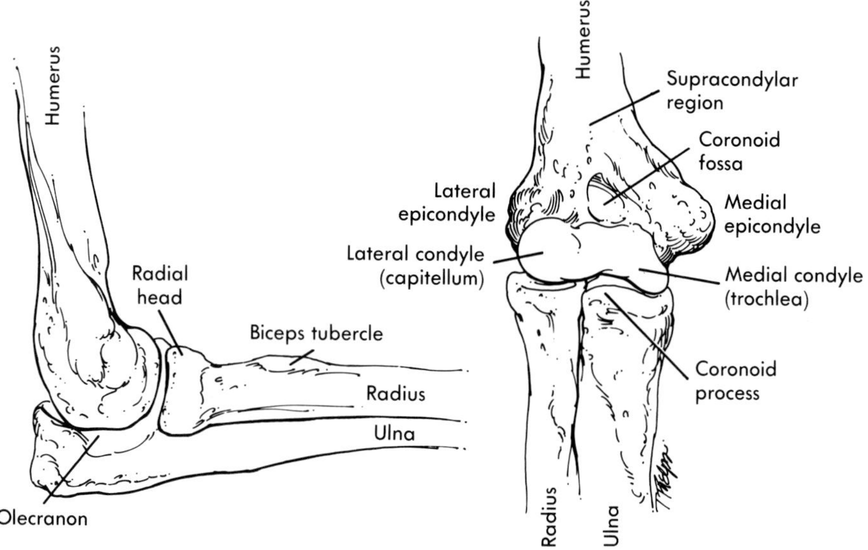

FIG. 16-1. Osseous anatomy of the elbow joint.

entire arch of flexion and extension of the elbow. The fan-shaped posterior oblique is less well developed, taut in flexion, and lax in extension. A small nonfunctional transverse ligament is present on the ulnar attachment of the medial collateral ligament. The medial collateral ligament complex is reinforced by the flexor muscle mass origin.

Medial collateral ligament components

- Anterior oblique—thick parallel fibers
- Posterior oblique—fan shaped
- Transverse—nonfunctional

The **lateral collateral ligament** has three components. The major component of the ligament originates from the lateral epicondyle and inserts into the annular ligament. The annular ligament encompasses the radial head with both origin and insertion on the proximal ulna at the radial notch. The annular ligament contains and restrains the proximal radial head during forceful flexion and supination. A smaller posterolateral collateral ligament has been described and takes origin from the lateral epicondyle. It inserts into the ulna at the base of the annular ligament. This entire complex is further reinforced by the anconeus muscle laterally[18] (Fig. 16-2).

Lateral collateral ligament complex

- Lateral collateral ligament
- Annular ligament
- Posterolateral collateral ligament
- Anconeus muscle

BIOMECHANICS OF ELBOW STABILITY

Biomechanically, valgus elbow stability primarily depends on the integrity of the medial collateral ligament, of which the primary stabilizing factor is the anterior oblique component.[21] This is present in response to the valgus load placed on the elbow in everyday activities and accentuated in throwing sports.

Restraints to valgus stress

- Medial collateral ligament—anterior oblique component
- Radiocapitellar joint—secondary restraint

Lateral joint stability has two components: the stability provided by the annular ligament, which maintains the relationship of the radial head to the proximal radioulnar joint (this ligament is critical in forceful flexion-supination activities), and the lateral collateral ligament, which is of less significance. Varus elbow joint forces are rare and therefore the lateral collateral ligament is not commonly stressed. The lateral ligament anatomy reflects this. The radiocapitellar joint acts as a secondary constraint to valgus stress.

Therefore the stability of the elbow joint is

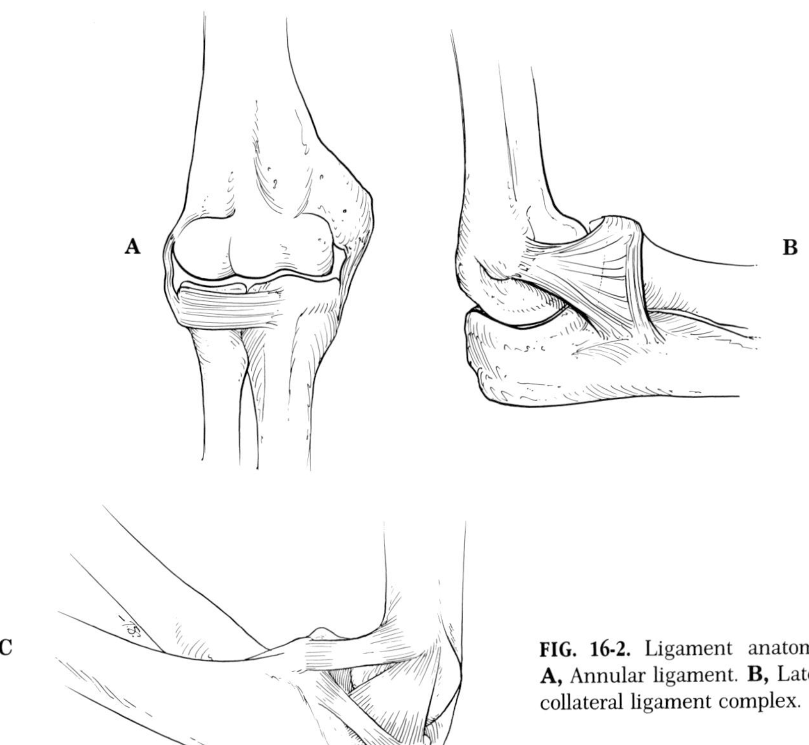

FIG. 16-2. Ligament anatomy of the elbow joint. **A,** Annular ligament. **B,** Lateral ligament. **C,** Medial collateral ligament complex.

contingent on the bony relationship of the radiocapitellar articulation, the trochlear-ulnar joint with its coronoid process, and an intact medial and lateral collateral ligament complex. Alterations in any of these elements may produce pain, weakness, limitation of motion, or instability.

Additional support about the elbow is formed by the muscle envelope, particularly the flexor and extensor tendon origins of the wrist. Various forms of acute overuse muscle strain exist (see Chapter 17). Medial epicondylitis, lateral epicondylitis, triceps tendinitis, and biceps tendonitis may result from an overload or overuse syndrome. Treatment consists of rest, brace or strap support, antiinflammatories followed by strengthening and range of motion programs. Initial ice treatment followed by heat modalities are beneficial. Cortisone injection to a specific site is used sparingly. In the athlete with chronic elbow pain, overuse injuries must be considered both as a primary diagnosis as well as in the differential diagnosis of elbow instability.

SKELETALLY IMMATURE ATHLETES

Children's elbow injuries are usually seen as a result of trauma to the elbow. The result is either fracture or dislocation. The diagnosis and treatment of these injuries are not within the scope of this chapter. It is sufficient to say that closed treatment is usually effective for reduction of the fractures or dislocations, followed by healing and range-of-motion recovery.

Little League Elbow

Little league elbow is an all-inclusive term that may encompass a variety of pathologic problems within the elbow.[2,6] Localized elbow pain at the medial epicondyle associated with a diminished ability to throw suggests a medial epicondyle stress lesion. Usually benign and responding to simple rest, it can, with continued valgus stress such as throwing or a fall, produce an epicondylar avulsion fracture.[28]

Medial Epicondyle Fractures

Medial epicondylar fractures in children may signify a greater problem of acute elbow instability. This fracture is usually associated with a fall and is often nondisplaced. If displacement is present, instability can exist. In the younger child the entire medial epicondylar fragment is avulsed and contains the medial collateral ligament. If the valgus

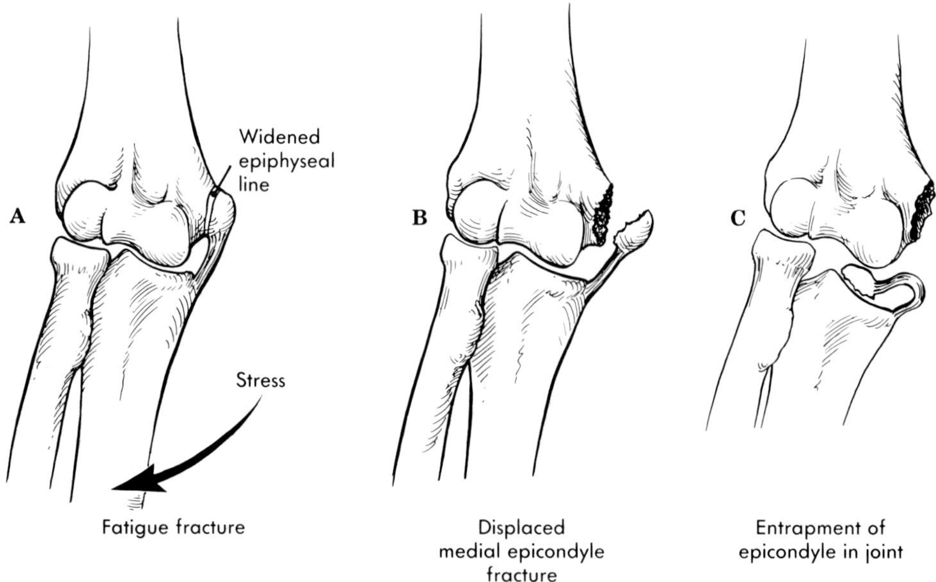

FIG. 16-3. Valgus stress lesions in children. **A,** Stress fracture. **B,** Fracture of epicondyle. **C,** Fracture displaced into joint.

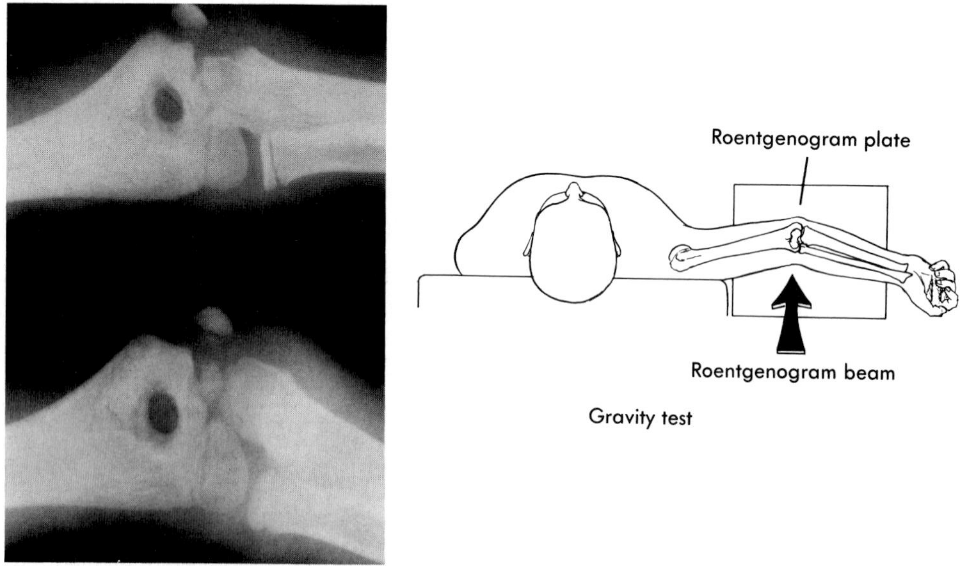

FIG. 16-4. Gravity valgus stress test.

gravity stress test is positive, then surgical repair is indicated.[28] Failure to obtain accurate replacement may result in marked instability of the elbow. Also the fracture fragment may become entrapped within the joint, preventing reduction. This is seen roentgenographically as a widened ulnar trochlear joint (Fig. 16-3).

In the older child, the epiphysis is in the process of closing. Avulsion fracture fragments may be small and may not necessarily involve the collateral ligament. Instability is less likely. Unless instability can be demonstrated with the gravity valgus stress test, these fractures may well be treated conservatively (Fig. 16-4). Acute valgus instability with demonstrated tear of the medial collateral ligament has been successfully treated conservatively. However, if return to competitive-level athletics is expected and the involved elbow is the dominant arm, performance may be better ensured with surgical

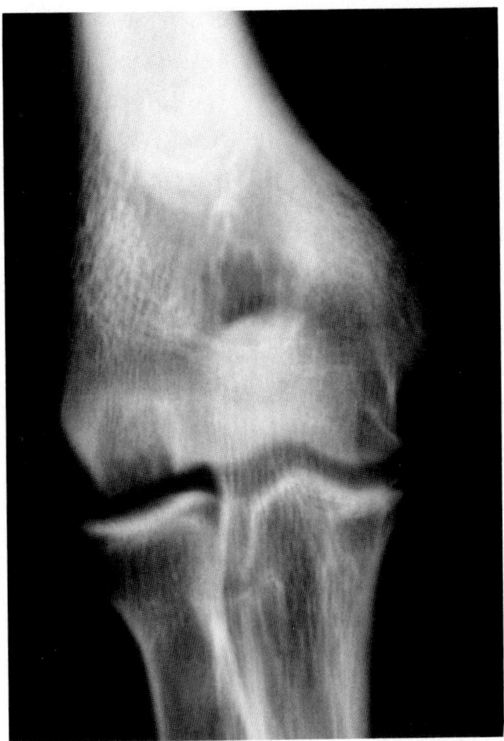

FIG. 16-5. Osteochondritis dissecans of the capitellum.

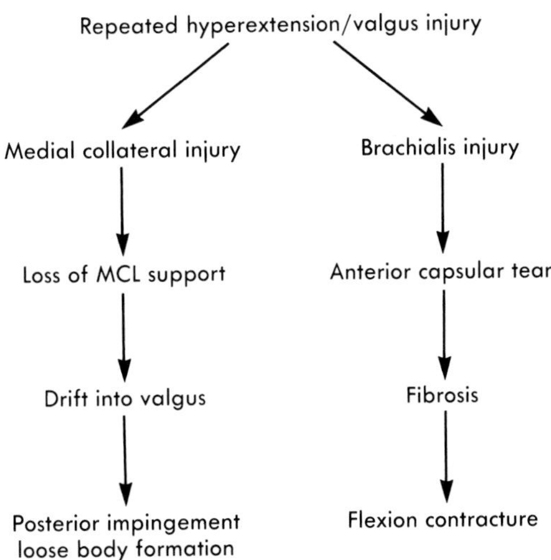

FIG. 16-6. Anterior elbow pain.

repair. Displaced epicondylar fractures are reattached with either Kirschner wires in the young child or malleolar screw in the adolescent. The medial collateral ligament is evaluated and repaired as indicated.

Lateral Elbow Pain

Lateral elbow pain in a child or young adolescent suggest lateral epicondylitis; however, this is relatively rare. More common is **osteochondritis dissecans** or osteochondrosis of the radiocapitellar joint.[20] The basic pathologic state is avascular necrosis of either the capitellum or radial head or both. The diagnosis is made by suspicion, the presence of an elbow flexion contracture, and roentgenographic findings. Treatment consists of rest and withdrawal from throwing activities. Continued throwing activities will deform the articular surfaces and can produce permanent joint irregularities or exfoliate loose bodies (Fig. 16-5).

Anterior/Posterior Pain

Pure anterior or pure posterior pain is rarely seen in the child or adolescent unless fracture dislocation is present.

ADULT INJURIES

Anterior Elbow Pain

As the adolescent matures and sports participation becomes more sophisticated, the injuries tend to be more localized and more severe (Fig. 16-6). Of these, anterior elbow pain associated with hyperextension injuries suggests brachialis muscle or anterior capsular tears with or without joint subluxation. In addition, a capsular flexion contracture may result from bleeding and fibrosis within the capsule. This anterior flexion contracture is often seen in professional baseball pitchers, resulting in part from compensatory hypertrophy of the flexor forearm mass and repeated injury to the anterior capsule and medial ligament structures of the elbow. As medial ligament support is lost, the forearm drifts into valgus and posterior impingement of the olecranon into the olecranon fossa may occur.[13] The result is loose body formation (Fig. 16-7).

> **Anterior flexion contracture in pitchers**
>
> - Repeated anterior capsule injury
> - Flexor mass hypertrophy
> - Repeated medial collateral ligament injury

Biceps Tendonitis/Rupture

Biceps tendonitis at the elbow level is rare. However, with hyperextension or repetitive forceful pronation-supination activities, the musculotendinous junction or tendon insertion on the radial tuberosity may be damaged.

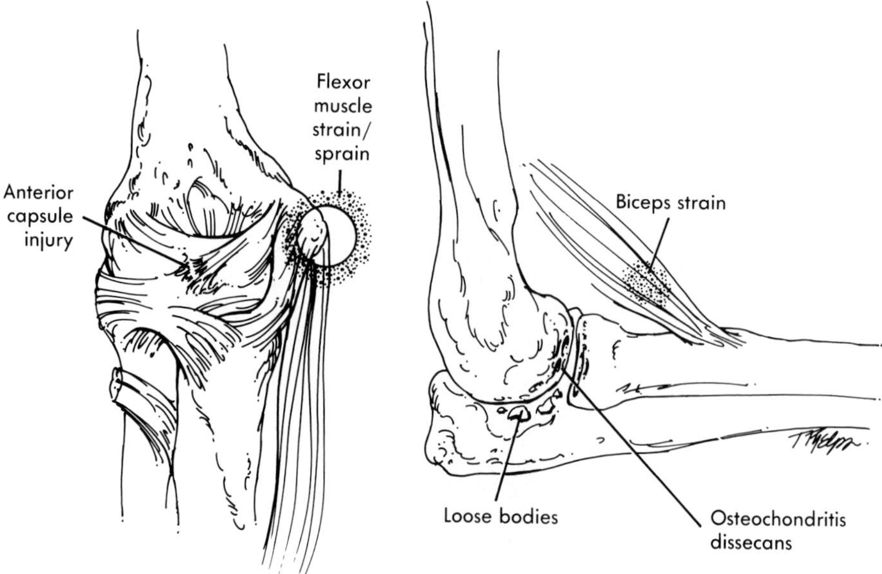

FIG. 16-7. Causes of anterior elbow pain.

Occasionally violent extension or forceful flexion against immovable objects produce a distal biceps tendon avulsion. This is easily identified by the loss of biceps tendon function and a palpable defect at the elbow. The characteristic loss of supination strength is present.

Diagnosis of distal biceps tendon rupture must be differentiated from a **disruption of the annular ligament** with anterior dislocation of the radial head. This also may occur after forceful flexion of the elbow against resistance. The diagnosis of dislocation is easily made roentgenographically.

Both conditions warrant surgical reconstruction. Pull-out wire reattachment of the avulsed biceps tendon to the radial tuberosity requires the forearm to be in supination and the elbow in greater than 90-degree flexion. Protection for 6 weeks is required. Following this, active flexion, active extension, and protected passive extension for an additional 2 weeks is recommended. A 3- to 6-month period is necessary before full activities are instituted.

Annular ligament tears are similarly protected to allow appropriate healing of the repaired or reconstructed annular ligament.

Medial Elbow Pain

Acute medial elbow pain may occur from either epicondylitis with bone or muscle lesions. Actual **rupture of the flexor forearm mass** is rare and limited almost entirely to the activity of throwing or elbow dislocation. Its diagnostic signs are ecchymosis and hemorrhage of the medial elbow with a palpable muscle defect.

Acute **rupture of the medial collateral ligament** has been reported in javelin throwers[25]; however, baseball pitchers and other throwing athletes can occasionally sustain this lesion. The clinical diagnosis is made by demonstrating instability of the elbow to valgus stress, associated with pain localized to the medial aspect of the elbow. This diagnosis may be confirmed by the use of elbow arthrography showing extravasation of dye along the torn ligament[9,16] (Fig. 16-8). However, stress roentgenographic examination of the elbow is usually adequate unless the instability to stress is masked by spasm of the intact forearm flexor muscle mass (Fig. 16-9).

Ulnar Neuritis

Repetitive medial elbow joint injury may occur from activities such as unrestrained throwing. This can result in an ulnar traction spur medially and secondary ulnar neuritis. Pain, numbness, tingling along the course of the ulnar nerve distribution, and (in severe cases) intrinsic muscle function loss may be present. Acute ulnar neuritis in the absence of other elbow pathology may be managed with rest, antiinflammatories, and protection. If the sensory deficits persist and interfere with competitive athletics, the diagnosis should be confirmed by nerve con-

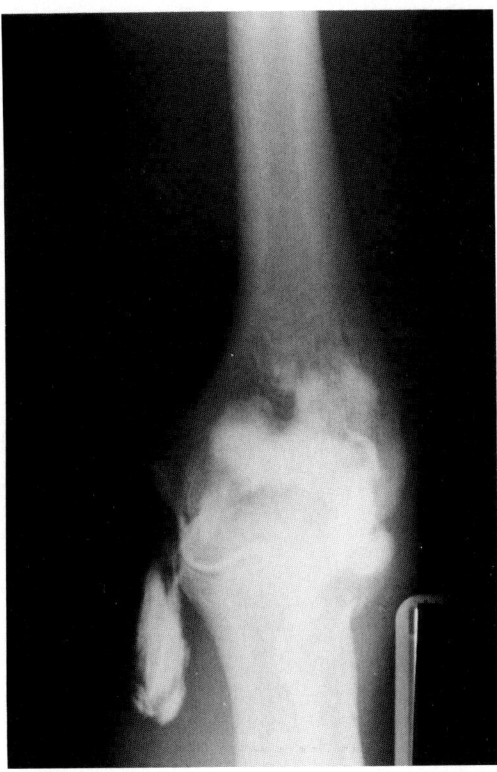

FIG. 16-8. Positive elbow arthrogram with acute medial collateral ligament tear.

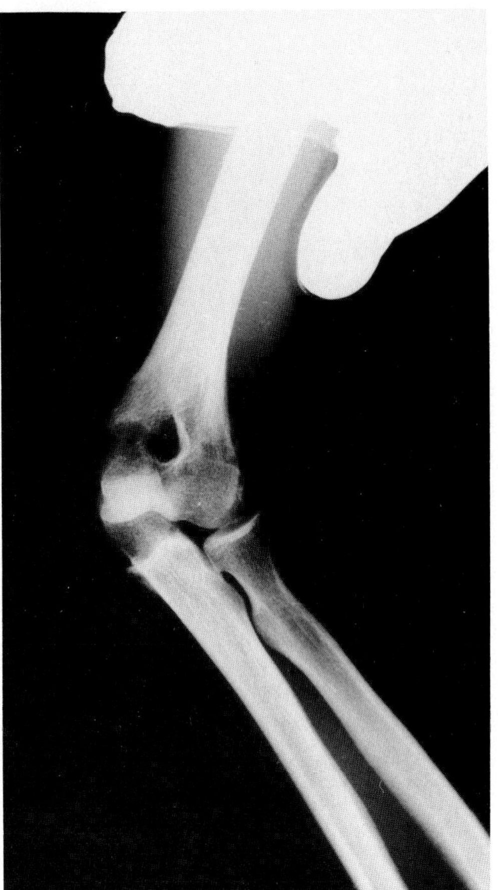

FIG. 16-9. Manual valgus stress roentgenogram.

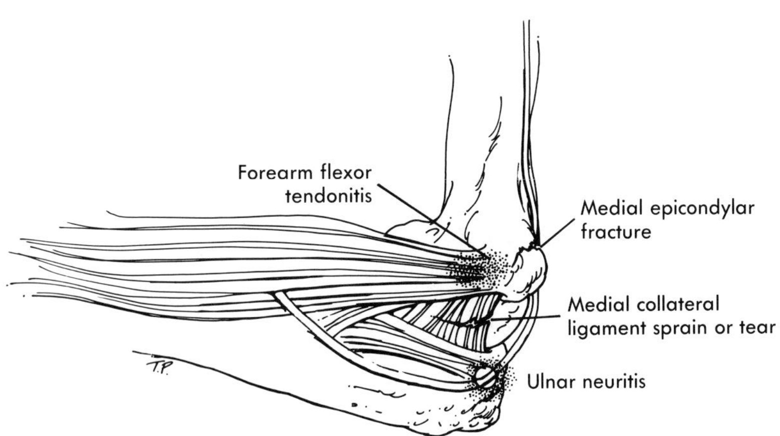

FIG. 16-10. Causes of medial elbow pain.

duction tests and electromyography (EMG). Decompression is indicated by clinical assessment and confirmed by electrodiagnostic studies. Ulnar nerve compression is treated by either simple fascial decompression of the ulnar nerve within the cubital tunnel or anterior transposition of the nerve either submuscularly or subcutaneously[7] (Fig. 16-10).

Acute Medial Stress Injuries

Acute medial stress injuries to the elbow may require medial reconstruction of either

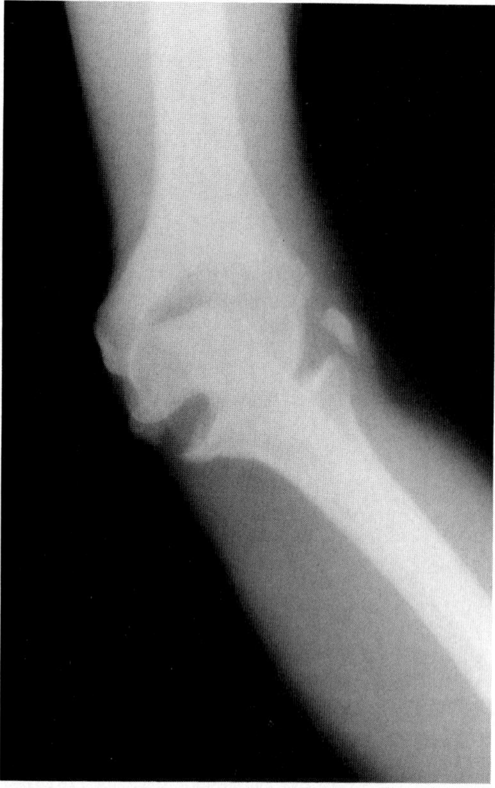

FIG. 16-11. Chronic medial elbow instability with intraligamentous heterotopic calcification.

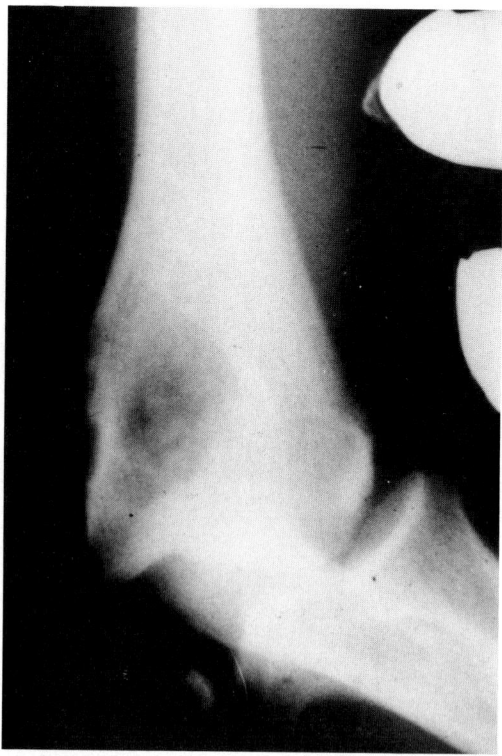

FIG. 16-12. Gross instability of the elbow after heterotopic calcification removal and medial collateral ligament disruption.

fractures and/or the medial collateral ligament.[8] In these instances, decompression of the ulnar nerve and anterior transposition is indicated to prevent damage to the nerve from acute bleeding, swelling, chronic scar fibrosis, and cubital tunnel compression.

Heterotopic Bone Islands

Medial joint line ossicles within the substance of the medial collateral ligament are seen in competitive throwing athletes. These ossicles do not represent loose body formation and in general should not be removed. Instead, they are heterotopic bone islands within the substance of the medial collateral ligament and represent healed incomplete medial collateral ligament tears (Fig. 16-11). If removal of these heterotopic bone islands within the medial collateral ligament is contemplated, extreme care should be taken to evaluate the status of the medial collateral ligament and to ensure that incompetency of the collateral ligament does not result following resection. This heterotopic lesion, left unmolested, does not usually restrict motion. We have unfortunately seen those patients who have had this procedure performed with resultant unstable elbows after "a loose body was removed." In fact, the entire medial collateral ligament complex was inadvertently resected (Fig. 16-12).

Heterotopic bone present in the anterior capsule may compromise range of motion. Actually it may form a bony bridge across the anterior capsule with a rigid contracture. The anterior lesion must be clearly distinguished from the medial ossicle.

Medial Collateral Ligament Rupture

Acute medial collateral ligament ruptures are seen normally in two instances: dislocations and throwing sports.[19] In both instances, the acute tear represents primary avulsion from its origin on the medial epicondyle in about 70% of the cases. In an additional 20%, the avulsion will be distal at the insertion of

Acute medial collateral ligament rupture

- Avulsion from epicondyle—70%
- Avulsion from ulna—20%
- Midsubstance tears—10%

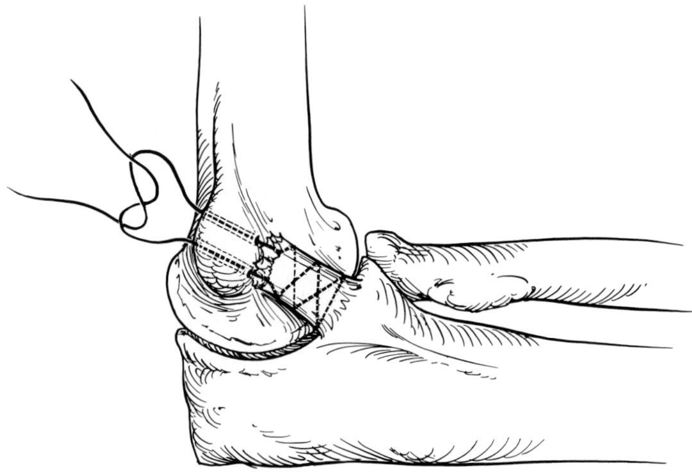

FIG. 16-13. Reattachment of the avulsed medial collateral ligament to the medial epicondyle.

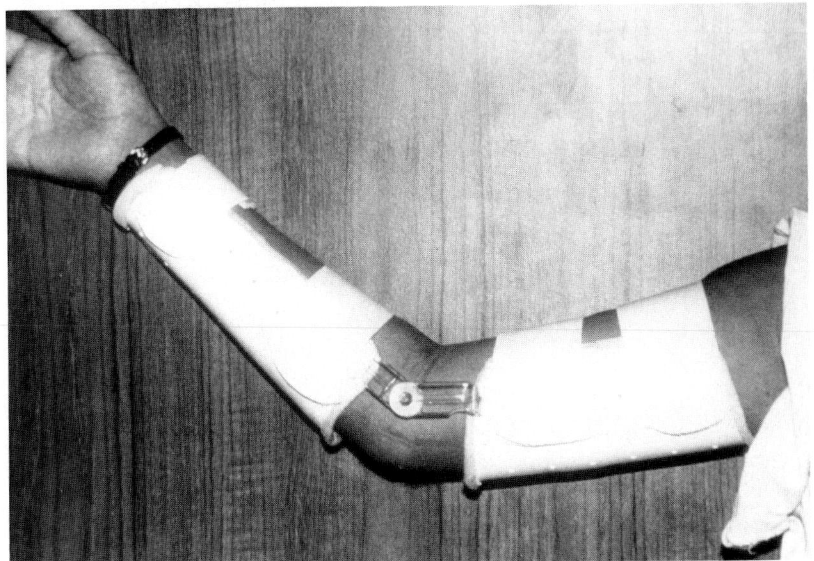

FIG. 16-14. Cast brace on the elbow.

the ligament on the ulna. The remaining 10% will be midsubstance tears.

Repair depends on the site and type of tear.[24] A medial epicondyle avulsion tear is repaired by the use of drill holes through the undersurface of the medial epicondyle after periosteal roughening of the medial epicondyle. The ligament is brought snugly to and tied over the epicondyle. Distal lesions are reattached using either drill holes and sutures or staples (Fig. 16-13).

Midsubstance tears are repaired with mattress or figure-eight sutures. In all instances, proper tension is restored by placing the elbow at 30 degrees of flexion and suturing the ligament in place. The forearm flexor mass is then reattached over the repaired ligament.

The ulnar nerve, if not symptomatic, is simply decompressed through the flexor carpi ul-

Medial collateral ligament repair techniques

- Epicondyle avulsion—repair through drill holes
- Midsubstance tear—mattress or figure-eight sutures
- Ulna avulsion—reattach through drill holes or staple
- Always—tension ligament at 30 degress

naris distally and proximally by resection of the intermuscular septum. If there is clinical evidence of ulnar neuropathy before surgery, then appropriate external neurolysis and anterior transposition is performed. With the anterior transposition, we prefer to position the nerve alongside the recessed reflected flexor forearm muscle mass rather than in the subcutaneous or submuscular position. The flexor mass is not sutured about the nerve.

The wound is drained and placed in a posterior splint for 7 days. A cast brace protecting varus-valgus stress but allowing flexion with extension block to within 30 degrees is used for 1 month. For 2 additional months, the cast brace is used but the extension block is removed. When full flexion-extension is achieved, strengthening exercises are allowed in the second 3-month period (Fig. 16-14). Resumption of throwing activities may begin at 6 months and be maximized over the course of a year. Return to competitive athletics is delayed for 1 year.

Postoperative regimen

- Posterior splint—7 days
- Cast brace (30—120 degrees)—4 weeks
- Cast brace (0—120 degress)—8 weeks
- Begin strengthening after range of motion returns (usually at 12 weeks)
- Resume throwing at 6 months

Varus Instability

Varus instability is rare; however, varus instability in association with anterior radial head dislocation and annular ligament disruption is seen occasionally. The athlete initially complains of a "popping" sensation on the lateral aspect of the elbow with associated pain. During forceful flexion or supination, the radial head dislocates anteriorly. There may also be an associated varus instability that can be demonstrated on varus stress roentgenograms (Fig. 16-15).

Acutely these injuries may be repaired by reattaching the annular ligament to its origin with sutures to bone or using the pull-out wire technique. In addition, the lateral collateral ligament complex of the elbow must be evaluated and reconstructed, when necessary, to either its epicondylar origin, the proximal ulna, or to the annular ligament. Radial head subluxation has been identified in association with incomplete radial head fractures and medial instability of the elbow. This will be discussed later in this chapter.

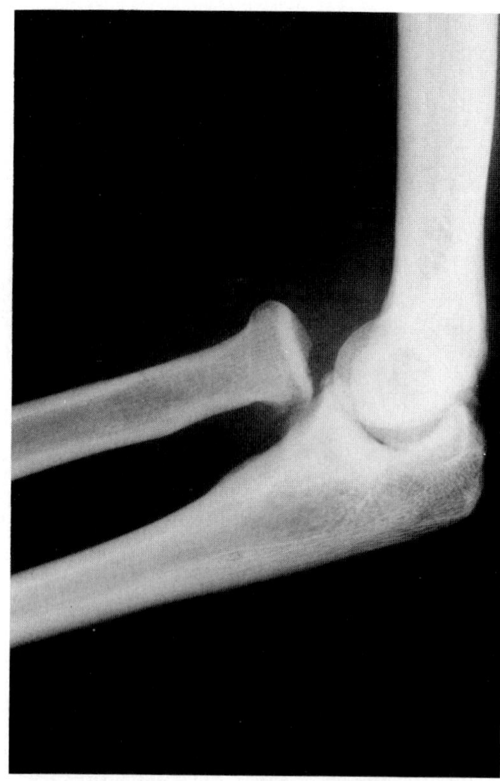

FIG. 16-15. Anterior dislocation of the radial head.

Lateral Muscle Injuries

Acute rupture of the lateral extensor muscle origin is associated with severe pain. A "pop" or "snap" about the elbow is described. In the competitive athlete these acute ruptures of the lateral extensor origin are best repaired surgically.

Interosseous Nerve Compression

Chronic lateral epicondylitis (tennis elbow) will not be discussed in this chapter (see Chapter 17). However, compression of the posterior interosseous nerve by the supinator arcade (the arcade of Frosche) must be differentiated from acute and chronic lateral epicondylitis. Acute entrapment or compression of the posterior interosseous nerve is associated with elbow fractures and/or massive soft tissue injuries. Swelling may produce nerve compression, which is reflected in an inability to extend the thumb and fingers. Since the posterior interosseous nerve is a motor nerve to the common finger extensor muscles and thumb extensor, a pure motor palsy results. Posterior interosseous nerve palsy in association with elbow fractures where compartment syndrome is not present is treated closed with the expectation that nerve recovery

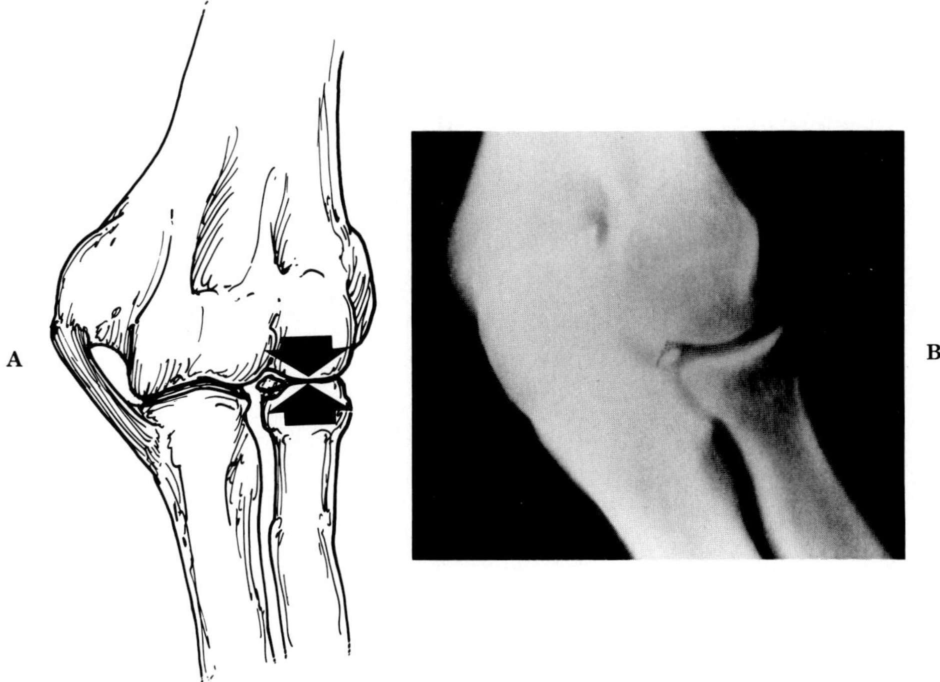

FIG. 16-16. Radial head–capitellum compression loose bodies. **A,** Drawing. **B,** Roentgenogram.

should follow. However, following open fracture fixation, particularly with proximal radius and radial head fractures, surgical identification of the posterior interosseous nerve is made. It is important to assess the possibility of nerve contusion versus transection or rupture.

Neural entrapment, particularly of the lateral antebrachial cutaneous nerve or the terminal portion of the musculocutaneous nerve, may present as lateral elbow pain and burning and should be differentiated from lateral epicondylitis and posterior interosseous nerve entrapment syndrome.

Loose Bodies

Bone changes may result from focal osteochondritis dissecans or diffuse avascular necrosis of the radial head or capitellar joint. When the medial collateral ligament is incompetent, compression of the lateral radiocapitellar joint may occur with loose body formation. These loose bodies in the lateral joint may cause a mechanical block to radial head rotation or a fixed flexion contracture. The loose body can be removed arthroscopically or by an open surgical procedure. Loose body excision rarely resolves the flexion contracture but may provide pain relief and correct joint locking (Fig. 16-16).

Arthroscopy of the elbow has been used for diagnosis of elbow pathology and also removal of loose bodies.[10] Currently it has not been expanded past this because of the very narrow anatomic confines of the joint. Chondroplasty, olecranon decompression ostectomy, or radial head decompression resection may be performed in selected cases.

Attenuated Medial Collateral Ligament

Chronic valgus instability is most commonly seen in the professional throwing athlete, specifically the professional baseball pitcher. Attenuation of the medial collateral ligament occurs because of chronic repetitive valgus load during the throwing act. The elbow carrying angle drifts into an increasing valgus position, which is documented in more than 30% of professional baseball pitchers. As this occurs, the medial tip of the olecranon process may impinge on the wall of the olecranon fossa, causing development of either osteophytes on the medial olecranon tip or loose body formation within the olecranon fossa.[13] Wilson[27] has described this as a valgus hyperextension overload in the pitching elbow. Joint débridement and olecranon impingement osteotomy may relieve the symptoms[27] (Fig. 16-17).

Similarly, valgus stress can cause an attenuated medial collateral ligament with resultant lateral radiocapitellar joint compression.

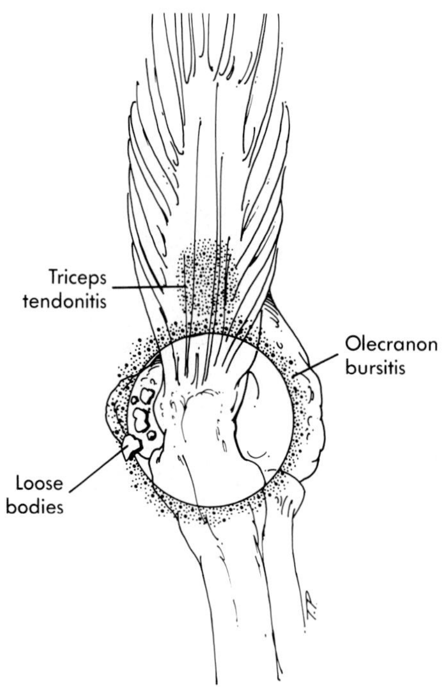

FIG. 16-17. Causes of posterior elbow pain.

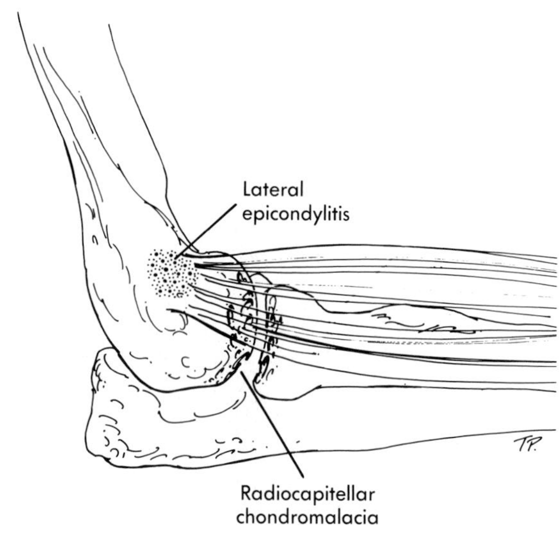

FIG. 16-18. Causes of lateral elbow pain.

Osteophytes and lateral loose bodies occur because the radiocapitellar joint acts as a secondary defense mechanism to valgus stress (Fig. 16-18). Open or arthroscopic joint débridement with loose body excision may be indicated.

Radial head or capitellar resection are done only with caution, because once significant bony alterations are performed within the elbow joint, an athlete's professional career may well be terminated. This is particularly true if medial ligament incompetency is missed and subsequent lateral elbow surgery further accentuates elbow instability.

ACUTE FRACTURES AND DISLOCATIONS

Anteroposterior stability of the elbow joint is the function primarily of an intact coronoid process and integrity of the medial and lateral collateral ligaments. The capsule offers little support against the stresses of acute flexion or extension. In addition, the anterior muscular groups (the brachialis and biceps) do little to maintain anteroposterior stability in the face of forced hyperextension.

Elbow dislocations are generally an injury of hyperextension.[26] The olecranon process is forced into the olecranon fossa and levers the trochlea over the coronoid process. In the course of this traumatic event, the medial collateral ligament is usually ruptured and the lateral collateral ligament may also be disrupted. If the dislocation is simple without associated fractures, reduction may result in a stable elbow if the forearm flexors, extensors, and annular ligament have maintained their continuity. In these cases early motion is resumed and the ultimate prognosis is good.[11,15]

Elbow dislocations that are complex and involve fractures of the bony stabilizing forces about the elbow present a much more difficult problem (Fig. 16-19). Medial collateral ligament rupture, when associated with radial head or capitellar fracture dislocation, creates a significant instability pattern that cannot completely be corrected on either the medial or lateral side of the elbow alone for maximum functional return. Attempts to preserve capitellar fracture fragments and radial head fracture fragments with internal fixation are performed (Fig. 16-20). Medial collateral ligament repair is performed. In severe comminuted cases of radial head fractures in which the radial head is removed, a silastic spacer may be used.[23] Silastic spacer alone

Silastic radial head spacers

- May be used in severe comminuted radial head fractures
- Do not provide adequate lateral stability against valgus stress if used alone and medial collateral ligament support is absent
- May cause silicone synovitis
- May go on to fatigue fractures

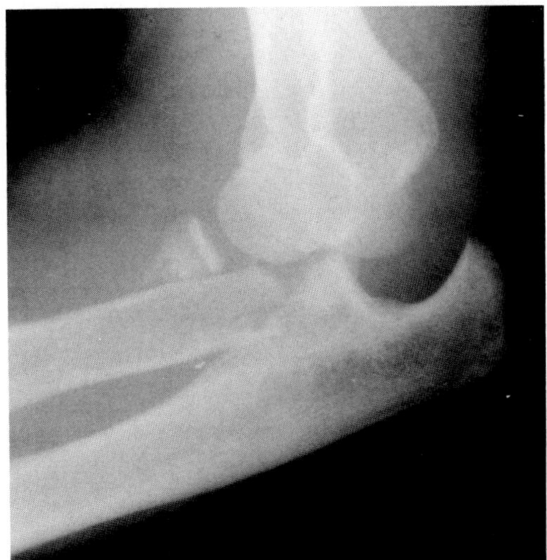

FIG. 16-19. Complex fracture dislocation of the elbow.

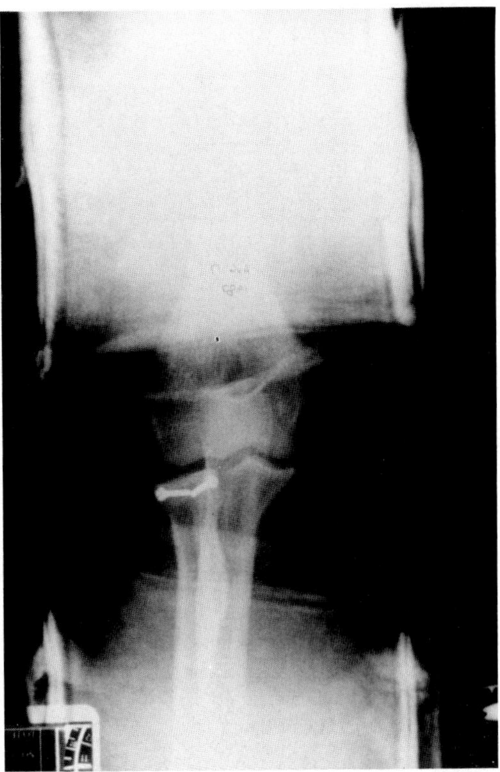

FIG. 16-20. Open reduction with internal fixation of a radial head fracture to preserve lateral elbow stability.

does not provide adequate lateral stability against valgus forces if medial collateral ligament support is absent. Silastic spacers also produce additional problems of particulate synovitis and fatigue fractures within the prosthesis. We use the silastic radial head as a lateral stint to support the medial collateral ligament repair in those cases where there is loss of both stabilizers.

Coronoid fractures additionally must be addressed in fracture dislocation injuries with reconstruction of the coronoid if it involves greater than the anterior 20%, which allows for the insertion of the capsule and brachialis. The remainder of the coronoid allows for the insertion of the anterior oblique ligament as a stabilizing factor in the elbow and must be reconstructed for stability (Fig. 16-21).

Acute **radial head fractures** must be managed appropriately with minimal immobilization and early motion for the nondisplaced or grade I type fracture. A grade II or III type fracture in the competitive athlete presents a more difficult problem. Many advocate open reduction and internal fixation (ORIF) using screw or pin fixation. This is followed by early motion. A type IV comminuted fracture dislocation often ends a career in competitive athletics. Removal of comminuted radial head fractures, stabilization of the elbow joint, and evaluation of the wrist joint for distal ulna dislocation is mandatory in these injuries. Prognosis is guarded, and chronic residual elbow pain as well as restriction of motion persists.

Radial head fractures in athletes

- Nondisplaced or type I—minimal immobilization and early motion
- Grade II—ORIF and early motion
- Grade III—ORIF and early motion if possible
- Grade IV (comminuted)—radial resection; check distal joint (Essex-Lopresti injury); guarded prognosis for sports

POSTERIOR ELBOW PROBLEMS

Posterior elbow pain may be seen with **olecranon bursitis,** which can be inflammatory or infectious. Generally these are managed conservatively with rest, protection, and antiinflammatories. If, however, aspiration is performed, it is recommended that the area be prepped surgically and a large bore needle, after xylocaine infiltration through the skin, be inserted through subcutaneous tissue into the olecranon bursa. This allows the needle tract to seal, decreases the incidence of infection, and also decreases the incidence of fistula formation through the thin skin. Chronic persistent bursitis or infected bursitis is surgically incised and drained or totally excised.

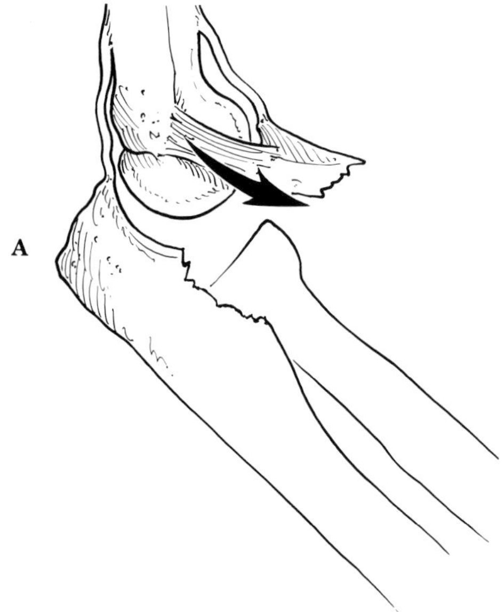

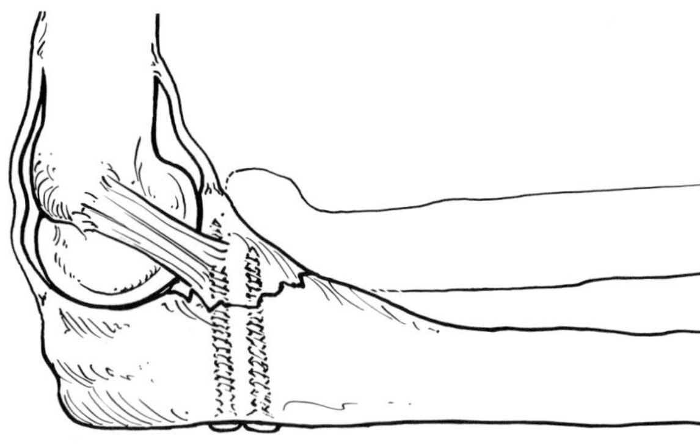

FIG. 16-21. A, Fracture coronoid with dislocation. **B,** Open reduction with internal fixation of a coronoid fracture for stability.

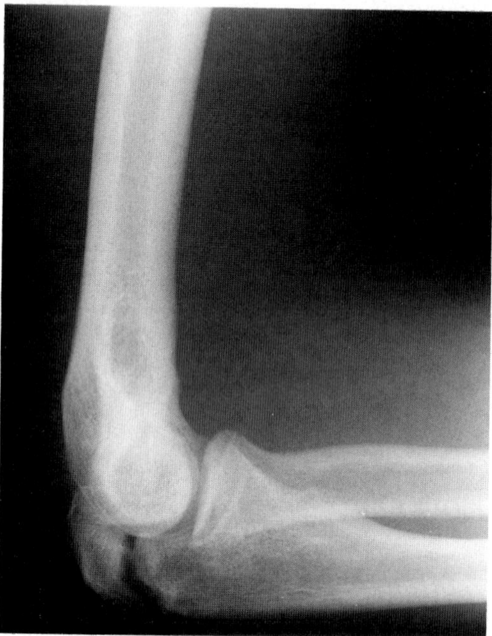

FIG. 16-22. Stress fracture olecranon in adolescent.

Triceps tendonitis with spur formation on the olecranon tip can be seen acutely as an overuse extension phenomenon. Additionally **valgus extension overload syndrome** produces posterior elbow pain because of olecranon impingement into the olecranon fossa of the distal humerus. Loose body formation may occur, causing pain and locking as well as blocking of motion. Surgical removal is indicated. At the same time decompression of the posterior olecranon may be performed.

Triceps rupture is uncommon but when seen should be reconstructed as the professional athlete with such a rupture will lose power extension. Reconstruction may be performed with repair of the triceps or by tendon-grafting procedures through the triceps tendon into the olecranon. Rehabilitation is similar to the biceps reattachment with protected active motion, and no resistive motion until satisfactory healing has occurred.

Olecranon fractures may be seen as stress fractures in the young athlete or as acute fractures in the mature athlete (Fig. 16-22). Olecranon fractures without concomitant injury about the elbow may be treated, if nondisplaced, with extension immobilization until healed. If displaced, then open reduction or internal fixation (Fig. 16-23) versus excision of the olecranon process are options[1,5] (Fig. 16-24).

VASCULAR INJURIES

Acute vascular insufficiency or rupture of the brachial artery is rare, however, in cases of supracondylar fractures or fracture dislocations of the elbow, consideration of vascular injury must be made[4,12] (Fig. 16-25). Appropriate monitoring of pulses, Doppler evaluation, and indicated arteriography will allow early diagnosis and treatment. Nerve entrapment may likewise occur and requires sur-

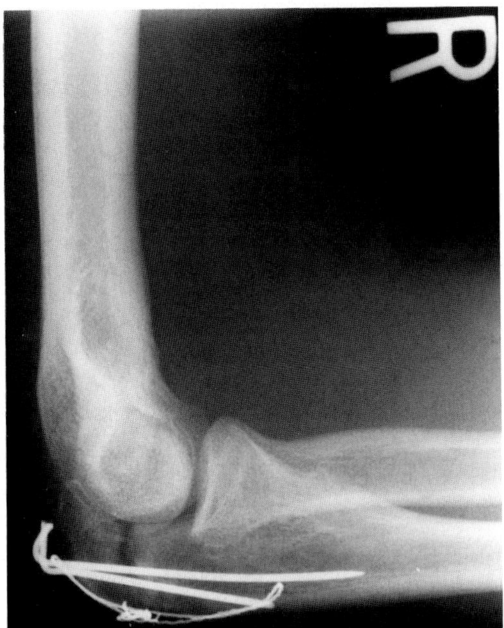

FIG. 16-23. Open reduction with internal fixation of a olecranon fracture with K-wire and tension-band technique.

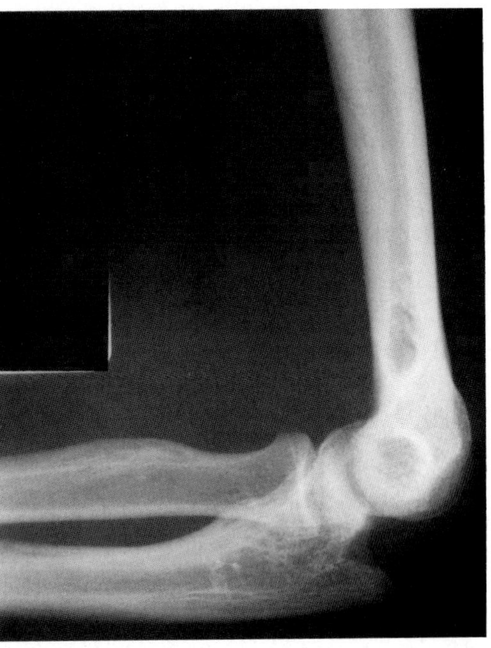

FIG. 16-24. Excision of olecranon with stable elbow because of preservation of the anterior oblique component of the medial collateral ligament.

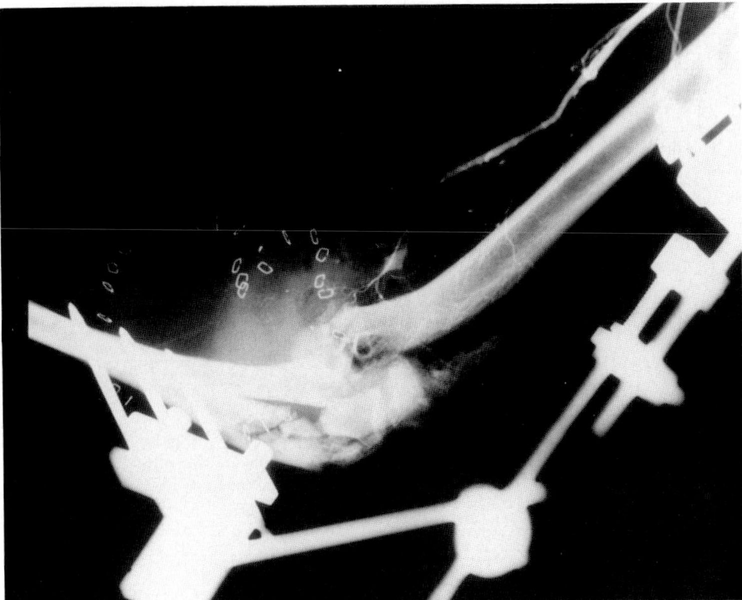

FIG. 16-25. Arteriogram with occlusion of the brachial artery in severe fracture about the elbow.

gical correction.[14] Compartment syndrome is evaluated through clinical examination and pressure monitoring of the compartments. Fasciotomies, extending up to the elbow, are indicated in the deteriorating patient or when there are appropritae pressure readings using either the wick catheter or the blood pressure gauge monitoring of intracompartmental pressures. At the level of the elbow, the brachial artery needs to be visualized and decompressed as does the median nerve, radial nerve, and, on occasion, the ulnar nerve.

REHABILITATION

Rehabilitation of the elbow varies according to the injury and the pathology involved. Medial and lateral epicondylitis rehabilitation programs have been extensively outlined in Chapter 19. Fracture rehabilitation programs likewise have been outlined. Ligament reconstruction stresses controlled mobilization while protecting against deforming forces.[8] Clinical and biomechanical factors as well as physiology of ligament and bone healing must be considered in the rehabilitation process. Maximized healing and motion must be obtained before competitive athletics is resumed.

Rehabilitation issues regarding the elbow must be specific for the injury, age of the patient, type of sports activity involved, and level of competition. Each reconstruction has a specific rehabilitation program and has been outlined under issues of rehabilitation in the individual sections of the chapter.

REFERENCES

1. Adler S, Fay GF, and MacAusland WR: Treatment of olecranon fractures, indications for excision of the olecranon fracture, repair of the triceps tendon, J Trauma 2:597, 1962.
2. Brodgon BG and Crow NF: Little leaguer's elbow, Am J Roentgenol 8:671, 1960.
3. DeHaven KE and Evarts CM: Throwing injuries of the elbow in athletes, Orthop Clin North Am 1:801, 1973.
4. Eliason EL and Brown RB: Posterior dislocation at the elbow with rupture of the radial and ulnar arteries, Ann Surg 106:1111-1115, 1937.
5. Gartsman GM, Sculco TP, and Otis JC: Operative treatment of olecranon fractures: excision or open reduction with internal fixation, J Bone Joint Surg 63(A)(5):718, 1981.
6. Gugenheim et al: Little league survey: the Houston study, Am J Sports Med 4:189, 1976.
7. Indelicato P et al: Correctable elbow lesions in professional baseball players, Am J Sports Med 7(1):72, 1979.
8. Jobe FW, Stark H, and Lombardo SJ: Reconstruction of the ulnar collateral ligament in athletes, J Bone Joint Surg 68(A)(8):1158-1163, Oct, 1986.
9. Johanson O: Capsular and ligament injuries of the elbow joint: a clincal and arthrographic study, Acta Chir Scand 287(Suppl):17-24, 1962.
10. Johnson LL: Arthroscopy of the elbow. In Diagnostic and surgical arthroscopy, St Louis, 1981, The CV Mosby Co, p 390.
11. Josefsson O, Johnell D, and Gentz CF: Long-term sequelae and simple dislocation of the elbow, J Bone Joint Surg 66(A)(6):927-930, July, 1984.
12. Kerin R: Elbow dislocation and its association: vascular disruption, J Bone Joint Surg 51(A)(4): 756, 1969.
13. King JW, Brelsford HF, and Tullos HS: Analysis of the pitching arm of the professional baseball pitcher, Clin Orthop 67:116, 1969.
14. Mannenfelt L: Median nerve entrapment after dislocation of the elbow: report of a case, J Bone Joint Surg 50(B):152, 1968.
15. Melhloff T et al: Treatment of simple elbow dislocation in the adult, ASES and AAOS, San Francisco, J Bone Joint Surg.70A:244,1988.
16. Mink JH, Eckardt JJ, and Grant TT: Arthrography in recurrent dislocation of the elbow, Am J Radiol 136:1242, 1981.
17. Morrey BF: Anatomy of the elbow joint. In Morrey BF, editor: The elbow and its disorders, Philadelphia, 1985, WB Saunders Co.
18. Morrey BF and An KN: Functional anatomy of the ligaments of the elbow, Clin Orthop 201:84-90, Dec, 1985.
19. Norwood LA, Shook JA, and Andrews JR: Acute medial elbow ruptures, Am J Sports Med 9:(1):16, 1981.
20. Pappa AM: Elbow problems associated with baseball during childhood and adolescence, Clin Orthop 164:30, 1982.
21. Schwab GH et al: Biomechanics of elbow instability: the role of the medial collateral ligament, Clin Orthop 146:42-52, 1980.
22. Slocum DB: Classification of elbow injuries from baseball players, Am J Sports Med 6:62, 1978.
23. Swanson AB, Jaeger SH, and LaRochelle D: Comminuted fracture of the radial head: the role of the silicone-implant replacement arthroplasty, J Bone Joint Surg 63(A):1039, 1981.
24. Tullos HS et al: Factors influencing elbow instability. In Murray DG, editor: AAOS: Instructional course lectures, Vol 8, St Louis, 1982, The CV Mosby Co, pp 185-199.
25. Waris W: Elbow injuries in javelin throwers, Acta Chir Scand 93:563, 1946.
26. Wheeler DK and Linscheid RL: Fracture dislocations of the elbow, Clin Orthop 50:95, 1967.
27. Wilson FD et al: Valgus extension overload in the pitcher's elbow, Am J Sports Med 11:83, 1983.
28. Woods GW: Elbow instability and medial epicondyle fractures, Am J Sports Med 5:23, 1977.

CHAPTER 17 Overuse Injuries of the Elbow

James C. Parkes

The material presented in this chapter represents what I have learned from many wonderful teachers. I would like to give them the credit they deserve for teaching me so very much. They are Dr. Frank Stinchfield, Dr. James Nicholas, Dr. Charles Neer, Dr. Robert Carroll, Dr. Alex Garcia, Dr. Frank Jobe, and Dr. John Marshall.

Injuries to the elbow are not at all uncommon. The elbow is a very vulnerable joint, located midway between the shoulder and the wrist. With proper treatment, technique and conditioning, the elbow can be made to perform satisfactorily. Overuse injuries can be divided into three groups: (1) musculotendinous, (2) those involving the joint itself (i.e., ligament, bone, and cartilage), and (3) neural entrapment lesions.

MUSCULOTENDINOUS INJURIES

Musculotendinous injuries are the most common elbow injuries in athletes. There are essentially four areas where overuse injuries can occur. These are defined by their anatomic location—lateral, medial, posterior, and anterior.

Musculotendinous injuries

- Lateral
- Medial
- Posterior
- Anterior

Lateral Musculotendinous Injuries

The common extensor muscles of the wrist and fingers, centered around the extensor carpi radialis brevis, span the wrist and elbow and originate on the lateral epicondyle of the humerus. This musculotendinous unit is very susceptible to injuries in racquet sports. The injured athlete most often is middle-aged, 30 to 50 years old. Improper stroke mechanics are commonly seen. For example, the athlete may begin the backhand stroke by leading with the elbow rather than the body and shoulder. This puts excessive stress on the common extensor origin and may lead to microscopic tears within the tendon. This in turn leads to inflammation and pain.

Clinical Picture

The patient complains of pain along the lateral aspect of the elbow. Tenderness is localized to the lateral epicondyle of the elbow. Passive volar flexion of the wrist with the elbow extended increases the pain, as does active dorsiflexion of the wrist against resistance. Roentgenograms of the elbow usually do not reveal any abnormalities. Occasionally a small calcific deposit over the epicondyle or a spur coming from the epicondyle can be observed. These are secondary to repetitive tension stresses placed on the common extensor tendon.

Treatment

The patient must understand that this is an "overstress" problem, and the physician should elaborate on this point. Once this is understood, the patient will be much more compliant with a comprehensive treatment plan. This plan begins with rest plus nonsteroidal antiinflammatory medicine. If this program does not bring about relief in 5 to 7 days, consideration is given to injecting the tender area with 0.5 ml of dexamethasone sodium phosphate or a comparable agent. The oral antiinflammatory agents are also continued. It is very important to note that repeated injections of steroids definitely lead to tendon destruction and complications; therefore each patient receives only a single injection in the course of his or her treatment program.

Within 1 to 2 weeks, the symptoms usually decrease and the patient is started on a physical therapy program designed to increase the strength and flexibility of the involved muscle group. The program also includes strength and flexibility exercises for the uninjured muscles about the elbow. Once strength and flexibility have returned to normal, the patient is returned to a competent tennis instructor for lessons on how to improve their stroke mechanics. The patient is urged to get a racquet with a larger head, medium tension on the strings (55 to 60 pounds), and a larger handle. In the authors experience, this program has been successful in over 90% of patients.

In the 10% of patients who fail to respond in 12 to 16 weeks, a surgical approach can be considered. The technique I have found most efficacious is a common extensor release. This is done on an outpatient basis with regional anesthesia. A 2-inch incision is made, centered over the epicondyle. The common extensor tendon is released from the epicondyle and allowed to retract distally. Any calcium or spurs that may be present are removed. The wound is closed with a continuous, running subcuticular suture, and a soft dressing is applied. The patient is started at once on gentle range of motion exercises and progressed in the rehabilitation of strength and flexibility as tolerated. Usually by 8 to 12 weeks the patient has regained full strength and flexibility and can resume playing. I have found that getting the patient to work with a registered physical therapist with a Cybex II equipment at high speed has been particularly helpful in preventing recurrence of problems. I think this strength at high speed is very helpful in games of skill such as tennis, baseball, golf, and racquet ball.

Return to tennis after musculotendinous injuries

- Larger head racquet
- Medium string tension
- Lighter racquet material
- Appropriate grip size

Medial Musculotendinous Injuries

Medial musculotendinous injuries are also very common. The flexor-pronator muscle tendon group consists of the pronator teres, flexor carpi radialis, flexor digitorum sublimis, and flexor carpi ulnaris. These muscles originate at the medial epicondyle. Like the lateral muscle tendon mass, it spans the elbow and wrist. This area receives particular stress in the act of serving in tennis and in the acceleration phase of ball throwing. This muscle tendon unit is the first line of defense in decreasing medial stress on the elbow. Because it spans two joints, it is very easy for its ability to elongate to be exceeded and microtrauma to occur, leading to inflammation and pain.

Flexor pronator muscles

- Pronator teres
- Flexor carpi radialis
- Flexor digitorum sublimis
- Flexor carpi ulnaris

Clinical Picture

The patient complains of pain on the inner aspect of the elbow, felt particularly when throwing a baseball or serving or hitting a forehand shot in tennis. Tenderness is found when palpating the medial epicondyle. The pain can be intensified by having the patient flex the wrist against resistance or by passively extending the wrist with the elbow in full extension. Roentgenographic evaluation usually does not reveal any abnormalities, but occasionally, as with the lateral side, calcific deposits or a spur coming from the medial epicondyle may be seen.

Treatment

Rest and nonsteroidal antiinflammatory agents are very important. Once again, if the pain is not markedly decreased in 5 to 7 days, one steroid injection (Decadron) into the tender area can be administered. When injecting, do not inject the steroid into the tendon but rather inject it on the surface. This surface technique, I have found, is much better for both relief of symptoms and sparing insult to the tendon. Usually, 1 to 2 weeks after the injection, one can begin a rehabilitation program to increase strength and flexibility of the medial flexor pronator group. It is very important once again to use the Cybex II at high speed. In my experience, this helps prevent further problems, because strength at high speed is an important component of sports participation.

In a rare instance, when this program fails, outpatient surgery may be the appropriate alternative. A medial flexor tendon release is performed with regional anesthesia. A 2-inch incision is made centered over the medial epicondyle, and the common flexor tendon is released from the epicondyle, and allowed to retract distally. Great care must be taken to stay superficial to the medial collateral ligament to avoid damaging it. The wound is closed with a continuous subcuticular suture, and a soft dressing is applied. Range of motion exercises are started at once, and the patient is rapidly progressed as tolerated. Usually by 8 to 12 weeks the patient can resume sports. Results have been quite good in the few patients who have not responded to a conservative treatment program.

Posterior Musculotendinous Injuries

The posterior region is not as commonly involved as the lateral and medial areas. The triceps muscle tendon unit is overloaded in sports that involve repetitive forceful extension of the elbow, such as throwing and racquet sports, gymnastics, shot putting, javelin throwing, boxing, and weight lifting.

Clinical picture

The patient's symptoms are referred to the posterior aspect of the elbow. On examination the patient has tenderness just superior to the attachment of the triceps on the olecranon or actually on the olecranon where the tendon attaches. There may also be some mild swelling over the tender area. If one has the patient try to forcefully extend the elbow against resistance, this increases the pain. Roentgenographic evaluation of the elbow does not generally reveal any significant findings.

Treatment

Rest and a short course of nonsteroidal, antiinflammatory medicine usually decreases the pain in 5 to 7 days. The patient then begins a program of rehabilitation to increase the strength and flexibility of the elbow extensor muscles. Steroid injections in this area are to be avoided, because experience has shown that this can lead to triceps tendon rupture. The physician should communicate with the athlete's coach so that proper mechanics training can be instituted. If this program is followed, the results are very successful.

Anterior Musculotendinous Injuries

The anterior area is the least commonly involved region about the elbow. However, injury in this area may be seen in athletes who participate in sports that require repetitive flexion with forced extension. This includes bowling, weight lifting, and gymnastics. In these sports, the biceps and brachialis muscle tendon units are repeatedly stressed and overloaded. This can lead to microtrauma and clinical problems.

Clinical Picture

The patient complains of pain along the anterior aspect of the elbow. Localized tenderness may be found along the course of the biceps tendon. Forced supination or flexion of the elbow increases the pain. Roentgenographic evaluation usually does not reveal pathologic findings. Steroid injections are avoided because of the potential of steroids to contribute to tendon rupture. Occasionally an acute distal biceps rupture may be suspected, often following steroid injections into the tendon. Anterior swelling and pain is found. A palpable gap can be noted in the usual location of the distal biceps tendon. Weakness of elbow supination and flexion is profound.

Treatment

For patients with symptoms of microtrauma and tendonitis, nonsteroidal antiinflammatory medicine, rest, and rehabilitation to increase the strength and flexibility of the flexor muscle mass are often very successful. With acute ruptures, we have used the Anderson-Boyd technique to repair them. However, high-level

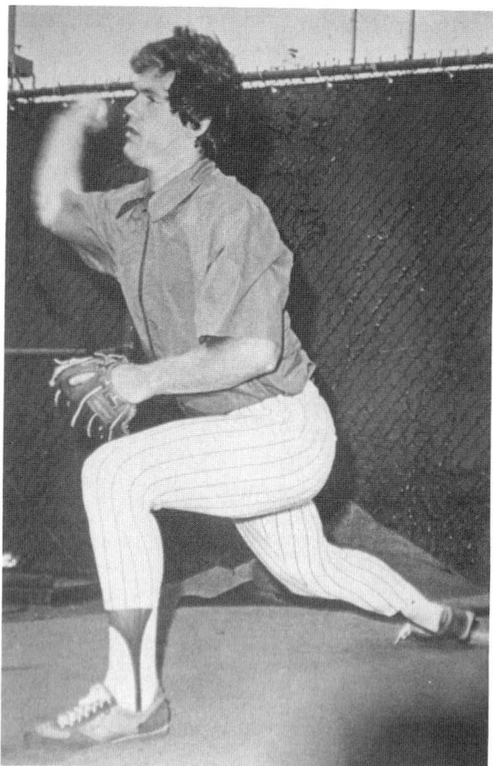

FIG. 17-1. Extreme valgus stress on the elbow as the pitcher is throwing in the mid acceleration phase. There is medial tension and lateral posterior compression stress. This combination leads to many clinical problems in the elbows of throwing athletes.

athletes can rarely return to their previous level of performance. Once again, steroid injections are to be avoided in this region because of the increased risk of subsequent tendon rupture.

BONE, LIGAMENT, AND CARTILAGE INJURIES

Injuries in this group involve the osseous structures, articular cartilage, and supporting ligaments of the elbow. This injury group is not as common as the musculotendinous injuries. Problems are usually seen medially, laterally, posteriorly, or in a combination of all these areas.

Medial Compartment Injuries

The medial aspect of the elbow is supported by the medial collateral ligament and the medial joint capsule. These deep structures are covered by the flexor-pronator muscle group. In throwing and racquet sports this area is subjected to intense valgus-tension stress (Fig. 17-1). The medial muscle group and medial collateral ligament attach to the medial epicondyle, which can also be injured by this valgus-tension stress.

Medial Epicondyle Injuries

The medial epicondyle serves as the origin for the flexor-pronator muscle mass as well as the medial collateral ligament. In sports such as javelin throwing, tennis, and pitching, the biomechanics of the elbow lead to tension forces on the medial epicondyle. This area is particularly prone to injury in young athletes before the medial epicondylar apophysis closes. The apophysis is a common site of tension stress injuries. Many studies have reported that radiographic changes in this region are noted in a significant number of little league athletes.

Clinical picture. Usually the patient is a young adolescent who has been throwing or playing racquet ball or tennis. He or she complains of pain along the inner aspect of the elbow. The discomfort is increased in intensity during athletic participation. Tenderness is found over the epicondyle.

Roentgenographs can demonstrate a number of abnormalities, including widening of the apophyseal line, enlargement of the apophysis, and fragmentation of the apophysis.

Roentgenographic findings in adolescent athletes with medial elbow pain

- Widening of the apophyseal line
- Apophyseal enlargement
- Fragmentation of the apophysis

Less commonly, the athlete experiences acute pain and will be unable to play. In this situation, examination will reveal the medial aspect of the elbow to be swollen and tender. Gentle valgus stress at 20 to 30 degrees of flexion will demonstrate instability when compared to the normal elbow. Roentgenographic examination will reveal partial or complete avulsion of the epicondyle.

Treatment. In the athlete with a chronic problem where no separation or less than 1 cm of separation is present, initial treatment includes nonsteroidal antiinflammatory medicine. This program will usually lead to decreased symptoms in 3 to 6 weeks. This should be followed by a rehabilitation program to increase strength and flexibility of the muscles about the elbow. Results of this treatment regimen are almost always successful.

In acute cases, where there is greater than 1 cm of separation of the epicondyle, open reduction and internal fixation with un-threaded K-wires is indicated. Once again, the results of these cases are quite successful.

Medial Capsuloligamentous Injuries

The medial capsule of the elbow, which spans from the humerus to the ulna, is reinforced by the medial (ulnar) collateral ligament. This ligament consists of anterior, oblique, and posterior bands. The anterior band is the most important, since it remains tight throughout the entire range of motion of the elbow because of its eccentric location. It extends from the medial epicondyle to the medial aspect of the coronoid process of the ulna. The posterior band is not as thick and is only tight when the elbow is flexed greater than 90 degrees. It originates from the medial epicondyle and runs to the medial margin of the ulna, which makes up the ulnar-trochlear joint. The oblique band runs from anterior to posterior on the ulna and does not have any apparent function.

When valgus stress occurs in sports such as tennis, baseball, racquet ball, and javelin throwing, tension on the medial capsule and ligament is generated (see Fig. 17-1). The overlying flexor pronator muscle group is the first line of defense against valgus stress and is more commonly injured, but repeated or violent stress can involve the deeper capsule and ligament. Also, the tension stress that the capsule and ligament puts on the ulna and humerus can lead to spur formation (Fig. 17-2). These spurs can compress the ulnar nerve, which lies directly on the medial capsule and ligament.

Clinical picture. The patient usually complains of pain along the inner aspect of the elbow during sports such as baseball, tennis, and racquet ball. On examination, tenderness is elicited over the medial aspect of the elbow joint below the medial epicondyle. This can be intensified by applying valgus stress to the elbow at 20 to 30 degrees of flexion. Most commonly, the patient will experience acute medial elbow pain of such intensity that he or she is unable to continue participating. Valgus stress applied to the elbow at 20 to 30 degrees of flexion when compared to the opposite elbow will reveal definite valgus laxity. This can be substantiated by stress roentgenographs. Routine roentgenographs often reveal spur formation on the ulna in the region of the coronoid process where the medial ligament attaches and ossification of the medial collateral ligament between the base of the epicondyle and the ulna.

Treatment. Treatment of athletes with chronic medial capsuloligamentous injury begins with rest and nonsteroidal antiinflammatory medicine. This will usually lead to decreased symptoms in 7 to 14 days. An intensive physical therapy program to increase strength and flexibility of the muscles about the elbow is then commenced. A review of the athlete's playing mechanics should be discussed with his or her coach or trainer.

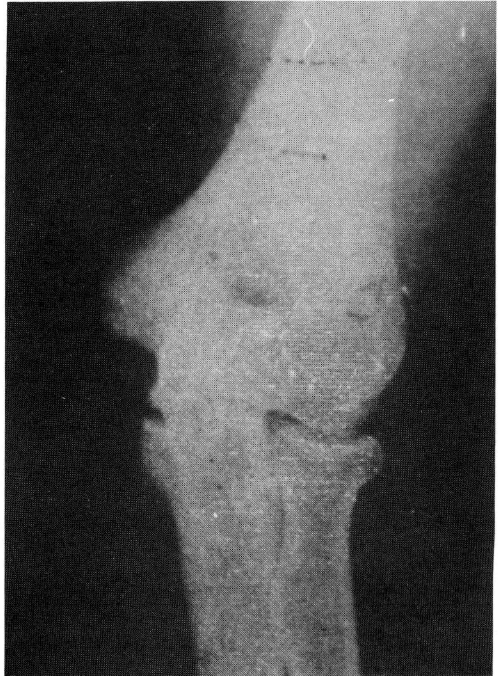

FIG. 17-2. Spurring of the ulna trochlear joint and calcification in the region of the medial collateral ligament. This is secondary to tension stresses placed on this aspect of the elbow. The ulnar nerve, which runs in the medial epicondylar groove, can be compressed by these structures.

In the case of an acute rupture, surgical repair is indicated. If the ligament is pulled off the base of the epicondyle, it can be repaired directly. However, in midsubstance tears, I have reinforced the repair using an autogeneous graft of the palmaris longus tendon. The ulnar nerve in all these cases should be transposed anteriorly. I have been successful in returning players to their sports using this technique.

Reconstruction of the medial collateral ligament can also be considered for those athletes with chronic medial instability. However, in the author's experience, results of late reconstruction are not as successful as those performed on acute injuries.

Lateral Compartment Injuries

The lateral compartment is subjected to significant compressive stress, particularly in

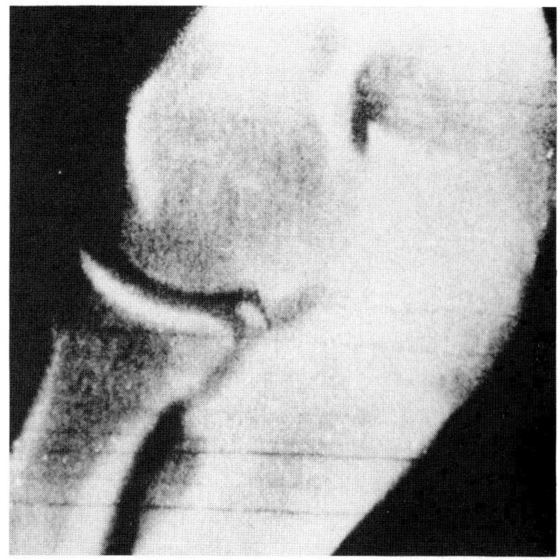

FIG. 17-3. Loose body in the lateral compartment, secondary to compression of the radial head against the capitellum.

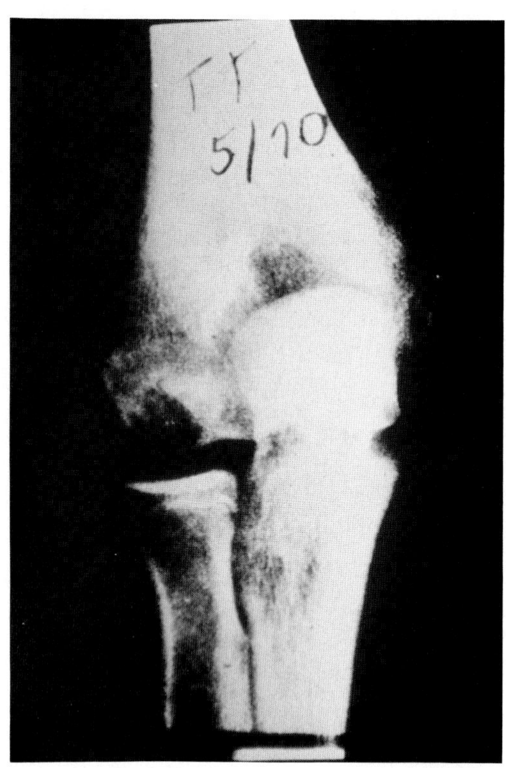

FIG. 17-4. Radiolucent area in the capitellum is secondary to repetitive compression stress of the radial head against the capitellum.

sports such as tennis, baseball, gymnastics, racquet ball, and javelin throwing. These activities tend to place a valgus stress on the elbow, causing tension forces medially and compression forces laterally. Lateral compression forces involve the radial head and the capitellum. This repetitive compressive stress across the radiocapitellar joint can lead to degeneration of the articular cartilage of the radial head, capitellum, or both. This in turn can create loose body formation (Fig. 17-3).

In children, the epiphyses are very sensitive to compression stress, and osteochondritis can develop. (Fig 17-4).

Loose Body Formation

Repetitive stress of the radial head against the capitellum can lead to injury of the articular cartilage surfaces. Loose body formation occurs as the fragments of articular cartilage break off into the joint. Loose bodies can arise from the surface of the radial head, capitellum, or both.

Clinical picture. The patient's chief complaint is pain in the elbow, which is associated with catching and clicking. No single traumatic event is usually recalled. However, some patients may experience a locking episode with the elbow "sticking" at a certain point in flexion. Often, they must shake or toggle it to regain motion from the fixed position.

Examination discloses crepitus during passive range of motion testing. Occasionally a loose body can be palpated laterally between the radial head and capitellum.

Roentgenographs reveal loose bodies anteriorly in the radiocapitellar joint (see Fig. 17-3). However, often when one surgically explores these patients, more fragments are found than are revealed on roentgenographs because of the large number of pure cartilage (unossified) bodies.

Treatment. Loose bodies can be successfully removed using a lateral surgical approach. If the loose bodies are small, an arthroscope can be used to remove them. This approach avoids trauma to the medial structures, which, during sports, are placed under the most severe stress. Recovery usually is much quicker using the lateral approach. Postoperatively the arm is placed in a soft dressing and motion is instituted at once. After approximately 6 weeks of active and passive range of motion exercises, a strengthening program can be started. First, isometric exercises are performed, followed by isokinetic exercises. Twelve to 16 weeks after surgery, the patient can begin to compete again. Unless the radiocapitellar joint has severe articular cartilage damage, the outlook for return to full activity is quite good.

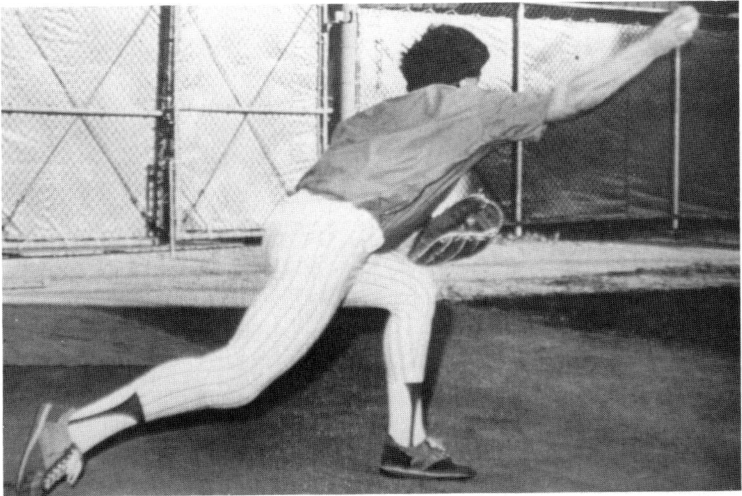

FIG. 17-5. In the follow-through and release phases of throwing, the elbow is forcefully extended, further compressing the olecranon into the olecranon fossa.

Osteochondral Fracture of the Radiocapitellar Joint

Occasionally an athlete will acutely stress the elbow with so much force that the impingement of the radial head against the capitellum will cause an acute osteochondral fracture. This is seen most commonly in gymnasts and weight lifters.

Clinical picture. The patient will experience acute pain in the elbow and will be unable to continue participation. On examination swelling and tenderness will be present most markedly over the radiocapitellar joint. Motion is quite painful and both flexion and extension are generally restricted. Routine plain roentgenographic views may not reveal the lesion. If a chondral or osteochondral fracture is suspected, special views such as oblique or tangential views chould be obtained. If these are negative, plain tomography or CT arthrography will identify the lesion. (See Chapter 14.)

Treatment. Removal of the osteochondral fragment can be done arthroscopically if the fragment is not too large. However, if a large fragment or multiple fragments are present, the open lateral approach may be necessary. The postoperative regimen is the same and the prognosis is usually excellent unless there is severe chondromalacia of the radiocapitellar joint, in which case the patient may not improve.

Osteochondritis of the Radiocapitellar Joint

Often referred to as little league elbow, osteochondritis of the radiocapitellar joint is seen in young athletes before physeal closure (see Chapter 30). I do not like this term because it fails to pin down exactly what the problem is, both in location and severity. Roentgenographic examination often reveals a lucency in the radial head and/or capitellum (Fig 17-4). Fragmentation and loose body formation may also be present.

Treatment. As long as no loose bodies are present, rest is the key to treatment. This is coupled with range of motion exercises. In 6 to 12 weeks, the patient usually has a marked decrease in symptoms, and a strengthening program can be instituted. In general, by 6 to 12 months healing of the soft tissues has taken place and the patient can resume activities without limitation. If loose bodies are present, they can be removed arthroscopically or by the open lateral approach, depending on the size and number of loose bodies and the condition of the radiocapitellar joint.

Posterior Compartment Injuries

In sports such as tennis, baseball, racquet ball, and javelin throwing, the elbow extends repetitively and the olecranon is repeatedly and forcefully driven into the olecranon fossa (Fig.17-5). Also in these sports, as the elbow extends, there is usually a valgus stress that forces the olecranon against the medial wall of the olecranon fossa. This repetitive compressive stress leads to bony osteophyte formation on the olecranon as well as loose body formation. The loose bodies arise from the olecranon striking the wall of the olecranon fossa and shearing off osteocartilaginous fragments. Less commonly, this repetitive impacting can lead to a stress fracture of the olecranon.

Loose Body and Spur Development

The repetitive impingement of the olecranon against the olecranon fossa can lead to enlargement of the olecranon, osteophyte formation, and loose body development.

Clinical picture. The patient complains of pain in the posterior aspect of the elbow. It may be associated with clicking and grating. Occasionally the elbow will lock in a fixed position and the patient will have to "shake it" to restore motion. On examination, crepitus can be felt over the posterior aspect of the elbow as the elbow is flexed and extended. Active extension is limited, because the osteophytes and loose bodies prevent full extension. Tenderness will be apparent posteriorly along the margins of the olecranon, and on occasion loose bodies may be palpable in the same area. Roentgenographic examination reveals marginal osteophytes and enlargement of the olecranon. In addition, one or more loose bodies can often be seen (Fig. 17-6).

Treatment. If no loose bodies are present, a period of rest plus judicious use of nonsteroidal antiinflammatory medicine can usually decrease the symptoms in 7 to 14 days. A complete rehabilitation program to increase strength and flexibility of the muscles about the elbow is begun when symptoms are improved. Generally, in 4 to 6 weeks, the patient can resume athletic participation. Once again, the coach should stress good mechanics to avoid a recurrence.

If symptoms persist or loose bodies are present, I have been very successful in removing the osteophytes and loose bodies through a lateral incision. This approach avoids violating the triceps tendon. A soft dressing is used for 2 weeks. Range of motion exercises are begun in the early postoperative period. In 2 weeks, the dressing is removed and progressive range of motion and strengthening exercises are instituted. Usually in 12 to 16 weeks the patient can resume athletic activity.

Stress Fracture of the Olecranon

A stress fracture is not a common injury but does occur in sports such as baseball, tennis, and racquet ball where repetitive forceful extension of the olecranon into the olecranon fossa occurs.

Clinical picture. The patient complains of a gradual onset of pain in the posterior aspect of the elbow. The pain steadily increases in severity to the point that performance is affected. At this point the patient usually seeks medical attention.

Tenderness is present over the olecranon and usually full extension is lacking. Forced extension against resistance usually increases the pain.

Findings on plain roentgenographs are usually negative. A bone scan will reveal an increased uptake in the olecranon, and lateral tomograms at that time usually will reveal the stress fracture line.

Treatment. Treatment consists of splinting the elbow for 4 to 6 weeks. This is followed by a progressive rehabilitation program to increase range of motion of the elbow and strengthen the muscles about it. Usually in 4 to 6 months the patient can return to full activity. If there is a nonunion, the area can be bone grafted, but this step is usually not necessary.

A
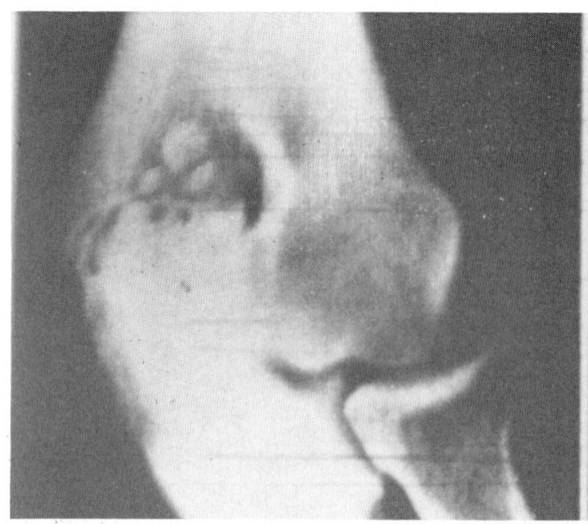
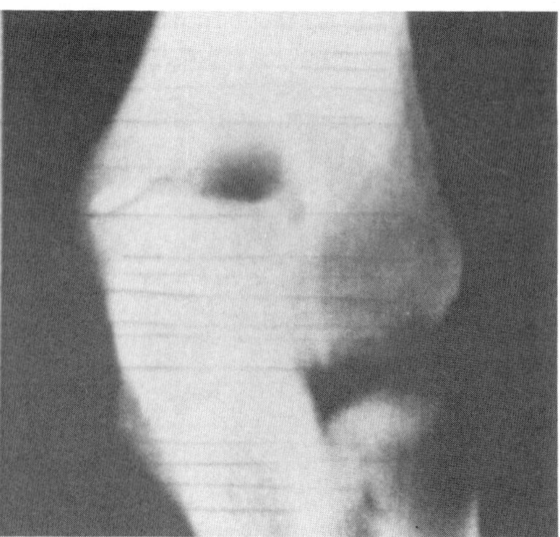
B

FIG. 17-6. A, Loose bodies in the posterior compartment. **B,** A fracture of a bony prominence on the medial aspect of the olecranon secondary to impaction of this region against the olecranon fossa.

NEURAL ENTRAPMENT LESIONS

Although neural entrapment lesions are not as common as musculotendinous and articular lesions, it is important to recognize them, because they are very treatable if recognized promptly.

Ulnar Nerve Entrapment

Ulnar nerve entrapment is often referred to as the *cubital tunnel syndrome*. The ulnar nerve passes along the medial aspect of the elbow after it has run its course down the medial aspect of the upper arm. As it passes along the inner aspect of the elbow, it enters the cubital tunnel. The floor of this tunnel is made up of the medial epicondylar groove. The roof is formed by a fascial band that extends from the medial epicondyle to the olecranon. Distally this tissue blends with the antebrachial fascia spanning the two heads of the flexor carpi ulnaris muscle. It is in this region that the nerve is most subject to the compression forces and tension stress most commonly seen in baseball, tennis, racquet ball, and javelin throwing.

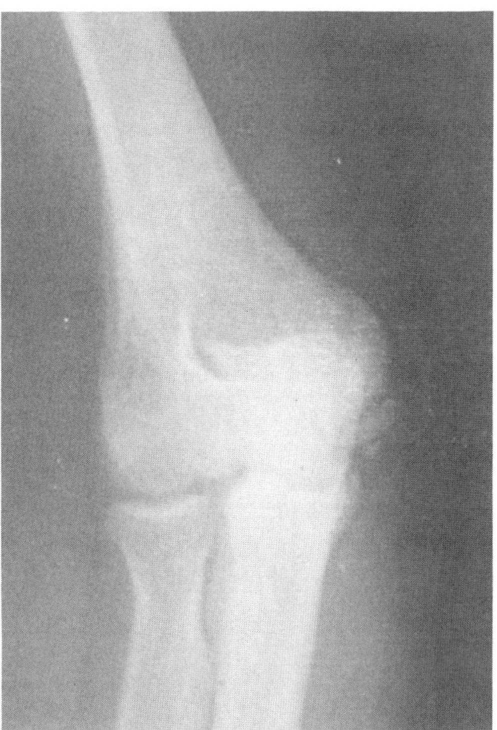

FIG. 17-7. Calcification inferior to the medial epicondyle, which can increase compression on the ulnar nerve as it lies in the medial epicondyle groove. These represent either avulsions from the medial epicondyle or calcifications in the medial collateral ligament or both.

Clinical Picture

The patient complains of pain along the inner aspect of the elbow. This is often associated with paresthesias in the distribution of the ulnar nerve in the hand (i.e., the fourth [ulnar aspect] and fifth fingers).

Tenderness can be found along the groove that is beneath the medial epicondyle. A positive Tinel's sign in this region can be elicited. Motor and sensory function can be diminished in the ulnar distribution in the hand, but often this is within normal limits. The presence of hypothenar atrophy should be noted. Nerve conduction in studies and electromyographic findings are positive only in about 40% to 50% of the cases. When they are positive, decreased conduction velocity of the ulnar nerve across the elbow and denervation changes in the ulnar intrinsic muscles of the hand are seen. Roentgenographic examination is often negative, but one may see some osteophyte formation on the coronoid process of the ulna and calcifications inferior to the medial epicondyle in the region of the medial collateral ligament (Fig. 17-7). The presence of these lesions further decreases the space available for the nerve in the cubital tunnel.

Treatment

If recognized early, rest and antiinflammatory medicine followed by a rehabilitation program to increase strength and flexibility of the muscles about the elbow, particularly the flexor pronator group, can be successful. However, if symptoms are present for greater than 12 to 16 weeks, the chances of a conservative program being successful are very poor. Tranposition of the ulna nerve anteriorly (the technique of Richard Eaton, M.D.)[21] will often yield a satisfactory result in these chronic or severe cases. (Figs. 17-8 and 17-9). This technique violates no major anatomic structures. I have performed it in over 50 elbows, and 90% of patients were able to return to full activity without restriction.

Radial Nerve Entrapment

Although not nearly as common as tendonitis on the lateral aspect of the elbow, radial nerve entrapment should always be considered in the differential diagnosis of what is often referred to as "tennis elbow." As the radial nerve approaches the elbow, it passes beneath the flexor carpiradialis brevis and at that point divides into a superficial sensory and posterior motor branch. The posterior interosseous branch passes beneath the flexor carpiradialis brevis and supinator. A portion of the supinator forms a very thick fibrous

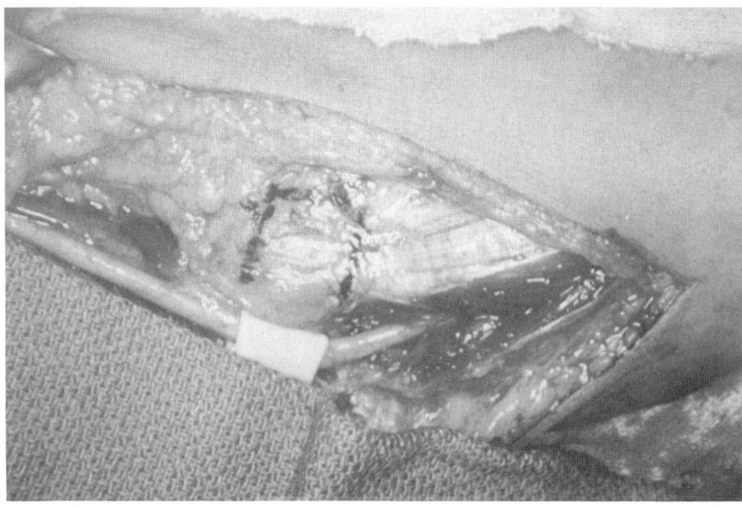

FIG. 17-8. The ulnar nerve has been freed up and is now ready to be transposed anterior to the fascial sling of Eaton (see Fig. 17-9).

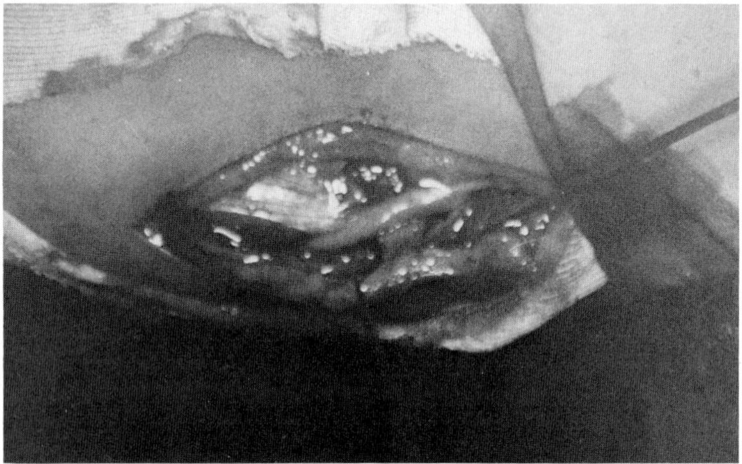

FIG. 17-9. The technique of Eaton: The ulnar nerve is positioned anterior to the fascial sling originating in the anterior aspect of the flexor pronator group where it attaches to the medial epicondyle. The fascial sling holds the nerve anterior to the epicondyle.

arcade that, as the forearm pronates, can compress on the posterior interosseous nerve. This anatomic arrangement predisposes the nerve to entrapment in tennis and racquet ball, in which repetitive pronation and supination of the forearm occurs.

Clinical Picture

The patient describes pain over the lateral aspect of the elbow. Often it is associated with sports such as racquet ball and tennis.

Tenderness is present over the anterior aspect of the elbow where the radial nerve courses over the radial head. The patient is not tender over the common extensor tendon on the lateral epicondyle, as one sees in the more common lateral tennis elbow syndrome. Active supination and passive pronation of the forearm increase the pain, as does forced extension of the third finger and wrist against resistance. These maneuvers tighten the fascial origin of the extensor carpiradialis brevis, and this creates compression on the sensitive radial nerve branch. Electromyography (EMG) usually yields negative findings, except in late cases in which degenerative changes can be seen in the radial nerve innervated muscles of the forearm. Nerve conduction studies frequently reveal delayed conduction of the radial nerve across the elbow.

Treatment

The vast majority of patients respond to a program of rest, nonsteroidal antiinflammatory medicine, and subsequent rehabilitation exercises to increase strength and flexibility of the elbow musculature. Emphasis is placed on conditioning of the extensor/supinator group. If symptoms persist despite the conservative program, exploration of the radial nerve anteriorly can be carried out. The nerve is decompressed by dividing the fibrous arcade in the region of the flexor carpiradialis brevis and supinator, which is referred to as the arcade of Frosch. However, this is necessary in less than 10% of all cases.

Pronator Teres Syndrome

As the medial nerve crosses the elbow anteriorly, just distal to the joint, it passes between the two heads of the pronator teres muscle where it is very vulnerable to entrapment in sports that involve repetitive pronation of the forearm such as baseball, racquetball, and tennis.

Clinical Picture

The patient complains of pain radiating from the elbow down the anterior forearm. This is often associated with numbness and tingling in the median nerve distribution in the hand (i.e., the thumb, index, and middle fingers). Forced pronation or passive supination tends to increase the pain. There is often a positive Tinel's sign where the medial nerve passes under the pronator muscle mass. In some patients one can detect decreased sensation in the thumb, index, and middle fingers, with associated weakness of the abductor pollicis brevis and flexor pollicis longus. Nerve conduction studies reveal decreased conduction of the median nerve in the upper forearm and normal conduction as it crosses the wrist, ruling out the more common carpal tunnel syndrome. Rarely, one may see denervative changes on EMG examination of the median nerve intrinsic muscles of the hand and the flexor pollicis longus.

Treatment

Rest, nonsteroidal antiinflammatory medicine, and subsequent exercises to increase the strength and range of motion of the muscles of the forearm and elbow, especially the flexor pronator group, is successful in most cases. In those rare cases that fail to respond, exploration of the median nerve via an anterior approach is performed. Neurolysis of the median nerve and releasing it from the constricting structures, particularly as it passes between the two heads of the pronator teres and under the flexor digitorum sublimis, can be successful.

SUMMARY

Overuse injuries of the elbow are common in athletes. *The best treatment is prevention.* The athlete should follow a good training program that includes endurance training, a balanced diet, and generalized flexibility and strength features. This is very important, because if the patient lacks endurance, is overweight, has tight back muscles and so on, mechanics will be affected, which in turn will affect the elbow. In addition, the athlete should engage in a good, ongoing program to maintain the strength and flexibility of the muscles of the dominant upper extremity used in the particular sport. If these guidelines are followed, the chances of injury are markedly decreased. If a problem does develop, rest, appropriate use of nonsteroidal antiinflammatory medicine, and subsequent participation in a good rehabilitation program have been successful in the vast majority of cases. In cases that have not responded to treatment and require surgery, the results have also been quite successful.

SUGGESTED READINGS

1. Adams JE: Injury to the throwing arm: a study of traumatic changes in the elbow of boy baseball players, Calif Med 102:127, 1965.
2. Adams JE: Bone injury in very young athletes, Clin Orthop 58:129, 1968.
3. Albright JA et al: Clinical study of baseball pitches: correlation of injury to the throwing arm with method of delivery, Am J Sports Med 6:15, 1978.
4. Allmon F et al: Tennis elbow: Who is most likely to get it and how, Phys Sports Med 3:43, 1975.
5. Appleberg DG and Larson SJ: Dynamic anatomy of the ulna nerve and the elbow, Plast Reconstr Surg 23:57, 1973.
6. Barnes DA and Tullas HS: An analysis of 100 symptomatic baseball players, Am J Sports Med 6:62, 1978.
7. Bennett GE: Shoulder and elbow lesions of the professional baseball pitcher, JAMA 117:510, 1941.
8. Bennett GE: Shoulder and elbow lesions distinctive of baseball players, Am J Surg 126:106, 1947.
9. Bennett GE: Elbow and shoulder lesions of baseball players, Am J Surg 98:484, 1952.
10. Brogdan GG and Brown NE: Little leaguer's elbow, AJR 83:671-675, 1959.
11. Brown R et al: Osteochondritis of the capitellum, Am J Sports Med 2:27, 1974.
12. Buchthal F, Rosenbalch E, and Trojaborg W: Electrophysiological findings in entrapment of the medial nerve at the wrist and elbow, J Neurol Neurosurg Psychiatry 37:340, 1974.
13. Capener N: Posterior interosseus nerve lesion: Proceedings of the Second Hand Club, J Bone Joint Surg 46B:361, 1964.

14. Childress AM: Recurrent ulna nerve dislocation at the elbow, Clin Orthop 108:168, 1975.
15. Clark CB: Cubital tunnel syndrome, JAMA 241:801, 1979.
16. Coonrad RW and Hooper WR: Tennis elbow: its course, natural history, conservative and surgical management, J Bone Joint Surg 55A:1177, 1973.
17. Cyriax JH: The pathology and treatment of tennis elbow, J Bone Joint Surg 18:921, 1936.
18. DeHaven KE and Evarts CM: Throwing injuries of the elbow in athletes, Orthop Clin North Am 4:801, 1973.
19. DeHaven KE et al: Throwing injuries to the adolescent elbow, Contemp Surg 9:65, 1976.
20. DelPizzo W, Jobe F, and Norwood L: Ulna nerve entrapment in baseball players, Am J Sports Med 5:182, 1977.
21. Eaton RE, Crowe JF, and Parkes JC: Anterior transposition of the ulna nerve using a non-compressing fasciodermal sling, J Bone Joint Surg 62A:820, 1980.
22. Feindel W and Stratford J: Cubital tunnel compression in tardy ulna palsy, Am Med Assoc J 78:351, 1958.
23. Feindel W, and Stratford J: The role of the cubital tunnel in tardy ulna palsy, Am J Surg 1:206, 1978.
24. Foster RJ and Edshage S: Factors related to outcome of surgically managed compressive ulna neuropathy at the elbow level, J Hand Surg 6: 181, 1981.
25. Francis R et al: Little league elbow a decade later, Phys Sports Med 6:88, April 1978.
26. Garden RS: Tennis elbow, J Bone Join Surg 43B:100, 1961.
27. Godshall RW: Traumatic ulna neuropathy in adolescent baseball pitchers, J Bone Joint Surg 53A:359, 1971.
28. Goldie, I: Epicondylitis lateralis humeri: a pathogenetical study, Acta Chir Scand (suppl) 399:1, 1964.
29. Grona WA: Pitcher's elbow in adolescents, Am J Sports Med 8:333-336, 1980.
30. Hanson MJ and Nareds S: Results of anterior transposition of the ulna nerve for ulna neuritis, Br Med J 1:27, 1970.
31. Hartz CR et al: The pronator teres syndrome, J Bone Joint Surg 63A:885, 1981.
32. Heller CJ and Wittre LL: Avascular necrosis of the capitellum, J Bone Joint Surg 42A:513, 1960.
33. Herasarva Y and Sadaheda M: Sports and peripheral nerve injury, Am J Sports Med 11:420, 1983.
34. Ilfeld FW and Freed SM: Treatment of tennis elbow: use of special brace, JAMA 195:67, 1966.
35. Indelicato PA et al: Correctable elbow lesions in professional baseball players: a review of 25 cases, Am J Sports Med 7:72, 1979.
36. Johnson RK et al: Median nerve entrapment syndrome in the proximal forearm, J Hand Surg 4:48, 1979.
37. Kaplan EB: Treatment of tennis elbow (epicondylitis), J Bone Joint Surg 41A:147, 1959.
38. Kerlon RK et al: Throwing injuries of the shoulder and elbow in adults, Am Pract Orthop Surg 6:41, 1975.
39. King JW and Tullas HS: Analysis of the pitching arm of the professional baseball pitcher, Clin Orthop 67:116, 1969.
40. Larson RL and McMahan RO: The epyphyses and the childhood athlete, JAMA 196:607, 1966.
41. Lipscomb BA: Baseball pitching injuries in growing athletes, Am J Sports Med 3:25, 1975.
42. Major HP: Lawn-tennis elbow, Br Med J 2:557, 1883.
43. Michele AA and Krueger FJ: Lateral epicondylitis of the elbow, Surgery 39:277, 1956.
44. Middleman IC: Shoulder and elbow lesions of baseball players, Am J Surg 2:627, 1961.
45. Nirschl RP: Good tennis = good medicine, Phys Sports Med 3:27, 1973.
46. Nirschl RP: Tennis elbow, Orthop Clin North Am 4:787, 1973.
47. Nirschl RP and Petrone F: Tennis elbow, J Bone Joint Surg 61A:832, 1979.
48. Nirschl RP and Sobel J: Conservative treatment of tennis elbow, Phys Sports Med 9:42, 1981.
49. Panetta CA and Jones JM: Epicondylitis of the humerus, Mayo Clin 33:303, 1958.
50. Peltokallo, P: Joint injuries in Finnish baseball players, J Sports Med Phys Fit 3:229, 1963.
51. Phalen GS: The cubital tunnel syndrome, Clin Orthop 83:29, 1972.
52. Rales MD and Mundsley RH: Radial tunnel syndrome, J Bone Joint Surg 543A:499, 1972.
53. Rales MC and Mundsley RH: Radial tunnel syndrome: resistant tennis elbow as a nerve entrapment, J Bone Joint Surg 54NA:499, 1972.
54. Slager RF: From little league to big league, the weak spot is the arm, Am J Sports Med 5:37, 1977.
55. Slocum DB: Classification of elbow injuries from baseball pitching, Tex Med 64:48-53, 1968.
56. Spencer GE Jr and Herndon CH: Surgical treatment of epicondylitis, J Bone Joint Surg 35A:421, 1953.
57. Staal A: The entrapment neuropathies, Handbook Clin Neural 7, 285, 1970.
58. Thompson WAL and Kopell HP: Peripheral entrapment neuropathies of the upper extremity, N Engl J Med 260:1261, 1959.
59. Targ JS: Little league: the theft of a careful youth, Phys Sports Med 8:73, 1978.
60. Targ JS and Mayer RA: Non-union of a stress fracture through the olecranon epyphyseal plate observed in an adolescent baseball pitcher, J Bone Joint Surg 59A:264, 1977.
61. Targ JS et al: The effect of competitive pitching on the shoulders and elbows of preadolescent baseball players, Pediatrics 49:267, 1972.
62. Trias A and Ray RD: Juvenile osteochondritis of the radial head, J Bone Joint Surg 45A:576, 1963.
63. Tullos HS: Lesions of the pitching arm in adolescents, JAMA 220:264, 1972.
64. Unverfirth LJ and Olix, ML: The effect of local steroid injections on tendons, Am J Sports Med 1:31, 1973.
65. Vonderpaal DW et al: Peripheral compression lesions of the ulna nerve, J Bone Joint Surg 503A:792, 1968.
66. Wadsworth TG: The external compression syndrome of the ulna nerve at the cubital tunnel, Clin Orthop 124:189, 1977.
67. Wares W: Elbow injuries of javelin throwers, Acta Chir Scand 93:564, 1946.
68. Werner C: Lateral elbow pain and posterior interosseous nerve entrapment, Acta Orthop Scand FM:1, 1979.
69. Wilson FD et al: Valgus extension overload in the pitching elbow, Am J Sports Med 11:83, 1983.
70. Woods WG and Tullos HS: The throwing arm (elbow injuries), Am J Sports Med 69:43, 1973.
71. Woods WG and Tullos HS: Elbow instability and medial epicondyle fractures, Am J Sports Med 5:23, 1977.
72. Zarens B, Andrews JR, and Carson W: Injuries of the throwing arm, Philadelphia, 1985, WB Saunders Co.

CHAPTER 18 Degenerative Joint Disease of the Elbow

John J. Brems

The elbow joint is a complex joint having freedom of motion along both the transverse and longitudinal planes. Despite its mechanical complexity and despite the tremendous biomechanical forces to which it is subjected in throwing sports, it is remarkably resistant to progressive degenerative joint disease. That degenerative arthritis of the elbow is extremely rare is testified to by the fact that less than 5% of the elbow arthroplasties performed at the Mayo clinic were done so for primary degenerative arthritis.[5,6] Goodfellow and Bullough[1] described the pattern of aging of the elbow articular cartilage and found consistent age-related findings at the radiocapitellar joint, but they found only limited changes at the articular cartilage of the humeroulnar joint.

Muscle strain, ligament sprains, and generalized overuse syndromes are frequent conditions encountered by the athlete but do not lead to degenerative joint disease. Loose bodies, frequently seen in the elbow, may lead to wear and degenerative changes and should not be ignored. Untreated loose bodies may lead to "three body wear" with severe rapid damage to the articular surfaces.[3]

HISTORY AND PHYSICAL EXAMINATION

The most consistent patient complaint is limitation of elbow motion, manifested primarily as a flexion contracture. This contracture may be either bone in origin as in olecranon impingement from hypertrophic spurring, or it may be soft tissue in origin from a tight anterior capsule or a contracted brachialis or biceps muscle.

Findings in elbow degenerative joint disease

- Flexion contracture
- Loss of terminal flexion
- Forearm atrophy
- Limitation of forearm rotation (variable)
- Crepitus

The athlete may complain of medial joint pain from a chronic inflammation or sprain of the medial ligament complex, consisting of the anterior and posterior oblique ligaments. Stretching of the ligaments may lead to increased compression at the radiocapitellar joint laterally. This may result in a fragmentation of the lateral joint articular surfaces with resultant formation of loose bodies and, later, degenerative disease. The patients may complain of pain posteriorly and along the medial olecranon border. Tullos et al[2] found a high incidence of degenerative changes in this area in baseball pitchers.

Forearm atrophy may be present on the affected extremity, but generally this is difficult to assess and is of limited value in patient evaluation.

When examining range of motion, in addition to the flexion contracture, there is usually loss of maximal flexion when compared to the uninvolved extremity (Fig. 18-1). In degenerative disease, this is most likely secondary to radial head osteophytes that impinge on the anterior distal humerus. A tight posterior capsule or triceps contracture may also limit flexion. Loose bodies and the pain

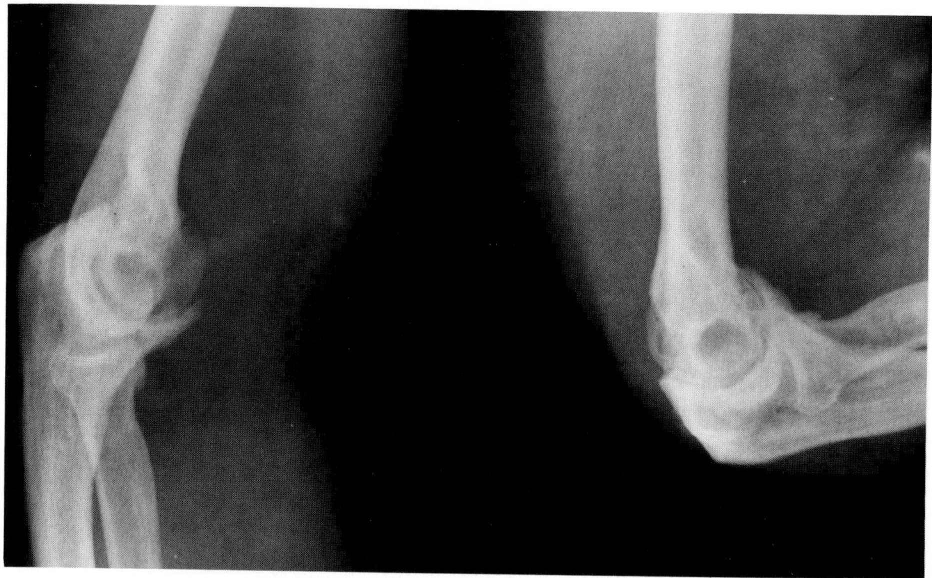

FIG. 18-1. Roentgenogram taken in the lateral projection shows the maximal extension and flexion obtained in this elbow with severe degenerative arthritis. The common cause of loss of extension is osteophytes on the olecranon process or loose bodies in the olecranon fossa. A tight anterior capsule or brachialis and biceps contractures also limit extension. Flexion is usually limited by osteophytes on the radial head and in the area of the coronoid process. Additionally, soft tissue contractures involving the triceps or posterior capsule can limit flexion.

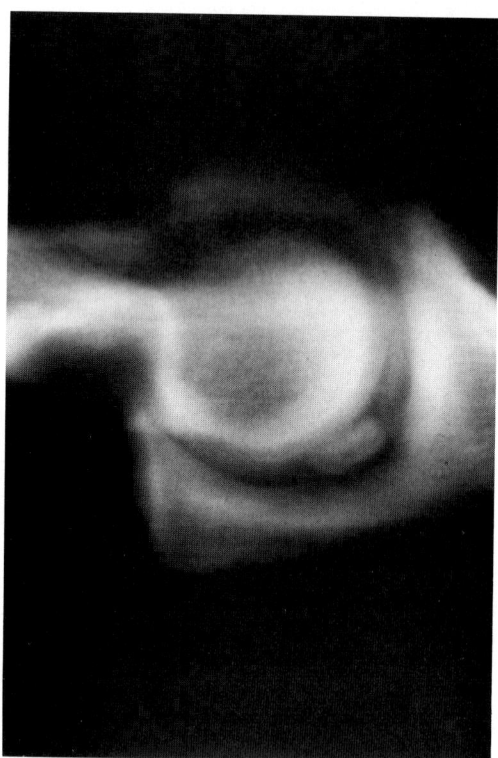

FIG. 18-2. Arthrotomogram of the elbow of a presently active NFL lineman. This technique is superior for defining the size and location of loose bodies. Not all loose bodies are calcified and ossified, and this technique of arthrotomography can demonstrate these types of cartilagenous loose bodies.

of joint incongruity may limit the observed motion (Fig. 18-2).

Pronation and supination motions may likewise be limited to varying degrees, depending on the location of the degenerative change. It is important for the examiner to initially measure the pronation and supination passively. Active motion causes increased compression of the articular surfaces and may increase pain, resulting in an apparent loss of motion greater in degree than would be seen with passive examination. Similarly, when evaluating the joint for crepitus, one must remember that active motion may increase the crepitus that may otherwise go undetected. Needless to say, a careful neurologic examination is mandatory.

ROENTGENOGRAPHIC EVALUATION

A minimum of anteroposterior (AP) and lateral views are required for evaluating the elbow. The AP view is performed with the elbow in extension and the lateral view with the elbow in 90 degrees of flexion. In degenerative joint disease, one looks for joint space narrowing and hypertrophic bone changes (Fig. 18-3). Occasionally a joint effusion may be seen by the presence of the anterior and posterior fat pad signs.

The most common area for joint space narrowing is at the radiocapitellar joint. Hyper-

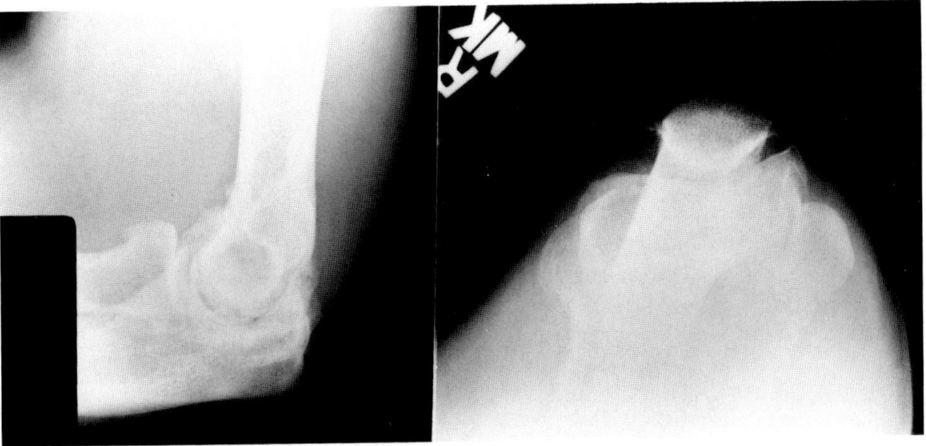

FIG. 18-3. Two views of an active NFL lineman, showing severe arthritis of the elbow. The most characteristic changes are osteophytes on the radial head and on the coronoid and olecranon processes. The axial view clearly shows the degenerative process involving the olecranon process.

trophic new bone may be seen at the articular margins of the radial head and neck and around the olecranon process, especially on its medial side. Loose bodies may be seen anywhere in the joint but most commonly are found in the olecranon fossa or on the lateral side of the joint. Double-contrast arthrotomography is especially helpful in identifying intraarticular loose bodies.

MANAGEMENT

Operative management is only rarely indicated for primary degenerative joint disease about the elbow. For the most severe cases where there is pain and disability unresponsive to nonoperative management, either fascial arthroplasty or arthrodesis may be indicated. The gross instability following resection arthroplasty makes this procedure unsatisfactory except in severe sepsis or tuberculosis. Total joint replacement or hemiarthroplasty has only limited use in the surgical management of degenerative disease of the elbow in the active athletic patient. Indications and contraindications are very well outlined in Morrey.[4] Arthroscopic joint debridement is in its infancy, and adequate data is not yet available to recommend its widespread use in the arthritic elbow (see Chapter 5).

Nonoperative management of degenerative joint disease of the elbow must initially attempt to control pain. Pain management may consist of antiinflammatory agents orally, together with splinting to decrease tissue edema. In more severe cases, intraarticular corticosteroids may be given. Once pain has abated, range of motion exercises and general

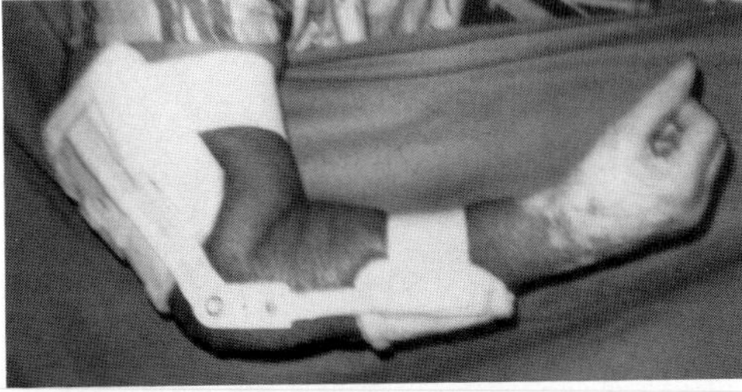

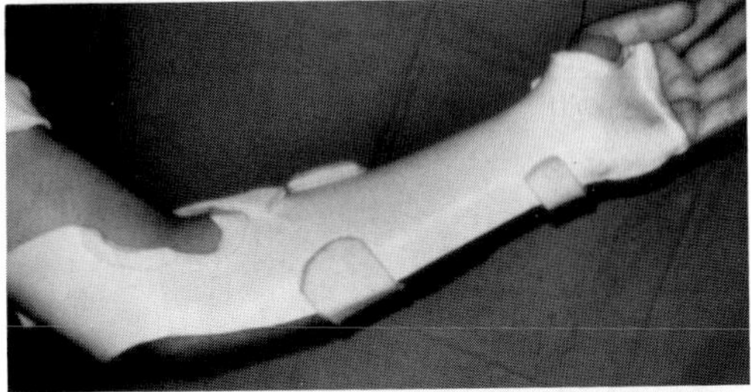

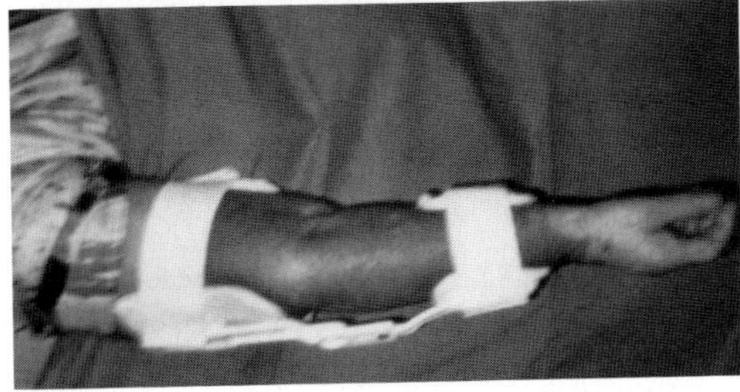

FIG. 18-4. Fabrication of thermoplastic splints in the fixed position or with hinges provide significant relief of pain in the arthritic elbow. They may be used as resting night splints, or, with hinges, they may be worn during certain activities to provide increased stability and to limit motion to the more painless arc.

muscle conditioning begins. Adjustable splints may be fabricated with thermoplastic materials in which range of motion in flexion and extension are controlled (Fig. 18-4). These splints should be worn at night and may be worn during activities to resist extremes of motion that may otherwise cause or aggravate symptoms.

When intraarticular corticosteroids are used, they are most easily instilled via the lateral side in the radiocapitellar joint. Physical therapy modalities include instruction in active range of motion exercises to the limit of pain and general muscle strengthening using isometric and isotonic techniques.

SUMMARY

Management of degenerative joint disease about the elbow fortunately is not a common problem. Few orthopaedic surgeons are faced with active patients who have advanced arthritis and the literature offers little guidance in their management. The vast majority appear to respond satisfactorily to nonoperative management, and surgical intervention should remain the management of last resort.

REFERENCES

1. Goodfellow JW and Bullough PG: The pattern of aging of the articular cartilage of the elbow joint, J Bone Joint Surg 49(B):175, 1967.
2. King JW, Brelsford HJ, and Tullos HS: Analysis of the pitching arm of the professional baseball pitcher, Clin Orthop 67:116, 1969.
3. Morrey BF: Loose bodies. In Morrey BF, editor: The elbow and its disorders, 1985, Philadelphia, WB Saunders Co, p 736.
4. Morrey BF: Reconstructive procedure of the elbow. In Morrey BF, editor: The elbow and its disorders, 1985, Philadelphlia, WB Saunders Co, p 530.
5. Morrey BF et al: Total elbow arthroplasty: a five-year experience at the Mayo Clinic, J Bone Joint Surg, 63(A):1050, 1981.
6. Ortner DJ: Description and classification of degenerative bone changes in the distal joint surfaces of the humerus, Am J Phys Anthrop 28:139, 1968.

CHAPTER 19 Rehabilitation of Elbow Injuries

Fred L. Allman
Carolyn A. Carlson

The basic power unit of performance is the musculotendinous unit; therefore most elbow problems that arise during or as a result of athletic activity are related to muscular activity. The main offender is a dynamic overload to the musculotendinous unit. The resulting injuries may be acute, subacute, or chronic. In addition, injuries may occur over an extended period of time as the result of the late effects of repetitive microtrauma.

Injuries to the elbow and subsequent rehabilitation must include restoration of all the basic qualities of muscle function. Clinically, there are three basic qualities of muscle function.

1. *Strength*—the ability of a muscle to contract
2. *Elasticity*—the ability of a muscle to give up contraction and to yield to passive stretch
3. *Coordination*—the ability of a muscle to cooperate with other muscles in proper timing and with appropriate power and elasticity

It is usually possible to explain a deficiency in muscle action as the consequence of one, two, or all three of these basic qualities of muscle function.

A muscle acts from an elongated position because the elastic force of the muscle augments a contractible force. A muscle contracts best from its full length. Overuse or overloading leads to fatigue, and with fatigue the muscle relaxes more slowly and more incompletely than normal. It then enters a state of myostatic contracture in which injuries are likely to occur. The resulting injury might be a minor strain to the muscle or tendon. If repeated strains occur, actual tears may take place in the muscle. Attempts at repair result in fibrosis, and this fibrosis may in turn result in a permanent loss of elbow extension.

Although rest, ice, and gentle massage are helpful, the main effort in treatment and rehabilitation should be directed to the cause of the condition rather than to the resultant effect. The musculotendinous unit must be slowly and gradually strengthened to withstand the stress of athletic participation without producing an undue overload. Rehabilitation therefore must consist primarily of restoration or improvement in the quality of the impaired muscle function. If the muscle is weak, it must be strengthened. If the muscle is inelastic, the elasticity must be improved. If the muscle has lost its proper timing and synchronous action, the goal should be to restore proper coordination. The problem may be related to all three qualities—strength, elasticity, and coordination.

For the athlete with an elbow injury, especially in the throwing and racquet sports, rehabilitation must extend beyond the upper extremity, trunk, and lower extremities, and rehabilitation must also be directed to these areas. An alteration of function involving any of these regions will likely lead to further and more prolonged problems. Therefore total body fitness must be one of the goals of rehabilitation.

RATIONALE FOR REHABILITATION FOR SPECIFIC ELBOW CONDITIONS

Tension Overload

These injuries occur in both throwing and racquet sports, as well as in weight training.

Medial Tension Overload

In baseball, the most common injury is a tear or partial avulsion of one of the tendons or muscle insertions, often the result of medial overload produced by the valgus strain on the elbow (see Chapter 16).

In football, the windup is less than in baseball, the forward fling is shorter, and the follow-through is in a different arc and not as powerful.

Hammer throwing and shot-putting place tremendous traction stress on the heavy muscles of the elbow and shoulder because of the momentum of the follow-through and the heavier projectile that is being propelled.

The javelin is released with a powerful extension of the elbow and with forcible pronation of the forearm. The pronation is extreme and it is necessary to prevent the whip of the javelin. In the follow-through the thrower may almost completely turn around.

Tension overload is seen frequently early in the season. Tightness develops on the medial aspect of the involved elbow. The medial muscle mass becomes tense and sore, and temporarily there is a loss of extension. If activity is allowed to continue while the athlete is in a state of myostatic contracture, then more serious injury is likely to occur, because fibrosis results from multiple tearing throughout the muscle with resultant permanent loss of elbow extension.

The aim of rehabilitation in this condition is to slowly and gradually strengthen the musculotendinous unit to withstand the stress without producing an undue overload.

Lateral Tension Overload

In tennis or other racquet sports, lateral tension overload is likely to occur. This is often referred to as "lateral epicondylitis." This condition is primarily caused by intrinsic and extrinsic overload at the extensor aponeurosis.

Lateral Compression Injuries

Lateral compression injuries are the result of impaction of the head of the radius against the capitellum in the act of throwing. Roughening and degeneration of the articular cartilage often result from repeated injury.

More than 50 years ago, Shands showed that trauma to hyaline cartilage produced a definite hyperplasia. The margins and the tip of the olecranon and the adjacent surfaces of the condyle of the humerus are constantly traumatized by the act of throwing. The result produces a definite osteochrondritis with exfoliation of the articular cartilage, which may in turn produce loose bodies, synovial thickening, and semiattached cartilaginous masses that obstruct and limit extension of the elbow.

Minor abnormalities in valgus-varus alignment of the ulna can result in impingement of the tip of the olecranon against the walls of the fossa as full extension is approached.

Rehabilitation for lateral compression injuries is very helpful in the early stages of injury but has considerable limitation after osteophytes, loose bodies, and articular cartilage damage has occurred. Therefore the aim should be to detect lateral compression injuries early and begin rehabilitation before more pronounced changes occur.

Extension Injuries

Extension injuries are relatively common in the throwing sports but especially so in pitchers. Extension injuries are probably secondary to medial tension and lateral compression in that, as noted previously, these two mechanisms cause increased valgus with abnormal wear and tear on the medial side of the olecranon process and articulate cartilage damage on the lateral side because of impaction.

Chronic intermittent overload by the extensor mechanism, however, can in itself result in hypertrophy of the ulna, the humerus, and the triceps muscle. If allowed to continue over a prolonged period of time, hypertrophy of the ulna and distal humerus results in a decrease in the size of the olecranon fossa, thus producing abnormal wear and loose body formation.

REHABILITATION PRINCIPLES

After injury or surgical procedure, initial rehabilitation is directed toward maintaining and regaining a normal range of motion. Gentle, active range of motion includes flexion, extension, pronation, and supination of the forearm. Gentle, slow, passive stretching for both extension and flexion is begun. For the elbow healing from surgery, or for those with major soft tissue or osseous damage such as dislocated elbows, care is taken to avoid early aggressive stretching because of the risk of traumatic myositis ossificans.

Forearm musculature flexibility is improved by passively stretching the extensor musculature (flexion with pronation) and the flexor-pronator group (passive extension with supination.)

Initial strengthening is achieved by low-resistance, high-repetition biceps and triceps curls. Pronation and supination are also improved through use of a hammer or similar tool to produce greater torque throughout the range of motion.

Proper technique is emphasized with the patient concentrating on number of repetitions rather than amount of weight lifted.

Finally, grip and shoulder exercises are initiated. For grip, patients may use a tennis ball for frequent isometric exercise. Many other grip devices are adequate as well. The shoulder may be exercised with free weights using a low-weight, high-repetition protocol. Strengthening exercises are conducted in straight anatomic and functional planes. For some individuals, primarily athletes, a well-structured machine program such as Nautilus may be used. Occasionally, in the late postoperative phase of rehabilitation, the elbow may require more aggressive stretching, especially for flexion contracture. Ideally the patient performs this independently, beginning with a good warm-up and then high-repetition exercise, followed by passive stretching with a dumbbell in the affected hand and positioning the elbow to allow for maximal flexor pronator stretch. As is the rule in the initial postoperative phase, ice is applied immediately after exercise.

Rehabilitation of the elbow focuses on strength and flexibility of the prime movers and stabilizers, as well as on conditioning of the entire upper extremity.

ELBOW REHABILITATION PROGRAMS

The Baltimore Therapeutic Equipment

The Baltimore Therapeutic Equipment (BTE) is a versatile, computerized system that may be used to provide quantitative analysis of:

1. Maximal isometric strength
2. Maximal work capacity (strength over time)
3. Maximal versus submaximal effort

This single compact instrument has a number of attachments and is designed to provide for specific repetitive motions against measurable resistances over a measurable period of time.

A number of different weight-lifting modes may be simulated as well as functional motions that are the key to athletic performance. The machine's capacity is limited only by the imagination of the clinician.

Regarding the elbow, the BTE may be used to:

1. Evaluate strength
2. Provide various strength and training modes
3. Simulate athletic activity before return to play

For the competitive athlete the BTE assists the clinician in providing a complete rehabilitation program, and it is an effective adjunct to free weights and machines.

Figs. 19-1 through 19-4 demonstrate the use of the BTE.

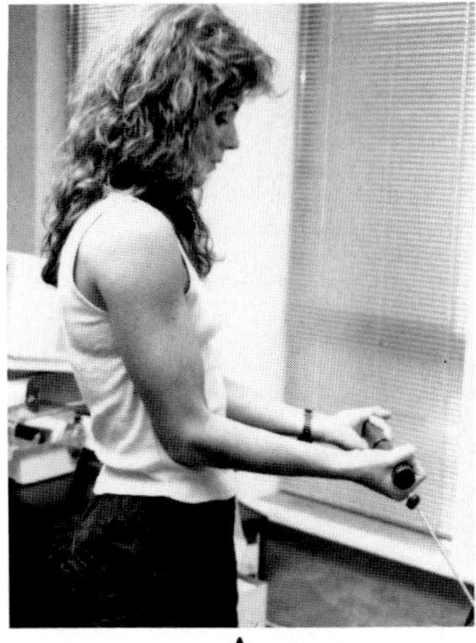
A

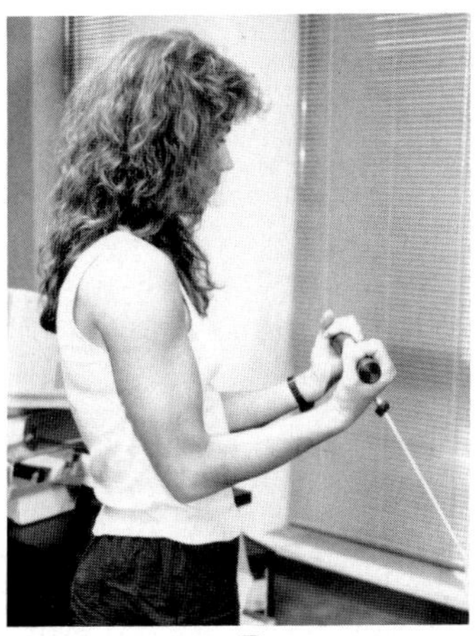
B

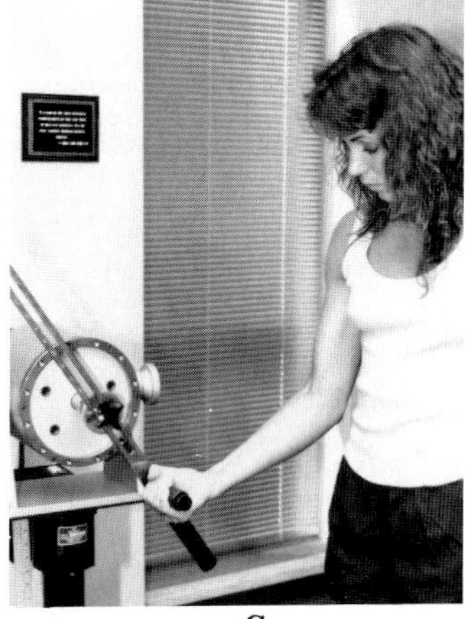
C

FIG. 19-1. A and **B,** Elbow flexion (pulley method) and **C,** elbow flexion (bar method) BTE evaluation.

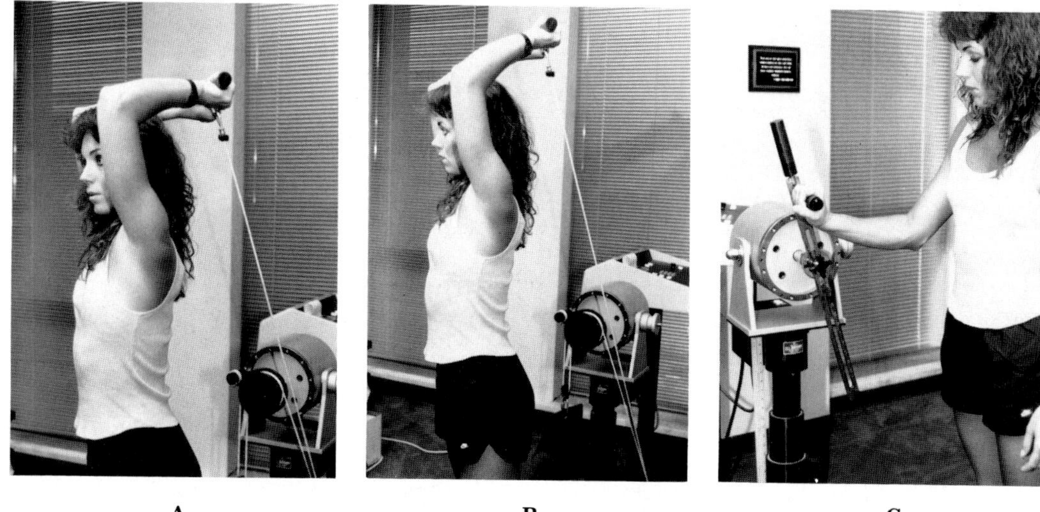

FIG. 19-2. A and **B,** Elbow extension (pulley method). **C,** Elbow extension (bar method) BTE evaluation.

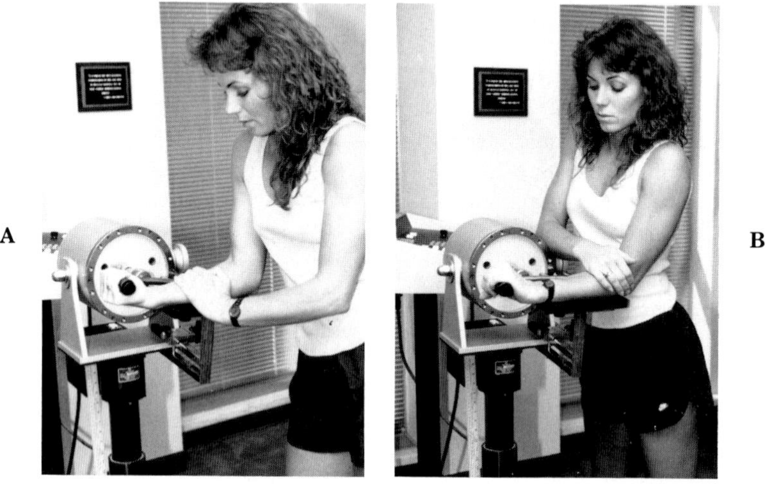

FIG. 19-3. A, Wrist flexion. **B,** Wrist extension (BTE evaluation).

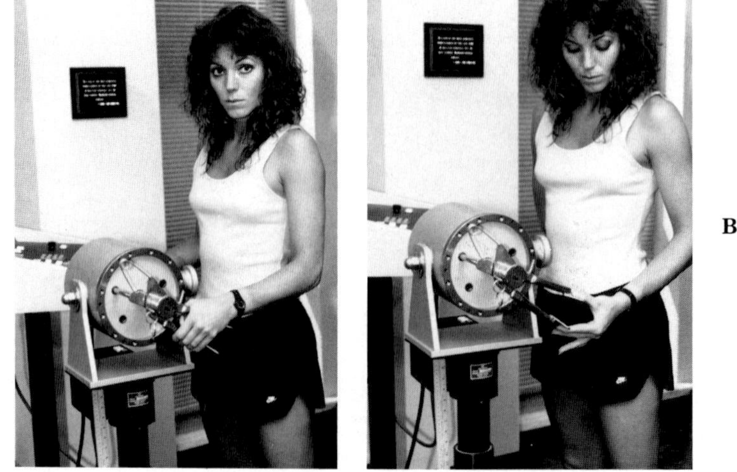

FIG. 19-4. A, Grip. **B,** Pinch-grip (BTE evaluation).

Proprioceptive Neuromuscular Facilitation (PNF)

PNF patterns for the upper extremity incorporate elbow, wrist, and hand motion in functional, repetitive, and concentric actions. These patterns allow application of graded resistance by the therapist in functional patterns not applicable by machines. In certain cases of elbow rehabilitation, PNF may be the initial means of beginning a strengthening program as well as providing motion and isometric exercise to other joints in the affected extremity.

REHABILITATION PROTOCOLS

Specific protocols exist to rehabilitate the competitive athlete, the recreational or weekend athlete, and the active "little league" athlete as well.

Program I is designed to rehabilitate the competitive athlete as quickly and effectively as possible through use of the BTE. This requires the patient to be seen in the clinic 3 times per week for intensive work on the BTE, free weights, and machines for total upper body conditioning. Other mechanical devices that can provide a variety of strength-training techniques can also be used.

Program II considers the recreational athlete and/or amateur who has access to a fitness facility or collegiate training room. In this situation athletes may use free weights at home and/or the gym, and they may also use upper body machines at the fitness facility.

Program III covers a home program for those individuals who do not have easy access to a fitness facility or training room and do not require intensive physical therapy.

Each program achieves the desired end result of greater strength, flexibility, and overall performance but is designed to meet the needs of the individual.

Elbow Rehabilitation Program I

I. *Initial evaluation*—includes history and mechanism of injury
   A. BTE strength assessment
      1. Elbow flexion, extension
      2. Wrist flexion, extension
      3. Forearm pronation, supination
      4. Grip
      5. Pinch grip
   B. Grip strength—Jamar hand dynamometer (see Fig. 19-5)
   C. Active range of motion (AROM)
      1. Elbow
      2. Wrist
      3. Fingers
   D. Girth—upper arm and forearm

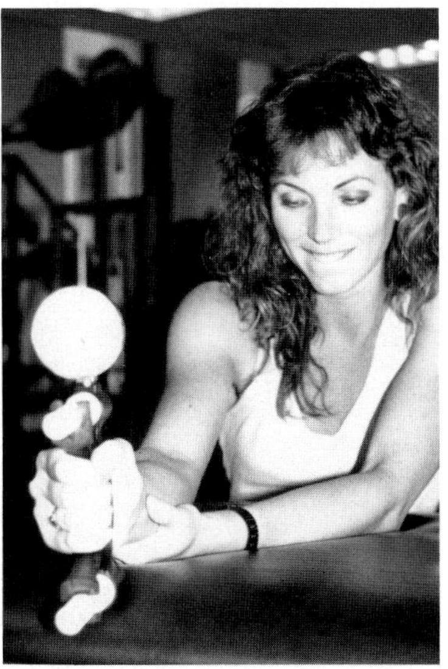

FIG. 19-5. Grip—Jamar hand dynamometer.

II. *Exercise program*
   A. Specific to elbow and forearm
      1. BTE—elbow flexion, extension
      2. BTE—forearm pronation, supination, flexion, and extension
         BTE—grip
         BTE—motion specific to sport (i.e., tennis, baseball, golf)
      3. Free weights—low-weight, high-repetition exercise (to alternate with BTE)
         a. Elbow flexion, extension—dumbbells 3 sets of 10 repetitions
         b. Wrist flexion, extension—light dumbbells, i.e., "heavy hands" 3 sets of 10 repetitions
         c. Forearm pronation, supination—hammer, tennis racquet, bar weighted at one end 3 sets of 10 repetitions
   B. General upper body conditioning
      1. Nautilus or exercise machines
         a. Shoulder—deltoids, trapezius, shoulder girdle musculature
         b. Chest—pectorals, anterior deltoid
         c. Arms—forearm curl machine
         d. Theraband exercises for shoulder rotator cuff
   C. Flexibility
      1. Forearm—extensors, flexors
         a. Gentle passive stretch
      2. Shoulder—anterior, posterior musculature

a. Overhead stretch (for latissimus and extensors)
b. Extension/pectoral stretch for anterior shoulder and chest muscles
c. Horizontal adduction stretch for posterior deltoid and rotator cuff muscles

III. *Modalities*
A. Heat
1. Before beginning exercise
2. Subacute or chronic phase
B. Ice
1. After exercise session for 20 minutes
2. Ice massage—directly to painful area using circular motion for approximately 5 to 10 minutes
3. As needed for pain and swelling control

IV. *Protocol specifics*
A. Frequency
1. Three times per week
B. Location
1. Sports medicine clinic or physical therapy department
C. Duration
1. Approximately 1½ hr visits
2. One month, then reevaluation
D. Reevaluation
1. BTE strength testing
2. Jamar grip testing
3. AROM measurements
E. Conditions necessary for return to play
1. Pain-free
2. Equal strength bilaterally
3. Equal AROM and/or girth (upper arm and forearm)

Elbow Rehabilitation Program II

I. *Initial evaluation*—includes history and mechanism of injury
A. BTE strength assessment
1. Elbow flexion, extension
2. Wrist flexion, extension
3. Forearm pronation, supination
4. Grip
5. Pinch grip
B. Grip strength—Jamar
C. AROM measurements
1. Elbow
2. Wrist
3. Fingers
D. Girth—upper arm and forearm

II. *Exercise program*
A. Specific to elbow and forearm
1. Free weights—low-weight, high-repetition
a. Elbow flexion, extension 3 sets of 10 repetitions
b. Wrist flexion, extension 3 sets of 10 repetitions (beginning with 1 or 2 lbs)
c. Forearm pronation, supination 3 sets of 10 repetitions (using a hammer, racquet or other end-weighted device)
2. Theraband exercises elbow flexion, extension, pronation, supination
B. Upper body conditioning (Fig. 19-6 and 19-7)
1. Nautilus or exercise machines
a. Shoulder—deltoid, trapezius, shoulder girdle musculature, compound shoulder, shoulder shrug, rowing torso combined pullover T/A
b. Chest—pectorals, anterior deltoid (combined chest machine)
c. Arms—biceps/triceps machine
2. Theraband—rotator cuff exercise
C. Flexibility—gentle passive stretching
1. Forearm—flexors and extensors
2. Shoulder—anterior and posterior musculature
D. Home program
1. Dumbbells/free weights
2. Theraband
3. Practice sports-specific motions before return to play

III. *Modalities*
A. Heat
1. Before exercise
2. Subacute or chronic phase
B. Ice
1. After exercise for 20 minutes
2. Alternative—ice massage to affected area 5 to 10 minutes
3. As needed for pain control

IV. *Protocol specifics*
A. Frequency
1. Daily home program every day at first; as weight increases, decrease to program three times per week
2. Clinic, training room, gym—three times per week
B. Location
1. Clinic, training room
2. Home
C. Duration
1. One-hour gym visits
2. Approximately 30 minutes home program

A

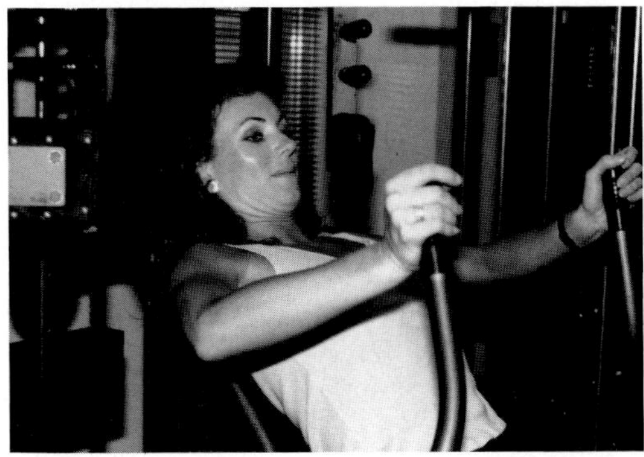

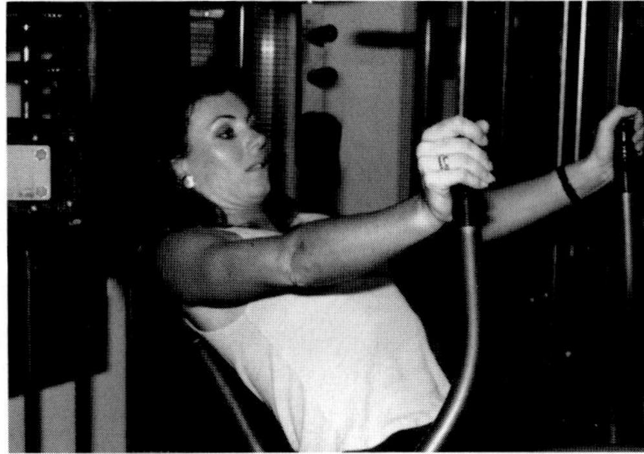

B

FIG. 19-6. A and **B** Chest press—Nautilus.

A

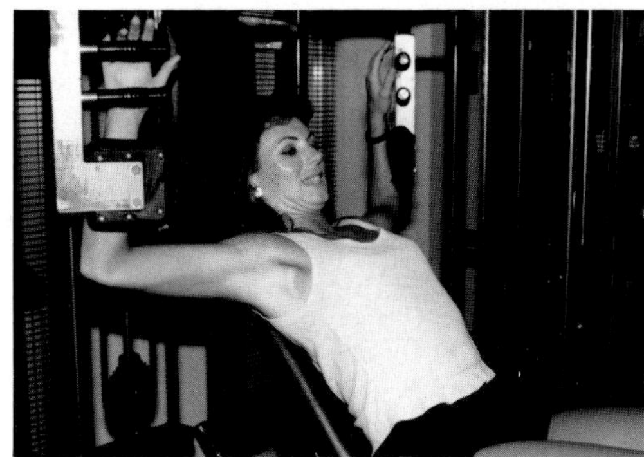

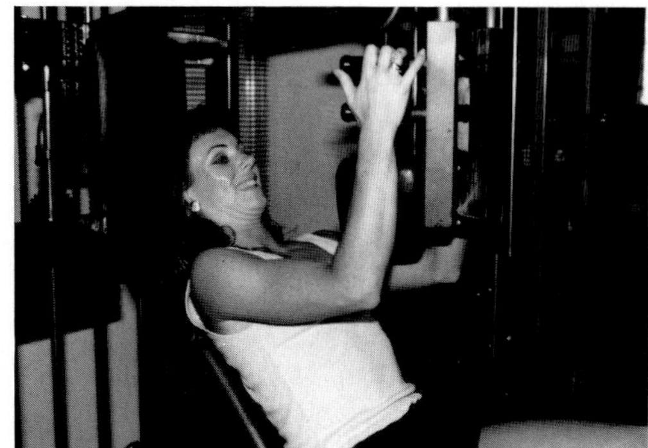

B

C

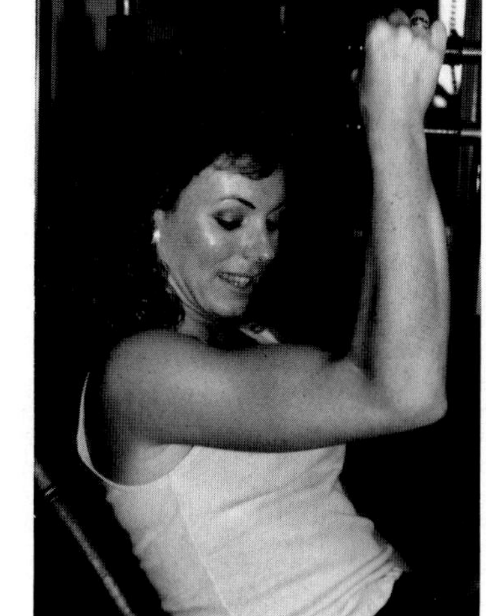

FIG. 19-7. A-C Pectoral flys—Nautilus.

D. Reevaluation
   1. BTE strength test
   2. Jamar grip testing
   3. AROM measurements
E. Conditions necessary for return to play
   1. Pain-free
   2. Equal strength bilaterally (or within 10%)
   3. Equal AROM and/or girth of upper arm and forearm

Elbow Rehabilitation Program III

I. *Initial evaluation*—includes history and mechanism
   A. BTE strength assesment—as time permits
      1. Elbow, wrist, forearm musculature
      2. Grip
   B. Jamar—grip strength
   C. AROM measurements
   D. Girth—upper arm and forearm
II. *Exercise program*
   A. Specific to elbow and forearm
      1. Free weights—low-weight, high-repetition dumbbells, "heavy hands"
         a. Elbow flexion, extension 3 sets of 10 repetitions (Fig. 19-8)
         b. Wrist flexion, extension 3 sets of 10 repetitions (Fig. 19-9)
         c. Forearm pronation, supination 3 sets of 10 repetitions (Fig. 19-10)
      2. Theraband—isometric resistive exercise
         a. Elbow flexion, extension 3 sets of 10 repetitions
         b. Forearm pronation, supination 3 sets of 10 repetitions
   B. Upper body conditioning
      1. Free weights
         a. Shoulder
            1. Super 7 PREs: active resistive straight plan range of motion
            2. Shrugs
      2. Theraband
         a. Rotator cuffs—internal and external rotation
   C. Flexibililty—gentle, passive stretching
      1. Forearm—flexors and extensors
      2. Shoulder—anterior, posterior musculature
   D. Sports
      1. Practice motion of sports-specific activity
      2. Gradual return to play
III. *Modalities*
   A. Heat—as needed before exercise or sport
   B. Ice
      1. After exercise or sport for 20 minutes
      2. Alternative—ice massage to affected area 5 to 10 minutes
      3. As needed for pain control

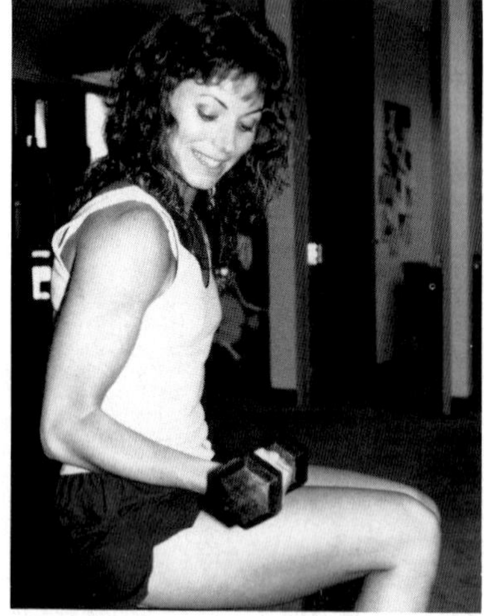

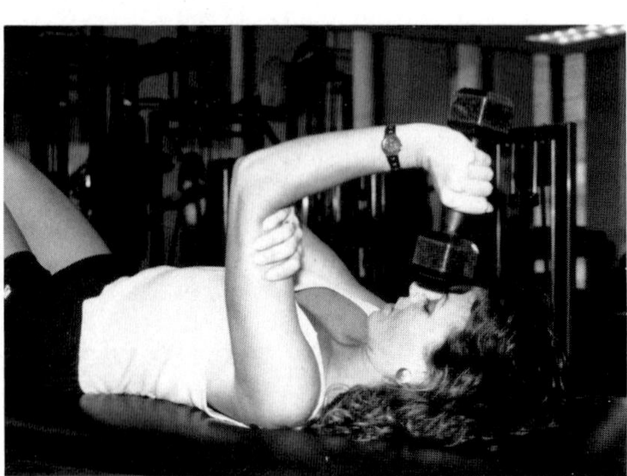

FIG. 19-8. A, Elbow flexion using free weights. **B,** Elbow extension using free weights.

A 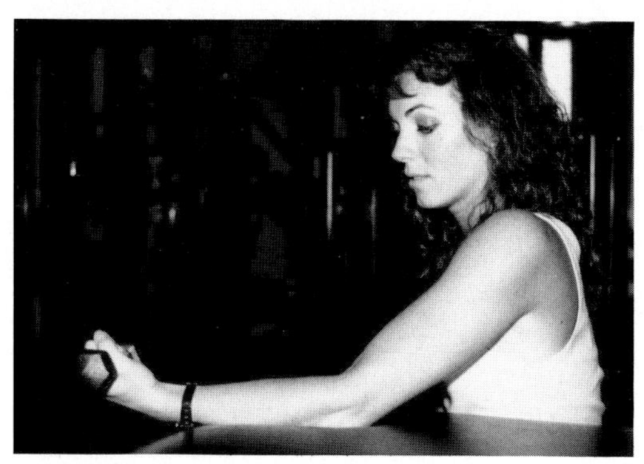 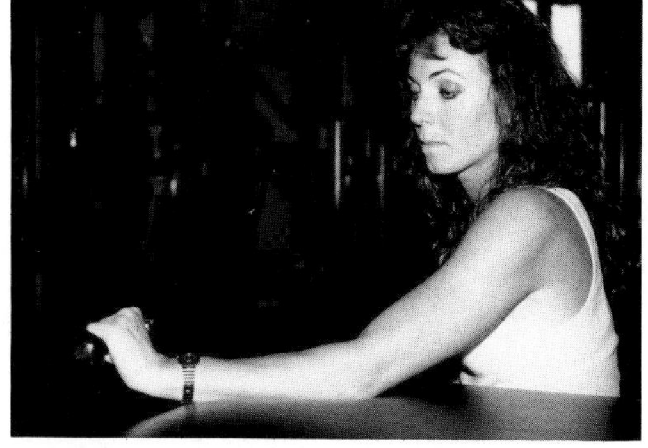 B

FIG. 19-9. A, Wrist flexion with free weights. **B,** Wrist extension with free weight.

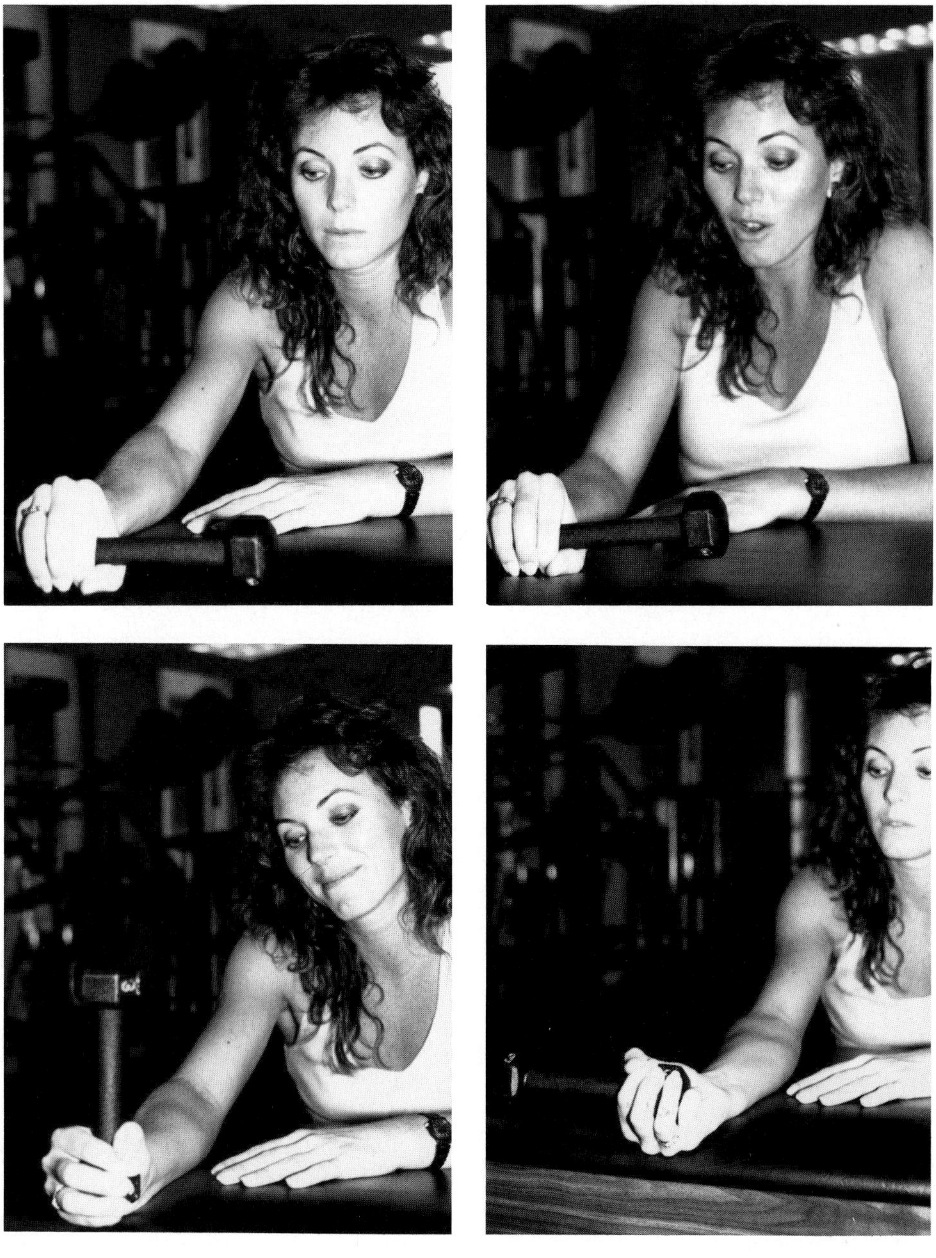

A B

C D

FIG. 19-10. Forearm exercises. **A** and **B,** pronation with free weights; **C,** forearm neutral; **D,** Supination with free weights.

IV. *Protocol specifics*
   A. Frequency
      1. Daily home program (daily initially; as weights increase, decrease frequency to three times per week)
   B. Location—home
   C. Duration
      1. Once per day, approximately 30 to 45 minutes
   D. Reevaluation
      1. BTE strength test (if performed initially)
      2. Jamar grip testing
      3. AROM measurements
   E. Conditions necessary for return to play
      1. Pain-free
      2. Equal strength bilaterally (or within 10%)
      3. Equal AROM and/or girth of upper arm and forearm

HOME REHABILITATION PROGRAMS

An important component of any elbow rehabilitation program is the home program. These programs are designed to allow the athlete to gain strength and flexibility with the use of minimal equipment. The home program reinforces the exercise regimen performed at the rehabilitation center and prevents regression of the athlete's progress by avoiding days in inactivity. Home programs are often designed to meet specific rehabilitation needs. Often a general program can be used and portions of it tailored to meet each patient's needs. A more specific program is often used for lateral tennis elbow.

General Home Elbow Program

1. *Elbow flexion (curls)*—Weight in hand; arm at side; slowly bend elbow, bring hand to the palm-up position. Hold 2 to 3 seconds, return to starting position. Three sets of 10 repetitions.

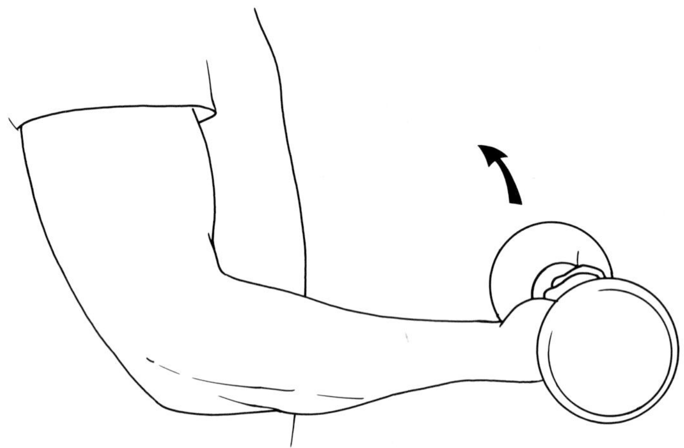

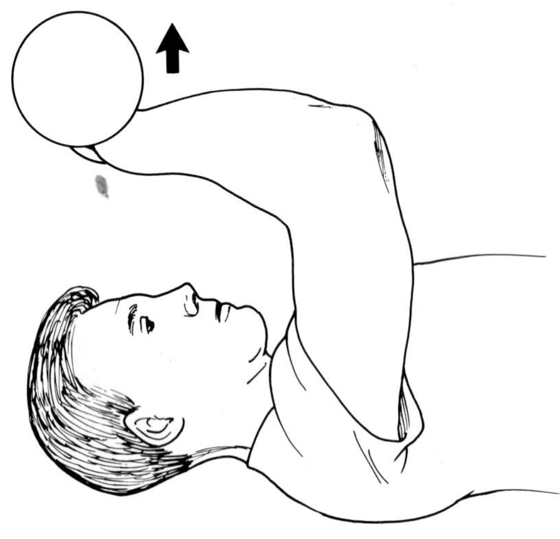

2. *Elbow extension (triceps curls)*—(Supine) arm raised toward ceiling; weight in hand; support arm with opposite hand. Slowly allow elbow to bend, then straighten elbow out; return to bent position to start again. Three sets of 10 repetitions (see Fig. 19-8, *B*.

3. *Forearm pronation/supination*—Grasp hammer (or similar light resistance); forearm supported; rotate hand to palm down position; return to starting position and rotate to palm-up position. Return to starting position; repeat 3 sets 10 repetitions (see Fig. 19-10).

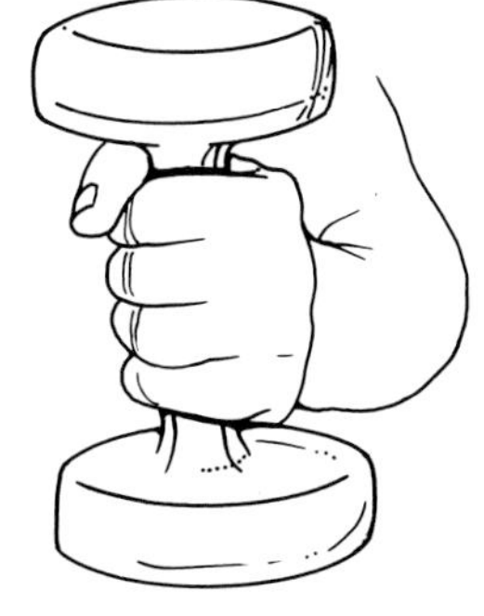

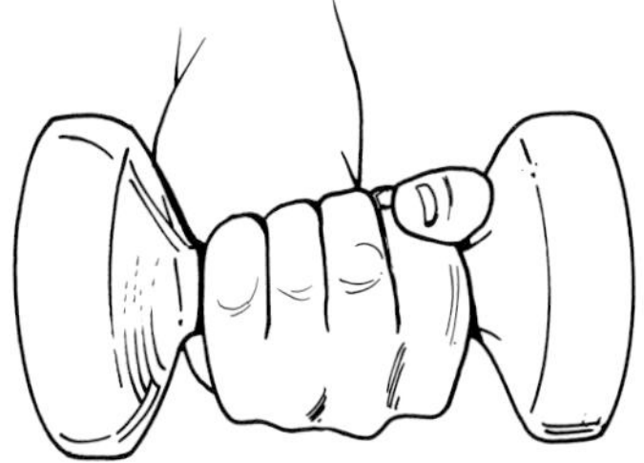

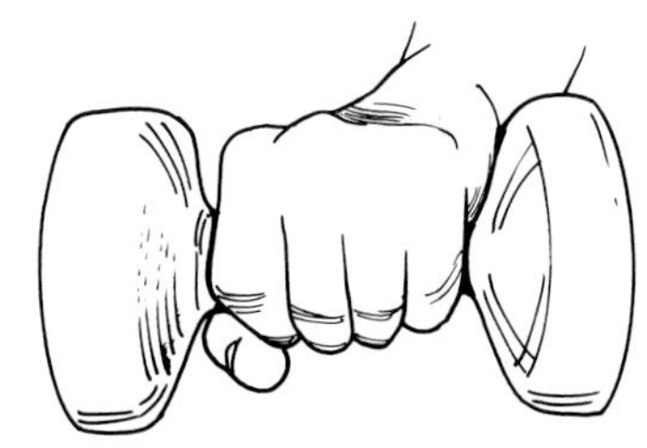

4. *Forearm stretching*—With arm in extended position, palm down, apply pressure to back of hand; feel stretch along top of forearm.

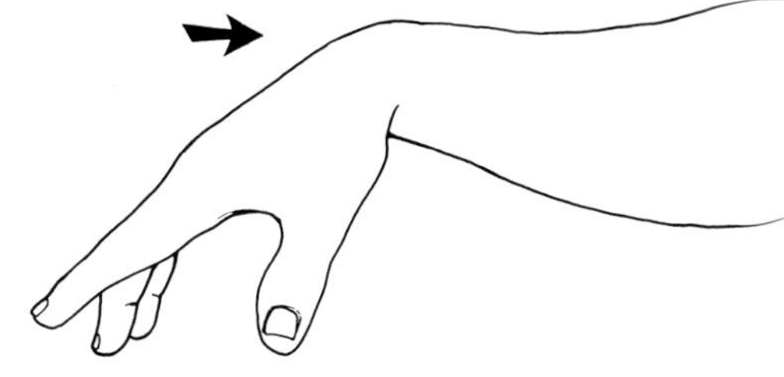

5. *Gripping exercise*—Carry an old tennis ball or other grip device and grip it frequently.

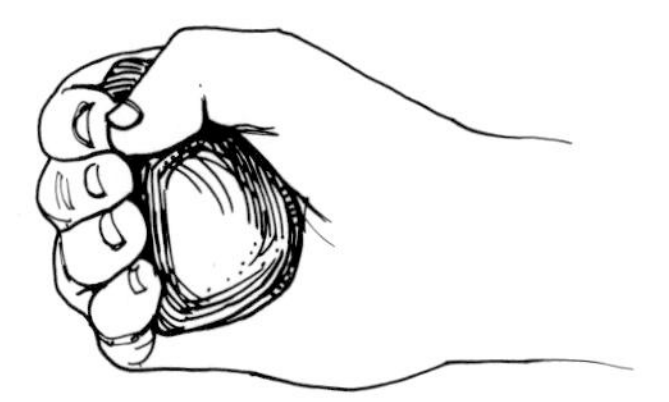

6. *Wrist curls and extensions*—Weight in hand, forearm supported, bend wrist in palm-up position, then palm down. Three sets 10 repetitions.
   Wrist flexion—Place the wrist in a palm-up position, supported at the edge of a table or on your knee, so that only the hand will be allowed to move. Grasp the weighted dumbbell (2 lbs pounds) or weighted bag. Perform the exercise as follows:
   1. Flex (bend upward) the wrist as far as possible.
   2. Hold 2 to 3 seconds.
   3. Lower fully; repeat up to 15 repetitions.
   4. Increase weight if 15 proper repetitions can be performed with no pain at the site of injury.

   Wrist extension—Performed in similar fashion to exercise 1 except palm faces down. Start with 2 lbs pounds.

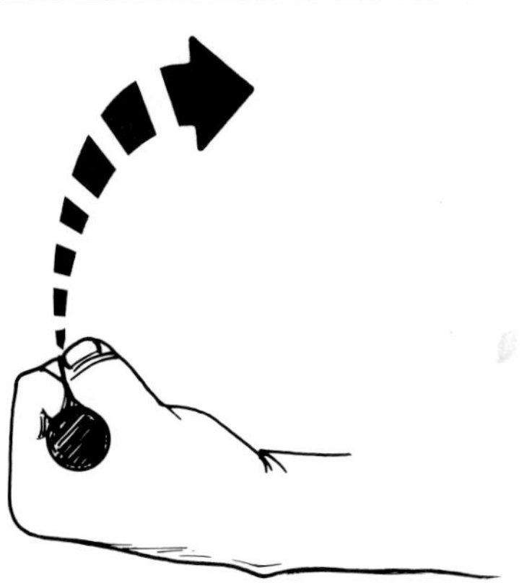

Home Rehabilitation for Tennis Elbow

Hot or Cold

Using either ice or moist heat can provide you with relief from pain. Both have similar physiologic responses that we desire. Therefore, use the modality in small time quantities, *though often.*

Ice is recommended for an acute, inflamed stage. Moist heat may be more comfortable for a chronic, sore period. (You can be in an acute stage even though the injury has been around for a long time.) Perform ice massage (water frozen in a Dixie cup) right on the area of pain for 5 minutes. Use moist heat (hot towels) as above for 5 minutes.

Stretching

Extend arm, straighten elbow. Let hand fall palm down. Grasp involved hand with noninvolved hand and pull down, bending wrist. You should feel a pull along the top of the forearm and into the area of pain. Hold for a count of 20, 5 times.

Exercise

Elbow bent, wrist supported.

1. Weight held in hand. Palm down. Raise wrist/hand up slowly and lower slowly.
2. Palm up. Bend wrist up slowly; lower slowly.
3. Thumb up. Bend wrist up.

All exercises—20 repetitions, 3 to 5 times a day. Begin with 1 pound and *increase as tolerated.*

Stretch again.

Ice again.

1. Also, squeeze tennis ball throughout the day.
2. Take lessons, if appropriate.
3. Check handle grip and size and weight of racquet.

PREVENTION OF ELBOW AND SHOULDER PROBLEMS

Over the years, we have developed a set of guidelines that we give to our throwing athletes to prevent elbow and shoulder problems. These apply for young athletes, recreational athletes, and professional athletes. These guidelines include the following:

1. Begin warm-up early enough to avoid being hurried.
2. Adjust warm-up period to weather conditions.
3. Gradually work up to maximal efficiency.
4. Concentrate on complete relaxation following each pitch.
5. Do not expose pitching arm to draft.
   a. Wear long-sleeved sweat shirt.
   b. Wear jacket when not pitching.
6. Do not attempt to pitch in presence of illness, injury, or when under undue mental tension.
7. Report shoulder or elbow pain immediately and discontinue pitching until after complete evaluation. (Under proper circumstances, you may be able to play another position.)
8. Do not practice throwing at home.
9. Don't shag fly balls and throw them in from the outfield if you are not properly warmed up.
10. Do not pitch more often than the league rules permit.
11. Do not pitch in more than one league.
12. After any layoff, regardless of cause or duration, be sure to resume activity gradually and do not attempt to throw hard or in a game until full recovery has been reached.

RETURN TO SPORTS CRITERIA

Return to sports activity follows a sequence much like the rehabilitation program. Initially the motion necessary for the specific sport is performed without weight, with the athlete monitoring technique in the mirror and paying close attention to detail. In the throwing sports, once pain is gone, throwing is allowed, with a gradual increase in the amount of time spent throwing. Again, technique is of the utmost importance in this phase. If over the course of several sessions pain does not recur, the athlete may begin to increase velocity. Throughout this final phase, as during early rehabilitation, there must be adequate warm-up, exercise (sport), and cool-down phases. The importance of a general conditioning program cannot be overemphasized. As early as possible with a given injury to the elbow, patients are strongly encouraged to maintain or increase their aerobic fitness and strength of the sound extremities. This facilitates a safe and rapid return to athletic competition or recreational activities.

SUMMARY

In conclusion, the elbow allows for fairly simple and direct methods of rehabilitation because four basic motions are present. On a more subtle level is the soft tissue response to trauma about the elbow. Hence the clinician must pay close attention to any change in level of pain, any reproducible pain, or minimal changes in range of motion. These may be indicators of early myositis ossificans, irritation of the ulnar nerve in the cubital tunnel, or the radial nerve in the arcade of Frohse. Most often, discontinuing the aggravating activity will resolve the pain.

CHAPTER 20 Athletic Training and Protective Equipment

Robert C. Reese, Jr.
T. Pepper Burruss
Joseph Patten

A variety of elbow injuries in the athlete can be managed with application of appropriate taping and protective padding. These techniques are an adjunct to the usual modes of treatment of both acute and chronic elbow injuries. Use of these modalities can permit an earlier return to sports if used in a judicious manner and monitored by trained sports medicine personnel.

TAPING TECHNIQUES

Athletic tape can be used at the elbow for hyperextension injuries or as part of treatment for mild valgus injuries. In both instances, tape is applied in order to restrict an undesired motion. For moderate to severe injuries, in which a significant limited range of motion is required, a plastic orthosis with hinges may be more appropriate.

In general, elbow-taping techniques work best after the swelling has resolved. Taping is then used to protect the athlete on return to participation. At all times, close supervision of the athlete is maintained because neurovascular problems can potentially arise with elbow injuries and their treatment.

Hyperextension Injuries

The hyperextension taping technique is designed to limit elbow extension after a hyperextension injury. It is a useful technique in mild injuries and provides mild restriction of elbow extension.

Technique

The arm is usually shaved from the shoulder to the wrist. A pad is placed in the crease of the elbow after petroleum jelly has been applied to the undersurface of the pad (Fig. 20-1). This lubricated pad prevents tape burns around the flexion crease of the elbow. Tape adhesive spray is next applied to the surrounding area to provide better adherence of the tape and underwrap material to the skin.

Underwrap material is placed circumferentially around the elbow, beginning distally at the midforearm and continuing proximally to the midarm (Fig. 20-2). Anchor strips are applied with elastic tape on the proximal and distal portions of the underwrap (Fig. 20-3).

The elbow is held at approximately 30 degrees and crossing strips (x-strips) of standard cloth adhesive tape are applied along the anterior (flexion) portion of the elbow (Fig. 20-4; *A*). These strips, which cross the elbow anteriorly, will limit elbow extension by virtue of their application with the elbow held in flexion. These crossing strips, or check reins, are applied in an alternating fashion until the anterior aspect of the elbow is covered (Fig. 20-4, *B*).

Anchor strips of cloth adhesive tape are now placed on the elbow in a circumferential fashion, at both the midpoint of the arm and midpoint of the foream, to anchor the check reins

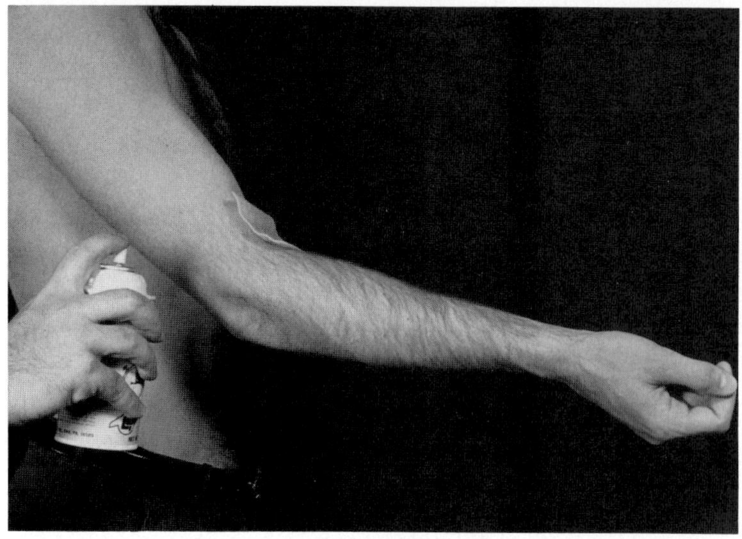

FIG. 20-1. Lubricated pad is placed in elbow flexion crease to prevent tape burns.

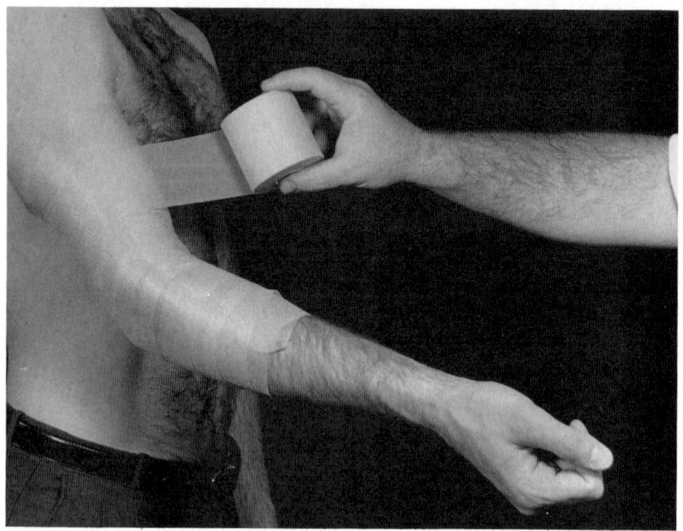

FIG. 20-2. Underwrap applied.

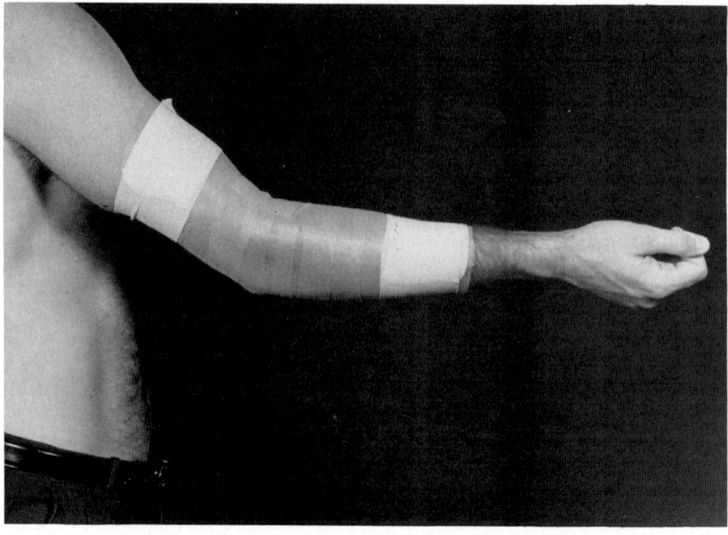

FIG. 20-3. Anchor strips at proximal and distal limits of tape area.

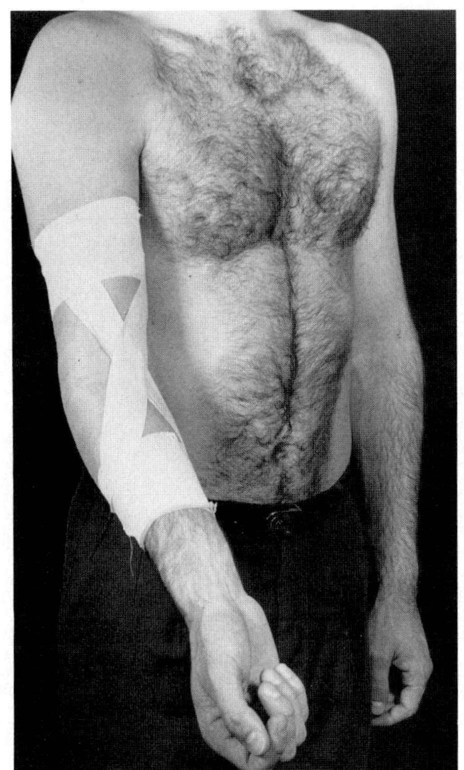

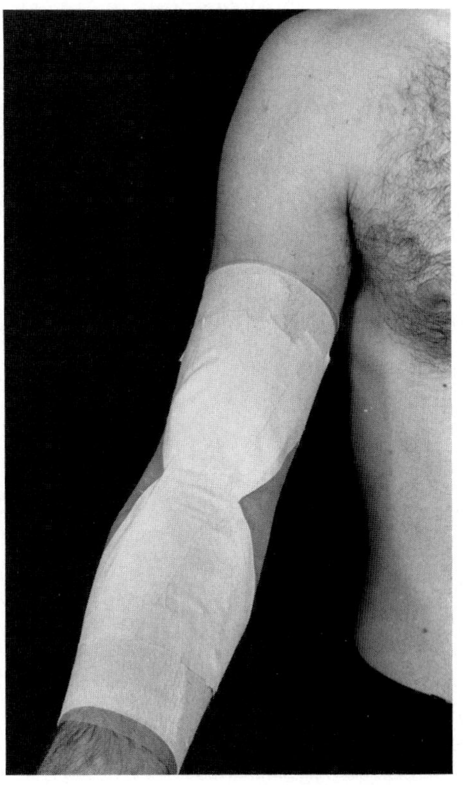

FIG. 20-4. A, Check reins (x-strips) applied anteriorly to limit extension. **B,** Elbow is covered anteriorly with a series of check reins.

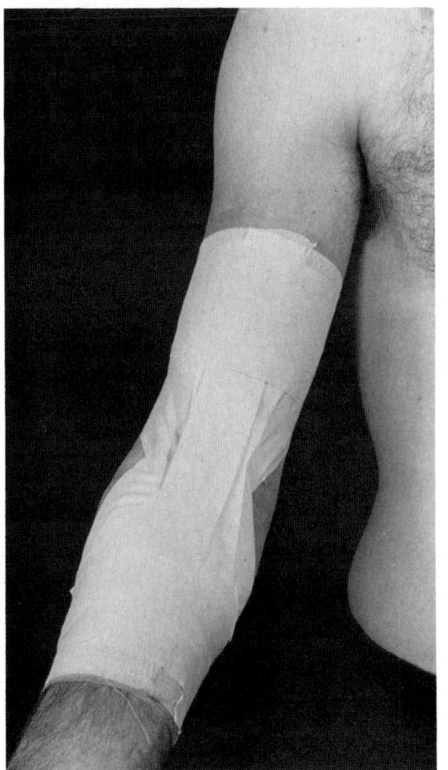

FIG. 20-5. Anchor strips applied at midpoint of arm and forearm to secure check reins.

at the proximal and distal limits of the tape job (Fig. 20-5).

A layer of elastic tape is now used to secure and solidify the entire tape application. The elastic tape is applied circumferentially from distal to proximal as one continuous, overlapping strip of tape (Fig. 20-6). A short piece of cloth tape is placed proximally to affix the elastic tape in place at the proximal portion of the tape job.

This completed taping technique will permit elbow flexion but limit elbow extension as a result of the cloth adhesive tape applied anteriorly on the elbow with the elbow in a flexed position.

Variations

The check rein pattern (cloth adhesive butterfly) can be prepared ahead of time to facilitate the application of the tape job in the locker room (Fig. 20-7). This is accomplished

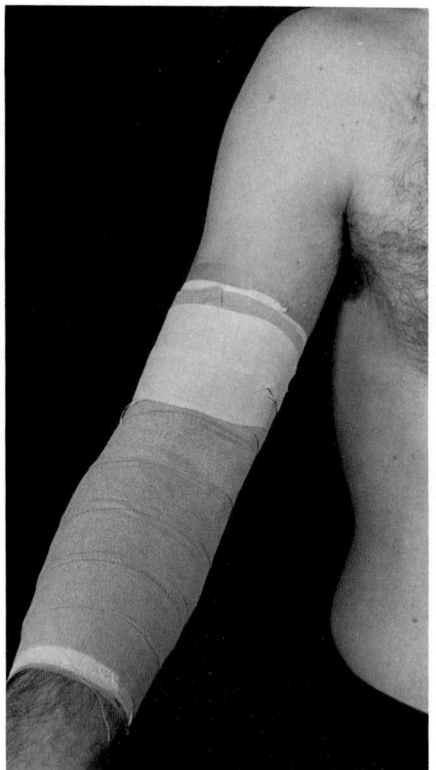

FIG. 20-6. Elastic tape is used to bind entire tape application.

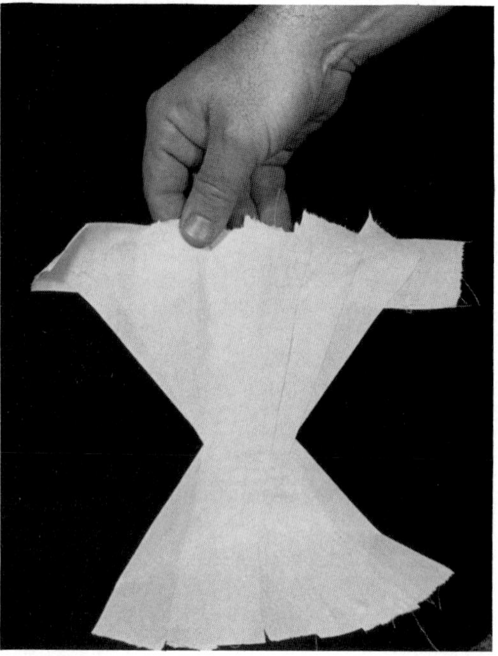

FIG. 20-7. Tape butterfly or x pattern of check reins can be prepared on a smooth, clean surface to facilitate application.

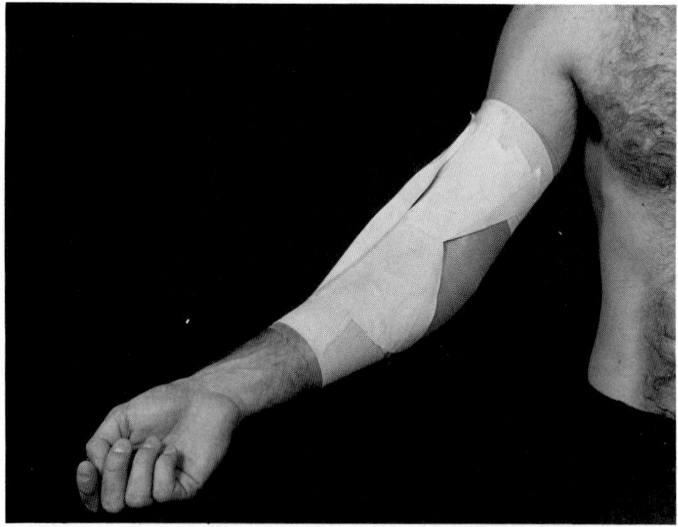

FIG. 20-8. Crimped adhesive tape applied anteriorly for additional strength.

by applying the adhesive tape in the crossing pattern onto a smooth, clean surface that will allow the tape to be carefully lifted off as a single unit after completion of the taping scheme. The entire check rein unit can then be applied directly to the arm and anchored in place as previously described.

Another technique variation includes the use of a crimped piece of cloth adhesive tape to provide additional bulk and strength to the tape technique. This crimped strip is placed longitudinally along the anterior aspect of the elbow (Fig. 20-8) and is secured with anchor strips at the proximal and distal por-

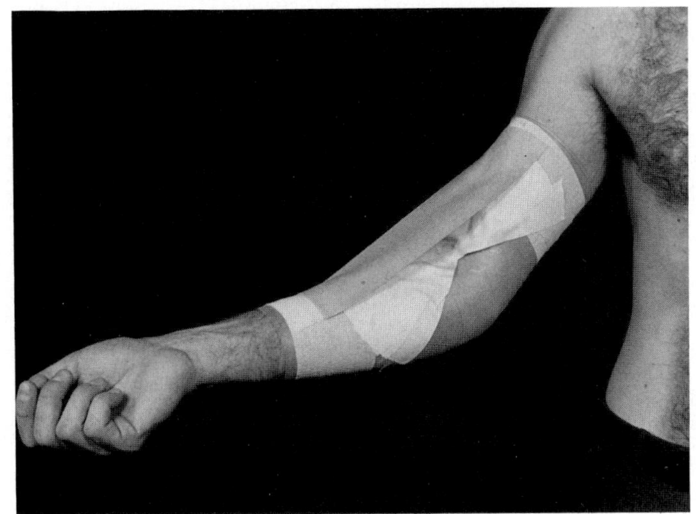

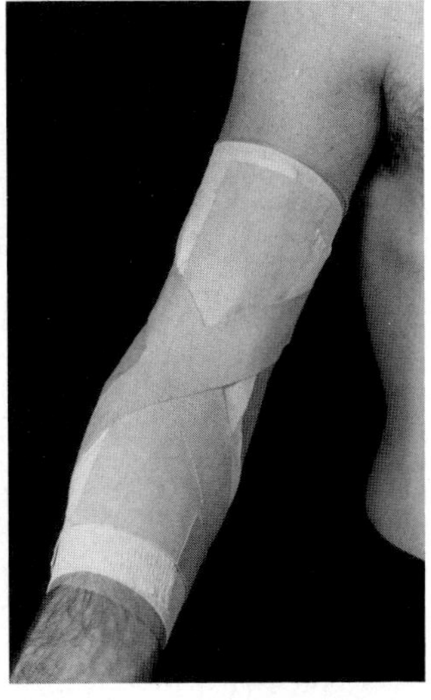

FIG. 20-9. A and **B,** Moleskin applied anteriorly for strength.

tions of the tape. A small space can initially be left between the body of the tape job and the crimped piece of tape. This crimped tape is then incorporated into the entire tape job.

The use of moleskin can also improve the ability of the taping technique to restrict extension. Moleskin can be costly, however, and its use is recommended when budget considerations will permit. The moleskin is applied as an anterior longitudinal check rein across the flexion crease (Fig. 20-9). After application of the moleskin, elastic tape is used circumferentially to hold the moleskin in place. The key to this technique is making certain the moleskin is well-anchored proximally and distally by cloth adhesive tape.

In addition to a direct longitudinal anterior strut, x-shaped check reins can also be fabricated out of 1½ inch moleskin. These are applied in a similar fashion as an x-shaped check rein made from cloth tape, but in a smaller number since the moleskin cannot conform as well as the less bulky elastic tape. The moleskin ends should overlap to have the moleskin adhere to the previous strip and provide integrity to the tape technique. As additional layers of moleskin are added, the flexibility of the elbow is diminished because of the bulk and strength of the moleskin. This will provide the greatest limitation of elbow extension possible with taping and will provide great stability and integrity of the taping technique. Of course, as with the use of moleskin in any fashion, elastic tape is applied to seal the entire tape job.

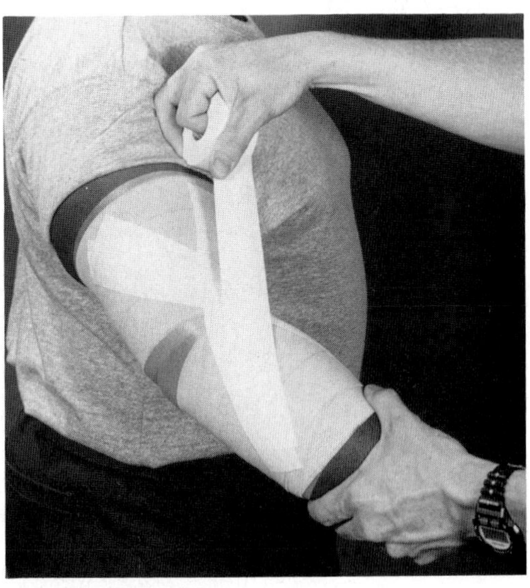

FIG. 20-10. Check reins applied medially or laterally can provide some support to resist varus or valgus stress.

Medial-lateral Elbow Support

Occasionally, elbow taping techniques can enhance treatment of mild valgus elbow injuries. This would be appropriate in situations in which minimal laxity is present, swelling is not readily apparent, and protective support without great bulk is desired.

For this technique, longitudinal strips (check reins) are applied along the medial or lateral aspect of the elbow. This is done after the standard preparation and prewrapping the elbow (Fig. 20-10). If protection against valgus forces is sought, the longitudinal strips are placed medially. If varus protection is the goal, the strips should be applied along the lateral side of the elbow. These strips can provide some support to the elbow when external valgus or varus loads are applied. For situations in which moderate or great forces are anticipated, however, more stability and protection are offered by a hinged orthosis, and the orthosis would be the better choice.

PROTECTIVE EQUIPMENT

Elbow Pads

Elbow pads are some of the most basic and frequently used protective pads in athletic participation (Fig. 20-11). Essentially, the pads provide cushioning for the portions of the elbow that can be injured by direct contact. Most commonly, the olecranon bursa is the site of the contusion and traumatic bursitis, so the bulk of the padding is concentrated posteriorly.

Most elbow pads are a combination of foam rubber and elastic. A variety of foam densities are available, from very light open and closed cell foam rubbers to dense viscoelastic polymers such as Sorbothane. Some pads incorporate donut-shaped foam rings that provide more protection to the region.

Occasionally, a hard shell pad that takes repeated contact over the proximal ulna and olecranon process is needed for an athlete. These can be custom fabricated with thermomoldable plastic, such as Orthoplast, and built with appropriate padding and relief areas (Fig. 20-12). They are fixed in place with circumferential elastic and cloth adhesive tape around the forearm. The shells are not taped proximal to the elbow flexion crease, so as to permit elbow motion.

Great care should be taken in selecting prefabricated elbow pads or in fabricating a hard shell for elbow protection. Ill-fitting pads provide little or no protection if they slip up or down the arm. Pads with too much bulk anteriorly limit elbow flexion and restrict the athlete. The choice of pads should ultimately take into consideration the sport, the athlete's size, and the athlete's needs in terms of protective capability.

Elbow Orthoses

Hinged elbow orthoses can be extremely useful in athletics. Most commonly, these

A

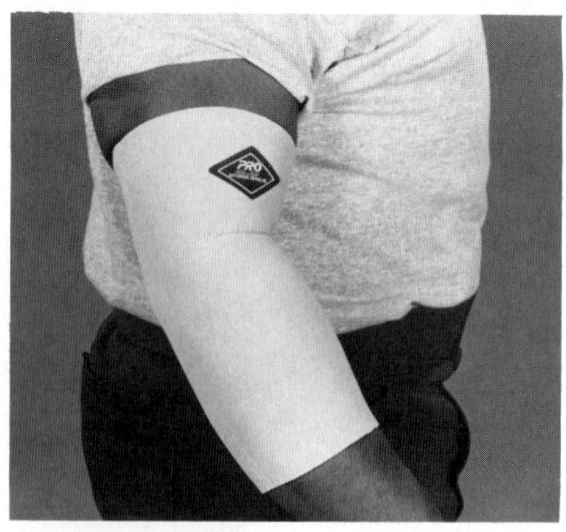

B

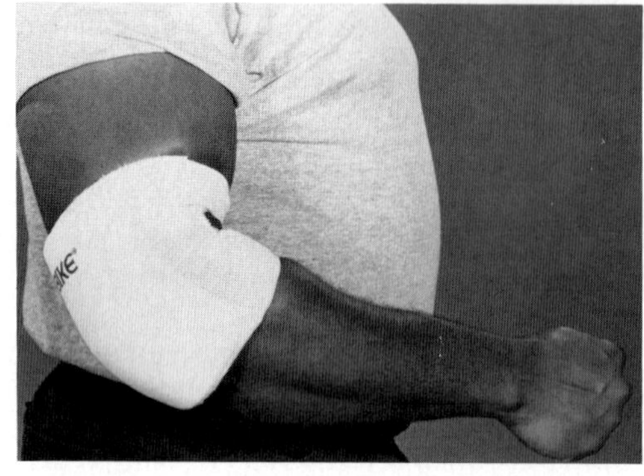

C

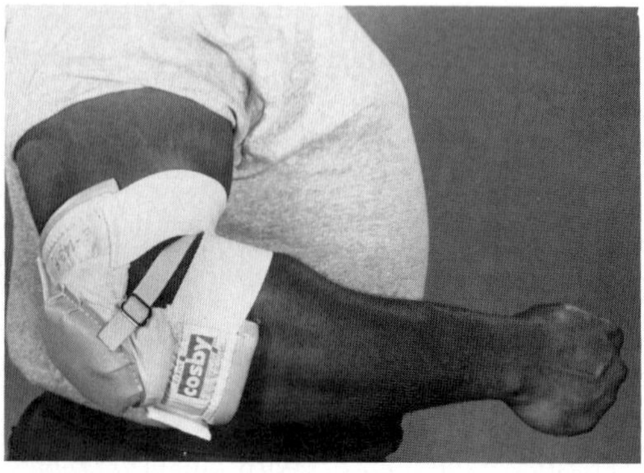

FIG. 20-11. Elbow pads are designed to protect the olecranon bursa and proximal ulna. **A,** Neoprene. **B,** Cloth and foam. **C,** Leather, foam, and cloth.

A 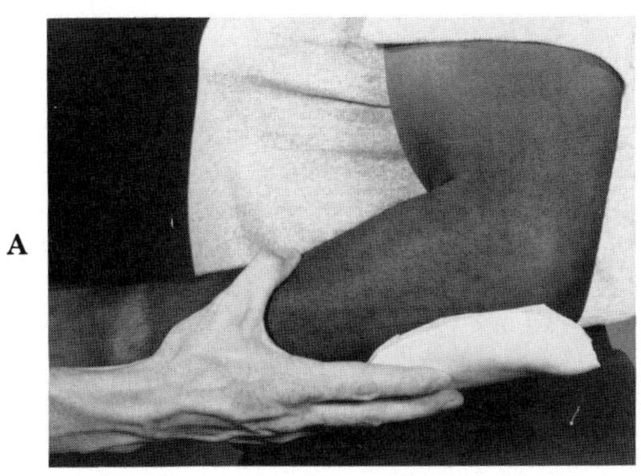 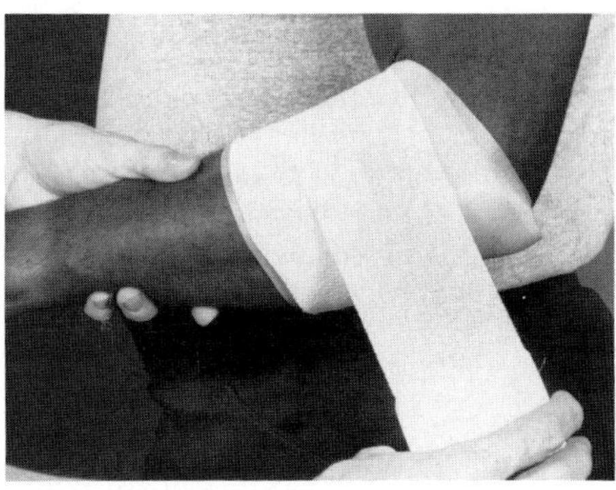 B

FIG. 20-12. A, Hard plastic shell can be fabricated to protect the proximal ulna. **B,** Care must be taken to allow elbow motion.

A 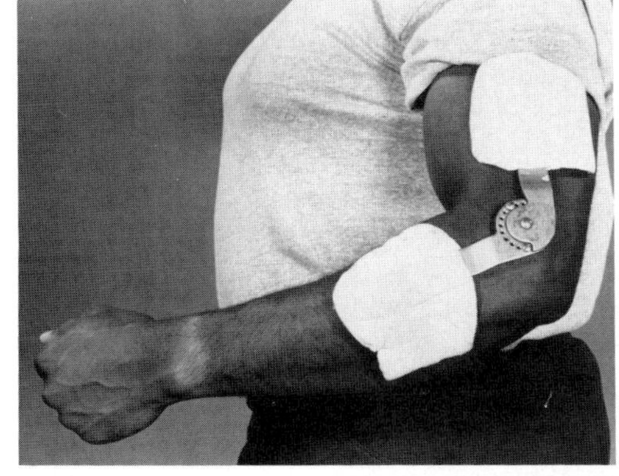 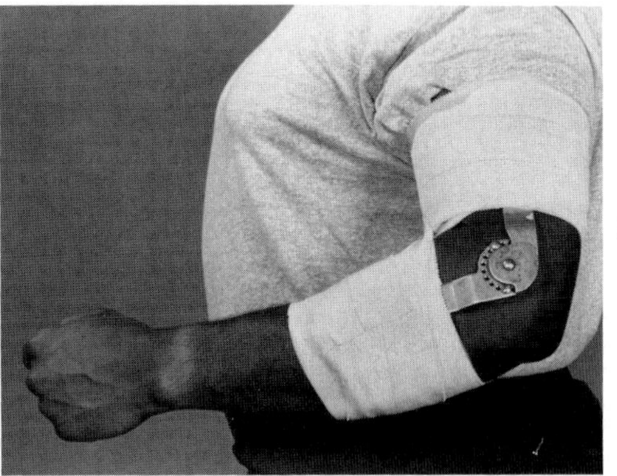 B

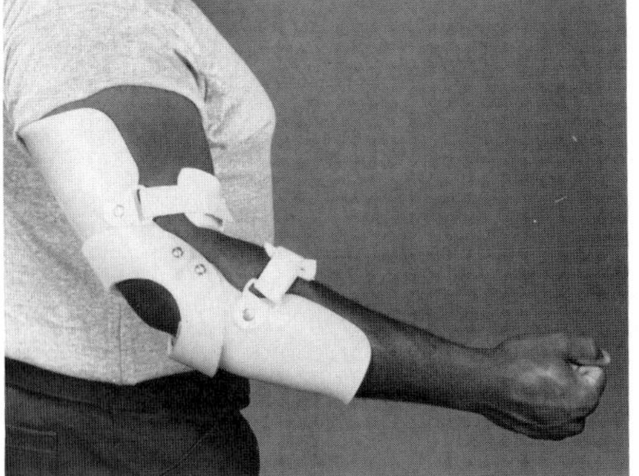 C

FIG. 20-13. Hinged elbow orthosis. **A,** Lateral hinge. **B,** Taped in place lateral hinge. **C,** Posterior hard shell with elbow hinge.

braces are used following a hyperextension sprain or a posterior elbow dislocation. In this setting, the orthosis can be used to permit flexion and limit elbow extension, protecting the anterior structures (capsule and tendons) from further injury.

Orthoses can be designed with medial and lateral hinges or with either a single medial or a single lateral hinge (Fig. 20-13). Double-hinged orthoses provide the most rigidity and are often used initially following injury. Often the medial hinge is removed to permit the athlete easier use of the arm, while the lateral hinge is left in place. In any case, these metal hinges need to be adequately padded to prevent injury to other athletes.

The hinges often are adjustable and the range of motion desired can be set by the treating individual. Hinged orthoses can be built as a unit, with permanently attached plastic shells for securing the hinge to the extremity. The hinge itself can be applied with underwrap and athletic tape if less bulk is desired.

PART IV Wrist and Hand

CHAPTER 21 Anatomy of the Forearm, Wrist, and Hand

George Bogumill

SKIN AND SUBCUTANEOUS TISSUE

Forearm

The skin of the forearm is thick and hairy on the dorsal radial aspect and fairly thin and hairless on the ulnar flexor aspect. The amount of subcutaneous fat varies greatly among individuals and is held loosely to the deep fascia by the vessels and nerves that penetrate the fascia to extend into the subcutaneous tissue and skin. The subcutaneous fat and overlying skin strip readily from the deep fascial layer. Most of the veins and lymphatics draining the hand travel in this subcutaneous layer, as do the superficial sensory nerves.

Dorsal Hand

The skin of the hand is frequently injured because of its exposed position; it is the most frequent unprotected point of contact of the body with the environment. The skin on the dorsum of the hand is loose and elastic to allow for the increased length needed for simultaneous flexion of wrist and digits. The larger surface area needed during flexion must be considered when placing skin grafts on the dorsum of the hand. The flexible elastic skin over the dorsum of the hand and fingers, particularly over the metacarpophalangeal (MP) joints, tears easily because of its thinness and lack of deep attachments. Between the skin and extensor tendons lies the subcutaneous space, a potential space with sparse fatty subcutaneous tissue that readily fills with lymphatic fluid and accounts for the major dorsal swelling following any trauma, infection, or other insult to the hand or fingers. In this subcutaneous space over the dorsum of the hand lie the dorsal venous arches; draining them are the major veins extending proximally into the forearm.

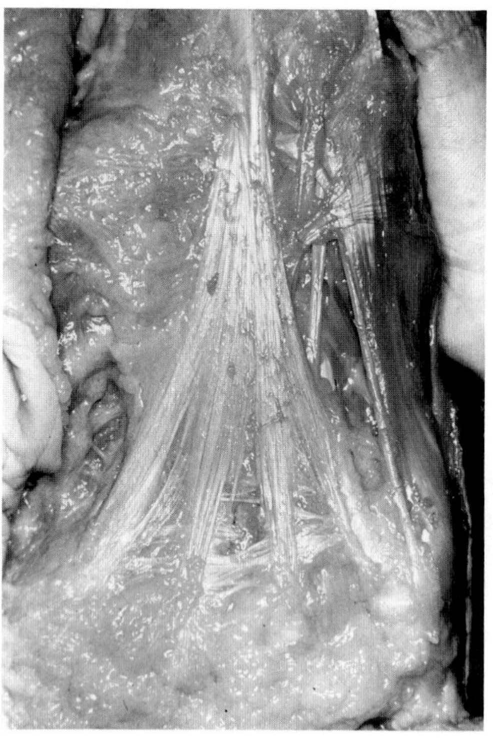

FIG. 21-1. Palmar aponeurosis. Longitudinal fibers begin as a continuation of the palmaris longus and end in the palmar skin over the metacarpophalangeal joint. Transverse fibers are present at the level of the distal palmar crease and the finger webs. The numerous small nubbins remaining on the anterior surface are the cut ends of septa and vessels that anchor and nourish the palmar skin.

Palmar Hand

On the palm of the hand the skin is thick, hairless, and usually callused to varying degree. It has numerous nerve endings and sweat glands. It is held in place during grasp by numerous short vertical fibrous septa extending from the palmar aponeurosis into the deeper layers of the skin (Fig. 21-1). The blood supply to palmar skin is conveyed by numerous short vessels that pass through the palmar aponeurosis with the fibrous septa. Skin loss is common after traumatic shearing or surgical elevation of palmar skin flaps for transposition.

The palmar aponeurosis has longitudinal fibers that run from the wrist crease to the skin of the distal palm with extensions to the side of the proximal phalanges. Eight septa pass from the deep surface to anchor the aponeurosis to the anterior interosseous fascia and form canals for lumbrical muscles, digital vessels, and nerves (see Fig. 21-7).

Digits

The palmar skin of the digits is also thicker and less distensible than the dorsal skin. It is held in place primarily by the retaining ligaments of the digits (Cleland[4] and Grayson[7]) on the midlateral line of the fingers.[11] The pulp of the finger in the distal segment is held in place by numerous septa and blood vessels connecting the skin to the periosteum of the distal phalanx. This effectively provides padding of the end of the finger without slippage of the skin during grasp. The skin of the fingertip has numerous nerve endings of different types, sensitive to pressure, light touch, and pain.

On the dorsum of the terminal segment of the finger is the nail bed and plate. The nail bed is thin, with its deeper layers continuous with the periosteum of the distal phalanx. The nail bed and matrix are readily torn when the phalanx is fractured, resulting in open contaminated fractures with the nail displaced over the eponychium.

BONES AND JOINTS

Forearm

The skeleton of the forearm is composed of radius and ulna, which are attached firmly to each other in a way that allows smooth rotation of the forearm through an arc of 180 degrees. At the proximal end they are attached by the annular and quadrate ligaments, which hold the radial head against the proximal ulna; the combination articulates with the humerus to form the elbow joint. They also articulate at their distal ends to form the distal radioulnar joint separated from the radiocarpal joint by the triangular fibrocartilage complex, (TFCC) (Fig. 21-2, *B*). A major component holding the two bones together in all positions of elbow flexion and forearm rotation is the interosseous membrane, recently demonstrated to have a thick condensation in its central portion that remains taut in all positions of forearm rotation.

There is intense interest at present in the relative lengths of the radius and ulna, particularly as related to Kienböck's disease, and many operations have been devised to adjust their length and relationship to the carpus and to each other. Whether these operations will stand the test of time is uncertain.

Wrist

The wrist is the region that connects the distal forearm to the hand. Its boundaries are somewhat imprecise, depending on the purposes of description. It consists of the distal

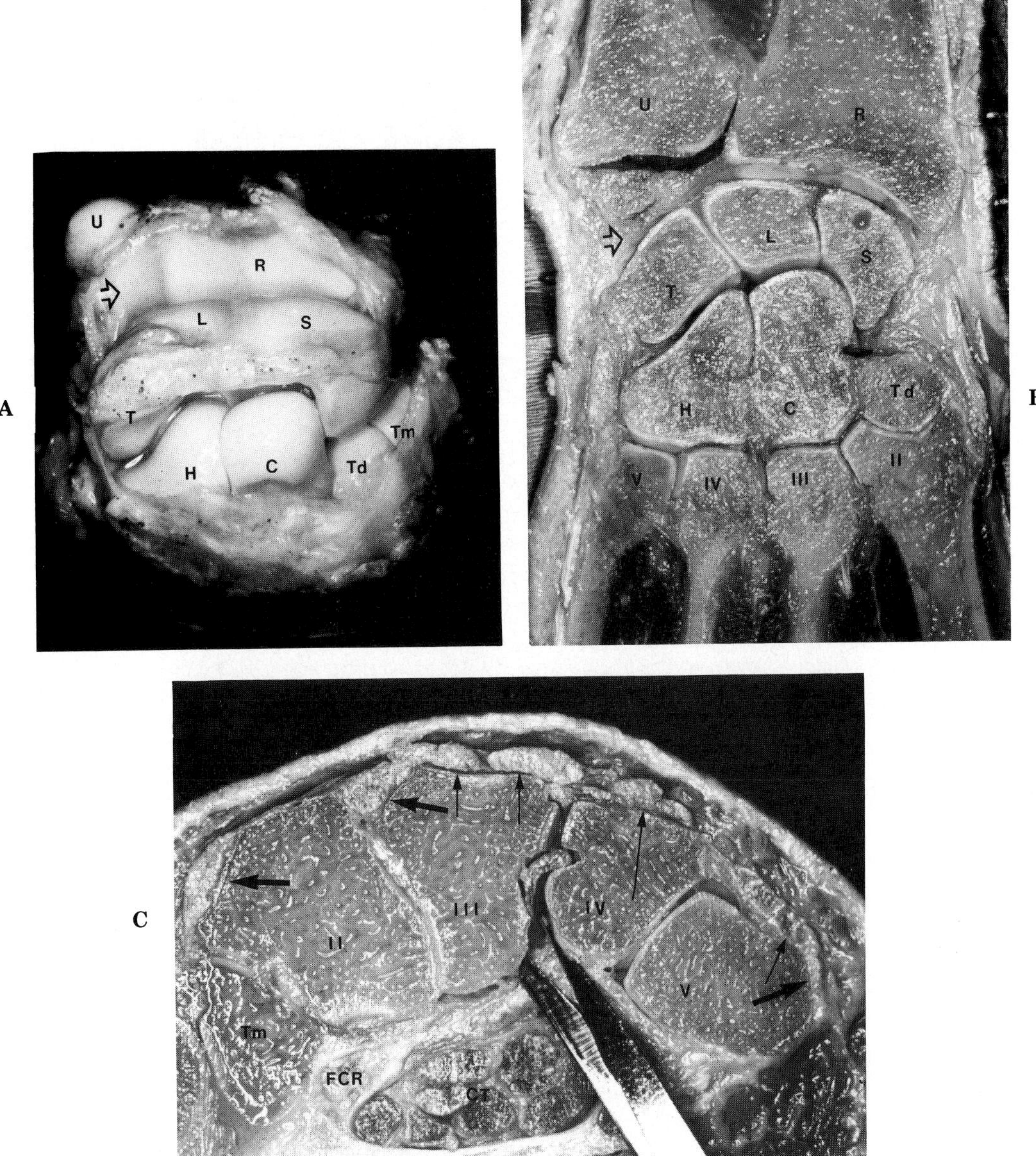

FIG. 21-2. A, Dorsal view of radiocarpal and midcarpal joints. Proximal surfaces of scaphoid, lunate, and triquetrum are joined by intercarpal ligaments that separate radiocarpal and midcarpal joints. **B,** Coronal section through midcarpus. Intercarpal ligaments bind carpals together in proximal and distal rows. Triangular fibrocartilage complex separates distal radioulnar from radiocarpal joint. Note ununited ulnar styloid. **C,** Transverse section through bases of second through fifth metacarpals to illustrate strong interosseous ligaments and proximal palmar arch. *C,* capitate; *CT,* carpal tunnel; *FCR,* flexor carpi radialis; *H,* hamate; *L,* lunate; *R,* radius; *S,* scaphoid; *T,* triquetrum; *Tm,* trapezium; *Td,* trapezoid; *U,* ulna; *heavy arrows,* wrist extensors; *light arrows,* finger extensors; *open arrow,* triangular fibrocartilage complex; *II* to *V,* metacarpals.

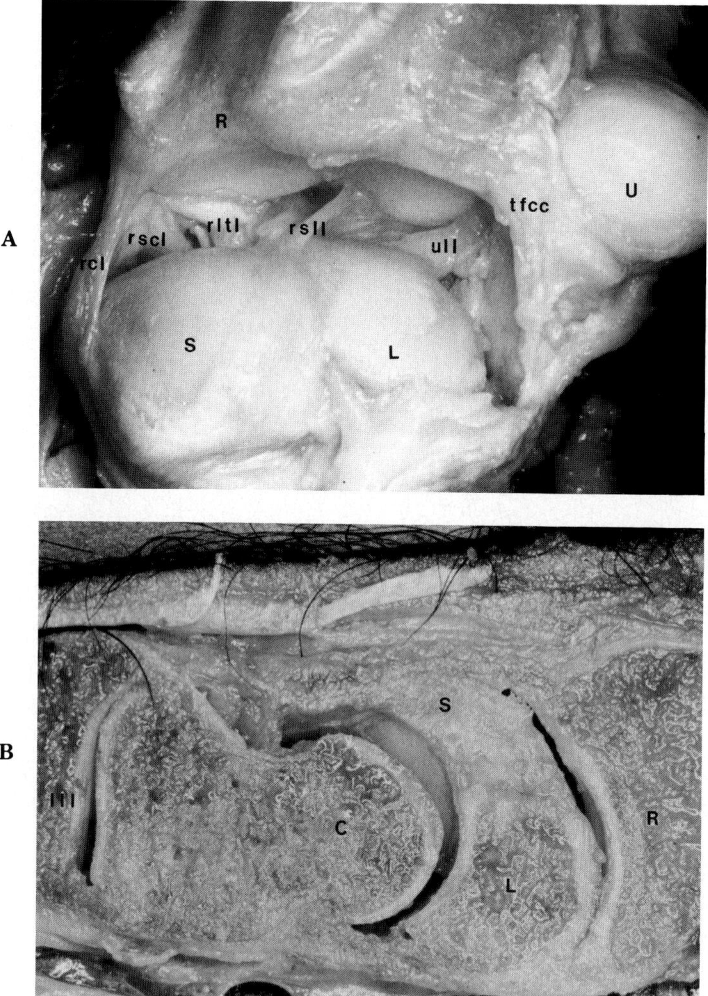

FIG. 21-3. A, Dorsal view of palmar radiocarpal ligaments. **B,** Sagittal section through center of capitate to illustrate thickness and attachments of palmar ligaments. *C,* Capitate; *L,* lunate; *R,* radius; *Rcl,* radial collateral ligament; *Rltl,* radiolunate triquetral ligament; *Rscl,* radioscaphocapitate ligament; *Rsll,* radioscapholunate ligament; *S,* scaphoid; *Tfcc,* triangular fibrocartilage complex; *U,* ulna; *Ull,* ulnolunate ligament.

radius and ulna, the proximal ends of the five metacarpals, and the intercalated carpal bones, eight in number, conventionally described in two rows of four bones each (Fig. 21-2, *A* and *B*). The eight bones also have been described and evaluated kinematically as being arranged in columns[16]; these are less obvious anatomically.

The carpal bones are bound to each other, and to the radius and metacarpals (Fig. 21-2, *B* and *C*), by a complex array of ligaments that are difficult to define (Figs. 21-3 and 21-4). These ligaments show a fair amount of variability from wrist to wrist and are given a variety of names by different authors.[9,14,17] The mobility of the wrist is determined by the shapes of the bones making up this complex, as well as by the attachments and lengths of the various ligaments.[10] This complex osteoligamentous array allows a large range of motion limited at the extremes by a combination of bony shape and ligamentous attachment. With the exception of the pisiform, there are no muscles originating or inserting directly onto the carpal bones. Therefore wrist movements are purely passive, being both permitted and restrained by the complex shape and ligamentous attachments of the various bones; the carpus acts as a freely moving intercalated segment between forearm and hand. The long wrist flexors and extensors cross the carpus to insert into the metacarpal

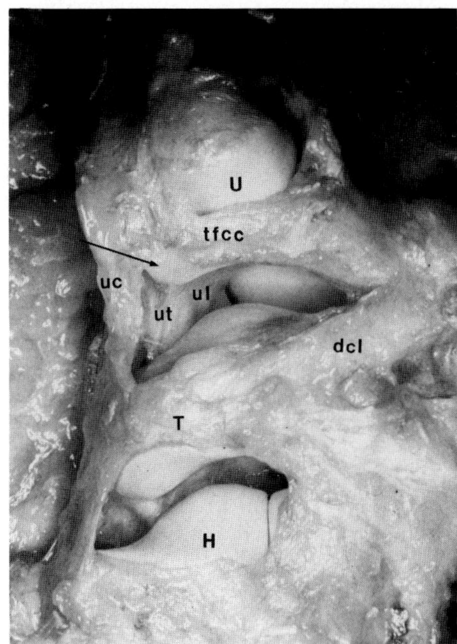

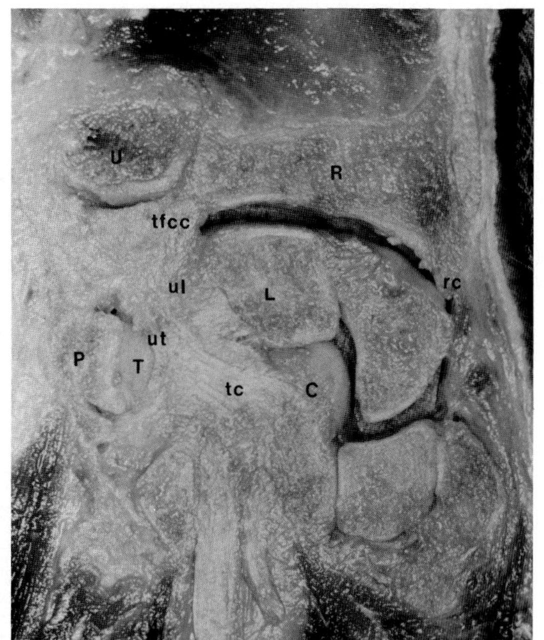

FIG. 21-4. A, Dorsal view of ulnar wrist joints and ligaments. **B,** Palmar aspect of ulnocarpal ligaments. *C,* Capitate; *Dcl,* dorsal radiocarpal ligaments; *H,* hamate; *L,* lunate; *P,* pisiform; *R,* radius; *Rc,* radial collateral ligament; *T,* triquetrum; *Tfcc,* triangular fibrocartilage complex; *Uc,* ulnar collateral ligament; *Ul,* ulnolunate ligament; *Ut,* ulnotriquetral ligament, continues as *tc,* triquetral capitate ligament; *arrow,* ulnar styloid.

bases. Thus the position of the wrist at any given moment depends on a summation of forces applied by muscle pull, external resistance, the osseous configuration, and ligament attachments.[8,17] The axes of flexion/extension and radial/ulnar deviation pass through the head of the capitate.

Large portions of the surface of the involved bones are covered with articular cartilage (Fig. 21-5). The ligamentous attachments are the sites for vascular access to nourish the individual carpal bones. When these ligaments are disrupted, the vessels frequently are also disrupted, with variable effects on the individual bones.

The fibrous capsule, lined by synovium, divides the complex into a series of joints that are separate from each other in the normal wrist but may communicate as the individual ages (e.g., distal radioulnar joint with the radiocarpal joint).[13]

Hand

The metacarpal region of the hand is somewhat longer than the carpal area and comprises most of the length and breadth of palm and dorsum of the hand. The first, fourth, and fifth metacarpals are quite mobile at their basilar attachment, whereas the second and third metacarpals are relatively immobile and constitute the so-called "fixed point of the hand." The shape of the metacarpals and their relationships to the carpus provide for a longitudinal arch as well as two transverse arches, one at the base of the metacarpals, which are firmly anchored to each other by short interosseous ligaments and joint capsules (see Fig. 21-2, C), and one at the metacarpal heads. These arches are primarily adaptive in function and allow the palm of the hand to be placed around objects of varying sizes and to still maintain contact and grasp. When the fingers are flexed individually, their tips are directed toward the tuberosity of the scaphoid, a useful bit of information that allows determination and control of rotation during fracture treatment. This distal transverse arch is flattened when all fingers are flexed simultaneously.

Digits

Metacarpophalangeal Joints

The phalanges are three in each finger and two in the thumb. The base of the proximal phalanx articulates with the metacarpal head to form the metacarpophalangeal joint. Although the head of the metacarpal is rounded and the base of the phalanx concave, the fit

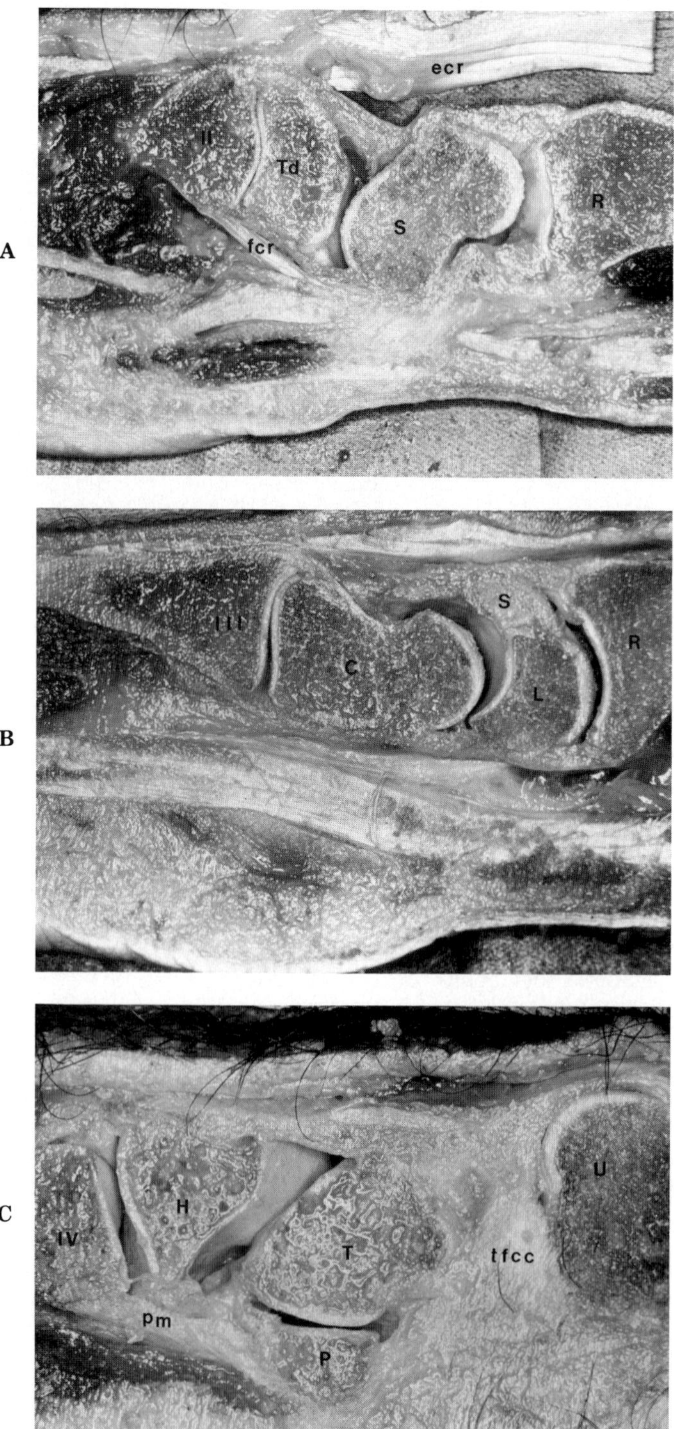

FIG. 21-5. Sagittal sections through radial, central, and ulnar thirds of wrist joint to illustrate carpal relationships and ligaments. **A,** Section through scaphoid. Note insertion of flexor carpi radialis into base of second metacarpal. **B,** Section through capitolunate joint. **C,** Section through triquetrohamate joint. *C,* Capitate; *ECR,* extensor carpi radialis longus and brevis; *FCR,* flexor carpi radialis; *H,* hamate; *L,* lunate; *P,* pisiform; *Pm,* pisometacarpal ligament; *R,* radius; *S,* scaphoid; *Td,* trapezoid; *T,* triquetrum; *Tfcc,* triangular fibrocartilage complex; *U,* ulna; *II, III,* and *IV,* metacarpals.

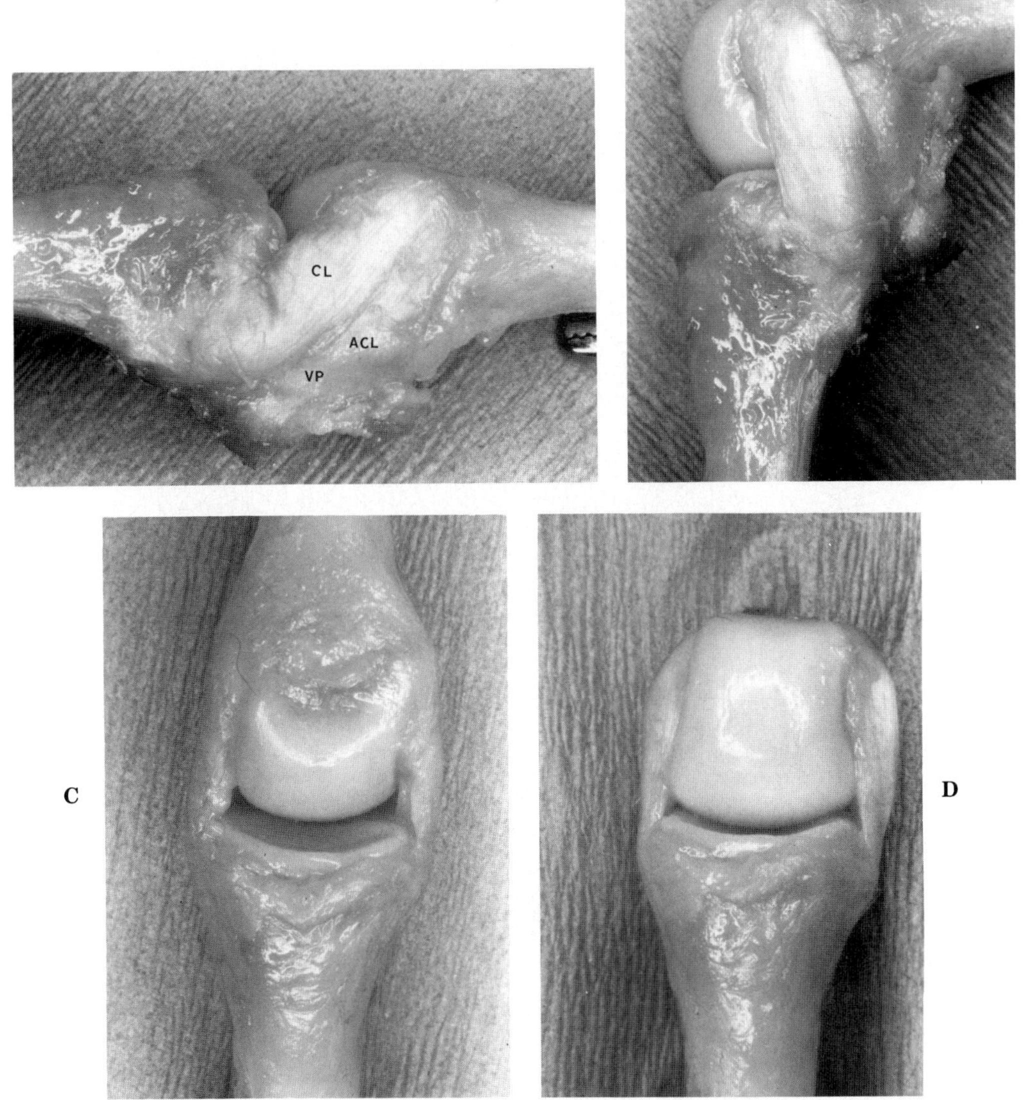

FIG. 21-6. Lateral and dorsal views of collateral ligaments of metacarpophalangeal joint of finger. Cord portion of ligament is lax in extension, allowing separation of joint surfaces (**A** and **C**) but becomes taut as the phalanx glides around the metacarpal head (**B** and **D**). The reverse is true for the accessory collateral ligament. *ACL,* Accessory collateral ligament attached to the volar plate; *CL,* collateral ligament (cord portion); *VP,* volar plate.

is not congruent but quite loose. The integrity of the joint is maintained by the collateral ligaments, volar plate, and joint capsule; motion is allowed in flexion, extension, abduction, adduction, and, to a limited extent, rotation. The proximal attachment of the collateral ligament to the head of the metacarpal is dorsal to the axis of flexion and extension (Fig. 21-6). The collateral ligament is relatively lax when the joint is extended, allowing distraction of the joint surfaces. As the phalanx glides toward the palm around the head of the metacarpal during flexion, the slack in the ligament disappears; when the joint is fully flexed, the ligament is at its maximal tension. Thus positioning the fingers in flexion is very useful to help reduce and control rotation of metacarpal fractures during healing. Fingers should be splinted in metacarpophalangeal joint flexion to prevent shortening of the lig-

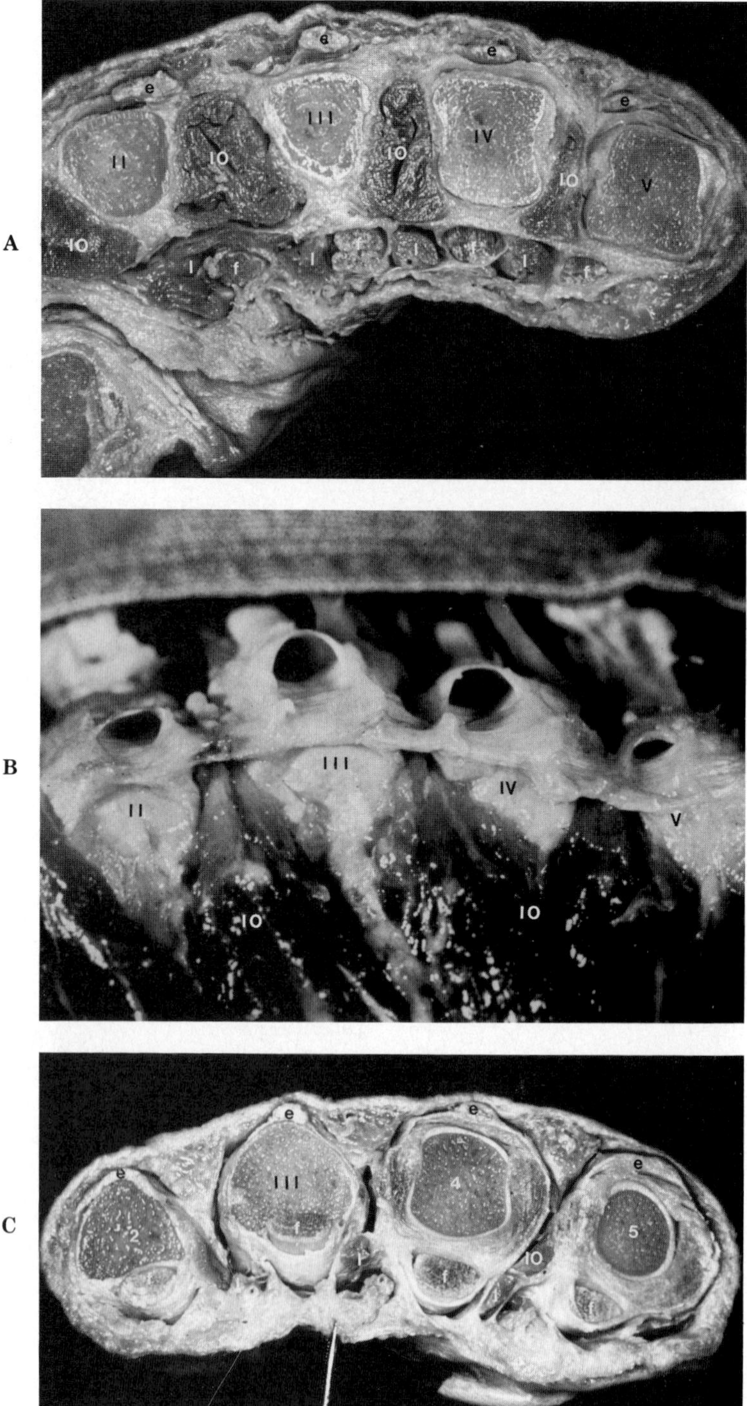

FIG. 21-7. Transverse sections through, **A,** distal palm; **B,** flexor tendon sheaths; and **C,** metacarpophalangeal joints. **A,** Section through distal metacarpal area. Note septa from deep surface of palmar aponeurosis to anterior interosseous membrane, creating compartments for lumbricals and digital nerves and vessels. These septa are commonly involved with Dupuytren's contracture but seldom with trauma. **B,** Dissection to illustrate relationship of volar plate of metacarpophalangeal joints to deep transverse metacarpal ligaments and A-1 pulleys. **C,** Transverse section through metacarpophalangeal joint level. Note extensor hoods, collateral ligaments, volar plate, and flexor pulleys, connected by deep transverse metacarpal ligaments. *e,* Finger extensor tendons; *f,* finger flexor tendons; *IO,* interosseous muscles; *l,* lumbrical muscles; *II* to *V,* metacarpals; *2, 4,* and *5,* proximal phalanges.

aments during the immobilization period with consequent loss of proximal phalangeal flexion.

The portion of the ligament that tightens with flexion is the cord portion attaching from bone to bone. The accessory collateral ligament, or fan portion, extends from the metacarpal heads to the sides of the volar plate and remains tighter in full extension than it does in full flexion. The volar plates attach firmly to the base of the proximal phalanx and, with the cord and fan portions of the collateral ligaments, form a pocket for articulation with the metacarpal head (Fig. 21-6). Also attaching to the sides of the volar plate, connecting the volar plate of one finger with the next, are the deep transverse metacarpal ligaments (Fig. 21-7, *B* and *C*). Joining this juncture are attachments of the A-1 flexor pulley, as well as the insertion of the transverse portion of the extensor hood. Thus at the sides of the volar plate we have an extensive array of fibrous bands, blending and mingling to provide a substantial structure.

Interphalangeal Joints

The proximal and distal interphalangeal joints have a different configuration than the metacarpophalangeal joint. The head of the proximal phalanx is almost circular in the sagittal plane but is broad and straight in the coronal plane. The cord and fan portions of the collateral ligaments remain taut in all positions of the joint and effectively restrict abduction and adduction. In the child they attach to the epiphysis and metaphysis, providing a measure of stability to the growth plate.[2] Extending proximally from the volar plate and the base of the proximal phalanx is a band of fibers that attaches to the shaft of the proximal phalanx at the attachment of the A-2 pulley. This band acts as a checkrein to prevent hyperextension of the proximal interphalangeal joint.[3] Hypertrophy of this band is commonly seen after injury to the proximal interphalangeal joint and results in severe flexion contractures. Passing beneath this fibrous band are transverse vessels from the digital arteries that extend to the distal end of the proximal phalanx and enter into the proximal interphalangeal joint.

Thumb Articulations

The thumb skeleton is considerably different from that of the fingers. The bones are shorter, broader, and heavier. They consist of one metacarpal and two phalanges, rather than three (Fig. 21-8). The **trapezial metacarpal joint** at the base of the thumb is reciprocally biconcavoconvex (saddle shaped), which allows for motion in flexion, extension, abduction, adduction, and also some rotation because the ligaments and fit of the joint are relatively loose. There is a significant volar/ulnar ligament that holds the base of the metacarpal to the base of the second metacarpal and trapezoid. It is this ligament that holds the smaller fracture fragment of an intraarticular Bennett's fracture in place. The orientation of the thumb is approximately 90 degrees pronated from the orientation of the rest of the digits; this can be increased to nearly 180 degrees so that the pulp of the thumb opposes the pulp of the index and middle fingers. The tip of the thumb can be brought to the tip, or even to the base, of each of the fingers by the ability of the thumb metacarpal to be rotated at its base.

The **thumb metacarpophalangeal joint** is an articulation between the rounded head of the metacarpal and the concave surface of the base of the proximal phalanx. This joint, too, is relatively lax but not as lax as the finger metacarpophalangeal joints. It has heavier radial and ulnar collateral ligaments. The volar plate contains two sesamoids at the insertions of the adductor pollicis, flexor pollicis brevis, and abductor pollicis brevis. Displacement of a sesamoid seen on a roentgenogram indicates serious disruption of the joint ligaments.

The **interphalangeal joint** of the thumb articulates with the rounded head of the proximal phalanx in such a manner that flexion provides for increasing pronation of the distal phalanx as flexion increases. The movement at this joint is primarily hinge because of the relatively broad shape of the joint surfaces in the coronal plane compared to the circular shape in the sagittal plane. There is often enough laxity of this joint to allow a variable amount of hyperextension from individual to individual. It usually flexes almost 90 degrees and can hyperextend from 15 to 90 degrees and still be entirely within a normal range. The metacarpophalangeal joint conversely has a variable amount of flexion from individual to individual; some persons have almost none, and others have a range from hyperextension to 90 degrees of flexion.

FLEXOR MUSCLE SYSTEM

Forearm

The flexor/pronator muscle group takes its origin from a common tendon attached to the medial epicondyle of the humerus, as well as from the numerous intermuscular septa between the various muscle groups. The muscle bellies are proximally located in the forearm with the tendons beginning in the substance

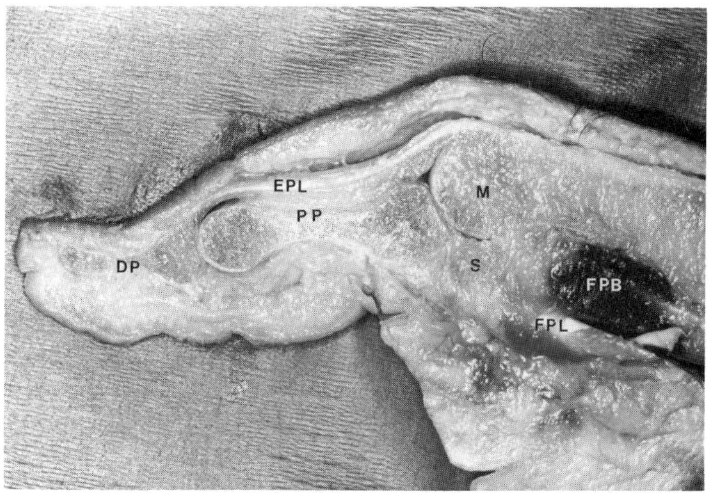

FIG. 21-8. Sagittal section of thumb. Volar plate of metacarpophalangeal joint is thickened by a sesamoid bone at the blended insertions of abductor pollicis brevis with flexor pollicis brevis into the volar plate and proximal phalanx. If the plate is displaced on roentgenogram, it usually indicates major disruption of the joint. *DP*, Distal phalanx; *EPL*, extensor pollicis longus; *FPB*, flexor pollicis brevis; *FPL*, flexor pollicis longus; *M*, metacarpal; *PP*, proximal phalanx; *S*, sesamoid.

of the muscle. In the distal third of the forearm much of the muscle tissue has been replaced by tendon (Fig. 21-9). This configuration is felt to account partly for the difference in success rates of replantations through the proximal versus distal forearm. The muscles are conventionally described in several layers, with the pronator teres, flexor carpi radialis, palmaris longus, and flexor carpi ulnaris being in the superficial layer; the flexor digitorum superficialis comprises an intermediate but still fairly superficial layer. The flexor pollicis longus, flexor digitorum profundus, and pronator quadratus remain deeply placed in the forearm, since they originate from the radius and ulna, respectively. Because of the inelastic nature of the fibrous septa between the muscle groups, any swelling of injured muscle will quickly result in worsening ischemia, most pronounced in the deepest muscles, that is, flexor pollicis longus and flexor digitorum profundus (Fig. 21-10).

Flexor muscle layers

Superficial
- Pronator teres
- Flexor carpi radialis
- Palmaris longus
- Flexor carpi ulnaris

Intermediate
- Flexor digitorum superficialis

Deep
- Flexor pollicis longus
- Flexor digitorum profundus
- Pronator quadratus

The **pronator teres,** the most proximal of this entire group of muscles, crosses obliquely from the medial epicondyle of the humerus to the middle of the shaft of the radius, where it ends in a fairly short broad tendon and inserts onto the radial aspect of the middle of the shaft, just distal to the insertion of the supinator. When using this muscle for transfer, the short tendon can be effectively elongated by raising some of the adjacent periosteum in continuity with the tendon; the muscle can thus reach the back of the forearm in the commonly used transfer to the extensor carpi radialis brevis for wrist extension in radial nerve palsies. It is innervated by the median nerve, which passes between the humeral and ulnar heads of this muscle to enter the proximal forearm.

The **flexor carpi radialis** ends near the middle of the forearm in a tendon that travels with the radial artery to the level of the wrist. Here it passes in a separate synovial-lined tunnel across the carpus, lying in a groove in the trapezium and inserting into the second metacarpal base with a frequent slip to the third.

The **palmaris longus** is present in approximately 85% of forearms. It ends as a long, flat, slender tendon that is inserted into superficial layers of the flexor retinaculum at the wrist. Its fibers continue into the palmar aponeurosis; it is innervated by the median nerve.

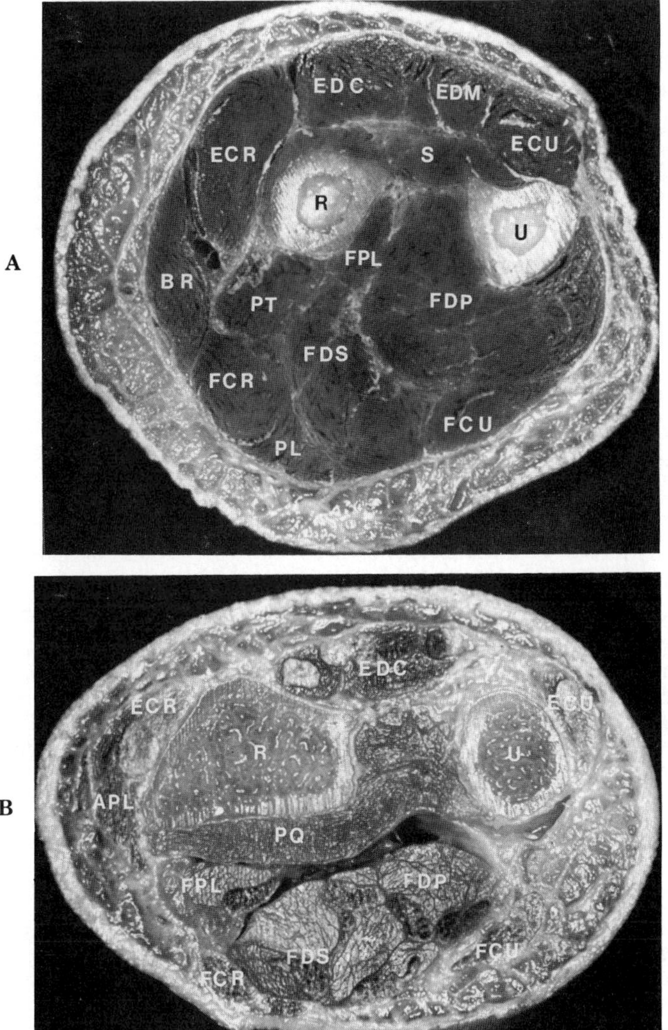

FIG. 21-9. Cross sections through, **A,** proximal and, **B,** distal forearm to illustrate relative size and position of flexor and extensor muscle groups. *APL,* Abductor pollicis longus; *BR,* brachioradialis; *ECR,* extensor carpi radialis brevis and longus; *ECU,* extensor carpi ulnaris; *EDC,* extensor digitorum communis; *EDM,* extensor digiti minimi; *EPL,* extensor pollicis longus; *FCR,* flexor carpi radialis; *FCU,* flexor carpi ulnaris; *FDP,* flexor digitorum profundus; *FDS,* flexor digitorum superficialis; *FPL,* flexor pollicis longus; *PL,* palmaris longus; *PQ,* pronator quadratus; *PT,* pronator teres; *R,* radius; *S,* supinator; *U,* ulna.

The **flexor carpi ulnaris** originates with the common tendon from the medial humeral epicondyle, as well as an extensive origin from the ulnar shaft and medial intermuscular septum. The muscle fibers extend almost to the wrist, a feature that makes it easy to distinguish the tendon from ulnar nerve when both are lacerated in the distal forearm. The flexor carpi ulnaris tendon inserts into the pisiform and from there, via the pisohamate and pisometacarpal ligaments, into the hamate and fifth metacarpal, respectively. The ulnar nerve enters the proximal forearm between the humeral and ulnar heads of origin of this muscle; at this point it is subject to compression by a transversely placed band of fibers connecting the two heads and attaching to the medial humeral epicondyle and olecranon. This band of fibers is lax in extension of the joint, but as the joint flexes the olecranon process moves away from the medial epicondyle and this fibrous band then becomes taut over the nerve.

The pisohamate ligament forms the floor of Guyon's canal, and the roof is formed by a prolongation of fibers from the transverse ret-

A

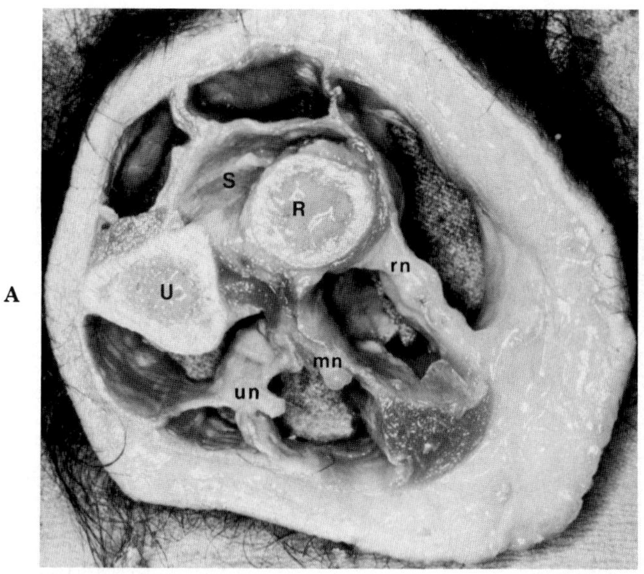

B

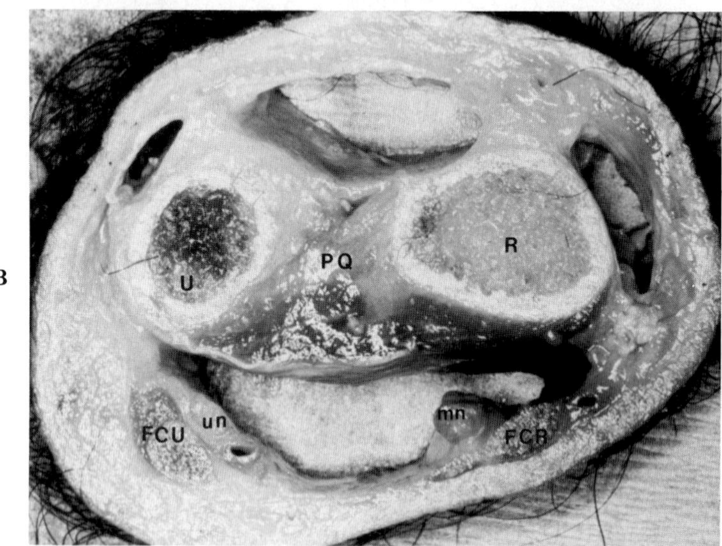

FIG. 21-10. Cross sections through proximal and distal aspects of forearm with most muscle bellies removed, to illustrate the intermuscular septa forming compartments that contain muscles, nerves, and vessels. The septa also serve to increase the surface area for origin of muscle fibers of the flexor and extensor muscle groups. Note vulnerability of nerves to expansion of muscles with increased pressure in compartments. **A,** Proximal forearm. Note median and ulnar nerves. **B,** Distal forearm, with fewer compartments because most muscle bellies have been replaced by tendons. *FCR,* Flexor carpi radialis; *FCU,* flexor carpi ulnaris; *Mn,* median nerve; *PQ,* pronator quadratus; *R,* radius; *Rn,* radial nerve; *S,* supinator; *U,* ulna; *Un,* ulnar nerve.

inaculum ligament. Guyon's canal transmits the ulnar artery, vein, and nerve from forearm to palm.

The **flexor digitorum superficialis, flexor pollicis longus,** and **flexor digitorum profundus** give rise to tendons in the middle of the forearm, which then traverse the carpal tunnel.

Carpal Tunnel

The carpal tunnel is formed on three sides by carpal bones forming a C on transverse section. The C is converted into a D by the flexor retinaculum, which closes the volar aspect (Fig. 21-11). The retinacular ligament is approximately 2.5 cm (1 inch) long from proximal to distal; it attaches to the triquetrum

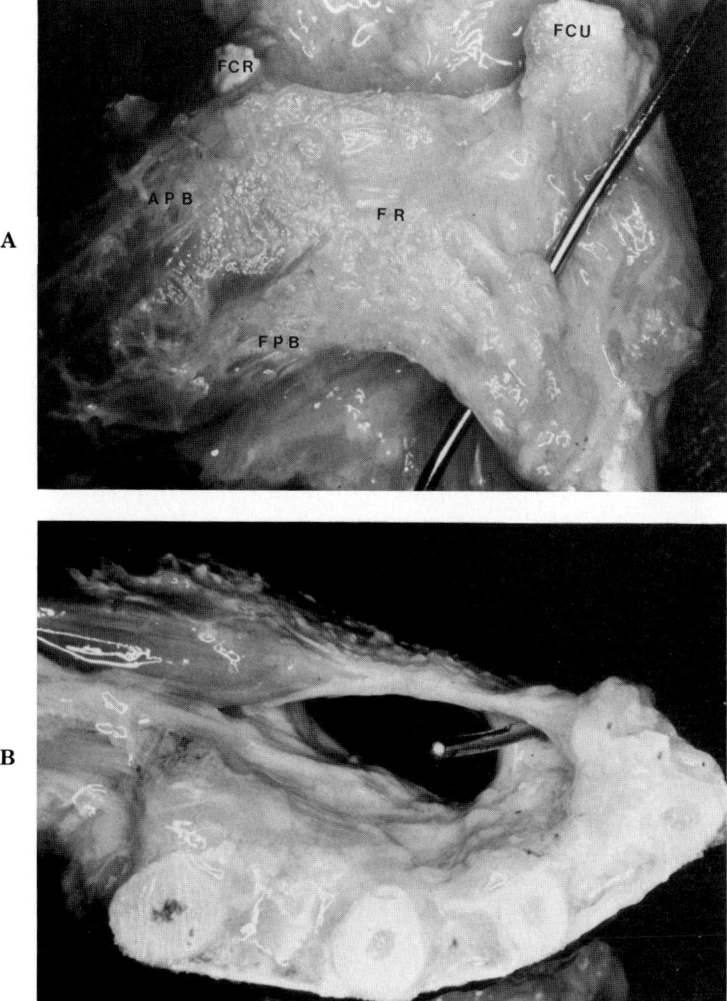

FIG. 21-11. (A), Anterior and, **(B),** transverse views of carpal tunnel. Probe lies in unnamed tunnel for deep branch of ulnar artery and nerve. *APB,* Abductor pollicis brevis; *FCR,* flexor carpi radialis; *FCU,* flexor carpi ulnaris; *FPB,* flexor pollicis brevis; *FR,* flexor retinaculum.

and hook of the hamate on the ulnar side and to the tuberosities of scaphoid and trapezium on the radial side. The carpus and flexor retinaculum thus form a rigid-walled tunnel lined by synovium, through which pass the nine tendons of the flexor digitorum superficialis, flexor digitorum profundus, and flexor pollicis longus muscles and the median nerve.

Palm and Digits

As the tendons of the finger and thumb flexors cross the palm, they lie on the anterior surface of the anterior interosseous membrane, a sheet of fascia that separates them from the interosseous muscles (see Fig. 21-7, *A*). The long thumb flexor and the flexors to the little finger each reside in a continuous digital tenosynovial sheath beginning proximal to the wrist and ending at the base of the terminal phalanx of the digit. The index, middle, and ring fingers have similar tenosynovial sheaths in the fingers, but the sheaths do not extend proximal to the level of the distal palm, forming a cul-de-sac just proximal to the A-1 pulley by reflecting from the pulley onto the tendon.

Each finger has a series of pulleys recently redescribed by Doyle[5] and others and designated annulus 1 through 5 and cruciate 1 through 3. Pulleys A-1 to A-3 are located at the level of the metacarpophalangeal joint volar plate (A-1), proximal phalanx (A-2), and volar plate of the proximal interphalangeal joint (A-3). The A-3 pulley is somewhat in-

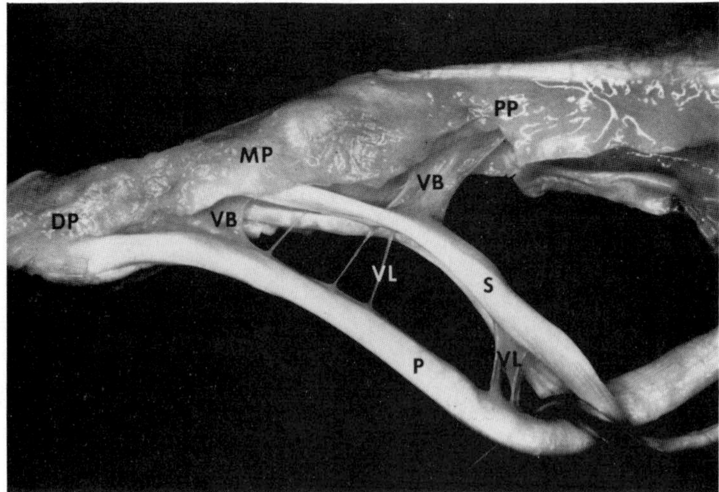

FIG. 21-12. Flexor tendon mechanism in the finger. The flexor digitorum superficialis tendon splits in distal palm to permit passage of flexor digitorum profundus; the two halves rejoin and decussate dorsal to the profundus at proximal interphalangeal joint level. The vincular vessels enter the tendons dorsally. *DP,* Distal phalanx; *MP,* middle phalanx; *P,* flexor digitorum profundus; *PP,* proximal phalanx; *S,* flexor digitorum superficialis; *VB,* vinculum breve; *VL,* vinculum longum. (From Pettrone, F, editor: Symposium of upper extremity injuries in athletes, St Louis, 1986, The CV Mosby Co.)

constant and seldom substantial. The A-4 pulley is attached to the middle phalanx, and the A-5 pulley, when present, is at the level of the volar plate of the distal interphalangeal joint.

Pulley sites in digits

- A-1: metacarpophalangeal joint
- A-2: proximal phalanx
- A-3: proximal interphalangeal joint
- A-4: middle phalanx
- A-5: distal interphalangeal joint

The pulleys are lined on their inner surface by the parietal layer of synovium, which reflects onto the tendon at the profundus insertion and just proximal to the A-1 pulley as a visceral layer of synovium. The space between is filled with synovial fluid to lubricate and nourish the tendons. A mesotenon conveys blood vessels to the tendons; it is discontinuous in the fingers and represented by the vincula longus and brevis of each tendon (Fig. 21-12). Vessels enter the tendons on their dorsal surface and remain in the dorsal half as they extend up and down the length of the tendon.[1,12] In the thumb there are two pulleys: a transverse one at the level of the metacarpophalangeal joint and an oblique one across the volar aspect of the proximal phalanx (Fig. 21-13, *B*).

Pulley sites in thumb

- Transverse: metacarpophalangeal joint
- Oblique: proximal phalanx

As the finger flexor tendons approach the A-1 pulley, the superficialis tendon is anterior to the profundus, but it divides to pass around either side of the profundus to become dorsal. At the distal end of the proximal phalanx, the fibers of each half of the superficialis rejoin and decussate with each other behind the profundus tendon in such a manner that the profundus cannot be compressed and hindered in its gliding by longitudinal pull on the superficialis. Each half of the superficialis tendon spirals around the profundus tendon, decussates dorsal to it at the proximal interphalangeal joint level, and inserts into the middle of the shaft of the middle phalanx, not to its base (Fig. 21-14, *A*). Thus fractures of the base of the middle phalanx are not displaced by muscle pull. The profundus passes through this decussation to reach its attachment to the volar base of the distal phalanx (Fig. 21-14, *B*); fractures of the volar lip of the distal phalanx often are displaced by muscle pull. The decussation is a very important part of the gliding mechanism for the flexor digitorum profundus and should not be re-

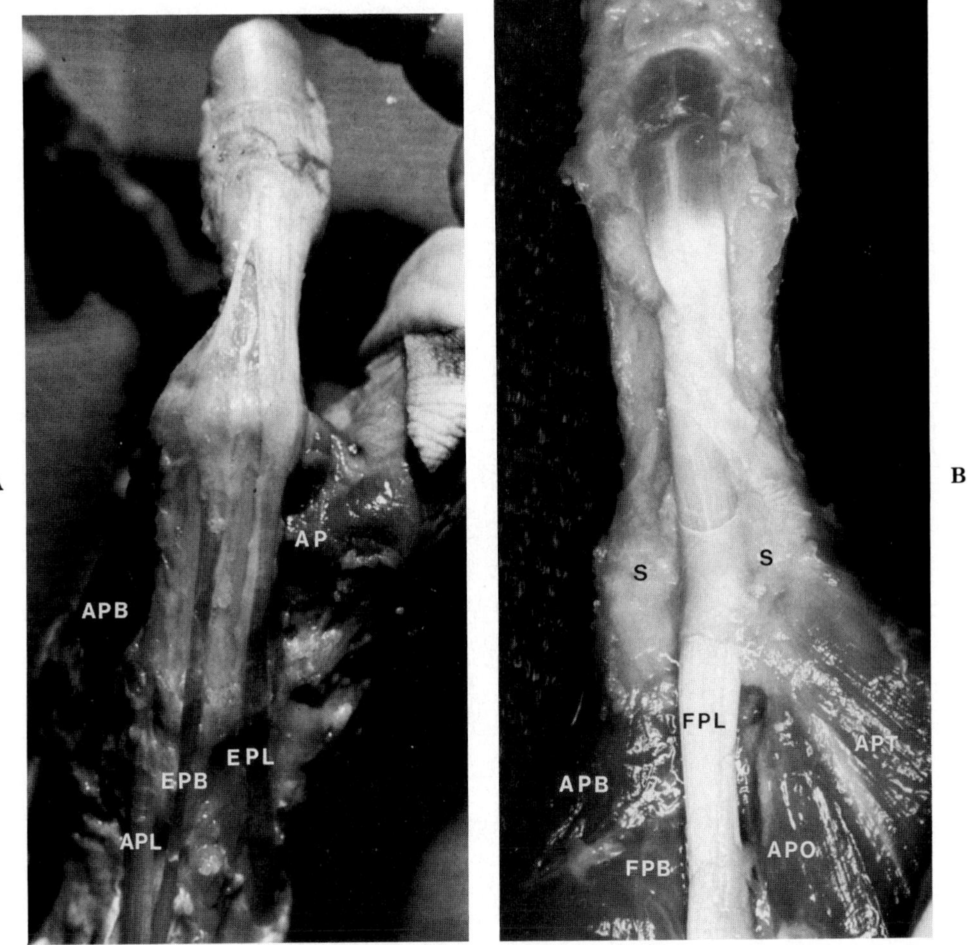

FIG. 21-13. A, Thumb extensors. **B,** Thumb flexors. Abductor pollicis brevis and adductor pollicis are primary flexors of metacarpophalangeal joint but send extensions into the extensor pollicis longus to form a hood over the proximal phalanx and assist extension of the interphalangeal joint. Note oblique flexor pulley over proximal phalanx, which must be avoided when doing trigger thumb release. Sesamoid bones are present in volar plate at conjoined sites of insertions of abductor and adductor with flexor pollicis brevis. *AP,* Adductor pollicis; *APO,* adductor pollicis, oblique head; *APT,* adductor pollicis, transverse head; *APB,* abductor pollicis brevis; *APL,* abductor pollicis longus; *EPB,* extensor pollicis brevis; *EPL,* extensor pollicis longus; *FPB,* flexor pollicis brevis; *FPL,* flexor pollicis longus; *S,* sesamoid bones in volar plate.

moved or damaged during tendon repair. The long thumb flexor passes through transverse and diagonal pulleys[6] and inserts closer to the terminal end of the distal phalanx than do the finger flexors (Fig. 21-14, *C*).

EXTENSOR MUSCLE SYSTEM

Forearm

The extensor/supinator muscles, like the flexors, take their origin as a partially differentiated muscle mass from the distal humerus. The brachioradialis and radial wrist extensors originate as muscular fibers without intervening tendon from the lateral aspect of the distal third of the humerus and lateral epicondyle. The brachioradialis is primarily an elbow flexor and has no direct function on the wrist or hand, although it may assist pronation or supination to the middle position of forearm rotation. The extensor carpi radialis longus and brevis muscles insert by large tendons into the dorsal radial aspects of the bases of the second and third metacarpals, respectively (see Fig. 21-2, *C*). They are active wrist extensors and radial deviators of the hand and contribute significantly to power grip. Wrist and finger motions are synergistic; to obtain maximal wrist extension, one must flex the fingers. Active wrist extension and stabiliza-

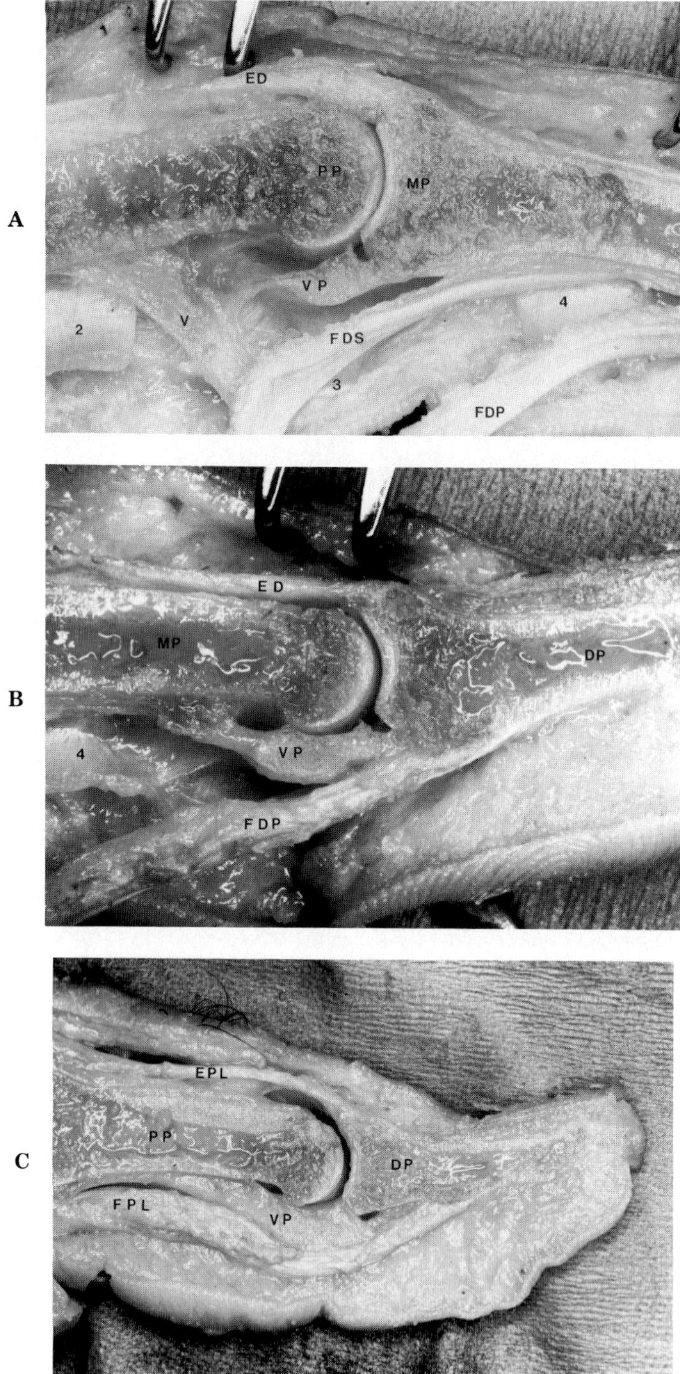

FIG. 21-14. A, Sagittal section through proximal interphalangeal joint of middle finger. Central slip of extensor blends with dorsal capsule and inserts into dorsal lip of middle phalanx. Flexor digitorum superficialis inserts into midshaft of middle phalanx. **B,** Sagittal section through distal interphalangeal joint of middle finger. Extensor and flexor insert into base of distal phalanx. **C,** Sagittal section through interphalangeal joint of thumb. Extensor pollicis longus inserts into dorsal base of distal phalanx, but flexor pollicis longus inserts well distal on shaft of distal phalanx. Note that volar plate contains a sesamoid bone. *2, 3,* and *4,* Annular flexor pulleys; *DP,* distal phalanx; *ED,* extensor digitorum; *EPL,* extensor pollicis longus; *FDP,* flexor digitorum profundus; *FDS,* flexor digitorum superficialis; *FPL,* flexor pollicis longus; *MP,* middle phalanx; *PP,* proximal phalanx; *V,* vinculum; *VP,* volar plate.

tion during power grip allow greater force to be applied by the finger flexors. When the wrist extensors are paralyzed, grip is markedly weakened. The brachioradialis and extensor carpi radialis longus and brevis are innervated by the radial nerve proximal to the elbow joint.

The remainder of the extensor muscles originate in the proximal forearm from a conjoined tendon attaching to the lateral epicondyle and from the radius, ulna, and interosseous membrane. There is also an extensive origin from septa between the individual muscle groups (see Figs. 21-10 and 21-11). Tendons originate from this muscle mass in the middle of the forearm and extend distally toward their insertions. As the tendons cross the wrist, they pass through compartments in the extensor retinaculum complex, which binds them to the dorsal radius and ulna (Fig. 21-15, *B*) and provides for function without bowstringing. At the wrist level the tendons are enclosed in synovial sheaths that extend a short distance proximal and distal to the retinaculum. Over the metacarpals a loose paratenon forms a mesotenon to convey blood supply to the tendons.

Extensor Retinaculum

The extensor retinaculum complex is a thickening of distal forearm fascia by transversely placed fibers that are attached to the radial aspect of the distal radius; they cross the distal radius and carpus dorsally to blend with the ulnar collateral ligament and the fascia of the hypothenar eminence. From the deep surface of the retinaculum pass a number of short strong fibrous bands (Fig. 21-15), attaching the retinaculum firmly to the distal

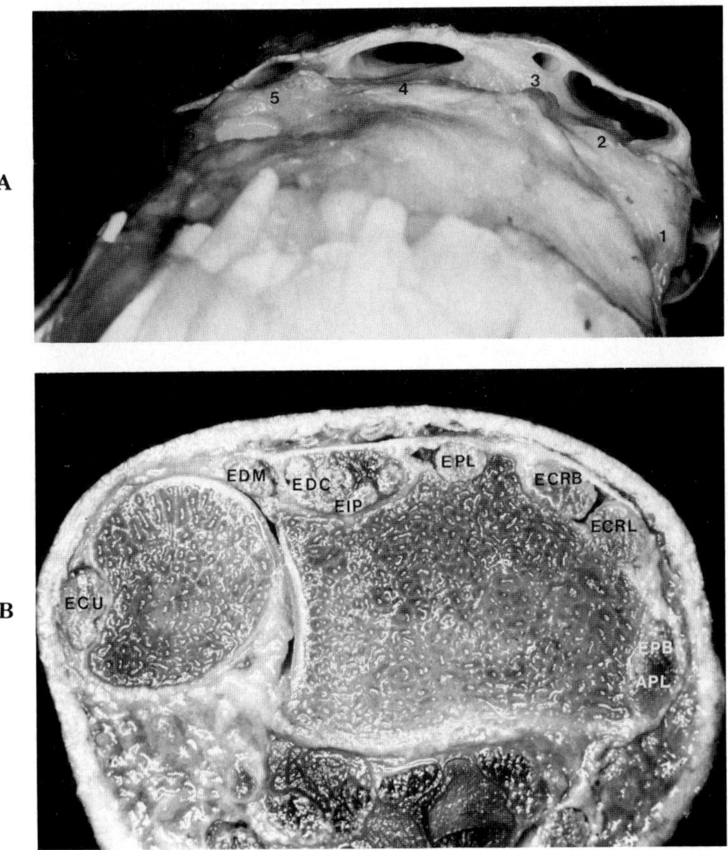

FIG. 21-15. A, Extensor retinaculum to illustrate septa and compartments after tendons have been removed. Note first compartment has a septum dividing it in half. **B,** Cross section through distal radioulnar joint to illustrate extensor compartments with tendons in situ. Compartments 1 through 5 are attached to the distal radius; compartment 6 with the extensor carpi ulnaris is attached to the ulna, and thus extensor carpi ulnaris functions as a wrist adductor when forearm is pronated. *APL,* Abductor pollicis longus; *ECRB,* extensor carpi radialis brevis; *ECRL,* extensor carpi radialis longus; *ECU,* extensor carpi ulnaris; *EDC,* extensor digitorum communis; *EDM,* extensor digiti minimi; *EIP,* extensor indicis proprius; *EPB,* extensor pollicis brevis; *EPL,* extensor pollicis longus.

radius and making a series of synovial-lined compartments or tunnels through which pass the extensor tendons.

The first compartment is the most radial, and through it pass the abductor pollicis longus and extensor pollicis brevis tendons. These may be as few as two in number or as many as six or seven because the abductor pollicus longus may have multiple tendon slips. The compartment may be a single large compartment or, more commonly, incompletely septate. The combination of multiple tendons and partial septations may be the cause of de Quervain's stenosing tenosynovitis.

Through the second compartment pass the two radial wrist extensors, and through the third compartment passes the extensor pollicis longus. The second and third compartments are separated by Lister's tubercle to which the extensor retinaculum is firmly attached, and just distal to which the second and third compartments become one.

Extensor compartments

1: Abductor pollicis longus
   Extensor pollicis brevis
2: Extensor carpi radialis longus
   Extensor carpi radialis brevis
3: Extensor pollicis longus
4: Extensor digitorum communis
   Extensor indicis proprius
5: Extensor digiti minimi
6: Extensor carpi ulnaris

Through the fourth compartment pass the tendons of the extensor digitorum communis superficially and the deeper extensor indicis proprius, which frequently has muscle fibers present almost to the level of the compartment.

The fifth compartment is attached to the distal radius or to the dorsal ligament of the distal radioulnar joint and transmits the double tendons of the extensor digiti minimi.

The sixth compartment is attached solely to the distal ulna where it covers a deep groove containing the extensor carpi ulnaris (Fig. 21-15, *B*). When the forearm is in supination, the tendon is on the dorsal aspect of the forearm. With pronation, as the radius rotates around the distal ulna carrying its attached hand, the extensor carpi ulnaris remains in place since the ulna does not rotate. Thus the tendon remains on the ulnar aspect of the wrist and is no longer a wrist extensor but functions as an adductor to stabilize the wrist when opening the thumb for grasp. The extensor carpi ulnaris inserts into the dorsal aspect of the fifth metacarpal base.

Dorsal Hand

As the extensors to the fingers traverse the dorsal aspect of the metacarpal area, they are bound together by a sheet of intertendinous fascia and also by tendon bundles (juncturae tendinum) that pass from one tendon to an adjacent one (Fig. 21-16, *A*). This combination creates an extensor plane that is bounded on superficial and deep surfaces by potential spaces that contain veins, lymphatics, and superficial nerves (Fig. 21-16, *B* and *C*) and can be easily distended by fluid. The space superficial to the tendons can be obliterated without significant alteration of function, because even though the skin becomes adherent to the tendons, they can glide and carry the adherent skin along. However, if the subaponeurotic space deep to the tendons is obliterated by infection or scar tissue, the tendons become adherent to the immobile bones or the fascia covering the interosseous muscle, and the tendons are no longer able to glide. This is frequently seen following burns or other trauma to the extensor tendons, resulting in an extension contracture of the metacarpophalangeal joints.

Extensor Hood Mechanism

When the extensor tendons reach the distal end of the metacarpal, they enter into the complex array of the extensor hood.[15] Sagittal fibers extend from the sides of each extensor tendon to pass toward the palm alongside the capsule of the joint and the collateral ligament and insert into the sides of the volar plate of the metacarpophalangeal joint (Fig. 21-17, *A* and *C*). Traction on these fibers produces extension of the proximal phalanx of the finger. Distal to the sagittal fibers are transverse and oblique fibers that originate from the interosseous and lumbrical muscles and blend into the sides of the extensor tendon over the proximal phalanx (Fig. 21-17, *A*, *B*, and *D*). These facilitate flexion of the metacarpophalangeal joint by forming a hood over the top of the proximal phalanx. As the extensor tendon complex approaches the proximal interphalangeal joint, the central group of fibers divides into three distinct portions, with the central slip continuing across the proximal interphalangeal joint and inserting into the dorsal base of the middle phalanx. The other two slips diverge to the radial and ulnar aspects of the joint, respectively, where they join fibers from the interosseous and lumbrical muscles to form the lateral bands. Oblique

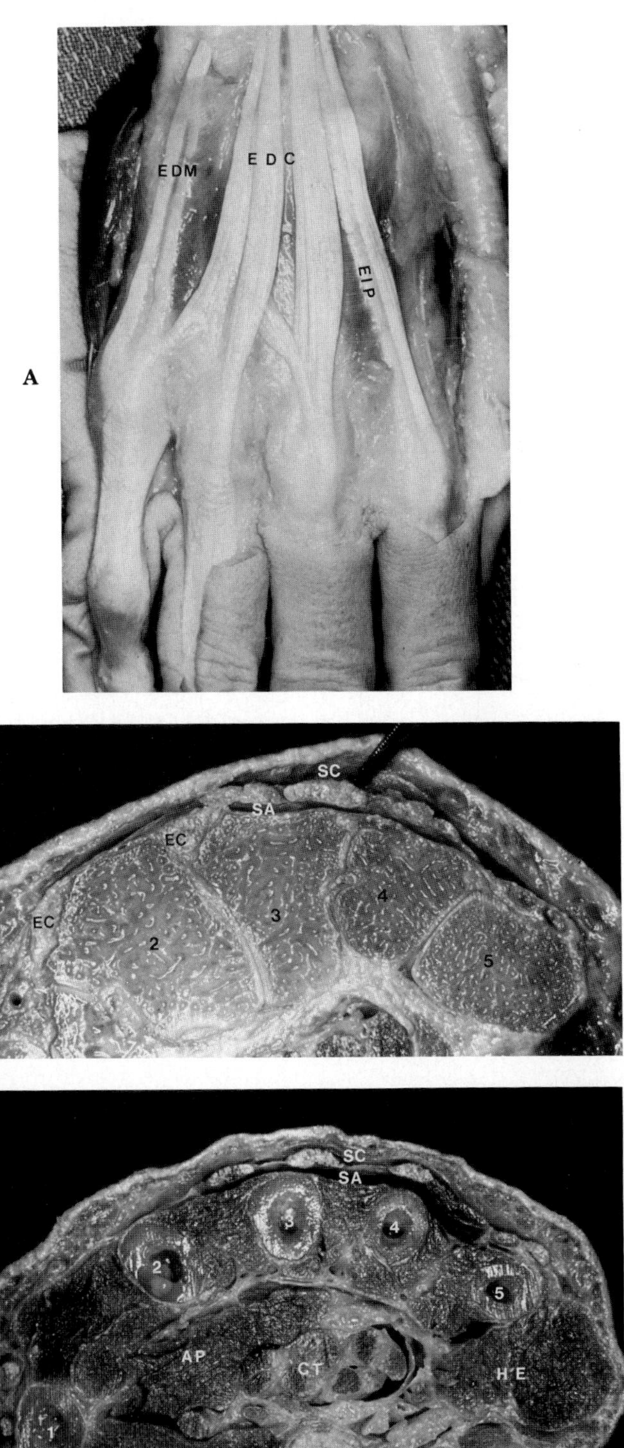

FIG. 21-16. A, Extensor tendon plane across dorsum of hand. Juncturae tendinum and fascia bind tendons into unit. Note that double tendon of extensor digit minimi coming through separate (fifth) compartment of extensor retinaculum is augmented distally by junctura from ring finger extensor. **B,** Cross section through bases of metacarpals to illustrate extensor tendon plane and subcutaneous (with probe) and subaponeurotic spaces. **C,** Cross section through midpalm. Note extensor plane and spaces allowing free gliding. *AP,* Abductor pollicis; *CT,* carpal tunnel; *EC,* extensor carpi radialis longus and brevis; *EDC,* extensor digitorum communis; *EDM,* extensor digiti minimi; *EIP,* extensor indicis proprius; *GC,* Guyon's canal; *HE,* hypothenar eminence; *SA,* subaponeurotic space; *SC,* subcutaneous space; *TE,* thenar eminence; *1* to 5, metacarpals.

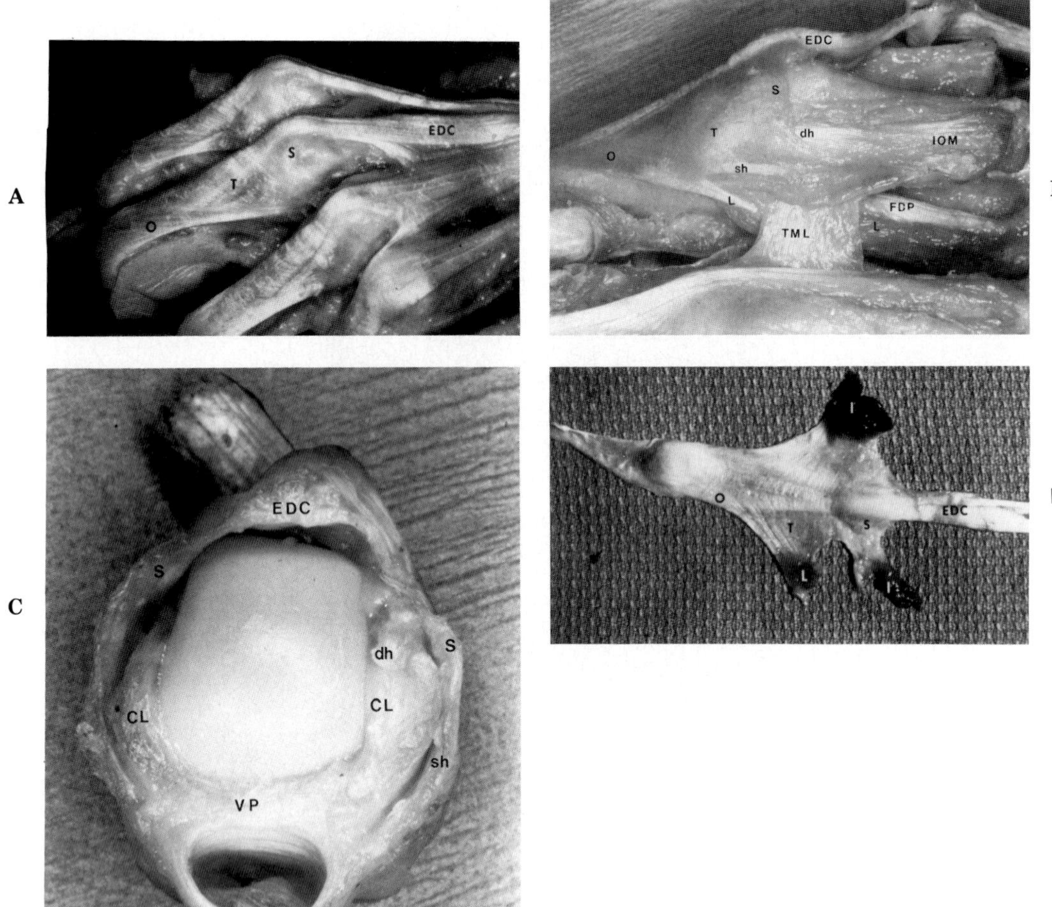

FIG. 21-17. Extensor hood mechanism of the fingers. **A,** Long extensor tendon blends with fibers from interossei and lumbricals to provide flexion and extension at metacarpophalangeal joint, as well as extension at interphalangeal joints. **B,** Radial view of metacarpophalangeal joint of long finger demonstrating deep and superficial portions of second dorsal interosseous muscle relationship to extensor hood. Deep portion inserts into proximal phalanx, and superficial portion blends into extensor hood and lateral band and lumbrical. **C,** End on view of long finger metacarpal head illustrating relationship of extensor hood, collateral ligaments, volar plate, and A-1 pulley. *D,* Dorsal view of an extensor hood illustrates blending of tendon fibers from extrinsic and intrinsic extensors. *A-1,* First annular pulley; *CL,* collateral ligament; *dh,* deep head, second dorsal interosseous muscle; *EDC,* extensor digitorum communis; *FDP,* flexor digitorum profundus; *IOM,* second dorsal interosseous muscle; *L,* lumbrical; *O,* oblique fibers from intrinsic muscle that extend interphalangeal joints; *S,* sagittal fibers from long extensor that extend proximal phalanx; *sh,* superficial head, second dorsal interosseous muscle; *T,* transverse fibers from intrinsic muscle that flex proximal phalanx; *TML,* transverse metacarpal ligament; *VP,* volar plate. (**A** and **D** from Petterone F, editor: Symposium of upper extremity injuries in athletes, St Louis, 1986, The CV Mosby Co.)

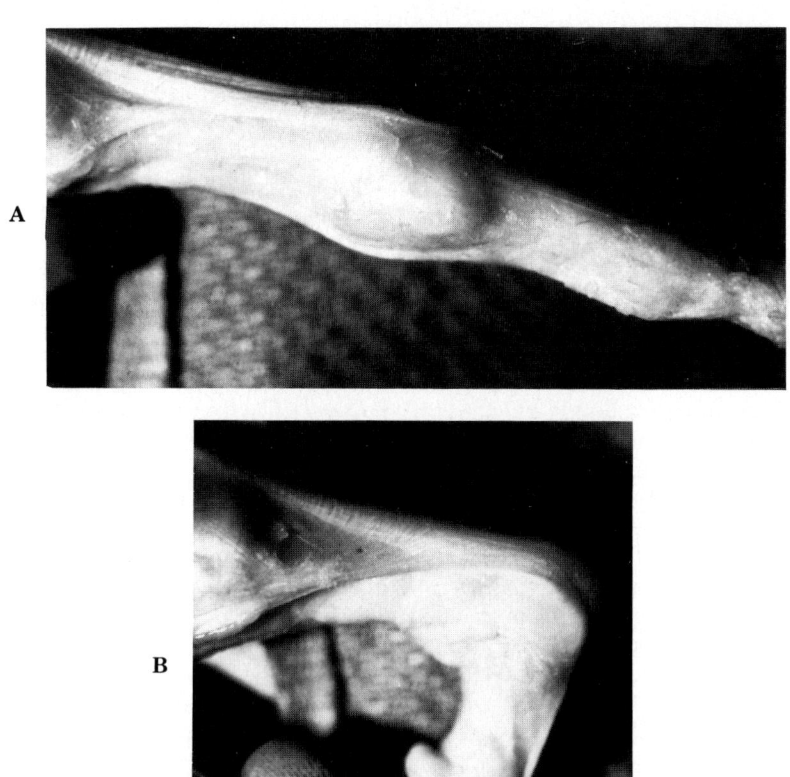

FIG. 21-18. Side view of extensor hood position over proximal interphalangeal joint. **A,** Extension. **B,** Flexion. Lateral bands normally slip volar during flexion; they may be retained there by the transverse retinacular ligament if central slip is ruptured.

fibers from interosseous and lumbrical muscles also separate and blend with the three portions of the central slip to compose a strong insertion into the proximal phalanx and continue as the lateral bands to attach into the dorsal lip of the proximal portion of the distal phalanx. These intersecting fibers do not contain elastic fibers, but by their basket-weave effect they allow for some give-and-take with movement of the different joints. At the proximal interphalangeal joint level the lateral bands lie dorsal to the flexion/extension axis and thus extend the proximal interphalangeal joint. The lateral bands slide toward the palm during flexion to permit simultaneous flexion of proximal and distal interphalangeal joints (Fig. 21-18). When the central slip is ruptured, the lateral bands slide anterior to the flexion/extension axis and are held there by fibers of the transverse retinacular ligament. They can no longer extend the proximal interphalangeal joint; when extension is attempted, the proximal interphalangeal joint flexes more and the distal interphalangeal joint receives all the extensor power producing the boutonnière deformity. With time, adhesions develop and the deformity is no longer passively correctable.

The interosseous muscles are short and bulky with limited excursion but excellent power. They are the primary flexors of the metacarpophalangeal joints and make up approximately 50% of the strength of power grip. On the radial side of the index and middle fingers, most of the first and second dorsal interosseous muscles insert directly into the proximal phalanx (see Fig. 21-16, *B*) and thus function as powerful abductors to resist thumb forces during pinch.

This intricate arrangement of the extensor hood permits the beautiful and complex interplay between extrinsic flexors and extensors and the interosseous and lumbrical muscles to provide the almost infinite variability in positioning the digital joints and segments for function. With the metacarpophalangeal joint flexed, the long extensor becomes the primary extensor of the proximal interphalangeal and distal interphalangeal joints, augmented by tenodesis effect and wrist position. If the metacarpophalangeal joint is extended or hyperextended, the long extensor of the finger no longer has enough excursion remaining to extend the interphalangeal joints. Conversely, if the interosseous muscles have used up their excursion by flexing the metacarpophalangeal joints fully, they no longer have enough remaining excursion to extend the interphalangeal joints fully. Thus there is a balance between the interosseous muscles and the long extensors of each digit that interact to provide the delicate balance available to have any degree of flexion or extension available to any joint of the finger, regardless of the position of more proximal and distal joints. This is the basis for the intrinsic plus or intrinsic minus configurations and contractures that develop when one set of muscles is paralyzed by radial or ulnar palsies.

The three thumb extensors are the abductor pollicis longus, which attaches into the base of the first metacarpal; the extensor pollicis brevis, which blends with the dorsal capsule over the metacarpophalangeal joint and inserts into the base of the proximal phalanx with a frequent contribution continuing to the distal phalanx; and the extensor pollicis longus, which passes the metacarpophalangeal joint on its ulnar aspect and inserts into the base of the distal phalanx (see Figs. 21-13, *A*, and 21-14, *B*). The extensor pollicis longus is augmented over the proximal phalanx by contributions from the abductor pollicis brevis and adductor pollicis to form an extensor hood over the dorsum of the joint, which functions much as the extensor hood of the fingers. The adductor pollicis and abductor pollicis brevis are flexors of the metacarpophalangeal joint of the thumb and extensors of the interphalangeal joint. This is the function that is often seen in opposition of the thumb and in pinch.

NERVES

Superficial Nerves

The forearm and hand are supplied by a number of cutaneous nerves, some of which are continuations of those supplying sensation in the arm and around the elbow while others limit their cutaneous distribution to the hand. The **musculocutaneous nerve** emerges at the lateral border of the biceps and continues into the forearm as the lateral antebrachial cutaneous nerve. It divides into dorsal and volar branches that supply sensation to the radial aspect of the forearm from elbow to wrist, where they blend with the cutaneous supply of the superficial radial nerve. Injuries of either nerve can cause similar symptoms of pain and paresthesias over the base of the thumb.

The **medial antebrachial cutaneous nerve** is a branch from the medial cord of the brachial plexus. It supplies the skin of the medial aspect of the forearm over the flexor muscle mass from elbow to wrist. It is important to realize that it is the medial antebrachial cutaneous nerve that supplies this area of the forearm because so often inexperienced persons assume that this area of the forearm is supplied by the ulnar nerve. Occasionally, one end of the ulnar nerve is sutured to an end of the antebrachial cutaneous nerve, not realizing that there should be two nerves repaired following a laceration above the elbow that results in anesthesia of the ulnar aspect of the forearm and hand.

The **superficial radial nerve** passes down the forearm deep to the brachioradialis muscle and emerges near the wrist on the dorsal aspect of the tendon of that muscle. It winds around the distal radial aspect of the wrist to supply the base of the thenar eminence on the palmar side, as well as the dorsal aspect of the thumb web and a variable area on the dorsum of the index, middle, and occasionally ring finger metacarpals and proximal phalanges. These branches cross the wrist superficially in the area of the anatomic snuffbox and are frequently injured during operations for deQuervain's stenosing tenosynovitis. They are easily visible, and one is usually palpable as it crosses the extensor pollicis longus tendon at the level of the snuffbox. The superficial radial nerve supplies most of the dorsum of the thumb to the eponychial level. On the fingers, the nerve extends approximately to the level of the proximal interphalangeal joint, dorsally. The distal two segments of the fingers are supplied with sensation by dorsal branches of the volar digital nerves, and thus a volar digital block would provide adequate anesthesia to operate on the nail bed or the distal interphalangeal joint.

The remainder of the dorsum of the hand has cutaneous innervation from the **dorsal branch of the ulnar nerve,** which originates several inches proximal to the wrist flexion crease in the volar forearm. The dorsal branch travels with the main ulnar nerve to the level of the ulnar styloid where it crosses the ulnar collateral ligament and extensor carpi ulnaris tendon to attain the back of the hand. Here it supplies the dorsum of the proximal segments of the ring and little fingers with a frequent contribution to the middle finger. It also supplies a variable amount of the skin over the ulnar metacarpals.

Deep Nerves

The deep nerves in the hand and forearm are three, each of which enters the forearm between two heads of one of the forearm muscles and supplies both motor and sensory innervation.

Radial Nerve

The radial nerve enters between the deep and superficial layers of the supinator muscle to reach the back of the forearm. As it exits the supinator it divides into a number of short nerves that pass directly posterior to enter the deep surface of the extensors of the fingers and the extensor carpi ulnaris. The remainder of this nerve continues as the posterior interosseous nerve, which travels on the posterior aspect of the interosseous membrane with the posterior interosseous artery to the level of the wrist, ending in the capsule of the wrist joint or in an extensor digitorum brevis manus if one is present. The posterior interosseous nerve provides motor innervation to the abductor pollicis brevis, extensor pollicis longus, extensor pollicis brevis, and extensor indicis proprius.

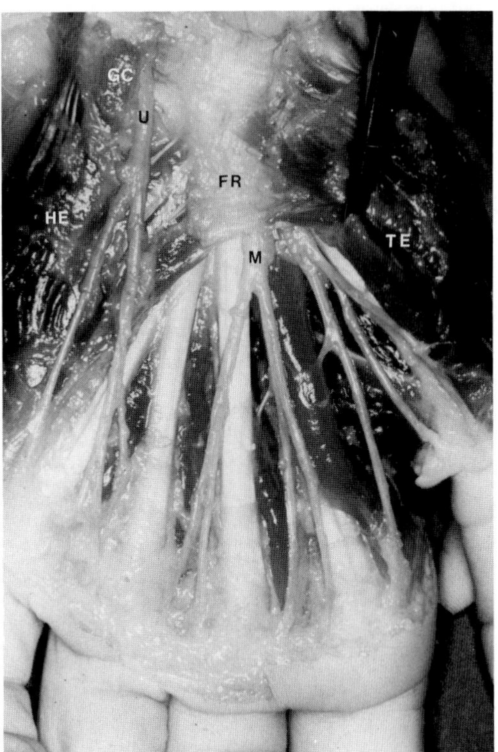

FIG. 21-19. Dissection of median and ulnar nerves in palm. Vessels have been removed. Note motor branches to first and second lumbricals from common digital nerves to index and middle fingers. Median nerve emerges from distal end of flexor retinaculum (carpal tunnel). Ulnar nerve is more superficial in Guyon's canal (opened). *FR*, Flexor retinaculum; *GC*, Guyon's canal; *HE*, hypothenar eminence; *M*, median nerve; *TE*, thenar eminence; *U*, ulnar nerve.

Ulnar Nerve

The ulnar nerve enters the forearm between the humeral and ulnar heads of the flexor carpi ulnaris. At this point, it is subject to compression by a transverse band between these two heads. It continues distally between the flexor carpi ulnaris and the flexor digitorum profundus muscle bellies, supplying both muscles with several branches, one in the proximal forearm and one more distally. It supplies the muscle bellies of the flexor digitorum profundus to ring and little fingers, occasionally to the middle finger, but seldom to the index finger. As the ulnar nerve approaches the wrist, it lies deep to the tendon of the flexor carpi ulnaris adjacent to the ulnar artery and vein. With these vessels, it enters Guyon's canal, where it divides into three major branches, one of which is sensory in the form of common and proper digital nerves to the two sides of the little finger and the ulnar side of the ring finger (Fig. 21-19). It frequently blends with a branch of the median nerve to supply the radial side of the ring finger. A second branch supplies the muscles of the hypothenar eminence, and a third branch winds around the hook of the hamate through a special unnamed canal in the flexor retinaculum (Fig. 21-11) and winds its way across the bases of the proximal metacarpals in company with the deep arterial arch. As it crosses the palm from ulnar to radial, it sends branches to the palmar and dorsal interosseous muscles of each space, to the lumbrical muscles of the same fingers supplied by the ulnar nerve in the forearm (i.e., to the ring and little fingers and possibly the middle finger). It passes between the two heads of the adductor pollicis to end in the first dorsal interosseous muscle.

Median Nerve

The median nerve passes beneath the lacertus fibrosus before it enters the forearm between the humeral and ulnar heads of the pronator teres, where it is subject to compression. It then passes beneath the proximal origin of the flexor digitorum superficialis as it originates from radius and ulna and a loop of intervening fascia; this could also be a site of nerve compression. The anterior interosseous branch arises from the medial aspect of the median nerve near the hiatus in the pronator teres and joins the anterior interosseous artery, to pass distally between the radius and ulna to its termination in the pronator quadratus and wrist joint capsule. Along the way, it sends muscle branches to the flexor pollicis longus and digitorum profundus to the index finger. The remainder of the median nerve passes distally in the forearm attached to the underside of the flexor digitorum superficialis. One must be aware of this fact when the muscle is injured or tendons are being taken for transfer, because the nerve mingles with the tendons in the distal part of the forearm and could be injured. The nerve then passes beneath the flexor retinaculum at the wrist, where it is frequently subject to compression, causing carpal tunnel syndrome. As it exits the carpal tunnel, a branch arises laterally and winds around or through the distal portion of the flexor retinaculum to enter the thenar muscles and supply the abductor pollicis brevis, opponens pollicis, and in most cases, one or both heads of the flexor pollicis brevis. The median nerve then terminates by forming a number of branches that become the common and proper digital nerves to the thumb, index, and middle fingers and one branch to the ring finger (Fig. 21-19). The branch to the radial aspect of the thumb passes directly across the metacarpophalangeal flexion crease in the volar midline of the thumb and can be easily injured in approaches for trigger thumb release. The more ulnar branch lies on the base of the thumb metacarpal. This is the nerve that may be traumated in bowlers and undergoes interstitial fibrosis.

The common digital nerves provide motor branches to index and middle finger lumbrical muscles (Fig. 21-19) before they divide in each web space to form proper digital nerves to each side of each finger. This division is proximal to the division of the common metacarpal arteries, which makes digital transpositions easier.

The proper digital nerves travel beside the flexor tendon sheaths to the same digit. At the level of the metacarpophalangeal joint, each volar digital nerve sends a branch obliquely across the sides of the proximal phalanx to reach the dorsal aspect of the terminal two segments of the digit. Thus the dorsal innervation to middle and distal phalanges of each finger is supplied by the proper digital nerve. This is not true for the thumb, where most of the supply of the dorsal aspect comes from the superficial radial nerve.

The common digital nerves travel with the digital arteries along the side of the finger, just below the midlateral line, where they are held in place by Cleland's and Grayson's ligaments. A midaxial incision would thus place the neurovascular bundle in the volar skin flap. This is a safe incision to use to approach the side of the finger or the flexor sheath except at the proximal portion of the proximal phalanx, where the dorsal branch is heading dorsally across the side of the digit.

VESSELS

Arteries

The **brachial artery** is a direct continuation of the axillary. It enters the forearm by passing beneath the laceratus fibrosus, where it may be compressed with injuries to the distal humerus or elbow. It divides into radial and ulnar arteries after giving off recurrent branches that join in the anastomosis about the elbow.

The **radial artery** crosses superficial to the pronator teres and progresses distally down the forearm on the volar aspect of the distal radius, providing a nutrient artery to the radius and a number of muscle branches. A dorsal branch passes toward the ulna at the level of the carpus and gives off several dorsal metacarpal arteries. As the radial artery turns dorsally to cross the anatomic snuffbox it divides into superficial and deep branches. The superficial branch crosses the thenar eminence to join the terminal end of the superficial branch of the ulnar artery in forming the superficial arterial arch in the palm. The deep branch continues through the anatomic snuffbox deep to the thumb extensors, where it is very vulnerable to injury in approaches to the scaphoid or in procedures on the basal thumb joint. It passes between the two heads of the first dorsal interosseous muscle at the proximal ends of the first and second metacarpals to enter the deep surface of the palm, where it gives proper digital branches to the thumb and the radial aspect of the index finger. It continues between the two heads of the adductor pollicis, travels across the bases of the metacarpals, sending branches into the carpal tunnel to supply the synovium and carpal bones, and joins the deep branch of the ulnar artery to make up the deep arterial arch. Extending distally from this arch are metacarpal branches that communicate with digital arteries from the superficial arch at the web space. This frequently is the route of arterial supply to the fingers when the ulnar artery is occluded, which often occurs in the hypothenar hammer syndrome.

The **common interosseous artery** originates from the ulnar artery soon after it arises as one of the terminal divisions of the brachial artery and travels to the upper end of the interosseous membrane. Here it divides into anterior and posterior interosseous arteries that pass distally on either surface of the interosseous membrane to the level of the wrist joint, where they may again communicate with each other and with other vessels in an anastomosis around the carpus.

The **ulnar artery,** after providing the common interosseous artery, progresses distally between the flexor carpi ulnaris and flexor digitorum profundus muscles in company with the ulnar nerve. At the level of the wrist joint it enters Guyon's canal, where it divides into superficial and deep branches. The superficial branch passes radially beneath the palmar aponeurosis just at the distal end of the carpal tunnel, where it ends by joining the superficial branch of the radial artery near the thenar eminence. Frequently this communication is absent and the ulnar artery takes an oblique course across the palm, ending in the common digital artery to the web space between the index and middle fingers. The superficial branch is subcutaneous for a short distance between its exit from Guyon's canal and the edge of the palmar aponeurosis. At this site it is subject to trauma in using the heel of the hand to strike objects. From the superficial arch arise several common digital arteries that then divide into proper digital arteries to supply each side of the fingers. The tip of the index finger may be supplied solely by a branch from the radial artery or entirely by a branch from the ulnar artery. In this situation, occlusion of the radial or ulnar artery might result in ischemic necrosis of a portion of the tip of the finger. The deep branch of the ulnar artery, given off in Guyon's canal, travels with the deep branch of the ulnar nerve through a canal in the origin of the hypothenar muscles from the hook of the hamate (see Fig. 21-11). It passes across the bases of the metacarpals to join the deep branch of the radial artery to form the deep arch that lies approximately 1 cm proximal to the superficial arch.

Veins

Veins are numerous in the fingers and thumb where they run longitudinally in the subcutaneous fatty tissue. When they approach the web spaces they pass dorsally onto the back of the hand and empty into a dorsal venous arch over the distal portions of the metacarpals. From the radial and ulnar ends of this arch larger collecting veins arise and traverse the radial and ulnar aspects of the forearm to the cubital area, where the more ulnar vein passes deep to join the brachial vein. The more radial vein crosses the cubital fossa as the antecubital vein and continues proximally as the cephalic vein. There is usually a large connection between these two at the level of the proximal forearm.

Lymphatics

Lymphatics tend to follow the veins and drain dorsally onto the back of the hand. There is an extensive network in the subcutaneous space on the back of the hand and forearm. Any insult to the fingers will quickly be reflected in edema of the back of the hand; this has to be carefully evaluated to avoid confusion with an abscess following a purulent tenosynovitis of a finger. There are no lymph nodes in the hand or forearm. There is a first node evident in the epitrochlear region above the medial epicondyle of the humerus, and then the major drainage is into the axillary nodes.

REFERENCES

1. Amadio PS, Jaeger SH, and Hunter JM: Nutritional aspects of tendon healing. In Hunter JM et al, editors: Rehabilitation of the hand, ed 2, St Louis, 1984, The CV Mosby Co.
2. Bogumill GP: A morphologic study of the relationship of collateral ligaments to the growth plate in the digits, J Hand Surg 8:74, 1983.
3. Bowers WH et al: The proximal interphalangeal joint volar plate. I. An anatomical and biomechanical study, J Hand Surg 5:79, 1980.
4. Cleland FRS: On the cutaneous ligaments of the phalanges, J Anat Physiol 12:526, 1878.
5. Doyle JR and Blythe W: The finger flexor tendon sheath and pulleys: anatomy and reconstruction. AAOS symposium on tendon surgery in the hand, St Louis, 1975, The CV Mosby Co.
6. Doyle JR and Blythe WF: Anatomy of the flexor tendon sheath and pulleys of the thumb, J Hand Surg 2:149, 1977.
7. Grayson J: The cutaneous ligaments of the digits, J Anat 75:164, 1940.
8. Mayfield JK: Wrist ligamentous anatomy and pathogenesis of carpal instability, Ortho Clin North Am 15:209, 1984.
9. Mayfield JK, Johnson RP, and Kilcoyne RF: The ligaments of the human wrist and their functional significance, Anat Rec 186:417, 1976.
10. Mayfield JK, Johnson RP, and Kilcoyne RF: Carpal dislocation: pathomechanics and progressive perilunar instability, J Hand Surg 5:226, 1980.
11. Milford L: Retaining ligaments of the digits of the hand, Philadelphia, 1968, WB Saunders Co.
12. Ochiai N et al: Vascular anatomy of flexor tendons. I. Vincular system and blood supply of the pro-

fundus tendon in the digital sheath, J Hand Surg 4:321, 1979.
13. Palmer AK: The distal radioulnar joint: anatomy, biomechanics and triangular fibrocartilage complex abnormalities, Hand Clin 3(1):31, 1987.
14. Palmer AK and Werner FW: The triangular fibrocartilage complex of the wrist: anatomy and function, J Hand Surg 6:153, 1981.
15. Smith RJ: Intrinsic muscles of the fingers: function, dysfunction, and surgical reconstruction. In AAOS instructional course lectures, vol XXIV, St Louis, 1975, The CV Mosby Co.
16. Taleisnik J: The ligaments of the wrist, J Hand Surg 1:110, 1976.
17. Taleisnik J: Wrist: anatomy, function and injury. In AAOS instructional course lectures, vol XXVII, St Louis, 1978, The CV Mosby Co.

SUGGESTED READINGS

Bogumill GP: Functional anatomy of the forearm and hand. In Pettrone FA, editor: AAOS symposium on upper extremity injuries in athletes, St Louis, 1986, The CV Mosby Co.

Bogumill GP: Anatomy of the wrist. In Lichtman DL, editor: The wrist and its disorders. Philadelphia, 1988, WB Saunders Co.

Kanavel AB: Infections of the hand: a guide to the surgical treatment of acute and chronic suppurative processes in the fingers, hand and forearm, ed 7, Philadelphia, 1939, Lea & Febiger.

Laudsmeer JMF: Atlas of anatomy of the hand, Edinburgh, 1976, Churchill Livingstone Ltd.

Spinner M, editor: Kaplan's functional and surgical anatomy of the hand, ed 3, Philadelphia, 1984, JB Lippincott Co.

Taleisnick J: The wrist, New York, 1985, Churchill Livingstone, Ltd.

Tubiana R, editor: The hand, vol I, Philadelphia, 1981, WB Saunders Co.

CHAPTER 22 Diagnostic and Surgical Arthroscopy of the Wrist

Terry L. Whipple

LOADING PATTERNS OF THE WRIST IN SPORTS

The wrist is a complex joint capable of motion in three planes. It provides the foundation for force transfer from the hand and postures the hand for fine motor activity and power grip.

In sports, the wrist may sustain injury through any of four principle mechanisms: throwing, weight bearing, twisting, and impact.[4]

Throwing

In all throwing activities, the wrist moves from a position of extension and radial deviation toward flexion and ulnar deviation—a motion also common to racquet sports, golf, and batting. The weight of a ball, club, or the hand itself applies traction to the wrist while in the motion of throwing or swinging. Most of this traction is applied through the abductor pollicis longus, extensor pollicis brevis, and the radial wrist extensors, while a counterforce is applied through the flexor carpi ulnaris. If a supinating motion is involved, as in throwing a curve ball or undercutting a tennis forehand, the extensor carpi ulnaris stretches through its retinaculum over the distal ulna. Overuse syndromes therefore usually relate to these specific muscle tendon units or to the ligaments that support the pisiform.[3,17,31,37,38] Excessive throwing or swinging of racquets, bats, or clubs may cause extensor carpi ulnaris tendonitis, de Quervain's stenosing tenosynovitis, or occasionally, sprains of the pisitriquetral ligament or stress fractures of the pisiform. Intraarticular injuries of the wrist are not commonly associated with throwing or swinging motions.[1,2,9,26,30]

Weight Bearing

In sports such as gymnastics, weight lifting, shotputting, and distance cycling the wrist bears heavy compression loads. Torque may also be applied during compression. In gymnastics, support of one's entire body weight through the wrist is required for floor exercises, parallel bars, vaulting, and aerial rings. In body building or competitive weight lifting, compressive loads through the wrist may greatly exceed body weight. These loads

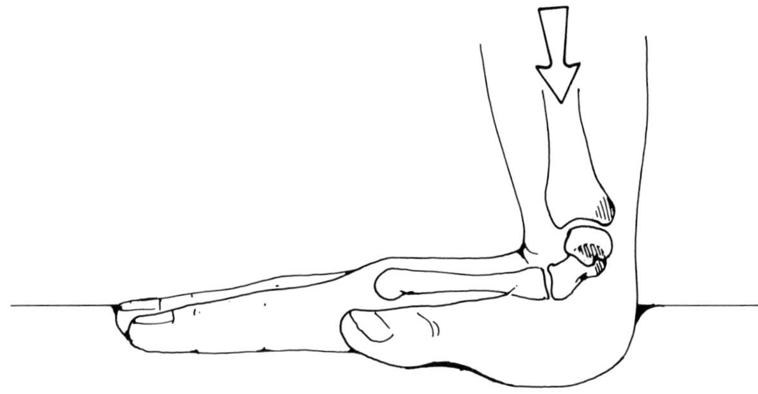

FIG. 22-1. Axial loading of the wrist in dorsiflexion. Axial loading cannot produce articular lesions on the volar lip of the radius or the dorsal aspect of the head of the capitate *(shaded areas)*.

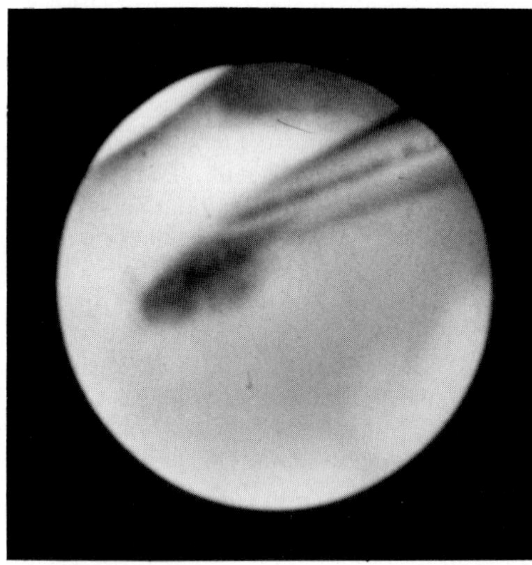

FIG. 22-2. Right wrist. Arthroscopic view of a linear tear in the volar aspect of the TFC articular disk. The tear runs parallel to the volar radioulnar ligament.

are usually transferred with the forearm pronated and the wrist in extension and radial deviation. Most of the stress is applied to the palmar structures, which include the flexor carpi ulnaris–pisiform–triquetrum complex, the volar ulnocarpal ligaments, the volar radiocarpal ligaments, and the thicker palmar aspect of the scapholunate ligament. Hyperextension of the wrist dorsiflexes the lunate but forces it in a palmar direction. Dislocation of the lunate may occur in weight-bearing activity as a result of rupture of the volar radiocarpal ligaments and the intrinsic ligaments of the proximal carpal row. The volar radiocarpal ligaments are well developed as an evolutionary reflection of our quadruped ancestors.

Articular lesions may develop on the head of the capitate or the volar lip of the radius (Fig. 22-1) and the volar ulnocarpal ligament is sometimes avulsed from the central disk of the triangular fibrocartilage complex (TFCC). Alternatively, tears through the central disk may occur parallel to its volar margin (Fig. 22-2 and Plate 13).*

Twisting

Most pronation and supination motions are a function of the elbow and forearm. The wrist translates this motion through the distal radioulnar joint, resulting in tension on the volar and dorsal radioulnar ligaments, which attach to the base of the ulnar styloid. These structures are at risk to excessive passive pronation or supination (Fig. 22-3).[21,22,25]

Twisting injuries are not uncommon in wrestling and gymnastics. Again, parallel bars, floor exercises, and aerial rings pose the greatest threat in gymnastics. Forceful pronation and supination are motions that are uncommon in other sports. Twisting injuries to the wrist are more often associated with industrial accidents involving rotating machinery or hand tools. If the force is dissipated distally, the volar ligaments between the triquetrum and hamate may tear, resulting in midcarpal instability. Disruption of the saddle joint between the hamate and triquetrum causes the hamate to drop palmarward in supination and causes the proximal pole of the hamate to cross the articular surface of the lunate in extreme ulnar deviation.[7,15,22] This injury can be devastating.

Impact

Obviously, the most unpredictable form of impact loading results from falls that can oc-

*References 5, 6, 8, 11, 15, 18.

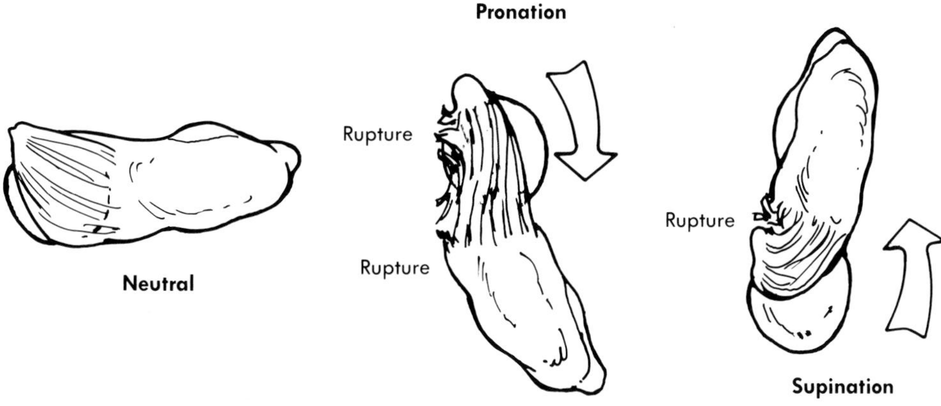

FIG. 22-3. When the wrist is forcefully pronated, injuries to the volar radioulnar ligament may occur. "Ulna dorsal" instability of the distal radioulnar joint may also be present. Hypersupination injuries may rupture the dorsal radioulnar ligament which is rolled at the base of the ulnar styloid.

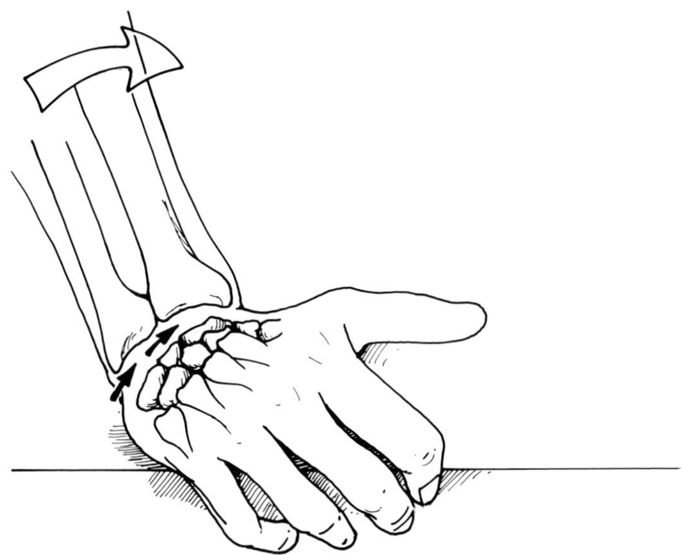

FIG. 22-4. Falls on the outstretched hand usually apply force through the ulnar side of the palm. As the elbow collapses into flexion, the forearm pronates on the fixed hand. The carpus shifts radialward. Resulting injuries caused by traction forces on the ulnar side of the wrist and compression forces on the radial side.

cur in any athletic activity. Falls on the outstretched hand usually load the palmar aspect of the wrist. A shearing force progresses from the ulnar to the radial side of the wrist as body weight is applied (Fig. 22-4). Virtually any structure of the wrist can be injured in a fall, but the most common injuries are fractures of the distal radius with or without disruption of the distal radioulnar joint, fractures of the ulnar styloid, fractures of the waist of the scaphoid, tears of the lunotriquetral or scapholunate ligaments, tears of the triangular fibrocartilage, and tears of the volar radiocarpal ligaments.* If the neck of the capitate articulates with the dorsal edge of the lunate in hyperextension of the wrist, excessive force may produce a transverse fracture of the capitate, although this is an infrequent occurrence.

Falls on the flexed wrist put stress on the dorsal side. Common injuries include avulsion of the dorsal capsule from the distal radius, tears of the scapholunate ligament, frac-

*References 5, 6, 13, 15, 18, 23.

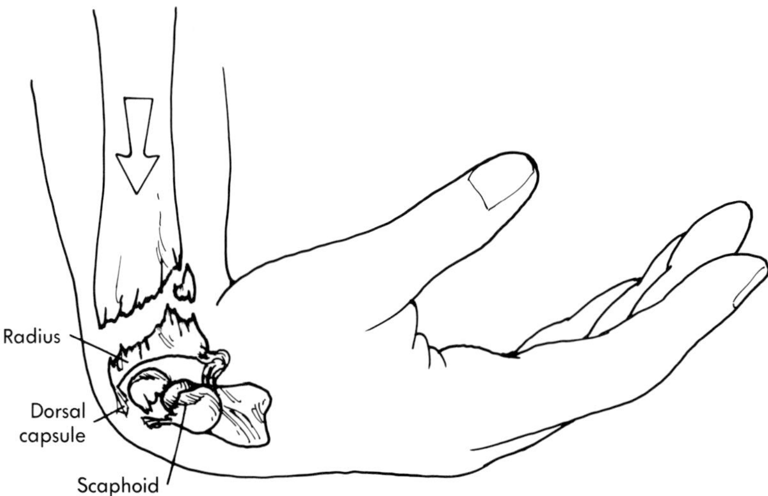

FIG. 22-5. Falls on the wrist in flexion produce dorsal soft tissue injuries or fractures of the distal radius, frequently with a volar butterfly fragment.

tures of the scaphoid, and flexion fractures of the distal radius (Fig. 22-5).[12,20,23]

Seemingly minor dorsal or volar capsule sprains may result in eventual ganglion formation through a process of mucoid degeneration.

More controlled impact loading to the wrist occurs with any sport in which the hands are used for offensive or defensive purposes. Examples include combat sports such as boxing or martial arts. In these sports the wrist is usually loaded in either of two ways. In boxing, axial loads through the metacarpals are transferred to the carpus through the capitate, lunate, and proximal pole of the scaphoid. If excessive, such forces may result in chondromalacic changes on the articular cartilage of the head of the capitate or on the convex surfaces of the lunate and scaphoid. The loading pattern is controlled by stabilization of the carpus with the extensor and flexor tendons. Forces applied with the wrist malpositioned or unstabilized load the intercarpal ligaments, especially the weaker dorsal aspect of the scapholunate ligament and the dorsal wrist capsule. Fractures of the proximal pole of the scaphoid may occur, or small bone fragments may be avulsed at the insertion of the scapholunate ligament.

Impact loading also occurs on the ulnar side of the wrist in combat sports. Most offensive actions load the palmar aspect of the ulnar side of the wrist along the base of the fifth metacarpal or in the region of the pisiform. Defensive maneuvers more often load the dorsal ulnar aspect of the wrist when absorbing or deflecting the blows of an opponent.

Palmar ulnar impact injuries may fracture the pisiform or tear its ligamentous attachment to the triquetrum (Fig. 22-6). The saddle joint of the triquetrum and hamate is also at risk, and fractures of the fifth metacarpal are common. Impact injuries applied directly to the base of the palm may fracture the hook of the hamate.[19]

Defensive injuries to the dorsal ulnar aspect of the wrist usually involve the extensor carpi ulnaris retinaculum, the ulnar styloid, and the lunotriquetral ligament. Less commonly, the dorsal ligamentous aspect of the TFCC may be torn or avulsed from the central articular disk.

Athletic injuries to the ulnar side of the wrist usually involve soft tissues. Injuries on the radial side are more likely to involve bone and articular cartilage.[6,8,22]

ARTHROSCOPY AND ITS ROLE IN WRIST DISORDERS

The value of wrist arthroscopy in sports injuries lies in its potential for achieving the most satisfactory long-term treatment results with decreased treatment morbidity when the alternative would be either a prolonged nonoperative treatment with less precise anatomic repair of injured tissues, or an extensive surgical exposure. Arthroscopy also has an advantage in the professional or high-performance amateur athlete in achieving a more rapid return to competition because it facilitates obtaining an earlier definitive diagnosis. When appropriate, arthroscopy also allows minimally invasive surgical techniques.

Wrist arthroscopy is a recently developed treatment modality. Although attempted spo-

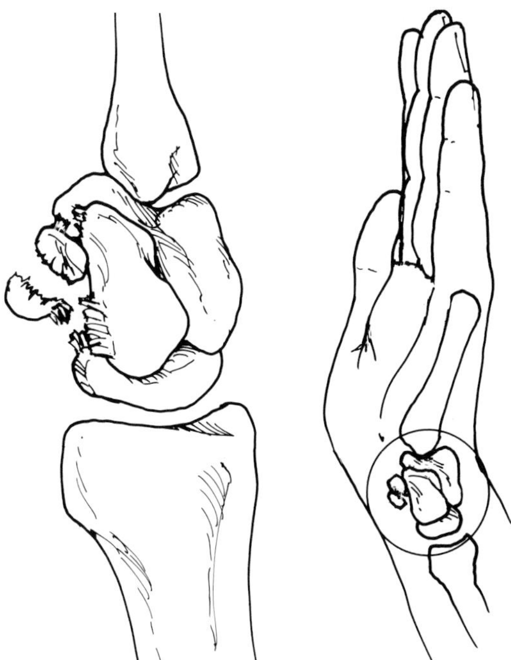

FIG. 22-6. Impact load applied to the palmar ulnar aspect of the wrist may fracture the pisiform or tear the pisotriquetral ligaments.

radically since 1975 in the United States and Japan, it was not until 1985 that the technique was refined sufficiently that diagnostic arthroscopic examination became a practical consideration, and that surgical procedures under arthroscopic control were attempted with predictable and favorable expectations.[24,35,36]

Equipment

Because the interosseous spaces between the radius and proximal carpal row and between the proximal and distal carpal rows are quite limited, an arthroscope with an outermost diameter of 3 mm or less is necessary for a comprehensive arthroscopic examination. In small athletes, especially petite females, smaller scopes with an outside sheath diameter of 2.5 mm or less are advantageous in the radiocarpal and midcarpal spaces because they enable examination of the joint thoroughly without traumatizing the articular surfaces. The smaller scopes are essential for inspection of the scaphoid-trapezium-trapezoid (STT) joint and the distal radioulnar joint.

With larger scopes in the 5 mm diameter range, a larger portal can be made to place the tip of the scope just inside the joint and view from side to side. This affords a larger field of view but provides very limited access to the volar structures and midcarpal articular surfaces. Larger scopes may be useful for an occasional wrist examination when the cost of smaller instruments is not warranted but is no substitute for the smaller scopes if wrist arthroscopy is to be practiced regularly.

Because the smaller diameter arthroscopes contain more fragile optics that can easily break, shorter arthroscope lengths are recommended to reduce the bending forces applied. High-sensitivity lightweight microchip video cameras are essential to provide a magnified image. The lighter weight microchip cameras place less force on the small-diameter arthroscopes than do heavier tube cameras, and the more sensitive microchip designs perform best with smaller diameter scopes carrying fewer fiberoptic light bundles.

Small grasping devices, cutting forceps, and miniature sharp knives are available to facilitate surgical procedures in the wrist. These tools make it possible to retrieve loose bodies or debride small fragments of tissue from the joint and can be used to excise portions of the triangular fibrocartilage articular disk (Fig. 22-7). Miniaturized tips that fit powered arthroscopic instrumentation are also available and are indispensible for ensuring a clear visual field and efficient removal of any thin or filmy tissue (Fig. 22-8).

Wrist arthroscopy equipment

- Small-diameter arthroscope (3 mm or less)
- High-sensitivity microchip video camera
- Small grasping devices, scissors
- Miniature sharp knives
- Miniature motorized equipment
- Cordless wire driver
- Disposable pinch inflow system

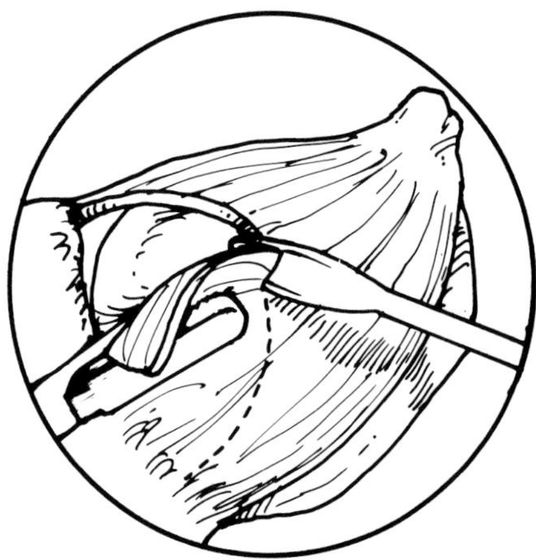

FIG. 22-7. Representation of arthroscopic excision of the radial central aspect of the TFC articular disk with a miniature banana blade arthroscopy knife and grasping forceps.

A small, preferably cordless wire driver can be used to stabilize carpal bones or fracture fragments under arthroscopic control.

A disposable inflow system has been developed with a specially designed pinch chamber in the sterile field that will introduce 2 to 3 mm of irrigant under pressure when needed (Fig. 22-9). This helps to keep the joint distended and obviates the need for cumbersome syringes and stopcocks. Expensive mechanized pumps have not been found necessary in this small joint.

Wrist arthroscopy is a technically demanding procedure. Appropriate instrumentation will definitely make the procedure easier and will enhance the surgeon's successful performance.

OPERATING ROOM ENVIRONMENT

The surgical team should be coordinated and well rehearsed when undertaking arthroscopy of the wrist. The patient is positioned supine with the shoulder abducted 60 to 90 degrees and supported on a hand table or an arm board (Fig. 22-10). The elbow is flexed 90 degrees with the forearm vertical. Sterile finger traps are applied to the index and long fingers for most procedures, but if a pathologic condition is suspected, on the ulnar side of the joint, the finger traps should be applied to the ring and little fingers to achieve greater distraction on the ulnar side. Sufficient traction is applied to the finger traps to lift the patient's elbow just off the arm board. This usually requires 7 to 10 pounds of distraction, depending on the patient's size. Distraction equal to the weight of the upper extremity, however, is usually sufficient to distract the radiocarpal and midcarpal spaces for good arthroscopic visualization. In patients who have inflammatory arthritis, all four digits may be placed in finger traps to distribute the traction forces and consideration should be given to using less weight.

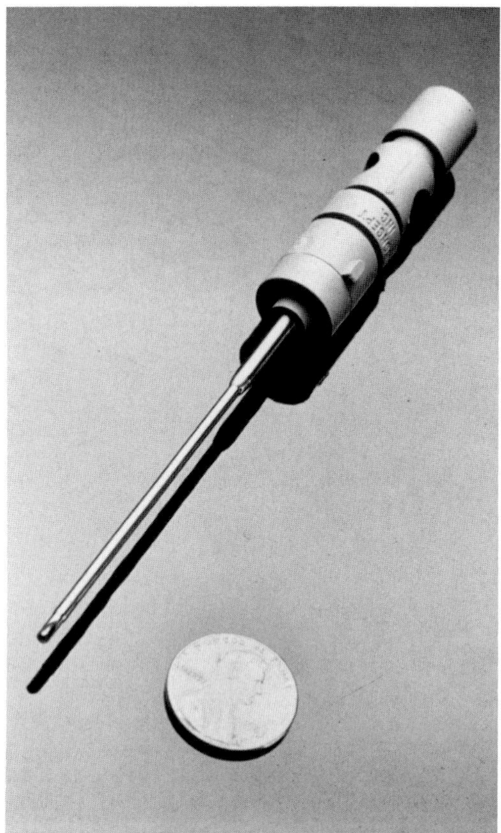

FIG. 22-8. This 2 mm shaver tip is helpful for the removal of small cartilage fibers and filmy synovial tissue from the joint (Concept, Inc, Clearwater, Fla).

Video equipment is positioned on the opposite side of the patient. The surgeon sits adjacent to the patient's head, facing the dorsum of the hand. The assistant sits opposite the surgeon at the patient's axilla, facing the palm. This allows the assistant easy access to instruments placed at the end of the hand table, as well as a good view of the video monitor, and the ability to steady the arthroscope and camera for the surgeon when necessary (Fig. 22-11).

WRIST TECHNIQUES

Arthroscopic portals for the wrist are most easily identified by the extensor compartments between which they lie.[36] There are five primary portals for the radiocarpal space (Fig. 22-12). The first portal is between the first

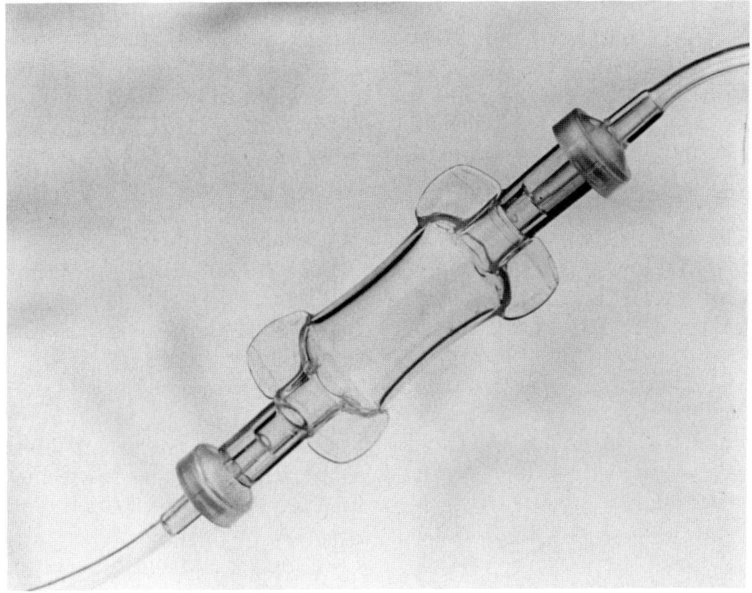

FIG. 22-9. This 2 mm pinch chamber near the end of the inflow tubing allows rapid introduction of additional irrigant when needed (Concept, Inc, Clearwater, Fla).

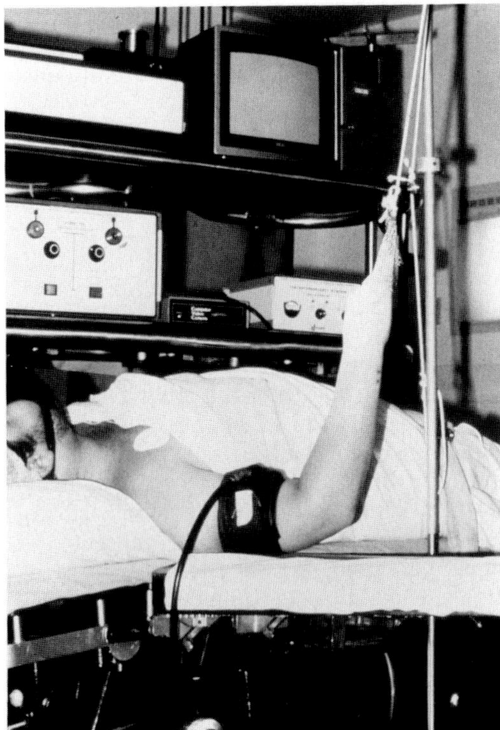

FIG. 22-10. Patient positioned for wrist arthroscopy with traction applied to the ring and little fingers through finger traps. Electronic and video equipment are arranged on the nonoperative side of the patient.

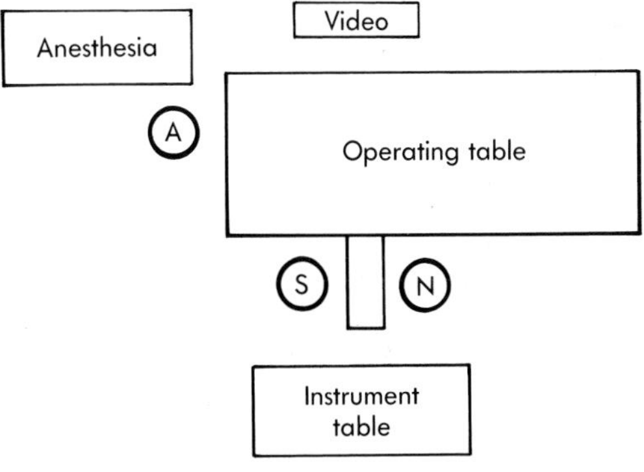

FIG. 22-11. Diagrammatic representation of convenient operating room arrangement. *A*, anesthesiologist, *S*, surgeon, *N*, nurse assistant.

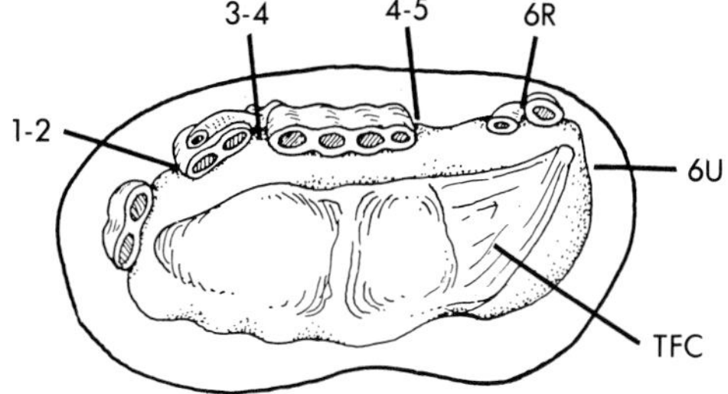

FIG. 22-12. Representation of the arthroscopy portals for the radiocarpal space for the left wrist. Portals are identified between the first and second extensor compartments *(1-2)*, the third and fourth extensor compartments *(3-4)*, the fourth and fifth extensor compartments *(4-5)*, and just to the radial *(6R)* and ulnar *(6U)* sides of the extensor carpi ulnaris.

and second extensor compartments *(1-2)*, just adjacent to the point of intersection of the extensor pollicis longus with the extensor carpi radialis longus. The most important portal for general radiocarpal examination lies between the third and fourth extensor compartments *(3-4)*. From here, most of the articular surfaces of the radiocarpal space and the entire triangular fibrocartilage can be visualized. Between the fourth and fifth extensor compartments *(4-5)* accessory instruments are introduced to facilitate examination or arthroscopic surgical procedures. Just to the radial side of the extensor carpi ulnaris (ECU) *(6R)* or to its ulnar side *(6U)*, an atraumatic plastic inflow cannula is placed. These two ulnar portals are also useful for the arthroscope or for cutting instruments when excising torn flaps of tissue from the triangular fibrocartilage.

There are three useful portals for the midcarpal space. The first lies about 1 cm distal to the 3-4 portal in line with the radial margin of the third ray. This is identified as the midcarpal radial portal (MCR). The scaphoid trapezium trapezoid (STT) joint can be seen from this portal, as can the articulations between the scaphoid and lunate and also between the lunate and triquetrum. A more ulnar portal between the extensor digitorum communis tendon to the little finger and the extensor digiti quinti is used for accessory or operating instruments. This portal is identified as the midcarpal ulnar portal (MCU). Finally, a useful portal occasionally used for accessory instruments in the STT joint interval lies in line with the second metacarpal, just distal to the extensor pollicis longus tendon. This portal is identified as the STT portal. Instruments should enter between the trapezoid and the distal pole of the scaphoid. The radial artery is protected by the intervening extensor carpi radialis longus tendon.

Arthroscopy portals

Radiocarpal space
- Between first and second dorsal compartments (1-2)
- Between third and fourth dorsal compartments (3-4)
- Between fourth and fifth dorsal compartments (4-5)
- Radial aspect ECU (6R)
- Ulnar aspect ECU (6U)

Midcarpal space
- Midcarpal radial (MCR)
- Midcarpal ulnar (MCU)
- Scaphoid trapezium trapezoid (STT) portal

The distal radioulnar joint can occasionally be entered with a small arthroscope through a portal at the metaphyseal flare of the distal ulna. With the forearm supinated, the dorsal capsule of the distal radioulnar joint is lax and most easily entered, but care must be taken not to injure the extensor tendon to the little finger. It is sometimes possible to advance the arthroscope from this position into the space between the head of the ulna and the proximal surface of the triangular fibrocartilage articular disk to retrieve loose bodies and to inspect or transfix fractures of the ulnar styloid.

The arthroscopic sheath and trocar should always be introduced with a twisting motion to separate the joint capsule fibers in an atraumatic manner. Other instruments should be inserted in a similar fashion. Preferred instruments have tapered or gently pointed tips. Care must be taken to avoid inadvertent introduction of any air bubbles into the joint, because they will impair visualization and may be difficult to absolve.[24,36]

DIAGNOSTIC ARTHROSCOPY

Arthroscopic examination of the wrist is most useful for soft tissue injuries that cannot be precisely diagnosed through conventional imaging techniques. As we gain more experience, it has become apparent that even definitive diagnoses based on arthrography can be further qualified by arthroscopic examination. Arthroscopic examination will also facilitate treatment planning. Leakage of contrast medium through the triangular fibrocartilage confirms communication between two normally separated spaces, but provides no useful information with respect to the mechanical significance or the chronicity of the defect. Tears in the scapholunate or lunotriquetral ligaments may or may not be repairable, but this determination cannot be made on the basis of arthrography alone. Arthroscopic examination is helpful, therefore, if plain roentgenograms are normal following the acute injury, yet there is reasonable clinical suspicion of an intraarticular soft tissue injury. Extraarticular tendons, nerves, and vessels cannot be evaluated arthroscopically, of course. Arthrography, isotope scanning, or magnetic resonance imaging may be helpful preoperatively in certain circumstances.[5,6,10]

In the radiocarpal space articular surfaces, volar wrist ligaments, and the dorsal wrist capsule can be inspected thoroughly for signs of trauma. The wrist should be flexed and extended while watching the motion relation-

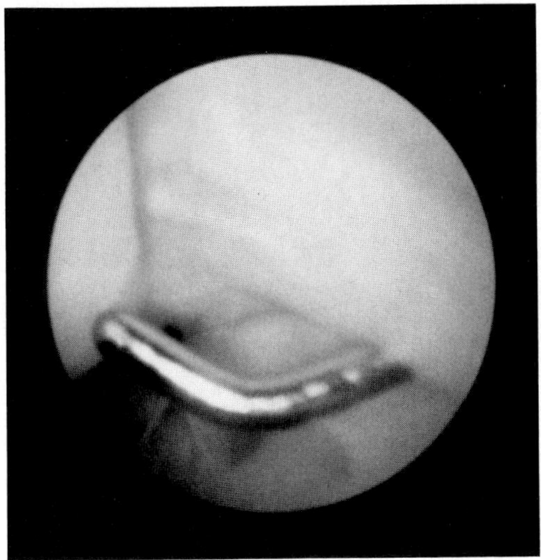

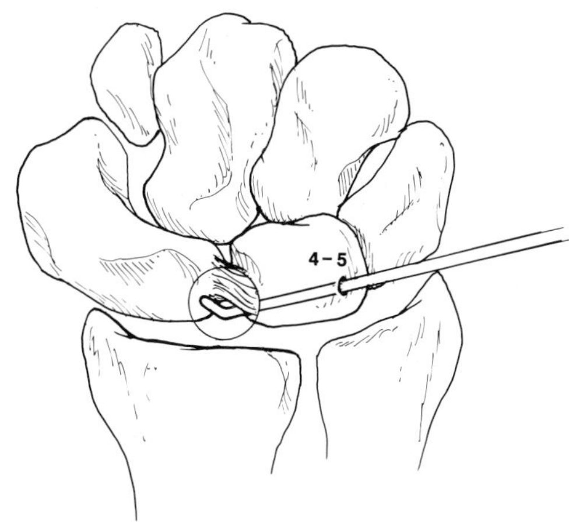

FIG. 22-13. Probe exploring the scapholunate ligament of a right wrist through the 4-5 portal.

ships between the scaphoid and lunate. The scapholunate ligament must be probed thoroughly from the 4-5 portal.

Articular surfaces, the scapholunate, and the lunotriquetral ligaments should be probed thoroughly from the 4-5 portal in search of softening or rupture (Fig. 22-13). Most tears of the scapholunate ligament originate dorsally where the ligament is thinner, and may progress to varying degrees toward the volar aspect.*

The triangular fibrocartilage is visualized well from the 3-4 portal or the 6R portal, but the latter vantage is most useful. A probe may be introduced through the 4-5, 6R, or 6U portals. It is often necessary to switch the portals for the arthroscope and probe to facilitate a thorough evaluation of the TFCC. Tears in the central articular disk may be found adjacent to the TFCC's attachment to the sigmoid notch (type 1) in the central portion of the articular disk as in cases of ulnocarpal impingement (type 2), or parallel to the dorsal or volar capsule attachments to the articular disk (type 3).[5,21,27]

In an acute injury, inspection of the volar radiocarpal ligaments may disclose hemorrhage or ligament laxity even in wrist extension (Fig. 22-14). Moving the wrist through flexion and extension during the course of arthroscopic examination, as well as extensive probing of the ligaments, will help to define the magnitude of these injuries.[6,27]

*References 6, 8, 10, 15, 18, 21, 34.

In the midcarpal space, the articular surfaces of the scaphoid and capitate can be examined well. In the STT joint, articular changes may be found on the distal pole of the scaphoid, at times severe enough to expose subchondral bone.[10]

Structures visualized by wrist arthroscopy

- Articular surfaces
- Volar wrist ligaments
- Dorsal wrist capsule
- Scapholunate ligament
- Lunotriquetral ligament
- Triangular fibrocartilage
- Intercarpal relationships
- Distal radioulnar joint

On the ulnar side of the midcarpal space, the tip of the hamate should be inspected thoroughly. It is normally smooth and glistening, and the interval between the hamate and triquetrum will permit only a glimpse of the volar ulnocarpal ligaments at best. If this space is widened, if the volar ligaments can be visualized well, and especially if there are erosive changes present on the proximal pole of the hamate, a midcarpal instability is almost certainly present. This injury is characterized by stretch or rupture of the volar ulnocarpal ligament complex extending between the triquetrum and the hamate. In ulnar deviation, at the completion of a golf swing, for example, the tip of the hamate will trip across the ulnar

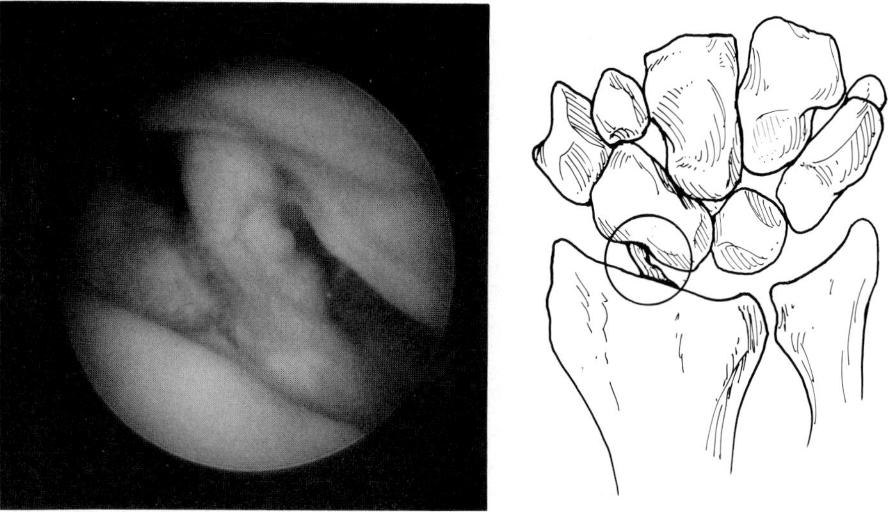

FIG. 22-14. Through the 3-4 portal, acute hemorrhage is seen adjacent to a lax volar radiocarpal ligament.

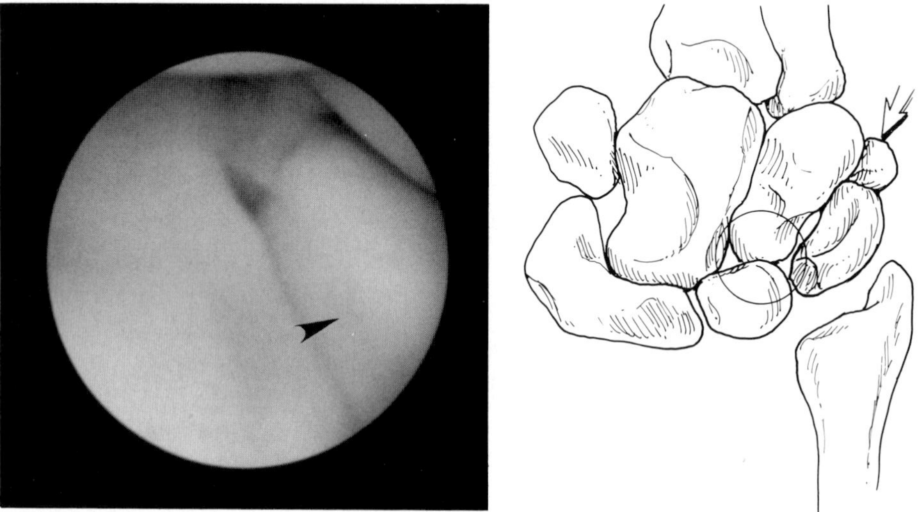

FIG. 22-15. In the midcarpal space of a right wrist, instability between the lunate and triquetrum is evidenced by excessive motion of the triquetrum when external pressure is applied. The lunate articular facet of the triquetrum is seen *(arrow)*.

edge of the lunate with a discernable "clunk." Midcarpal instability is usually associated with rupture of the lunotriquetral ligament as well.[7,10,14,15]

Finally, from the midcarpal space the orientation of the lunate to the scaphoid and the triquetrum should be examined. Each of these carpal bones may be palpated dorsally to test for abnormal anterior-posterior translation motion. When all intercarpal ligaments are intact, slight flexion and extension is possible between the scaphoid and lunate and between the lunate and triquetrum. However, this motion is constrained so that the distal articular surface of the proximal row is never grossly irregular. Normally there should be no exposure of the articular surfaces between the lunate and the triquetrum, nor between the scaphoid and the lunate (Fig. 22-15).[6,8,15]

The distal radioulnar joint should be examined if there is suspicion of a pathologic condition. This is a difficult joint to examine arthroscopically. With some experience, the degree of distal radioulnar dissociation can be appreciated from translational movements between the bones in extremes of pronation and supination. Loose bodies are occasionally found in this joint as well (Fig. 22-16).[10,15,22]

The volar ulnocarpal ligaments originate from the fovea of the head of the ulna and extend distally blending with the volar edge of the triangular fibrocartilage to form a complex. Avulsion of the ulnocarpal ligaments can sometimes be seen proximal to the triangular fibrocartilage at the base of the ulnar styloid. This injury usually occurs in association with extremes of forceful extension and radial deviation.

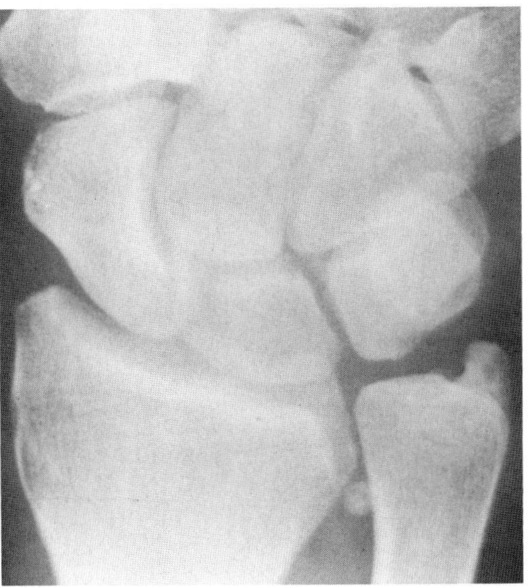

FIG. 22-16. Loose bodies seen in the distal radioulnar joint of the right wrist.

ARTHROSCOPIC SURGERY

Arthroscopic surgery is not a new surgical procedure. It is a minimally invasive technique for accomplishing traditional, tested surgical procedures for a variety of wrist disorders, many of which are commonly encountered in athletes. With the reduced morbidity of minimally invasive arthroscopic technique, the indications for surgical treatment of certain disorders might be influenced by the possibility of shortened recuperation periods. Many disorders of the wrist are amenable only to open repair; type III tears of the TFCC and instability of the distal radioulnar joint are such examples. However, with developing skills and instrumentation, some wrist disorders have become treatable with minimally invasive techniques under arthroscopic control.[32,33]

Articular Cartilage

There is no definitive means of repairing or reversing injuries to hyaline cartilage. The potential for autogenous repair appears to be dependent on the health and responsiveness of remaining chondrocytes and the degree of severity of the injury. Arthroscopic shaving of Outerbridge grade II and grade III articular lesions in the knee has been shown to have no reparative benefit for the articular surface. This procedure is believed to be beneficial to the joint, however, by decreasing the inflammatory reaction that is caused by shedded fragments of hyaline cartilage. This procedure has equal therapeutic potential for grade II and grade III articular lesions of the wrist which are common following repeated impact loading or compression loading of this joint. Surface debridement can be accomplished easily with miniaturized shaver tips for motorized instrumentation with virtually no recuperation required. At the same time, hypertrophic or inflamed synovial membranes can be removed.

Full-thickness articular lesions exposing subchondral bone have no potential for autogenous recovery. It has been demonstrated in other joints, however, that exposure of intraosseous circulation to the surface of the defect will produce granulation tissue formation on the exposed subchondral bone. If protected, this granulation tissue can mature into reasonably firm fibrocartilage and provide some reduction in friction during motion of opposing joint surfaces. This procedure, known as **abrasion arthroplasty,** is a more logical procedure in non–weight-bearing joints of the upper extremity. Short-term results of abrading full-thickness defects on articular surfaces of the radius, distal pole of the scaphoid, and proximal tip if the hamate has produced symptomatic relief. However, a return to sports that involves weight bearing or impact loading on these surfaces should not be recommended.

Small powered burrs or curettes are used for removal of superficial subchondral surfaces. Vascular elements are abundant in the distal radius, but are apparently sparse in the subchondral bone of the carpals. Drilling exposed carpal surfaces with 0.045-inch K-wires is recommended to access intraosseous vascularity and to minimize removal of normal bone contours (Fig. 22-17).

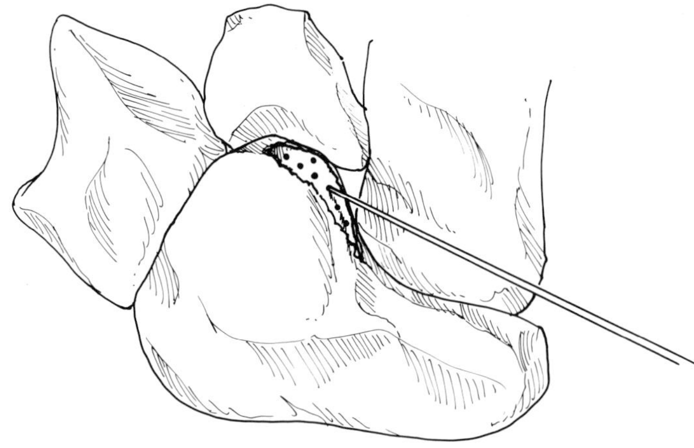

FIG. 22-17. Representation of drilling the subchondral bone in a full-thickness articular defect on the distal pole of scaphoid with a smooth K-wire.

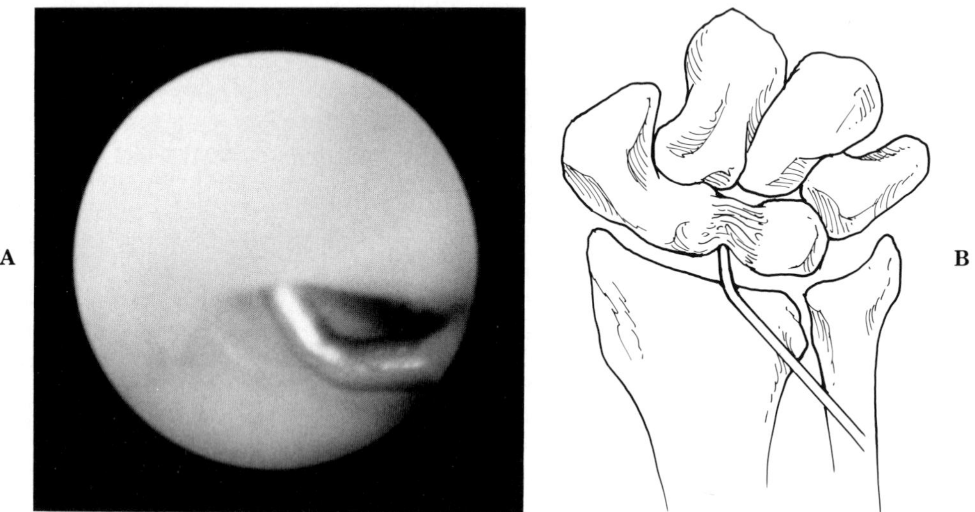

FIG. 22-18. Probe demonstrating a stretch injury to the scapholunate ligament of a right wrist. **A,** arthroscopic view, **B,** artist's perspective.

Intercarpal Ligaments

Many procedures have been devised for chronic severe rotatory subluxation of the scaphoid. Invariably, this condition results from a neglected tear of the scapholunate ligament. The radioscaphoidcapitate ligament over which the scaphoid flexes may also be torn or stretched. Rarely do acute injuries result in complete disruption of the scapholunate articulation. Adequate intervention in the acute stage of scapholunate disruption may prevent the eventual consequences of more severe instability. Widening of the scapholunate interval on anterior-posterior roentgenograms or angulation of more than 15 degrees between the capitate and lunate axes on lateral roentgenograms is evidence of major scapholunate instability. These changes are rarely seen following acute injury, however, and may reflect chronicity of the scapholunate instability.

Localized tenderness dorsally over the scapholunate junction following an acute injury should raise suspicion of scapholunate ligament disruption. If acute tenderness persists after 3 to 4 weeks of immobilization, an arthrogram is indicated. If contrast material flows from the radiocarpal to the midcarpal space through the scapholunate interval, a tear in the scapholunate ligament is confirmed. A negative arthrogram, however, is of little clinical significance. The scapholunate membrane can be stretched enough to cause instability of this joint without complete lig-

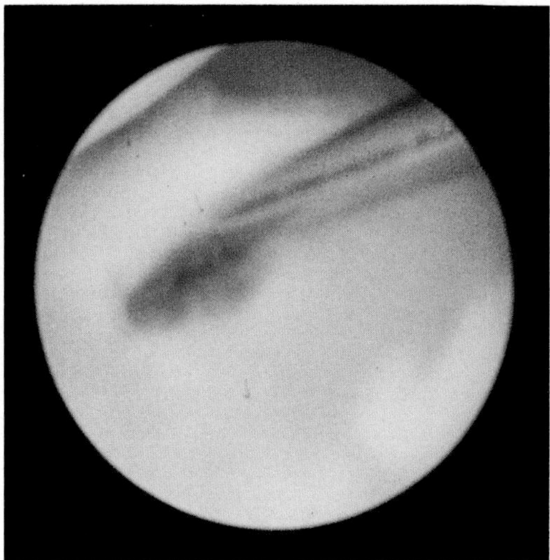

PLATE 13. Right wrist. Arthroscopic view of a linear tear in the volar aspect of the TFC articular disk. The tear runs parallel to the volar radioulnar ligament.

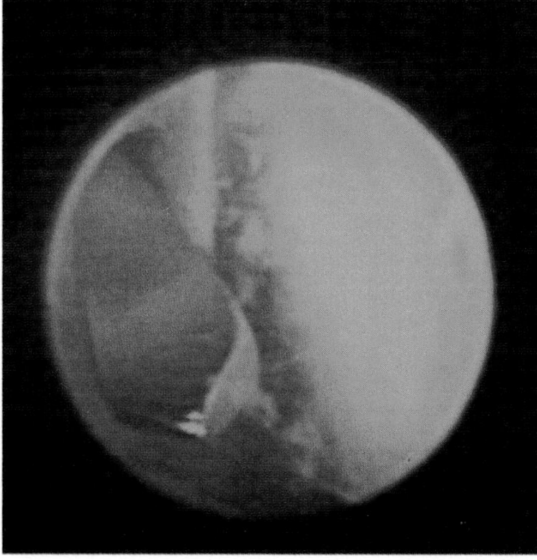

PLATE 14. Arthroscopic view of .045-inch smooth K-wire entering the radial wrist capsule adjacent to the proximal pole of the scaphoid.

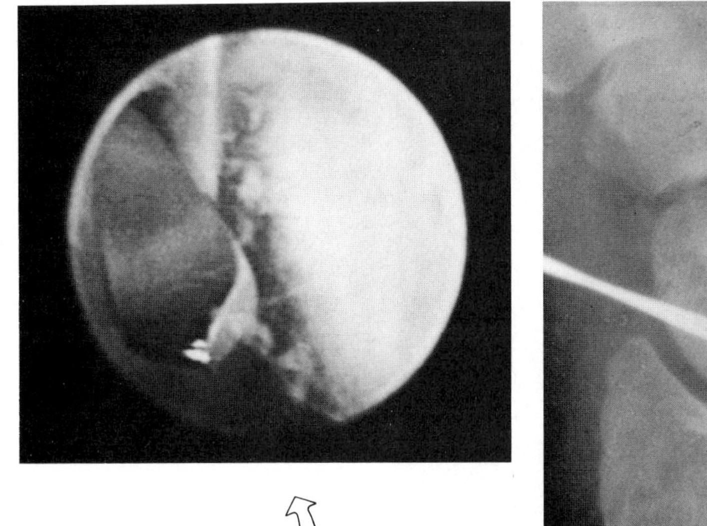

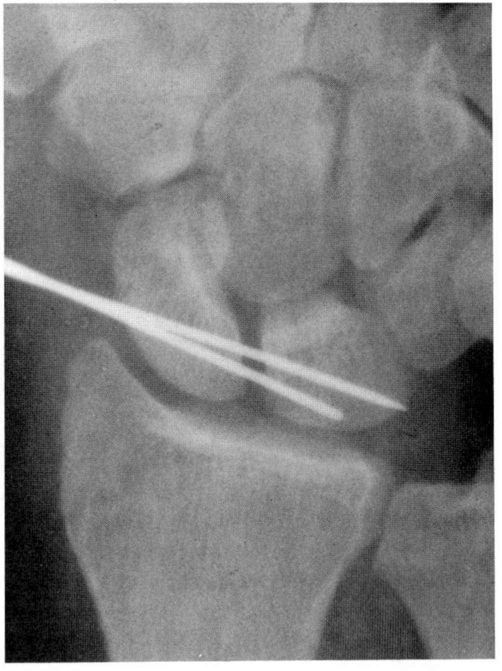

FIG. 22-19. Illustration of the technique for arthroscopic reduction internal fixation of an acute scapholunate dissociation injury of the right wrist. **A,** Arthroscopic view of .045-inch smooth K-wire entering the radial wrist capsule adjacent to the proximal pole of the scaphoid. **B,** Representation of two K-wires drilled into the proximal pole scaphoid to aid with manipulation and reduction before fixation of the scapholunate interval. **C,** Postoperative roentgenogram with the scapholunate joint reduced and two K-wires properly positioned to stabilize the joint.

ament disruption, just as similar stretch injuries occur in the knee, ankle, and shoulder. If the injury is reduced and immobilized early, healing of the scapholunate ligament is possible. Injury to the scapholunate ligament is confirmed by examination and probing through the 3-4 and 4-5 radiocarpal portals (Fig. 22-18).

To reduce and stabilize the scapholunate interval, two 0.045-inch K-wires are placed transcutaneously into the proximal pole of the scaphoid from the radial side aiming toward the lunate (Fig. 22-19 and Plate 14). The arthroscope is then placed in the midcarpal radial portal to observe the volar articular margins of the scaphoid and lunate in the midcarpal space. The wrist is extended and deviated to the ulnar side to stand the scaphoid vertically. This will reduce the scapholunate joint in most cases. Minor adjustment can be accomplished by manipulating one or both of the K-wires, or by applying pressure to the scaphoid tubercle. When the articular margins of the scaphoid and lunate are perfectly matched, the K-wires are advanced across the joint into the lunate. Three to four pins should be placed across the scapholunate interval. Arthroscopic inspection of the midcarpal space and the radiocarpal space will confirm that other articular surfaces have not been violated. An intraoperative roentgenogram is used to ensure that the pins have been satisfactorily placed. The pins are cut short and the wrist is protected with a cast for 8 weeks.

Although this treatment approach to scapholunate dissociation has not been evaluated by follow-up arthroscopic examination or arthrograms in large numbers of cases, it is presumed that fibrosis between the scaphoid and lunate along the pin tracks provides sufficient stabilization of this interval. Watson has described this concept as a beneficial fibrous union.*

Similar principles are applied for arthroscopic reduction and pin fixation of acute tears of the lunotriquetral ligament and the hamatetriquetral ligament. In these cases, K-wires are introduced on the ulnar side of the wrist into the triquetrum, and are advanced into the lunate or the hamate as necessary. At least three pins are recommended to avoid rotation of the carpals around the pin

*References 6, 7, 8, 10, 15, 20, 24, 32, 33, 34.

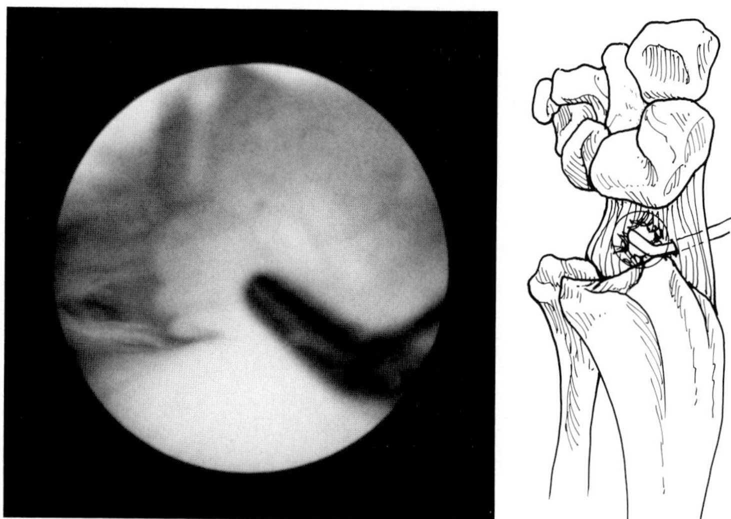

FIG. 22-20. Viewed from the 1-2 portal. Disrupted fibers in the dorsal capsule of a right wrist are probed through the 3-4 portal. Acute injuries demonstrate edema and hypertrophic synovium as well as disrupted fibers.

axes and to evoke a sufficient fibrous response.*

Volar and Dorsal Ligament Injuries

As previously discussed, hyperextension or hyperflexion injuries to the wrist may tear or avulse the palmar or dorsal radiocarpal ligaments, respectively. In our experience, palmar ligaments are more likely to stretch or rupture, because dorsal capsular ligaments are more commonly avulsed from their attachment to the radius. Examination of these ligaments is best accomplished through the 1-2 radiocarpal portal with the assistance of a 4-5 placed hook probe.[6,24,35]

Volar radiocarpal ligament injuries are treated by manipulating the wrist under arthroscopic examination to find the position of greatest ligament laxity—usually flexion and slight radial deviation. The wrist is then immobilized in this position for 4 to 6 weeks. A protective, removable gauntlet is recommended thereafter for 3 months, and the wrist should be taped for any athletic endeavor for 6 to 12 months, depending on the severity of the ligament injury. Although experience is insufficient at this time to predict with certainty, neglect of these volar radiocarpal ligament injuries may reasonably be expected to cause dorsal intercalated segmental instability (DISI) posturing of the lunate.[2,6,14]

Dorsal capsular injuries are treated somewhat differently, as they usually entail avulsion from the radius. With the wrist in dorsiflexion, it is usually possible to visualize the site of avulsion. The dorsal capsule gains attachment to the radius and the carpals immediately adjacent to the articular surface. If there is any undermining of capsule adjacent to the articular margin, ligament avulsion should be suspected. Localized hemorrhage is evident in more acute injuries (Fig. 22-20).

In subacute injuries, with the arthroscope in the 1-2 portal and an accessory burr or curette in the 4-5 or 6R portal, the exposed bone can be abraded to produce bleeding. The wrist should then be positioned in extension with a well-molded cast to relax the dorsal capsule in contact with the freshly abraded bone. Immobilization is recommended for 6 weeks, followed by a protective gauntlet and spica splinting for athletic activities.[18,27]

Triangular Fibrocartilage Complex

Injuries to the triangular fibrocartilage complex (TFCC) resulting from impact loading or excessive torque are treated in ways analogous to meniscus tears in the knee. The TFCC provides an opposing articular surface for the ulnar half of the lunate and the triquetrum. By virtue of the insertion of dorsal and volar ulnocarpal ligaments onto the triangular fibrocartilage, this structure also participates in ulnocarpal stability, though the precise mechanism is not well understood. The TFCC has also been credited with contribution to the stability of the distal radioul-

*References 6, 7, 8, 10, 15, 20.

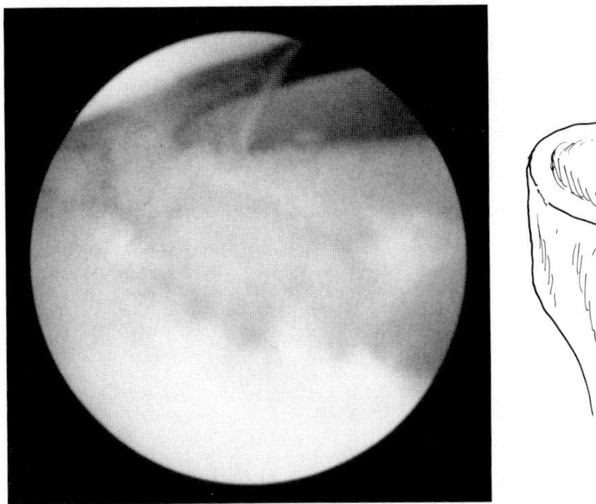

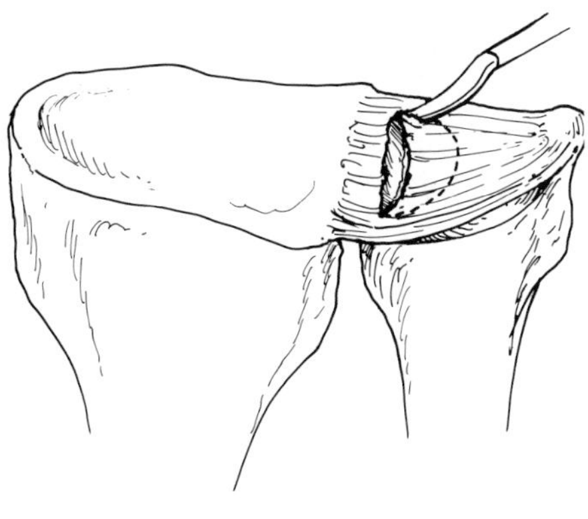

FIG. 22-21. A, Arthroscopic view of miniature banana blade knife excising the unstable portion of a type I tear in the TFC articular disk, right wrist. **B,** Representation of a type I tear and the intended line of tissue resection.

A

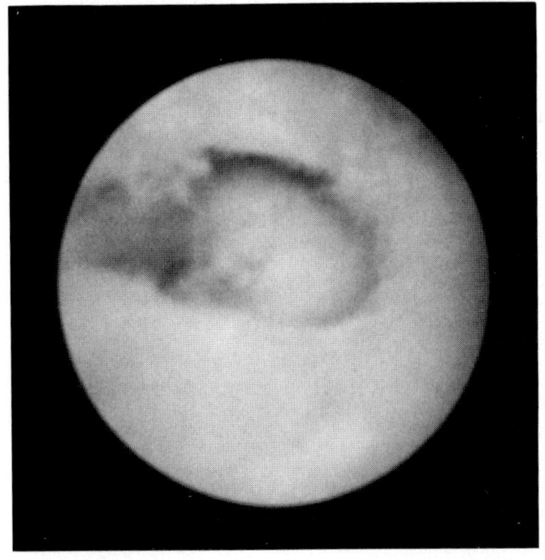

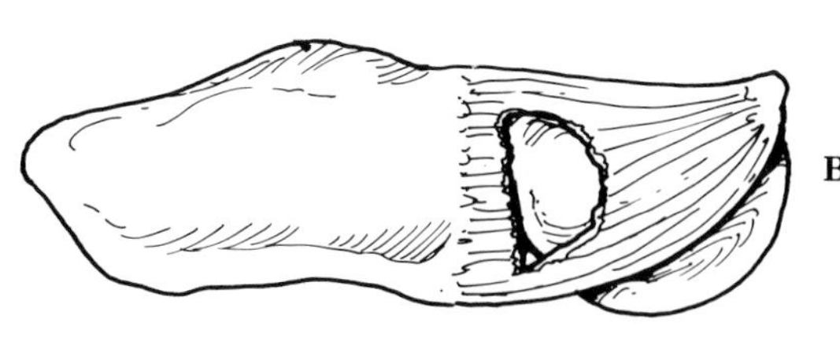

B

FIG. 22-22. Resected central portion of TFC articular disk. Ulnar head is visible through the defect. **A,** Arthroscopic view. **B,** Artist's perspective.

nar joint, although selective cutting studies have challenged this concept.

Central perforations of the triangular fibrocartilage that do not disrupt the peripheral ligamentous attachments or the insertion of the TFCC onto the radius are of little mechanical consequence. The edges of these injuries can be trimmed smoother if necessary, but little definitive treatment is required.

By contrast, type I and type III injuries to the central disk of the triangular fibrocartilage should be treated more aggressively. Angular type I tears that create flaps of articular disk may interfere mechanically with wrist flexion and extension or with ulnar deviation. With the arthroscope placed in the 6R portal or the 3-4 portal, unstable flaps of tissue can be excised from the triangular fibrocartilage using miniaturized arthroscopic knives, basket forceps, punches, or certain motorized shaver tips. All unstable tissue should be removed from tears of the central articular disk of the triangular fibrocartilage. This may in many cases convert type I tears to stable central perforations of the articular disk (Figs. 22-21 and 22-22).

The wrist may be splinted postoperatively for comfort for a few days, but there is other-

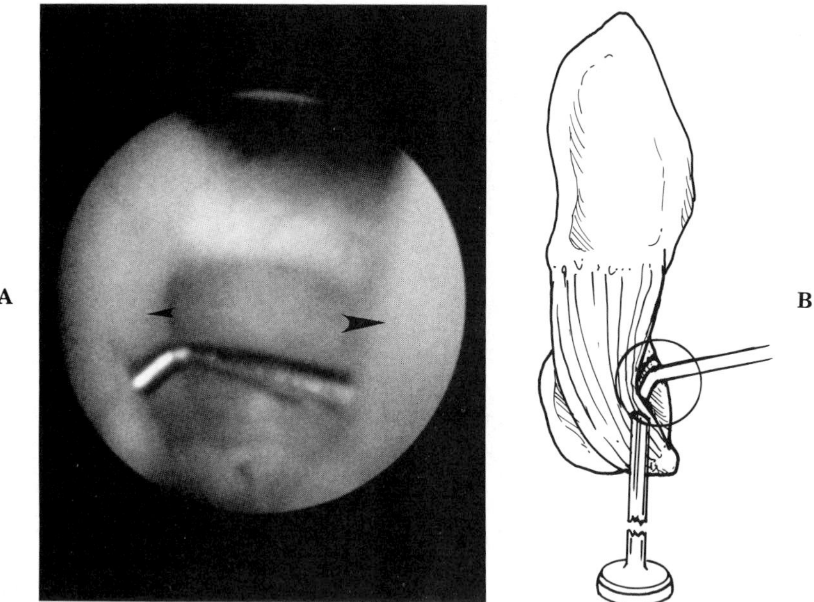

FIG. 22-23. View from the 6R portal of a type III separation of the articular disk *(large arrow)*. **A,** Arthroscopic view. **B,** Artist's perspective.

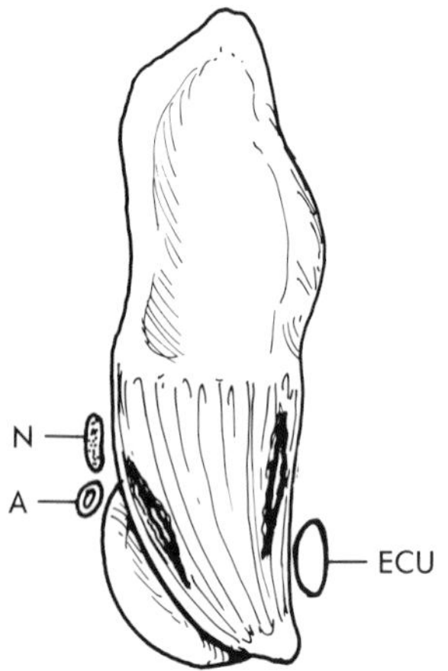

FIG. 22-24. Type III tears of the TFCC are not amenable to arthroscopic repair because of the overlying extensor carpi ulnaris *(ECU)* tendon dorsally, the ulnar nerve *(N)*, and artery *(A)* volarly.

wise no contraindication to early return of functioning and competition with protective taping.

Type III tears greater than 3 or 4 mm in length should be treated with open suture repair (Fig. 22-23). Arthroscopic repair is probably not feasible, because the ulnar nerve and artery lie immediately adjacent to the volar wrist capsule, and the extensor carpi ulnaris tendon overlies the dorsal tears (Fig. 22-24). Precise approaches to the torn complex can be achieved by marking the tear under arthroscopic control with a hypodermic needle. A longitudinal miniature arthrotomy can then be made to directly access the tear by following the path of the needle.[5,15,22,28]

Intraarticular Fractures

There is no substitute for anatomic reduction of articular surfaces in the treatment of intraarticular fractures. To preserve joint mechanics and low friction contact and to decrease formation of adhesions, all fracture fragments containing articular cartilage should be precisely positioned as if assembling a three-dimensional jigsaw puzzle. Arthroscopy has provided a great advantage in the treatment of such fractures of the distal radius. Athletes are susceptible to distal radial fractures from falls on the upper extremity in almost every sport. High-speed or collision sports impart even greater energy with increased risk of fracture comminution. Many fracture fragments have inadequate capsule or ligament attachment to allow manipulative reduction with closed techniques. This problem is typified by the so-called "die-punch" fracture in which the dorsal portion of the lunate facet of the radius is depressed proximally and impacted.

These fractures are amenable to treatment under arthroscopic control by precise reduction and K-wire fixation of the fracture fragments. This is a tedious procedure, however, and should not be undertaken casually.

Guided by good-quality preoperative roentgenograms and CT scans of the articular sur-

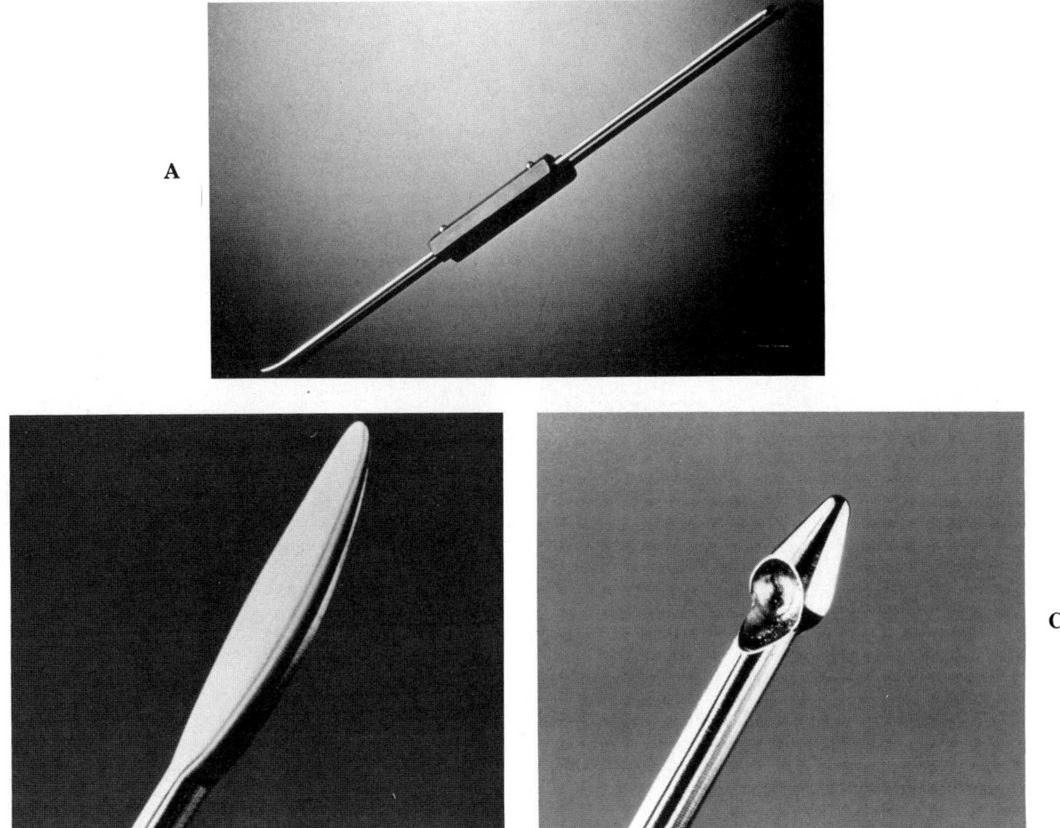

FIG. 22-25. A, Double-ended tool for small-joint arthroscopy. **B,** Curved, flat dissector on one end. **C,** Curette with tapered point on opposite end (Concept, Inc, Clearwater, Fla).

face if necessary, the distal radius is visualized arthroscopically through the 3-4 or 1-2 portal. Large-volume irrigation is required to evacuate the hemarthrosis. The forearm should be wrapped snugly with a sterile compressive bandage to minimize fluid extravasation into the muscular compartments through fracture planes. This is a precautionary measure, although the risk is not as great as it might seem. It is important that the irrigation fluid should never be introduced with an inflow rate that is greater than the outflow system from the joint can accommodate. This will provide adequate lavage of the joint space without forced extravasation into the soft tissues.

Lactated Ringer's solution is recommended, not only because it is the most physiologically compatible solution for articular cartilage, but also because it is readily absorbed from soft tissue compartments if extravasated. By clisis, lactated Ringer's solution is absorbed within minutes. Compartment compression syndromes resulting from closed fractures are usually caused by intramuscular bleeding, producing increased pressure for sustained periods. Arterial perfusion must be compromised for 3 to 4 hours before ischemic changes become irreversible. It is unlikely such compartmental pressure could be maintained by the extravasation of lactated Ringer's solution through articular fracture planes, although awareness of this potential risk should not be underemphasized.

Through accessory portals, small forceps or brushes can be used to remove the fibrin clot that may obscure fracture surfaces. When all fracture lines are well visualized, reduction of the fracture is centered around the largest articular fragment. Smaller fragments are repositioned as much as possible with the assistance of traction and periarticular pressure. Small, smooth K-wires are drilled into fragments that contain minimal soft tissue attachment and cannot be otherwise manipulated. These K-wires are then used to maneuver the fragments into position to reassemble the articular surface. When fragments are impacted, it may be necessary to free them from one another with a small blunt dissector placed in the fracture planes as a lever (Fig. 22-25). As each fragment is reduced, a K-wire is advanced into the major adjacent fragments

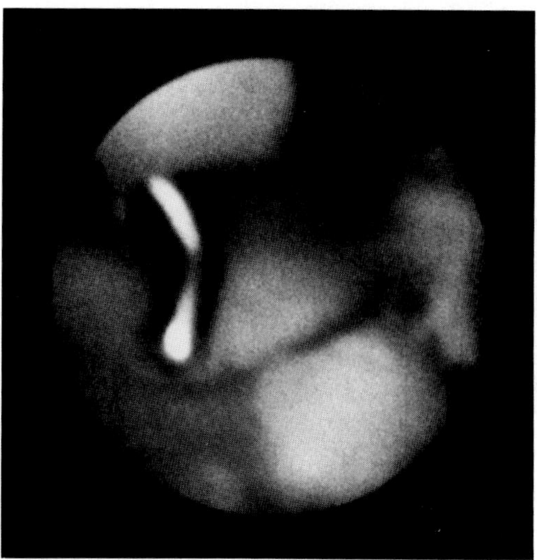

FIG. 22-26. Arthroscopic view of a reduced articular fracture of the distal radius. Intraarticular probe is used to assist with reduction of fragments.

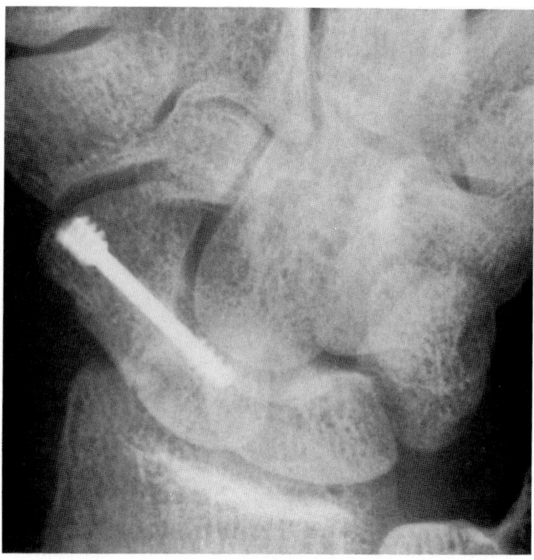

FIG. 22-27. Intraosseous compression screw placed arthroscopically in a nondisplaced fracture of the waist of the scaphoid in a football player, right wrist.

to stabilize the fragments. These wires are discreetly placed between tendons so as not to impair finger movement (Fig. 22-26).

When the entire articular surface has been reassembled, an intraoperative roentgenogram is taken to confirm fracture reduction, joint surface contour, and pin placement. There need be no concern for voids beneath articular surfaces because they will fill in during fracture healing with cancellous bone, making grafting unnecessary.

A cast is applied for 2 to 4 weeks, which is then converted to a splint that can be removed for early controlled motion exercises. This regimen facilitates remodeling of the articular surface, mobilizes adjacent joints early, decreases the possibility of intraarticular adhesions, and preserves tendon function. Long-term results from accurate reconstruction of the articular surface following such fractures justifies the surgical efforts required.

Nondisplaced fractures of the waist of the scaphoid have been treated successfully with arthroscopic placement of intraosseous screws (Fig. 22-27). The advantage of screw fixation is the early return of the athlete to competition while the fracture is healing without the need for rigid wrist immobilization. Undoubtedly, these fractures would heal otherwise in the vast majority of cases, but may require 6 to 12 weeks of cast immobilization. Many contact sports leagues will not permit a player to wear hard casts, however, and the practicality of repeatedly applying latex casts is questionable. Intraosseous screws provide compressed immobilization of fractures of the scaphoid, and permits the athlete to return to competition with simple tape splinting.

The cannulated Concept intraosseous screw or the Herbert screw are both suitable for this treatment. The Concept compression jig is easier to use under arthroscopic control, and preliminary K-wire fixation allows one to confirm the intended placement of the screw with intraoperative roentgenograms before drilling the bone.

This treatment modality is recommended for those athletes who are not permitted to wear casts and desire to return to competition at the earliest possible time. There appears to be little risk and definite advantage to early surgical intervention and internal fixation in properly selected cases of minimally displaced and nondisplaced scaphoid fractures.

Loose Bodies

Osseous loose bodies resulting from acute or repetitive wrist trauma can usually be diagnosed by conventional radiographs. Unossified cartilaginous loose bodies are radiolucent, and may present with symptoms of intermittent interference with wrist motion. At arthroscopy, mechanically significant loose bodies can be located and removed with a cup forceps (Fig. 22-28). Care should be taken to explore by palpation and probing all visible recesses within the joint such as the prestyloid recess and the space of Poirier.

Removal of loose bodies that interfere with

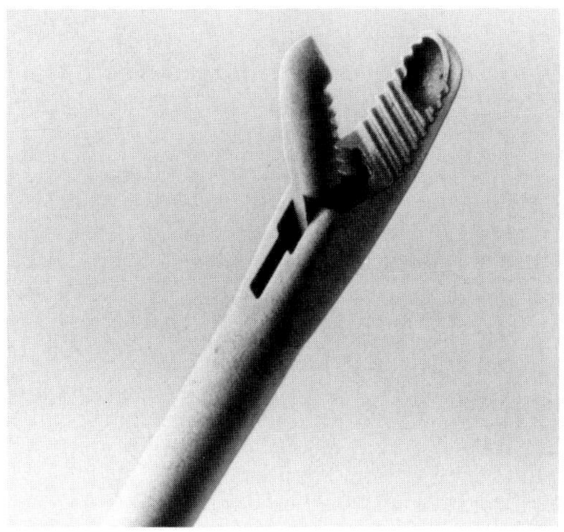

FIG. 22-28. These 2.2 mm cupped grasping forceps are helpful for removing osteocartilaginous loose bodies from the wrist (Concept, Inc, Clearwater, Fla).

the wrist function brings immediate symptomatic relief. Recuperation entails only healing of the skin punctures which occurs readily within 3 to 7 days. Acute osteocartilaginous fracture fragments too small to be replaced can be removed under arthroscopic control, but the site of origin should be freshened with a curette or burr, and the wrist should be protected for 6 to 8 weeks to allow satisfactory fibrosis of the fracture site. Fracture fragments that are of ample size should be anatomically replaced, which usually requires an arthrotomy. Long-term functional results depend on the preservation of normal joint contours.[29]

SUMMARY

The indication for wrist arthroscopy in athletes is primarily for soft tissue intraarticular injuries, but also includes intraarticular fractures, and cases where conventional imaging techniques have failed to delineate the etiology of wrist pain. Surgical intervention with minimally invasive techniques are advantageous in cases of acute intercarpal ligament injury, especially lesions of the scapholunate joint and the lunotriquetral joint. Midcarpal instability and disruption of the triquetral hamate joint occur less frequently but may be problematic for the athlete. Arthroscopic reduction and internal fixation of mild to moderate carpal instability can produce arthrofibrosis sufficient to stabilize these small joints. Arthroscopic reduction and internal fixation of intraarticular fractures is of great advantage in the anatomic restoration of joint surfaces with minimally invasive techniques. This treatment approach facilitates early mobilization of the joints in many cases.

It must be emphasized that arthroscopic surgery of the wrist is not a new procedure, but only an advantageous, minimally invasive technique for applying well-established surgical principles of treatment to wrist injuries in appropriately selected cases.

REFERENCES

1. Allum R: Skateboard injuries: a new epidemic, Injury 10:152, 1978.
2. Bergfeld JA, Weiker GC, and Andrish JT: Soft playing splint for protection of significant hand and wrist injuries in sports, Am J Sports Med 10:293, 1982.
3. Burkhart S and Woods M: Post-traumatic recurrent subluxation of the extensor carpi ulnaris tendon, J Hand Surg 7A:1, 1982.
4. Burton RL: Overview for athletic upper extremity injuries. In Injuries of the upper extremity in the competitive athlete, pp. 297-299.
5. Coleman HM: Injuries of the articular disc of the wrist, J Bone Joint Surg 42B:522, 1960.
6. Culver JE: Instabilities of the wrist, Clin Sports Med 5:725, 1986.
7. Dobyns JH, Sim FH, and Linscheid RL: Sports stress syndromes of the hand and wrist, Am J Sports Med 6:236, 1978.
8. Dobyns JH et al: Traumatic instability of the wrist. In AAOS instructional course lecture, vol 24, St Louis, 1975, The CV Mosby Co, pp 182-199.
9. Golfer's Wrist, editorial, Br Med J, December 24-31, p 1622, 1977.
10. Green DP: The sore wrist without a fracture. In AAOS Instructional course lecture, St Louis, 1977, The CV Mosby Co, pp. 300-313.
11. Gumbs V and Segal D: Bilateral distal radius and ulnar fractures in adolescent weight lifters, Am J Sports Med 10:375, 1982.
12. Heiple KG, Freehafer AA, and Van't Hof A: Isolated traumatic dislocation of the distal end of the ulna or distal radioulnar joint, J Bone Joint Surg 44A:1387, 1962.
13. Lichtman DM, Noble WH, and Alexander CE: Dynamic triquetrolunate instability, case report, J Hand Surg 9A:185, 1984.
14. Lichtman DM et al: Ulnar midcarpal instability—clinical and laboratory analysis, J Hand Surg 6A:515, 1981.
15. Linscheid RL and Dobyns JH: Athletic injuries of the wrist, Clin Orthop 196:141-151, 1985.
16. Linscheid RL et al: Traumatic instability of the wrist: diagnosis, classification, and pathomechanics, J Bone Joint Surg 54A:1612, 1972.
17. Lipscomb A: Baseball pitching injuries in growing athletes, J Sports Med 3:25, 1975.
18. Mayfield JK: Mechanism of carpal injuries, Clin Orthop 149:45, 1980.
19. McCue F and Baugher H: Hand and wrist injuries in the athlete, Am J Sports Med 7:275, 1979.
20. Palmer AK, Dobyns JH, and Linscheid RL: Management of posttraumatic instability of the wrist secondary to ligament rupture, J Hand Surg 3:507, 1978.
21. Posner M: Injuries to the hand and wrist in athletes, Orthop Clin North Am 8:593, 1977.
22. Rainey R and Peautsch M: Traumatic volar dis-

location of the distal radioulnar joint, Orthopedics 8:898, 1985.
23. Rose-Innes AP: Anterior dislocation of the ulna in the inferior radioulnar joint: case reports, with a discussion of the anatomy of rotation of the forearm, J Bone Joint Surg 42B:515, 1960.
24. Roth JH, Poehling GG, and Whipple TL: Arthroscopic surgery of the wrist. In Bassett FH III, editor: Instructional course lectures, vol XXXVII, Park Ridge, Ill, 1988, American Academy of Orthopaedic Surgeons.
25. Snook GA et al: Subluxtion of the distal radio-ulna joint by hyperpronation, J Bone Jont Surg 51A:1315, 1969.
26. Stark HH et al: Fracture of the hook of the hamate in athletes, J Bone Joint Surg 59A:575, 1977.
27. Taleisnik J: The ligaments of the wrist, J Hand Surg 1A:110, 1976.
28. Tehranzadeh J: Ganglion cysts and tear of the triangular fibrocartilage of both wrists in a cheerleader, Am J Sports Med 11:357, 1983.
29. Tehranzadeh J and Labosky D: Detection of loose osteochondral fragments by double contrast wrist arthrography, Am J Sports Med 12:77, 1984.
30. Torisu T: Fracture of the hook of the hamate by golf swing, Clin Orthop 83:91, 1972.
31. Traumatic tenosynovitis of the wrist, Br Med J, March 9, p 528, 1977, editorial.
32. Watson HK: Limited wrist arthrodesis, Clin Orthop 149:126, 1980.
33. Watson HK and Hempton RF: Limited wrist arthrodesis: the triscaphoid joint, I, J Hand Surg 5A:320, 1980.
34. Weeks P and Young V: A case of painful clicking wrist: a case report, J Hand Surg 4A:522, 1979.
35. Whipple TL: Arthroscopic surgery of the wrist. In Chapman MW: Operative orthopaedics, Philadelphia, 1988, JB Lippincott Co.
36. Whipple TL, Marotta JJ, and Powell JH III: Techniques of wrist arthroscopy, Arthroscopy 2:244, 1986.
37. Wood MB and Dobyns JH: Sports-related extra-articular wrist syndromes, Clin Orthop 202:93, 1986.
38. Wood MB and Linscheid RL: Abductor pollicis longus bursitis, Clin Orthop 93:293, 1973.

SUGGESTED READINGS

Bell R and Hawkins R: Stress fracture of the distal ulna, Clin Orthop 209:169, 1986.

Burton RI and Eaton RG: Common hand injuries in the athlete, Orthop Clin North Am 4:809, 1973.

Carr D and Johnson R: Upper extremity injuries in skiing, Am J Sports Med 9:378, 1981.

Dauphine RT and Linscheid RL: Unrecognized sprain patterns of the wrist, J Bone Joint Surg 57A:727, 1975 (abstract).

Dobyns JH and Linscheid RL: Fractures and dislocations of the wrist. In Rockwood CA Jr and Green DP, editors: Fractures, ed 2, Philadelphia, 1975, JB Lippincott Co., pp 345-440.

Ellsasser J and Stein A: Management of hand injuries in a professional football team, Am J Sports Med 7:178, 1979.

Flatt AE: Athletic injuries of the hand, J La State Med Soc 119:425, 1967.

Howard NJ: Peritendinitis crepitans: a muscle-effort syndrome, J Bone Joint Surg 19:447, 1937.

Kalenak A and Graham W et al: Athletic injuries of the hand, Am Fam Physician 14:136, 1976.

Mayfield JR, Johnson RP, and Kilcoyne RF: The ligaments of the human wrist and their functional significance, Anat Rec 186:417, 1976.

Mino DE, Palmer AK, and Levinsohn EM: The role of radiography and computerized tomography in the diagnosis of subluxation and dislocation of the distal radioulnar joint, J Hand Surg 8:23, 1983.

Mosher JF: Current concepts in the diagnosis and treatment of hand and wrist injuries in sports, Med Sci Sports Exerc 17:48-55, 1985.

Percy EC: Injuries to the elbow, wrist, and hand, Symposium on Athletic Injuries, September, 1967, p 744.

Rayan G: Recurrent dislocation of the extensor carpi ulnaris in athletes, Am J Sports Med 11:183, 1983.

Reagan DS, Linscheid RL, and Dobyns JH: Lunotriquetral sprains, J Hand Surg 9A:502, 1984.

Rettig A: Stress fracture of the ulna in an adolescent tournament tennis player, Am J Sports Med 11:103, 1983.

Roser L and Clawson D: Football injuries in the very young athlete, Clin Orthop 69:219, 1970.

Sprague B and Justis E: Nonunion of the carpal navicular, Arch Surg 108:692, 1974.

Strauss R and Lanese R: Injuries among wrestlers in school and college tournaments, JAMA 248:2016, 1982.

Wilson D: The perilous skateboard, Br Med J November 19, 1977, p 1349, (letter).

Youm Y et al: Kinematics of the wrist: I. An experimental study of radial-ulnar deviation and flexion-extension, J Bone Joint Surg 60A:423, 1978.

CHAPTER 23 Fractures of the Wrist

Charles P. Melone, Jr.

An increasing fund of knowledge regarding wrist anatomy, kinematics, and pathomechanics has led to important concepts that have considerably enhanced management of the athlete's fractured wrist. Prominent among these is that normal wrist function depends largely on preservation of specific shapes and relationships of multiple bony links (Fig. 23-1). The cuplike and colinear arrangement of the radius, lunate, and capitate (the primary **central links**) coupled with the skiff-shaped and oblique orientation of the scaphoid (the principal **radial link**) permits a wide but well-constrained range of flexion and extension distributed over multiple joints. Similarly, integrity of the pyramidal triquetrum (the key **ulnar link**) and its helicoid articulation with the hamate is essential for intercarpal rotation, as well as the synchronous translation that normally occurs between the carpal rows during radial and ulnar deviation. Further, because of their multiple articulations, the bony links are largely covered with hyaline cartilage; hence this vital surface area must remain undisturbed for normal kinematics. Clearly, any fracture that disrupts the relatively complex and unique chondro-osseous structure of the wrist poses a serious threat to unimpaired mobility and stability. When fracture occurs, the cardinal rule is to promptly restore normal configurations and anatomic relationships of the critical bony links.

Bony links of the wrist

Central link	Radial link	Ulnar link
Radius	Scaphoid	Triquetrum
Lunate		Hamate
Capitate		

Recognition that precise restoration of skeletal integrity is an absolute prerequisite for maximal recovery after wrist fracture has proved especially beneficial to the injured athlete. In the past, a tendency existed to consider most wrist fractures as trivial incidents with minimal morbidity. Often, a potentially disabling fracture was spuriously dismissed as an innocuous bone "bruise" or "chip"—often without the benefit of roentgenograms. Like the terminology, treatment was imprecise and recovery predictably compromised. That highly coordinated, powerful "flick of the wrist" characteristic of the skilled athlete rapidly deteriorated to a painfully weak clunk with the inability to throw, hit, or shoot with strength and dexterity. For some, the long-term consequences proved even more devastating, because the more serious fractures resulted in the inevitable sequence of painful

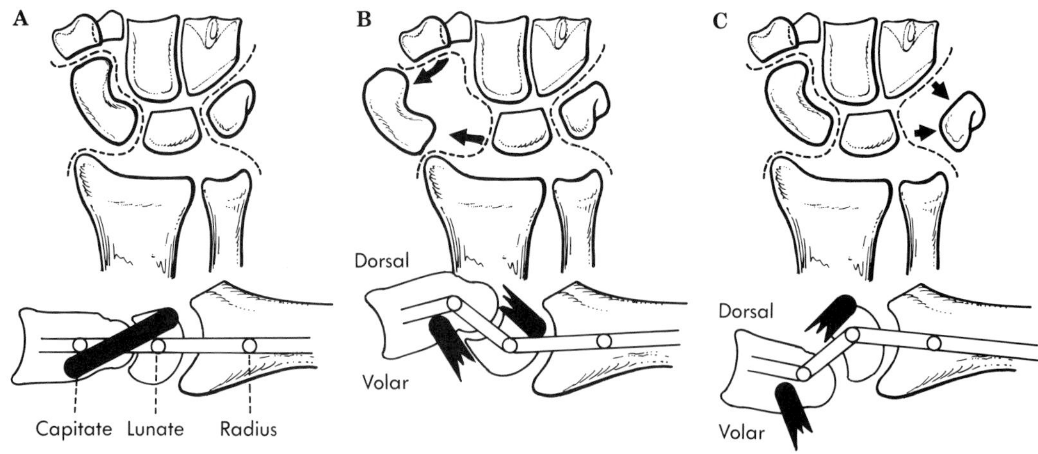

FIG. 23-1. A, Normal wrist function depends largely on preservation of specific shapes and relationships of critical bony links. Integrity of all skeletal components maintains the colinear relationship of the central links as viewed in the sagittal plane. **B,** With destabilization of the scaphoid by fracture, the link system collapses into a predictable dorsal intercalated segment instability (DISI) deformity with excessive dorsal tilting of the lunate. **C,** With destabilization of the triquetrum, the system tends to collapse into a volar intercalated segment instability (VISI) deformity. When wrist fracture occurs, the cardinal rule is to restore anatomic configurations of the disrupted bony links. (Modified from Nathan R, Lester B, and Melone CP, Jr: The acutely injured wrist: an anatomic basis for operative treatment, Orthop Rev 16:80, 1987.)

wrist instability followed by disabling arthritis. More recently, because of a heightened awareness of the functional significance of the intact wrist and of the serious complications associated with neglected fractures of the carpus and distal radius, such instances of unsatisfactory management have precipitously declined. A casual attitude toward wrist fractures among athletes has been supplanted by an intense concern for precision in diagnosis and treatment. No longer is a rapid return to competition the primary goal of either the sports physician or the injured athlete.

This chapter first discusses fundamental principles of management and then describes techniques that have consistently facilitated treatment of specific fractures incurred by athletes. The objective is to provide rational guidelines for treatment of those fractures prevalent among this highly skilled, select group.

PRINCIPLES OF MANAGEMENT

Clearly, the acute injury affords the opportune time for restitution of the fractured wrist. In contrast to the unpredictable and often disappointing results of delayed treatment, the prospects for maximal recovery are greatly improved by prompt, skillful management. In the vast majority of cases, the prevailing causes of fracture complications—delayed diagnosis, unrecognized fracture displacement, faulty immobilization, and premature return to competition—can be avoided by observing basic principles of optimal management.

Diagnostic Considerations

An accurate diagnosis begins with a detailed account of the injury as described by the athlete. The mere mention of certain sports activities should immediately arouse suspicion of specific fractures. For example, football is notorious for the occurrence of scaphoid fractures, skating for distal radius fractures, and stick-handling sports—baseball, golf, tennis, and hockey—for hamate hook (hamulus) fractures. The sport per se is often the first clue to the diagnosis.

Awareness of consistent patterns of injury also facilitates the diagnosis (Fig. 23-2). The usual mechanism is a forcible fall on the outstretched hand that induces a multidimensional force comprising hyperextension, axial compression, ulnar deviation, and intercarpal or radiocarpal supination. In many cases the force impacts on a selective site, causing an isolated fracture of either the carpus or distal radius. Occasionally a similar force results in a simultaneous fracture of the tubercle and waist of the scaphoid or of the scaphoid and the distal radius. In other cases a greater magnitude of force disrupts wider but predictable zones of wrist anatomy.[29,35,36] The greater arc injury, initially traversing the scaphoid, results in transscaphoid or transscaphoid-transcapitate perilunate fracture-dislocation; the lesser arc pattern disrupts the major ligamen-

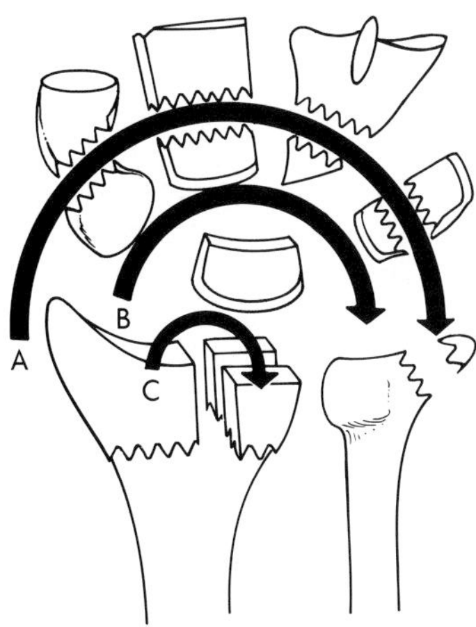

FIG. 23-2. A multidimensional force comprising hyperextension, ulnar deviation, and intercarpal or radiocarpal rotation causes consistent patterns of wrist fracture. **A,** The greater arc injury results in the transscaphoid, transcapitate fracture-dislocation. **B,** The lesser arc injury, traversing the perilunar zone, leads to perilunate or lunate dislocation often associated with fracture of the triquetrum. **C,** A violent compression force transmitted by the carpus disrupts the distal radius articular surface, resulting in predictable types of fracture.

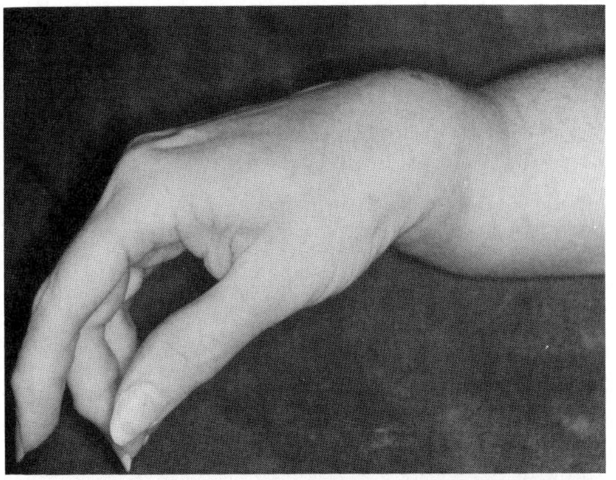

A

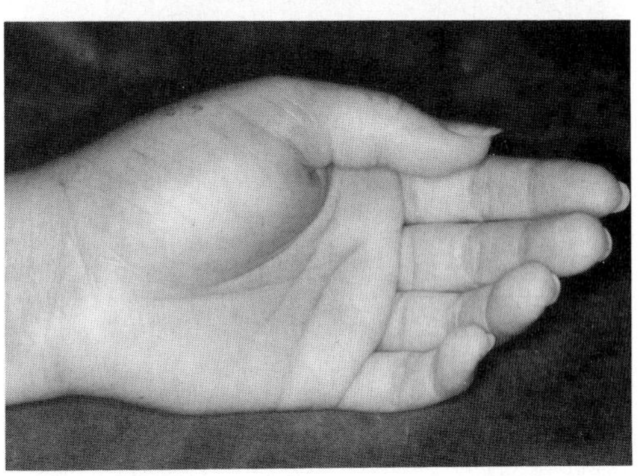

B

FIG. 23-3. A, Displaced fractures of the distal radius as well as those associated with perilunate injuries often result in readily apparent, characteristic deformity. **B,** Most carpal fractures, however, are associated with minimal disfigurement; nonetheless, careful examination of the carpal surface anatomy invariably pinpoints the site of the pathologic condition. In this case, swelling, bruising, and bony tenderness localized to the thenar eminence are highly suggestive of trapezium fracture.

tous support of the wrist, causing perilunate or lunate dislocation, often in association with avulsion fracture of the triquetrum or ulnar styloid. Thus, when a violent fall results in a painfully swollen wrist, one must suspect not only an isolated scaphoid or distal radius fracture but also a more extensive injury that may require treatment of multiple skeletal and soft tissue components. Similarly, one must recognize that a seemingly insignificant triquetrum fracture may be the only obvious evidence of a serious perilunate disruption that requires surgery for restoration of carpal stability.

Another common mechanism of injury is a direct blow to the palm.[9,37,45,54] A frequent result of this pattern is the hamate hook fracture, incurred when the handle of a baseball bat, golf club, tennis racket, or hockey stick forcibly strikes the hypothenar eminence. Less frequently, the trapezial ridge fracture results from a similar force transmitted to the base of the thumb. Since both fractures are elusive to routine roentgenography, they are apt to be overlooked at the time of injury. This problem is considerably lessened with recognition of the common mode of injury, as well as the need for special roentgenographic views to demonstrate the fracture.

The clinical findings of swelling, tenderness, and limited mobility make the diagnosis increasingly apparent. Perilunate fracture-dislocations and distal radius fractures are characterized by an unmistakable deformity with a pronounced loss of wrist motion (Fig. 23-3). In contrast, most carpal fractures are associated with less obvious, often minimal disfigurement and derangement; localized swelling or bruising with discrete bony tenderness is their distinctive feature. Like the classic example of anatomic snuff box swelling and tenderness as presumptive evidence of a scaphoid waist fracture, hypothenar or ulnar wrist swelling and point tenderness indicate hamate hook or pisiform fractures. Similar findings localized to the thenar eminence suggest a trapezial ridge or scaphoid tubercle fracture. A meticulous examination of the carpal surface anatomy invariably pinpoints the site of the pathologic condition.

Clear visualization of the fracture with appropriate roentgenograms of good quality confirms the diagnosis. Unlike those of the radius or ulna, acute fractures of the carpus are not readily demonstrated with routine wrist roentgenography. Special projections are thus an essential part of the standard evaluation (Fig. 23-4). In addition to posteroanterior, oblique, and lateral views, roentgenograms for a suspected scaphoid fracture should include radial and ulnar deviation studies and a clenched fist anteroposterior projection. Ulnar deviation and axial compression induced by the clenched fist exert distraction forces on the scaphoid fragments to illustrate better the fracture, whereas radial deviation, like the oblique view, enhances visualization of fragment displacement. Fracture displacement resulting in carpal instability is best detected on the lateral view that displays abnormal tilting of the lunate with loss of colinear relationships. With minor, albeit signif-

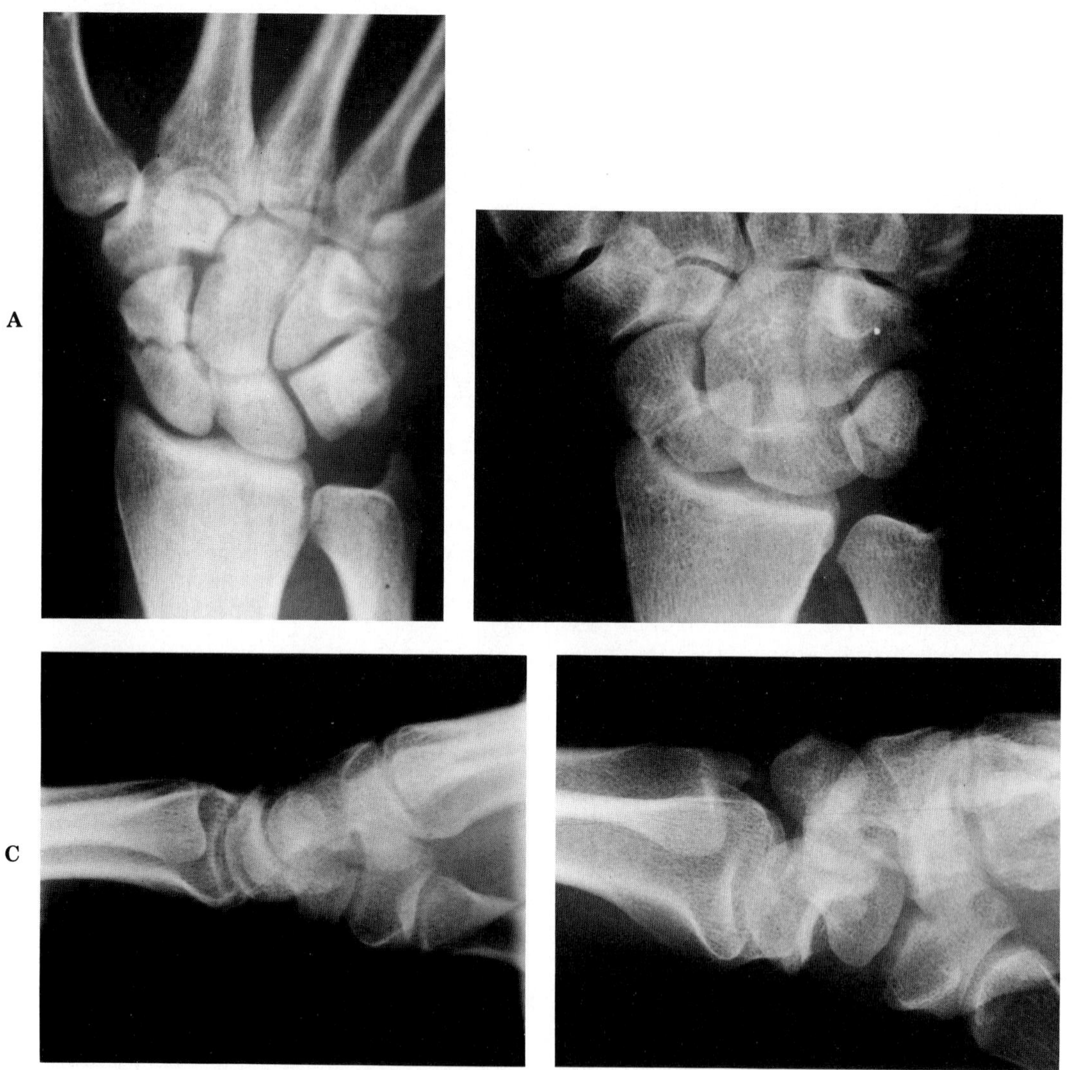

FIG. 23-4. Scaphoid roentgenography. **A,** Ulnar deviation, by virtue of its distraction effect on the scaphoid, enhances visualization of the fracture. **B,** The radial deviation view clearly demonstrates fracture instability with displacement of the fragments. Carpal instability resulting from scaphoid displacement is best illustrated on the lateral projection that displays abnormal tilting of the lunate. **C,** Mild dorsal tilting of the lunate is subtle evidence of fracture instability with displacement. **D,** In contrast, excessive volar tilting of the lunate with its empty articular concavity facing anteriorly (the spilled teacup sign) is a constant feature of the unstable transscaphoid perilunate fracture-dislocation. The distal scaphoid fragment displaces dorsally with the capitate, but the proximal pole remains attached to the volarly situated lunate. In all cases of scaphoid fracture displacement, prompt open reduction with internal fixation is necessary to restore osseous integrity and carpal stability.

Special roentgenographic techniques

Suspected scaphoid fracture
- Radial deviation, anteroposterior view
- Ulnar deviation, anteroposterior view
- Clenched fist, anteroposterior view

Suspected hook of hamate fracture
- Carpal tunnel view
- Oblique in radial deviation
- Lateral with thumb abducted

Suspected trapezial ridge fracture
- Carpal tunnel view

icant, scaphoid displacement, this finding is subtle; however, with the transscaphoid perilunate fracture-dislocation, normal relationships are grossly disturbed and the lateral projection graphically depicts the tilted lunate as a "spilled teacup" (Fig. 23-4, *C* and *D*).

The hamate hook fracture is confirmed by one of several techniques requiring careful positioning of the wrist: a carpal tunnel profile, an oblique view taken with the wrist radially deviated and semisupinated, or a lateral view projected through the first web space with the thumb abducted (Fig. 23-5). Occa-

A

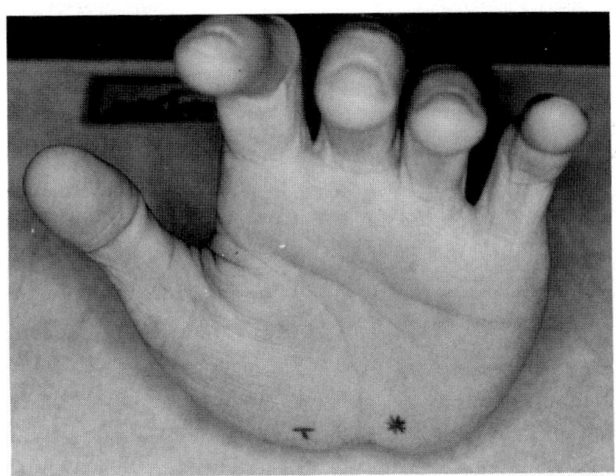

B

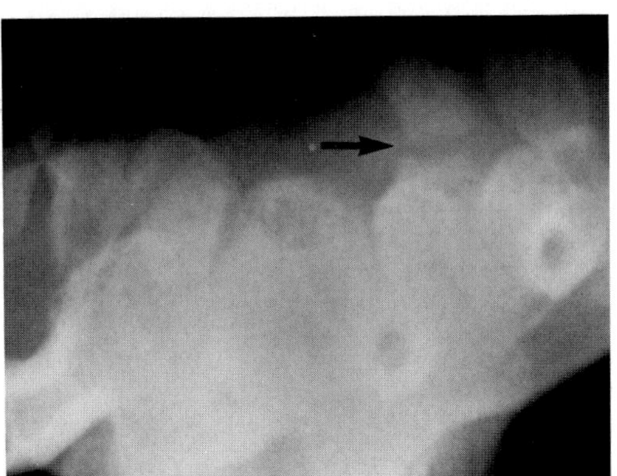

C

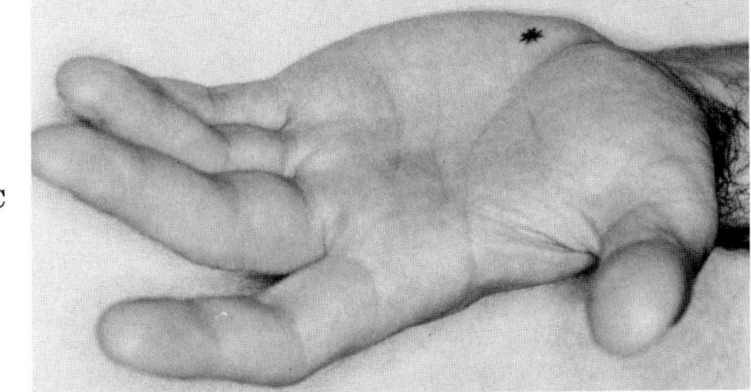

D

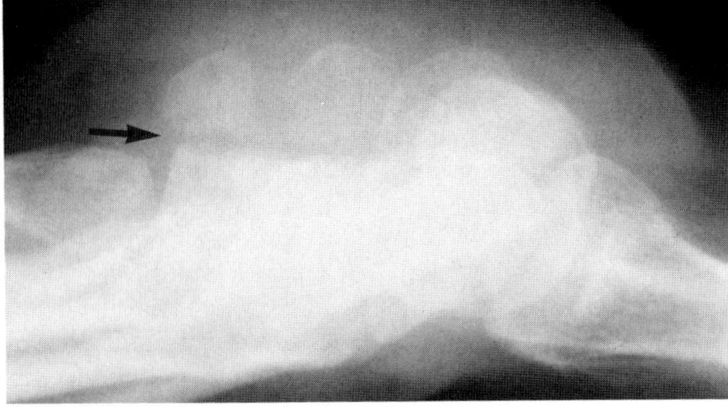

FIG. 23-5. Special roentgenographic projections are necessary to detect the hamate hook fracture *(arrows)*. **A** and **B,** The carpal tunnel profile taken with the wrist hyperextended. **C** and **D,** The oblique view obtained with the wrist radially deviated and semisupinated.

Continued.

E

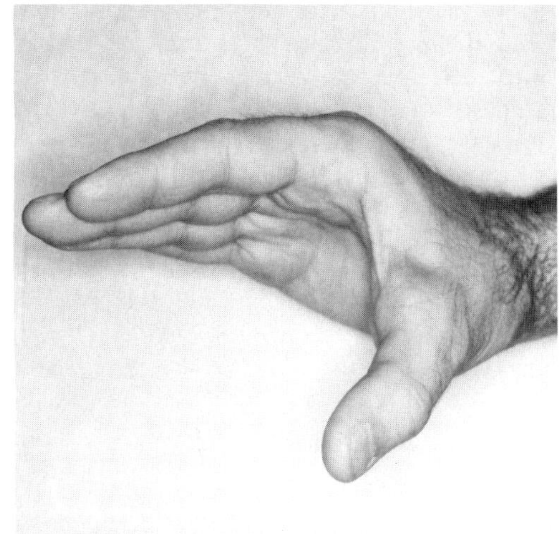

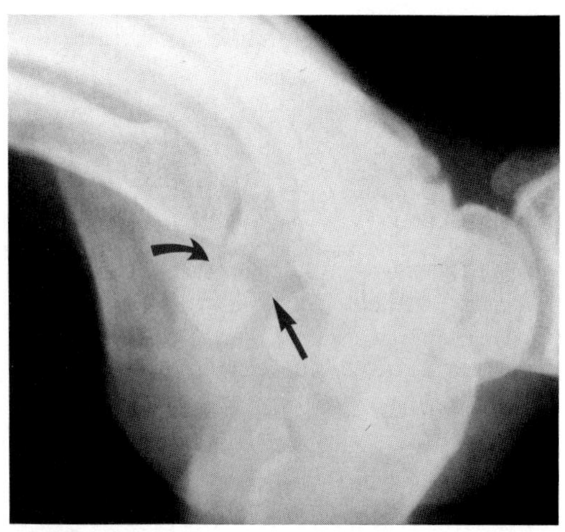

F

FIG. 23-5, cont'd. E and **F,** The lateral view projected through the first web space with the thumb widely abducted.

sionally, lateral tomography may be required to visualize the entire base of the hook. These views occasionally reveal the somewhat confusing presence of a bipartite hamulus—a malformation resulting from separate ossification centers that fail to unite (Fig. 23-6). This incidental finding is distinguished by a discrete, smooth ossicle, usually present bilaterally near the apex of the hook, and should not be mistaken for the fracture that invariably occurs at the base of the hook. The same techniques will clearly visualize a suspected pisiform fracture; the carpal tunnel projection is the essential view for diagnosis of the trapezial ridge fracture (Fig. 23-7).

Careful application of these standard roentgenographic techniques provides sufficient information for optimal management of the vast majority of fractures; nonetheless, uncertain situations are occasionally encountered. In such instances both polycyclic (trispiral) tomography and computed tomography have proved highly accurate methods of diagnosis* (Fig. 23-8). Tomography has also served as a precise means of assessing fracture union in cases with inconclusive plain roentgenograms. In contrast to the efficacy of selective roentgenography and tomography, invasive diagnostic studies are seldom, if ever, warranted for evaluation of the acutely fractured wrist. With awareness of characteristic mechanisms of injury, physical findings, and roentgenographic features, the overlooked "occult" wrist fracture of the athlete is an infrequent occurrence.

*References 4, 6, 8, 12, 19, 48.

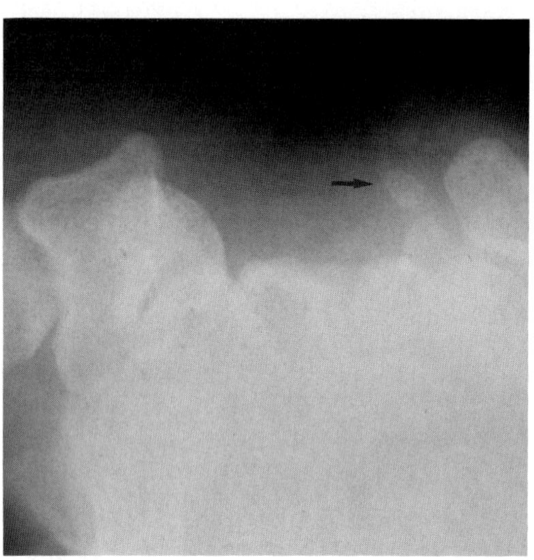

FIG. 23-6. The congenital bipartite hamulus is characterized by a smooth, oval ossicle *(arrow)* located near the apex of the hook and should not be mistaken for a fracture, which invariably occurs at the base of the hook.

Fracture Displacement

The importance of early recognition and correction of fracture displacement cannot be overstated. Displacement, the hallmark of the unstable fracture, retards healing and is the major factor predisposing to the serious complications of nonunion, malunion, wrist instability, and degenerative arthritis. Fracture stability must be promptly secured by anatomic reduction coupled with either external or internal fixation. For the more severe wrist fractures open treatment is mandatory for resto-

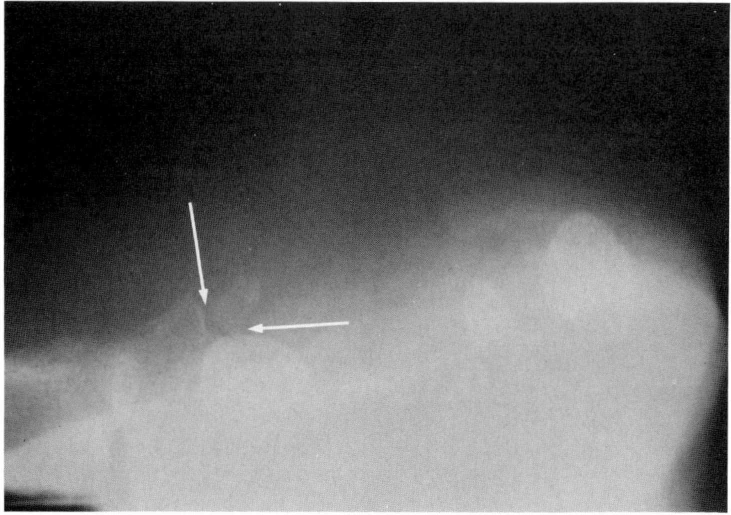

FIG. 23-7. The carpal tunnel profile is the key view for detecting the elusive trapezial ridge fracture *(arrows)*.

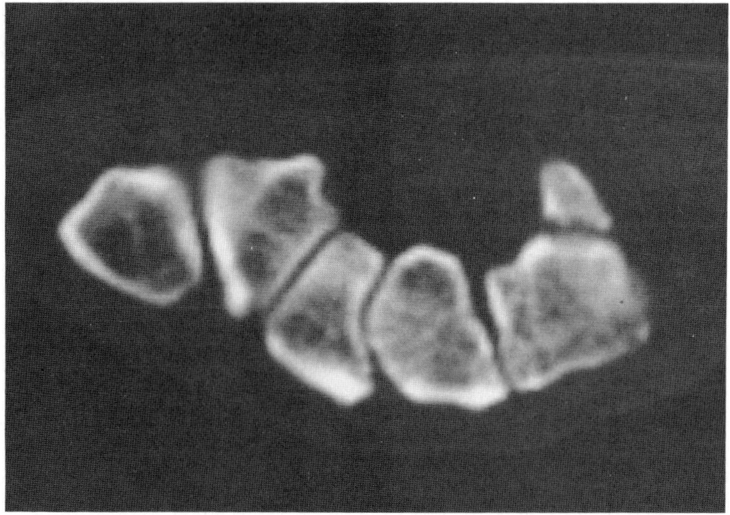

FIG. 23-8. In cases with inconclusive plain roentgenography, computed tomography is a highly accurate method of demonstrating the hamate hook fracture, which in this case is distracted.

ration of osseous integrity and wrist stability. Also, the fundamental principle that displaced articular fractures require open reduction and internal fixation for preservation of joint congruity applies to a considerable number of scaphoid, capitate, trapezium, and distal radius fractures.

Uncomplicated healing of either acute or chronic scaphoid fractures relies on exact apposition of fracture fragments. Even 1 mm of displacement indicates an unstable injury prone to nonunion. Cooney et al[12] reported that 6 (46%) of 13 acute fractures with 1 mm or more displacement failed to unite when treated by closed reduction and cast immobilization. Weber,[62] also employing closed treatment, found a 55% failure rate for 11 acute fractures with greater than 1 mm offset. Eddleland et al[18] experienced an even greater failure rate (92%) for 25 similarly displaced fractures treated with cast immobilization only. Further, Cooney and co-workers,[13] in their extensive review of 90 scaphoid nonunions treated with bone grafting, cited residual fragment displacement as the primary cause of failure. The implication of these experiences is clear: *precise open reduction with internal fixation is the best means of ensuring scaphoid healing for both the acutely displaced fracture and the chronically displaced nonunion.*

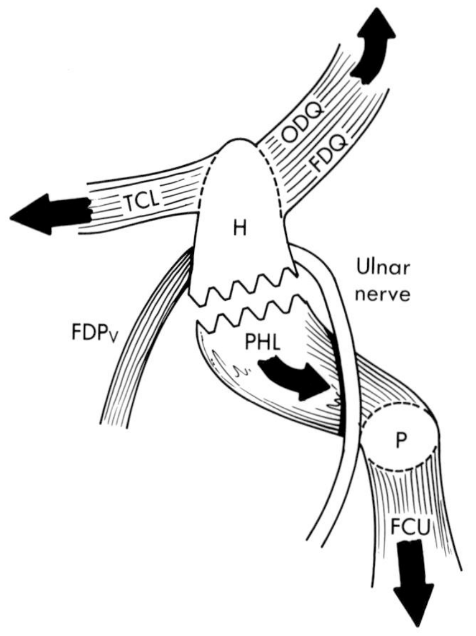

FIG. 23-9. The hamate hook is subject to a multitude of detrimental forces favoring fracture displacement and prejudicing healing. The flexor carpi ulnaris via the pisohamate ligament, the opponens digiti quinti, the flexor digiti quinti, and the transverse carpal ligament exert continuous distraction forces that essentially preclude union of unstable fractures. Because of proximity to the deep motor branch of the ulnar nerve and the deep flexors to the ring and small fingers, the chronic nonunion is prone to cause both compression neuropathy and attritional tendon rupture.

For the scaphoid, as well as the capitate, the degree of fracture displacement is proportional to concurrent ligamentous disruption. The widely displaced scaphoid fracture is a key component of the transscaphoid perilunate fracture-dislocation, whereas the markedly rotated capitate neck fracture invariably is associated with the transscaphoid-transcapitate perilunate fracture-dislocation, termed the "scaphocapitate syndrome." Both types of injury cause a massive derangement of wrist anatomy that must be rectified for preservation of carpal stability. In contrast to increasing dissatisfaction with the results of closed reduction for these transcarpal injuries, evidence is accumulating that a superior recovery can be effected by early open treatment.[1,26,44,48,60] Direct visualization facilitates reduction of the displaced fractures and permits meticulous repair of the disrupted ligaments.

The hamate hook fracture is subject to a multitude of deleterious forces that favor displacement and bias healing. This bony projection provides an insertion for the pisohamate ligament, an origin for the opponens digiti quinti as well as the flexor digiti quinti, and an ulnar purchase for the transverse carpal ligament (Fig. 23-9). Because of these strong soft tissue attachments exerting continuous distraction forces, displacement of the hamate hook is a frequent occurrence. A similar but less common problem occurs with the trapezial ridge fracture because of the distraction force transmitted by the radial attachment of the transverse carpal ligament. In such cases with fracture displacement, union is essentially precluded and prompt excision of the displaced fragment is undoubtedly the best means of affording a rapid, uncomplicated recovery.*

Unstable fractures of the distal radius typically demonstrate fragmentation and collapse of its articular surfaces. Resultant radial shortening creates a major disturbance of both radiocarpal and radioulnar joints. Lidström[33] has demonstrated that radial shortening of only 6 mm is apt to compromise wrist function, and others[46] have indicated that even smaller discrepancies in radial and ulnar length may cause serious articular derangement. Although an unsatisfactory reduction occasionally results in satisfactory function, malunion must be recognized as the common factor predisposing to an unfavorable recovery. Clearly, complications are lessened by restoration of radial length. For most unstable distal radius fractures of the athlete, continuous skeletal traction employing a method of external fixation is necessary to maintain an accurate reduction. For some, open treatment is essential for reduction and fixation of widely displaced articular surfaces, as well as repair of concurrent injury to vital periarticular structures.

In many cases persistent fracture displacement profoundly compromises wrist stability. Chronic instability of the key bony links leads to predictable collapse deformities of the wrist, which have been categorized on the basis of lunate displacement[34] (see Fig. 23-1). With destabilization of the scaphoid, capitate, or distal radius, the dissociated lunate usually shifts dorsally and the wrist is distorted in a characteristic posture termed **dorsal intercalated segment instability** (DISI) deformity. With destabilization of the triquetrum the lunate assumes an excessive volar tilt and the system collapses into a **volar flexion intercalated segment** (VISI) deformity. With either deformity, kinematics are seriously altered and dysfunction is considerable. This

*References 6, 9, 37, 45, 54, 64.

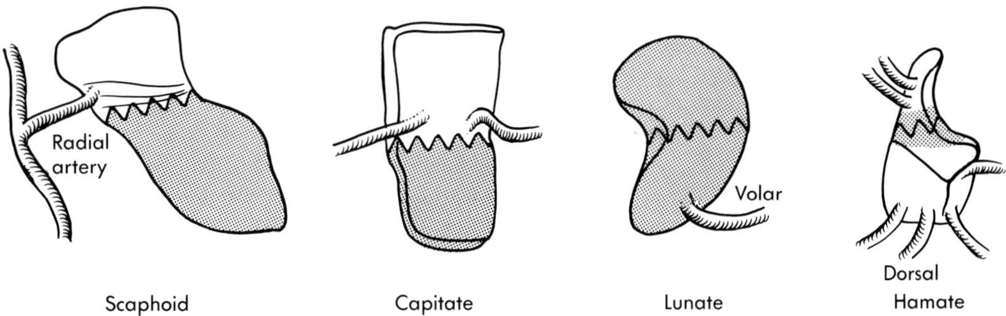

FIG. 23-10. Fracture vascularity. Because of insufficient circulation, the proximal two thirds of the scaphoid, the proximal capitate, the lunate, and the base of the hamate hook *(shaded areas)* are vulnerable to ischemia and avascular necrosis after fracture. Vascular insufficiency is the basis for the prolonged healing time so frequently associated with carpal fractures.

inevitable sequela of uncorrected fracture displacement, namely, instability with disabling deformity, can be prevented by precision management of the acutely injured wrist.

Chronic fracture displacement also poses a serious risk to the integrity of the vital soft tissues traversing the wrist. Owing to alterations in critical anatomic relationships, distal radius malunion and hamate hook nonunion may result in median and ulnar neuropathy.[11,28,41,54] Similarly, chronically malpositioned or ununited bone fragments are apt to cause attritional ruptures of the flexor or extensor tendons.[6,9,10,16,41] Continuous fraying with ultimate rupture of the small finger flexors is a significant complication of chronically ununited hamate hook fractures; ruptures of the deep flexors to the thumb and index finger are associated with malunited distal radius fractures; and rupture of the extensor pollicis longus is liable to result from any malunion or nonunion, which causes a synovitis over the dorsoradial aspect of the wrist. For these ruptures seldom is a totally satisfactory solution available. The frayed, retracted tendon ends generally preclude direct repair, and restoration of tendon integrity usually requires either intercalated grafts or local transfers—procedures limited in their capacity to restore normal function. The delayed occurrence of predictable soft tissue injuries must be recognized as an additional consequence of suboptimal primary care.

Fracture Vascularity

The blood supply of the carpus has been extensively studied by numerous investigators employing varying techniques.[23,24,31,47,58] Although controversy still exists over certain patterns of flow, a consensus prevails that the vascular anatomy of the carpus is a major prognostic factor of fracture healing. Because of relatively insufficient circulation, the proximal two thirds of the scaphoid, the proximal capitate, the entire lunate (in a significant percentage of persons), and the base of the hamate hook are vulnerable to ischemia and avascular necrosis after fracture (Fig. 23-10). Vascular insufficiency is, in fact, the basis for the characteristically prolonged healing time of carpal fractures.

Areas vulnerable to avascular necrosis

- Proximal two thirds of the scaphoid
- Proximal capitate
- Lunate
- Base of hamate hook

Fracture ischemia, however, should not be considered an insuperable obstable to healing nor should avascular necrosis (as evidenced by increased radiodensity of the affected area) be regarded as an irreversible process of carpal destruction.[40,48] With prompt and continued treatment, union can be expected in the vast majority of cases and will be followed by revascularization (see Fig. 23-14, *H* and *I*). Fracture healing with vascular ingrowth and new bone formation provides the basis for reconstitution of the devitalized area. Following union, the opaque area of necrosis gradually regains its normal density over a period of several months.

The major blood supply of the scaphoid arises from the radial artery and enters principally the waist or dorsoradial ridge of the bone. Although the distal scaphoid has an independent circulation, the proximal two thirds of the bone relies on an intraosseous retrograde blood flow and is therefore prone to ischemia with all fractures at or proximal to the waist. Because about 80% of scaphoid fractures occur in this vulnerable area, prolonged healing should be anticipated in most cases. Also, because of the retrograde perfusion, the more proximal the fracture, the greater will be the interference with circulation and the time of healing. Union of optimally managed waist fractures averages about 3 months, whereas fractures of the proximal one third or one fourth rarely unite in less than 4 months. In contrast, fractures of the tubercle are generally united within 6 weeks and those of the distal one third within 8 weeks.

The proximal capitate is also dependent on an intraosseous retrograde blood supply. Like the proximal scaphoid, the head and neck of the capitate are subjected to a major vascular disruption when fractured; hence, healing is similarly prolonged, often requiring several months of continuous immobilization. It is estimated that between 8% and 26% of lunates receive their nutrition from one artery, usually entering the volar surface of the bone.[24,31] This paucity of circulation in a substantial number of persons places the fractured lunate at a high risk for pronounced ischemia with an excessive healing time.

Panagis and co-workers[47] have defined the base of the hamate hook as another potentially high risk site for ischemia following trauma. The major portion of the hook and the body of the hamate derive their blood supply from separate sources that demonstrate few, if any, intraosseous connections. The base of the hook (the usual site of fracture) has no independent nutrient vessels and, devoid of an intrinsic vascular network, essentially is an avascular area with a limited capacity for healing. The lack of vascularity at this critical site unfavorably affects the prospects for union, and, at best, a lengthy healing process should be anticipated for undisplaced hamate hook fractures.

Fracture vascularity is also an important factor in the formulation of plans for surgery. Mainly because of concern about jeopardizing circulation, opinions vary regarding the best approach to the scaphoid. Some surgeons favor a dorsal exposure, whereas others advocate a volar approach for open reduction and internal fixation as well as bone grafting.* Ample evidence now exists that neither approach adversely affects the blood supply provided the critical vascular leash arising from the radial aspect of the bone and attaching to the waist is not disturbed. A direct radial approach through the anatomic snuff box, however, should be avoided, because it not only causes a serious threat to the critical blood supply but also precludes extensile exposure. The capitate, like the scaphoid, can be safely exposed from either its dorsal or volar surface as long as the crucial and clearly visible vascular network at the distal end of the bone is not sacrificed. In contrast, the dorsal approach to the lunate is preferentially employed, since it avoids the key palmar artery and affords superior exposure. The dorsal approach also averts interruption of the volarly situated radiocarpal ligaments, the major soft tissue stabilizers of the wrist.

Fracture Immobilization

Providing prompt effective immobilization and avoiding premature discontinuance of immobilization are absolute prerequisites for successful fracture union. Although some debate persists as to what constitutes optimal casting techniques, clearly, the mechanism of injury, the type of fracture, and the potential deforming forces must be carefully considered in developing logical guidelines for effective immobilization.

With scaphoid fractures, excessive thumb motion, wrist hyperextension, and ulnar deviation induce forces predisposing to displacement that must be eliminated. This is accomplished by employing a thumb spica cast maintaining the mildly flexed wrist in radial deviation. In addition to impacting the fracture fragments and reducing stress on damaged volar soft tissues, this position of wrist immobilization induces flexion of the lunate, thereby counteracting its tendency for instability with dorsal tilting so frequently associated with scaphoid fractures. The length of the cast is determined by the level and plane of fracture. Most fractures at or proximal to the waist are oblique to the longitudinal axis of the wrist—an arrangement rendering them particularly susceptible to shearing forces created by forearm rotation and transmitted to the scaphoid by the obliquely oriented radiocarpal ligaments. The deleterious effect of pronation and supination is minimized by extending the cast to incorporate the humeral epicondyles (Fig. 23-11, *A*). Thus effective immobilization for fractures of the proximal two thirds of the scaphoid must include the following features: (1) incorporation of the humeral epicondyles to block forearm rotation, (2) incorporation of the thumb to its interphalangeal (IP) joint, and (3) maintenance of the wrist in slight palmar flexion and radial deviation. Fractures of the distal third

*References 13, 26, 27, 40, 44, 51.

A 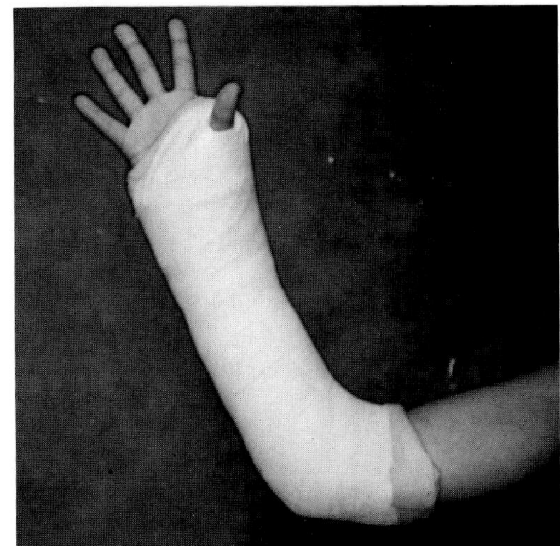

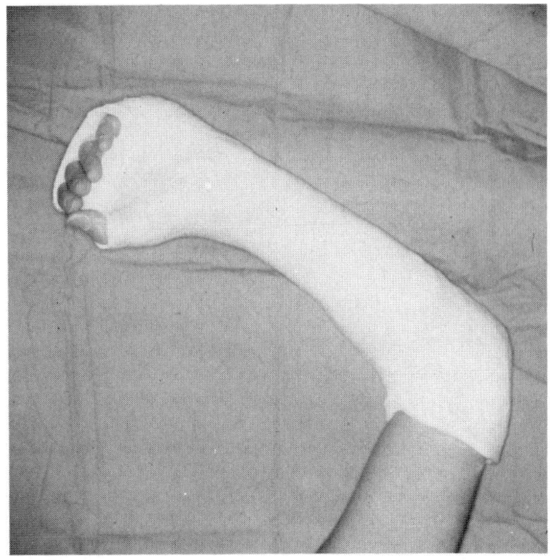 B

FIG. 23-11. A, Effective immobilization for fractures of the proximal two thirds of the scaphoid maintains the wrist in mild palmar flexion and radial deviation, incorporates the humeral epicondyles to block forearm rotation, and includes the thumb to its interphalangeal joint. **B,** Incorporating the finger metacarpophalangeal joints reduces the enormous compression forces generated by grasping—forces that are especially detrimental to healing of the fractured lunate.

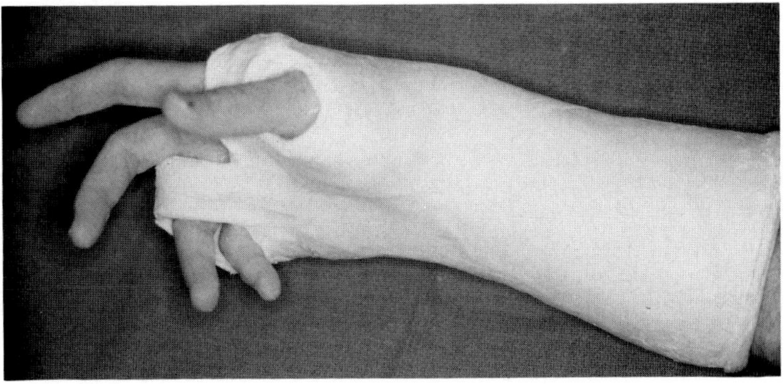

FIG. 23-12. Effective casting for undisplaced hamate hook fractures must neutralize the deforming forces of multiple soft tissue attachments. The wrist is maintained in mild flexion and the metacarpophalangeal joints of the ring and small fingers in acute flexion. The base of the thumb is also immobilized to prevent distraction forces transmitted via the transverse carpal ligament.

of the scaphoid, as well as those of the tubercle, have a much more adequate blood supply and are subject to far less stress. For these injuries that require less protection, a below-elbow cast provides sufficient immobilization.

The lunate fracture, even if undisplaced, should always be considered a precursor of avascular necrosis, fragmentation, and Kienböck's disease. Immobilization must afford maximal protection of this potentially fragile bone. In addition to the same criteria for fractures of the proximal scaphoid, casting of the lunate should include the flexed metacarpophalangeal joints of the fingers (Fig. 23-11, *B*). Incorporation of the most proximal finger joints substantially reduces the enormous compressive forces generated by grasping. These forces, unconstrained and continually absorbed by an ischemic lunate, constitute a major threat to further devitalization with fragmentation.

With hamate hook fractures the deforming forces created by the multiple soft tissue attachments (see Fig. 23-9) need to be neutralized. Comprehensive immobilization is provided by casting the wrist in slight flexion and the metacarpophalangeal (MCP) joints of the ring and small fingers in acute flexion. The cast also includes the base of the thumb, thereby preventing the distraction force evoked by the thenar musculature and transmitted to the hook via the transverse carpal ligament (Fig. 23-12).

Displaced extraarticular fractures of the

distal radius successfully manipulated by closed techniques rely heavily on precise casting for postreduction stability. A well-molded cast is essential to prevent the frequent problem of redisplacement. The cast holds the wrist in mild flexion and incorporates the base of the thumb as well as the humeral epicondyles to militate against detrimental forces occurring at the fracture site. Stability is augmented by selective positioning of the forearm: pronation is employed for Colles' fractures and supination for Smith's fractures. In contrast, extreme positioning of the wrist must be avoided as a potential source of major complications; for example, forced palmar flexion (the Cotton-Loder position) is notorious for causing median nerve compression and disastrous joint contractures of the wrist and digits.

As a basic rule, immobilization must be continued until thorough healing is demonstrated on the roentgenograms. The essential criterion for union is bony trabeculation across the fracture site with obliteration of the fracture line as illustrated on all roentgenographic views (Figs. 23-13, *F*, 23-14, *I*, and 23-15, *H*). For distal radius or ulna fractures the healing process is clearly visible; carpal fractures, in contrast, have no appreciable periosteal component to healing, so conspicuous callus formation is seldom present. If the quality of union cannot be ascertained with plain roentgenograms, an accurate assessment requires tomograms. Since healing is slow in wrist fractures, the time of immobilization often entails a minimum of 8 weeks. The considerable frustration evoked by this lengthy period must be alleviated by repeated reinforcement to the athlete that compliance with appropriate casting is an investment consistently rewarded by a favorable outcome.

Return to Competition

Strict guidelines for returning to unrestricted activities are difficult to establish for the athlete who is always vulnerable to injury. A rational decision requires careful consideration of many factors: the type of fracture, the thoroughness of healing, the extent of rehabilitation, and the patient's age, sport, special skills, and level of competition. For fear of reinjury with growth disturbance, an adolescent football player with a distal radius epiphyseal fracture should not resume contact until healing and remodeling of the growth plate are completed and normal function is demonstrated—a period as long as 4 months. In contrast, a professional baseball player might return to the lineup 4 weeks after excision of a hamate hook fracture with minimal risk of further damage.

Certain exceptions notwithstanding, the basic requisites for returning to competition are complete healing of the fracture as well as any concomitant soft tissue injuries and thorough rehabilitation with restoration of a painless, functional arc of wrist motion and near-normal strength. Only with maximal recovery can the risk of reinjury with further impairment be minimized. Also, because of its constant exposure to violent forces, the rehabilitated wrist, whenever possible, should be protected from further trauma. Gloves and rubber casts are usually permissible at all levels of competition, whereas plastic splints and even fiberglass or plaster casts are often allowed in the professional ranks. Custom-fit devices that enhance security against injury yet permit the desired degree of wrist mobility are now available and have become standard equipment for many sports.[3,5,38] With continual improvement in materials and designs, protective gloves and splints will undoubtedly decrease the incidence of wrist fracture and refracture among athletes. For example, a glove with precise contouring and padding of the palm is likely to minimize hamate hook or trapezial ridge fractures; it also will lessen the possibility of reinjury at sites previously requiring surgery.

Attempting to lessen the prolonged morbidity so frequently associated with the athlete's fractured wrist, an increasing number of physicians have permitted an early return to sports activities after certain undisplaced fractures. If the fracture has been judged stable and the acute symptoms of injury have resolved, the athlete resumes competition in a carefuly molded silicone wrist cast. Repeated cast changes are necessary to maintain effective immobilization, and careful roentgenographic surveillance is essential to ensure preservation of fracture stability and uncomplicated healing. With skillful and judicious employment of these techniques, uncompromised healing has been reported for various wrist fractures, including those of the scaphoid.[5,39,50] It needs to be emphasized, however, that for the majority of athletes, unrestrained activity before fracture union constitutes an unacceptable risk of serious complications that should be avoided. Further, even the foremost advocates of early competition with protective casts would agree that unstable wrist fractures requiring internal fixation should not be prematurely subjected to excessive forces. Despite protection afforded by fiberglass or plaster casts, hardware breakage or fracture displacement is apt to occur.

SPECIFIC INJURIES

Scaphoid Fractures

Experience bears out that with precise management of this most frequently injured and troublesome carpal bone, namely, the scaphoid, uncompromised healing can be achieved in greater than 95% of the cases.* Undisplaced fractures invariably respond to early continuous immobilization. Even in cases treated as late as 2 months after injury union can be expected if the fracture is stable and the immobilization effective. It needs to be emphasized, however, that since the slightest displacement essentially precludes healing, one must carefully assess the roentgenograms before concluding that the fracture is undisplaced and suitable for continuous casting. Also, because seemingly stable fractures may subsequently displace after the onset of treatment, continual roentgenographic surveillance is important during the relatively lengthy period of immobilization. The athlete must recognize that a term of relative inactivity approaching 6 months may prove necessary for optimal treatment and that patient compliance is critical to successful recovery.

The concept of an early return to competition with protective casting for unhealed, undisplaced fractures is attractive to those physicians and athletes experiencing the frustrations so frequently associated with the prolonged treatment of scaphoid injuries. Although the dual objective of active participation and concurrent fracture union has been accomplished in some instances,[50] the ununited scaphoid, regardless of protection, is always vulnerable to the hazardous and unpredictable forces of competitive sports. For the majority of athletes, the substantial risk of nonunion with its serious consequences clearly eclipses the transient benefits of a speedy return to sports. As policy consistent with sound judgment, the return to competition employing custom-fit devices for protection of the unhealed scaphoid should be reserved for highly select cases of stable fractures in athletes competing with either minimal risk of further damage or under exigent circumstances. Active participation of a professional athlete with an undisplaced distal third fracture might be permissible, whereas that of a high school football player with a potentially unstable proximal pole fracture is ill advised.

A consensus exists that displaced fractures require open reduction and internal fixation in an anatomic position. For the acute injury uncomplicated by carpal instability a volar approach (see Fig. 23-13) between the flexor carpi radialis and the radial artery affords ex-

*References 13, 18, 29, 40, 51, 56, 64.

Position for scaphoid fracture immobilization

- Slight wrist volar flexion and radial deviation
- Cast incorporates humeral epicondyles
- Thumb incorporated (to IP joint)

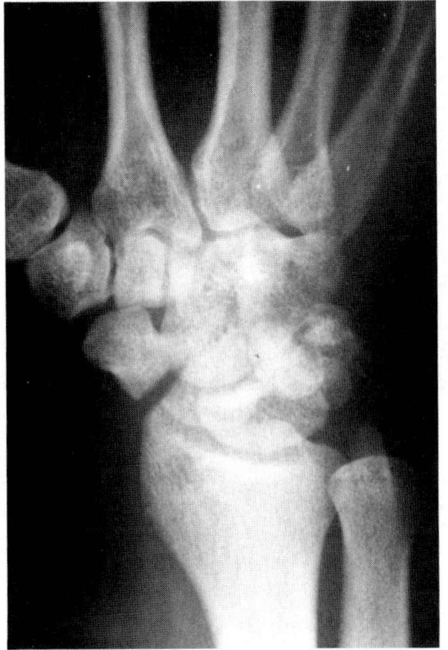

FIG. 23-13. A, An acutely displaced scaphoid fracture treated by prompt open reduction with Kirschner wire fixation. **B,** A volar approach between the flexor carpi radialis (FCR) and the radial artery provides excellent exposure for precise reduction and stabilization.

Continued.

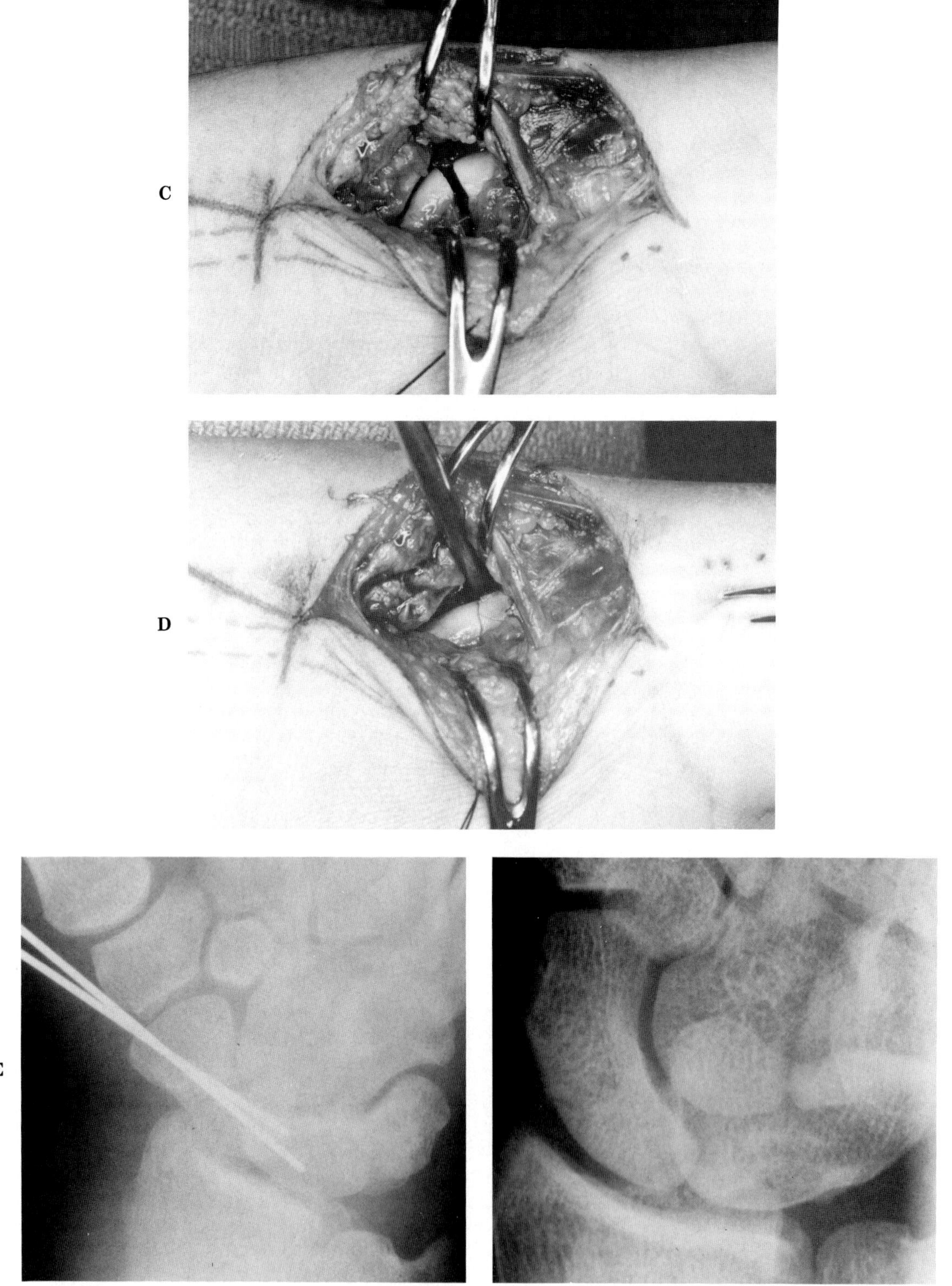

FIG. 23-13, cont'd. C, Judicious reflection of the wrist joint capsule permits clear visualization of widely displaced fracture fragments, which are, **D,** anatomically reduced. **E,** Securely fixed with fine wires. **F,** Twelve weeks after surgery roentgenographic union is demonstrated.

cellent exposure for reduction and stabilization, as well as repair of concomitant scapholunate ligament injury that is apt to occur with the more proximal fractures. Because of longstanding favorable experience, the majority of surgeons prefer conventional Kirschner wires for fixation. Despite renewed enthusiasm for rigid screw fixation,[27] this technique is difficult without substantially adding to damage in the area that is prone to compromise healing. Moreover, even with technical success, the fractured scaphoid should not be prematurely subjected to the deleterious forces created by early motion and active sports competition. The use of screw fixation for the athlete's acutely displaced scaphoid remains a controversial topic.

Personal experience with 21 acutely displaced fractures sustained by highly competitive athletes affirms the efficacy of prompt open reduction and internal fixation with Kirschner wires. Uncomplicated roentgenographic union has occurred, on the average, 10 weeks after surgery; rapid and thorough rehabilitation has been the rule, and return to competition has averaged 15 weeks postoperatively.

For displaced fractures associated with carpal dislocation (transscaphoid perilunate fracture-dislocation) combined volar and dorsal exposures provide optimal access to the extensive osseous and soft tissue damage (see Fig. 23-14). Through the dorsal approach an anatomic reduction of the scaphoid as well as the disrupted carpal articulations is achieved and stability is maintained by Kirschner

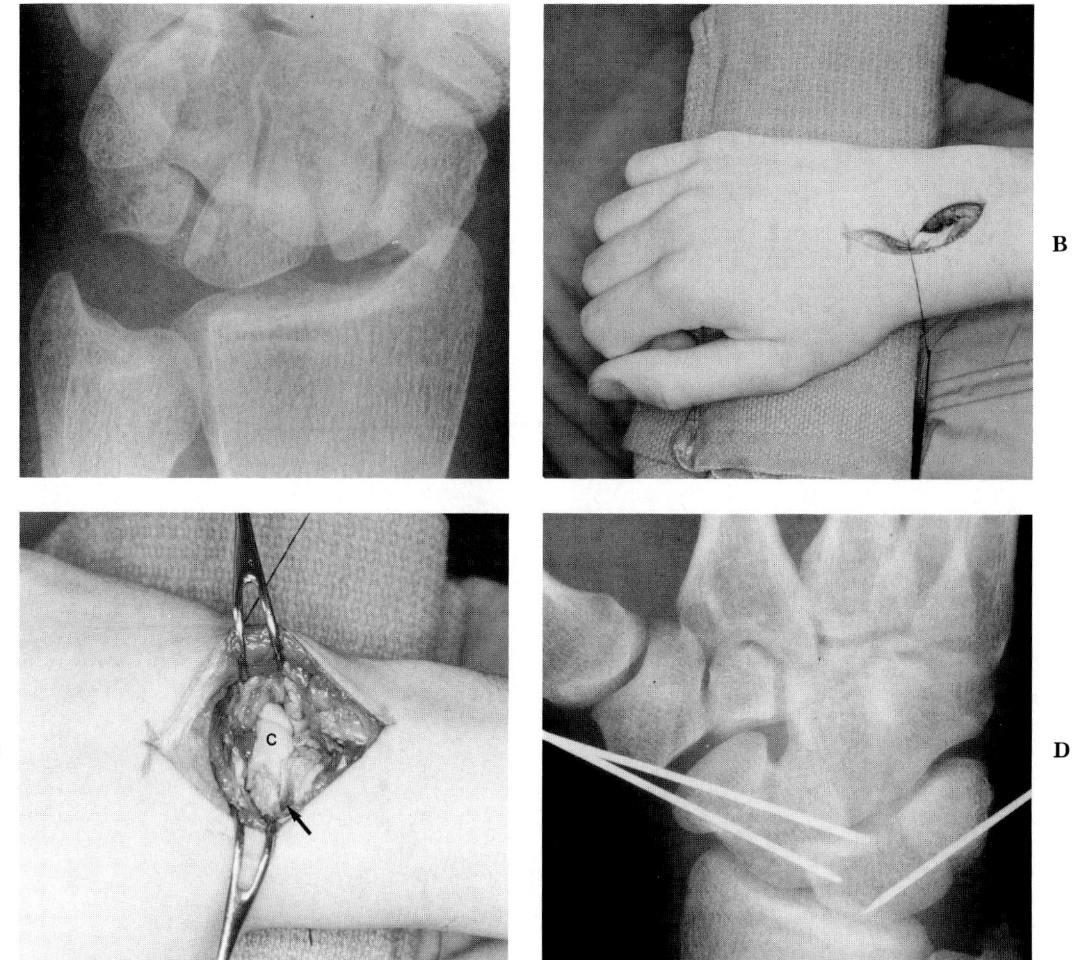

FIG. 23-14. A, Marked scaphoid displacement associated with the transscaphoid perilunate fracture-dislocation. As a preliminary step that considerably facilitates patient comfort and alleviates pressure on contused nerves, the midcarpal dislocation is reduced by closed manipulation. Fracture displacement as well as residual carpal dissociation is then corrected by combined dorsal and volar operative approaches. **B,** The dorsal approach. **C,** The displaced scaphoid *(arrow)* and the residual carpal subluxation *(C)* are clearly identified. **D,** Reduction and stabilization with Kirschner wires.

Continued.

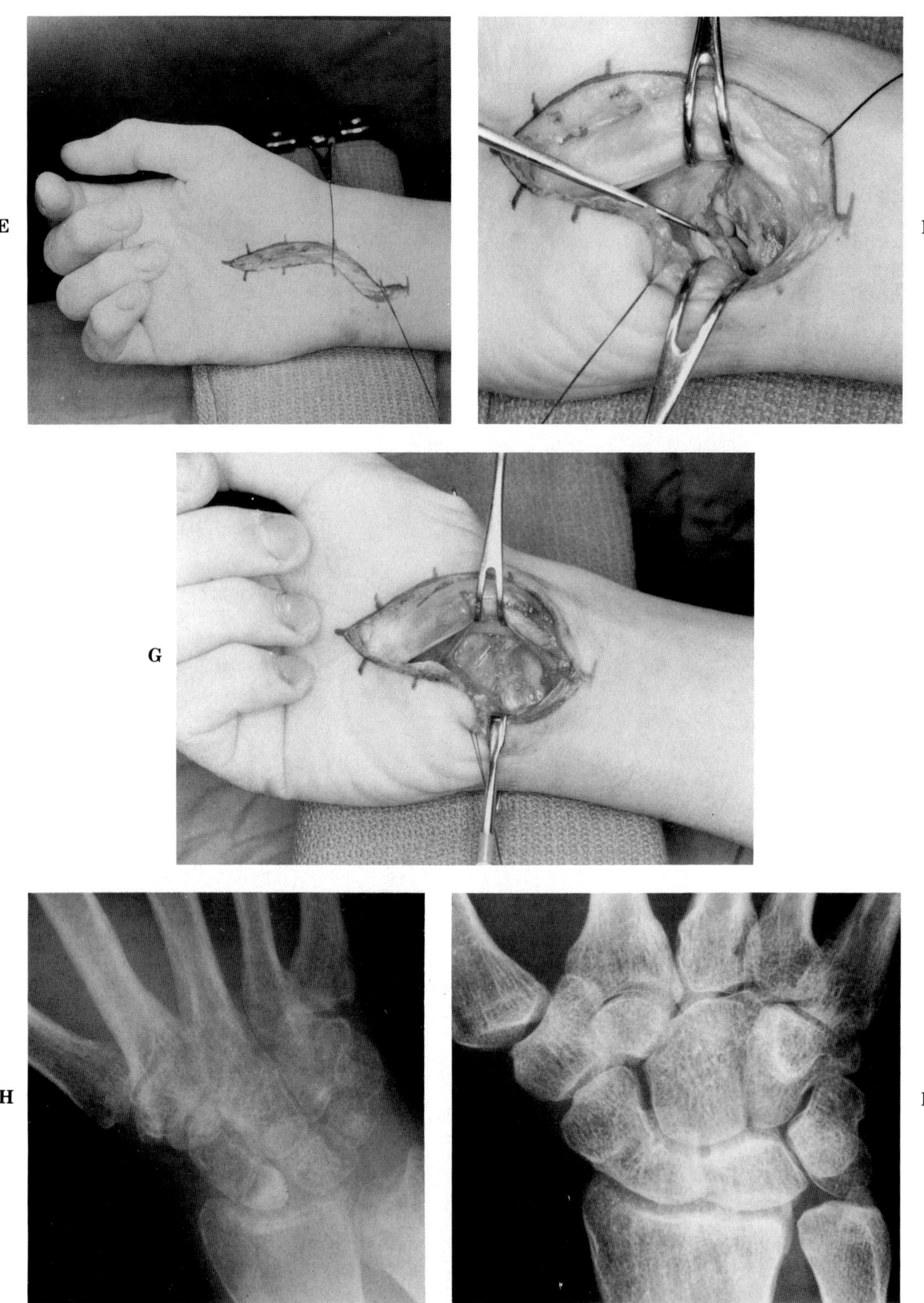

FIG. 23-14, cont'd. E, The volar exposure permits thorough decompression of contused nerves. **F,** The volar exposure also provides access to the critical soft tissue injury that invariably involves the major substances of the perilunar ligaments (at the tip of the probe). **G,** Meticulous repair of the disrupted volar ligamentous structure ensures maximal restitution of midcarpal and lunotriquetral stability. **H,** Eight weeks after surgery the scaphoid proximal pole demonstrates increased radiodensity indicative of avascular necrosis; however, **I,** continuous immobilization results in fracture union with revascularization and preservation of carpal relationships.

wires. The volar approach permits repair of the critical soft tissue injury that invariably involves the major substance of the key radiocarpal ligaments. In my experience, this combined surgical approach has consistently resulted in scaphoid union with preservation of carpal stability and a favorable functional recovery. Despite the enormous magnitude of this injury with its inevitable loss of some wrist mobility, most persons are able to resume their former activities after completing a comprehensive therapy program. However, the interval between injury and return to activity often exceeds 9 months, and in no case should this seriously injured wrist be prematurely subjected to excessive force.

Bone grafting as an osteogenic stimulus is indicated principally for the displaced fracture initially treated 6 or more weeks after injury and for the chronic nonunion of 4 or more months' duration. Once nonunion is detected, operative treatment should be recommended as the only reliable means of obtaining healing and preventing ultimate osteoarthritis. Neither small proximal fragments nor avascular necrosis contraindicates the procedure, which in most cases can be electively planned to cause the least interference with the athlete's career. The operation is performed through a volar zigzag incision that provides excellent access to both the scaphoid nonunion and the distal radius as the bone graft donor site (Fig. 23-15). Fibrous tissue is excised and sclerotic

A

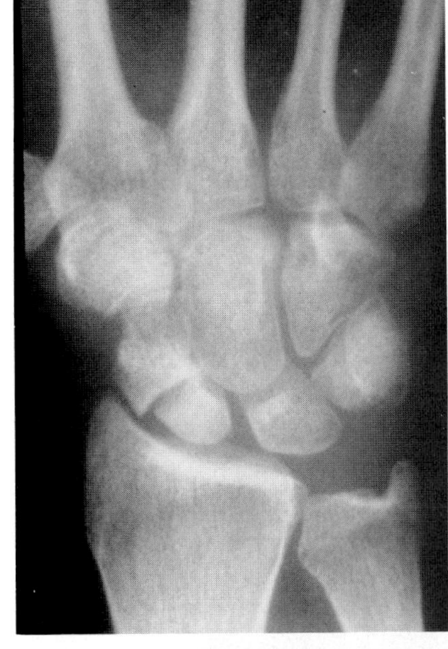

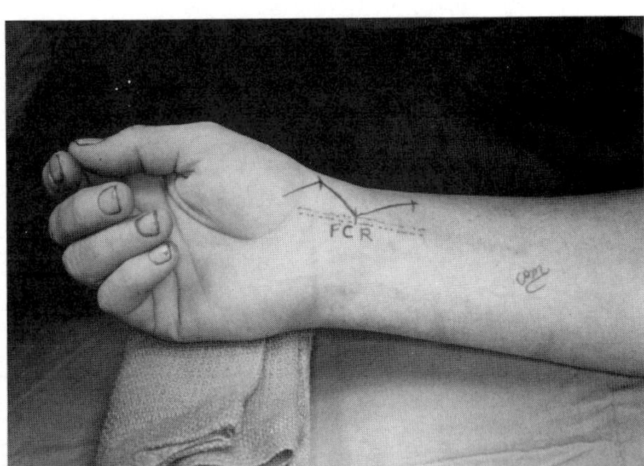

B

C

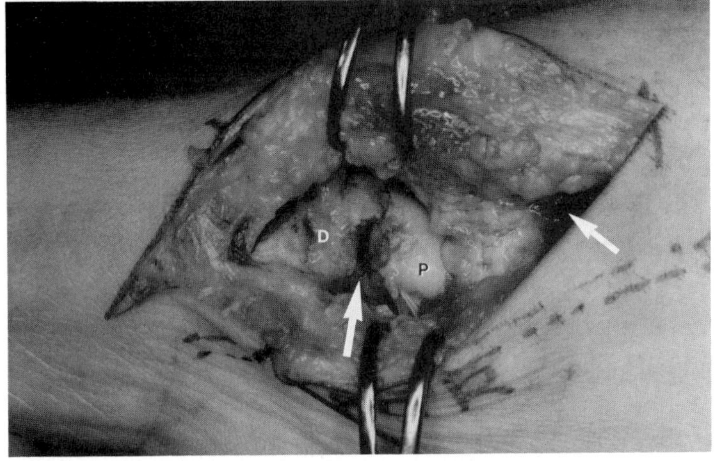

FIG. 23-15. A, Sixteen-month-old scaphoid nonunion treated by bone grafting and adjunctive postoperative pulsing electromagnetic fields. **B,** A volar zigzag incision provides excellent access to both the nonunion and the distal radius as a bone graft donor site. **C,** A wide gap *(left arrow)* filled with fibrous tissue and synovial fluid separates the proximal *(P)* and distal *(D)* fragments. The arrow to the right identifies the distal radius donor site.

Continued.

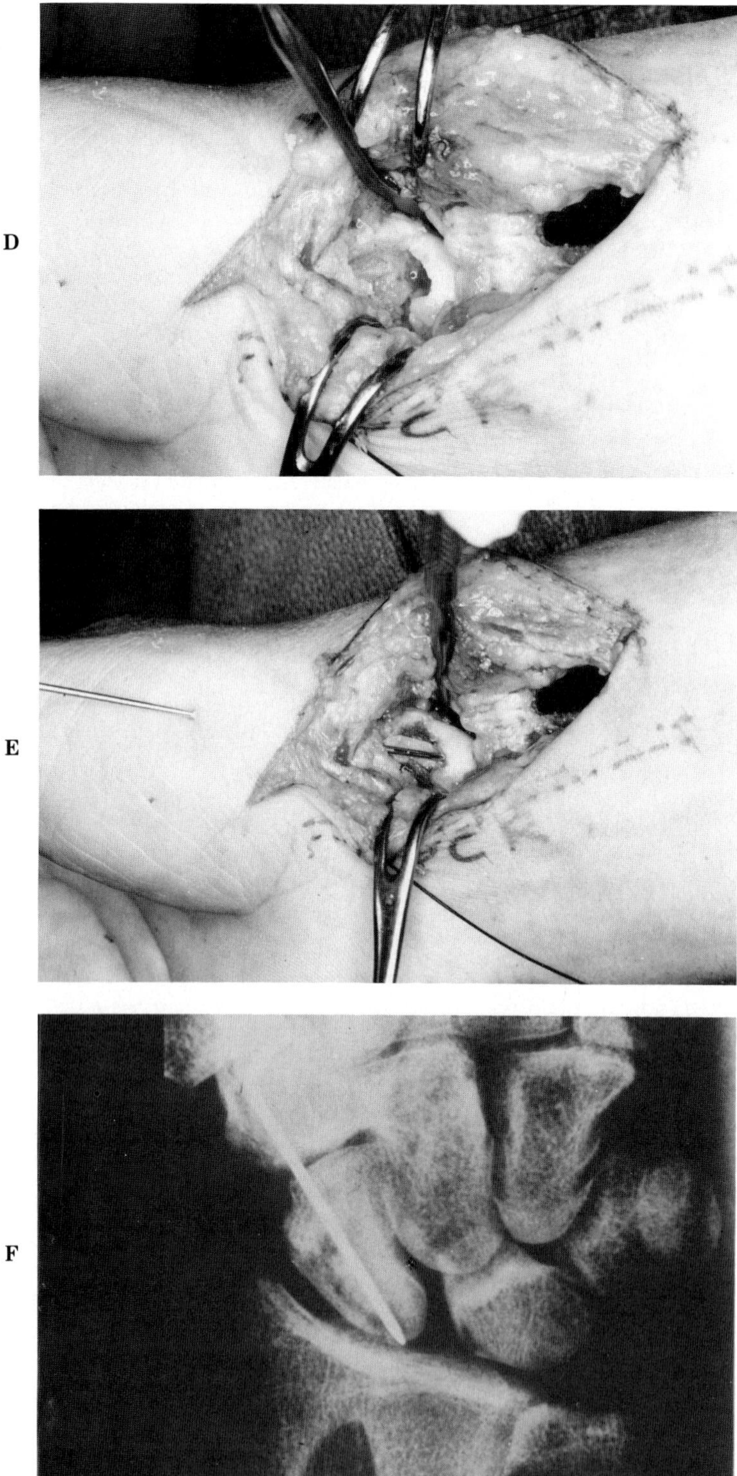

FIG. 23-15, cont'd. D, The fragments have been anatomically reduced and excavated for insertion of the bone graft. **E,** Cancellous bone is packed around a corticocancellous strut, and secure fixation is achieved with a Kirschner wire. **F,** The roentgenogram taken after surgery demonstrates an anatomic reduction and obliteration of the fracture with the graft.

G 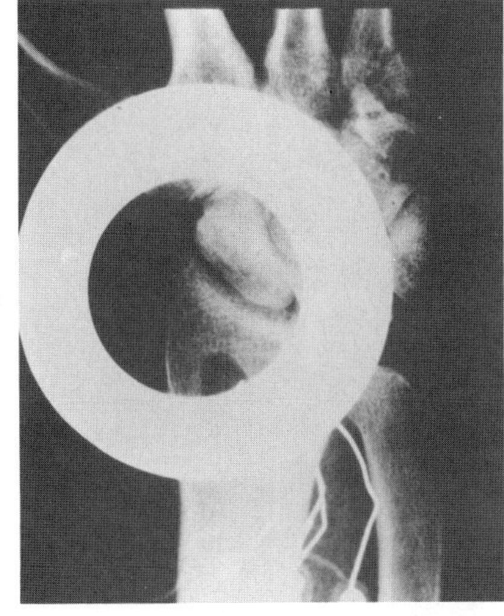

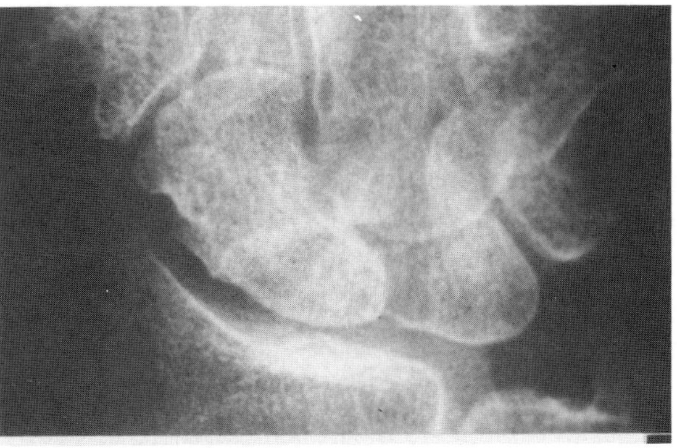 H

FIG. 23-15, cont'd. G, Five weeks postoperatively the wire has been removed and coils for application of electrical stimulation have been incorporated in the cast. **H,** Seventeen weeks after surgery the roentgenogram demonstrates incorporation of the graft and union.

bone debrided at the juncture of the ununited fragments. Both fragments are then excavated, creating a healthy host bed for insertion of the bone graft. The critical and most difficult step of the procedure is an anatomic reduction of the fragments, which are then secured with Kirschner wires. A perfect reduction is essential for uncomplicated endosteal healing, and stable fixation minimizes motion between the graft and its bed, thereby promoting rapid revascularization and union. Postoperatively, cast immobilization must be continued until roentgenographic union is clearly evident. In a personal series employing these techniques for 70 consecutive nonunions, with a 12-month average interval between fracture and surgery, union has occurred in 65 (93%) of the cases. Healing has averaged 5 months and consistently has been followed by a return to sports 3 to 4 months thereafter. Recently, in an effort to accelerate the recovery process, noninvasive electrical stimulation employing pulsing electromagnetic fields (PEMFs) has been added to the postoperative regimen. An analysis of 18 such cases indicates that adjunctive electricity, by virtue of its synergism with bone grafting, significantly reduces the time to union. Patients receiving PEMFs have healed more rapidly regardless of fracture location or the presence of avascular necrosis. This preliminary experience suggests that the use of adjuvant electricity in the treatment of scaphoid nonunion can safely expedite the athlete's recovery.

Indications for bone grafting

- Chronic nonunion greater than 4 months
- Displaced fractures receiving initial treatment 6 or more weeks after injury
- Acute, displaced comminuted fracture

When confronted with an ununited scaphoid, one should make every attempt to preserve osseous integrity of this vital carpal link. In the management of the injured athlete there is virtually no place for such procedures as styloidectomy, carpectomy, implant arthroplasty, or arthrodesis. These are salvage operations reserved for select cases of irreparable scaphoid injury complicated by osteoarthritis.

Hamate Hook Fractures

Any athlete who forcibly swings a sports device is liable to sustain the impact of the handle against the hypothenar eminence, thereby fracturing the vulnerable hook. Since the wrist nearest the handle is susceptible, the nondominant side is typically affected among baseball players and golfers, whereas the dominant side is affected in racquet sports.* The hamate hook fracture truly is a sports-specific problem that undoubtedly can be lessened by preventive measures: coaching to enhance one's stick- or racquet-handling ability, devising more secure grips on sports equipment, and fabricating precisely contoured protective gloves. Nonetheless, the hook fracture remains a frequent occurrence

Editor's note: These fractures also can result from a sudden, forceful contraction of the hypothenar intrinsic muscles.

A

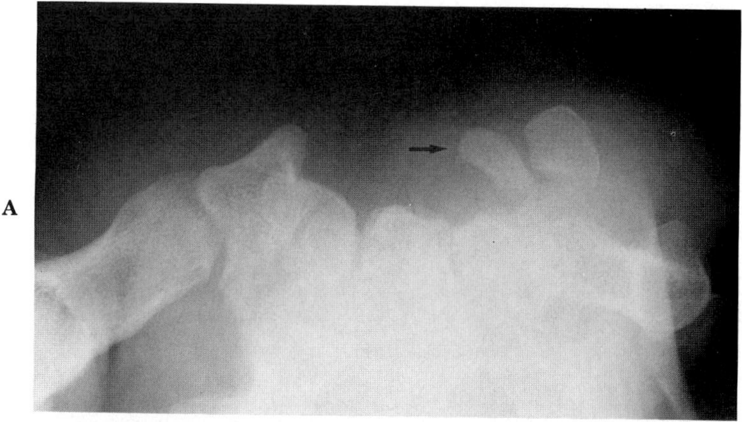

B

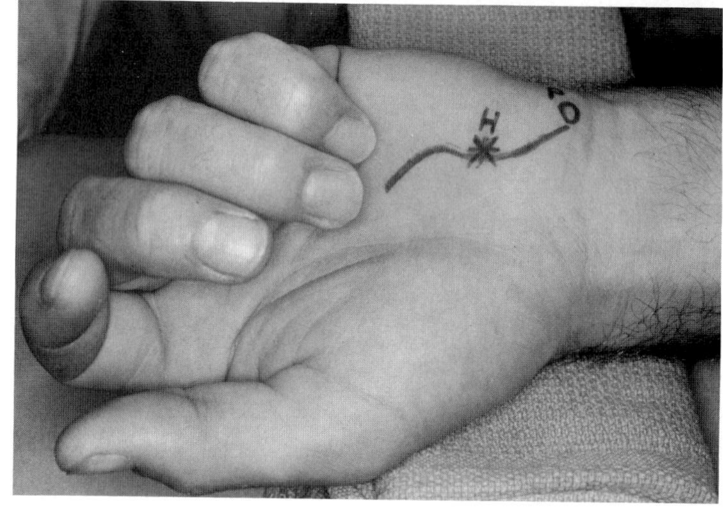

FIG. 23-16. A, Displaced hamate hook fracture *(arrow)*. **B,** Exposure is through a curved palmar incision extending from the hamate *(H)* to the pisiform *(PO)*.

Continued.

that requires prompt treatment to avert the disabling complications of painful nonunion, neuropathy, and tendon injury.

Immobilization position for hook of hamate fractures

- Wrist flexion
- MCP joint (ring and small fingers) in acute flexion
- Include base of thumb

Personal experience as well as that of others[6] confirms that healing of undisplaced fractures can occur with continuous casting, and thus a trial of immobilization is warranted for stable injuries. As anticipated, the healing process is prolonged and averages about 10 to 12 weeks. Even minimal distraction impedes this process, and, like that of the scaphoid, the hook fracture treated with casting requires continual roentgenographic or, preferably, tomographic surveillance to ensure exact apposition of the fracture fragments. Lateral tomograms provide an excellent view of the entire hook and are well suited for following fracture healing.

With fracture displacement, union is precluded, and for the athlete prompt excision of the hook is the best means of achieving a rapid, uncomplicated recovery.[6,9,19,54,64] The displaced fragment is exposed through a curved incision extending from the pisiform to the proximal palm along the radial border of the hypothenar eminence (Fig. 23-16). The adjacent soft tissues are carefully preserved as the hook is subperiosteally excised. Throughout the operation the highly vulnerable deep motor branch of the ulnar nerve must be clearly visualized and protected. The raw fracture surface is covered with adjacent periosteal tissues as well as the redundant pisohamate ligament, and soft tissue connec-

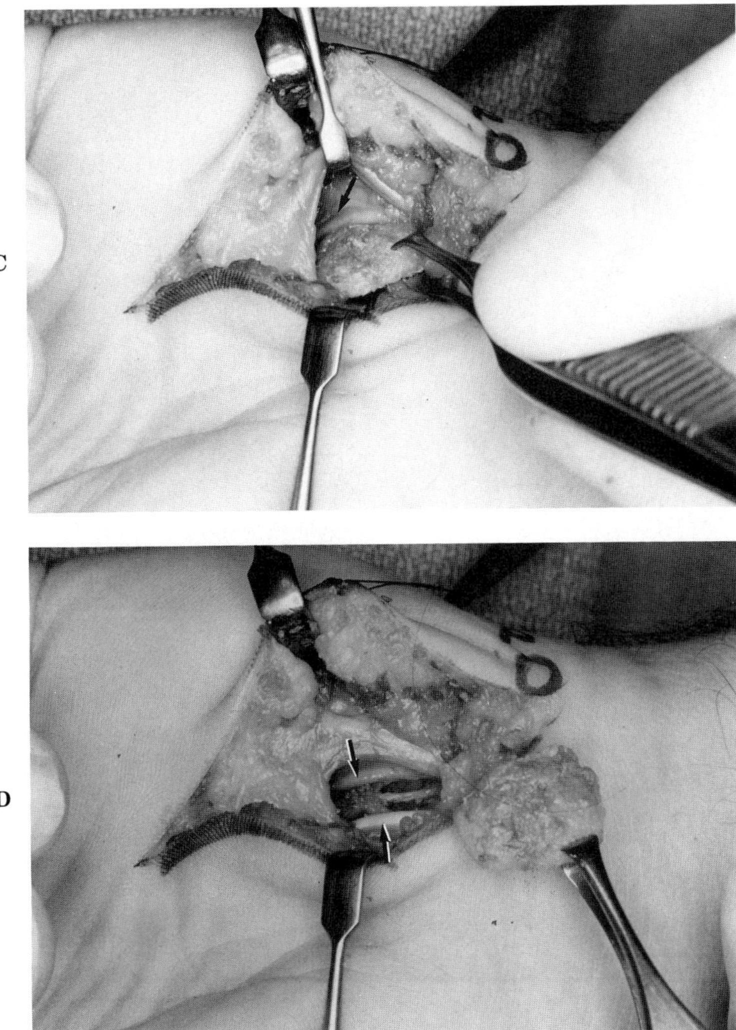

FIG. 23-16, cont'd. C, The highly vulnerable motor branch of the ulnar nerve *(arrow)* must be clearly visualized and protected throughout the procedure. **D,** The ununited hook fragment is excised subperiosteally without disturbing the adjacent nerve *(upper arrow)* or flexor tendons to the small finger *(lower arrow)*.

tions are restored by suturing the ulnar edge of the transverse carpal ligament to the fascial origin of the hypothenar muscles. These adjuvant repairs not only reconstitute important soft tissue attachments but also lessen postoperative wound sensitivity.

After hook excision sports participation with one's preinjury level of skill depends largely on the resolution of hypothenar pain and tenderness, symptoms that tend to persist for several months. The use of custom-fit gloves considerably lessens this problem and facilitates an earlier return to competition.

Triquetrum Fractures

Triquetrum fractures constitute the second or third most common group of carpal fractures.[2,7,8,32,64] The dorsal marginal fracture resulting from either soft tissue avulsion or bony impingement is most prevalent among athletes (Fig. 23-17, *A* and *B*) and, despite its frequent failure to unite, seldom requires more than 4 weeks of splint immobilization. At this point the wrist usually is asymptomatic and this relatively innocuous injury can be safely managed by protective splinting or casting, thereby permitting many athletes to resume their sport with minimal risk of further damage. For the occasional case of symptomatic nonunion, excision of the painful ossicle is the remedy.

In contrast to injuries of the dorsal surface, fractures of the radiovolar margin as well as those through the body of the triquetrum usu-

A
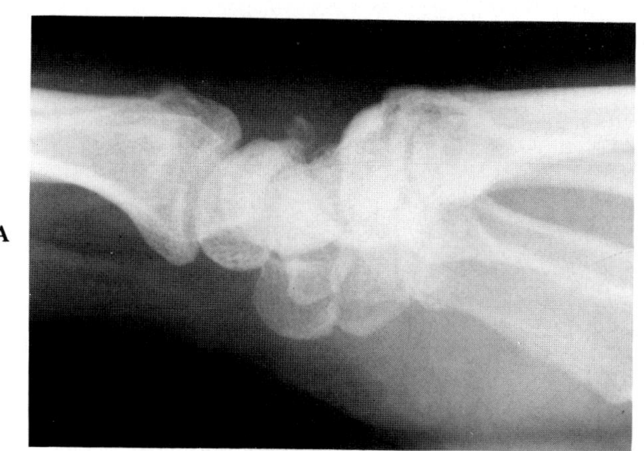
B
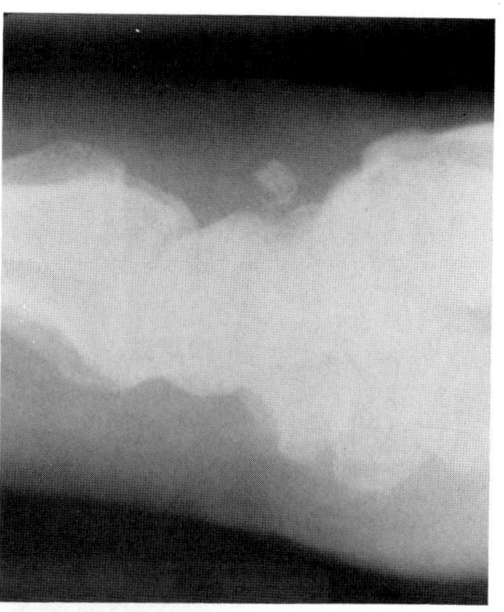
C
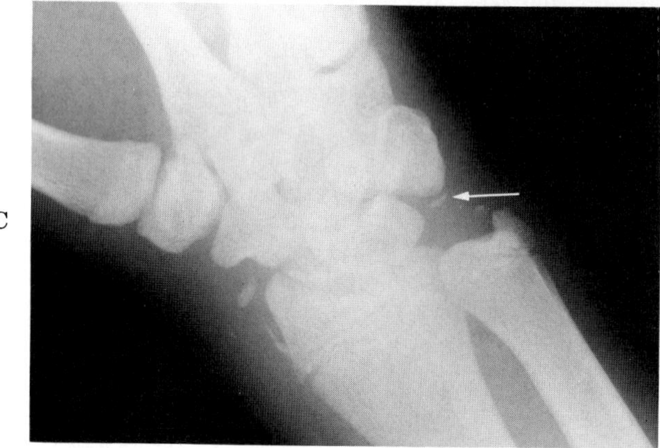

FIG. 23-17. Fractures of the triquetrum. **A,** This dorsal marginal fracture was clinically healed after 4 weeks of splinting. The concept of custom-fit protective casting with an early return to sports often is applicable to this injury, which rapidly becomes asymptomatic and causes no significant alteration of wrist function. **B,** A similar fracture resulting in nonunion. The ununited fragment usually is asymptomatic and has no adverse effect on wrist function. For the occasional painful nonunion, excision of the fragment is the remedy, and several weeks later competition with protection is permissible as tolerated. **C,** In contrast to the relatively innocuous dorsal fracture, the radiovolar marginal fracture *(arrow)* is a frequent component of serious perilunate fracture-dislocations that require surgery for restoration of carpal stability.

ally are associated with perilunate dislocation or fracture-dislocation[35,36] (Fig. 23-17 *C*). These serious disruptions of carpal anatomy generally require open treatment for reduction of fractures and repair of critical soft tissues. An essential part of the operation is stabilization of the triquetrum by open reduction and internal fixation or, more frequently, excision of the small radiovolar fragments and direct repair of the disrupted lunotriquetral capsuloligamentous structure (see Fig. 23-14, *F* and *G*). Following these serious injuries the athlete's name should remain on the disabled roster for a minimum of 4 months.

Other Carpal Fractures

Lunate Fractures

Sheltered by the enclosure of the radial fossa, the lunate is perhaps the carpal bone least vulnerable to fracture. Stewart and Cross,[57] in their extensive review of lunate injuries, most of which were dislocations, indicated that the acute fracture is rare. Beckenbaugh and associates,[4] however, identified fracture in 31 of 38 lunates with established Kienböck's osteonecrosis and postulated a causal relationship between the lunate fracture that fails to unite and irreversible avascular necrosis. Although this hypothesis is

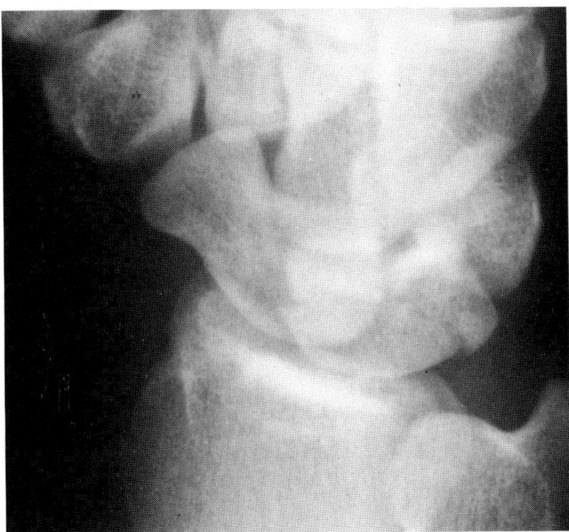

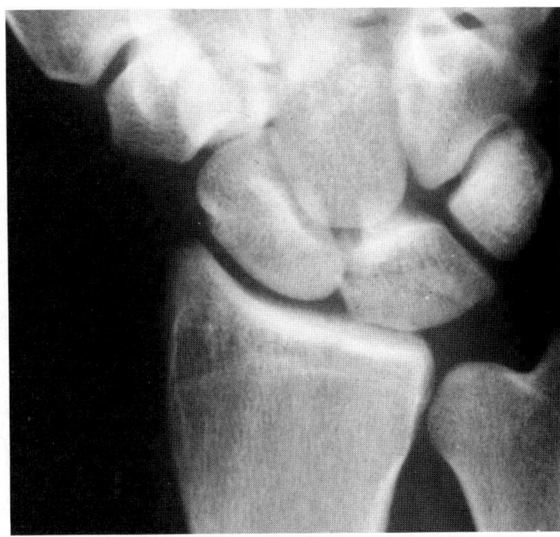

FIG. 23-18. Undisplaced fracture of the lunate in a young athlete with ulnar minus variance. This injury should always be considered a precursor to ischemia, fragmentation, and Kienböck's disease and requires anatomic alignment with prompt immobilization that must be continued until union is certain. In this case, follow-up roentgenograms demonstrated thorough healing with no evidence of progressive devitalization or fragmentation.

controversial and the acute fracture is infrequently encountered among athletes, the sports physician must recognize the potential danger of isolated trauma to the lunate, especially in that highly susceptible group with vascular insufficiency and ulnar minus variance. Lunate fractures should be promptly aligned, securely immobilized, and protected from further injury until union is certain (Fig. 23-18). Also because Kienböck's disease is apt to result from repeated trauma, the athlete with a healed fracture requires protective splinting or casting during subsequent sports participation and constant clinical surveillance.

Trapezium Fractures

Two basic types of trapezium injury are being diagnosed with increasing frequency.[8,15,22,37,45] The **vertical body fracture** is nearly the mirror image of the Bennett fracture-dislocation (Fig. 23-19, *A* and *B*). Instead of the ulnar lip of the thumb metacarpal fracturing, the radial aspect of the trapezium body is split and displaced proximally with the attached metacarpal, disrupting and dislocating the thumb carpometacarpal joint. Through an anterior approach with subperiosteal reflection of the thenar musculature the fracture is reduced and the capsular tissues are repaired, thereby restoring articular congruity and stability. Internal fixation is achieved with either Kirschner wires or small screws.

The **anterior ridge fracture** is analogous to the hamate hook fracture, because minimal distraction precludes healing with cast immobilization and chronically unhealed fractures are apt to result in neuropathy—in this instance involving the median nerve within the adjacent carpal tunnel. Fraying with inflammation or ultimate rupture of the flexor carpi radialis may prove an additional problem. An uncomplicated recovery is facilitated by early excision of the displaced ridge fragment, also employing anterior exposure (Fig. 23-19 *C* to *F*). In chronic cases with neuropathy or tendonitis the adjacent median nerve and flexor carpi radialis can be decompressed

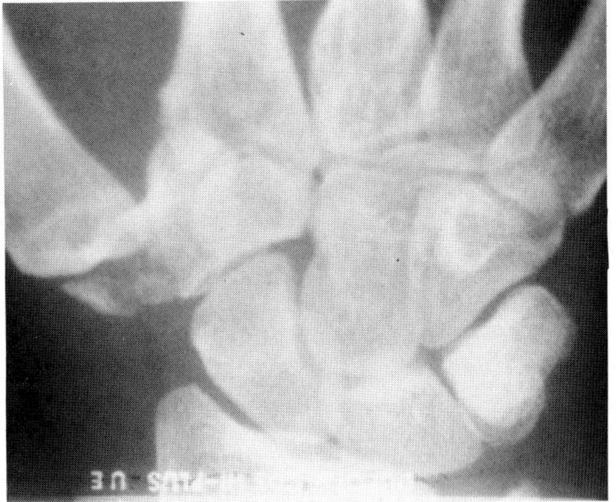

A

FIG. 23-19. Fractures of the trapezium. **A,** The vertical body fracture resulting in disruption with dislocation of the thumb carpometacarpal joint requires open treatment for both fracture reduction and capsular repair. *Continued.*

B

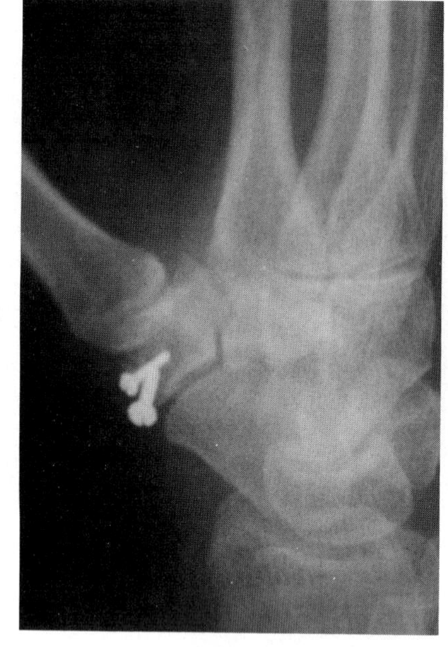

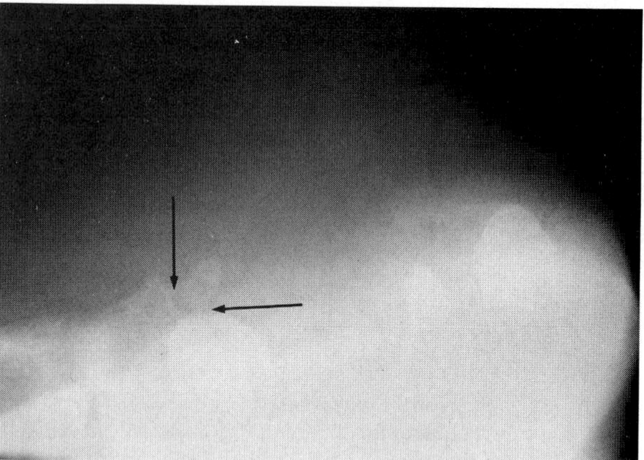

C

D

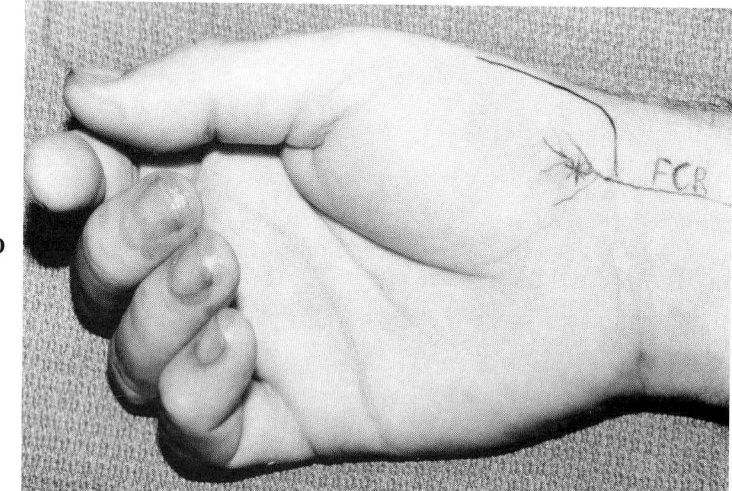

FIG. 23-19, cont'd. B, Internal fixation with 2 mm lag screws restores fracture stability and joint congruity. **C,** The distracted anterior ridge fracture *(arrows)* is optimally managed by early excision. **D,** An anterior approach bordering the thenar eminence.

simultaneously. Not infrequently, a considerable degree of wound sensitivity persists for several months after operation and is apt to compromise function. Impairment can be minimized by the use of protective gloves.

Potential complications of trapezial anterior ridge fracture

- Nonunion
- Median neuropathy
- Flexor carpi radialis attrition

Capitate Fractures

Fractures of the head or neck may occur as isolated events or more frequently as a key component of the transscaphoid-transcapitate perilunate fracture-dislocation (scaphocapitate syndrome). In either instance even minor displacement indicates instability that must be corrected by prompt open reduction.[21,26,48,55,60] The scaphocapitate syndrome is characterized by variable displacement of the scaphoid and marked rotation of the capitate head so that its articular surface usually faces the body of the capitate rather than the lunate

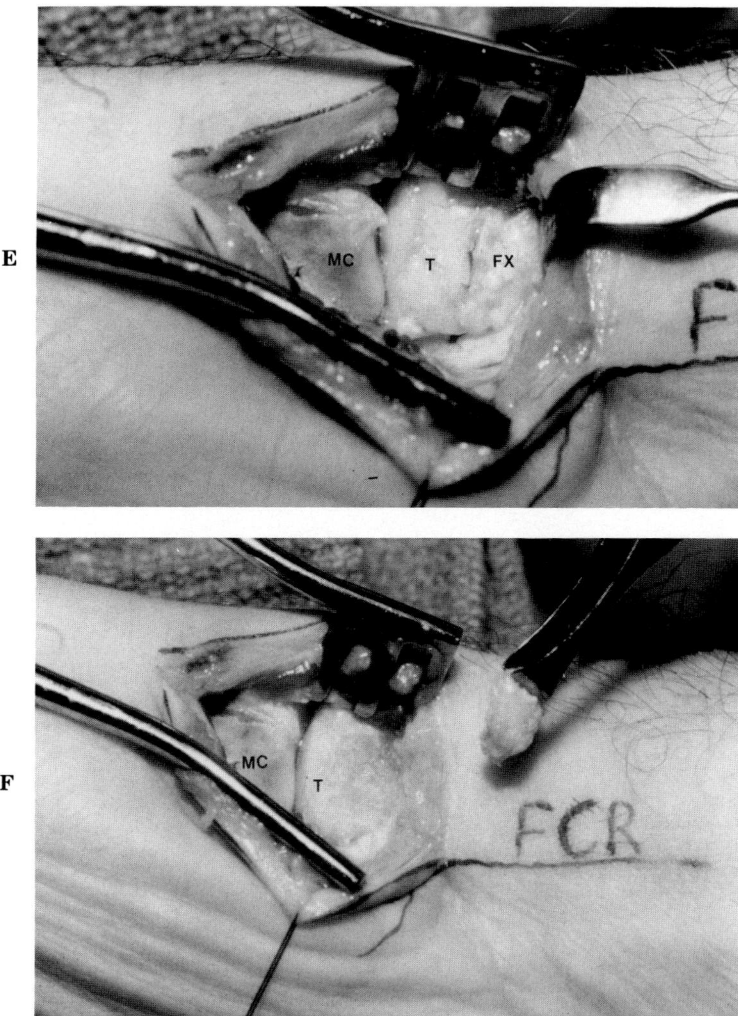

FIG. 23-19, cont'd. E, Subperiosteal reflection of the thenar musculature clearly identifies the fracture. *MC*, Metacarpal of the thumb, *T*, trapezium; *FX*, trapezial ridge fracture. **F,** The ununited fragment (held with the forceps) is excised, and the raw surface of the trapezium is smoothed to minimize postoperative tenderness.

(Fig. 23-20). The resultant squared-off appearance of the proximal capitate is a constant roentgenographic feature of this serious injury that always requires open treatment for restoration of osseous integrity and carpal stability. Through a dorsal approach the proximal capitate is first derotated and stabilized with Kirschner wires, thereby facilitating anatomic alignment and internal fixation of the scaphoid.[60] Although both bones are substantially devitalized and transient ischemia is frequently demonstrated on the roentgenograms, an accurate reduction consistently leads to successful union and a favorable outcome. However, a prolonged period, in excess of 6 months, is required for thorough healing and rehabilitation.

Pisiform Fractures

If undisplaced, pisiform fractures, which occur infrequently, are successfully treated by 3 to 6 weeks of immobilization in a cast similar to that used for undisplaced hamate hook fractures (Fig. 23-21). Excessively comminuted fractures or fracture-dislocations causing disruption of the pisotriquetral joint are prone to inadequate healing with persistent pain and are optimally managed by early pisiformectomy.[8,61] Through a small curved incision at the base of the hypothenar eminence the ul-

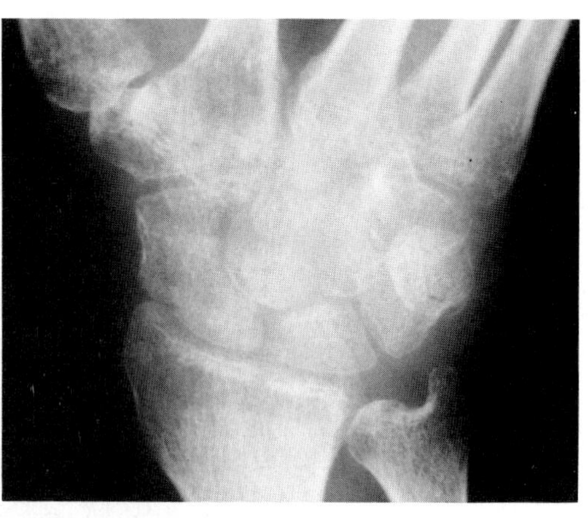

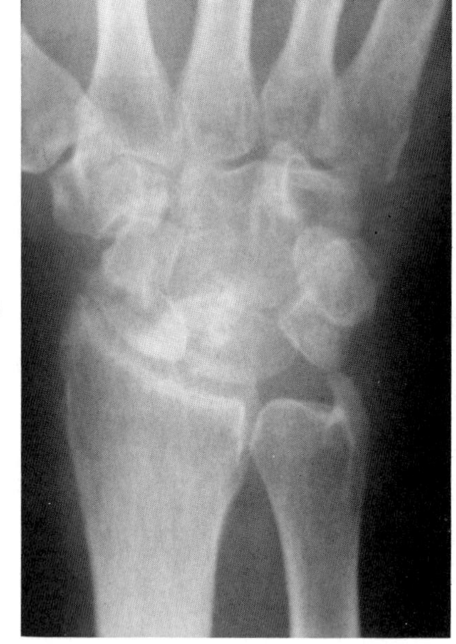

FIG. 23-20. The scaphocapitate syndrome. **A,** Typically the scaphoid fracture is displaced and the capitate head is rotated 180 degrees. The squared-off appearance of the proximal capitate is characteristic of this injury that always requires prompt open reduction and internal fixation for restoration of the severely disrupted carpal anatomy. **B,** Despite transient ischemia of the proximal capitate and scaphoid, both bones united favorably. **C,** In contrast, this untreated scaphocapitate injury resulted in persistent fracture displacement with avascular necrosis and the inevitable sequence of nonunion, carpal collapse, and arthritis.

nar nerve and artery are carefully protected and the pisiform is subperiosteally excised from the substance of the flexor carpi ulnaris. The tendon is repaired, and the wound is protected for several weeks postoperatively.

The pisiform fracture, like the dorsal marginal fracture of the triquetrum, causes only a minor interruption of the athlete's career. Following short-term casting of either the undisplaced fracture or the comminuted fracture requiring excision, the injury can be safely managed by protective devices that alleviate residual wound tenderness and permit an early resumption of activity.

Trapezoid Fractures

Trapezoid fractures, like those of the capitate or hamate body, are usually associated with violent injuries that include a major disruption of the adjacent carpometacarpal joint. Operative treatment is indicated for restoration of articular congruity as well as reduction of displaced carpal fragments. The rarely encountered isolated fracture of the trapezoid requires only a short term of immobilization, because osseous circulation is excellent as is the prospect for prompt union.

A

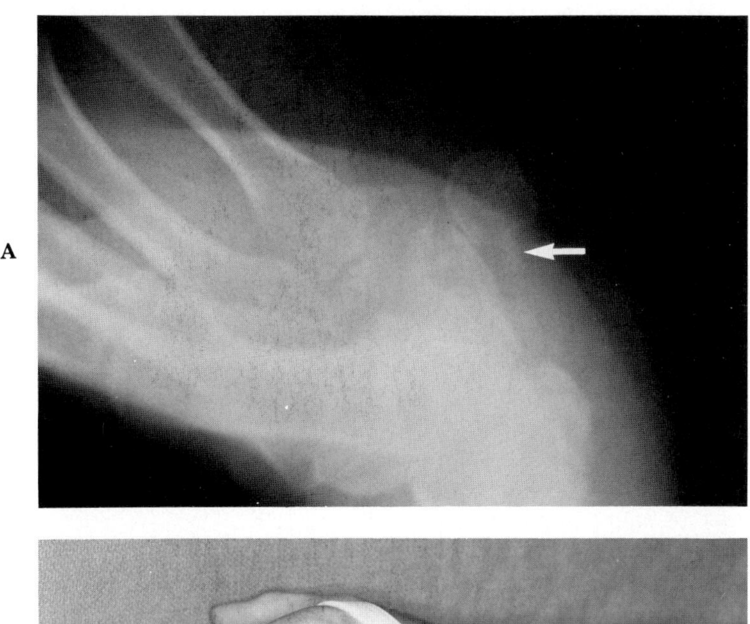

B

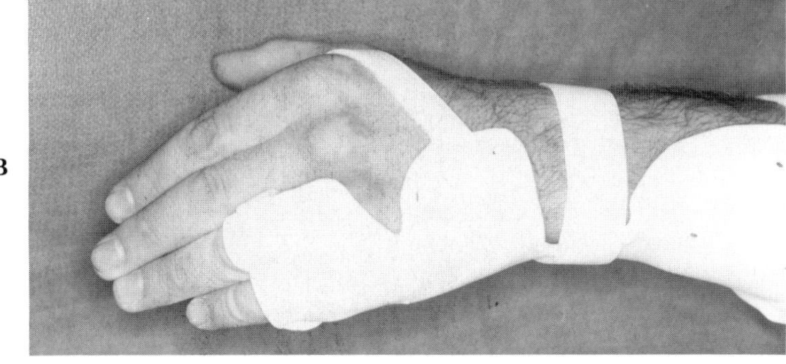

FIG. 23-21. A, Minimally displaced avulsion fracture of the pisiform *(arrow)*. **B,** Fracture was successfully treated with a contoured splint immobilizing the wrist in mild flexion and the metacarpophalangeal joints of the ring and small fingers in acute flexion. Four weeks after injury a custom-fit rubber cast safely permitted an early return to competition.

Distal Radius Fractures

Optimal management of distal radius fractures requires differentiation of the relatively low-energy metaphyseal injuries, traditionally termed "Colles' fracture" and "Smith's fracture," from the more violent injuries that disrupt the distal radius articular surfaces. The articular fractures are prevalent among physically active persons whose wrists are subjected to severe compression forces prone to occur during sports-related activities. The magnitude of force not only disrupts both the radiocarpal and distal radioulnar joints but also is apt to result in serious concomitant periarticular soft tissue and skeletal injury. Prominent among these concomitant injuries are contusions of the median and ulnar nerves, fractures of the scaphoid and distal ulna, and rupture of the scapholunate interosseous ligament. For the more severe articular fractures a method of accurate skeletal fixation is essential for securing fracture stability and ensuring uncomplicated healing, and in some cases open treatment is the only means of restoring the disrupted articular surfaces as well as repairing the critical periarticular damage.[11,30,41,42,63]

Articular Fractures

Axial compression is the key component in the mechanism of the distal radius articular injury (see Fig. 23-2, *C*). The carpus, principally the lunate, forcibly impacts the radial articular fossae, causing predictable patterns of fragmentation and displacement.[41] Despite variable comminution, articular fractures comprise four basic components: the radial shaft, the radial styloid, a dorsal medial fragment, and a palmar medial fragment. To underscore their pivotal position as the cornerstone of both the radiocarpal and radioulnar joints, the medial fragments along with their strong ligamentous attachments to the carpus and the ulnar styloid have been termed the "medial complex." Displacement of this complex always causes a serious biarticular disruption of the distal radius and is the basis for a classification of articular fractures into four types (Fig. 23-22).

Components of distal radius articular injury

- Radial shaft
- Radial styloid
- Dorsal medial fragment
- Palmar medial fragment

Classification and treatment. Type I fractures are minimally displaced, are stable, and are effectively treated by a relatively short period of continuous cast or splint immobilization (usually 4 weeks) followed by a program of progressive remobilization and strengthening supplemented with protective splinting until rehabilitation is complete.

The type II fracture is most frequently incurred by the athlete. In contrast to the type I injury, this fracture is characterized by extensive comminution and marked displacement with resultant fracture instability. The fracture is also prone to median or ulnar nerve contusion, which is apt to occur in nearly 20% of the cases. Displacement of the articular fragments is either dorsal, the die punch pattern,[41,53] or less frequently, volar—a fracture pattern analogous to the Smith type II or volar Barton's fracture-dislocation.[20,59] It is important to recognize that regardless of the direction of displacement the key medial fragments are not widely separated and are conducive to reduction by traction and manipulation with stabilization by external pins incorporated in either a plaster cast or an external fixation device.* Successful traction with external pin fixation, also termed "ligamentotaxis," is contingent on the strength of the ligamentous component of the medial complex, which usually remains intact despite extensive osseous fragmentation.[17] Maintaining these soft tissues under constant tension affords stability to the attached articular fragments.

For type II fractures in athletes pins and plaster have consistently proved a successful method of treatment. In the vast majority of cases accurate restitution of disrupted articular surfaces has been followed by uncomplicated fracture healing, a highly favorable recovery of wrist function, and, invariably, complete resolution of concomitant neuropathy over a period ranging from several weeks to several months. Owing to the excellent healing capacity of the distal radius as well as an unparalleled rehabilitative process, many athletes have returned to competition as early as 3 months after surgery.

Classification of distal radius articular fractures

Type I
Minimally displaced
Stable

Type II
Displaced medial complex
Extensive comminution
Unstable

Type III
Displaced medial complex
Displaced radial shaft fragment
Unstable

Type IV
Wide separation of medial fragments
Extensive soft tissue and periarticular damage
Unstable

Despite the conceptual simplicity of pins and plaster, it needs to be emphasized that skillful pin insertion and cast application are essential to success. Faulty techniques will result in a high rate of serious complications with loss of reduction and compromised recovery. The procedure employs two smooth 3/32-inch Steinmann's pins for skeletal fixation, distal and proximal to the fracture site (Fig. 23-23). The distal pin is passed through the base of the second and third metacarpals while the thumb and fingers are held in maximal abduction, thereby preventing web space narrowing with subsequent contracture and facilitating early digital motion. The proximal pin is passed dorsally, through the bare bone interval of the radius, engaging both radial cortices but projecting only several millimeters beyond the volar cortex, thus avoiding the critical soft tissues of the distal forearm. Precise insertion of the pins with a low-speed, high-torque drill avoids excessive reaming of the pin holes, minimizing such complications as pin loosening, pin tract infection, and pin site fracture or osteomyelitis. Attaching the distal pin to an overhead traction bow and applying a 2.3 kg (5-lb) countertraction weight over the well-padded arm effects ligamentotaxis, and gentle manipulation completes the reduction. Occasionally percutaneous Kirschner wires are used to augment

*References 14, 25, 30, 41, 53, 63.

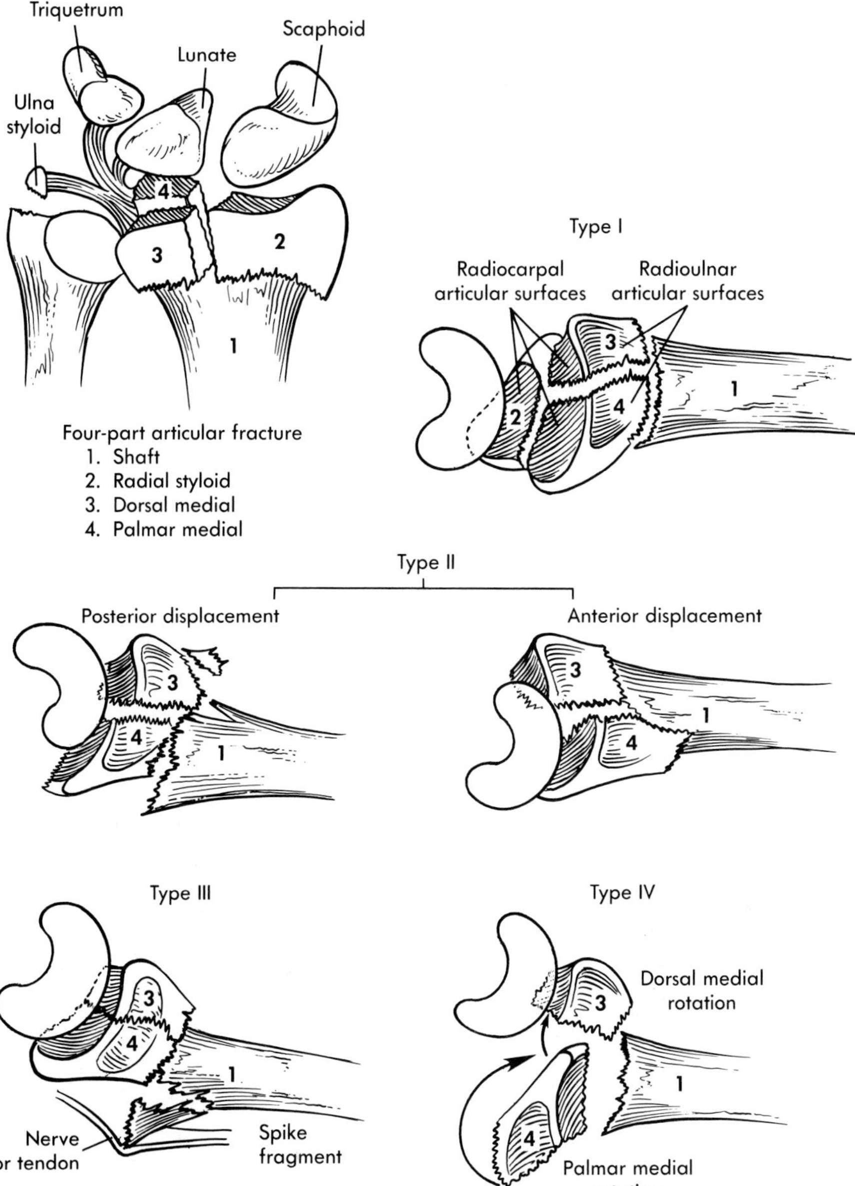

FIG. 23-22. Articular fractures of the distal radius consist of four basic components: (1) the radial shaft, (2) the radial styloid, (3) a dorsal medial fragment, and (4) a palmar medial fragment. The key medial fragments and their strong ligamentous attachments to the carpals and ulnar styloid have been termed the "medial complex." Displacement of this complex is the basis for classification of articular fractures into four types. The unstable type II fracture is most frequently encountered among athletes. (From Melone CP, Jr: Unstable fractures of the distal radius. In Lichtman DM, editor: The wrist and its disorders, Philadelphia, 1987, WB Saunders Co.)

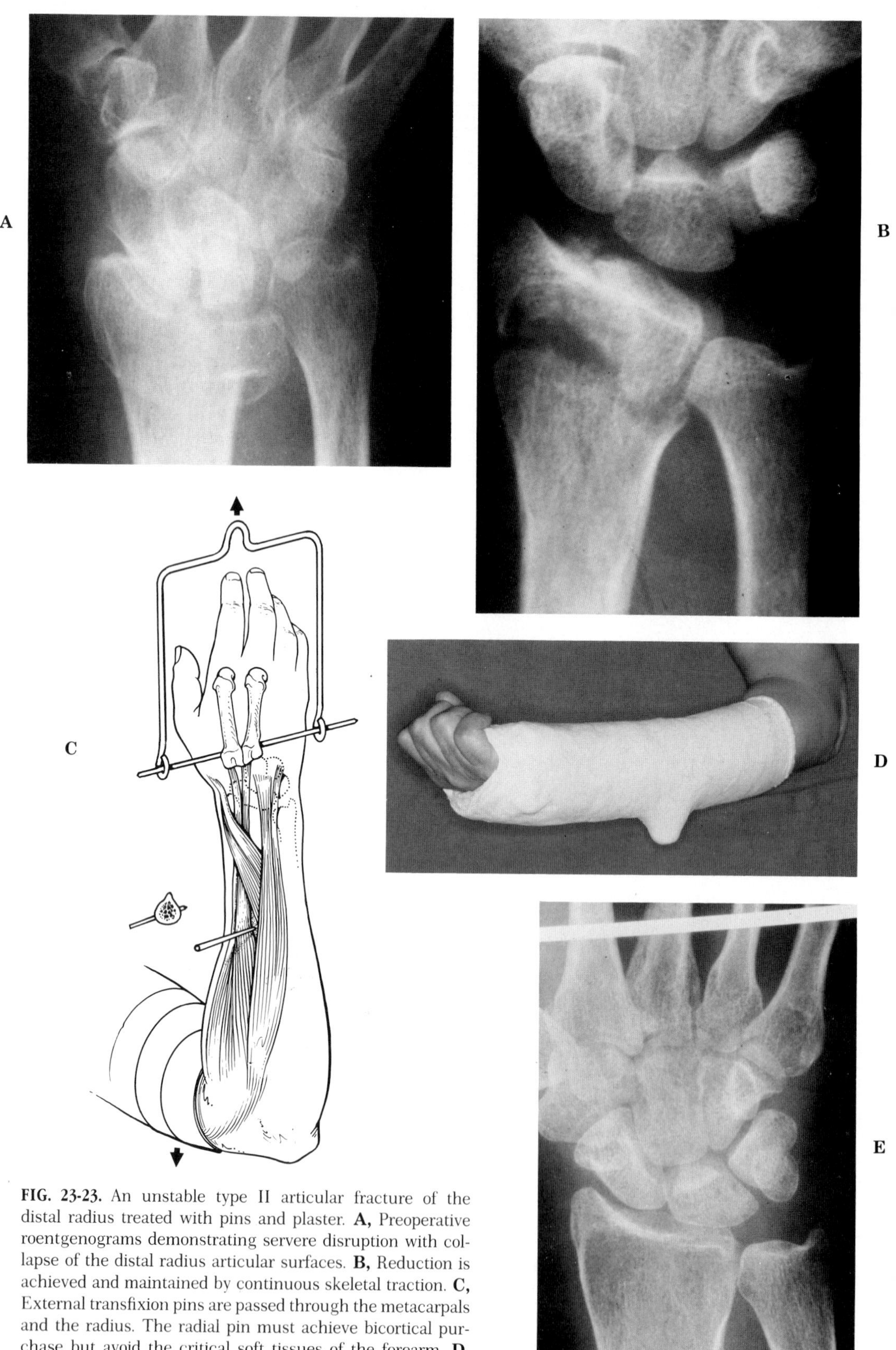

FIG. 23-23. An unstable type II articular fracture of the distal radius treated with pins and plaster. **A,** Preoperative roentgenograms demonstrating servere disruption with collapse of the distal radius articular surfaces. **B,** Reduction is achieved and maintained by continuous skeletal traction. **C,** External transfixion pins are passed through the metacarpals and the radius. The radial pin must achieve bicortical purchase but avoid the critical soft tissues of the forearm. **D,** After accurate reduction, the pins are incorporated in a short arm cast that permits immediate active motion of the thumb, fingers, and elbow. **E,** Uncomplicated union with preservation of the articular surfaces is demonstrated 8 weeks after surgery.

stability of the articular fragments as well as other concomitant skeletal injuries. After roentgenographic confirmation of an accurate reduction, the external pins are incorporated in a carefully molded short arm cast, leaving the fingers, thumb, and elbow free for immediate active motion. Although minor settling of the comminuted fragments is inevitable, a skillfully applied system will exert continuous traction and maintain the reduction for as long as 8 weeks, at which time roentgenographic union usually is demonstrated and the pins and plaster are removed.

Compared to pins and plaster, external fixators require more complex, invasive techniques; are prone to a considerably higher rate of complications; and, owing to their relative bulk with continual exposure, are apt to cause problems with patient acceptance.* The principal applications of these devices has been for open fractures associated with substantial soft tissue or bone loss, situations infrequently encountered with athletic injuries.

Type III and type IV injuries demonstrate more profound fracture instability that is apt to result from sports trauma. The type III fracture is characterized by displacement of the medial complex as a unit, as well as displacement of an additional spike fragment from the comminuted radial shaft. Typically this bony spike projects anteriorly, contusing the median nerve and adjacent tendons. Although the medial fragments can be successfully managed by external fixation, the spike fragment is irreducible by closed methods and necessitates open reduction with internal fixation.

The type IV fracture constitutes the most severe disruption of the distal radius articulations and is always associated with extensive periarticular damage. Characteristically the medial fragments are widely separated or rotated and cannot be accurately realigned by closed manipulation or traction. Open treatment is necessary for restoration of the articular surfaces and repair of concomitant soft tissue or skeletal injuries (Fig. 23-24).

Inasmuch as the major fracture displacement of both type III and type IV injuries usually is palmar and the soft tissue injury occurs within the flexor compartment of the wrist, an anterior approach extending from the carpal tunnel to the ulnar aspect of the wrist is the preferential means of surgical exposure. In cases with widely displaced radial styloid fragments, irreducible dorsal medial fragments, displaced scaphoid fractures, carpal dissociation, or extensor tendon injuries, extensile exposure requires a second incision over the dorsum of the wrist. Although the small, comminuted fracture fragments generally are not suitable for techniques of rigid

*Editor's note: Pins and plaster, a standard technique for these injuries, has in our practice as well as other hand surgeons, been supplanted by the use of external fixators. Although uncomplicated to apply at the time of the acute injury, we have found the post-treatment care quite difficult. If swelling becomes a problem, bivalving or splitting the cast is necessary and the pins can be disturbed with loss of fracture position or excessive pressure placed on the skin. External fixation generally will avoid these problems.

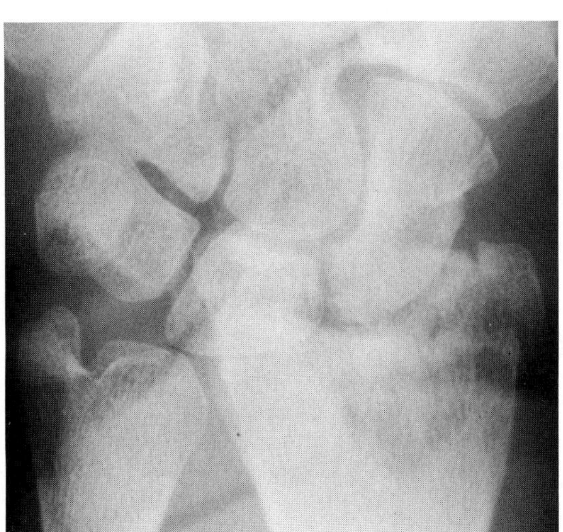

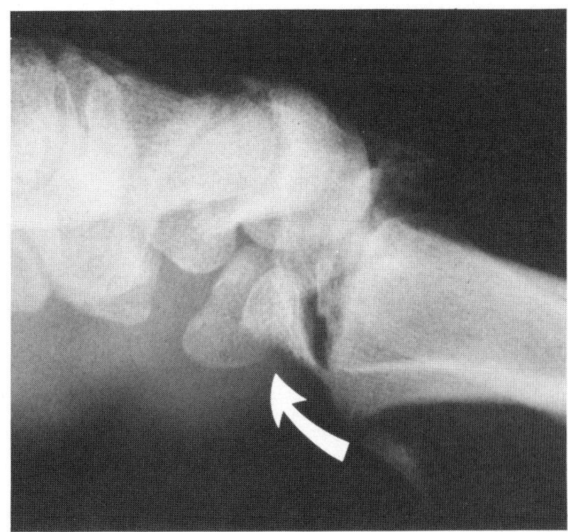

B

FIG. 23-24. Type IV distal radius articular fracture. **A,** Roentgenogram demonstrating severe biarticular disruption. **B,** Roentgenogram showing the palmar medial fragment *(tip of arrow)* rotated 180 degrees.

Continued.

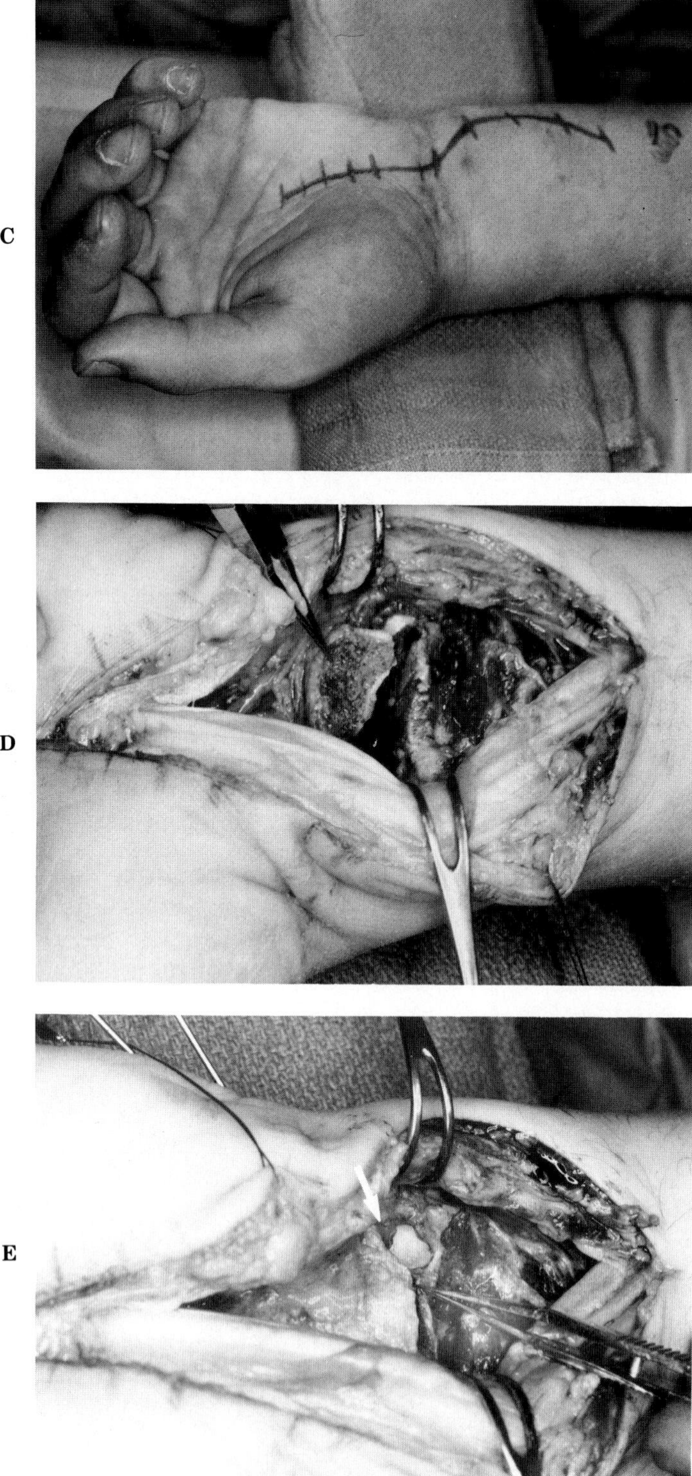

FIG. 23-24, cont'd. C, Open reduction is required for accurate restoration of the articular surfaces and is best achieved through an anterior approach that affords direct access to the displaced fragments, as well as any damaged soft tissues. **D,** The widely displaced palmar medial fragment (at the tip of the forceps) is to be, **E,** derotated, reduced, and stabilized with wires to adjacent fragments for restitution of radiocarpal and radioulnar *(arrow)* congruity.

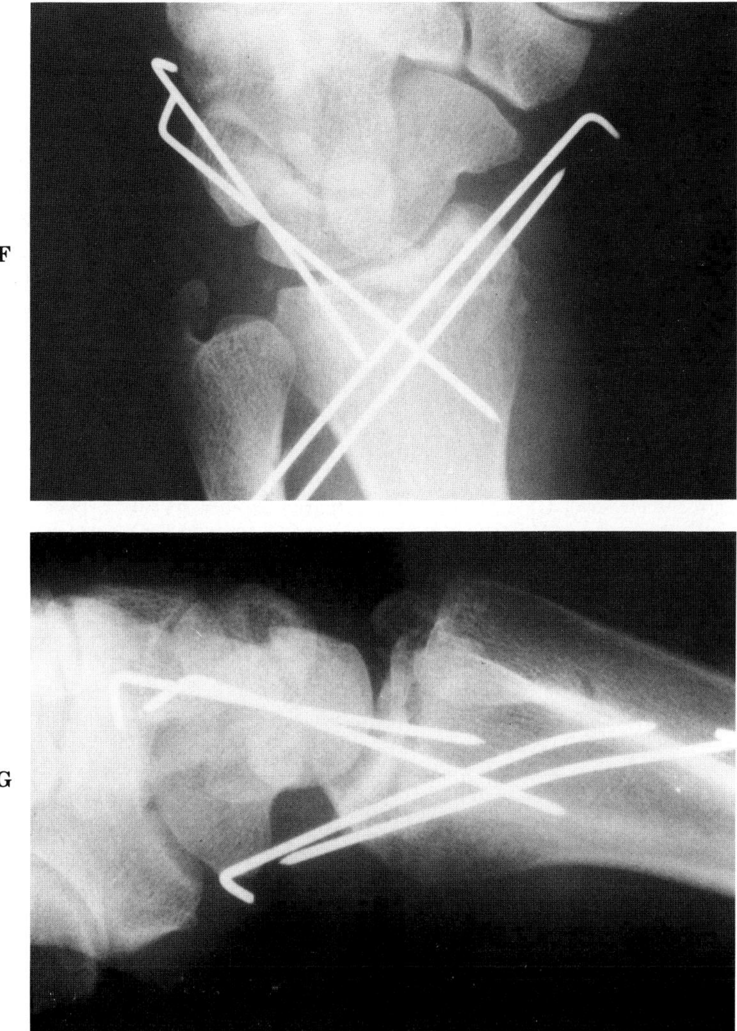

FIG. 23-24, cont'd. F and **G,** Following secure stabilization with multiple wires, postoperative roentgenograms demonstrate an accurate restoration of the distal radius articulations. (From Isani A and Melone CP, Jr: Classification and management of intra-articular fractures of the distal radius, Hand Clin 4:349, 1988.)

fixation, secure stabilization can be achieved with multiple Kirschner wires. In those instances with severe comminution, primary bone grafting augments fracture stability and enhances security against collapse of the articular surfaces. Experience bears out that even for these most serious articular fractures precise reduction and stabilization of every fracture component in conjunction with meticulous repair of all concomitant injuries are consistently rewarded by a favorable recovery.[42]

Another intraarticular fracture pattern which can occur is the volar Barton's fracture. In this situation the carpus is volarly subluxed with the fractured volar aspect of the distal radius. Volar Barton's fractures are grossly unstable and generally cannot be managed by a closed technique or techniques such as pins and plaster or external fixator. These injuries require open reduction and internal fixation with a buttress plate applied volarly.

Extraarticular Fractures

Metaphyseal fractures. In contrast to articular fractures, extraarticular injuries principally result from tension forces and tend to be stable after closed reduction and cast immobilization. Facilitated by a regional anesthetic, manipulation of Colles'-type fractures is accomplished by axial traction followed by palmar flexion, ulnar deviation, and pronation of the wrist. Smith-type fractures are reduced by traction and supination. Clearly, a stable reduction hinges on the restoration of an intact cortical buttress, either posterior or anterior.

If both radial cortices are extensively comminuted, the injury is inherently unstable, and without supplementary fixation, loss of reduction is inevitable. In such cases, techniques of external fixation, identical to those used for unstable articular fractures, are needed to maintain an accurate reduction.

Epiphyseal fractures. Prevalent among adolescent athletes are injuries of the distal radius epiphysis. An excessive tension force applied to the extended wrist characteristically causes a type II epiphyseal fracture, or separation. The plane of disruption traverses the growth plate through the zone of cell hypertrophy, and an intact epiphysis along with an attached small metaphyseal fragment (the Thurston-Holland sign) separates from the radial shaft[52] (Fig. 23-25). Since the critical germinal layer of the physis is essentially undisturbed, the prognosis for normal growth after a prompt, accurate reduction is excellent.

Successful reduction can be consistently achieved by gentle closed manipulation and cast immobilization employing techniques similar to those used for adult extraarticular injuries. The fundamental criteria for successful reduction are restoration of normal radial length and preservation of normal configurations of the distal radial epiphysis and radioulnar joint as viewed on the posteroanterior roentgenograms. In the assessment of normal radial length and contour, inspection of comparable roentgenograms of the uninjured wrist is essential to avoid misinterpretation caused by variations in anatomy or differences in roentgenographic techniques. In cases with fulfillment of these criteria, the reduction, regardless of persistent sagittal displacement as viewed on the lateral roentgenograms, should be recognized as satisfactory. One must remember that epiphyseal injuries can only occur in an immature skeleton that always has the potential for considerable remodeling after fracture. As long as radial length is accurately restored, type II fractures demonstrating as much as 50% displacement on the lateral roentgenogram will consistently remodel to a normal-appearing epiphysis (Fig. 23-25, *D* and *E*). Cast immobilization usually can be discontinued after 4 weeks, but the vulnerable, young athlete should not compete in contact sports until fracture remodeling and rehabilitation are complete, about 3 or 4 months.

Distal Ulna Fractures

Fractures of the ulnar styloid, head, or epiphysis seldom occur as isolated events. In the majority of cases they constitute a component of injury that includes a major fracture of the adjacent radius. As a general rule, successful treatment of the fractured radius results in accurate reduction and uncomplicated healing of the ulnar component with a favorable recovery of radioulnar and ulnocarpal joint function. A frequent example of this distinctive fracture pattern is the avulsion fracture of the ulnar styloid that occurs with nearly 90% of unstable distal radius fractures. In such cases the tip of the styloid is avulsed as the distal radius is displaced. Inasmuch as the major attachment of the triangular fibrocartilage complex at the base of the styloid remains intact, neither the small styloid fragment nor its frequent failure to unite appreciably affects recovery, provided the more serious radius fracture is accurately reduced and stabilized.

Less frequently, avulsion of the entire styloid with the attached triangular fibrocartilage occurs, usually in conjunction with either distal third (Galeazzi) or proximal (Essex-Lopresti) fractures of the radius. In cases with clinical and roentgenographic evidence of distal ulna instability, optimal management must include anatomic reduction and internal fixation of the displaced styloid for restoration of triangular fibrocartilage integrity and radioulnar stability. Secure fixation of the styloid fragment is achieved with either fine Kirschner wires or small screws. For the chronically unstable injury with an ununited, deformed ulnar styloid, excision of the bony fragment and direct suture of the triangular fibrocartilage through drill holes into the distal ulna remnant are the best means of restoring radioulnar stability.

Epiphyseal injuries of the distal ulna, unlike those of the distal radius, are prone to result in type III or IV fractures (Fig. 23-26). These serious growth plate disruptions invariably occur in association with displaced distal third fractures of the radius; hence, the injuries have been termed Galeazzi-equivalent lesions.[43,49] The radial component of the lesion is clearly visualized on routine roentgenographic projections and usually can be managed by closed manipulation. In contrast, the magnitude of injury to the ulnar component is less apparent but may preclude closed methods of treatment. If careful scrutiny of postreduction roentgenograms reveals residual epiphyseal displacement, prompt and precise open reduction and internal fixation with fine Kirschner wires are essential to prevent a disabling deformity of the ulna.

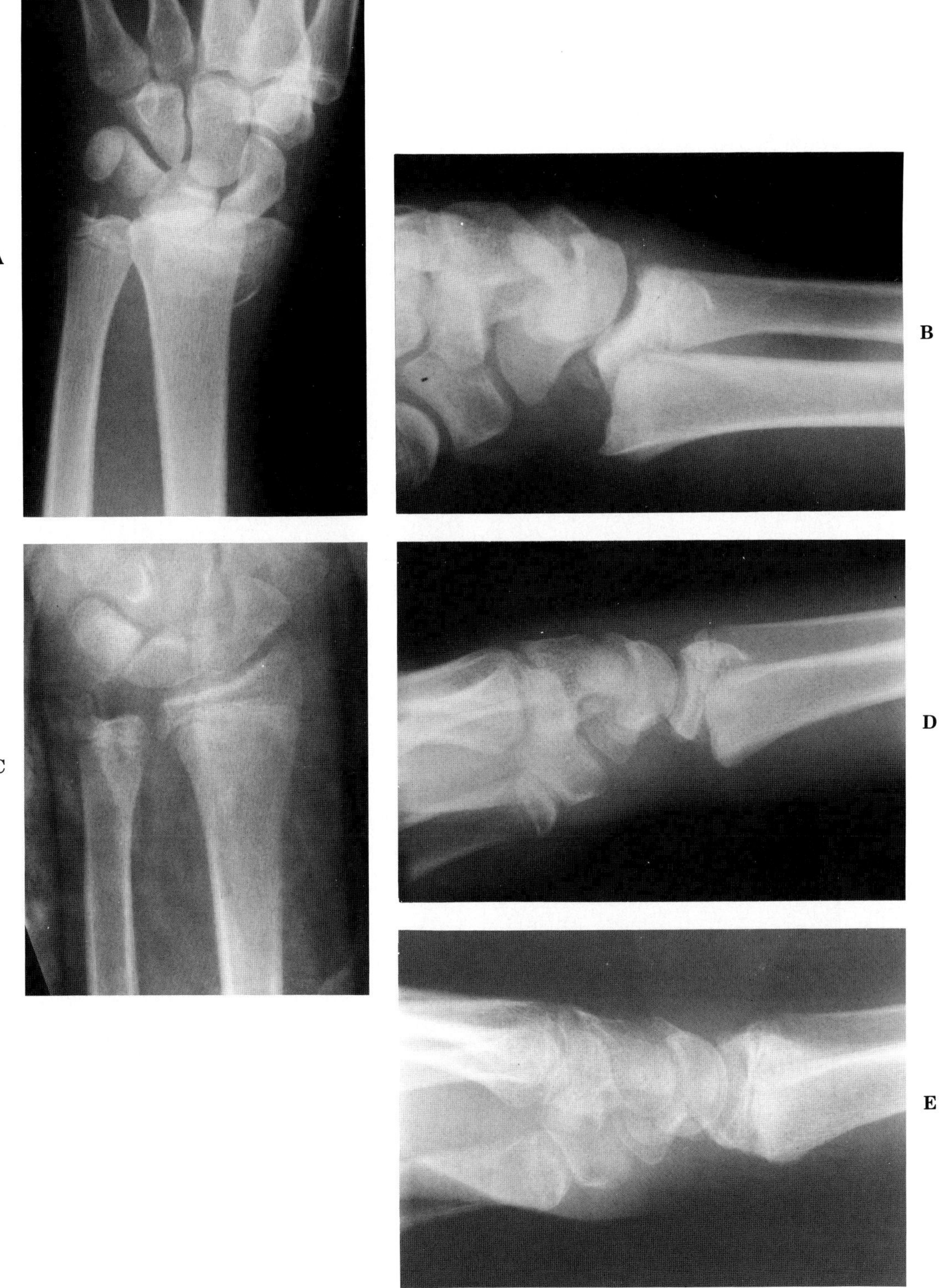

FIG. 23-25. A and **B,** Type II epiphyseal fracture of a 16-year-old football running back. **C,** Closed reduction successfully restores radial length and the normal epiphyseal configuration as viewed on the posteroanterior roentgenogram. **D,** Despite persistent sagittal displacement, this is a satisfactory reduction that does not require additional and potentially harmful manipulation. **E,** Over several months the remodeling process results in uncomplicated union with restitution of normal radial contours. (From Melone CP, Jr, and Grad JB: Fractures of the distal ends of the radius and ulna. In Pettrone FA, editor: American Academy of Orthopaedic Surgeons symposium on upper extremity injuries in athletes, St Louis, 1986, The CV Mosby Co.)

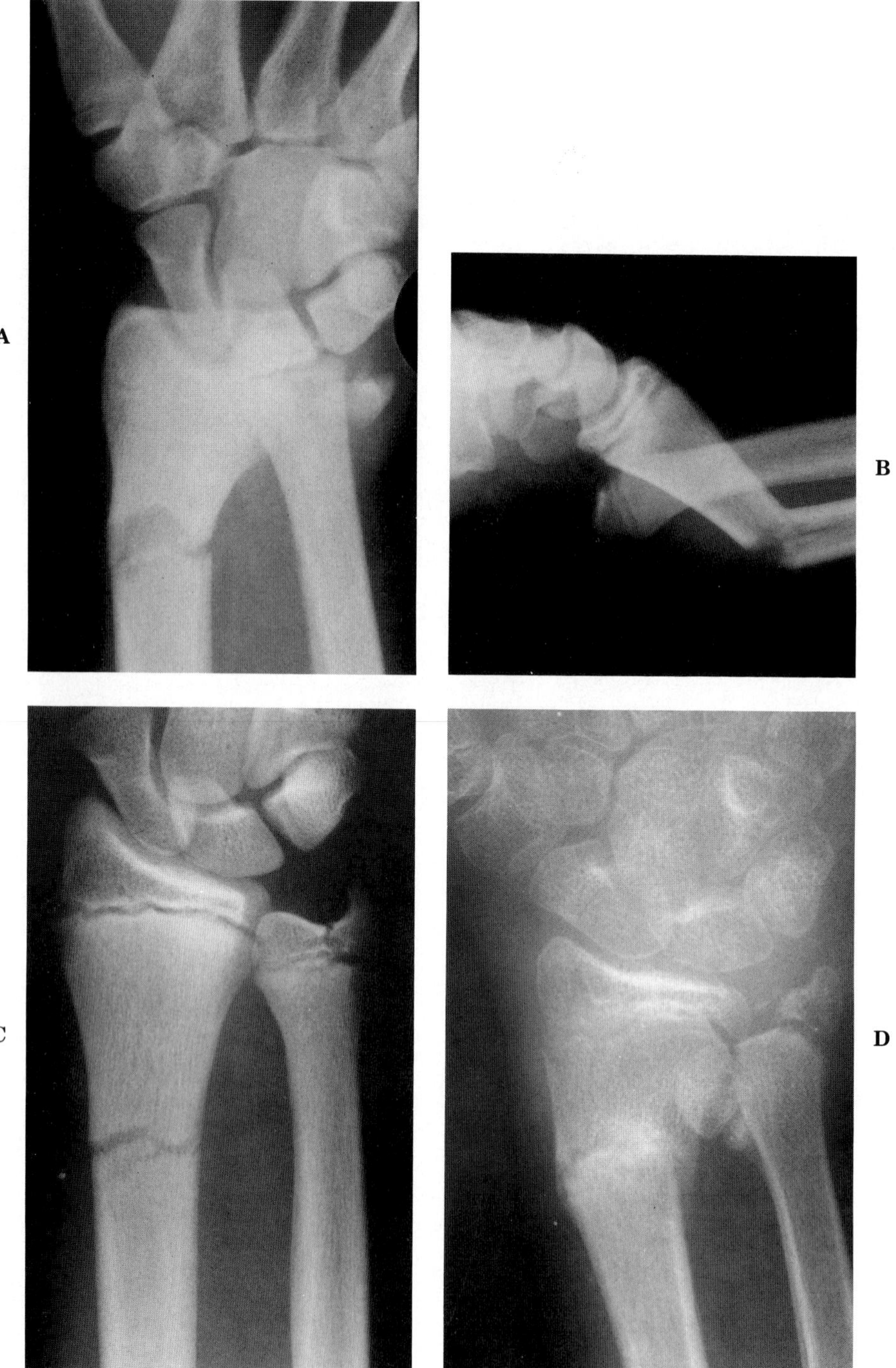

FIG. 23-26. A and **B,** Markedly displaced Galeazzi-equivalent fracture with a type III epiphyseal injury of the distal ulna incurred by an adolescent hockey player. **C,** Closed reduction results in an anatomic reduction. Roentgenographic surveillance, however, is mandatory to ensure stability, because even minimal epiphyseal displacement requires prompt open reduction with internal fixation. **D,** An untreated Galeazzi-equivalent fracture with a type IV distal ulna epiphyseal injury resulting in malunion and ultimately growth disturbance with deformity. For this injury, optimal treatment comprises prompt open reduction with internal fixation of the disrupted epiphysis. (From Melone CP, Jr, and Grad JB: Fractures of the distal ends of the radius and ulna. In Pettrone FA, editor: American Academy of Orthopaedic Surgeons symposium on upper extremity injuries in athletes, St Louis, 1986, The CV Mosby Co.

SUMMARY

Certain exceptions notwithstanding, the primary requisites of optimal management for the athlete's fractured wrist are prompt diagnosis, accurate and stable reduction, effective immobilization until healing is thorough, and comprehensive rehabilitation of the injured parts. Fulfillment of these fundamental criteria consistently leads to a highly favorable outcome with minimal risk of reinjury. In contrast, a compromise of these principles, especially for the sake of a speedy return to sports, invariably results in suboptimal recovery and, not infrequently, a permanent loss of skills.

The exceptions to the cardinal rule that successful treatment of wrist fractures requires precise restoration of anatomic relationships are specific: displaced hamate hook fractures, displaced trapezial ridge fractures, and comminuted pisiform fractures. In such instances, successful union essentially is precluded, and early excision of the displaced fragments is the logical means of facilitating an uncomplicated recovery.

Fractures treated by early excision

- Displaced hook of hamate
- Displaced trapezial ridge
- Comminuted pisiform

For some athletes the return to competition can be safely expedited by the use of custom-fit protective gloves, splints, or casts. For most, however, the treatment regimen usually entails a minimum of 3 or 4 months. Although the healing and rehabilitation process is often lengthy and may seem costly, particularly in terms of time lost from competition, seldom do athletes regret the investment once they return to their highly skillful activities unencumbered by wrist impairment. Never does the sports medicine physician regret compliance with the principles of optimal care.

REFERENCES

1. Adkinson JW and Chapman MW: Treatment of acute lunate and perilunate dislocations, Clin Orthop 164:199, 1982.
2. Bartone NF and Grieco RV: Fracture of the triquetrum, J Bone Joint Surg 38A:353, 1956.
3. Bassett III FH, Malone T, and Gilchrist RA: A protective splint of silicone rubber, Am J Sports Med 7:358, 1979.
4. Beckenbaugh RD et al: Kienböck's disease: the natural history of Kienböck's disease and consideration of lunate fractures, Clin Orthop 149:98, 1980.
5. Bergfeld JA et al: Soft playing splint for protection of significant hand and wrist injuries in sports, Am J Sports Med 10:293, 1982.
6. Bishop AT and Beckenbaugh RD: Fracture of the hamate hook, J Hand Surg 13A:135, 1988.
7. Bonnin JG and Greening WP: Fractures of the triquetrum, Br J Surg 31:278, 1944.
8. Bryan RS and Dobyns JH: Fractures of the carpal bones other than lunate and navicular, Clin Orthop 149:107, 1980.
9. Carter PR, Eaton RG, and Littler JW: Ununited fractures of the hook of the hamate, J Bone Joint Surg 59A:583, 1977.
10. Clayton ML: Rupture of the flexor tendon in carpal tunnel (non-rheumatoid) with special reference to fracture of the hook of the hamate, J Bone Joint Surg 51A:798, 1969.
11. Cooney WP, Dobyns JH, and Linscheid RL: Complications of Colles' fractures, J Bone Joint Surg 62A:613, 1980.
12. Cooney WP, Dobyns JH, and Linscheid RL: Fractures of the scaphoid: a rational approach to management, Clin Orthop 149:90, 1980.
13. Cooney WP, Dobyns JH, and Linscheid RL: Nonunion of the scaphoid: analysis of the results from bone grafting, J Hand Surg 5:343, 1980.
14. Cooney WP, Linscheid RL, and Dobyns JH: External pin fixation for unstable Colles' fractures, J Bone Joint Surg 61A:840, 1979.
15. Cordrey LJ and Ferrer-Torells M: Management of fractures of the greater multangular, J Bone Joint Surg 42A:1111, 1960.
16. Crosby EB and Linscheid RL: Rupture of the flexor profundus tendon of the ring finger secondary to ancient fracture of the hook of the hamate: review of the literature and report of two cases, J Bone Joint Surg 56A:1076, 1974.
17. DePalma AF: Comminuted fractures of the distal end of the radius treated by ulnar pinning, J Bone Joint Surg 34A:651, 1952.
18. Eddeland A et al: Fractures of the scaphoid, Scand J Plast Reconstr Surg 9:234, 1975.
19. Egawa M and Asai T: Fractures of the hook of the hamate: report of six cases and the suitability of computerized tomography, J Hand Surg 8:393, 1983.
20. Ellis J: Smith and Barton's fractures: a method of treatment, J Bone Joint Surg 47B:724, 1965.
21. Fenton RL: The naviculo-capitate fracture syndrome, J Bone Joint Surg 38A:681, 1956.
22. Freeland AE and Finley MD: Displaced vertical fracture of the trapezium treated with a small cancellous lag screw, J Hand Surg 9A:843, 1984.
23. Gelberman RH and Menon J: The vascularity of the scaphoid bone, J Hand Surg 5:508, 1980.
24. Gelberman RH et al: The vascularity of the lunate bone and Kienböck's disease, J Hand Surg 5:272, 1980.
25. Green DP: Pins and plaster treatment of comminuted fractures of the distal end of the radius, J Bone Joint Surg 57A:304, 1975.
26. Green DP and O'Brien ET: Open reduction of carpal dislocations: indications and operative techniques, J Hand Surg 3:250, 1978.
27. Herbert TJ and Fisher WE: Management of the fractured scaphoid using a new bone screw, J Bone Joint Surg 66B:114, 1984.
28. Howard FM: Ulnar-nerve palsy in wrist fractures, J Bone Joint Surg 43A:1197, 1961.
29. Johnson RP: The acutely injured wrist and its residuals, Clin Orthop 149:33, 1980.

30. Knirk JL and Jupiter JB: Intra-articular fractures of the distal end of the radius in young adults, J Bone Joint Surg 68A:647, 1986.
31. Lee MLH: Intraosseous arterial pattern of the carpal lunate bone and its relationship to avascular necrosis, Acta Orthop Scand 33:43, 1963.
32. Levy M et al: Chip fractures of the os triquetrum, J Bone Joint Surg 61B:355, 1979.
33. Lidström A: Fractures of the distal end of the radius: a clinical and statistical study of end results, Acta Orthop Scand (Suppl) 41:1, 1959.
34. Linscheid RL et al: Traumatic instability of the wrist: diagnosis, classification and pathomechanics, J Bone Joint Surg 54A:1612, 1972.
35. Mayfield JK: Mechanism of carpal injuries, Clin Orthop 149:45, 1980.
36. Mayfield JK, Johnson RP, and Kilcoyne RF: Carpal dislocations: pathomechanics and progressive periulnar instability, J Hand Surg 5:226, 1980.
37. McClain EJ and Boyes JH: Missed fractures of the greater multangular, J Bone Joint Surg 48A:1525, 1966.
38. McCue FC and Miller GA: Soft-tissue injuries to the hand. In Pettrone FA, editor: Symposium on upper extremity injuries in athletes, St Louis, 1986, The CV Mosby Co.
39. McCue FC et al: Hand and wrist injuries in the athlete, Am J Sports Med 7:275, 1979.
40. Melone CP, Jr: Scaphoid fractures: concepts of management, Clin Plast Surg 8:83, 1981.
41. Melone CP, Jr: Articular fractures of the distal radius, Orthop Clin North Am 15:217, 1984.
42. Melone CP, Jr: Open treatment for displaced articular fractures of the distal radius, Clin Orthop 202:103, 1986.
43. Mikić ZK: Galeazzi fracture-dislocations, J Bone Joint Surg 57A:1071, Dec 1975.
44. Moneim MS, Hofammann KE III, and Omer GE: Transscaphoid perilunate fracture-dislocation: result of open reduction and pin fixation, Clin Orthop 190:227, 1984.
45. Palmer AK: Trapezial ridge fractures, J Hand Surg 6:561, 1981.
46. Palmer AK and Werner FW: The triangular fibrocartilage complex of the wrist: anatomy and function, J Hand Surg 6:153, 1981.
47. Panagis JS et al: The arterial anatomy of human carpus. II. The intraosseous vascularity, J Hand Surg 8:375, 1983.
48. Rand JA, Linscheid RL, and Dobyns JH: Capitate fractures: a long-term follow-up, Clin Orthop 165:209, 1982.
49. Reckling FW: Unstable fracture-dislocation of the forearm (Monteggia and Galeazzi lesions), J Bone Joint Surg 64A:857, July 1982.
50. Riester JN et al: A review of scaphoid fracture healing in competitive athletes, Am J Sports Med 13:159, 1985.
51. Russe O: Fracture of the carpal navicular: diagnosis, non-operative treatment, and operative treatment, J Bone Joint Surg 42A:759, 1960.
52. Salter RB and Harris WR: Injuries involving the epiphyseal plate, J Bone Joint Surg 45A:587, April 1963.
53. Scheck M: Long-term follow-up of treatment of comminuted fractures of the distal end of the radius by transfixation with Kirschner wires and cast, J Bone Joint Surg 44A:337, 1962.
54. Stark HH et al: Fracture of the hook of the hamate in athletes, J Bone Joint Surg 59A:575, 1977.
55. Stein F and Siegel MW: Naviculocapitate fracture syndrome. A case report: new thoughts on the mechanism of injury, J Bone Joint Surg 51A:391, 1969.
56. Stewart MJ: Fractures of the carpal navicular (scaphoid): a report of 436 cases, J Bone Joint Surg 36A:998, 1954.
57. Stewart MJ and Cross H: The management of injuries of the carpal lunate with a review of sixty cases, J Bone Joint Surg 50A:1489, 1968.
58. Taleisnik J and Kelly PJ: The extraosseous and intraosseous blood supply of the scaphoid bone, J Bone Joint Surg 48A:1125, 1966.
59. Thomas FB: Reduction of Smith's fracture, J Bone Joint Surg 39B:463, August 1957.
60. Vance RM, Gelberman RH, and Evans EF: Scaphocapitate fractures: patterns of dislocation, mechanisms of injury and preliminary results of treatment, J Bone Joint Surg 62A:271, 1980.
61. Vasilas A, Grieco RV, and Bartone NF: Roentgen aspects of injuries to the pisiform bone and pisotriquetral joint, J Bone Joint Surg 42A:1317, 1960.
62. Weber ER: Biomechanical implications of scaphoid waist fractures, Clin Orthop 149:83, 1980.
63. Weber SC and Szabo RM: Severely comminuted distal radial fracture as an unsolved problem: complications associated with external fixation and pins and plaster techniques, J Hand Surg 11A:157, 1986.
64. Zemel NP and Stark HH: Fractures and dislocations of the carpal bones, Clin Sports Med 5:709, 1986.

CHAPTER 24 Ligamentous Injuries of the Wrist in Athletes

John F. Jennings
Clayton A. Peimer

Because of their functional role in athletic activities, the hand and wrist are particularly vulnerable to injury. Diagnosis and treatment of these injuries are especially complex in that the wrist is probably the most complicated joint in the body because of the integrated, multiple articulations of radius, ulna, and carpals.[22,73] To obtain the best possible outcome and maximal function, early diagnosis and appropriate treatment are crucial.[38]

The historically common diagnosis of a wrist ligament "sprain" after an injury is often spurious. Such a diagnosis can actually be

The authors thank Fran Sherwin, M.A., for her editorial assistance.

dangerous because it ignores possible structural derangement, and as a consequence chronic instability may develop secondary to an undiagnosed ligament injury. Every effort should be made to diagnose the wrist injury accurately so that proper treatment can be instituted promptly to preserve the athlete's skills at an optimal level.[16,83] The surgeon who would treat such problems needs a thorough understanding of wrist anatomy and biomechanics as well as of diagnostic and treatment modalities.

This chapter describes the anatomy of the hand and wrist with respect to the bony structures and ligaments, as well as their kinematics. The mechanism and patterns of carpal instabilities are detailed, and the diagnostic (including roentgenographic studies) and treatment protocols for specific injuries are presented.

ANATOMY

Osseous Anatomy

There are two rows of carpal bones. Beginning radially, the proximal row consists of the scaphoid, lunate, triquetrum, and pisiform bones, although the last is really a sesamoid of insertion for flexor carpi ulnaris. The distal row includes trapezium, trapezoid, capitate, and hamate bones. Structurally, the wrist positions the hand and transmits forces between the hand and forearm.[16] Wrist function requires a coordinated interaction of bones independently and as groups, dependent on their osseous anatomy and soft tissue attachments.

All the muscles that initiate wrist motion insert at a site distal to the wrist, making the carpus an intercalated segment, as described by Landsmeer.[29,47] In fact, since the distal carpal row moves in syndesmotic union with the hand, it is really just the proximal row that is an intercalated segment.[102]

Scaphoid

The scaphoid, the only bone that traverses the midcarpus, acts as a link between the proximal and distal carpal rows. Gilford[29] in 1943 and later Linschied et al[50] note that the two carpal rows should be unstable in compression either by extrinsic forces or by (intrinsic) muscle loads, unless they are secured by a mechanical stop, a function supplied by the bridging effect of the scaphoid.[42,52,86]

Lunate

The lunate bone is wedge shaped in sagittal section. The volar (palmar) pole is longer than the dorsal.[42] This configuration makes the lunate tend toward dorsiflexion (i.e., the distal surface points dorsally). The lunate articulates proximally with the radius and distally with the capitate, serving to transmit forces between them.

Triquetrum and Hamate

The triquetrum articulates with the lunate radially and the hamate distally. The surface facing the hamate has an inferior, shallow, paddle-shaped facet. The hamate has a helicoidal medial articular facet.[92] In ulnar deviation, therefore, the triquetrum "descends" beneath the hamate as if going down a spiral staircase and moves distally toward the fifth metacarpal, allowing the ulna to move closer to the hand. In radial deviation the reverse occurs; the triquetrum "ascends" this inclined plane and moves proximally into the space between the ulna and fifth metacarpal.

Trapezium, Trapezoid, and Capitate

These three bones are syndesmotic. They, as well as the hamate, support the metacarpals at the mobile (first, fourth, and fifth) and immobile (second and third) carpometacarpal joints, and they transmit forces to the forearm via the bones of the proximal carpal row.

Ligamentous Anatomy

The volar ligaments of the wrist are the major stabilizers. Taleisnik[90] has divided them into two major groups: extrinsic ligaments, which connect the carpus and radius or metacarpals, and the intrinsic ligaments, which originate and insert entirely on the carpal bones (Fig. 24-1).

Volar wrist ligaments

Extrinsic
- Carpus to radius
- Carpus to metacarpus

Intrinsic
- Intercarpal

Volar Radiocarpal Ligaments

There are two layers of volar radiocarpal ligaments, one superficial and one deep.[57,90] The superficial fibers assume an inverted V-shape with apex at the capitate, and from radial to ulnar, these fibers consist of the radioscaphocapitate, radiolunate, and radioscapholunate ligaments. The radial collateral ligament is the most lateral of the volar radio-

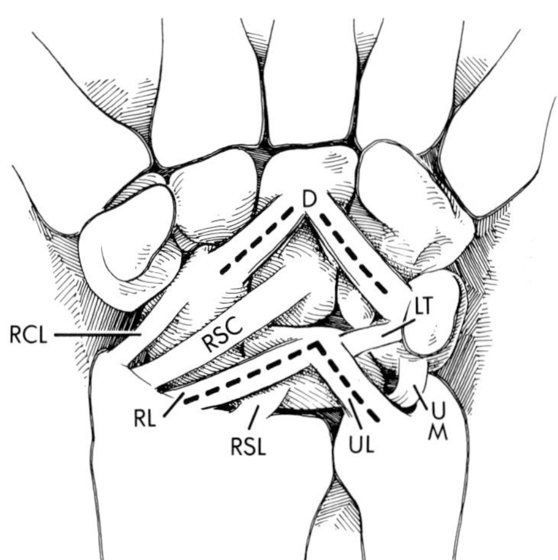

FIG. 24-1. Schematic drawing of volar wrist ligaments. *RSL,* radial collateral ligament; *RSC,* radioscaphocapitate ligament; *RL,* radiolunate ligament; *RSL,* radioscapholunate ligament; *LT,* lunotriquetral ligament; *UL,* ulnolunate ligament; *UM,* ulnocarpal meniscus homologue; *D,* deltoid or "V" ligament.

carpal ligaments, and since it is actually more volar than lateral, it probably does not truly function as a collateral ligament. In lower primates the ulna styloid articulates with the triquetrum. In humans a cartilaginous structure, the **ulnocarpal meniscus homolog,** is interposed between the ulna and triquetrum; there is no direct ligamentous connection between the ulna and the carpus.[48,90] This cartilage meniscus is separate from the **triangular fibrocartilaginous complex** (TFCC), although both attach to the dorsoulnar corner of the radius. The TFCC is connected to the carpus by the ulnolunate ligament, which secures the dorsoulnar radius to the volar carpus. The volar and radial corner of the radius is connected to the carpus by the deep (volar) radiocarpal ligaments. Therefore the carpus can be seen as "suspended" from the radius; the head of the ulna is not really part of the wrist joint itself.[27,74,90,97] The ulnar collateral ligament represents a thickening of joint capsule on the ulnar side rather than a true ligament.[46]

Volar radiocarpal ligaments

- Radioscaphocapitate
- Radiolunate
- Radioscapholunate
- Radial collateral

Intrinsic Ligaments

The intrinsic ligaments of the wrist originate and insert on the carpal bones. These volar ligaments, which are thicker and stronger than the dorsal ligaments, are further divided into short, intermediate, and long ligaments.

The **short intrinsic ligaments,**[98,90] which include the trapeziotrapezoidal, the trapeziocapitate, and the capitohamate, bind together the four bones of the distal row into a single, functional whole.

Intrinsic wrist ligaments

Short
- Trapeziotrapezoidal
- Trapeziocapitate
- Capitohamate

Intermediate
- Scaphoid-trapezium
- Scaphoid-lunate
- Lunate-triquetral

Long
- Deltoid

The **intermediate intrinsic ligaments**[39,90] connect the trapezium to the scaphoid and then to the bones of the proximal carpal row. These include the scaphoid-trapezium, the scaphoid-lunate, and the lunate-triquetral ligaments. The triquetrum is more firmly secured than the scaphoid to the lunate, permitting transmission of a dorsiflexion force from triquetrum to lunate and causing secondary lunate dorsiflexion with ulnar deviation.

Of the two **long intrinsic ligaments**[57,90,92] the volar (which is more important) has been referred to as the "deltoid," "radiate," "arcuate," and "V" ligament. The volar ligament stabilizes the capitate and may fan out proximally (from the capitate) to the scaphoid, lunate, and triquetrum. Often the central point of this "deltoid" fan ligament is absent, and there are attachments only to the scaphoid and triquetrum, forming an inverted "V" with the distal lunate in the middle of the opening.

Dorsal Radiocarpal Ligament

The dorsal radiocarpal ligament, or radiolunate triquetrum ligament, originates on the dorsal rim of the radius and inserts on the scaphoid, lunate, and triquetrum.[92] Further support is provided by the extensor tendon compartments.

Dorsal Intercarpal Ligament

The dorsal intercarpal ligament originates from the triquetrum and inserts dorsally into the scaphoid and trapezium.[92]

Summary

In summary, the major ligaments of the wrist are volar and intracapsular and cannot be readily visualized by the surgeon.[33,48,57] These volar ligaments are arranged in a double "V," with the capitate at the apex of the broad "V" and the lunate at the apex of the smaller "V." Between these, there may be an area of potential weakness, the **space of Poirier,** which is not present in persons with deltoid or radiate ligaments connecting the capitate to the lunate. Navarro[67,92] believed that this lunocapitate ligament "defect" might explain carpal subluxation. In individuals with systemic articular laxity or hypermobility syndromes, patterns of carpal instability can be produced as a consequence of volar or dorsal stress in the "normal wrist."[43,88,92]

KINEMATICS

The kinematics of the normal wrist has been studied and reported by many investigators.* The wrist is functionally more complex than might be inferred by the fact that it is characterized by two (transverse) rows of carpal bones. There are different perspectives on functional anatomy, and the clinician needs to understand them. The traditional concept was simply that the carpus was made up of two rows of carpal bones traversed by the scaphoid. Gilford[29] noted that this "link joint" would be unstable in compression were it not for the scaphoid's bridging across the midcarpus.

In 1935 Navarro proposed his theory of the "columnar carpus",[68] noting that the wrist is not made of transverse articulations but of three separate longitudinal columns (Fig. 24-2, *A*). He postulated that there is a central

*References 2, 9, 19, 41, 52, 58, 84, 96, 97, 105, 107.

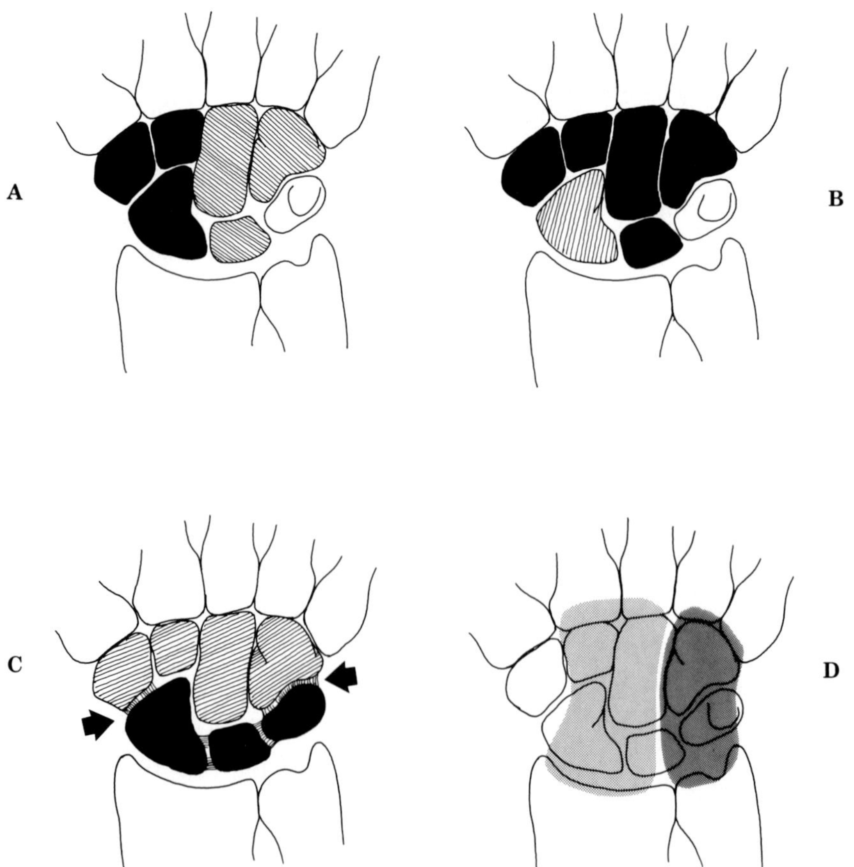

FIG. 24-2. Schematic concepts of carpal bone kinematic ralationships. **A,** Navarro "columnar wrist" theory.[71] **B,** Taleisnik's columnar wrist model.[94] **C,** Lichtman et al oval ring concept of carpal links.[52] **D,** Weber's longitudinal columnar theory of carpal mechanics.[104]

"flexion-extension column" composed of the lunate, capitate, and hamate; a lateral "mobile column" constituted by the scaphoid, trapezoid, and trapezium; and a medial "rotatory column" made up of the triquetrum (and pisiform). Navarro, who agreed with Destot,[23,92] stressed the fundamental role of the medial column and hand rotation. Taleisnik[90] modified this theory by suggesting that the central column should be expanded to include the lunate *and* all the bones of the distal carpal row (since they are intimately connected by the short intrinsic ligaments and move as one unit) (Fig. 24-2, *B*). He eliminated the pisiform from the medial column because it does not participate in integrating carpal motion. As a result of these modifications of theory, the central column is thought to be the main link of flexion and extension; the mobile scaphoid is still believed to stablize the midcarpus when dorsiflexed and to allow mobility with volar flexion; triquetral motion on the hamate functions as the pivot around which carpal rotation occurs.

In 1980 Lichtman and co-workers[49] studied several cases of ulnar midcarpal instability. They proposed an "oval ring" theory, conceptualizing the carpus as a dynamic ring (Fig. 24-2, C). They thought the lunate should not be considered part of the rigid central column, since there is considerable mobility between the scaphoid and lunate in all wrist motions. They believed that the movement of the proximal carpal row was synchronous at the scapholunate joint, that ulnar deviation is initiated at the triquetrohamate joint, and that radial deviation is initiated at the scaphotrapezial joint. Therefore their physiologic model would be a ring with two mobile links—the scaphotrapezial joint and the rotatory triquetrohamate joint—and any break in this ring (across bone *or* ligament) would result in destabilization and abnormal motion ("carpal instability").[8,49]

Weber[107] introduced the "longitudinal columns theory" in 1984, combining bone and ligament supports into two columns (Fig. 24-2, *D*). The **force bearing column** consists of the distal radius, the proximal two thirds of the scaphoid, the trapezoid, and the bases of the second and third metacarpals. The **control column** consists of the distal ulna, TFCC, triquetrum, hamate, and bases of the fourth and fifth metacarpals. He points out that the forces generated by the hand are ultimately directed radially via bony and ligamentous anatomy, first toward the scaphoid and lunate, and then to the distal radius. (Forces applied from an ulnar position are also directed in this fashion.) The medial control column depends on the triquetrohamate articulation, with movement at the helicoidal hamate surface causing dorsiflexion or volar flexion of the remainder of the proximal carpal row, which is accommodated at the scaphotrapezio-trapezoidal (STT) joint.

In summary, the radiocarpal and midcarpal joints both contribute in total flexion-extension and deviation.* Flexion-extension motions require that the lunate and capitate move together (i.e., in the same direction). For radial deviation to occur, the first metacarpal approaches the radius, and the scaphoid must *volar flex* (i.e., it becomes *vertical*), and the triquetrum moves proximally up the hamate. For ulnar deviation to occur, the scaphoid extends (i.e., it becomes horizontal) and the triquetrum descends distally beneath the hamate to narrow the space between the fifth metacarpal and ulna. The proximal carpal row is connected by the scapholunate and triquetrolunate interosseous ligaments, and therefore these bones move in the same direction. For example, in ulnar deviation when the triquetrum descends under the hamate, it actually dorsiflexes and thereby causes dorsiflexion of the lunate, which causes the scaphoid to dorsiflex (become horizontal). Therefore radial deviation places the scaphoid, lunate, and triquetrum in volar flexion, while the distal carpal row and hand are dorsiflexed. Ulnar deviation causes the opposite to occur.[92]

MECHANISM AND PATTERNS OF CARPAL INSTABILITIES

Watson[104] noted that if the carpal bones were unencumbered by ligamentous constraints, they would *not* assume the "normal" wrist position. Because of its larger volar pole, if alone, the lunate would tend to remain dorsiflexed, but the unlinked scaphoid would tend to remain volar flexed (vertical). Bony anatomy is constrained in such a way that the ligaments maintain predetermined interactive vectors. In a large sense, instability problems arise because of the difference between "constrained normal" and "bony neutral" anatomy. A specific injury results from several nonindependent factors. These include the characteristics of the injuring force, its magnitude, rate of loading, and direction; the position of the hand at impact, including all secondary angulatory and rotatory changes produced by temporal progression of the injury; and the relative strengths of the carpal bones and lig-

*References 57, 84, 92, 106, 107.

aments.[92] In general, the most frequent carpal injuries and dislocations are caused by an axial load directed proximally onto the palm (as in a fall), which produces combined hyperextension, ulnar deviation, and intercarpal supination and results in destruction of the radial bones and/or ligaments.[16,49,54-56] Instabilities in the ulnar carpus are likely to be caused by destructive forces applied to the ulnar side of the wrist, and these are believed to be associated with palmar flexion and intercarpal pronation.[99,102]

Factors in carpal injuries

- Magnitude of injury force
- Rate of load application
- Force direction
- Position of hand
- Angulatory and rotatary changes as injury develops
- Bone strength
- Ligament strength

Carpal injuries represent a spectrum of bony and ligamentous damage, and the terminology describing them depends on whether or not there are fractures associated with ligament disruption(s). If there is a major carpal dislocation without fracture, it is typically either a dislocation of the carpus around the lunate, with the lunate remaining in alignment (dorsal or volar *peri*lunate dislocation) or a dislocation of the lunate that is palmar (or, rarely, dorsal) to the radius. When there is a fracture associated with the dislocation, descriptive (diagnostic) terminology includes the name of the bone *fractured* (i.e., *transcaphoid* perilunate, *transcaphoid transcapitate* perilunate, etc.) Although perilunate and lunate injuries were historically considered separate entities, they are actually part of a continuum; the final roentgenographic picture depends on the aggregate of all forces (Fig. 24-3). The anatomic and biomechanical data show that there is "progressive perilunar instability" generally seen as four stages, each associated with further ligamentous injury as the carpus in progressively torn from the lunate.[54-56]

The instability patterns may be separated functionally into "static" and "dynamic" deformities.[34,91,92] Static or dissociative instabilities are apparent roentgenographically. Misplaced and widened intercarpal spaces are possibly as easy to find as a missing tooth—if only one takes the time to look. The dynamic or nondissociative instabilities may not be readily seen and will only be reproduced with the wrist in motion (patients may often assume such positions at will).[91] Routine roentgenograms from such patients will be normal, and at the least, static views in maximal deviation or cineradiographs (i.e., videofluoroscopy) are needed to reveal this group of (possibly incomplete) carpal instabilities.[2,31,91]

We find that Taleisnik's classifications based on columnar carpus theory are useful for grouping different injuries. We generally follow his terminology in discussing the di-

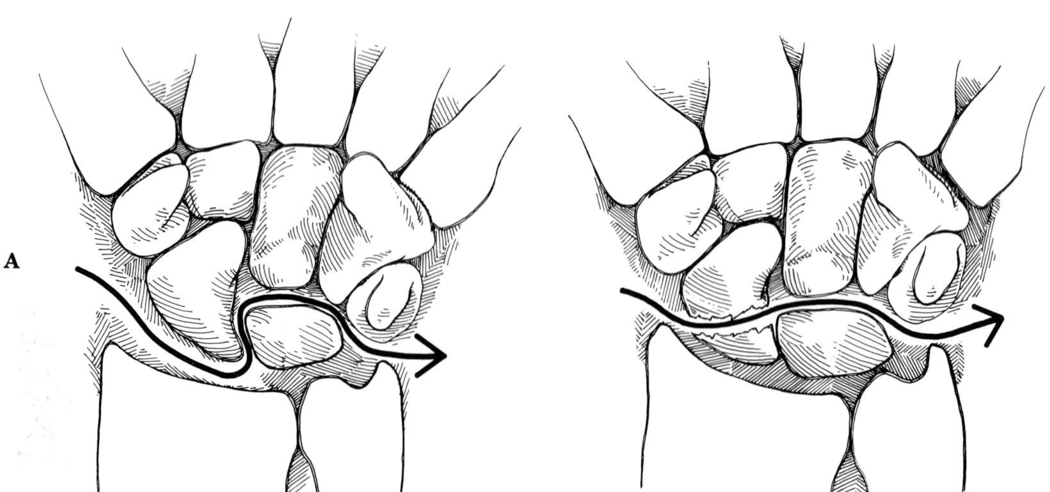

FIG. 24-3. Destructive forces are spent through the ligamentous and bony anatomy depending on exact position of hand at impact, rate of loading, and secondary peritraumatic events. **A,** Pure ligamentous "perilunate" disruption. **B,** Transosseous (transscaphoid, in this case) perilunate osteoligamentous disruption.

agnosis and management of wrist ligament pathology.

DIAGNOSIS

Athletic wrist injuries vary greatly. The physician who cares for the athlete faces the entire spectrum of injuries, from the acute ones sustained in a sudden fall, perhaps secondary to contact, to annoying, chronic wrist pain. Establishing a diagnosis, particularly for the latter patient, can be challenging. We believe it is essential to employ a logical, sequential approach to establish the diagnosis.

History and Physical Examination

The single most useful means of achieving the correct diagnosis is by taking a careful history. One needs to ascertain both the mechanism and hand/wrist position at injury[4] (e.g., "Was the hand extended or flexed?") and the current functional and symptomatic complaints (e.g., "What motion reproduces the pain?" or "Does pain occur during down swing or follow through?").

Next, inspection of the injured wrist may reveal areas of swelling, synovitis, hematoma, or ecchymosis that can give important clues to the underlying pathologic condition. Careful, sometimes tedious, palpation of topographic anatomy is essential. Particular attention must be directed to sites of pain, clicks, and snaps, especially in those patients with chronic problems. A logical and thorough (circumferential) pattern is most important, and the use of a pencil eraser may help localize complaints precisely to individual bony interspaces.[4,93]

The final step in the physical examination is an attempt to stress each symptomatic joint to reproduce the patient's symptoms, comparing "positive" findings to the unaffected, opposite side. Asking the patient to perform whatever motion produces the symptoms while listening *and* gently palpating for abnormal crepitance or bony motion may also be helpful. One may inject an isolated carpal joint with xylocaine in a further effort to localize complaints and confirm with the athlete the site of chronic discomfort, noting changes in symptoms or static grip strength after injection (grip strength is an important measure of pain and dysfunction). The history and physical examination serve to localize injuries. A variety of diagnostic imaging modalities may then be employed to verify or achieve a diagnosis.

Roentgenographic Assessment

Routine Wrist Survey

Initially, four standard views of the wrist should be taken, including posteroanterior (PA), lateral, radial oblique, and scaphoid axial projections.[30] The PA view allows a careful look at bone contours, uniformity of intercarpal spaces, and the "carpal arcs," as aggregate projections of the distal and proximal rows (respectively). A broken arc often indicates disruption of carpal joint integrity. The true lateral view with the wrist in neutral position (zero extension) is the sine-qua-non to verify axial alignment. The radius, lunate, and capitate are normally collinear; deformities are not collinear. A volar-flexed lunate and palmarly translocated capitate (e.g., in volar intercalated segment instability) or dorsiflexed lunate (e.g., in dorsal intercalated segment instability) indicate instability patterns.

Standard wrist views for assessment of ligament injury

- Posteroanterior (PA)
- Lateral
- Radial oblique
- Scaphoid axial

On a true lateral projection with the wrist in neutral, there are three angles, which can be measured, that may assist in making a roentgenographic diagnosis. The **scapholunate angle** is formed by the longitudinal axes of the scaphoid and lunate, and in normal wrists it can range from 30 to 60 degrees. Angles of over 65 to 70 degrees are consistent with scapholunate dissociation, and angles of less than 30 degrees often represent ulnar instabilities.[16,50] (Fig. 24-4). The **capitolunate angle,** formed by the longitudinal axes of the capitate and lunate, is normally zero (i.e., collinear). An angle of more than 15 degrees (dorsal or volar) indicates instability (Fig. 24-5). The **radiolunate angle** is formed by the longitudinal axes of the radius and lunate (also collinear) and measures the amount of dorsiflexion or palmar flexion of the proximal carpal row on the radius.[50] (Fig. 24-6).

In the recent literature, wrist instability has been further classified and clarified by Linscheid and Dobyns,[50] who divided instabilities into dorsal and volar intercalary segment instability patterns, based on the capitolunate angle as seen on true lateral roentgenographs.

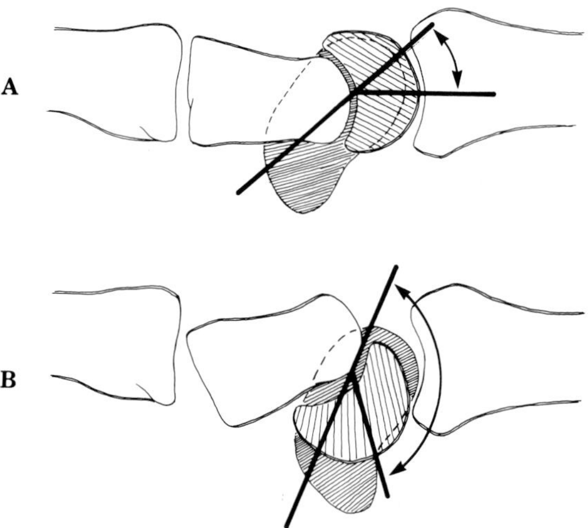

FIG. 24-4. Scapholunate angle measurement is made on the lateral roentgenograph. **A,** Normal scapholunate angle is 30 degrees to 60 degrees. **B,** Pathologic scapholunate angle where with scaphoid is vertical and lunate subluxated palmarward measure over 65 degrees.

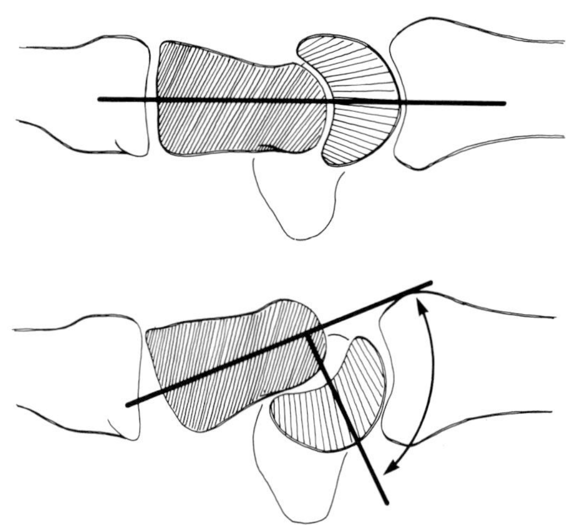

FIG. 24-5. The capitolunate angle is best measured on lateral roentgenographs. **A,** Normal capitolunate angle is 0 degrees to 15 degrees and in this view with the wrist neutral, the capitate, lunate, and radius are collinear (0 degrees). **B,** Pathologic capitolunate angle of more than +15° (as in this view of a DISI deformity) or greater than −15° with the lunate volar flexed (in VISI deformity, not shown).

Dorsal intercalated segmental instability (DISI) occurs when the lunate (the intercalated segment being the lunate) is dorsiflexed and the capitate is translocated dorsal to the radius (and no longer columnar) (Fig. 2-7). The opposite condition is the **volar intercalated segmental instability (VISI).** The lunate is found on roentgenograms to be volar flexed, and the longitudinal axis of the capitate is translocated volarward to the radius.

Linscheid and Dobyns later observed that **ulnar translocation** occurred when the (proximal) carpus was shifted toward the ulna, leaving a widened space between the radial styloid and scaphoid. They also found that **dorsal subluxation** occurred if the entire carpus was translocated dorsal to the (articular surface of) the radius.[23,91]

It is important to look for soft tissue swelling on such films.[17,18,37] Fracture of the volar lip or styloid of the radius disrupts continuity of the important volar ligaments and should make the physician wary of potential associated instability.[33] There is a strong association of ulnar minus variance (ulna shorter than radius) and potential ligament injury. In all cases the roentgenograms should reveal symmetric and uniform interspaces, unbroken contours, and bony architecture.*

*References 20, 31, 32, 50, 106, 107.

Supplementary Static Views

Specialized views should be obtained if a suspicious area is not sufficiently detailed with the routine survey or if obviously symptomatic joints appear benign. These additional static views may include a carpal tunnel projection to delineate the hamulus, oblique views between neutral and full pronation to visualize the ulnar side of the carpus, and a 30-degree semisupinated view to show the

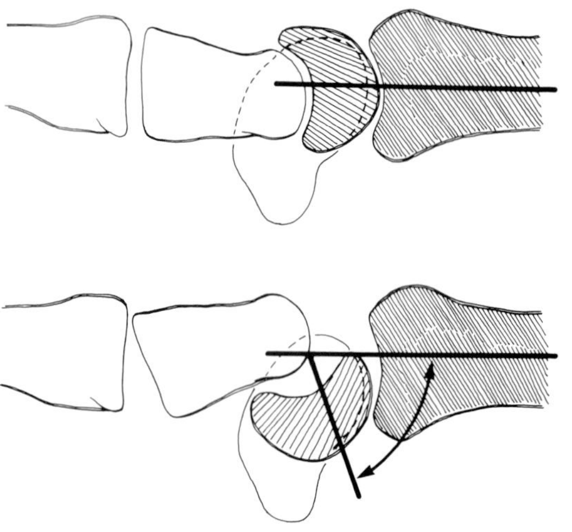

FIG. 24-6. The radiolunate angle is measured on true lateral roentgenographs. **A,** Normal radiolunate angle with the wrist neutral and the bones collinear. **B,** In DISI deformity, the lunate is subluxated palmarward and dorsiflexed; the angle is greater than 30 degrees.

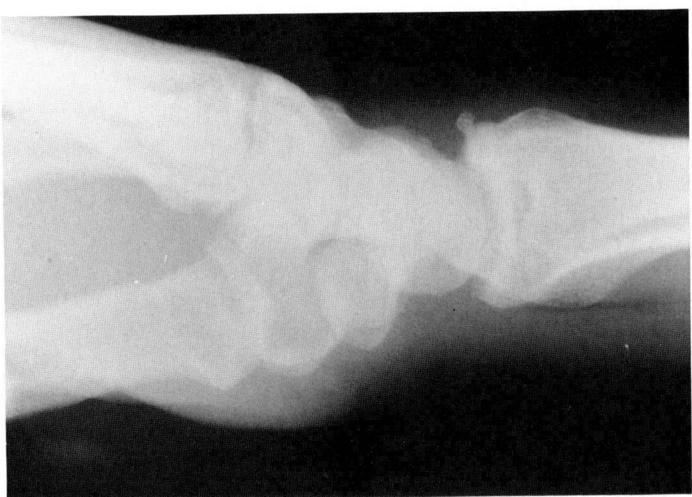

FIG. 24-7. The DISI deformity seen on this lateral roentgenograph includes dorsal subluxation of the capitate, lunate dorsiflexion with palmar subluxation, and a vertical scaphoid (the scaphoid is, technically speaking, volar flexed); the scapholunate, capitolunate, and radiolunate angles are all abnormal.

A

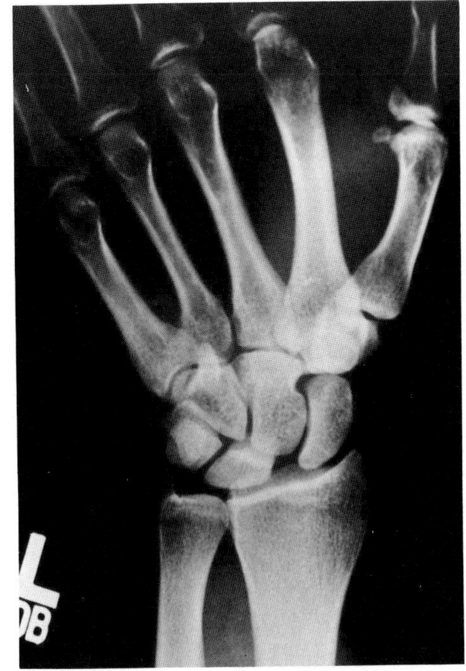

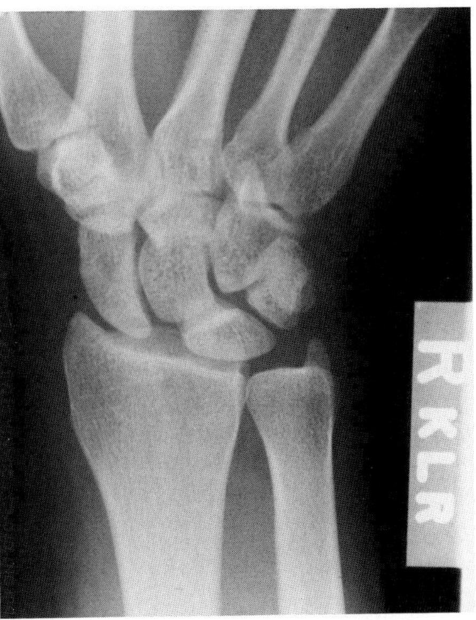

B

FIG. 24-8. A, Posteroanterior roentgenograph of the left wrist in a 27-year-old soccer player who fell and landed on his left palm and complained of pain; note abnormal widening of the scapholuante interval. **B,** Comparison views of the right wrist were obtained demonstrating the same David Letterman sign of over 3 mm scapholunate separation in this uninjured wrist. He recovered with only splint support.

Supplementary static projections

- Carpal tunnel view
- Oblique views
- 30-degree semisupinated view

palmar aspect of the triquetral surface, pisiform, and pisotriquetral joints.

If there is any question of potential carpal dissociation, we generally proceed with a modification of Gilula's "ligament instability" series.[31,32] These include the PA in neutral, radial deviation, and ulnar deviation; laterals in neutral, full radial deviation, and ulnar deviation; plus bilateral anteroposterior (AP) views with the fist actively clenched. The PA views delineate carpal arcs, scapholunate, lunotriquetral, and radiocarpal relationships. The laterals reveal DISI and VISI deformities not readily seen on the PA projections. The "grip view" actively loads the capitate onto the proximal row and accentuates potential scapholunate separation (dissociation). We do not routinely order full bilateral instability series but correlate any positive findings with those of the opposite wrist if needed (Fig. 24-8).

Ligament instability series

- PA (neutral, radial deviation, ulnar deviation)
- Lateral (neutral, radial deviation, ulnar deviation)
- Bilateral AP clenched fist

Videofluoroscopy

Motion studies provide the opportunity to observe nondissociative (dynamic) instability not apparent on the static films. Instability may be further elucidated with the wrist in motion and with stress applied to reveal often transient dissociations, which can be missed during the physical examination.[31,69] Studying videotapes in slow motion may also yield subtle signs of irregularity in the normally smooth motion of various carpal joints.[16]

Arthrography

Arthrography is a useful technique in delineating chronic ligamentous injuries, and is also useful in evaluating an acute situation as well.[65] Normally, there is no communication between the radiocarpal, midcarpal, and radioulnar joints. Injection of dye into a compartment can be followed (fluoroscopically) with and without wrist motion to evaluate the flow of dye across the compartments to indicate the presence of a ligamentous defect. It is best to videotape the actual injection to observe the flow of the dye. After injection the wrist is actively ranged to identify dynamic leaks. The digital subtraction technique allows the effective sequential injection of a series of joints (e.g., radiocarpal, then midcarpal, etc.) so that individual ligament tears can be evaluated (Fig. 24-9). However, Green reminds us that the significance of very small defects (which allow dye leakage) remains in doubt.[33]

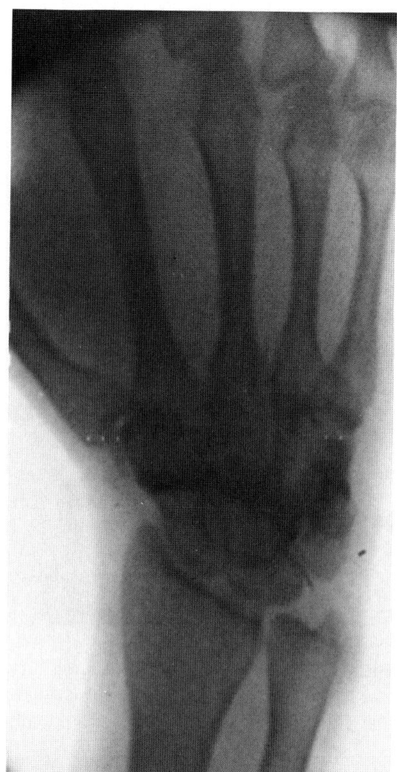

FIG. 24-9. Digital subtraction arthrogram following midcarpal injection in this 19-year-old cheerleader with chronic ulnar wrist pain following a fall from a pyramid reveals abnormal dye leakage via a lunotriquetral ligament tear. Subsequent radiocarpal and radioulnar injections were normal.

Tomograms, Bone Scans, and CT Scans

Tomograms and bone scans are not particularly helpful in diagnosing ligamentous injury, although they may be beneficial in defining or excluding osseous injuries (such as hamulus fracture) not revealed on plain roentgenographs. However, since many ligamentous injuries occur in association with fractures, these techniques are useful in visualizing an occult fracture in suspected association with ligamentous instability. The CT scan is the standard for evaluating distal radioulnar joint alignment and congruity.[78]

Arthroscopy

The use of the arthroscope as a diagnostic tool is still being assessed. Chapter 22 discusses wrist arthroscopy in detail. If conventional diagnostic imaging techniques have failed to provide a diagnosis, or if the significance of the diagnosis requires visual verification, for example, in the case of small dye leaks, the arthroscope has a definite role. Arthroscopic exploration of wrist ligaments and the TFCC produces less morbidity than arthrotomy.[15,104] In addition, the articular surfaces can be inspected by use of arthroscopy for evidence of damage that might change a proposed operative approach to an unstable wrist. We have used the arthroscope to evaluate and treat acute injuries associated with ligamentous disruption. The arthroscope allows us to exclude suturable ligament lesions. The restoration of anatomic alignment of the carpus in such cases can be percutaneously stabilized and verified both roentgenographically and by vision.[104] As hand surgeons gain more experience with the arthroscope, its role and definition with respect to both diagnosis and management of ligamentous wrist pathology will continue to expand (Fig. 24-10).

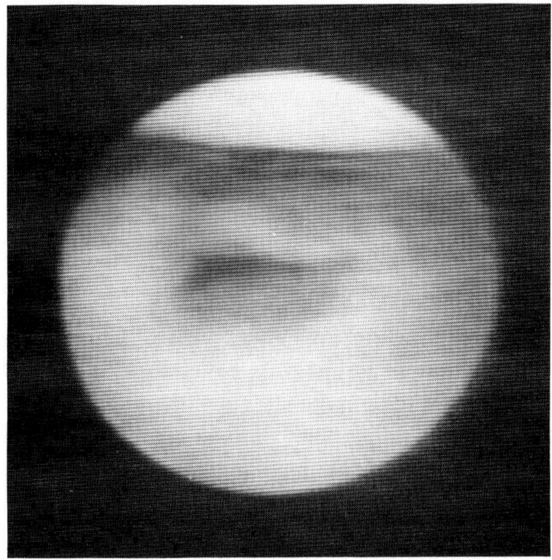

FIG. 24-10. Arthroscopic view of partial midbody TFCC tear in a symptomatic 19-year-old basketball player following a twisting injury while slam dunking (the lunate is seen at the top). This lesion was successfully treated by arthroscopic debridement.

MECHANISM, DIAGNOSIS, AND TREATMENT OF SPECIFIC INJURIES

This section defines and describes specific pathologic problems with respect to their anatomy and kinematics, diagnosis and imaging, and recommended treatment. Acute injuries of the wrist should be reduced and stabilized. The authors' own experience, as well as many reports in the literature, do not support open repairs rather than accurate percutaneous pinnings of purely intraarticular ligament tears in all cases.

Scapholunate Dissociation Instability

The most frequently identified carpal instability is scapholunate dissociation. Scapholunate ligamentous injuries may be as common as scaphoid fractures. The most significant problem with these injuries is a delay in making the diagnosis.[16,38,40,91] Treatment often does not begin until several months after injury, when full-blown static instability has developed. In the meantime, potential degenerative changes or ligament scarring may have already occurred, and the possibility of restoring normal wrist function has dramatically diminished.[16,34,38,40] We cannot overemphasize the importance of *suspecting* scapholunate dissociation, making the diagnosis promptly, and thereby greatly improving the ultimate outcome of these injuries.

Kinematics

The scaphoid ("mobile column") palmar flexes (becomes vertical) to permit normal radial deviation. The scaphoid is linked to the lunate by the scapholunate interosseous and radioscapholunate ligaments, and the lunate also is brought into palmar flexion as the capitate moves relatively palmar (muscle load-induced compression further assists to tilt the lunate).[84] As long as the triquetrolunate ligament is intact, the triquetrum moves from its "low" (dorsiflexed) position on the hamate upward into palmar flexion. There is disagreement as to whether these forces initiate mechanically at the scapho-trapezio-trapezoidal or at the triquetrohamate joint. A break in the scaphoid-to-lunate link still allows the scaphoid-to-palmar flex in response to loads, gravity, and radial deviation, but the lunate (which has the natural tendency to dorsiflex) would not be moved. The result is a palmar flexed (vertical) scaphoid and a dorsiflexed lunate and triquetrum. (The capitate rides high on the lunate, dorsal to the axial plane of the radius.) The lunate is now an intercalated segment that is dorsiflexed. The scaphoid is vertical and usually described on the lateral roentgenogram as a part of the dorsal intercalated segment instability (DISI) or as "rotatory scaphoid subluxation." Other forms of lateral instabilities include the rare primary STT dissociation[94] and scaphoid dislocations; however, these instabilities generally appear only as single case reports.[25,46,53,89]

Mechanism

The mechanism of injury is most frequently described as a fall on an outstretched hand, with impact at the thenar eminence, which results in hyperextension, ulnar deviation, and intercarpal supination.[6,54,55,92] With strong axial compression, the capitate becomes a "battering ram," driving proximally between scaphoid and lunate.[6,46,53] In experiments involving wrist loading, the scapholunate joint is known to be the first carpal joint injured. The scapholunate interosseous and radioscapholunate ligaments are capable of elongating before failure, so that there can be variations in injury patterns.[54,55] Such "stretched" ligaments may account for the acute dynamic instability patterns. With time and further attenuation, recognized static patterns develop. Complete dissociation of the scapholunate joint does not occur until the radioscaphoid portion of the radioscapholunate ligament ruptures.[4,34,51,54] Therefore, *any athlete complaining of radial wrist pain after a fall on an outstretched hand must be carefully evaluated for both scaphoid fracture and ligamentous injury.*

Kinematic Stages (Fig. 24-11)

1. As the wrist is loaded in dorsiflexed ulnar deviation and intercarpal supination, the scapholunate interosseous and radioscaphoid ligaments rupture, resulting in scapholunate dissociation.
2. Further loads rupture the radiocapitate ligament, resulting in capitolunate joint dislocation through the space of Poirier.
3. The triquetrum dissociates from the lunate as a consequence of radiolunotriquetral ligament rupture.
4. Disruption of the dorsal radiocarpal ligament occurs as the rest of the carpus loads downward onto its dorsal surface. The lunate dislocates volarward, leaving it suspended by its volar radial and ulnar ligamentous attachments. At this point, the distal surface faces palmar, but further carpal motion forces the lunate through the space of Poirier and rotates it (on the intact volar ligament) to face proximally.

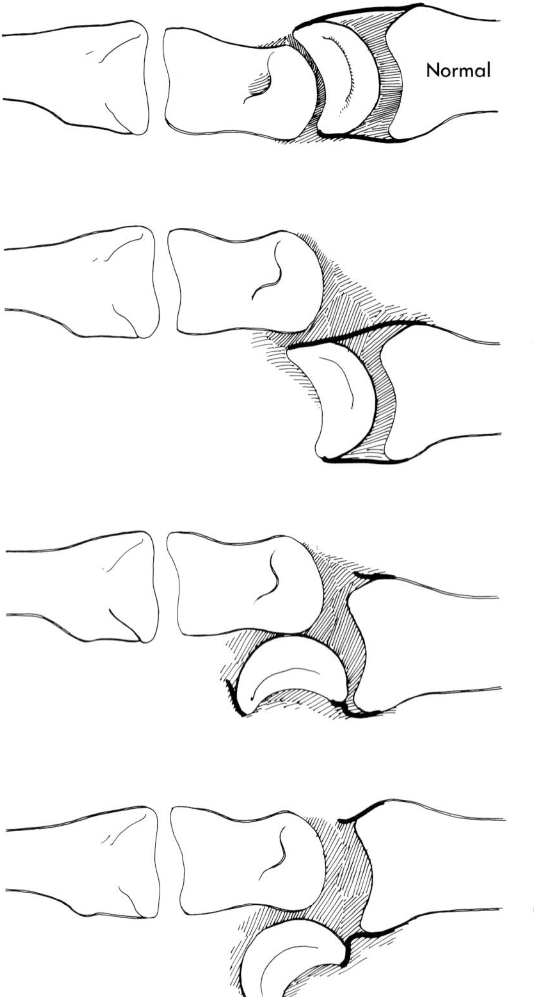

FIG. 24-11. Kinematic stages of progressive disruption (pure ligament and osteoligamentous) in perilunate and lunate disruption. **A,** Perilunate. **B,** Transition from perilunate to lunate dislocation. **C,** True lunate dislocation.

Variations can occur as some ligaments may elongate or attenuate, producing milder degrees of instability, permitting spontaneous reduction, and leaving little or no evidence on routine roentgenograms.[55] In 1943, Gilford and his colleagues[29] stressed the importance of the scaphoid as the connecting rod bridging the carpus to prevent the "link joint" from collapse. Most important, these authors noted that a scaphoid fracture often produces secondary carpal malalignment and collapse (Fig. 24-12). Fisk[26] later expanded on this theme, describing the zigzag pattern "concertina deformity" of wrist collapse typical of both scaphoid fractures and Kienböck's disease.

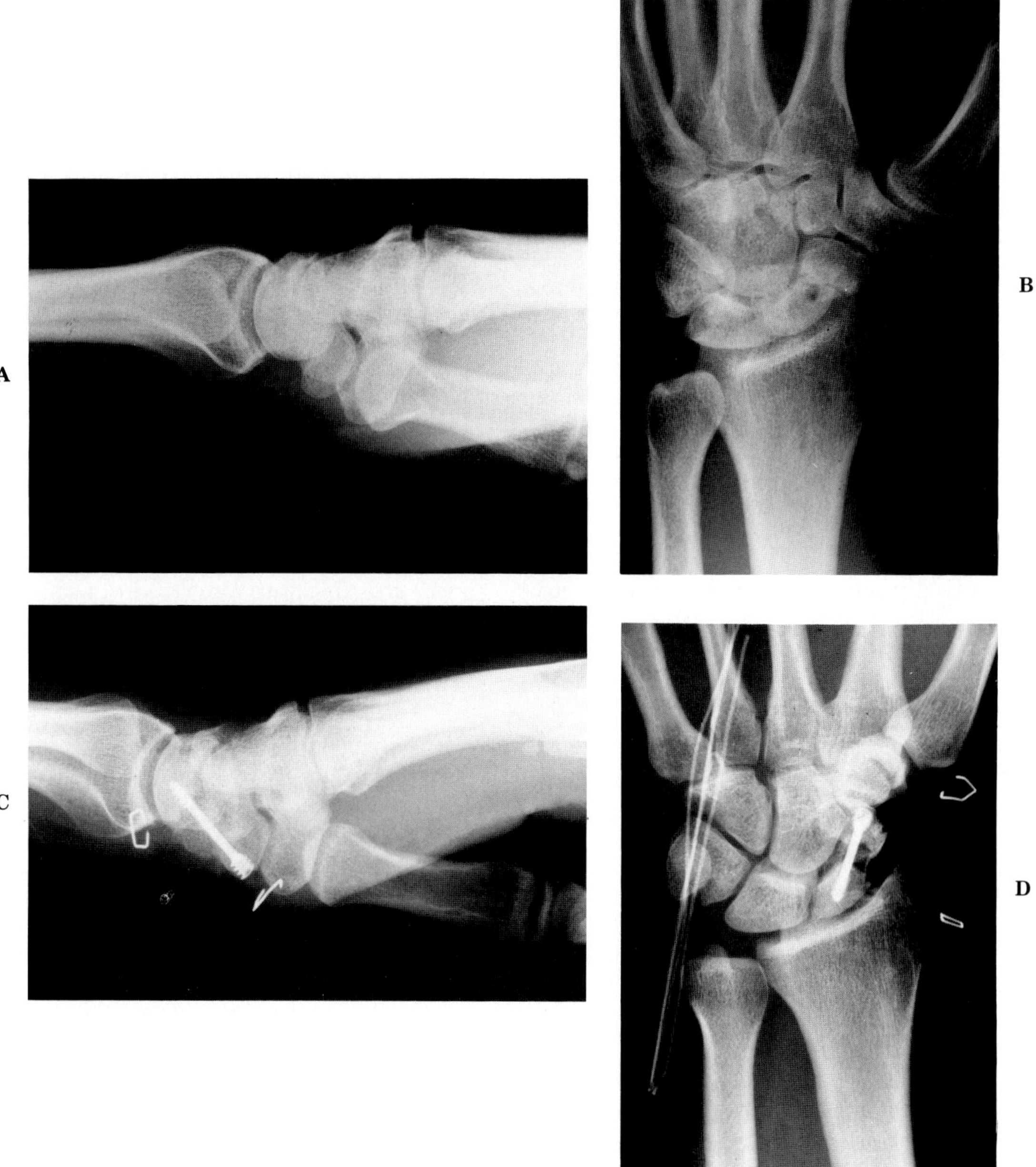

FIG. 24-12. A, and **B,** Lateral and PA roentgenographs demonstrate secondary carpal collapse when the scaphoid "link-joint" connecting rod is disrupted by fracture; including the DISI deformity seen on the lateral, but with scaphoid malangulation caused by fracture rather than a vertical position. **C,** and **D,** Following scaphoid osteotomy and iliac (wedge) bone graft with the fixation by Herbert compression screw, (Zimmer USA, Inc., Warsaw, IN) there has been consequent intercarpal reduction and restoration of normal bone relationships.

Diagnosis

Chronic problems are generally associated with (milder) intermittent symptoms related to certain activities, especially those requiring rotation or deviation of the wrist. Palmer[71] noted that 100% of his patients who had diagnosed ligamentous disruption experienced wrist pain, 91% had decreased grip strength, 71% demonstrated decreased motion, and one third experienced clicking of the wrist. The clicking has been described as a "catch-up" clunk—as the wrist moves from radial to ulnar deviation, the lunate and triquetrum move synchronously, but the scaphoid is "left behind" in palmar flexion.[41,37,99] As the radial side of the carpus elongates further, the scaphoid suddenly jumps into place, "catching up with" the lunate. Many patients with ligamentous instability have been found to have a diffuse ligamentous laxity of many joints, including those of the opposite extremity.[92]

Dynamic instabilities can often be diagnosed using **Watson's scaphoid test:** the examiner places four fingers of one hand on the distal radius and the thumb on the scaphoid tuberosity while the wrist is postured in ulnar deviation (elongating the scaphoid). Pressure is directed dorsally with the thumb at the volar scaphoid, while the wrist is radially deviated. Pressure on the scaphoid, which prevents it from becoming vertical, drives the proximal pole dorsally if the ligaments are not intact. Pain is the hallmark of a positive test, although sometimes the dorsal movement of the scaphoid can actually be seen to move dorsally.

Roentgenographic Assessment

There are several roentgenographic methods for diagnosing scapholunate dissociation. However, we recommend the "instability series" as especially helpful. Suggestive findings on PA projections include a scapholunate space greater than 2 to 3 mm (in any event, not greater than other intercarpal spaces). Marked gaps are obvious and are remembered when termed a "David Letterman" sign or "Terry-Thomas"[28] and "Leon Spinks" sign[37] (see Fig. 24-8). The scaphoid may appear foreshortened and have a superimposed cortical "ring" because of the end-on projection of its now vertical proximal pole.

Roentgenographic signs of scapholunate dissociation

- Scapholunate interval > 2-3 mm
- Foreshortened scaphoid
- Cortical "ring" sign
- Scapholunate angle > 65 degrees

On lateral films (see Figs. 24-4 to 24-7), the capitate, third metacarpal, and radius are normally collinear, with the scaphoid at 30 to 60 degrees. From this perspective, with the lunate in dorsiflexion (DISI), the scaphoid is in a vertical position (>65 to 70 degrees).[50] Motion studies reveal the abnormal "catch-up clunk," and the lunate remains dorsiflexed throughout motion, since the palmar flexing influence of the scaphoid has been lost. Arthrograms offer some information for cases that are otherwise difficult to diagnose.[73] We have begun to use diagnostic arthroscopy on those patients with suspected injuries but equivocal roentgenographic findings.

Treatment

Acute injuries. Controversy exists regarding proper management of acute scapholunate dissociation. Many authors feel strongly that only open treatment is proper.[36] Others, including the authors, believe that closed reduction (sometimes with arthroscopic verification) and Kirschner wire (K-wire) fixation are effective, if properly performed and if followed by maintenance with gauntlet cast support for 8 weeks.[34,79] Those who advocate open treatment argue the merits of a dorsal approach alone versus combined dorsal and volar approaches. The two incision approach allows the surgeon to both evaluate the reduction dorsally and repair the volar ligament through a separate volar incision.[37] The paradox[56] is that while wrist dorsiflexion is the position of bony reduction, this configuration further produces separation and displacement of the palmar ligaments. The problem is overcome by reducing the scaphoid in wrist dorsiflexion, pinning it to the capitate and/or lunate, but then immobilizing the wrist in mild palmar flexion to facilitate apposition of the torn ligaments.[37,92] Hand therapy is begun 8 weeks after repair/reduction, but impact loading is restricted for another 8 weeks.

After reduction of perilunate or lunate dislocations, rotatory scaphoid subluxation frequently becomes apparent in follow-up roentgenograms. We prefer to pin most cases acutely to avoid this complication. If diagnosed late, open reduction may often be required. In the presence of transosseous perilunate dislocations, the dynamic tendency to instability resulting from the "ligamentous disruption" is a likely cause of scaphoid nonunion.[66]

Chronic injury. Treatment of chronic

scapholunate dissociations can be difficult. Operations to stabilize the carpal architecture have been described.* The use of tendon grafts to reconstruct the radioscapholunate ligament has been described by several authors, but this approach has not been uniformly successful; therefore most surgeons have abandoned it.[23,42,71,92] Blatt[6] proposed reconstruction (especially for nondissociative instabilities) using a dorsal wrist capsular flap sutured to the distal pole of the scaphoid. The purpose of this procedure is to achieve more motion than can be expected from limited intercarpal arthrodeses. He performs this operation when a relatively unblemished scaphoid can be reduced easily to anatomic position at surgery. A thumb spica is used for immobilization for 2 months, and then hand therapy is initiated. No forceful stress is permitted for 4 to 6 months postoperatively. We have limited experience with this operation and can neither advocate nor condemn it for long-term efficiency in a vigorous population. More recently, Conyers[14] has reported a volar osteoligamentous stabilization for the subacute static DISI deformity.

Many authors now prefer limited intercarpal fusions to treat chronic scapholunate dissociation† (Fig. 24-13). In reconstructing the "force-bearing column," Weber believes it would make sense to link the scaphoid to the lunate in order to transfer force from the capitate to the radius. However, a sucessful scapholunate arthrodesis is most unusual, because of the small contact surface area and the considerable forces applied to the segments. In 1967 Peterson and Lipscombe[77] proposed scaphoid-trapezium-trapezoid (STT) fusion. Later popularized by Watson et al,[101] this procedure is used to reconstruct the scaphoid as a midcarpal strut, to restore carpal height, and to retain triquetral lunate motion (thus keeping more carpal motion).[37,44,45] The key is accurate reduction of the scaphoid to the level of the dorsiflexed lunate and restoration of the scapholunate unit to its normal position before pinning the scaphoid to the capitate. Since the entire distal carpal row is a single bony unit and the objective is to transmit forces from capitate through scaphoid and lunate to the radius, it makes equal mechanical sense to fuse the scaphoid to the capitate.[24,60] We prefer a scaphocapitate fusion since it is easier to perform than other intercarpal fusions. The joint is also in the operative area where most of the

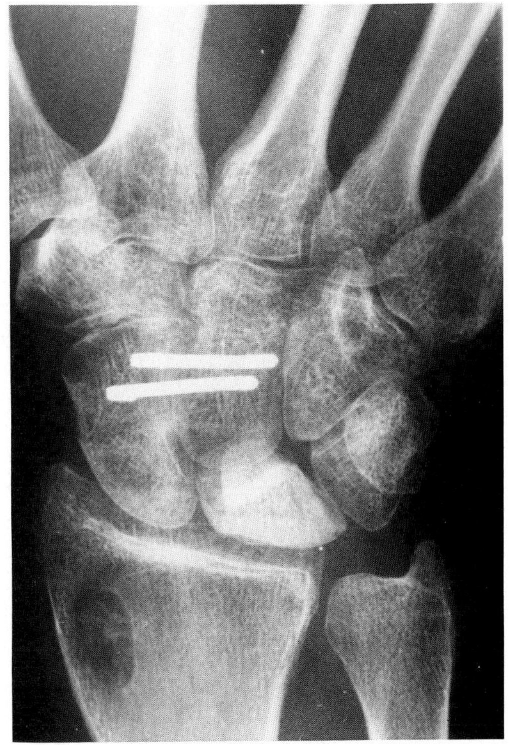

FIG. 24-13. PA roentgenographs of successful scaphocapitate arthrodesis in a 22-year-old squash player with Stage II Kienbock's disease.

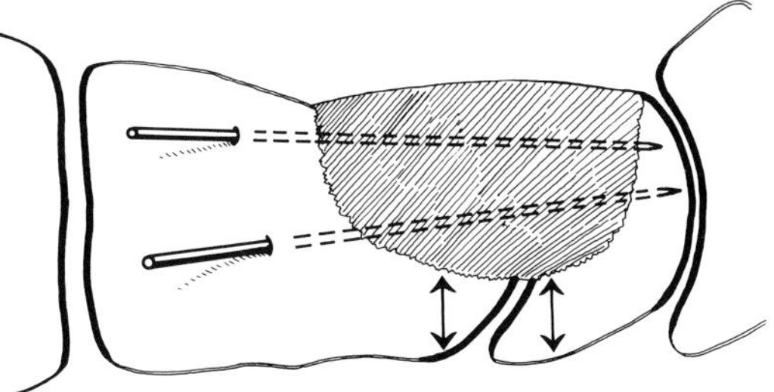

FIG. 24-14. Diagramatic representation of generic intercarpal arthrodesis, preserving original (reduced) intercarpal spaces by retaining the palmar third of cortex and cartilage, but tightly packing the curetted interspace generously with autogenous bone graft.

*References 3, 6, 23, 44, 45, 71, 98.

†References 36, 77, 78, 94, 101.

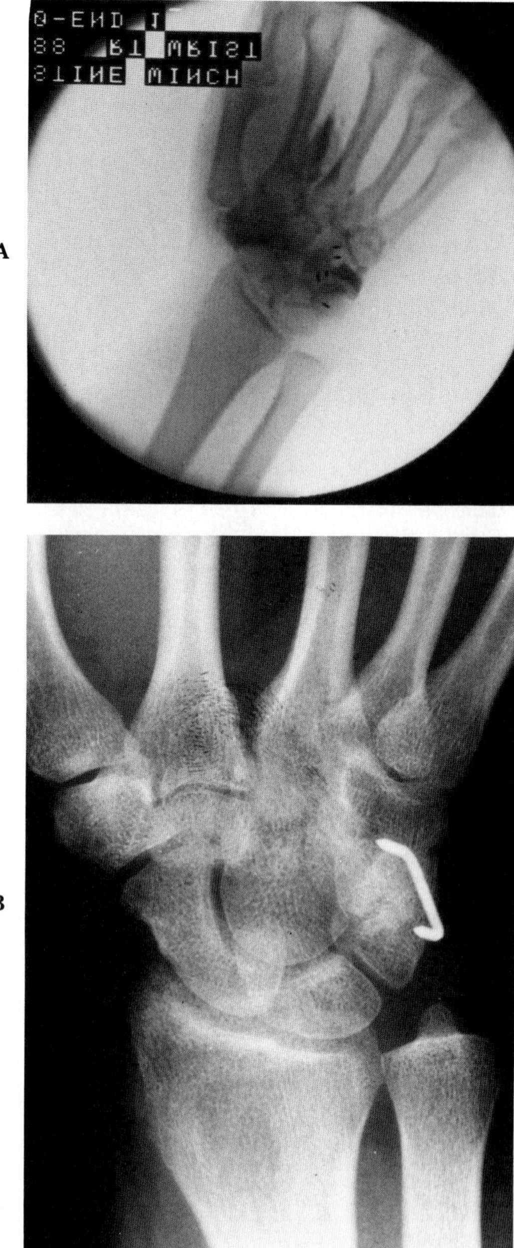

FIG. 24-15. A, Abnormal digital subtraction arthrogram following midcarpal injection demonstrating dye leakage across the hamotriquetral joint. **B,** This young female gymnast was successfully treated by HT intercarpal arthrodesis.

surgical dissection takes place.[78] For all limited arthrodeses, it is essential to preserve original intercarpal spaces by retaining the palmar third of cortex and cartilage but by tightly packing each curetted interspace with a generous bone graft (Fig. 24-14). We initially stabilize these bones with K-wires and power bone staples (3M Company, Minneapolis) and remove the wires at about 6 weeks. The use of titanium staples allows us to mobilize these wrists sooner, even as bone bridging is progressing, because of the stability added by the internal fixation (see Figs. 24-13 and 24-15, *B*).

When the scaphoid is allowed to remain chronically malpositioned vertically in palmar flexion, the transmission of forces takes alternate pathways across incongruent surfaces, resulting initially in localized osteoarthritis. Arthritic changes typically seen between radial styloid and scaphoid and also between capitate and lunate are referred to as **SLAC wrist** (scapholunate advanced collapse).[98] Since the radiolunate joint is spared in such former athletes, consideration should be given to performing radial styloidectomy or partial scaphoid excision plus lunocapitate arthrodesis. The use of silicone carpal implants in vigorous individuals of any age is clearly contraindicated because of the high potential for microfragmentation and secondary "silicone synovitis."[10,76]

Medial Carpal Instabilities

Medial instabilities involve the ligaments attached to the medial or rotatory column in Taleisnik's kinematic model, including triquetrolunate and triquetrohamate or midcarpal instability. Although the lateral (radial) carpus is bridged by the scaphoid (control rod of Gilford), the ulnar carpus lacks such a bony bridge and relies on the volar arcuate "V" ligament for stabilization.[29,57,90] In normal ulnar deviation, the triquetrum descends and the hamate moves distally and changes its position to one of dorsiflexion. Because of the lunotriquetral ligaments, this movement forces the remainder of the proximal row to dorsiflex synchronously. Sectioning the lunotriquetral ligament would exclude the secondary dorsiflexing influence of triquetrum to lunate. The resulting volar flexed lunate and scaphoid seen with a dorsiflexed triquetrum is the typical VISI pattern deformity seen only on lateral roentgenograms. This deformity may be dynamic, visualized only in such cases with axial compression, or as a static deformity in those with severe or chronic injuries.[92] In the presence of midcarpal instabilities, it is the loss of influence of the bony geometry of the hamate on the lunate that allows VISI deformity to develop.[1]

Triquetrohamate (Midcarpal) Instabilities

Mechanism

Most authors think that this injury is produced by impact on the medial side of the hand and hyperpronation.[35] However, many patients do not recall a specific injury, and many have asymptomatic ligamentous laxity in the opposite wrist.*

Diagnosis

Lichtman reports that his patients complained of a painful click with ulnar deviation and pronation of the wrist. The click was also reproduced upon axial compression (but may be asymptomatically produced on the opposite side as well).[1] Tenderness is present with palpation at the midcarpus, either in the capitolunate or triquetrohamate interspaces.

Triquetrolunate rupture, TFCC tears, ulnar abutment syndrome, and subluxation of the distal radioulnar joint potentially may also produce painful clicks on the ulnar aspect of the wrist.[8] After completion of the history and physical examination, roentgenographic studies will be warranted.

Causes of "clicks" in the ulnar area

- Triquetrohamate instability
- Triquetrolunate rupture
- TFCC tears
- Ulnar abutment syndrome
- Distal radioulnar joint subluxation

Roentgenographic Assessment

Because medial carpal instabilities are frequently dynamic, standard (static) PA, lateral, radial, and ulnar deviation views are often within normal limits. The most helpful diagnostic tool in evaluating midcarpal instabilities is the cineroentgenogram (videofluoroscopy).[1,8] Typically, in these cases, as the patient moves from the volar flexed "physiologic VISI" of radial deviation toward the ulna, there is a sudden "snap" of the proximal carpal row into DISI nearing the limits of ulnar deviation. The failure of a smooth transition from phys-

*References 1, 8, 36, 49, 88, 99.

iologic VISI to physiologic DISI is typical of midcarpal instability. Tears may also be demonstrated by arthrogram (Fig. 24-15, *A*).

Treatment

Patients with chronic, mild triquetrohamate instabilities may have an associated synovitis that does not require surgery. For athletes seen early after injury, antiinflammatory medications and local injections of steroids are justified only if frank dissociation cannot be definitely diagnosed.[1,49,92] The defined acute tear may be treated by percutaneous pinning and gauntlet cast or by a long arm cast (forearm in supination and wrist in neutral) for 6 to 8 weeks; we prefer pins in most instances.

Authors have various opinions regarding surgery for chronic pathologic conditions. Taleisnik[92] recommends capsulodesis (tenodesis) for patients who will not place excessive loads upon the wrist or for those whose grip strength is less than 40 kg and who will not have frequent, high loads applied, criteria that are rarely met in the injured athlete (we do not recommend lunotriquetral or triquetrohamate ligament reconstruction). Lichtman advocates triquetrohamate arthrodesis, because his ligamentous reconstructions proved ineffective[8] (Fig. 24-15, *B*). Patients and physicians must understand that up to a third of (aggregate) motion in the injured wrist compared with the noninjured wrist will be lost. However patients rarely complain since pain is reduced and power increases.[8,31,78]

During an operation for arthrodesis, the triquetrohamate joint is approached from the dorsum. The dorsal half to two thirds is decorticated, and the bones are reduced and pinned. With direct vision, one must verify that the midcarpal subluxation has been eliminated as the wrist goes through a full passive range of motion. Autogenous radius metaphyseal bone graft is harvested (through a separate incision) and densely packed to obliterate the interspace. We prefer this technique, but Taleisnik has suggested performing radiolunate arthrodesis with the lunate in neutral position and aligned with the radius or lunotriquetral-hamate-capitate fusion. Experimental data reveal that such operations markedly diminish wrist mobility.[24,60] The basic principle of limited arthrodeses is always the same: restore but do not change the normal spacial relationships between carpal bones with fusion[100] (see Fig. 24-14).

Triquetrolunate Instabilities

The triquetrum is securely tethered to the lunate by the triquetrolunate ligament. Triquetral descent on the hamate in ulnar deviation causes dorsiflexion, and the ligamentous connections among the bones of the proximal carpal row dorsiflex in the direction of both scaphoid and lunate synchronously (the "physiologic DISI"). Attenuation or rupture of the triquetrolunate ligament eliminates the controlling influence of the triquetrum, and the naturally volar flexing scaphoid, with its intact scapholunate ligament, brings the lunate into a volar flexed attitude, thereby creating the typical VISI deformity. On the lateral roentgenogram of such cases, the volar flexed lunate and scaphoid are seen concurrently with a dorsiflexed triquetrum in *both* radial and ulnar deviation.

Mechanism

The exact mechanism of injury is uncertain. Isolated triquetrolunate injury may result from hyperpronation of the hand on the forearm.[37,56,92] Weber[102,103] believes that such injuries are caused by impact on the dorsum of a palmar flexed hand and that, characteristically, the palmar fibers (radiolunotriquetral ligament) are spared. He presumes that these palmar fibers become the rotational axis as a VISI deformity develops. If the lunate is free to flex in a palmar direction at the same time as the scaphoid, the triquetrum dorsiflexes as it is forced by the capitate to move ulnarly and down the hamate; under such circumstances, a static VISI deformity may develop.

Diagnosis

Diagnosis can be difficult soon after injury, before a VISI pattern develops roentgenographically. The athlete may recount a history that includes falling on an outstretched hand in radial deviation. Or he or she may tell of being struck on the back of the hand and seeking treatment for pain along the ulnar side of the wrist. One may elicit tenderness at the triquetrolunate joint, frequently with associated weakness, but there may not be a click produced by passively loading the wrist and moving from ulnar to radial deviation.[1,82,102,103] The "lunatotriquetral ballotement test"[82] requires stabilization of the lunate with the examiner's thumb and index finger and shucking the pisiform and triquetrum palmarward and dorsally with the other hand to determine the presence of laxity, pain, and crepitance. Like diagnoses of midcarpal instabilities, differential diagnoses include TFCC tears, triquetrohamate tears, subluxation or dislocation of the radioulnar joint, subluxation of extensor carpi ulnaris (ECU) tendon, and ulnocarpal abutment.

Roentgenographic Assessment

Standard films are typically normal; however, an associated VISI deformity on the lateral view must be identified where both the scaphoid and lunate are volar flexed, but the triquetrum is dorsiflexed and distal on the hamate. The PA view shows a break in continuity in the carpal arcs at the triquetrolunate joint.[82,92] We find that the most useful test is an arthrogram, which will usually demonstrate the ligament tear (leak) and associated pathologic condition. In questionable cases, arthroscopy can play a role in achieving a definitive diagnosis or in distinguishing small and kinematically insignificant tears noted only as slow or one-way leaks on an arthrogram (see Fig. 24-9).

Treatment

Athletes who have acute partial tears, including significant injuries that do not yet show static VISI deformity on roentgenogram, should be immobilized for 6 to 8 weeks with a long arm cast positioning the wrist in ulnar deviation and dorsiflexion. The plaster should be molded to apply palmar pressure on the pisiform.[82,84,87]

In the presence of static VISI deformity, the scaphoid and lunate must be immobilized in a dorsiflexed position to match the triquetrum and consequently to reverse the clinical deformity. Acute complete disruptions should be fixed internally. Although open ligament repair is sometimes advocated,[1,82] we believe that percutaneous pinning under fluoroscopic control is sufficient if maintained for 8 weeks. For chronic cases, we agree with Lichtman, who recommends triquetrolunate arthrodesis for static deformities or nondissociative instabilities unresponsive to conservative care.

Proximal Carpal Instabilities (Ulnar Translocation)

Ulnar translocation has been found after trauma.[50,54,92] Recently Rayhack et al[81] described several cases in detail, in which three of eight patients were injured during athletics.

Diagnosis

Hyperextension associated with substantial torque, possibly pronation of the forearm on a fixed hand, is postulated as a mechanism for ulnar translation.[81] Cadaver dissections by Rayhack et al[81] revealed that the carpus could not be translocated toward the ulna until all insertions of the palmar radiocarpal ligaments are disrupted. At examination, acute injuries are associated with massive swelling and striking loss of strength. The carpus may be obviously unstable because of radio/ulnar pressure directed to the second metacarpal or triquetrum; redisplacement occurs with release of pressure (Fig. 24-16).

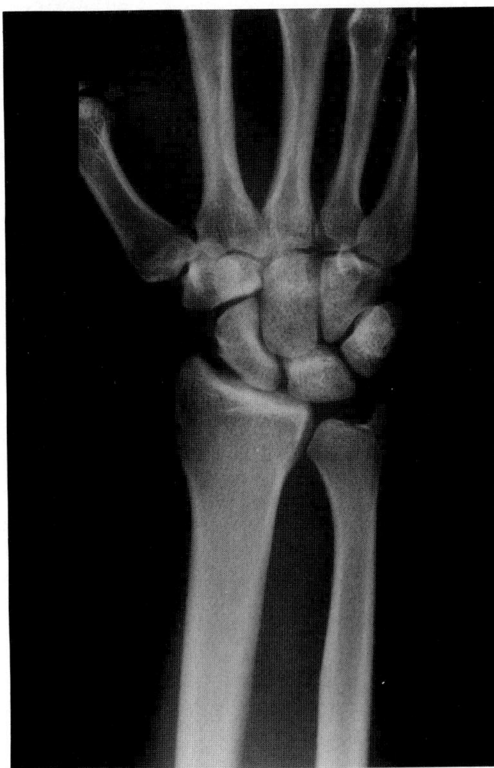

FIG. 24-16. Acute radiocarpal shift (with ulnar translation) in a 19-year-old girl who fell while competitively skateboarding. Note the increased radioscaphoid space. She was treated by open reduction, pinning of the scaphoid and lunate to the radius, plus repair of the dorsal and volar ligaments and capsule.

Roentgenographic Assessment

The diagnosis of ulnar translocation cannot be determined by clinical means alone; specific roentgenographic findings include ulnar displacement of the carpus on the radius with less than half of the lunate within the lunate fossa. The distance between the radial styloid and scaphoid is increased, and the lunate blocks ulnar deviation. Most important, McMurtry[58,107] and Chamay[11] described the measurement of the "carpal ulnar distance" or the "carpal translation index." If an erroneous diagnosis of scapholunate dissociation is made, an associated increase in the scapholunate interval influences the treatment and outcome.

Treatment

Initially, the injury should be reduced and the reduction should be held in a cast or splint until plans for surgery have been made. Closed reduction alone is inadequate. Primary ligament repair and internal stabilization is highly recommended. For chronic cases, radiolunate arthrodesis is performed because ligamentous stabilizations have proved futile.[37,71,92]

Dorsal and Palmar Subluxations

There are few reports of palmar translocation in the literature, and none pertain to athletic activities.[5] Dorsal translocation is frequently secondary to malunited fractures of the distal radius or rheumatoid arthritis. Treatment should be directed at correcting the malangulation of the articular surface of the radius by osteotomy if the articular surface is intact. If the articular surface is noncongruent or degenerated, limited fusion of involved joint(s) is best.

Diagnosis

Lateral roentgenograms demonstrate that the lunate and capitate are dorsal or volar to the articular surface of the radius, differing from perilunate dislocations, which are characterized by an intact radiolunate relationship except that the capitate is dorsal.

Treatment

When isolated and not associated with radial fractures, this injury needs open reduction, pinning, and ligament repair or reconstruction. Late cases will undoubtedly require radius–proximal row arthrodesis to achieve adequate stabilization.

Ligamentous Disruptions of the Distal Radioulnar Joint

Although ligamentous disruptions of the distal radioulnar joint have been recognized for nearly two centuries, only in the past decade have we gained a detailed understanding of the anatomy and biomechanics of this joint. The additional information should lead to improved treatment of athletes who sustain injuries to it. Besides the causative athletic endeavor, it is important to consider the patient's vocational and avocational goals as future treatment may depend on them.

Mechanism

The triangular fibrocartilage complex (TFCC) which is the major stabilizer of the distal radioulnar joint, is composed of the triangular fibrocartilage, ulnar meniscus homolog, ulnar collateral ligament, dorsal and volar radioulnar ligaments, the ulnolunate and ulnotriquetral ligaments, and the extensor carpi ulnaris tendon sheath.[74,75] Because many of these individual structures are poorly defined in the clinical setting, they have been grouped into one "complex" which arises from the ulnar aspect of the lunate fossa[7,75] and suspends the carpus from the distal radius. The complex inserts into the base of the ulnar styloid, and the volar aspect of the TFCC is very strongly attached to the lunotriquetral interosseous ligament and triquetrum. The TFCC is thick along its dorsal and volar edges, but thin in the center in the region of the lunate/TFCC articulation[75] (Fig. 24-17).

The forearm can rotate approximately 150 degrees at the distal radioulnar joint. The radius (and hand) rotates about the ulnar head, which is not immobile during this rotation, as was once believed. Ray et al[80] demonstrated that the distal ulna abducts 8 to 9 degrees with pronation and adducts with supination.

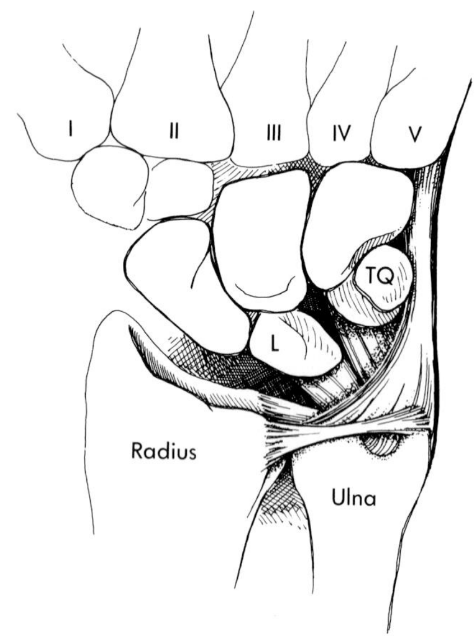

FIG. 24-17. The triangular fibrocartilage complex is comprised of the triangular fibrocartilage, ulnar meniscus homologue, ulnar collateral ligament, dorsal and volar radioulnar ligaments, ulnolunate and ulnotriquetral ligaments, and extensor carpi ulnaris; it is a major stabilizer of the distal radioulnar joint.

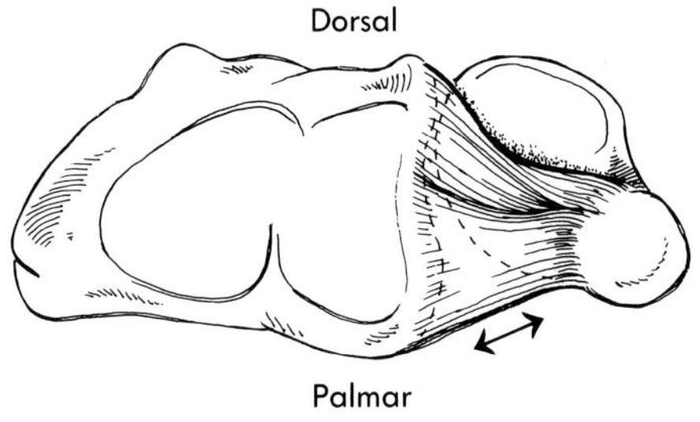

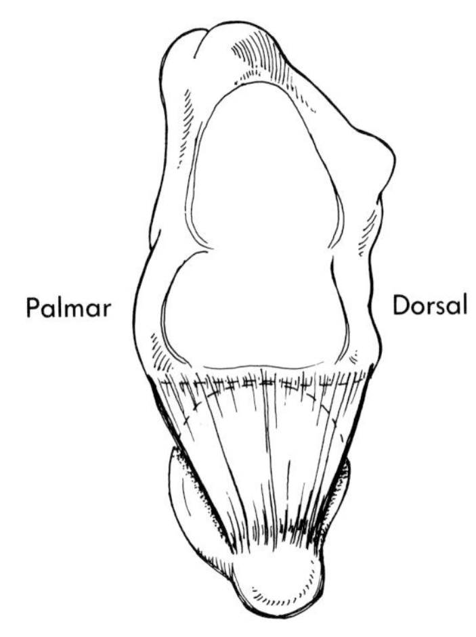

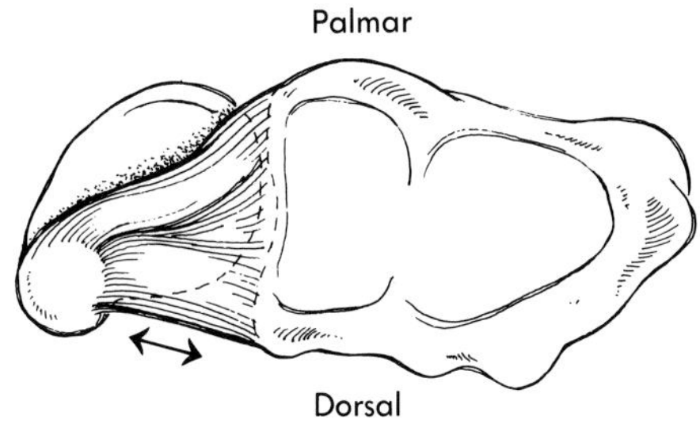

FIG. 24-18. The distal radioulnar joint stabilizing ligaments (TFCC) some fibers which are taut in any (all) forearm position such that injury of the volar fibers allows dorsal displacement while the ulna is in pronation; and the reverse in supination.

The ulnar head moves dorsally in pronation and volarward in supination.[95] In addition, Palmer[72] has demonstrated that the ulnar head moves distally with pronation and proximally with supination. Pronation therefore causes the ulna to abduct and to move dorsally and distally and supination causes the distal ulna to adduct and move volarward and proximally in relation to the radius. Stability throughout a range of motion and axial loading is dependent on both TFCC integrity and bony congruence. The volar aspect of the TFCC is taut in pronation and relaxed in supination; the reverse is true for its dorsal aspect, which is taut in supination and relaxed in pronation, thereby resisting subluxation (with the ulnocarpal ligaments) throughout forearm rotation (Fig. 24-18).

Triangular fibrocartilage complex

- Triangular fibrocartilage
- Ulnar meniscus homolog
- Ulnar collateral ligament
- Dorsal and volar radioulnar ligaments
- Ulnolunate ligament
- Ulnotriquetral ligament
- Extensor carpi ulnaris tendon sheath

Distal radioulnar joint mechanics

Pronation
- Distal ulna abducts
- Ulnar head moves dorsally
- Ulnar head advances distally

Supination
- Distal ulna adducts
- Ulnar head moves volarward
- Ulnar head advances proximally

The TFCC, the pronator quadratus, and the interosseous membrane are also important in cushioning and transmitting ulnar axial loads. Disruption of a portion of the TFCC may allow instability, and excision of the entire TFCC causes nonphysiologic increases in loading of the radius. Palmer[74] demonstrated that ulnar variance (the relative length of the ulna compared to that of the radius) also has dramatic effects on the amount of load borne by the ulna. Shortening the length of the ulna by 2.5 mm decreases the force borne by the distal ulna from 20% to 4% of the total force of the forearm. Increasing the length of the ulna by 2.5 mm increases the force borne by the ulna to 42% of the total. Such changes in transmission of load are significant in the development of early arthrosis at contact points.

Diagnosis

A history of wrist extension and forearm hyperpronation is commonly described by those who can recall the events leading to the injury. Typical examples of the incidents affecting athletes involve falling on the outstretched hand or "straight arming" an opponent in football or rugby.[35] In the presence of an acute injury, instability of the ulnar head, swelling, crepitance, or pain with volar-directed compression of the ulna can be observed. If there is no acute injury, it is necessary to localize the site of the pathologic abnormality by palpating the area. The differential diagnosis includes radioulnar or radiocarpal arthritis, extensor carpi ulnaris subluxation, ulnocarpal impingement, and medial and midcarpal instabilities. The athlete should describe when his or her pain occurs, and the physician should then attempt to reproduce the circumstances with manipulation. In the presence of instability, most often dorsal subluxation of the ulna (whatever the anatomic basis), a painful clunk will often accompany the passive maneuver. There are now a variety of imaging techniques that can assist in achieving an accurate diagnosis.

Roentgenographic Assessment

The lack of "truly standardized" PA and lateral views for evaluation of the distal radioulnar joint has contributed to the difficulty in evaluating films identifying dorsal or volar subluxation if the diagnosis is not clinically obvious. Bowers[7] recommends that the PA film be taken with the shoulder abducted to 90 degrees, elbow flexed 90 degrees, and the hand flat on each set. Both radial and ulnar styloids should be at the extreme medial and lateral edges on the roentgenogram. The lateral is taken with the shoulder at zero degrees abduction, with the elbow flexed to 90 degrees, and with the x-ray tube at right angles to the wrist. Besides looking for evidence of fracture or subluxation **ulnar variance** should be assessed because it may influence diagnosis and care. *Positive variance* is more often associated with TFCC injury and impingement, and *negative variance* is associated with Kienböck's disease and posttraumatic carpal instability. Trispiral tomograms can be helpful in identifying small fractures not seen in plain films.

We find that the CT scan is the most reliable method for assessing distal radioulnar joint congruence. Mino, Palmer et al[63,64] compared roentgenograms to CT scans for evaluating the distal radioulnar joint. The CT scan obviates the problem of achieving neutral wrist rotation on a plain film. The wrist of an acutely injured athlete can thereby be evaluated while still splinted, without regard to wrist position. MRI is now being used with some effectiveness in demonstrating the site and severity of TFCC disruption; but further refinements of this expensive technique will permit increased definition of its diagnostic value.[59]

Arthrography

Arthrography is an excellent method for identifying defects (tears) in the TFCC. Many patients have degenerative tears in the TFCC that were not caused by acute trauma. Degenerative defects and secondary ulnolunate abutment develop into synovitis secondary to cartilaginous erosion.[61,74] Wrist pain may be secondary to impingement (abutment), which is the real problem that needs to be addressed (not the "tear," which may well be asymptomatic). At the time of an acute injury the TFCC may be avulsed from the ulna, and contrast will leak into the subcutaneous tissues around the ulna or from the triquetral recess proximally across the TFCC into the distal radioulnar joint.[35,70] Central TFCC tears also are usually easy to demonstrate. Avulsion at the radial margin of the TFCC is clearly appreciated following both radiocarpal and distal radioulnar injections.

Arthroscopy

Improved equipment and techniques over the past several years permit more frequent use of the arthroscopic evaluation of the distal radioulnar joint. In many instances arthroscopy can be used not only for diagnostic purposes but for therapeutic debridement of symptomatic partial (flap) tears in the absence of abutment (see Fig. 24-10).

Treatment

The TFCC has three important functions: it is a major stabilizer of the distal radioulnar joint; it serves as a cushion or load-bearer for transfer of ulnar axial loads; and it is a major stabilizer of the ulnar carpus and hand on the forearm. Posttraumatic clinical assessment should address which functions have been altered, and treatment should proceed accordingly.

If an athlete has sustained an acute injury and seeks treatment with a fresh history and physical examination suggestive of subluxation or dislocation of the distal ulna, primary treatment should focus on achieving and maintaining reduction. Such injuries usually result from avulsion of the TFCC from the ulnar styloid base or from the distal radius, and therefore the forearm should be immobilized. If dorsal ulnar subluxation has occurred, the forearm is placed in full supination with the elbow at 90 degrees. For a volarward dislocated ulna the wrist is immobilized in pronation and the elbow at 90 degrees. Joint congruity in the cast must be checked with CT scan. If closed reduction is not successful, operative intervention is warranted. If the ulnar styloid is fractured *and* if it is a large enough fragment, it may be approximated with tension band wires or compression screw; the TFCC itself can be reapproximated with sutures or intraosseous wires.[8] The lunotriquetral ligament in all these cases should be evaluated to exclude associated injury.[74]

Acute perforations of the central portion of the TFCC are believed to be rare.[35,61,70] Those that are seen usually have neutral or positive ulnar variance.[62,70] Most will become asymptomatic with conservative care. However, some patients will complain of persistent wrist pain and "clicking." In such patients, we find that positive arthrograms are best followed by arthroscopic evaluation with debridement of the flap (and that is all that is necessary). If the physician is not skilled with the wrist arthroscope, open debridement may be performed although recovery is prolonged. Ulnar shortening by step-cut diaphyseal osteotomy may be indicated in those with arthroscopically verifiable abutment from positive ulnar variance.[70]

Treatment of the "older athlete" who has chronic wrist pain secondary to (an old) TFCC tear, is initially conservative, consisting of splint support, nonsteroidal antiinflammatory drugs (NSAIDs), and local injection. If these measures are not successful, arthrography followed by arthroscopic debridement of the tear (flap) should be performed. If there is arthroscopically verifiable ulnolunate impingement (the patient is ulnar neutral or positive), step-cut ulnar resection osteotomy should be performed concomitantly. Some authors advise complete excision of the disk,[13] but based on the functions of the TFCC, we feel that total excision should be avoided if at all possible. Bowers[7] has described many of the soft tissue approaches used in reconstruction of the chronically unstable distal radioulnar joint, using portions of flexor carpi ulnaris, extensor carpi ulnaris, and extensor retinaculum, but we have not been consistently pleased with long-term results of such procedures for younger athletes. Accurate initial assessment will prevent such difficult and unsatisfactory choices in the vigorous athlete. For athletes with chronic injuries and degenerative changes of the articular surfaces, we prefer a partial or complete (Darrach) ulnar head resection, although in certain cases some authors advise ulnar shortening and lunotriquetral fusion.[70]

SUMMARY

Although they involve a wide spectrum of anatomy and pathologic conditions, acute carpal ligament injuries can be accurately diagnosed and effectively treatable. Restoration of optimal function requires a careful and detailed examination in conjunction with proper imaging studies to establish the site and degree of damage. Healthy athletes deserve our best efforts. With early treatment and supervised rehabilitation, most will be able to resume their previous activities.

REFERENCES

1. Alexander CE, and Lichtman DM: Ulnar carpal instabilities, Orthop Clin N Am 15:307, 1984.
2. Arkless R: Cineradiography of normal and abnormal wrists, Am J Roentgenol 96:837, 1966.
3. Armstrong GWD: Rotational subluxation of the scaphoid. Can J Surg 11:306, 1968.
4. Beckenbaugh RD: Accurate evaluation and management of the painful wrist following injury, Orthop Clin N Am 15:289, 1984.
5. Bellinghausen HW, et al: Posttraumatic palmar carpal subluxation, J Bone Joint Surg 65A:998, 1983.
6. Blatt G: Capsulodesis in reconstructive hand surgery—dorsal capsulodesis for the unstable scaphoid and volar capsulodesis following excision of the distal ulna, Hand Clin 3:81, 1987.
7. Bowers WH: The distal radioulnar joint. In Green DP, editor: Operative hand surgery, ed 2, New York, 1988, Churchill-Livingstone, Inc.
8. Brown DE, and Lichtman DM: Midcarpal instability, Hand Clin 3:135, 1987.
9. Brumfield RH, and Champoux, JA: A biomechanical study of normal functional wrist motion, Clin Orthop Rel Res 187:23, 1984.
10. Carter PR, Benton LJ, and Dysert PA: Silicone rubber carpal implants: a study of the incidence of late osseous complications, J Hand Surg 11A:639, 1986.
11. Chamay A, Pellasanta D, and Vilaseca A: Radiolunate arthrodesis: factors of stability for the rheumatoid wrist, Ann Chir Main 3:5, 1983.
12. Coll GA: Palmar dislocation of the scaphoid and lunate, J Hand Surg 12A:476, 1987.
13. Coleman HM: Injuries of the articular disc at the wrist, J Bone Joint Surg 42:522, 1960.
14. Conyers DJ: Volar wrist ligament reconstruction and carpal stabilization through a palmar approach, Orthop Trans Proc Am Soc Surg Hand 1989 (In press).
15. Craig SN: Wrist arthroscopy, Clin Sports Med 6:551, 1987.
16. Culver JE: Instabilities of the wrist, Clin Sports Med 5:725, 1986.
17. Curtis DJ: Injuries of the wrist: an approach to diagnosis, Radiol Clin N Am 19:625, 1981.
18. Curtis DJ, et al: Importance of soft tissue evaluation in hand and wrist trauma: Statistical evaluation, Am J Radiol 142:781, 1984.
19. Cyriax EF: On the rotatory movements of the wrists, J Anat 60:199, 1926.
20. Czitrom AA, Dobyns JH, and Linscheid RL: Ulnar variance in carpal instability, J Hand Surg 12A:205, 1987.
21. Destot E: Injuries of the wrist: a radiological study, London, 1925, Ernest Benn.
22. Dobyns JH, and Linscheid RL: Editorial comment: carpal bone injuries, Clin Orthop Rel Res 149:2, 1980.
23. Fisk GR: An overview of injuries of the wrist, Clin Orthop Rel Res 149:137, 1980.
24. Douglas DP, Peimer CA, and Koniuch MP: Wrist motion after simulated limited intercarpal arthrodesis—an experimental study, J Bone Joint Surg 69A:1413, 1987.
25. England JPS: Subluxation of the carpal scaphoid, Proc R Soc Med 63:581, 1970.
26. Fisk G: Carpal instability and the fractured scaphoid, Ann R Coll Surg 46:63, 1970.
27. Gilford WW, Bolton RH, and Lambrinudi C: The mechanism of the wrist joint with special reference to fractures of the scaphoid, Guy's Hosp Rep 92:529, 1943.
28. Frankel VH: The Terry-Thomas sign, Clin Orthop Rel Res 129:121, 1977.
29. Gilula LA, et al: Roentgenographic diagnosis of the painful wrist, Clin Orthop Rel Res 187:52, 1984.
30. Gilula LA: Carpal injuries: analytic approach and case exercises, Am J Radiol 133:503, 1979.
31. Howard FN, Fahey T, and Wojcik E: Rotatory subluxation of the navicular, Clin Orthop Rel Res 104:134, 1974.
32. Gilula LA, and Weeks PN: Post-traumatic ligamentous instability of the wrist, Radiology 129:641, 1978.
33. Green DP: Carpal dislocations and instabilities. In Green DP, editor: Operative hand surgery, ed 2, New York, 1988, Churchill Livingstone, Inc.
34. Green DP, and O'Brien ET: Classification and management of carpal dislocations, Clin Orthop Rel Res 149:55, 1980.
35. Hamlin C: Traumatic disruption of the distal radioulnar joint, Am J Sports Med 5:93, 1977.
36. Kauer JMG: The interdependence of carpal articulation chains, Acta Anat 88:481, 1974.
37. Howard FN, et al: Symposium: carpal instability, Contemp Orthop 4:107, 1982.
38. Isani A, and Melone CP: Ligamentous injuries of the hand in athletes, Clin Sports Med 5:757, 1986.
39. Johnston HM: Varying positions of the carpal bones in the different movements at the wrist. I. Extension, ulnar and radial flexion, J Anat 41:109, 1907.
40. Jones WA: Beware the sprained wrist—the incidence and diagnosis of scapholunate instability, J Bone Joint Surg 70B:293, 1988.
41. Dobyns JH, et al: Traumatic instability of the wrist, AAOS Instructional Course Lectures, vol 24, St. Louis, 1975, The CV Mosby Co, p. 182.
42 Kauer JMG: Functional anatomy of the wrist, Clin Orthop 149:9, 1980.
43. Kirk JA, Ansell BN, and Bywaters EGL: The hypermobility syndrome, Ann Rheum Dis 26:419, 1967.
44. Kleinman WB: Management of chronic rotatory subluxation of the scaphoid by scapho-trapezio-trapezoid arthrodesis—rationale for the technique, postoperative changes in biomechanics, and results, Hand Clin 3:113, 1987.
45. Kleinman WB, Steichen JB, and Strickland JW: Management of chronic rotatory subluxation of the scaphoid by scaphotrapezio-trapezoid arthrodesis, J Hand Surg 7:125, 1982.
46. Kuth JR: Isolated dislocation of the carpal navicular: a case report, J Bone Joint Surg 21:479, 1939.
47. Landsmeer JMF: Studies in the anatomy of articulation, Acta Morphol Neerl Scand 3:287, 1961.
48. Lewis OJ, Hamshere RJ, and Bucknill TN: The anatomy of the wrist joint, J Anat 106:589, 1970.
49. Lichtman DM, et al: Ulnar midcarpal instability—clinical and laboratory analysis, J Hand Surg 6:515, 1981.

50. Linscheid RL, et al: Traumatic instability of the wrist diagnosis, classification and pathomechanics, J Bone Joint Surg 54A:1612, 1972.
51. Loeb TM, Urbaniak JR, and Goldner JL: Traumatic carpal instability: putting the pieces together, Orthop Trans 2:163, 1977.
52. MacConaill MA: The mechanical anatomy of the carpus and its bearings on some surgical problems, J Anat 75:166, 1941.
53. Maki NJ, Chuinard RG, and D'Ambrosia R: Isolated complete radial dislocation of the scaphoid: a case report and review of the literature, J Bone Joint Surg 64A:615, 1982.
54. Mayfield JK: Patterns of injury to carpal ligaments: a spectrum, Clin Orthop Rel Res 187:36, 1984.
55. Mayfield JK: Wrist ligamentous anatomy and pathogenesis of carpal instability, Orthop Clin No Am 15:209, 1984.
56. Mayfield JK, Johnson RP, and Kilcoyne RF: Carpal dislocations: pathomechanics and progressive perilunar instability, J Hand Surg 5:226, 1980.
57. Mayfield JK, Johnson RP, and Kilcoyne RF: The ligaments of the human wrist and their functional significance, Anat Rec 186:417, 1976.
58. McMurty R et al: Kinematics of the wrist: an experimental study of radial/ulnar deviation and flexion–extension, J Bone Joint Surg 60A:423, 1978.
59. Melone CP, and Leber C: Triangular fibrocartilage complex disruption: correlation between preoperative magnetic resonance imagery and operative pathology, Orthop Trans Proc Am Soc Surg Hand 1989 (In press).
60. Meyerdierks EM, Mosher JF, and Werner FW: Limited wrist arthrodesis: a laboratory study, J Hand Surg 12A:526, 1987.
61. Mikic ZDJ: Age changes in the triangular fibrocartilage complex of the wrist joint, J Anat 126:367, 1978.
62. Milch H: Cuff resection of the ulna for malunited Colles' fracture, J Bone Joint Surg 23:311, 1941.
63. Mino DE, Palmer AK, and Levinsohn EN: The role of radiography and computerized tomography in the diagnosis of subluxation and dislocation of the distal radioulnar joint, J Hand Surg 8:23, 1983.
64. Mino DE, Palmer AK, and Levinsohn, EN: Radiography and computerized tomography in the diagnosis of incongruity of the distal radio-ulnar joint, J Bone Joint Surg 67A:247, 1985
65. Moneim MS, and Omer GE: Wrist arthrography with acute carpal injuries, Orthopaedics 6:299, 1983.
66. Monsivais JJ, Nitz PA, and Scully TJ: The role of carpal instability in scaphoid non-union: casual or causal? J Hand Surg 11B:201, 1896.
67. Navarro A: Anales del Instituto de Clinica Quirurgica y Cirugia Experimental, Imprenta Artistica de Dornaleche, 1935, Montevideo.
68. Navarro A: Anatomia y fisiologia del carpo, An Inst Clin Quir Cir Exp, 1935, Montevideo.
69. Nielson PT, and Hedeble J: Post-traumatic scapholunate dissociation detected by wrist cineradiography, J Hand Surg 9A:135, 1984.
70. Palmer AK: The distal radioulnar joint: anatomy, biomechanics, and triangular fibrocartilage complex abnormalities, Hand Clinics 3:31, 1987.
71. Palmer AK, Dobyns JH, and Linscheid RL: Management of post-traumatic instability of the wrist secondary to ligament rupture, J Hand Surg 3:507, 1978.
72. Palmer AK, Glisson RR, and Werner FW: Ulnar variance determination, J Hand Surg 7:376, 1982.
73. Palmer AK, Levinsohn EN, and Kuzma GR: Arthrography of the wrist, J Hand Surg 8:15, 1983.
74. Palmer AK, and Werner FW: The triangular fibrocartilage complex of the wrist—anatomy and function, J Hand Surg 6:153, 1981.
75. Palmer AK, and Werner FW: Biomechanics of the distal radioulnar joint, Clin Ortho Rel Res 187:26, 1984.
76. Peimer CA, et al: Reactive synovitis after silicone arthroplasty, J Hand Surg 11A:624, 1986.
77. Peterson HA, and Lipscomb PR: Intercarpal arthrodesis, Arch Surg 94:127, 1967.
78. Pisano SM, et al: Scaphocapitate intercarpal arthrodesis, Orthop Trans Proc Am Soc Surg Hand 1989 (In press).
79. Rask MR: Carponavicular subluxation: report of a case treated with percutaneous pins. Orthop 2:134, 1979.
80. Ray RD, Johnson RJ, and Jameson RN: Rotation of the forearm: an experimental study of pronation and supination, J Bone Joint Surg 33A:993, 1951.
81. Rayhack JN, et al: Post-traumatic ulnar translation of the carpus, J Hand Surg 12A:180, 1987.
82. Reagan DS, Linscheid RL, and Dobyns JH: Lunotriquetral sprains, J Hand Surg 9A:502, 1984.
83. Ruby LK: Common hand injuries in the athlete, Clin Sports Med 2:609, 1983.
84. Ruby LK, et al: Relative motion of selected carpal bones: A kinematic analysis of normal wrist, J Hand Surg 13A:1, 1988.
85. Sarrafian SK, Melamed JL, and Goshgarian GN: Study of wrist motion in flexion and extension, Clin Orthop Rel Res 126:153, 1977.
86. Sebald JR, Dobyns JH, and Linscheid RL: The natural history of collapsed deformities of the wrist, Clin Orthop Rel Res 104:140, 1974.
87. Sherlock DA, and Phil D: Traumatic dorsoradial dislocation of the trapezium, J Hand Surg 12A:262, 1987.
88. Sutro CJ: Hypermobility of bones due to "over lengthened" capsular and ligamentous tissues, Surgery 21:67, 1947.
89. Tachakra SS: A case of trapezio-scaphoid subluxation, Br J Clin Pract 31:163, 1977.
90. Taleisnik J: The ligaments of the wrist, J Hand Surg 1:110, 1976.
91. Taleisnik J: Post-traumatic carpal instability, Clin Orthop Rel Res 149:73, 1980.
92. Taleisnik J: The wrist, New York, 1985, Churchill Livingstone, inc.
93. Taleisnik J: Pain on the ulnar side of the wrist, Hand Clin 3:51, 1987.
94. Uematsu A: Intercarpal fusion for treatment of carpal instability: a preliminary report, Clin Orthop Rel Res 144:159, 1979.
95. Vesely DG: The distal radio-ulnar joint, Clin Orthop Rel Res 51:75, 1967.
96. VonBonin G: A note on the kinematics of the wrist joint, J Anat 63:259, 1919.
97. Volz RG, Leib N, and Benjamin J: Biomechanics of the wrist, Clin Orthop Rel Res 149:112, 1980.
98. Watson HK, and Ballet FL: The SLAC wrist: scapholunate advanced collapse pattern of degenerative arthritis, J Hand Surg 9A:358, 1984.
99. Watson HK, and Black DN: Instabilities of the wrist, Hand Clin 3:103, 1987.

100. Watson HK, Goodman ML, and Johnson TR: Limited wrist arthrodesis. II. Intercarpal and radiocarpal combinations, J Hand Surg 6:223, 1981.
101. Watson HK, and Hempton RF: Limited wrist arthrodeses. I. The triscaphoid joint, J Hand Surg 5:320, 1980.
102. Weber ER: Concepts governing the rotational shift of the intercollated segment of the carpus, Orthop Clin N Am 15:193, 1984.
103. Weber ER: Wrist mechanics in association with ligamentous instabilities. In Lichtman DM, editor: The wrist and its disorders, Philadelphia, 1988, WB Saunders Co.
104. Whipple TL: Clinical application of wrist arthroscopy. In Lichtman DM, editor: The wrist and its disorders, Philadelphia, 1988, WB Saunders Co.
105. Wright RD: A detailed study of the movement of the wrist joint, J Anat 70:137, 1935.
106. Youm Y, and Flatt AE: Kinematics of the wrist, Clin Orthop Rel Res 149:21, 1980.
107. Youm Y, et al: Kinematics of the wrist. I. An experimental study of radial-ulnar deviation and flexion-extension, J Bone Joint Surg 60A:423, 1978.

SUGGESTED READINGS

Arkless R: Rheumatoid wrists: cineradiography, Radiol 88:543, 1967.

Fernandez DL, and Ghillani R: External fixation of complex carpal dislocations: a preliminary report, J Hand Surg 12(3)A:335, 1987.

Gieck JH, and Mayer V: Protective splinting for the hand and wrist, Clin Sports Med 5:795, 1986.

Goldberg B, and Heller A: Dorsal dislocation of the triquetrum with rotary subluxation of the scaphoid, J Hand Surg 12A:119, 1987.

Mayer V, and Gieck JH: Rehabilitation of hand injuries in athletes, Clin Sports Med 5:783, 1986.

CHAPTER 25 Wrist Pain

E.F. Shaw Wilgis
Adolph Y. Yates, Jr.

The injured wrist of the athlete deserves careful evaluation. Many vague wrist "sprains" improve with temporary and conservative therapy and with no more specific diagnosis. Wrist "sprain," however, should be a diagnosis of exclusion and one that is used less often as sophistication with wrist evaluation improves. The missed scaphoid fracture or undiagnosed ligamentous instability can lead to prolonged impairment and the need for more protracted intervention. The identification of a specific pattern of injury can lead to better-directed treatment and, when appropriate, more aggressive and immediate intervention. The results should be an earlier and a safer return to the patient's avocation and avoidance of permanent disability.

The complexity of the wrist makes it uniquely vulnerable to many modes of injury. Anatomically, the wrist includes the region between the metacarpals and the distal radius and ulna. Its functions are to position the hand in space and to transmit forces to and from the hand and forearm[8]; few sports do not make demands on these functions. The wrist is required to provide multiaxial motion while bearing forces across its many joints. At the same time, it acts as the narrow conduit for the nerves, vessels, and tendons of the most important human organ of function—the hand.

There are many etiologic factors associated with wrist symptoms. A direct blow or overuse trauma can yield an articular or extraarticular injury, resulting in a painful wrist. Successful treatment requires a correct diagnosis. Therefore a thorough knowledge of these pathologic conditions is paramount.

HISTORY

A careful history is the beginning of any evaluation of a wrist injury. Often the examiners must rely on the history to pinpoint the site, type, and degree of pain and any motions that exacerbate the discomfort. Previous injury to the wrist should be elicited; injuries whose scale is out of proportion to the mechanism of injury may be the result of an old underlying instability. An example would be carpometacarpal dislocation from light contact in a patient with a previous injury to the same joint from a higher-energy accident. What causes or exacerbates the pain of the acute injury can help establish its dynamic components.

A more chronic presentation needs careful questioning about any intervening therapy, its success, and any waxing and waning of the pain. The exact mechanism of injury may not be available. A history of the patient's sports involvement, including athletic participation in other seasons, as well as work activity is necessary. Most articular injuries result from excessive loading of the wrist, such as a fall while in dorsiflexion, ulnar deviation, and carpal spination. Thus it is important to ascertain a traumatic event, however trivial it may seem. The wrist may also absorb injury by excessive use of muscle, be it a single overuse trauma or repetitive activity. Certain sports are associated with specific injuries, such as handlebar palsy,[11,27] catcher's hand,[5,17] and bowler's thumb.[10] The patient's position in team sports should be determined. Riester and associates' study of football players[25] showed a 1 in 100 incidence per season of scaphoid fractures; interestingly, they also showed an 8:3 ratio of defensive to offensive players.

PHYSICAL EXAMINATION

Guided by a careful history, the physician begins examination of the wrist with inspection. The contralateral wrist should be inspected for comparison and should be included throughout the examination as a reference for the involved wrist. Areas of swelling and deformity should be observed, as well as small puncture wounds, lacerations, and old scars. The examiner should record active and passive flexion, extension, pronation, supination, and radioulnar deviation and compare these motions to the contralateral wrist. A careful neurovascular examination is also essential, using two-point discrimination; observation of changes in color, temperature, perspiration, and pulse; and Allen's test. The paths and sensory distributions of the sensory branch of the radial nerve, the dorsal branch of the ulnar nerve, and the palmar cutaneous branch of the median nerve should be checked for neuromata or dysesthesias to light touch.

The history should guide the palpation of the injured wrist. It is important to localize the anatomic point of maximal tenderness. This site can guide the examiner toward anatomic derangements. Each of the carpal bones, the distal radius and the ulna, and the base of the metacarpals should be palpated both volarly and dorsally; as well as the anatomic snuffbox, lunate, hamate, triquetrum, distal ulna, distal radioulnar joint, distal pole of the scaphoid, and pisiform. Palpation of the carpal tunnel with its median nerve and flexor tendons should be coupled with palpation of the ulnar nerve and artery in Guyon's canal. The remaining flexor and extensor tendons should also be palpated in their various routes for tenderness, crepitus, or subluxation.

Passive and active range of motion should be observed, as well as the limitations imposed by pain. Palpation over the radioulnar, radiocarpal, ulnocarpal, intracarpal, and carpometacarpal joints during motion can reveal clicks and hesitations. A click alone does not mean a pathologic condition; however, a painful click may have clinical significance, often reflecting carpal instabilities. A painful click as the wrist is forced into palmar flexion and radial deviation is associated with the proximal pole of the scaphoid subluxing dorsally over the rim of the radius, a sign of scapholunate dissociation. The clicks associated with ulnar instability usually occur with ulnar deviation and rotation.

Special tests can be useful in wrist examination. **Finkelstein's test** is used to evaluate the first dorsal compartment (containing the abductor pollicis longus and extensor pollicis brevis) for tendonitis. The examiner holds the thumb flexed and abducted and then deviates the wrist ulnarward stretching those tendons. A positive test elicits pain over the first dorsal compartment.

Wrist examination: special tests

- Finkelstein's test
- Phalen's test
- Watson's test
- Injection tests

Phalen's test consists of permitting the wrist to drop into a palmarflexed position for 60 seconds to duplicate the symptoms of carpal tunnel syndrome when Tinel's sign is inconclusive. **Watson's test** has been described by several authors[3,13] and involves using the fingers to apply pressure over the distal dorsal radius while using the thumb to apply pressure over the palmar distal pole of the scaphoid. The wrist is then put through radial deviation. A painful click in the area of the scaphoid denotes a positive test; the click is secondary to dorsal subluxation of the scaphoid and is considered a sign of scapholunate instability.

Another important diagnostic tool is the injection of a local anesthetic at the point of greatest tenderness. Generally, 1% to 2% lidocaine injected into the point of tenderness can help localize the anatomic derangement and dictate therapeutic options. The examiner should assess the range of motion and grip strength before and after injection. Steroid injections, when appropriate, can accompany such injections.[13]

ROENTGENOGRAPHY

Roentgenograms are the next step in evaluating the wrist. The importance of routine posterioanterior (PA) and lateral roentgenograms in the neutral position cannot be overemphasized.

Roentgenographic normal limits

- Scapholunate gap (PA): <3 mm
- Scapholunate angle (lateral): 30 to 70 degrees

With **PA roentgenograms,** the scaphoid and the distance between the carpal bones can be assessed. A gap of 3 mm or more between the scaphoid and lunate is abnormal and indicates a tear of the scapholunate interosseous ligament. A supinated, clenched-fist AP roentgenogram will accentuate this gap. A "foreshortening" of the scaphoid and the "ring sign," which is the distal tubercle seen head-on, both suggest palmar flexion of the scaphoid. A widened space between the lunate and triquetrum may denote a tear of the lunotriquetral ligament.

On the **lateral roentgenogram,** an angle between the long axis of the scaphoid and the lunate greater than 70 degrees is abnormal and consistent with scapholunate dissociation. An angle of 30 degrees or less is also abnormal and could signify ulnocarpal instability. Lateral roentgenograms in full flexion and extension complement PA roentgenograms in radial and ulnar deviation when the examiner is assessing carpal instability.[13] Comparison roentgenograms of the contralateral wrist are valuable.

Special plain roentgenograms can further elucidate pathologic conditions. A **carpal tunnel view,** which is a roentgenogram with the wrist in full extension, fingers extended, and the beam in front of the third metacarpal, helps to visualize fractures of the hook of the hamate. The pisotriquetral area can be better seen with lateral roentgenograms of the hand and forearm in 10 to 15 degrees of supination.[13] **Couno and Watson's special view**[9,13] offers better visualization of the carpometacarpal joints; this is a lateral view taken with 30 degrees of supination and 20 to 30 degrees of ulnar deviation.

Additionally, **fluoroscopy** and **cine roentgenograms** allow one to view the wrist while it is in motion and are the best techniques for demonstrating dynamic instability patterns. Coupling fluoroscopy with **arthrography** is also useful. In this instance, contrast is inserted into the radial styloid recess. It is important that the exact passage of the contrast be observed to determine whether any communication with the midcarpal area is from the discontinuity of the scapholunate or the lunotriquetral ligaments. Communication with the radioulnar joint may help diagnose tears in the triangular fibrocartilage complex. **Double-contrast arthrography** has been described as useful in diagnosing loose foreign bodies.[30]

With vague wrist complaints, **bone scans** are a useful screening device. A positive scan can localize lesions and dictate further diagnostic workup, whereas a negative scan will confirm the absence of articular pathologic conditions. It should be noted, however, that scans are often nonspecific and can have overlying incidental findings.

Trispiral tomography has replaced laminar tomography for more careful evaluation of possible fractures or cases of avascular necrosis.[24] Acute and chronic fractures of the scaphoid and the hamate, and the early sclerotic or cystic changes of avascular necrosis of the scaphoid, lunate, and hamate are often seen on such tomographic views when not visualized on plain roentgenograms. It is important that the clinician specify that both anteroposterior and lateral views are needed. An alternative approach is the use of computed tomography; this depends on the availability and the quality of the scanner and its resolution. It offers much of the same information as above and is probably the best way to evaluate the distal radioulnar joint.[22]

Magnetic resonance imaging (MRI) of the wrist is still evolving but has the advantage of soft tissue definition and no radiation exposure. It has been shown effective in evaluating ganglion cysts, fractures of the hamate, nonunions of the scaphoid, and even the compression of the median nerve in carpal tunnel syndrome.[32] **Cine MRI** as a research tool has been used by Mandelbaum to find subtle dynamic instabilities in the distal radioulnar joint in gymnasts.[18]

The various modalities of roentgenography available require the clinician to consider time and cost and to use the history and physical examination to selectively guide decisions. Incidental and misleading findings are possible in any study, especially arthrography and bone scans, and must be coupled with a leading diagnosis and not obtained in shotgun fashion.

ARTHROSCOPY

Diagnostic and therapeutic arthroscopy can be used in the patient with acute or chronic wrist pain. Effective instrumentation would include a 2.7 mm scope, a mini shaver, and a probe. In the acute situation, if conventional examinaton and roentgenographic technique fail to reveal the pathologic condition, an arthroscope can be inserted in the radiocarpal region between the digital extensor tendons and wrist extensor tendons in the fluid-filled and distracted wrist joint in an appropriately anesthetized patient. Appropriate visualization of the articular surface of the radius and ulna and triangular fibrocartilage complex can be made. The scaphoid and interligamentous structures between the scaphoid and lunate and triquetrum can be inspected and probed through a probe inserted on the ulnar aspect of the wrist. The arthroscope can then be introduced deeply, and the volar ligaments can be inspected. Small ligamentous tears can be shaved, and synovium can be removed with a mini shaver.

The midcarpal joint can also be inspected arthroscopically and the ligaments probed for diagnostic purposes.

For chronic pain, diagnostic arthroscopic surgery can be combined with therapeutic arthroscopic surgery if necessary. Therapeutic surgery for the most part consists of synovectomy and a shaving of ligamentous tears. This has been a valuable addition for the patient with unexplained or undiagnosed wrist pain and, in many cases, can help evaluate the situation before planning definitive treatment. For example, if one is considering a procedure within the wrist joint, such as an intercarpal arthrodesis, the articular surfaces should be inspected and a prediction made as to whether the treatment would be appropriate on a long-term basis. We have found this to be particularly useful in evaluating the treatment of scaphoid nonunion and concomitant radioscaphoid arthritis. Visualizaton of the radioarticular surface will direct our treatment depending on the presence or absence of articular damage.

DIFFERENTIAL DIAGNOSIS OF WRIST PAIN

The following is not an exhaustive listing of pathologic conditions of the wrist. It will review the more common problems of the wrist likely to occur from trauma or overuse, especially in a sports setting. To simplify the array of conditions, the derangements will be catalogued into two broad groups. Articular injuries will include all bony and ligamentous conditions isolated to the carpus, whereas extraarticular injuries pertain to lesions of the tendons, nerves, and vessels that cross the carpus.

Fractures

Scaphoid

The most common of the carpal bones to be fractured is the scaphoid, accounting for approximately 70% of carpal fractures.[2] It occurs in a 1:10 ratio to fractures of the distal radius but occurs more frequently in the younger sports-related population.[7] Waist fractures of the scaphoid have been shown to be caused by pressure to the radial aspect of the palm with the wrist in dorsiflexion.[31] The scaphoid bridges the two carpal rows, making it more prone to injury with falls onto the outstretched distal palm.[31] Diagnosis of this fracture begins with heightened suspicion. Any pain in the radiocarpal area should be suspected of being a scaphoid fracture. Palpable tenderness of the scaphoid, either on the volar side or in the anatomic snuffbox, necessitates 2 weeks' immobilization, even with normal roentgenograms. At both the initial presentation and the 2-week follow-up, the scaphoid series as described above is the first line of x-ray evaluation. If a fracture is not seen on plain roentgenograms at that time and if the patient continues to have tenderness, then tomograms or possibly bone scan or MRI can be obtained to confirm the diagnosis.

The reason for such concern with this fracture is its predilection to go on to delayed union or nonunion and, more importantly, to the high incidence of avascular necrosis (AVN) associated with scaphoid fractures. The scaphoid has a single interosseous artery, and 70% of the blood supply to the proximal pole depends on one dorsal branch of the radial artery.[12] As a result, 30% of middle-third fractures and close to 100% of proximal fractures go on to AVN.[12,34]

Scaphoid fractures can be classified by the timing of their presentation, their anatomic location, their configuration, and the amount of initial displacement. The fracture that is seen 2 hours after injury differs from the one that is seen 2 weeks after injury and differs even more from the one that is seen 2 months after injury. Anatomically, 70% of scaphoid fractures occur through the middle third; 20% proximally; and 10% through the distal third.[26] Some authors have classified the fracture by its configuration, either being a horizontal oblique, transverse, or vertical oblique fracture; the clinical significance is that the last of these three is considered unstable.[26] Another commonly used criterion for stability is the degree of initial displacement.

Distribution of scaphoid fractures

- Middle third: 70%
- Proximal third: 20%
- Distal third: 10%

The significance of the various classifications is both prognostic and therapeutic. Prognostically, a delayed presentation, a proximal-third fracture, or one that is displaced has a higher likelihood of going on to nonunion or AVN. These types of fractures may warrant more prolonged immobilizaton, long-arm casting, and possibly more aggressive early surgical intervention (Fig. 25-1). The nondisplaced, stable fracture can be initially treated with a short arm–thumb spica cast in slight palmar flexion and slight radial deviation.[7,34] The cast should be changed every 3 to 4 weeks to assure a good fit, and roentgenograms should be frequent as well to guarantee adequate position. Average duration of immobilization is about 3 months.[7,34] The displaced fracture first needs reduction through longitudinal traction and is then casted in a long arm spica cast.[7] If the reduction is adequate, the same stipulations apply as above, and the long-arm cast can be converted to a short-arm cast at about the sixth or eighth week. Inability to reduce the fracture is an indication for surgery. Once the fracture is thought to be healed, the patient can resume activity wearing a rigid splint for at least the first 2 months.[34] Riester and associates,[25] Cabrera and McCue,[5] and Bergfield and associates[1] have all reported successful treatment of football players with acute scaphoid fractures in soft but rigid Silastic or silicone casts that allowed them to continue their sports participation. The decision to allow contact sports during the period of initial immobilization should be individualized not only to the fracture pattern, but also, more importantly, to the needs and level of competition of the athlete, with his or her full participation in the decision and understanding of the risks involved.

Prognostic factors for nonunion or AVN

- Delayed presentation
- Proximal-third fracture
- Displacement

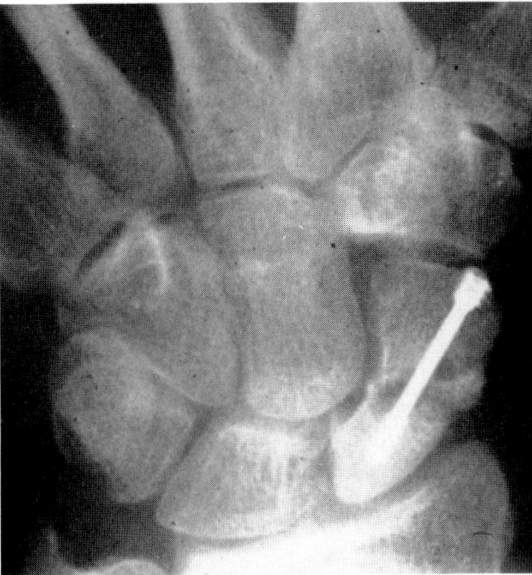

FIG. 25-1. Scaphoid fracture internally fixed with a Herbert screw.

Triquetrum

The triquetrum is the second most fractured carpus.[2] Chip or avulsion fractures are the most common. Body fractures are unusual in the athlete.[34] The dorsal chip fracture is most common and is thought to be secondary to hyperflexion, ulnar deviation, and impingement on the ulnar styloid.[4,16] Splinting for 4 to 6 weeks is usually sufficient and allows the patient to return to sports.[4,34] Occasional nonunions of the chip fracture types require excision when symptomatic.[4]

Hamate

The hamate is a less frequently fractured carpal bone. The hook of the hamate, however, is particularly prone to injury in club and racquet sports such as golf, baseball, and ten-

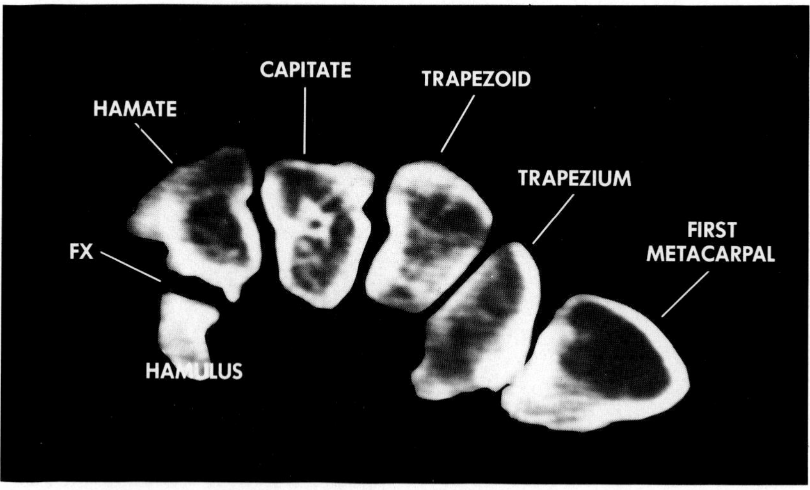

FIG. 25-2. CT scan depicting fracture of the hook of the hamate.

nis. The classic and often seen example of method of injury is the "dubbed" golf swing; the force of the swing is blocked by the ground, transmitted up the shaft of the club, and levered against the hypothenar area of the top of the hand, causing a hook of the hamate fracture.[4,34] A history of such an injury or pain in the hypothenar area should lead to special views such as the carpal tunnel view. An oblique view with the wrist in supination can show a lateral profile of the fracture. Both CT and MRI have been used to show this fracture as well[32] (Fig. 25-2). Although fractures of the body of the hamate heal quite readily with splinting, many authors recommend early excision of the hook fragment, which allows return to activity in as early as 6 weeks.[4,6,28,34]

Hook of hamate evaluation

- Carpal tunnel view
- Oblique view with wrist in supination
- Computed tomography
- Magnetic resonance imaging

Lunate

Fractures of the other carpal bones are less common, but certain aspects should be considered. Compression fractures of the lunate from repetitive trauma that interrupts the blood supply have been suggested as the cause of Kienböck's disease, or avascular necrosis of the lunate. The diagnosis is indicated by well-localized pain over the lunate and a secondary decrease in the range of motion in the involved wrist. Early roentgenograms may appear normal, despite definitive symptoms; tomograms and bone scans are the next step and will often uncover early changes despite normal plain roentgenograms. Treatment of Kienböck's disease is beyond the scope of this chapter. However, patients with suspected and unconfirmed Kienböck's disease can be treated with a short-arm cast for several weeks. The definitive surgical therapy of this entity is controversial.

Pisiform

Fractures of the pisiform are usually secondary to direct trauma.[4,34] These are usually best treated with a short-arm cast for 3 to 6 weeks.[4,34] Occasionally posttraumatic arthrosis may necessitate excision, with postoperative recovery lasting about 8 weeks.[34]

Trapezium

The trapezium is usually injured by a blow to the adducted thumb or a fall on the hyperextended wrist in radial deviation.[4,34] Nondisplaced avulsion or vertical fractures can be treated conservatively with casting; displaced vertical fractures, however, are best treated by internal fixation either by percutaneous pinning or by open reduction, the choice depending on the size and reducibility of the fracture.[4,34]

Capitate

Capitate fractures can occur as an isolated entity; they may, however, be a sign of scaphocapitate fracture as the result of continuing deforming hyperextension after the more typical fracture of the scaphoid and subsequent impingement of the radius.[29] For isolated capitate fractures, conservative therapy consisting of splinting or casting will suffice.[4] If reduction is not possible, then open reduction and internal fixation are necessary.[34] The capitate is another of the carpal bones at risk for AVN after fracture. Both AVN and posttraumatic arthrosis may require midcarpal arthrodesis.[4]

Trapezoid

The trapezoid is the least frequently fractured carpus. It responds well to casting for 3 to 6 weeks. Again, late posttraumatic arthrosis may indicate fusion.[4]

Ligament Injuries and Instability

The intercalated wrist is without intrinsic musculature. Its dynamic and static stability depends on intracapsular ligaments, interosseous ligaments, and the inherent stability of the different joint configurations. The major volar intracapsular ligaments are the radiocapitate, the radiotriquetral, and the radioscaphoid; the important dorsal intracapsular ligament is the dorsal radiocarpal ligament.[8,19] The interosseous ligaments run circumferentially around each carpal row, primarily giving rotational stability from one carpal bone to another.[8]

Wrist instability from injury to these ligaments is an intricate topic. The instability may be seen on examination as tenderness in a certain area alone or as a painful click such as in Watson's test, described previously. If static instability exists, then plain roentgenograms will reveal gaps in the carpal rows, particularly the scapholunate area or the triquetrolunate area on AP or oblique views. On normal lateral views, the lunate lies within a 0- to 15-degree arc of longitudinal alignment between the radius and the capitate. A collapse that results in dorsiflexion of the lunate is referred to as a dorsal intercalated segmental instability (DISI). When the instability results in palmar flexion of the lunate, it is referred to as a volar intercalated segmental instability (VISI). Such angulations reflect disruption of the interosseous ligaments on either side of the lunate responsible for rotational control. In a DISI configuration, the failed ligament is the scapholunate ligament, which allows volar tilt of the scaphoid and dorsal angulaton of the lunate. The opposite is true of the triquetrolunate ligament, or sometimes the triquetral hamate ligament, the failures of which can cause the VISI configuration. These are gross simplifications of what can be more complicated injuries involving many other structures or fractures. These injuries can be arranged into (1) radial instabilities, which center around injuries to and around the scaphoid; and (2) ulnar instabilities, which involve the lunotriquetral or midcarpal joints.[8]

Bridging the two types of instability is a sequence of injuries known as progressive perilunar instability.[8,19,20] This sequence is a result of progressive hyperextension, ulnar deviation, and supination, causing circumferential injury to the ligaments surrounding the lunate, starting with the scapholunate ligament, which is stage 1.[8,19,20] The next ligament to be injured is the capitolunate or stage 2, followed by the triquetrolunate. Stage 3 permits dorsal perilunate dislocation. Stage 4 is disruption of the dorsal radiocarpal ligament; this allows volar dislocation of the lunate itself.[8,19,20]

If plain roentgenograms or motion roentgenograms fail to show the instability, options still include cine and fluoroscopy. If strong clinical suspicion exists for wrist instability, then arthrography can be useful in showing disruptions of the proximal row interosseous ligaments. Once the particular instability has been demonstrated, care must be taken to rule out any associated nondisplaced fractures.

The care of the acutely unstable wrist is controversial, with recommendations ranging from simple immobilization to percutaneous fixation, to open reduction and ligament repair (Fig. 25-3). A conservative approach would be to reduce and hold the wrist immobilized in a cast for 6 to 12 weeks, relying on frequent roentgenograms to assure continued reduction; pin fixation would be reserved for failure to hold position.[8] Green feels that neither is stable enough for successful treatment of the acute scapholunate dissociation, and he recommends immediate surgical repair of the ligament.[13]

If such an injury is seen later or if it becomes a chronic instability, splinting with the soft cast as described by Bergfield and associates[1] and other authors can provide symptomatic relief. For chronic instability, nonsteroidal antiinflammatory drugs (NSAIDs) and steroid injections may provide significant relief. Surgery is indicated for those patients for whom conservative treatment fails. The various ligament repairs and arthrodeses are beyond the scope of this discussion.

Radioulnar Joint

Injuries to the radioulnar joint are easily confused with radiocarpal and carpocarpal complaints. Rotation that causes pain in this area, especially forced resisted pronation that

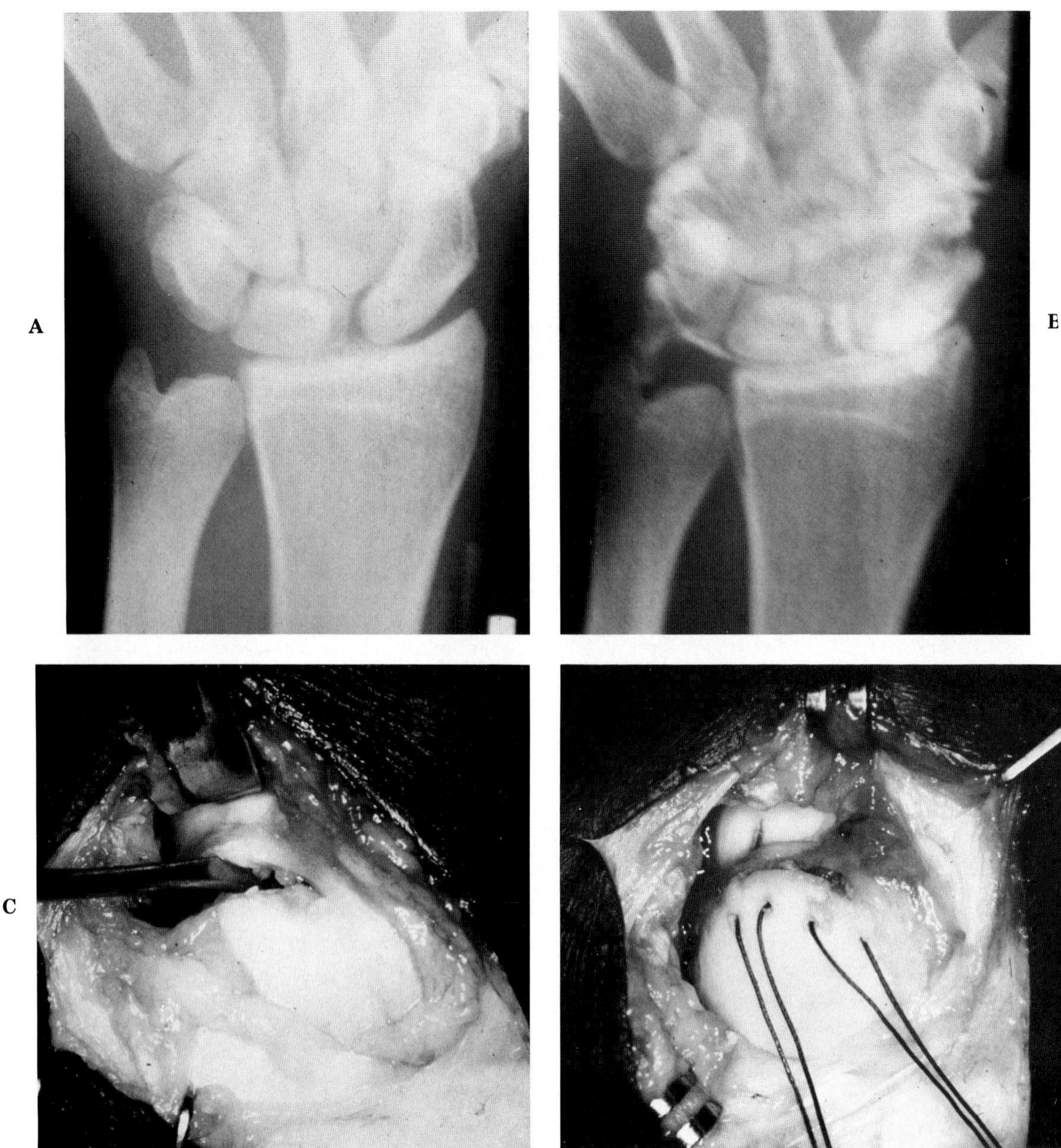

FIG. 25-3. A, Scapholunate ligament rupture. **B,** Arthrogram showing dye in the scapholunate space. **C,** The ligament rupture at surgery. **D,** Operative repair of the scapholunate ligament.

re-creates the patient's complaint, suggests injury to the radioulnar joint.[13,22] It needs to be distinguished from ulnocarpal impingement in ulnar-positive wrists, as well as ulnocarpal pathologic conditions. In addition to actual fractures through this area and radioulnar dissociations, the triangular fibrocartilage complex can be torn, causing pain. The triangular fibrocartilage complex is the complicated harness that radiates from the lunate fossa of the radius to the ulna and up to the edges of the ulnar wrist and fifth metacarpal[22]; it acts as a sling, "supporting the distal ulnar carpus and radius from the distal ulna."[22,23]

Diagnostic studies that can aid in evaluating the distal radioulnar joint include CT scans to evaluate possible dissociation; bone scans to help validate clinical suspicions of arthrosis in this area; and arthrograms to help diagnose tears in the triangular fibrocartilage complex. Extrusion of contrast into the radioulnar area is a frequent incidental finding and should not be considered pathognomonic unless coupled with a strong clinical suspicion based on history and examination.[13]

Radioulnar dissociation, ulnocarpal arthrosis, ulnar impingement, and questions of ulnar-positive or -minus wrists can be addressed as chronic problems; they are best treated symptomatically and with splints before entertaining the option of surgery such as arthroplasty or Darrach or Lauenstein procedures. The chronic triangular fibrocartilage complex tear that does not improve may benefit from surgery and debridement either through the arthroscope or open operative procedure. Of more immediate importance is the athlete with a suspected acute triangular fibrocartilage complex tear. Green feels that this is unlikely to have predictably good results if treated operatively at a later time; thus he recommends immediate long-arm casting for 4 to 6 weeks, regardless of the time of athletic season.[13]

Carpometacarpal Injuries

The ulnar four carpometacarpal joints are not commonly involved in sports-related injuries. Their sturdy ligaments and capsules are more likely to be injured in more violent events such as motor vehicle accidents and industrial injuries.[14] Dislocations of these joints are reducible but frequently require open pinning to guarantee stability.[14] Chronic sprains of the same joints can be pinpointed with lidocaine injections.[13,14] The lateral carpometacarpal view is described above and may be helpful in identifying small fractures, arthritis, and subluxation.[9] Although splints may help symptomatically, the procedure of choice is arthrodesis.[14]

Tendinous Injuries

Repetitive motion of the wrist in throwing, lifting, and contact sports can result in various forms of tendonitis, tenosynovitis, and tendon subluxation. Clinically, there is tenderness localized to the involved tendon. Pain is accentuated by passive stretch of the involved tendon. Roentgenograms are usually normal except for occasional calcifications around the involved tendon sheath.

Dorsal Tendonitis

Dorsal tendonitis is usually secondary to overuse, not infrequently from the backhand of racquet sports. It is manifested by swelling, erythema, and pain with resisted motion over the tendons involved.[5,33] The second dorsal compartment, containing the radial wrist extensors, and the sixth compartment, containing the extensor carpi ulnaris, are the most common sites of such inflammation after the first compartment (de Quervain's disease).[5,33] Treatment consists of splinting, NSAIDs, activity modification, and eventually strengthening of the involved muscles and is usually effective. Special care should be taken with tendonitis of the third compartment, especially with a history of previous injury; the inflammation may be secondary to posttraumatic deformity of Lister's tubercle following fracture and requires surgery to avoid rupture of the extensor pollicis longus.[33]

de Quervain's Disease

de Quervain's disease represents tenosynovitis of the first dorsal compartment. The first dorsal compartment contains the abductor pollicis longus and extensor pollicis brevis. These tendons are particularly prone to tendonitis from repetitive hand and wrist motions; bowling is a common example. On physical examination, there is tenderness and swelling at the radial styloid. There may be a thickened, inflamed cyst over the first dorsal compartment as well. A positive Finkelstein's test is highly suggestive for this condition. If de Quervain's disease is treated early, the treatment is the same as for other dorsal compartments, consisting of rest, splinting, and oral NSAIDs. Steroid injections, if coupled with rest, can also be effective. If conservative therapy fails or if the condition is allowed to progress to a chronic state, surgical decompression becomes necessary. During surgery, a search for anatomic abnormalities is important; failure to recognize a separate canal for the extensor pollicis brevis or multiple slips of the abductor pollicis longus may yield an unsatisfactory result.

Recurrent Subluxation of the Extensor Carpi Ulnaris Tendon

Subluxations of the extensor carpi ulnaris rarely are seen as an acute injury.[5] They represent tears of the retinacular restraints of the sixth dorsal compartment, allowing the extensor carpi ulnaris to repeatedly escape its groove and producing "snapping symptoms."[13,33] Such a snapping sensation can be felt by palpation over the sixth compartment when the wrist is supinated while in ulnar deviation. Various authors recommend surgical reconstruction of the tendon's restraints if conservative therapy fails.[13,33]

Intersection Syndrome

Intersection syndrome is described well by Wood and Dobyns[33] and is suggested by pain, crepitus, and a "squeaky" sensation in the area of the radial dorsal forearm where the abductor pollicis longus and the extensor pollicis brevis cross over the radial wrist extensors. It is common among weight lifters and various types of rowers.[33] The treatment is the same as with other tendonitis problems (i.e., rest, NSAIDs, splinting, and when needed, steroid injection) and is usually effective.[33] It is mentioned here to be distinguished from the tendonitis of the more proximal dorsal compartments.

Flexor Tendonitis

The flexor carpi ulnaris is the most common of the flexor tendons to be afflicted with tendonitis.[33] The treatment for this tendon as well as other flexor tendons is similar to that of the extensor tendons, namely, rest, splinting, and NSAIDs.

The flexors of the digits, because of their location within the carpal tunnel, can both mimic and cause carpal tunnel syndrome. Conservative treatment can be successful, but the workup should also consider median nerve compression. If there is no relief of symptoms, both carpal tunnel release and synovectomy of the flexors may be necessary.[5,33]

Nerve Compression

Carpal Tunnel Syndrome

Any sports activity requiring repeated hand and wrist motion can cause carpal tunnel syndrome and compression of the median nerve. Symptoms usually consist of pain in the wrist area radiating to the radial three and one-half digits; there may also be complaints of paresthesias in the same area, often with nocturnal intensification. On examination, positive Tinel's sign over the carpal tunnel, positive Phalen's test, decreased sensation over the median nerve distribution, and signs of thenar motor weakness are all diagnostic. Conservative therapy, consisting of splinting and NSAIDs, can be curative. However, if there is no improvement or if there is any question as to the diagnosis, electromyography and nerve conduction studies can be useful. Persistent symptoms despite treatment and signs of motor weakness are indications to proceed with operative decompression.

Guyon's Canal Syndrome

The ulnar nerve corollary to the carpal tunnel is Guyon's canal. This is another site of potential nerve compression, although less commonly seen. It is a problem seen with cyclists because of the compression of their grips, thus the name "handlebar palsy."[11,27] Although the ulnar nerve does not have to share this small space with the many flexor tendons that sometimes compress the carpal tunnel, it does course through this area with the ulnar artery, and pathologic conditions of the ulnar artery can either mimic or cause ulnar nerve compression. Positive Tinel's sign (paresthesias of the ulnar one and one-half digits) with or without signs of motor branch involvement is diagnostic. Treatment should initially be conservative, including modification of activity, splinting, and NSAIDs. Again, electromyograms and nerve conduction studies may be useful, especially when there is a possibility of more proximal involvement. Failure to respond to conservative treatment is an indication for surgical decompression.[5,33]

Other Causes of Wrist Pain

Vascular Injuries

Repetitive trauma to the ulnar artery along its course through Guyon's canal to its digital branches can cause both thrombosis and aneurysm; this has been called "catcher's hand,"[5,17] but it is also seen in cyclists[21] and handball players.[5] A careful vascular examination, with the use of Doppler ultrasound, can usually make the diagnosis without arteriography.[5] This condition can be asymptomatic but most often occurs with paresthesias in the ulnar nerve distribution. Vasospastic or vasoocclusive symptoms that afflict the digits may also exist. Treatment is surgical, usually with resection of the involved segment.[5,33] Reanastomosis is made if there is no tension,[5] but this and grafting remain controversial.[33] Both the radial artery and persistent median artery can be seen with traumatic thrombosis or aneurysm, the latter causing median nerve neuritis; these are rare injuries.[33]

Ganglions

Ganglions can occur from either intraarticular or extraarticular origins. Diagnosis is usually from palpation, but pain without mass may be the presenting complaint of an occult dorsal ganglion; articular injection with lidocaine can help make this diagnosis but not definitively.[13] There has been a recent report of the use of MRI to locate ganglions, and this may be of use in such a situation.[32] Extraarticular ganglions most frequently arise from the flexor carpi radialis tendon sheath, the digital extensors, and the roof of the first dorsal compartment.[33] Treatment involves rest and splinting, but again, if there is no improvement, surgical excision may be necessary.

SUMMARY

The preceding discussion of wrist injuries is not unique to athletes. On the contrary,

TABLE 25-1 Wrist injuries and initial treatment in the athlete

Injury	Treatment
Fractures	
Scaphoid, nondisplaced	Short arm–thumb spica cast; possible cast
Scaphoid, displaced	Long arm thumb spica cast; possible surgery with Herbert screw
Triquetrum (chip)	Splint for 4-6 wk
Hamate (body)	Splint for 4-6 wk; open reduction internal fixation (ORIF) if displaced
Hamate (hook)	Consider early excision if symptomatic
Lunate	Short arm cast
Trapezium, nondisplaced	Cast for 6 wk
Trapezium, displaced	Pin, possible ORIF
Capitate	Splint or cast for 6 wk
Trapezoid	Cast for 3-6 wk
Ligamentous Injuries	
Acute DISI, VISI, perilunate injuries	Controversial; options include (1) reduction with cast, (2) pin, (3) ligament repair
Chronic DISI, VISI, perilunate injuries	NSAIDs, splint, injection; consider limited fusion
Acute triangular fibrocartilage complex	Long arm cast for 4-6 wk
Chronic triangular fibrocartilage complex	Splint, NSAIDs, possible flap debridement
Carpometacarpal Dislocation	
	Pin, possible ORIF
Tendinous Injuries	
Dorsal and volar tendonitis, de Quervain's disease	NSAIDs, splint, rest
Nerve Injuries	
Carpal tunnel, Guyon's canal	NSAIDs, splint, rest
Ulnar Artery Thrombosis	Excision of segment
Ganglion	
	Splint, NSAID

nonathletic injuries to the wrist in each of the above categories far outnumber sports-related ones. There is no dramatic and uniquely sports-related injury in the wrist, such as the anterior cruciate ligament of the knee or the recurrent dislocation of the shoulder. There is, however, a shift in the spectrum of injury because of the younger age of the population involved; the athlete will fracture the scaphoid or injure one of its tendons in a fall rather than suffer Colles' fracture; he or she is more prone to tendonitis from overuse than from underlying arthritis. Expectations are different as well; the athlete's demands for full and immediate functional recovery of the injured part are greater than the industrial-related accident or the same injury in the elderly.

The vast majority of the injuries described can be treated conservatively, and even contact sports can be resumed wearing the soft casts described.[1,5,25] Certain exceptions must be kept in mind. Green feels that injuries to the distal radioulnar joint, in particular a tear in the triangular fibrocartilage complex, should be placed in a long arm cast immediately; he also feels that disruption of the scapholunate ligament deserves immediate surgical repair.[13] More than one author agrees that hook of the hamate fractures can cause prolonged disability unless they are simply excised on presentation, thus allowing full recovery in as soon as 6 weeks.[4,6,28,34] The return to full contact with a soft cast for a football player with a scaphoid fracture is proposed by some,[1,5,25] but this remains controversial.[15,34] Table 25-1 outlines various injuries of the wrist, conservative versus more immediate surgical therapy, and recommendations as far as return to activity.

The most important point in taking care of the athlete with a wrist injury is recognition of those injuries that carry possible long-term disability without dramatic initial deformity. Wrist "sprains" do exist but should remain a diagnosis of exclusion.

REFERENCES

1. Bergfield JA et al: Soft playing splint for protection of significant hand and wrist injuries in sports, Am J Sports Med 10:293, 1982.

2. Borgeskov S et al: Fracture of the carpal bones, Acta Orthop Scand 37:276, 1966.
3. Brown DE and Lichtman DM: The evaluation of chronic wrist pain, Orthop Clin North Am 15:185, 1984.
4. Bryan RS and Dobyns JH: Fractures of the carpal bones other than lunate or navicular, Clin Orthop Rel Res 149:107, June 1980.
5. Cabrera JM and McCue FC III: Nonosseous athletic injuries of the elbow, forearm and hand, Clin Sports Med 5:681, Oct 1986.
6. Carter PD, Eaton RO, and Littler JW: Ununited fracture of the hook of the hamate, J Bone Joint Surg 59A:583, 1977.
7. Cooney WP, Dobyns JH, and Linscheid RL: Fractures of the scaphoid: a rational approach to management, Clin Orthop Rel Res 1949:90, June 1980.
8. Culver JE: Instabilities of the wrist, Clin Sports Med 5:725, Oct 1986.
9. Cuono CB and Watson HK: The carpal boss: surgical treatment and etiologic considerations, Plast Reconstr Surg 63:88, 1979.
10. Dobyns JH et al: Bowler's thumb: diagnosis and treatment: a review of seventeen cases, J Bone Joint Surg 54A:751, 1972.
11. Finelli PF: Handlebar palsy (letter), N Engl J Med 292:702, 1975.
12. Gelberman RH et al: The arterial anatomy of the human carpus. I. The extraosseous vascularity, J Hand Surg 8:367, 1983.
13. Green DP: The sore wrist without a fracture. In Stauffer ES, editor: Instructional course lectures, vol. XXXIV, St Louis, 1985, The CV Mosby Co.
14. Gunther SF: The carpometacarpal joints, Orthop Clin North Am 15:259, April 1984.
15. Habeck T: Commentary on reference 1, Am J Sports Med 10:295, 1982.
16. Levy M et al: Chip fracture of the os triquetrum, J Bone Joint Surg 61B:355, 1979.
17. Lowrey CW, Chadwick RO, and Waltman EN: Digital vessel trauma from repetitive impact in baseball catchers, J Hand Surg 1:236, 1976.
18. Mandelbaum B: Wrist pain. In Gymnasts. The Bennett lecture, sports medicine symposium, Johns Hopkins, June 1987.
19. Mayfield JK: Wrist ligamentous anatomy and pathogenesis of carpal instability, Orthop Clin North Am 15:209, 1984.
20. Mayfield JK, Johnson RP, and Kilcoyne R: Carpal dislocation: pathomechanics and progressive perilunar instability, J Hand Surg 5:226, 1980.
21. Nullander LH, Nalebuff EA, and Kodson E: Aneurysms and thrombosis of the ulnar artery in the hand, Arch Surg 105:686, 1972.
22. Palmer AK: The distal radioulnar joint, Orthop Clin North Am 15:321, April 1984.
23. Palmer AK and Werner FW: The triangular fibrocartilage complex of the wrist: anatomy and function, J Hand Surg 6:153, 1981.
24. Posner MA and Greenspan A: Trispiral tomography for the evaluation of wrist problems, J Hand Surg 13A:175, 1988.
25. Riester JN et al: A review of scaphoid fracture healing in competitive athletes, Am J Sports Med 13:159, 1985.
26. Russe O: Fracture of the carpal navicular, J Bone Joint Surg 47A:759, 1980.
27. Smail DF: Handlebar palsy (letter), N Engl J Med 292:322, 1975.
28. Stark HH et al: Fracture of the hook of the hamate in athletes, J Bone Joint Surg 59A:575, 1977.
29. Stein F and Siegel MW: Naviculocapitate fracture and syndrome: a case report and new thoughts on the mechanism of injury, J Bone Joint Surg 51A:391, 1968.
30. Tehranzadeh J and Labosky DA: Detection of intra-articular loose osteochondral fragments by double contrast wrist arthrography: a case report of a basketball injury, Am J Sports Med 12:177, 1984.
31. Weber ER and Chao EY: An experimental approach to the mechanism of scaphoid waist fractures, J Hand Surg 3:142, 1978.
32. Weis KL, Beltran J, and Lubbers LM: High-field MR surface coil imaging of the hand and wrist. II. Pathologic correlations and clinical relevance, Radiology 160:147, 1986.
33. Wood MB and Dobyns JH: Sports related extra-articular wrist syndromes, Clin Orthop Rel Res 202:93, Jan 1986.
34. Zemel NP and Stark HH: Fractures and dislocations of the carpal bones, Clin Sports Med 5:705, Oct 1986.

CHAPTER 26 Hand Injuries

Martin A. Posner

The hand, by virtue of its wide range of functional activities and vulnerable anatomic position, is susceptible to a wide variety of sports related injuries. The incidence of these injuries is difficult to determine, because there are little available data. Even in those segments of the population in which statistics have been compiled, the accuracy of the statistics is questionable. In organized college sports, for example, statistics have been collected for injuries considered to be "significant", that is preventing the athlete from participating in a sport for at least 1 week.[98] However, many athletes with a variety of serious injuries, to the hand continue to play with a cast or brace. These athletes are therefore not considered technically disabled, so the available data underestimate the true incidence of injury. However, these data are helpful in indicating those college sports in which the hand is particularly at risk, including football, gymnastics, wrestling, and basketball.

Sports with highest risk of hand injury

- Football
- Gymnastics
- Wrestling
- Basketball

Regardless of the patient's age or level of proficiency—occasional recreational athlete, serious amateur competitor, or paid professional—all hand injuries require a careful medical evaluation, including appropriate roentgenograms. Without early and accurate assessment, treatment is delayed. A relatively simple problem that could be successfully treated with a splint or cast may progress to a chronic condition requiring complicated surgery. More important, the surgery necessitated by this delay may fail to restore normal mobility or strength. This may prevent the athlete from ever being able to resume full sport participation.

A wide variety of injuries ranging from skin abrasions to displaced intraarticular fractures can affect the hand in athletics. Even common abrasions or contusions should not be quickly dismissed as trivial. Local swelling, ecchymoses, and tenderness may indicate a more serious injury to underlying structures. This chapter will discuss serious injuries involving muscle-tendon units, ligaments, and bones at specific anatomic regions of the fingers and thumb.

Fingers

CARPOMETACARRPAL JOINT AREA

Anatomy

The carpometacarpal joints of the fingers comprise the articulations between the trapezoid, capitate, and hamate, and the bases of the second through fifth metacarpals. Though the trapezium articulates with the radial aspect of the second metacarpal, it is primarily involved with the stability and mobility of the first metacarpal and will therefore be discussed in the section on the thumb.

The anatomic configuration of the ligaments and the articular surfaces of the finger metacarpals and their contiguous carpal bones form two functional units, one being stable and the other mobile. The carpometacarpal joints of the index and middle fingers are stable, and their metacarpals make up the lingitudinal arch of the hand. The carpometacarpal joints of the ring and little fingers are mobile, with the fifth metacarpal having greater mobility than the fourth. The differences in mobility are caused by the unique configuration of the articular surfaces of the joints. The articular surface of the base of the fourth metacarpal is divided into a radial and ulnar portion by a proximal ridge. The ulnar portion articulates with the hamate at a facet that has a quadrangular or semilunar outline and is flat in the transverse axis.[50] The ulnar portion of the hamate is shallow and articulates with the base of the fifth metacarpal, which is convex in the volar-dorsal axis and concave in the radial-ulnar axis. The corresponding surfaces of both the hamate and fifth metacarpal resemble the saddle configuration at the basal joint of the thumb. This accounts for the greater mobility of the fifth metacarpal, particularly with respect to flexion and extension.[154]

The functional aspects of the stable and mobile components of the carpometacarpal joints are easily appreciated when the position of the metacarpal heads is observed during finger motions. In complete extension, the metacarpal heads are in the same plane, allowing the palm to be placed flat against an object or surface. When the fist is clenched, the heads of the second and third metacarpals remain stable. However, there is progressive flexion of the heads of the fourth and fifth, resulting in a curved arch. The heads of all of the finger metacarpals make up the transverse arch. The curvature of the transverse arch is similar to that of the proximal transverse arch, which is rigid and composed of the distal and carpal bones.

Muscle-Tendon Injuries

Strains are injuries to muscle-tendon units. Strains can be divided into acute and chronic types, depending on the nature of the forces and the duration of their application. When the cause of injury is a single forceful contraction of the muscle against resistance (overexertion) or when the muscle is suddenly stretched beyond its normal extensile range (overstretching), the result is an acute strain. A chronic strain is caused by excessive use beyond the muscle fatigue quotient.

Acute strains are classified as first, second, or third degree, depending on the magnitude of the injury to the muscle-tendon unit. Rarely is the tendon itself damaged, provided it is healthy. More commonly, damage is to the muscle belly, the musculotendinous junction, or the site of the tendon's insertion into bone.[126] In a first-degree, or mild, strain, there may be local muscle or tendon irritation, but no loss of strength or mobility. Treatment is primarily symptomatic and consists of rest and avoidance of active motion. A second-degree, or moderate, strain occurs when there is actual damage to a portion of the muscle-tendon unit that compromises its strength. There may be a partial tear of the muscle itself or a partial avulsion of the tendon at its bone insertion. Protection is important in this type of injury to prevent further damage. A third-degree strain is the most severe and is characterized by a complete rupture of a portion of the muscle-tendon unit.

Chronic strains are caused by overuse, which usually occurs over a prolonged period; however, the strains may also occur following a single, prolonged activity. Though by definition a chronic strain is not caused by an acute injury, it may be initated by one that is not adequately treated. The symptoms of a chronic strain are varied and depend on the area of the muscle-tendon unit that is affected. If the muscle itself is fatigued, a myositis develops, which leads to secondary spasm. Similar irritation can occur to the musculotendinous junction, anywhere along the course of the tendon, or at the site of the tendon's insertion into bone. If the tendon is irritated in its course through a sheath where it is surrounded by tenosynovium, tenosynovitis develops. Initially, there may be local tenderness and swelling over the sheath. In more severe cases, a fluid exudate develops which may cause adhesions between the tendon and its sheath and interfere with the normal gliding motion of the tendon. Crepitation, sometimes referred to as "snowball" crepitation, can often be palpated with active tendon motion in such cases.[141] If untreated, tenosynovitis can progress until the tendon becomes entrapped within its sheath and affects the mobility of the joint.

In the wrist, it is important to differentiate tenosynovitis from an underlying problem involving the wrist ligaments or carpal bones. This is relatively simple when dealing with deQuervain's tenosynovitis of the abductor pollicis longus and extensor pollicis brevis tendons. The problem becomes more difficult when tenosynovitis involves one of the wrist extensors, particularly the extensor carpi ulnaris. Local pain and tenderness may not be confined to the tendon sheath because of a concomitant problem involving the triangular fibrocartilage complex. Injection of the tendon sheath with lidocaine helps differentiate between a tendon and ligament problem in this area.

Accurate and early diagnosis of tenosynovitis of the digital extensors is important. This is particularly true when the extensor pollicis longus is affected, because this tendon tends to rupture. This complication is rarely seen with a tenosynovitis of any other extensor tendon. An exception might be tenosynovitis of the extensor digiti quinti proprius, which is more likely to occur in a chronic arthritic disorder such as rheumatoid arthritis than after an injury. The extensor pollicis longus is vulnerable because it is a relatively thin tendon that passes through a narrow curved tunnel around Lister's tuburcle. If the swelling that occurs with tenosynovitis within its sheath persists it can damage the blood supply to the tendon and lead to rupture. Usually this problem occurs after a Colles' fracture, more commonly when the fracture is minimally or even nondisplaced than when there is severe displacement of the fragments.[59] The explanation for this seeming paradox is that in a nondisplaced fracture of the distal end of the radius, the tendon sheath remains intact and the swelling compromises circulation to the tendon. Conversely, with a severely comminuted and displaced fracture, the sheath is more likely to be torn. This allows greater freedom of the tendon, and the sheath is therefore less likely to be affected by the local swelling. Though an extensor pollicis longus tenosynovitis usually results from chronic overuse, resulting in the so-called drummer boy's palsy, it can also be initiated by an acute injury. It has been observed in a tennis player who, while practicing his serve for many hours, repetitively snapped his wrist into flexion (Fig. 26-1). Though the interval between activity and tendon rupture was hours in this

A

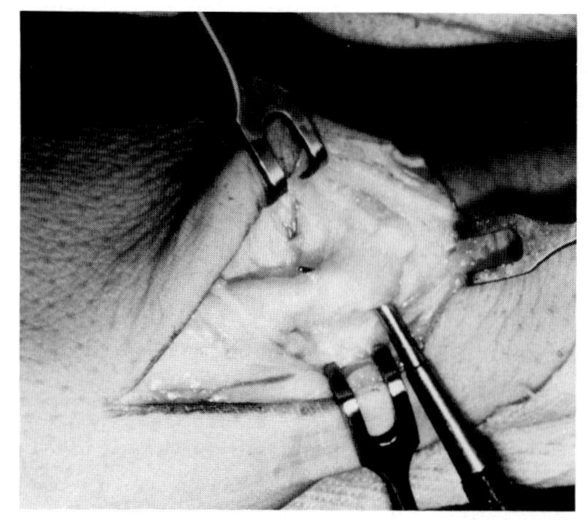

B

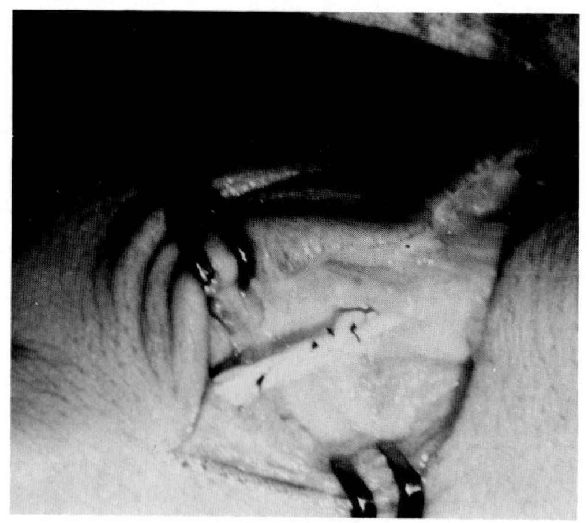

C

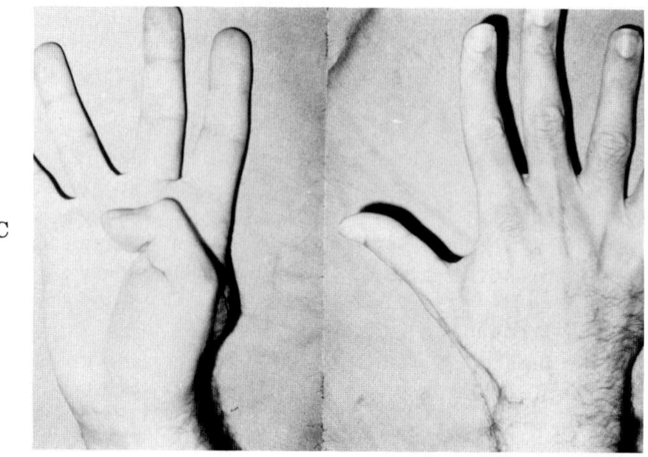

FIG. 26-1. A, A 30-year-old tennis player reported practicing his tennis serve for many hours. Within several days, he developed swelling over the dorsal aspect of his wrist and then noted inability to extend the interphalangeal joint of his thumb. At surgery, the extensor pollicis longus tendon had ruptured and the tendon ends were joined by an area of scarred tenosynovium. **B** and **C,** A tendon transfer using the extensor indicis proprius to the distal stump of the ruptured tendon was carried out. This restored excellent thumb mobility.

particular individual, the interval is more likely to be days or weeks. Prompt recognition of tenosynovitis in the wrist is important in prevention of tendon rupture.

Regardless of the tendon involved or the area of the muscle-tendon unit that is irritated, treatment for a chronic strain is basically rest. The use of a wrist splint as well as nonsteroidal antiinflammatory medication is also helpful. Injection of a steroid into the involved tendon sheath may also be effective. Soluble steroids such as dexamethasone are preferable to insoluble steroids, which tend to leave a deposit. Repeated injections should be avoided. It is questionable whether the treatment should be used for tenosynovitis of the extensor pollicis longus, because the steroid itself may contribute to a tendon rupture. If conservative measures fail and the tenosynovitis persists, surgery is necessary to release the tendon sheath and excise any hypertrophic tenosynovium. For deQuervains's tenosynovitis, the sheath is unnecessary and should be excised. This ensures that any septum enclosing the extensor pollicis brevis is also released. Similar treatment for tenosynovitis of the extensor carpi ulnaris would be ill-advised, because excising the tendon sheath over the sixth dorsal compartment would likely result in subluxation of the tendon with forearm rotation. The sheath should be closed following tenosynovectomy of this compartment, but in a fashion that avoids restricting the gliding movement of the tendon.

Inflammation of the flexor tendons is also common, and the clinical presentation depends on the area that is involved. Flexor tenosynovitis within the carpal tunnel would not only cause pain and limited mobility of the fingers, but would also result in compression of the median nerve. This problem has been observed in athletes whose sport requires repetitive pulling (i.e., rowing) or pressure applied to the palms of the hands for prolonged periods (i.e., cycling). The most effective treatment is cessation of the activity and rest. Flexor tenosynovitis usually subsides fairly rapidly, which also relieves the symptoms of the median nerve compression. In athletes whose carpal tunnel is developmentally shallow or whose problem is chronic, improvement following conservative treatment may be limited. If symptoms persist or weakness develops in the the intrinsic muscles, surgical decompression and neurolysis of the nerve are required.

With overuse of the wrist flexors, it is usually the flexor carpi ulnaris that is strained. Inflammation of its tendon causes symptoms and physical findings that can be dramatic, particularly when there is a calcific deposit. Clinically, there is redness, increased warmth, and swelling that may extend into the hand and proximally into the forearm. Local tenderness is usually intense and the diagnosis is often confused with cellulitis or lymphangitis (Fig. 26-2). However, there is never any local lymphadenopathy or other general signs of infection, such as a fever. The diagnosis is established by a roentgenogram that shows a calcific deposit, usually near the insertion of the tendon into the pisiform.[33,129] The most effective roentgenographic projection is an oblique view of the wrist that permits the pisiform bone to be seen in profile. There is no correlation between the intensity of the patient's symptoms and clinical signs and the size of the calcium deposit. The cause of the calcification remains unclear. Some believed that there is an area of necrotic tissue in the tendon caused by some minor trauma, and that into this area of decreased vascularity calcium salts are precipitated. Treatment consists of needling the deposit with a short 25-gauge needle and injecting a local anesthetic mixed with a soluble steroid. Care must be taken to avoid traumatizing the ulnar artery or nerve during this injection. It is questionable whether the steroid increases the efficacy of needling the deposit, though it may aid in reducing the local inflammation. Clinical improvement is usually rapid, with pain, tenderness, and erythema subsiding within 24 to 48 hours. Repeat roentgenograms 1 week later usually show a significant, if not complete, resorption of the deposit. Surgical ex-

A

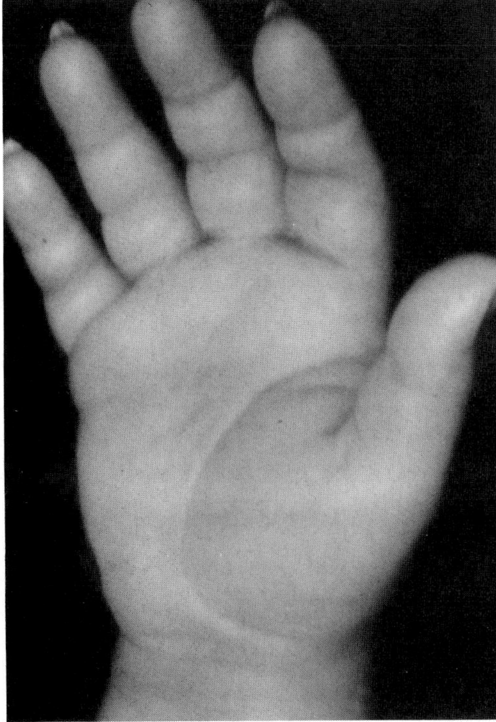

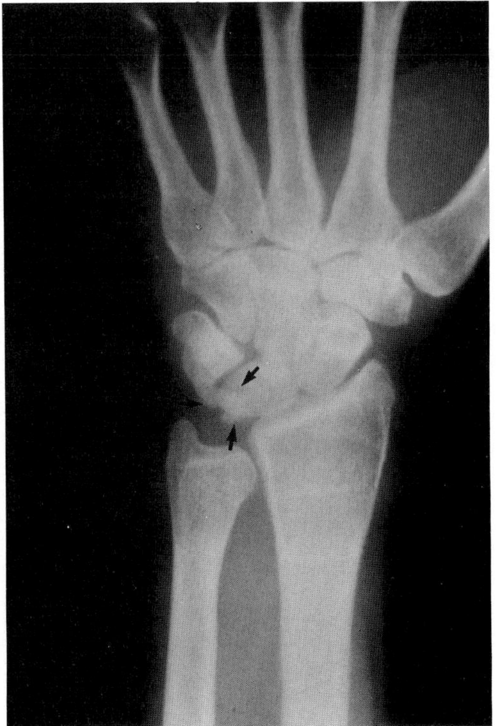

B

FIG. 26-2. A and **B** Swelling of the entire hand with marked tenderness and erythema in the area of the pisiform. Roentgenograms show a large calcific deposit *(arrows)*.

cision of the calcium deposit is rarely necessary.

Ligament Injuries

Acute Injuries

Ligament injuries at the carpometacarpal joints are usually associated with subluxations or dislocations. Avulsion fractures of the bases of the metacarpals or adjacent carpal bones frequently accompany these injuries. There is usually marked swelling over the dorsal aspect of the hand; however, there may be no obvious deformity, and the severity of the injury may initially go unrecognized. Routine anteroposterior and lateral roentgenograms may fail to demonstrate the pathologic condition. Oblique roentgenograms in different projections are often required to profile the injured joint(s) adequately. The vast preponderance of these dislocations are dorsal and, if recognized early, can be easily reduced by manipulation. However, the propensity for redislocation is high, particularly for the second and third metacarpals, because of contraction of the extensor carpi radialis longus and brevis tendons.[164] The fourth and fifth metacarpals tend to be more stable after reduction, though they may also redislocate. Plaster immobilization is inadequate as the sole method of treatment after reduction, and percutaneous Kirschner pin fixation of the injured joint(s) is recommended (Fig. 26-3). Care must be taken in the placement of the pins to avoid injuring the extensor tendons to the fingers, the sensory branches of the radial nerve, or the dorsal sensory branch of the ulnar nerve. The pins need not transfix the radiocarpal joint. If possible, they should also avoid trans-

A

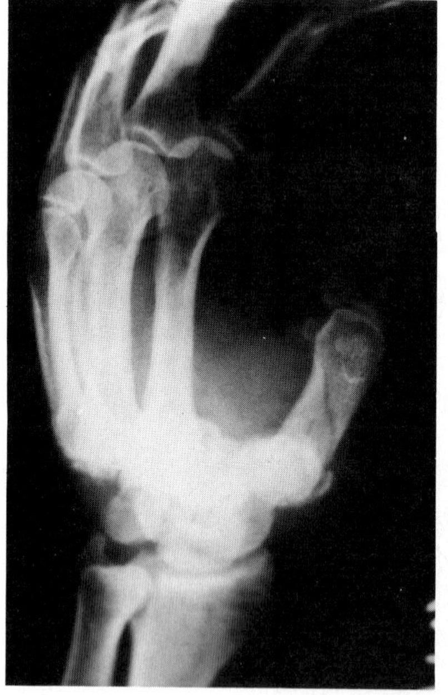

B

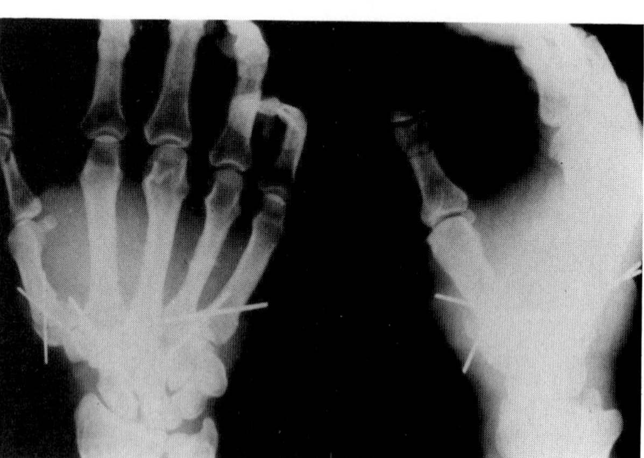

C

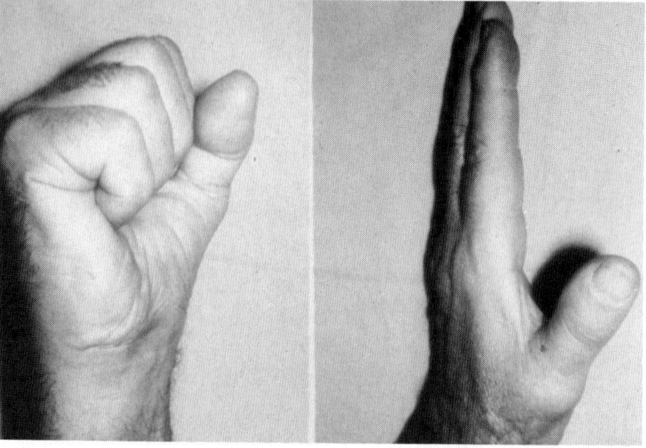

FIG. 26-3. A, Acute dislocation to the carpometacarpal joints of all fingers and a fracture of the first metacarpal. **B,** Following closed reductions, the carpometacarpal joints were stabilized using Kirschner pins which were inserted percutaneously. Open reduction and internal fixation were necessary for the fractured first metacarpal. **C,** Active range of motion exercises were started soon after surgery, and the patient regained complete digital mobility.

fixing of the midcarpal joint. The wrist is splinted, but the splint is removed several times each day for active range of motion exercises. Unrestricted movements for the digits are encouraged immediately after reduction and pin fixation. The pins are left in place for a minimum of 8 weeks. Close follow-up is required for months after removal of the pins, because later subluxations can occur.

Subluxation or dislocation of the carpometacarpal joint of the little finger may be accompanied by a comminuted fracture at the base of the metacarpal. If there is displacement of the metacarpal, it is usually more ulnar than dorsal, because of the direction of pull of the extensor carpi ulnaris. Operative reduction and internal fixation of these fractures are required to restore articular congruity and reduce the risk of later arthritis.[15]

Chronic Injuries

Injuries to the carpometacarpal joints that are not adequately treated at the time of the acute trauma frequently lead to chronic instability and/or arthritis, which is likely to compromise hand function seriously. There is pain and deformity at the involved joint(s), which seriously weaken grip strength (Fig. 26-4). With involvement of the index and middle metacarpals, arthrodeses will restore stability to joints that normally are functionally stable (Fig. 26-5). When secondary arthritic changes develop at the carpometacarpal joint of the little finger, resectional arthroplasties have been recommended to maintain mobility.[130] However, arthrodeses eliminates pain more predictably, and does not cause any significant funtional impairment if the joint is fused in flexion. Fusing the joint in this position will maintain the normal curvature of

A

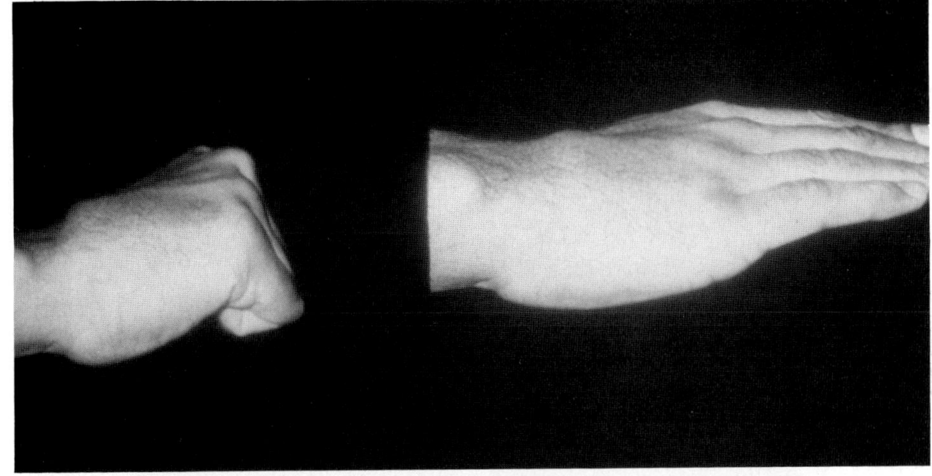

B

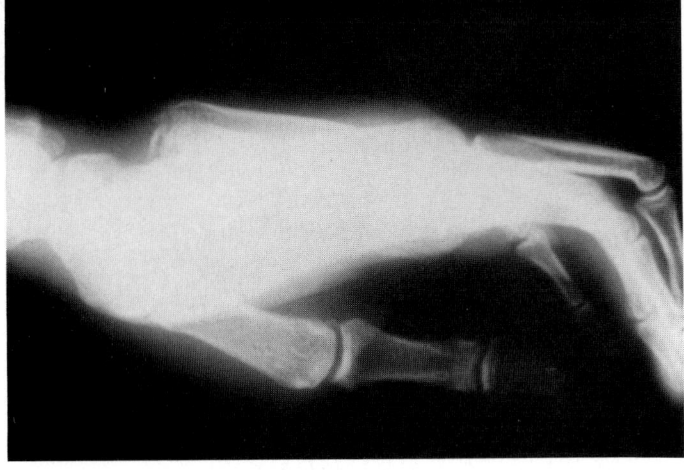

FIG. 26-4. Chronic dislocations (more than 1 year) involving the carpometacarpal joints of the ring and little fingers in a 19-year-old college wrestler. The patient never had any treatment at the time of his injury and his present complaints were pain, weakness of grasp, and an obvious deformity.

A

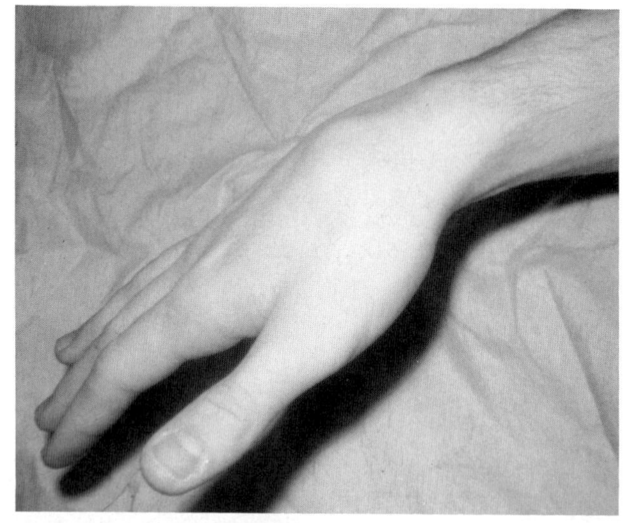

B

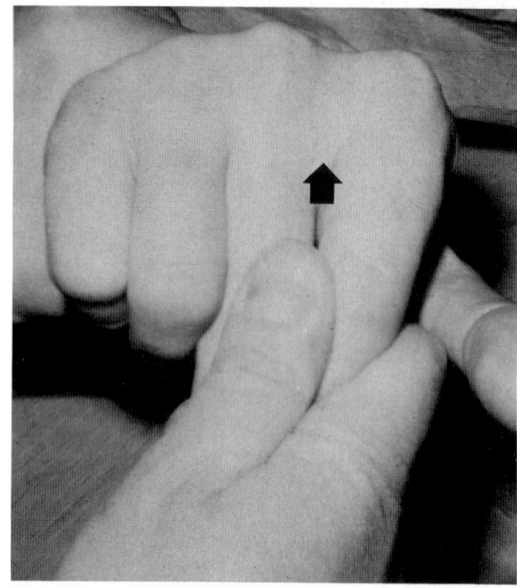

C

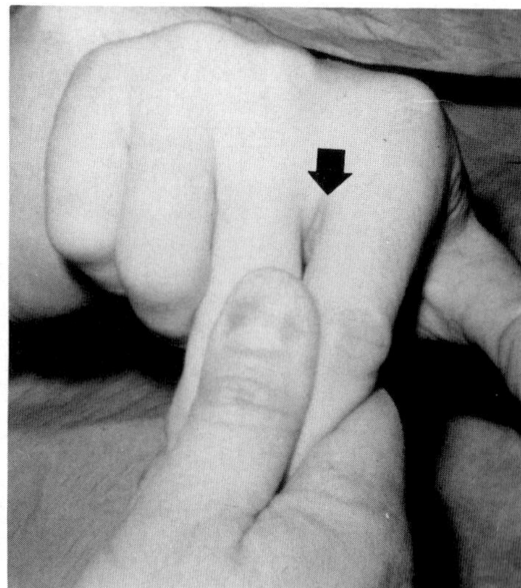

FIG. 26-5. A, A 24-year-old professional football player complained of pain at the carpometacarpal joints of his index and middle fingers. He recalled an injury to the area 1 year earlier that was never treated. Both joints were tender, and the bases of the second and third metacarpals were dorsally subluxed. **B,** and **C** Instability at the affected carpometacarpal joint was readily apparent by upward and downward pressure on the flexed fingers. The normal curvature of the transverse metacarpal arch was distorted with downward pressure on the fingers.

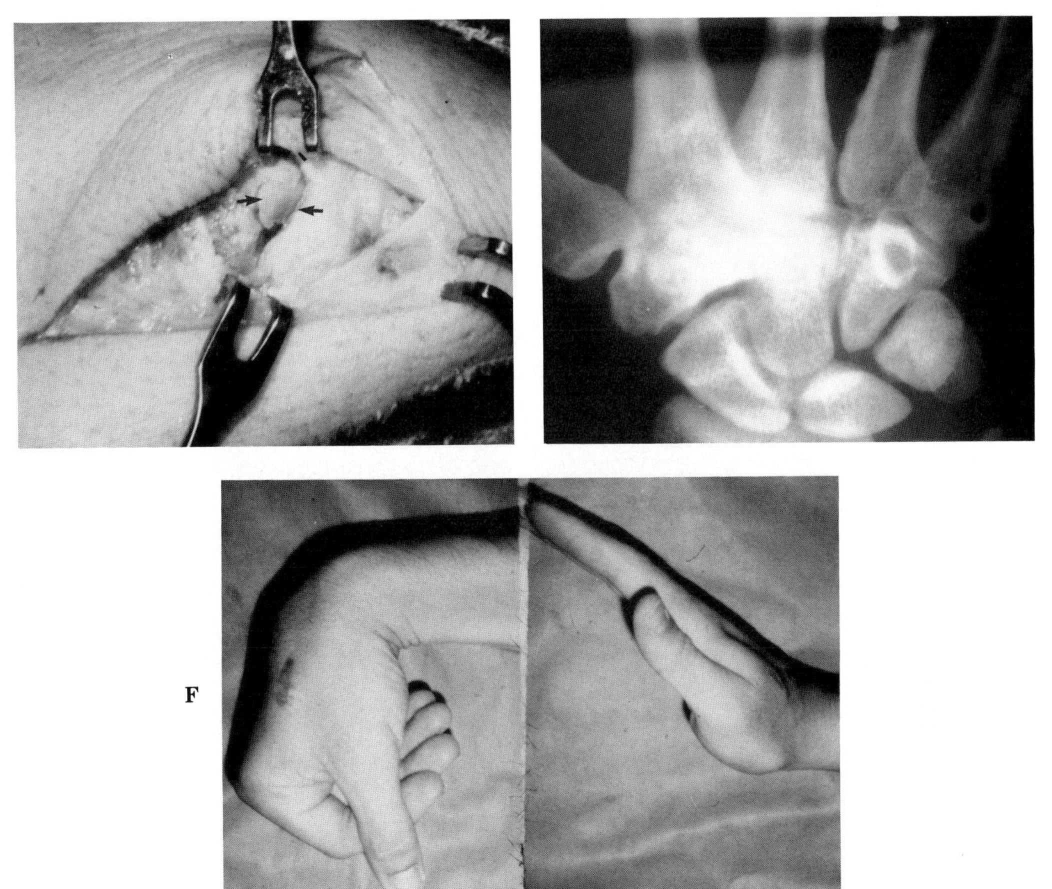

FIG. 26-5, cont'd. D, At surgery, there were arthritic changes with erosive changes in the cartilaginous surfaces of the joints. **E** and **F,** Both joints were arthrodesed, eliminating the previous pain. Postoperative wrist motions were only slightly impaired.

the distal transverse metacarpal arch with the clenched fist. Though the patient will be unable to completely flatten the palm with finger extension, this rarely causes functional impairment (Fig. 26-6).

METACARPAL AREA

Anatomy

The second, third, fourth, and fifth metacarpals function as stabilizers between the carpus and fingers. They form a functional unit that is separate from the role of the first metacarpal. The longitudinal axis for all the finger metacarpals is slightly bowed with a dorsal convexity, but each bone has distinct characteristics in shape and size. Though the head of the third metacarpal is frequently the most prominent with the clenched fist , it is not necessarily the longest metacarpal. The second metacarpal is usually as long as, if not longer than, the third.[154] The apparent greater length of the third metacarpal is because its articulation with the carpus is at a more distal level than the other metacarpals. The fourth metacarpal is shorter than the third, and the fifth is the shortest. Each metacarpal is stabilized proximally by the carpometacarpal ligaments, distally by the deep transverse metacarpal ligaments, and contrally by the interossei muscles. A fracture to a single metacarpal is therefore inherently stable, particularly when one of the central metacarpals (third or fourth), is injured because it receives addtional support from its adjacent border metacarpal (second or fifth). The interossei muscles provide a muscular environment for the bones, which accomodates posttraumatic edema to a greater degree than in the finger itself. It serves to protect the gliding of the flexor and, more notably, the extensor tendons. This is because viscoelastic tissue resistance usually does not develop to the degree that would result in tendon adherence. Fractures of the metacarpals are therefore considered to be more "benign" than phalangeal fractures.[185] Nevertheless, trauma to this area of the hand is serious and requires careful attention.

A

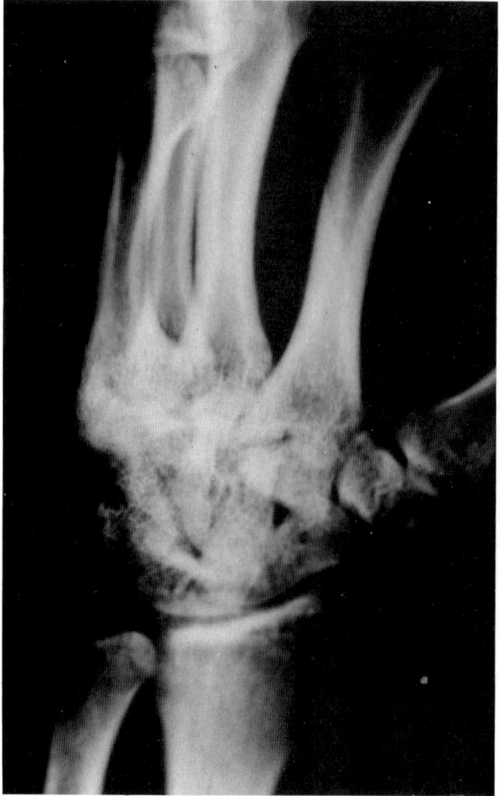

B

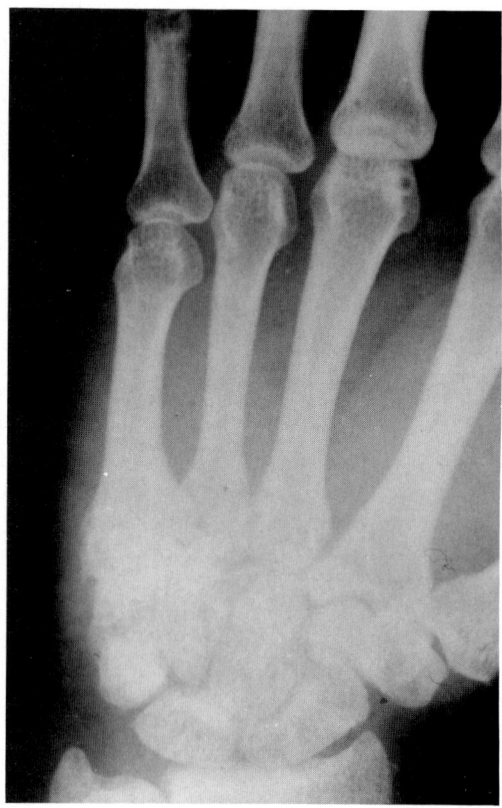

FIG. 26-6. A, Traumatic arthritis of the carpometacarpal joints of the ring and little fingers after untreated intraarticular fractures of the bases of the fourth and fifth metacarpals. Mobility at both joints was limited and painful. **B,** Arthrodeses of both joints were carried out, eliminating both pain and the deformity.

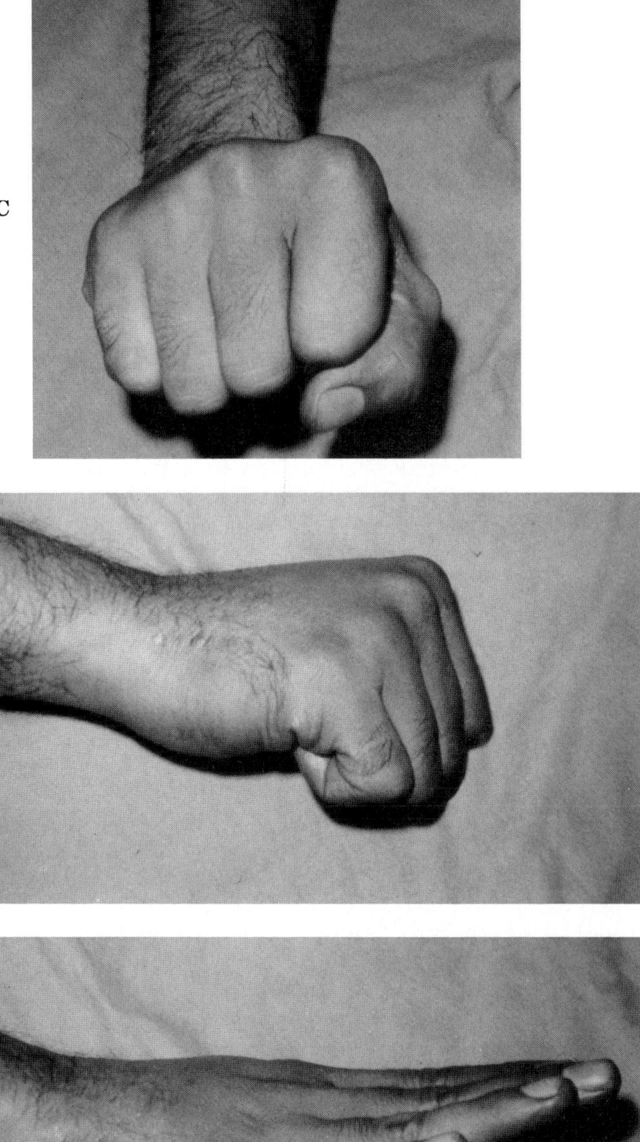

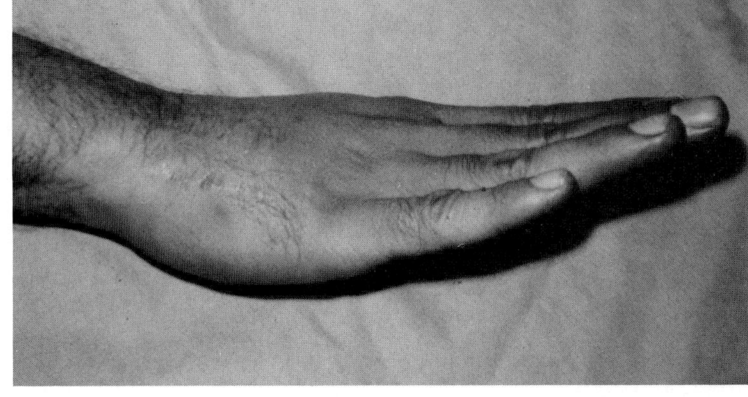

FIG. 26-6, cont'd. C, The joints were fused in flexion to avoid flattening of the transverse metacarpal arch when the patient clenched a fist. **D,** The patient regained full digital mobility. **E,** In extension he could not completely flatten his palm, which did not cause any functional impairment.

Muscle-Tendon Injuries

Extrinsics

Acute injuries. Injuries to the muscle-tendon units affect either the tendons of the extrinsic forearm muscles or the intrinsic muscles which are located entirely in the hand. Acute extrinsic strains usually involve the flexor tendons and follow sudden overstretching. The tendon most commonly fails at its bony insertion, but ruptures in the palm do occur. Though tendons that rupture within their substance can rarely be successfully repaired, an exception is sometimes seen with rupture of a flexor profundus in the area of origin of its lumbrical muscle. The frayed tendon ends can sometimes be excised without sacrificing too much tendon length and the repair site covered using the lumbrical.

Chronic injuries. Chronic extrinsic strains are caused by overuse and are commonly manifested by tenosynovitis at the wrist level, which was discussed in the previous section (see p. 497).

Intrinsics

Acute injuries. Strains of the intrinsic muscles in the palm usually result from overuse. These injuries predominate over similar strains to the extrinsics. Strains of the intrinsics are common in sports that require repetitive gripping, such as tennis, golf, and rowing.[56] Initially, the athlete with intrinsic muscle fatigue complains of "aching," "tiredness," or "cramping" in the hand. Recovery is usually prompt with rest and cessation of the activity, and there are usually no residual sequelae. Continued overuse, however, may lead to more severe and persistent symptoms and, in some cases, can actually result in fibrosis and contractures of the injured muscle(s). Acute intrinsic muscle injuries can also result from closed direct trauma, particularly to the most vulnerable dorsal aspect of the hand. There may be swelling and even hemorrhage within the muscles. Early recognition is important. As soon as the acute swelling subsides, exercises are started to reduce the likelihood of later contractures. The objective of the exercises is to stretch the intrinsic muscle. This can be accomplished by two methods: either by holding the metacarpophalangeal joint(s) in maximum extension and having the patient actively and passively flex the interphalangeal joints; or by holding the interphalangeal joints in flexion, usually with an elastic strap, and having the patient actively and passively extend the metacarpophalangeal joint(s). The assistance of a hand therapist is important in fabricating the necessary exercise devices and in monitoring the patient's compliance with the program.

Chronic injuries. If unrecognized, intrinsic muscle injuries can progress to fibrosis, resuting in contractures. The classic deformities of an intrinsic hand with flexion contractures of all metacarpophalngeal joints and extension contractures of all interphalangeal joints are more commonly encountered after severe crush or burn injuries than after athletic injuries. The type of intrinsic contractures seen in the athlete is rarely as severe. The findings are apt to be subtle, sometimes with no obvious deformity to the finger(s). The patient may even be able to move the finger(s) completely, but complains of "stiffness" or "tightness" with flexion. The intrinsic contractures in these cases may involve just a few muscles, sometimes those within a single intermetacarpal area. Such contractures frequently result from a fracture of a single metacarpal, but they can also occur in the absence of fracture. The realization that isolated contractures occur and may exist even in the presence of complete digital mobility is imporant to make the diagnosis.

The contracture must be demonstrated by physical examination. For example, an injury to the area between the third dorsal and fourth metacarpals can damage the third dorsal and second volar interossei muscles. Contractures of these two intrinsics would affect the function of the middle and ring fingers. When testing for the presence of intrinsic contractures, the excursion of the intrinsics to either side of these fingers must be compared. For the middle finger, this involves maximally extending or hyperextending the proximal phalanx and then deviating it radially before evaluating the degree of passive flexion of the proximal interphalangeal joint. With contracture of the third dorsal interosseous, passive flexion of the joint would be limited.

Excursion of the uninvolved second dorsal interosseous is then evaluated by deviating the proximal phalanx ulnarly while maintaining the metacarpophalangeal joint in hyperextension and again passively flexing the proximal interphalangeal joint. A similar procedure is carried out for the ring finger to compare the excursion of the second volar interosseous on the radial side of the digit, which may be contracted, with the excursion of the fourth dorsal interosseous on the ulnar side, which is probably unaffected. If surgery is required, limiting the release to the tendons of the contracted intrinsic muscles should correct the problem. Isolated contractures of the first dorsal interosseous on the radial side of the index or of the intrinsics in the hypothenar area are less common. Because these muscles are bounded by a metacarpal on only one side, they are not as confined as the intrinsics in the intermetacarpal areas. They are therefore not as susceptible to the effects of swelling and hemorrhage.

Fractures

A variety of forces can produce a fracture of the metacarpal shaft, including indirect compression, torsion, or a direct blow that damages the overlying soft tissues. Careful clinical examination is the essential first step in treatment and should always precede roentgenographs. Rotation, angulation, and/or shortening at the fracture site can often be diagnosed by simply observing the resting position of the injured finger as well as its relationship to the adjacent fingers at rest and during gentle active motion. This is particularly true when there is malrotation, which may not be evident on routine roentgenograms. It has been estimated that *for each degree of malrotation at the fracture site as much as 5 degrees of malrotation will occur at the finger tip.*[142] Thus a fracture that is rotated only 5 degrees can result in 1.5 cm of digital overlap, an obviously unacceptable condition that requires correction.[58]

The vast majority of metacarpal fractures can be successfully managed by closed measures. Though circular plaster casts are frequently applied in hospital emergency departments for these fractures, they are unnecessary and often troublesome to deal with in follow-up visits. Effective immobilization for the acute fracture is more easily provided by applying a padded aluminum splint on the volar aspect of the injured digit and then incorporating it into a plaster splint with the wrist held in slight dorsiflexion. The splint is applied with the patient's forearm in supination and the wrist resting on a gauze roll to achieve the desired position of slight wrist dorsiflexion. The aluminum splint is bent to conform to the position of the wrist and finger, with the metacarpal joint in acute flexion to minimize the risk of a later extension contracture. The splint is sandwiched between a sufficient number of plaster splints, which stabilizes both the splint as well as the wrist joint. The aluminum splint is always molded to the finger and never the reverse. The normal capsular laxity of a metacarpophalangeal joint in extension may permit a malrotated or angulated fracture to appear to be "reduced" if the finger is manipulated to a splint that has been molded to conform to the position of the adjacent uninjured fingers. The improvement in alignment or rotation of the injured finger would be illusory, because when the splint was removed the deformity would persist. With stable fractures, active range of motion exercises can be started within 7 to 10 days. The splint is removed several times each day for these execises and then reapplied and worn at all other times. With less stable fractures, the total period of immobilization may have to be longer before active exercises are begun but should *never* exceed 3 weeks. If immobilization for longer than 3 weeks is necessary, the fracture should have been treated with some type of internal fixation.

With each follow-up visit, the clinical appearance of the finger and the roentgenograms are checked to determine if there has been any displacement at the fracture site. Splint immobilization is continued, allowing for periodic daily exercises, until there is roentgenographic evidence of complete healing. The initial aluminum and plaster splint can be changed to a plastic splint, which is lighter in weight and easier for the patient to remove for the exercise program. Immobilization of uninjured fingers during the healing process should be avoided.

Oblique/Spiral Fractures

Metacarpal fractures are classified as oblique/spiral, transverse, or comminuted. Oblique/spiral fractures are the most common type. These fractures result from a rotational force on the bone and have a tendency to displace, resulting in overriding of the fragments and shortening. The displacement may not be present at the time of acute injury, but occur a week or two later. Therefore these fractures require attentive follow-up care. When there is displacement, various techniques have been recommended for internal fixation. Kirschner pins probably are the most popular. Two or more parallel pins drilled across the fracture site will provide rigid fixation (Fig. 26-7). Percutaneous insertion of the pins at either the fracture site or through the head of the bone and down its medullary cavity has been suggested.[16,34,113,157] With respect to percutaneous pin fixation at the fracture site, the technique is safer for oblique fractures of the second and fifth metacarpals than for similar fractures of the third and

Metacarpal fracture patterns

- Oblique/spiral
- Transverse
- Comminuted

fourth metacarpals, in which there is greater danger of impaling an extensor tendon(s) with the pin. Drilling the pin down the medullary cavity of the bone can cause scarring of the joint capsule and extensor tendon hood and, unless other pins are inserted across the fracture, may not control rotation.[150,151] If longitudinal pins are used, they should be inserted at the sides of the metacarpal head in the area of origin of the collateral ligaments, thus avoiding damage to its articular surface.[139] The most effective method of pin placement is surgery. The risk of an open procedure is far outweighed by clear visualization

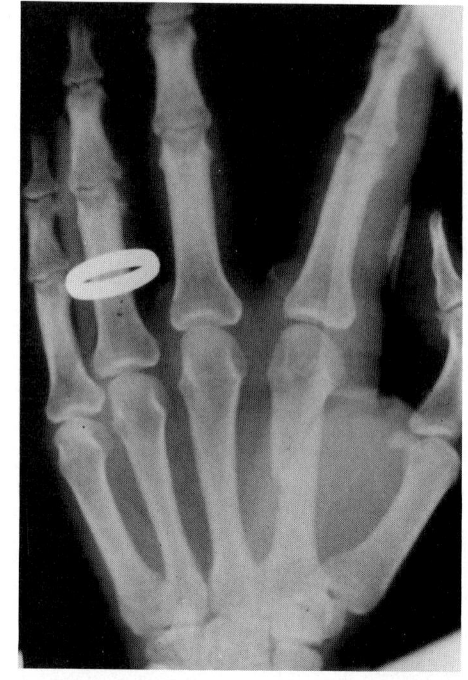

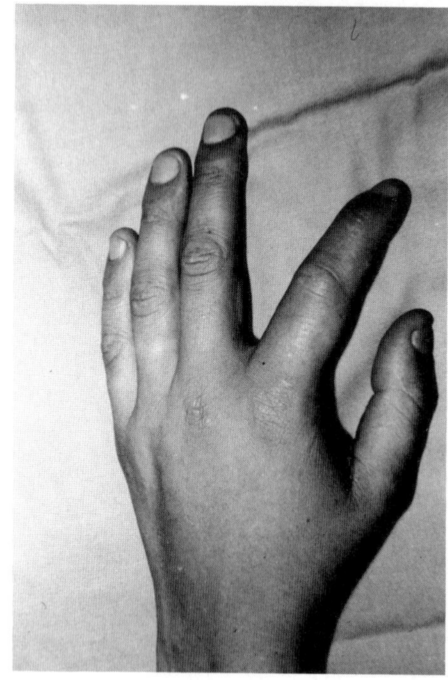

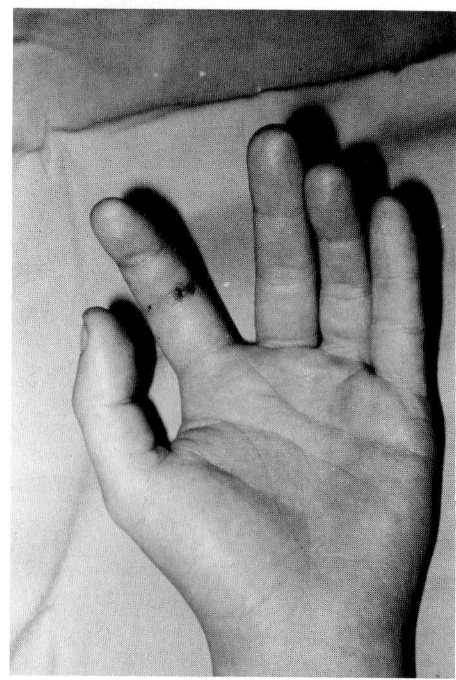

FIG. 26-7. A to **C,** Oblique fracture of the second metacarpal causing an obvious rotational deformity of the finger.

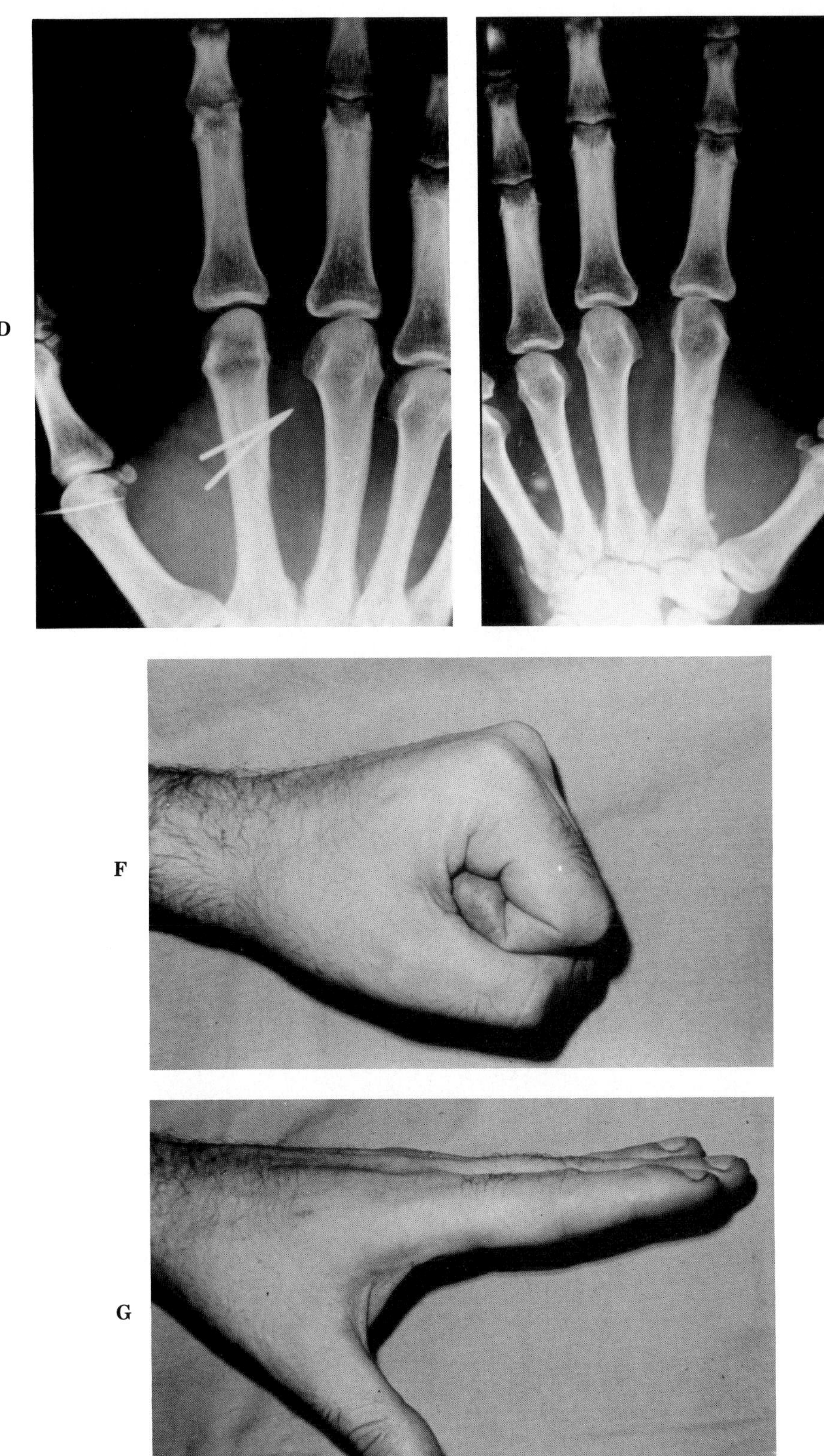

FIG. 26-7, cont'd. D and **E,** Rigid internal fixation was obtained using multiple Kirschner pins, which resulted in healing within 8 weeks. **F** and **G,** The patient started active range of motion exercises within 10 days of surgery and regained complete digital mobility.

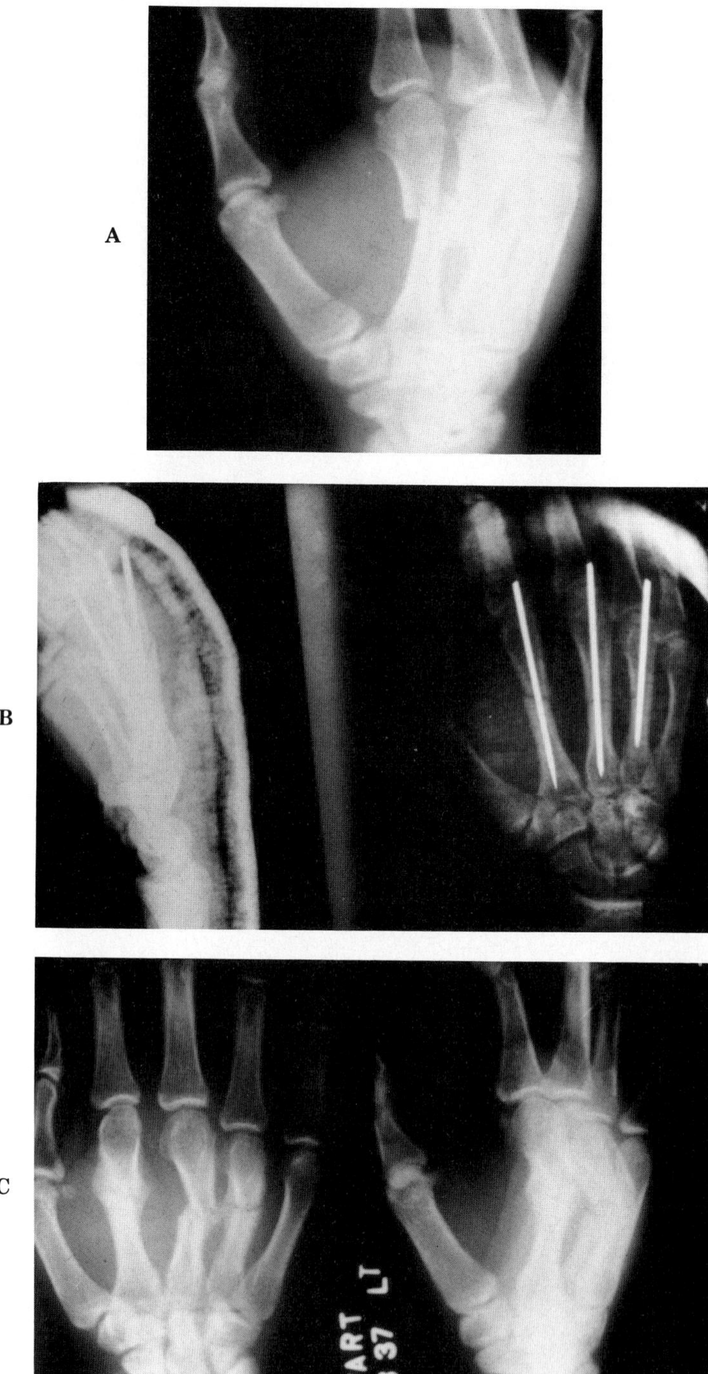

FIG. 26-8. A and **B,** Transverse fractures of the second, third, and fourth metacarpals were stabilized using intramedullary pins inserted through the metacarpal heads. Though the fractures were successfully stabilized using this technique, inserting pins through joints will result in capsular scarring and lead to joint stiffness. It is a method of treatment that should be avoided. The surgeon who treated this patient was apparently aware of the risks of the procedure and, in an attempt to minimize them, removed the pins after only 6 weeks. **C,** The fractures had not sufficiently healed and collapsed. Transverse fractures in the diaphyseal portion of a metacarpal take longer to heal than similar fractures in the metaphyseal area of the bone. Stabilizing the fractures with small plates and screws would have been the preferred method of treatment.

of the fracture, obtaining of an anatomic reduction and precise insertion of the pins. The use of two or more small lag screws is also an effective method of fixation for this type of fracture, provided the length of the fracture is at least twice the width of the bone.[58] Shorter fractures can also be treated with a lag screw, but must be supplemented with a neutralization plate.

Transverse Fractures

Transverse fractures differ from oblique or spiral fractures in several ways. They tend toward greater overriding, which accentuates the deformity; however, once reduced, they are more stable because the fracture ends are compressed together. Another difference may be the rate of healing, which is slower for a transverse midshaft fracture, because the fracture surfaces are small and in the cortical diaphyseal portion of the bone (Fig. 26-8). These fractures may also result in angulation, which is usually dorsal. Though this angulation rarely interferes with gliding of the extensor tendons, it can cause an imbalance at the metacarpophalangeal joint, producing a claw-type deformity with finger extension. In addition, the head of the fractured metacarpal becomes more prominent in the palm and may interfere with grasp. Opinions vary as to the degree of angulation that is acceptable for each metacarpal. Up to 10 degrees of angulation for the second and third metacarpals is tolerated by some authors. Acceptable angulation for the mobile fourth and fifth metacarpals ranges from 20 degrees for the fourth to 35 degrees for the fifth.[55,171] Shortening is generally not a significant problem for a single shaft fracture because of the tethering effect of the deep transverse metacarpal ligaments, which are attached to the adjacent intact metacarpals. Some authors claim that shortening never poses a functional problem,[12,28] whereas others recommend that it be corrected.[74]

Though the published figures for what is considered acceptable angulation and shortening provide convenient reference points, they should not be applied to every case. Each patient's fracture must be treated with a complete understanding of the demands placed on the athlete's hand in the particular sport. For the amateur or professional boxer, any angulation of a fractured metacarpal, whether it be the stable second or mobile fifth, requires correction. The tremendous compressive forces applied to the hand in boxing will likely refracture the metacarpal if it is allowed to heal in angulation. Shortening of a metacarpal would be equally detrimental to individuals in whom precision and coordinated finger movements are important. Pianists, the ultimate athletes with respect to dexterity and endurance in hand function, fall into this category.

Most transverse fractures can be successfully managed by closed manipulation. If closed reduction cannot be achieved, surgery is necessary. As with oblique fractures, various methods for internal fixation are available, including Kirschner pins, wiring, or a plate.[68,80,116,187,188] A plate applied to the dorsal surface of the bone provides excellent rigidity and is particularly useful for multiple fractures.[139]

Comminuted Fractures

In severely comminuted fractures, the problems of fixation are increased. These fractures may require stabilization by drilling pins into the adjacent intact metacarpals.

METACARPOPHALANGEAL JOINT AREA

Anatomy

The metacarpophalangeal joints of the fingers are the most proximal joints in a series of four separate triarticular chains that face the palm and thumb to achieve prehension. Though the joints within each triarticular chain have structural differences, they function as a unit to facilitate flexion and prevent hyperextension.[45] The metacarpophalangeal joint is formed by an asymmetric spheroidal head of the metacarpal, which articulates against the broad, concave base of the proximal phalanx. It is a multiaxial condyloid joint that permits flexion, extension, abduction, adduction, and, to a slight degree, circumduction. The asymmetry of the head is apparent when it is viewed in different projections: it is flattened transversely and wider volarly than dorsally. In the frontal plane, the head curves smoothly on its radial side but stops abruptly on its ulnar side (Fig. 26-9). This asymmetry is most obvious in the second and third metacarpals and is responsible for the tendency of the proximal phalanges of these two fingers to drift ulnarly with flexion.[45] Flexion-extension movements of the metacarpophalangeal joints do not occur about a single axis, but rather about a series of axes, which lie on an arc that moves in a palmar direction with increasing joint flexion.

The supporting structures for each joint consist of a capsule dorsally; a glenoid fibrocartilage plate volarly, and a combination of ligaments, sagittal bands, and intrinsic tendons laterally. The dorsal capsule is thin and

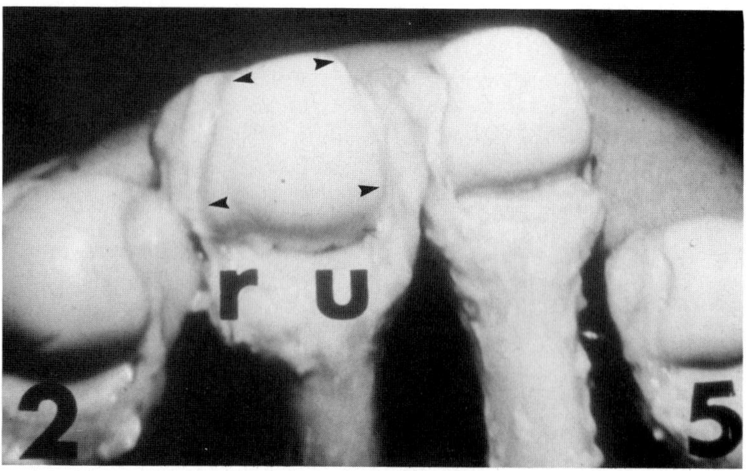

FIG. 26-9. Frontal view of the metacarpophalangeal joints of the fingers. The metacarpal heads are trapezoidal in configuration. They are narrower dorsally than volarly, and the collateral ligaments are shown to be taut in full flexion.

is reinforced by fibers from the overlying extensor tendon(s). These fibers permit gliding of the extensor apparatus and stabilize the tendon in a midline position over the joint.[154] The capsule is lax to facilitate a wide range of flexion, and it forms a large bursa that extends proximally for a distance of 15 to 20 millimeters along the dorsal aspect of the metacarpal. At the joint line, the synovial membrane of the capsule folds inward to form a meniscal cushion. Its function is unknown. It may prevent the dorsal capsule from being trapped between the joint surfaces during extension, or it may improve the joint congruity in an area where the surface of the phalangeal head is small.[45]

The volar aspect of the capsule consists of a thick fibrocartilaginous structure, the volar plate. Its distal portion is thick, rigid, and cartilaginous and moves volar to the head with flexion and extension. It is firmly anchored into the volar surface of the proximal phalanx. Proximally, the plate is thin, flexible, and membranous. With joint flexion, it folds like the bellows of an accordion between the metacarpal head and the cartilage portion of the plate. The anterior part of the plate forms the posterior wall of the fibrous tendon sheath at the level of the A-1 pulley. The volar plates are interconnected by the deep transverse metacarpal ligaments.

Laterally, the ligament support for the metacarpophalangeal joint is composed of two parts, the collateral ligaments and the accessory collateral ligaments (Fig. 26-10). The collateral ligaments arise from eccentrically located tuberosities on the sides of the metacarpal head and insert on lateral tuberosities on the proximal phalanx, near its volar surface. Asymmetry exists in these ligaments as in the metacarpal head. The radial fibers are thicker and stronger and run in a more oblique direction than the ulnar fibers. These differences produce passive axial rotation of the finger, which goes from supination in the extended position to pronation as it is flexed. This contributes to the tendency for the finger to deviate in an ulnar direction.[105] Both collateral ligaments are dorsal to the flexion-extension axis for these joints. Because this axis moves volarly with joint flexion, the collateral ligaments are lax in extension and become increasingly taut as the proximal phalanx flexes. They must also diverge to accommodate the wider width of the metacarpal head on its volar side, which is another reason they become taut with joint flexion. Therefore lateral movement is greatest in extension and becomes increasingly limited with progressive flexion. The collateral ligaments also stabilize the joint in its flexion-extension arc. Without these ligaments, the tremendous flexion force on the proximal phalanx supplied by the extrinsic flexor tendons and intrinsic muscles (interossei and lumbricals) would result in volar subluxation of the joint.[54,171]

The accessory collateral ligaments originate on the sides of the metacarpal head volar to the origins of the collateral ligaments. They insert on the borders of the glenoid fibrocartilage plate. The accessory collateral ligaments are volar to the flexion-extension axis of the joint. They are lax in flexion and taut

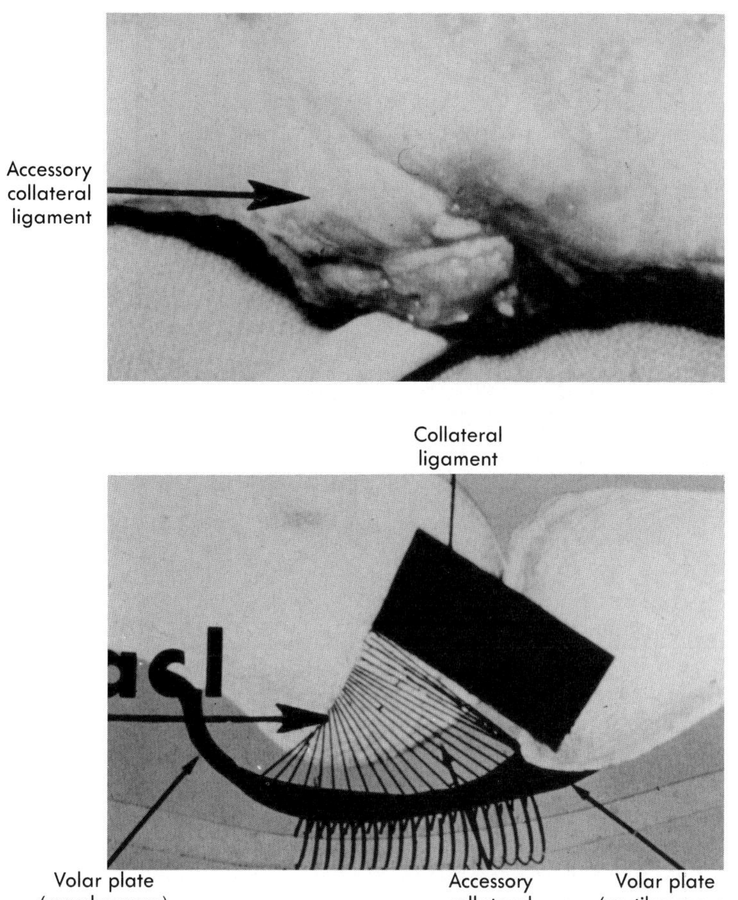

FIG. 26-10. Anatomic and diagrammatic views of the lateral aspect of a metacarpophalangeal joint.

in extension, the reverse for the collateral ligaments. The accessory collateral ligaments, by their suspensory action on the volar plate, stabilize the flexor tendons with joint flexion. Additional lateral stability for the metacarpophalangeal joints is provided by the intrinsic muscles and sagittal fibers of the dorsal tendon mechanism.

Tendon Injuries

Subluxation of the extensor tendon from its midline position over the dorsal aspect of a metacarpophalangeal joint usually results from forceful deviation of the finger in an ulnar direction. The middle finger is most frequently affected because of the unique anatomic relationship of its extensor tendon to the dorsal hood. There is not the intimate connection between tendon and the transverse fibers of the hood that exists for other fingers; rather, the extensor tendon in the middle finger lies on top of the hood, to which it is only loosely connected. Consequently, there is a defect in continuity between the radial intrinsic muscle and the extensor tendon, which leaves the tendon vulnerable to displacement. The force required to cause this displacement is greatest in full extension and full flexion and decreases during the first 60 degrees of flexion.[99]

An extensor tendon subluxation can also occur from a direct blow, such as striking a hard object with the clenched fist. Involvement of the middle finger and displacement of the tendon in an ulnar direction is also seen with this type of injury, but not with the same frequency as with sudden forceful deviation of the finger. Regardless of the mechanism of injury, the diagnosis requires a careful examination, because swelling over the injured joint may obscure the position of the tendon and its displacement may go unrecognized. Even when there is swelling and the tendon cannot be palpated, subluxation should be suspected. The examiner follows the direction of the tendon from its more proximal portion over the metacarpal, where it can be more easily palpated. Once the diagnosis is established, there are two treatment options. If the tendon is relocated with extension of the metacarpophalangeal joint, a volar splint can be used for 3 to 4 weeks, with the fingers immobilized in full extension. The interphalangeal joints should not be immobilized. A soft, wide catheter can be placed to the displaced side of the tendon to help maintain it in its correct position. The other treatment option is surgery, which is indicated for severe subluxation of the tendon, particularly when it remains subluxed with extension. Repair of the torn sagittal fibers will effectively restore the tendon to its normal position.[78,99]

In chronic cases, direct repair of the torn fibers may also be possible after excision of the scar tissue at the site of hood disruption (Fig. 26-11). If necessary, a relaxing incision is made on the ulnar side of the tendon to relocate it into its proper position. If the radial portion of the hood is so deficient or scarred as to preclude repair, some form of tether must be used to centralize the tendon. Various techniques have been proposed including rerouting a juncturae tendinum or splitting the extensor tendon and rerouting that tendon slip around the radial collateral ligament or lumbrical muscle.[32,118,192] Regardless of which procedure is carried out, care must be taken to ensure that the repair is secure enough to resist recurrence of the subluxation when the finger is passively flexed at surgery.[42]

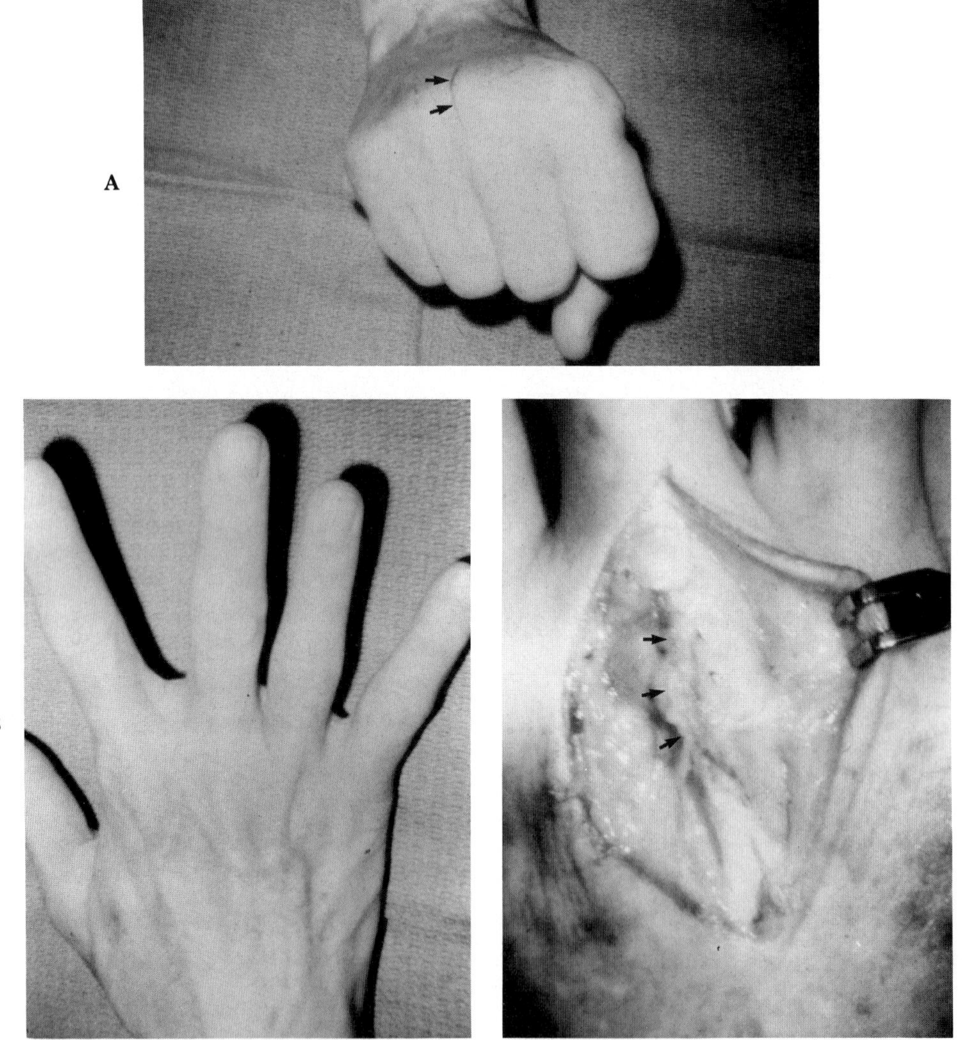

FIG. 26-11. A and **B,** Chronic ulnar subluxation of the extensor tendon to the middle finger, which is obvious with the joint in full flexion. Even in extension there was slight ulnar deviation of the finger, because the extensor tendon was not in its normal midline position. **C,** The hood is explored through a curved incision and the sagittal fibers *(arrows)* repaired, restoring the tendon to its normal midline position.

D

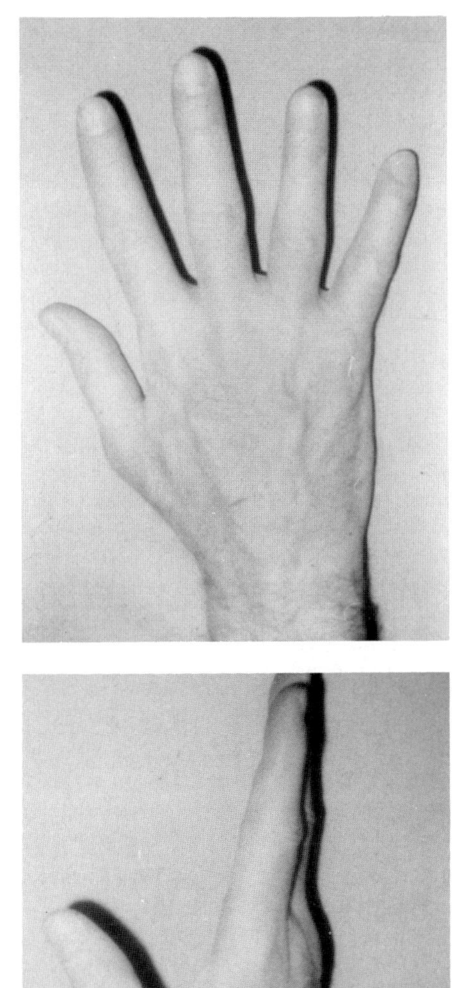

E

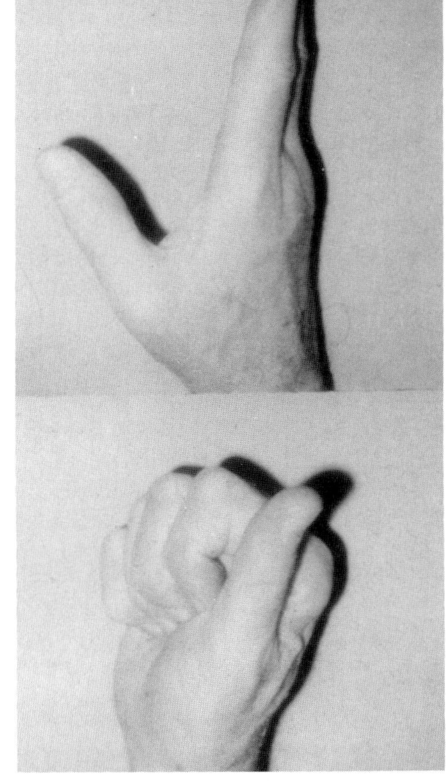

FIG. 26-11, cont'd. D and **E,** Postoperatively, the tendon was restored to its normal position over the joint, and the previous ulnar deviation of the finger in extension was eliminated.

Ligament Injuries

In general, ligaments in the mobile joints of the hand have two important functions: to permit normal joint motion and to provide stability against abnormal motions. When the force toward an abnormal motion exceeds the power of the ligament to prevent it, a sprain occurs. Sprains therefore result from overstress, as opposed to contusions, which result from a direct blow to a ligament. When stress is applied to a ligament, it initially tenses to withstand the force. However, at some point it fails, resulting in damage to its fibers. The extent of damage depends on the force and duration of its application.

There are three categories of sprains. **First-degree sprain** is the mildest. Only a few fibers of the ligament are damaged, and the strength of the ligament is not compromised. It is therefore unnecessary to protect the ligament and treatment is entirely symptomatic. The patient is usually able to resume full activities within 1 to 2 weeks. In **second-degree sprain,** or moderate sprain, a greater portion of the ligament is torn. Some functional loss usually results. The joint is stable with active motion, but some laxity can be demonstrated with stress testing. Because part of the ligament remains intact, treatment is directed toward protection. If the joint is immobilized, the damaged portion of the ligament should be expected to heal, because the torn fibers are probably in close proximity to each other. In spite of adequate protection, some second-degree sprains do not heal and, though there may be no appreciable joint instability, the patient may have a significant disability. Surgery is sometimes necessary for these cases. The **third-degree sprain,** or severe sprain, occurs when the ligament is completely torn, either within its substance or at one end of its bony attachments. If it is damaged at either attachment, it may have avulsed with a bone fragment. This is sometimes referred to as a "sprain-fracture."[141] Though a fracture is technically present, the injury is primarily to the ligament, and it is to the ligament which treatment must be directed. With third-degree sprains, the stabilizing function of the ligament is lost and the joint is unstable. Subluxations or dislocations with clinical and/or roentgenographic evidence of joint incongruity are obvious third-degree sprains. Frequently, the initial subluxation or dislocation spontaneously reduces, leaving a joint that is stable with active motion and has no incongruity. Stress testing in these cases will demonstrate gross instability.

Though the treatment for third-degree sprains depends on the specific ligament disrupted, several general principles should be followed. The primary objective is to restore stability. Therefore it is advisable to immobilize the joint for several weeks. This is followed by active range of motion exercises and protection for 2 to 3 months. Avoidance of immobilization to reduce the likelihood of later joint stiffness may succeed, but at the risk of continued instability. If stiffness develops after treatment, it is preferable to instability and usually easier to treat.[21]

Surgery is required for third-degree sprains in the following situations. The first is failure to restore normal articular congruity after reduction of a subluxation or dislocation. This will be evident on anteroposterior and/or lateral roentgenograms. A second indication is unstressed instability. If the joint fails to remain in alignment with active motion, then there are interposed tissues within the joint or the disruption of capsular structures is of such magnitude that it requires surgical exploration and repair. A third indication for surgery is an articular fracture fragment that remains widely displaced. In all likelihood, the avulsed ligament is attached to this fragment, and its displaced position usually precludes the possibility of healing with stability.

Volar Plate

Ligament injuries to the metacarpophalangeal joints are uncommon, but when they occur they usually follow sudden hyperextension, which results in a dorsal dislocation. The index finger is involved most commonly,[6,134] followed by the little finger. The volar plate ruptures at its membranous connection to the metacarpal and shifts dorsally with the proximal phalanx, to which it remains attached. The plate becomes entrapped behind the dorsal aspect of the metacarpal head. The metacarpal is further trapped by taut structures on both radial and ulnar sides of its neck. In dislocation of the index finger, the lumbrical muscle is radial and the flexor tendons are ulnar; in dislocation of the little finger, both the lumbrical muscle and flexor tendons are to the radial side and the conjoined tendon of the hypothenar intrinsic muscles to the ulnar side.[5,95] Rarely, the torn volar plate, while still attached to the dislocated phalanx, is not displaced behind the metacarpal head but remains volar to it. A closed reduction is readily achievable in these situations. First the wrist is flexed to relax the tendons. Then pressure is applied to the dorsal aspect of the base of the proximal phalanx in a distal and volar direction, sliding the joint into flexion. Care must be taken not to apply traction on the joint or to hyperextend the digit initially, because

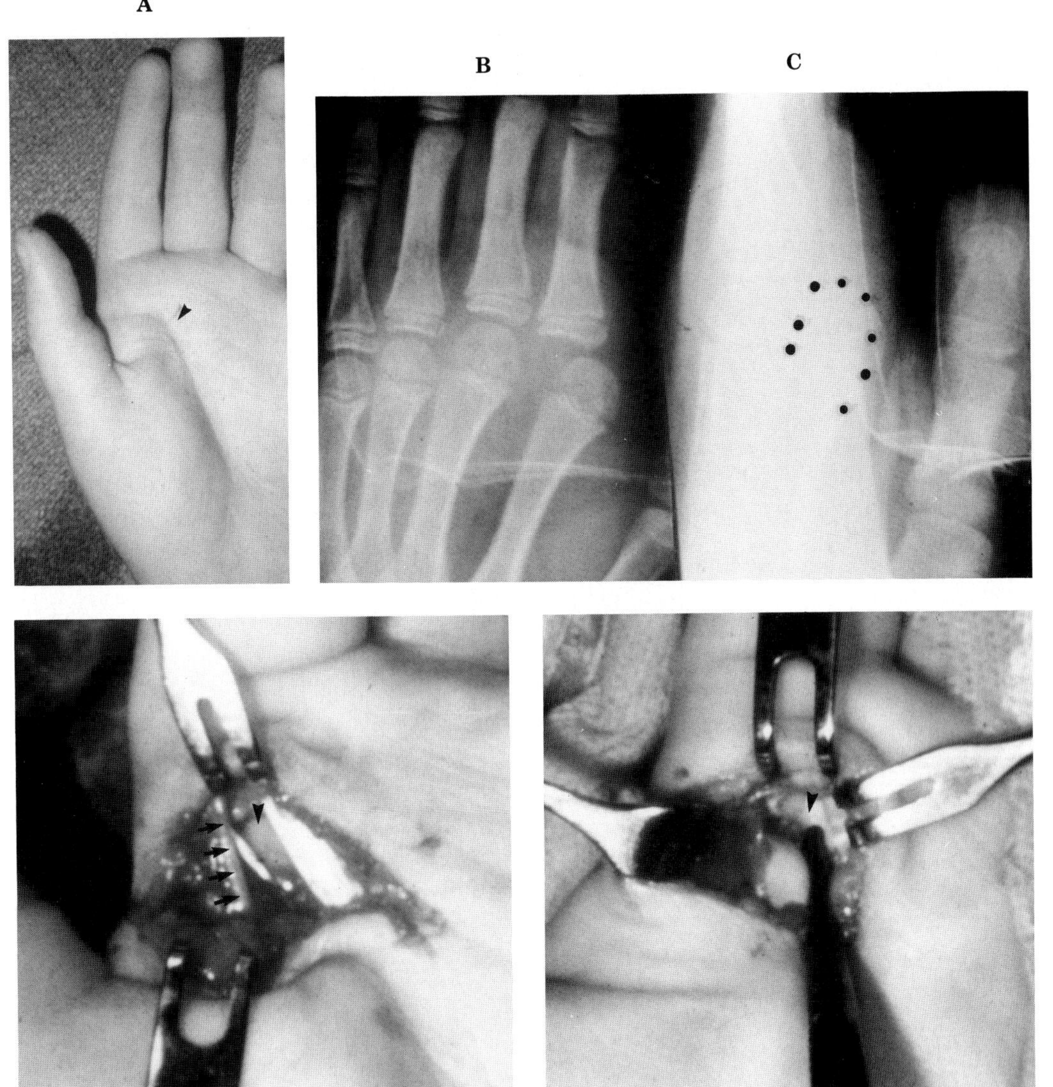

FIG. 26-12. A, Dorsal dislocation of the metacarpophalangeal joint of an index finger. The index finger was adducted against the adjacent middle finger and the palmar skin was puckered *(arrow)* in the palmar crease. **B** and **C,** Lateral roentgenograms show the proximal phalanx to be dorsal to the metacarpal head. In the oblique view, there is abnormal widening of the joint space. **D,** At surgery, care must be taken when making skin incisions because the radial neurovascular bundle *(small arrows)* is tented over the head of the metacarpal *(large arrow)* and can easily be inadvertently cut. **E,** The volar plate *(arrow)* is displaced posterior to the head of the metacarpal and is the major structure that prevents reduction.

this maneuver might shift the plate distally. The plate could then pass behind the metacarpal head, converting an incomplete subluxation into a complete and irreducible dislocation.[43]

Complete dislocation, often termed "complex" because of the number of anatomic structures that block its reduction, was first described by Farebeuf in 1876 and introduced into the English literature by Barnard in 1901. It was not until 1957 that Kaplan published his classic article describing its clinical and anatomic features.[95] The finger is flexed at the interphalangeal joints and slightly hyperextended at its metacarpophalangeal joint (Fig. 26-12). The finger is also deviated toward the adjacent fingers. The palmar skin is characteristically dimpled or puckered at the proximal palmar crease. Dorsally, a defect can be palpated proximal to the phalanx. In an incomplete subluxation there is no lateral deviation of the finger, because the proximal phalanx, which may be hyperextended up to 90 degrees, lies directly dorsal to the metacarpal head.[72] Roentgenograms show widening of the joint space on the anteroposterior view and an obvious dislocation on the lateral view. Because the sesamoid bones of the fingers are embedded within the volar plate, their presence within the joint on the lateral roentgenographic view is pathognomonic of a complex dislocation.[138,184] The original surgical approach recommended by Farebeuf was dorsal, and though some contemporary surgeons have advocated this approach,[14] the preferred method is a midaxial incision along the side of the joint (radial for the index finger and ulnar for the little finger), which is then curved into the palmar crease. Meticulous care must be taken with the skin incision because of the risk of severing the neurovascular bundle, which is tented over the metacarpal head. The radial neurovascular bundle is vulnerable for the index finger dislocation, and the ulnar neurovascular bundle is vulnerable for the little finger dislocation. The structure that is most important in preventing relocation is the volar plate, which is interposed between the base of the phalanx and the metacarpal head. The plate must be removed from this position before reduction can be achieved. The first step is to relieve the tension of the overlying flexor tendons, and this is accomplished by releasing the A-1 pulley of the tendon sheath. With the tendons retracted, an attempt is made to extricate the plate with the aid of a probe. This is possible if, at the time of the dislocation, the plate tears not only from its proximal attachment but also from its lateral connection to the adjacent deep transverse metacarpal ligament. Frequently, the lateral attachment does not tear completely, and the portion that remains intact must be released by an incision along the lateral edge of the plate. The plate can then be restored to its normal position. It is unnecessary to reattach the plate to the periosteum at the neck of the metacarpal. Active exercises must begin on the first postoperative day because of the inverse relationship between the time of postoperative immobilization and the ultimate range of motion for the joint.[125] A dorsal block splint is used to protect against hyper extension for the first 2 weeks. If there is still any concern about redislocation, a dynamic flexion splint is used for an additional week or two. The elastic cord on the splint should be of sufficient tension to prevent hyper extension, but not full extension, during exercises.

Collateral Ligaments

Collateral ligament sprains of the metacarpophalangeal joints are rare for several reasons. The joints are protected by their recessed position in the palm and support is provided by adjacent fingers. In addition, the anatomic configuration of the ligaments permits the fingers to deviate in extension. The mechanism of injury is forced lateral deviation, almost always in an ulnar direction and usually with the joint in some flexion. The degree of joint flexion at the moment of injury is a determining factor in the severity of the sprain. In full extension, normal ligament laxity will more likely dissipate a laterally or ulnarly directed force than if that same force is applied to the joint in full flexion when the ligament is taut.

The diagnosis of collateral ligament sprain is frequently delayed. The patient, though experiencing pain, often does not appreciate the seriousness of the injury if joint motions are not impaired. After weeks and sometimes months of discomfort, the patient will finally seek medical attention. By that time there will be little if any swelling, and the joint will appear deceptively benign. However, careful examination will show tenderness over the injured ligament and, more importantly, instability with stress testing. The evaluation is carried out by passive motion of the joint radially and ulnarly, in full extension as well as full flexion. Though there will be normal laxity in full extension, there should be none in full flexion. Slight or gross instability in the flexed position demonstrates a second- or third-degree sprain (Fig. 26-13). In some third-degree sprains, the diagnosis will be obvious by simple observation of the deviated position of the finger (Fig. 26-14). Arthrography is also a useful diagnostic technique.[86]

Ligament injuries of these joints have received scant attention in the literature and, though they have been reported to occur most frequently in the ring and little fingers, they may occur in any finger.[44,86] Surgery is usually necessary when there is gross instability. If possible, the torn collateral ligament is reinserted into the bone from which it avulsed, which may be either the phalanx or metacarpal (Figs. 26-15 and 26-16). In some situations, particularly chronic cases, it may be necessary to reconstruct a new ligament using a tendon graft (i.e., palmaris longus). Care must be taken to reestablish the normal configuration of the ligament. Reconstruction so that the ligament is taut in full extension must be avoided, because this will result in an extension contracture of the joint. Though this might not pose a problem to the athlete whose fingers are often in an extended position (e.g., the basketball player or football pass receiver), it would be disabling to the athlete whose sport requires grasping with the clenched fist. It is preferable to reconstruct the ligament in

Text continued on p. 526.

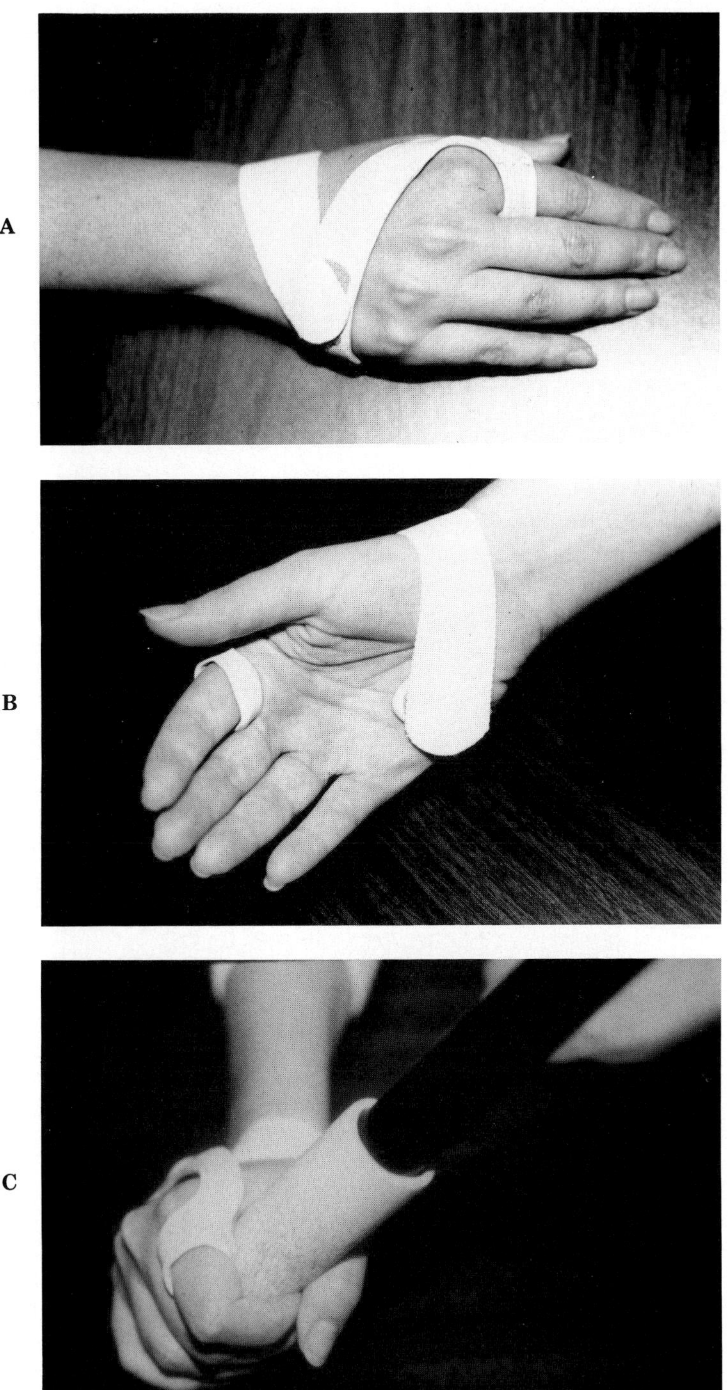

FIG. 26-13. A, A second-degree injury to the radial collateral ligament of the metacarpophalangeal joint of the finger treated with a protective splint. **B** and **C,** The splint prevents ulnar deviation of the index finger and can be worn under a mitten, permitting the patient to resume skiing.

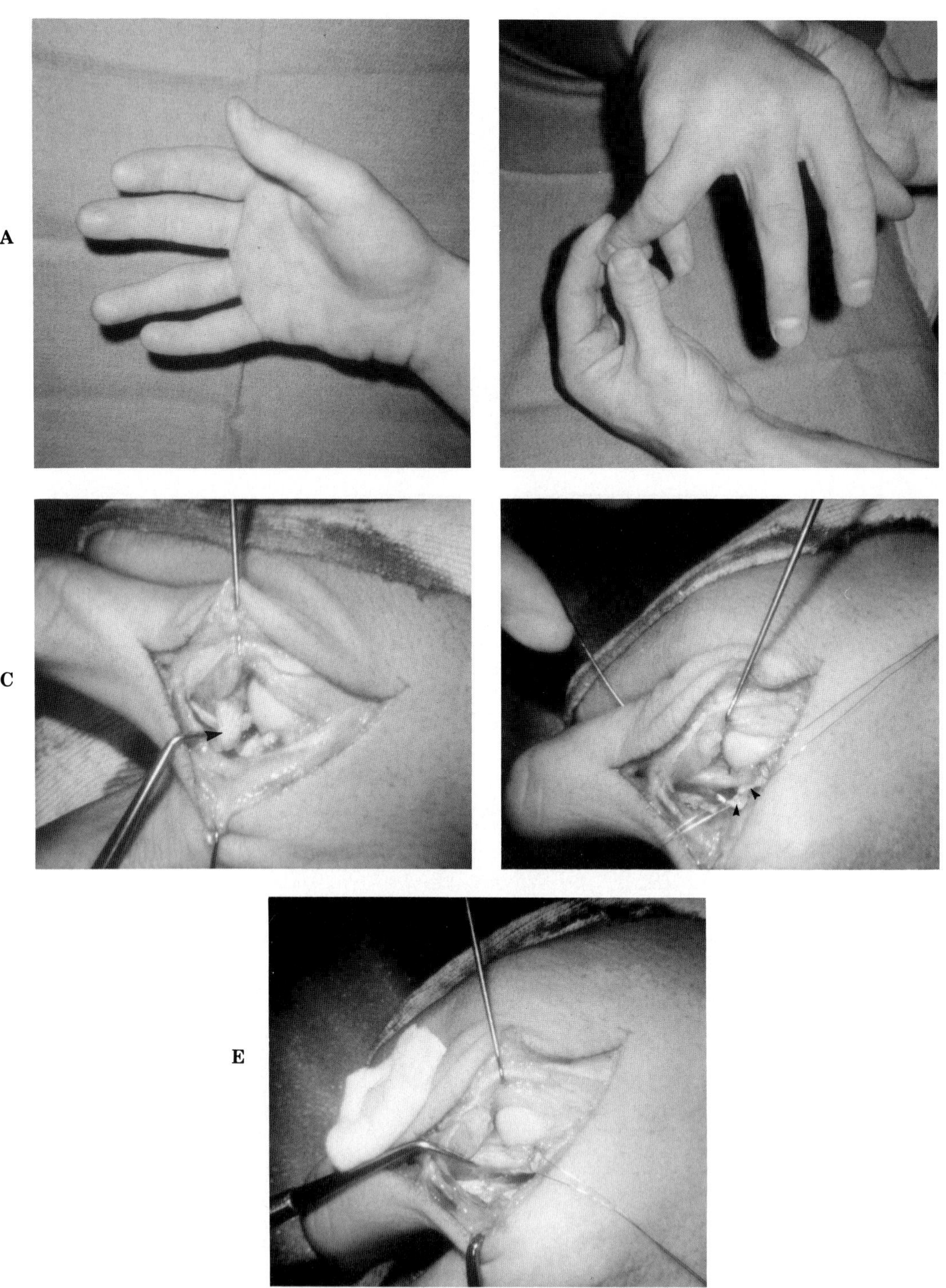

FIG. 26-14. A and **B,** A 28-year-old professional basketball player ruptured the radial collateral ligament to the metacarpophalangeal joint of his right ring finger. At rest, the finger deviated toward the little finger. Stress testing with the joint flexed showed marked instability. **C** to **E,** At surgery, the volar two thirds of the ligament *(large arrow)* ruptured proximally and was reattached to the metacarpal. The dorsal one third of the ligament *(small arrow)* was reattached using a pull-out wire suture into a slot made in the proximal phalanx. Padding was placed beneath the button to avoid skin ulcer.

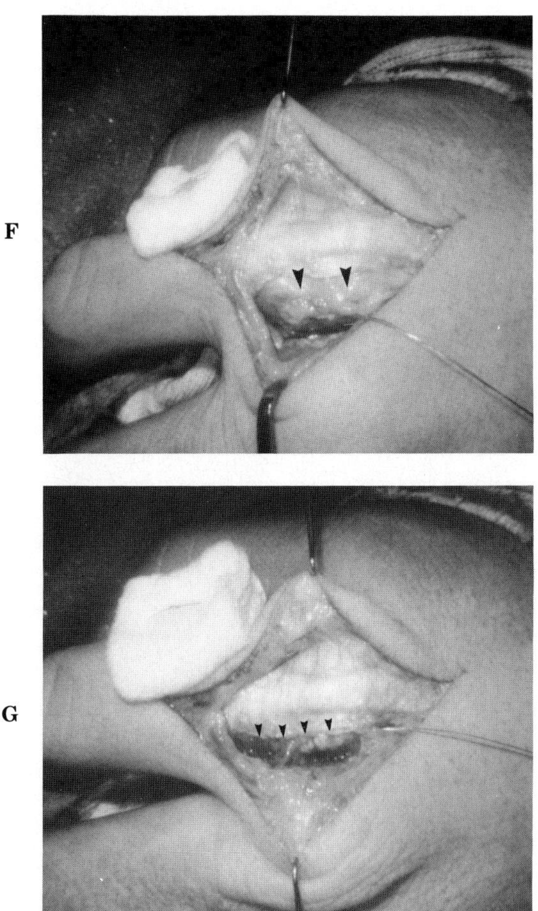

FIG. 26-14, cont'd. F and **G,** The dorsal capsule *(arrow)* was then sutured to the repaired ligament. This was followed by closure of the dorsal hood.

Continued.

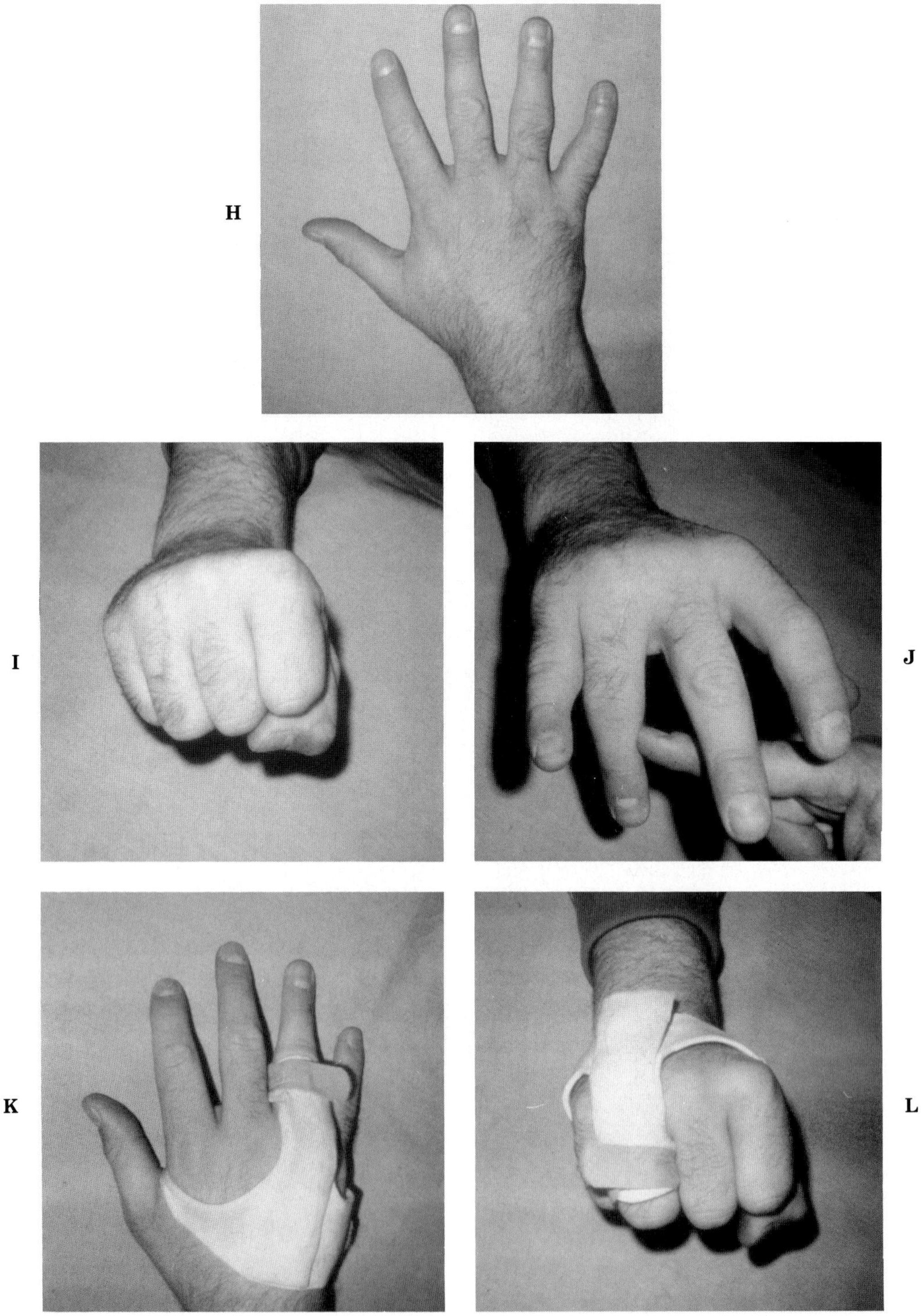

H

I

J

K

L

FIG. 26-14, cont'd. H to **L,** The patient regained complete mobility and stability of his finger. He was allowed to play basketball within 1 month of his surgery wearing a small splint that blocked full extension as well as lateral deviation of the finger.

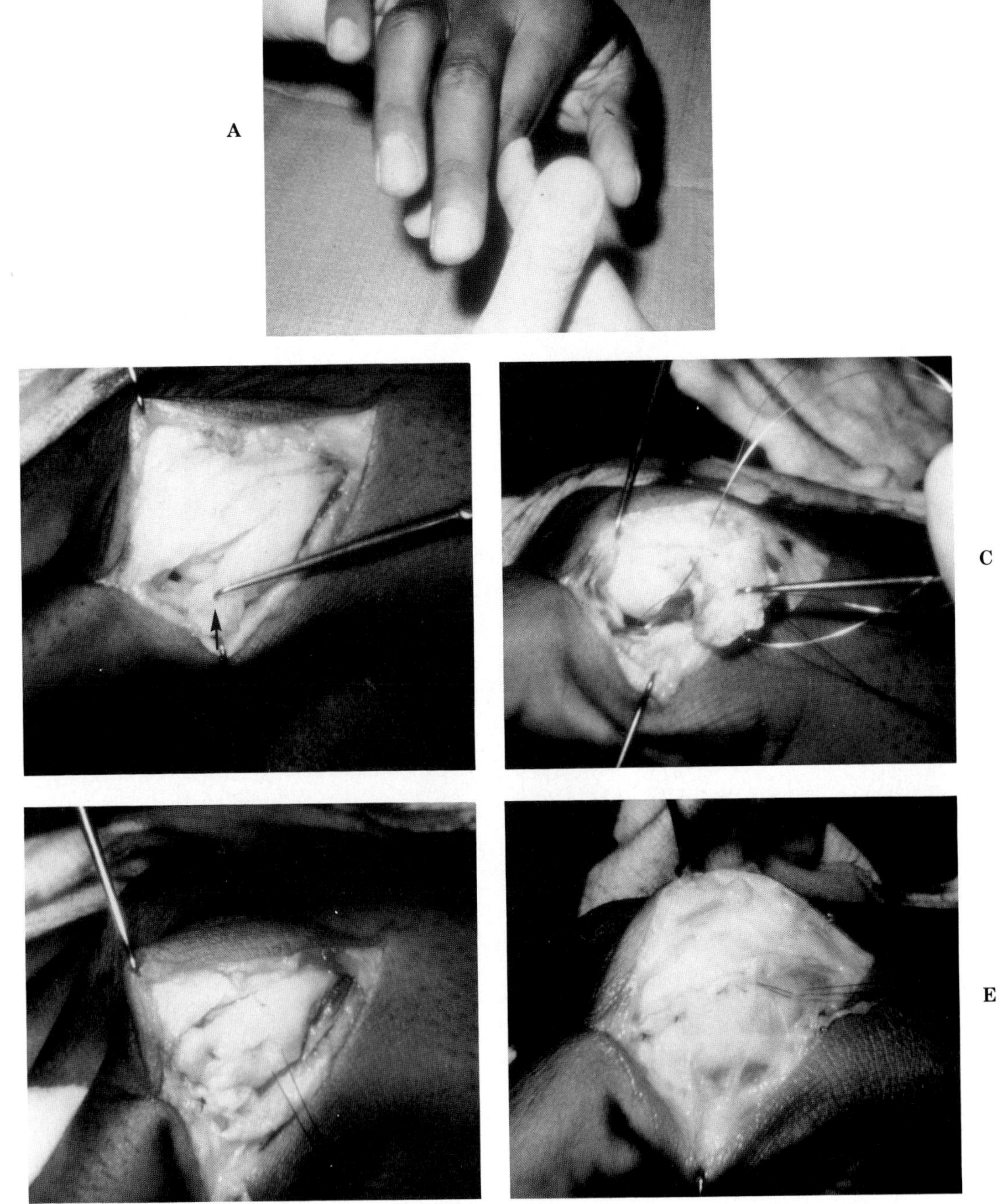

FIG. 26-15. A, Chronic instability of the metacarpophalangeal joint of the index finger in a 28-year-old professional football player. **B, C,** and **D,** The ligament *(arrow)* had ruptured from the proximal phalanx and was reinserted into the bone using a pull-out wire suture. **E,** The dorsal hood was then repaired. *Continued.*

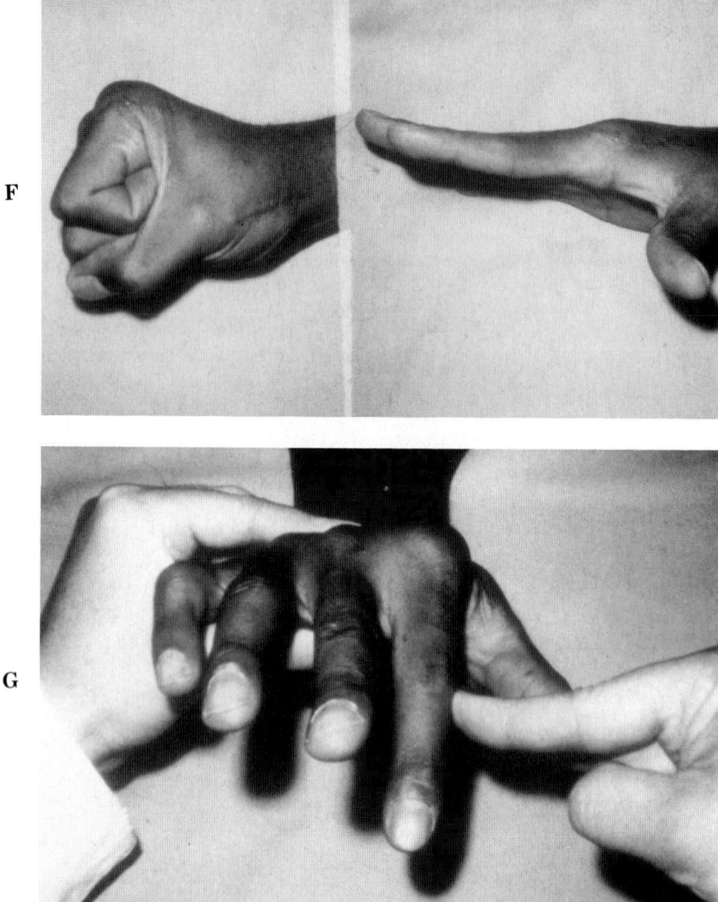

FIG. 26-15, cont'd. F and **G,** Because this patient was a pass receiver, care was taken to avoid producing a flexion contracture, because extension of the joint was more important than flexion. He regained excellent mobility as well as stability of the finger.

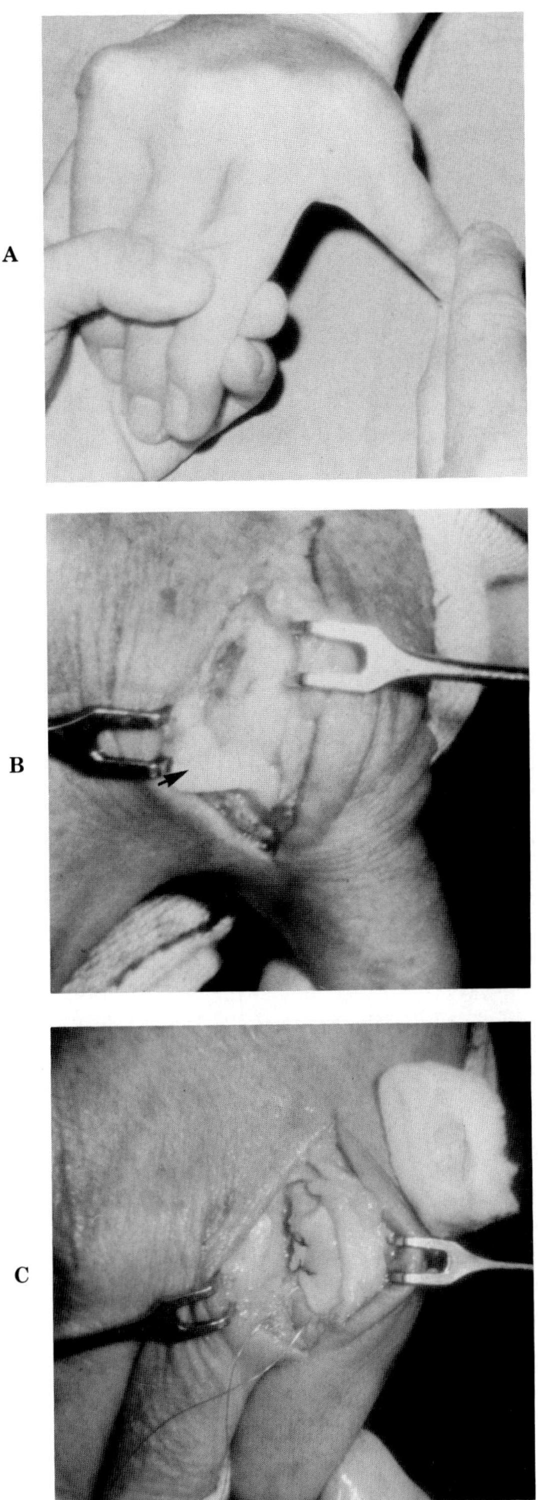

FIG. 26-16. A, Chronic instability of the metacarpophalangeal joint of the little finger caused by a rupture of the radial collateral ligament. **B** and **C,** At surgery, the ligament had ruptured proximally and was reinserted into the metacarpal using a pull-out wire suture. The dorsal capsule *(large arrow)* was then repaired and the dorsal hood closed *(small arrows)*.

Continued.

D

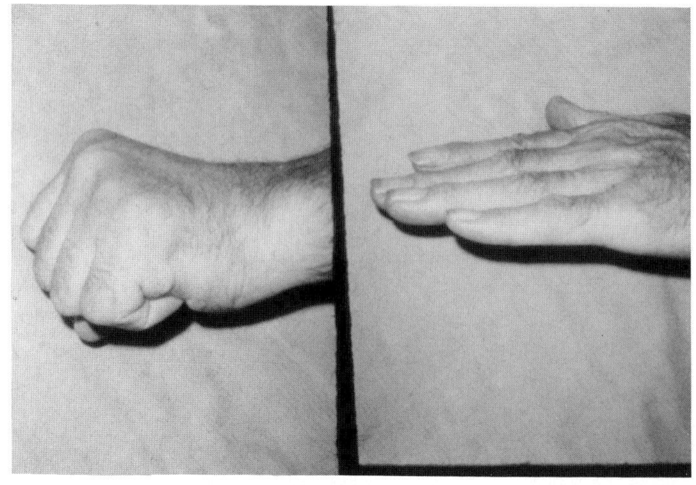

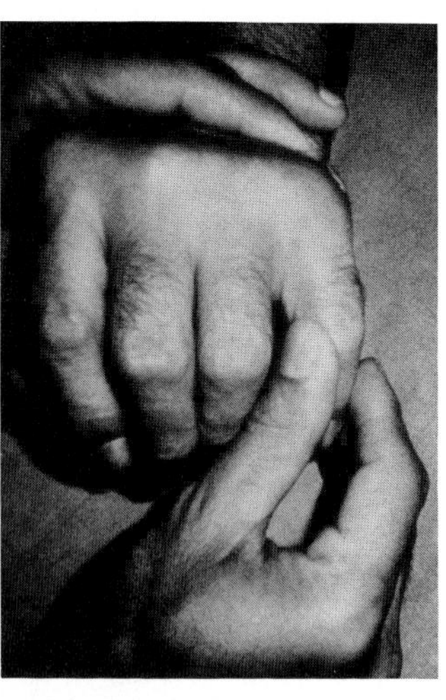

E

FIG. 26-16, cont'd. D to **E** Postoperatively, the patient regained complete mobility and stability.

such a way that it is taut with the joint in about 60 degrees of flexion.

Dorsal Capsule

Direct trauma to the dorsal aspect of a knuckle is common and usually causes a contusion, which heals within a week or two. With greater trauma, there is a tear in the dorsal hood involving either the radial or ulnar sagittal fibers. If the radial sagittal fibers are torn, the extensor tendon would be displaced in an ulnar direction. This would resemble the tendon subluxation that occurs with forced ulnar deviation of a finger, as previously discussed. An even more severe blow to the knuckle or repetitive blows occuring during one episode or over a long period can damage the underlying dorsal joint capsule and actually cause it to rupture. These injuries can occur in any sport in which the knuckles are subjected to local direct trauma, such as amateur and professional boxing and karate.[153]

It is important to differentiate a capsular tear from the less severe injury to the sagittal fibers of the underlying dorsal hood. Though an injury to the dorsal hood may respond to nonoperative treatment, particularly if there is only slight displacement of the tendon, a dorsal capsular tear usually requires surgery (Fig. 26-17). The position of the extensor tendon may aid in the differential diagnosis. In some situations when the capsule is torn on its ulnar aspect, the tendon is deviated radially. This would be exceedingly rare if the injury was confined to the hood. The most important clinical finding is a palpable defect over the joint, which represents the site of the tear. This is a consistent finding even when the tear is in the midline and the tendon is not subluxed. In these situations, the tendon can be shifted to one side, usually the radial, to allow palpation of the defect (Fig. 26-18). At surgery, there is scarring either over the tendon itself, or more commonly in the radial or ulnar sagittal fibers. An incision is made in the scarred area of the hood, which is then retracted to permit inspection of the underlying capsule. Though the torn edges of the capsule may be retracted and adherent to the hood, they can be mobilized by sharp dissection and brought together for repair. Contractures of the torn capsule have not been ob-

FIG. 26-17 A, A 21-year-old Olympic gold medal winner in boxing complained of chronic pain over the metacarpophalangeal joint of his middle finger. The extensor tendon *(arrow)* was displaced ulnarly, and there was a palpable defect directly over the head of the underlying metacarpal. **B,** At surgery, a curved incision was made over the joint, and when skin flaps were mobilized the metacarpal head was clearly visible *(probe)*. **C,** The tear in the hood was incised further proximally and distally to visualize the joint capsule, which was torn *(small arrows)* over a distance of more than 2.0 cm. **D,** The capsule, which was adherent to the underlying dorsal hood, was mobilized and then repaired with fine 4-0 nylon sutures. **E,** The dorsal hood was then repaired. **F,** The patient regained full digital flexion and continued with his successful professional career, becoming world champion.

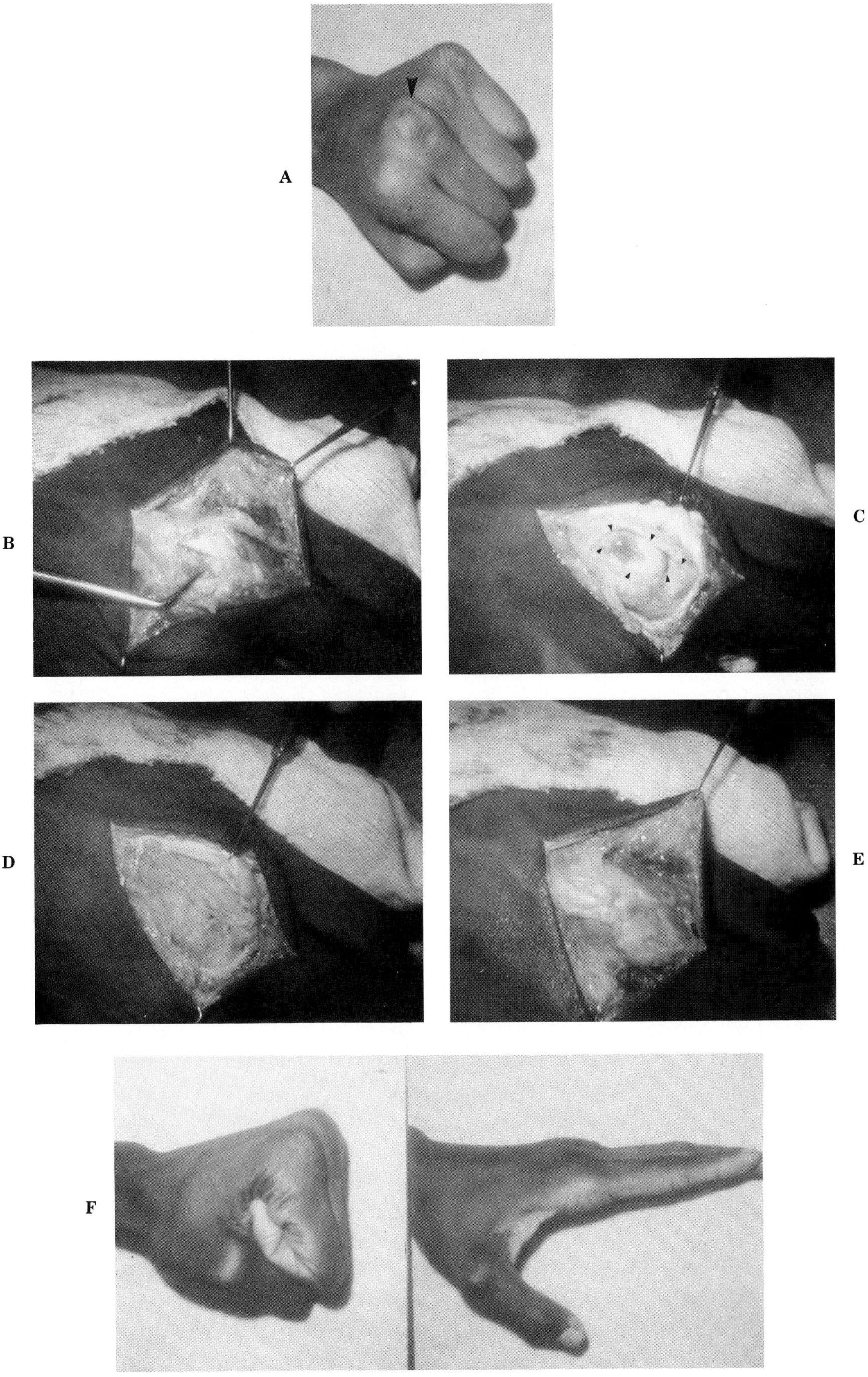

A

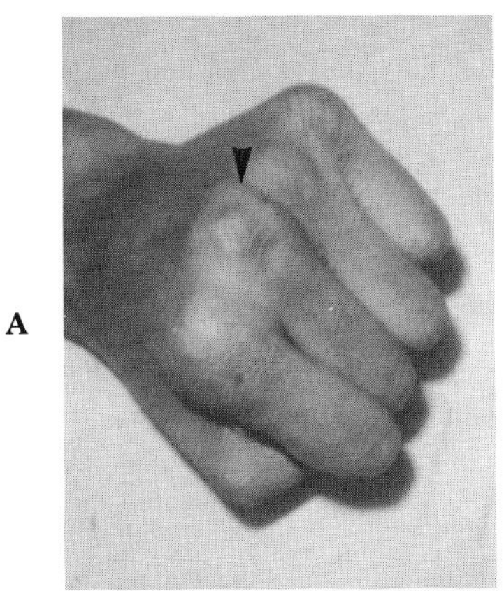

B

C

D

E

F

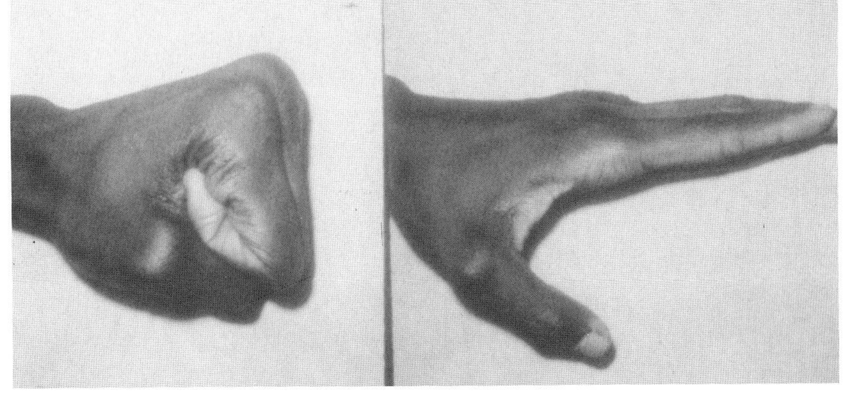

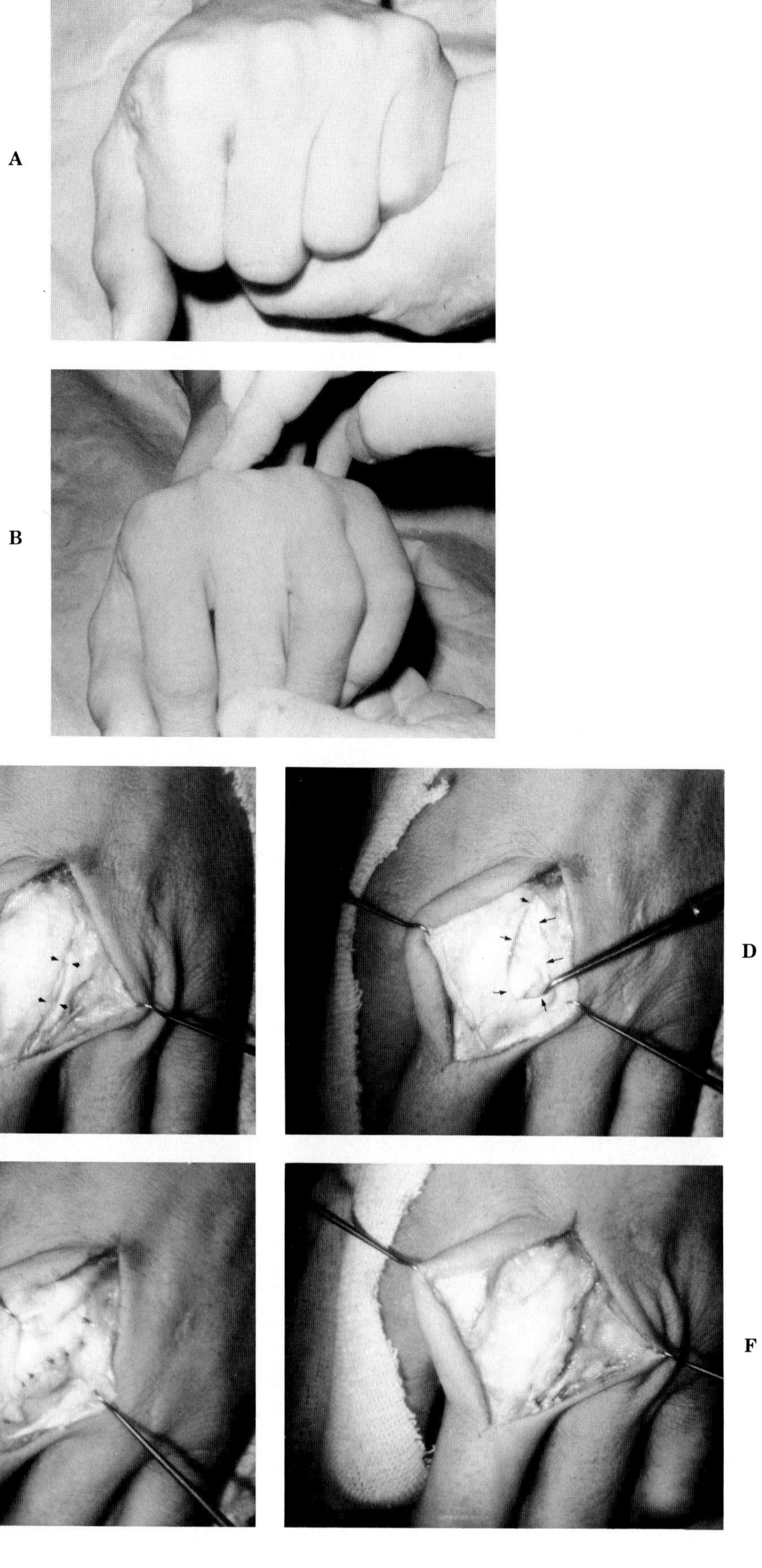
A
B
C
D
E
F

FIG. 26-18. **A** and **B,** A 22-year-old professional boxer complained of pain of more than 1 year's duration over the metacarpophalangeal joint of his middle finger. Following each bout, he reported pain and swelling that took weeks to subside. Though the extensor tendon was in its normal midline position at rest, it was easily shifted radially, and a defect was palpable in the underlying capsule. **C,** At surgery, an incision *(arrows)* was made to the radial side of the extensor tendon through a scarred, but intact, dorsal hood. **D,** With the hood retracted, there was a large defect *(arrows)* in the capsule. **E** and **F,** The capsule was repaired and the dorsal hood closed.

served, probably because the tears are always in a longitudinal or slightly oblique direction. Any ragged edges of the capsule are sharply excised; however, before this is done care must be taken to ensure that the capsule can be repaired and still permit full joint flexion. Following capsular repair with fine nonabsorbable sutures, the incision in the sagittal fibers is closed, and, if necessary, the extensor tendon is relocated into its normal midline position. Postoperatively, the joint is immobilized in acute flexion. This position is particularly important for boxers, though a residual flexion contracture would not pose any functional impairment in making a fist, a mild extension contracture might end the athlete's career. Active exercises are started 3 weeks after surgery, and punching is avoided for at least 6 months. In athletes for whom clenching a fist is not as important, the joint is immobilized in less flexion postoperatively.

Fractures

Fractures of the distal portion of a metacarpal are more likely to involve the neck of the bone than its intraarticular head. A fracture of the metacarpal neck usually results from a direct blow with the clenched fist. Typically the fracture is angled dorsally because of the direction of the impact and the deforming force of the interossei muscles. The angulation can result in several problems: the head, which is tilted volarly, can cause a painful prominence in the palm that interferes with grasp; there may be a tendon imbalance similar but less severe, to that which occurs with angulated fractures in the midshaft of the bone; and finally, extension at the metacarpophalangeal joint is restricted equivalent to the degree of tilt.[185] The latter problem is usually of little functional significance, because the normal hyperextension of the metacarpophalangeal joints that exists in many patients negates any loss of extension. As with the indications for treatment of angulated shaft fractures, various figures have been proposed as being an acceptable deformity for a particular metacarpal neck fracture. Greater angulation can generally be tolerated for the fourth and especially the fifth metacarpal because of the mobility of their carpometacarpal joints, which diminishes the effect of the palmar protrusion of the heads of the bones during grasp. The acceptable degree of angulation depends not simply on a numeric value but on the specific functional requirements of each patient. Though slight angulation in a fourth or fifth metacarpal neck fracture may not be annoying to a basketball or football player, it may compromise the effectiveness of a baseball pitcher and have dire consequences for a boxer.

Problems stemming from residual angulation of metacarpal neck fractures

- Metacarpal head in palm—painful and interferes with grip
- Tendon imbalance
- Loss of metacarpophalangeal extension

Frequently, metacarpal neck fractures can be treated by closed reduction and external immobilization. The metacarpophalangeal joint of the injured finger is flexed completely, which relaxes the deforming force of the intrinsic muscles. This maneuver also tightens the collateral ligaments, which stabilizes the fractured metacarpal head. Upward pressure on the proximal phalanx levers the head back into alignment. First recommended by Jahss,[87] this is an effective technique for reducing a fracture; however, it should never be used as a method for immobilization, because it will result in proximal interphalangeal joint stiffness or even pressure necrosis over the extensor mechanism at that joint. If closed reduction is not successful or if the reduction is unstable, surgery is necessary. Kirschner pin fixation of the fracture is an effective method, either alone or in combination with a dorsal tension band wire.

Though intraarticular fractures are less

common than metacarpal neck fractures, they are potentially more serious and often lead to joint stiffness. These fractures are most commonly seen in athletic injuries and can be classified depending on anatomic involvement. This classification includes small osteochrondral fragments; intraarticular fractures that are oblique (sagittal), vertical (coronal), or horizontal (transverse); comminuted fractures, or those associated with ligament avulsions.[124] Avulsion fractures may be small, and special roentgenographic views may aid in their visualization, including the Brewerton view.[106] This view, which was originally designed to demonstrate early erosive changes in the metacarpal heads in patients with rheumatoid arthritis, is taken with the dorsal aspects of the fingers on the roentgenographic cassette, the metacarpophalangeal joints flexed 65 degrees, and the roentgen beam angled from a position 15 degrees to the ulnar side of the hand.[24] Treatment for intraarticular fractures frequently requires surgery to restore articular congruity. The use of Kirschner pins is an effective method of fixation. Postoperatively, the joint is immobilized in flexion, and active range of motion exercises are started within a week or two to minimize joint stiffness. In severely comminuted fractures of the metacarpal head, skeletal traction through the proximal phalanx may be required to maintain the length of the bone.

Intraarticular fracture patterns

- Osteochondral fragments
- Oblique (sagittal)
- Vertical (coronal)
- Horizontal (transverse)
- Associated with ligament avulsions

PROXIMAL PHALANGEAL AREA

Anatomy

In contradistinction to the metacarpal area of the palm, the phalangeal areas in the fingers are not protected by overlying muscles and are in closer contact with the tendons. At the proximal phalangeal level, the bone is virtually encircled by the flexor tendons on their volar aspect and the extensor tendon mechanism laterally and dorsally. A cross-section through this level demonstrates the intimate association between bone and tendon and the limited area through which the tendons glide. Any disturbance in these gliding pathways will cause tendon adherence and subsequent loss of mobility. The area is therefore vulnerable to the pernicious effects of edema.

Tendon Injuries

Aside from lacerations, tendon problems in this area are usually caused by closed trauma. The normally restricted area in which the tendons glide can easily become more limited by adhesions, which may develop with or without a concomitant fracture. The problems are magnified with a fracture because of the likelihood for greater scarring and the fact that even slight bony displacement may further interfere with the gliding pathways of the tendons. Adhesions may involve the extrinsic or intrinsic components of the dorsal tendon mechanism, or they may affect the flexor tendons on the volar aspect of the digit.

Scarring of an extrinsic extensor tendon is most likely to occur as the tendon passes under the retinaculum at the wrist level or over the dorsal aspect of the hand, where it may become adherent to a metacarpal. At these locations, the limited excursion of the tendon prevents simultaneous flexion of the metacarpophalangeal and proximal interphalangeal joints of a finger. The dorsal tenodesis prevents flexion of the proximal interphalangeal joint when the metacarpophalangeal joint is actively or passively flexed. When the proximal interphalangeal joint flexes, the reverse situation occurs, and the metacarpophalangeal joint goes into extension or even hyperextension. Clinically, the patient is able to actively flex the proximal interphalangeal joint if the metacarpophalangeal joint is extended and vice versa. Simultaneous flexion of both joints is impossible. When the extrinsic extensor becomes adherent over the proximal phalanx, the tenodesis affects flexion at only one joint, the proximal interphalangeal joint. Scarring of the dorsal tendon mechanism may also involve or be limited to its intrinsic components, the lateral bands. Clinically, the test for intrinsic tightness will be positive. As discussed in the section on intrinsic contractures at the metacarpal level, testing for tight intrinsics is a passive examination, and it is important that the patient not try to assist the examiner by actively flexing the finger. Active flexion of the finger may mask a mild degree of intrinsic tightness, and the problem may go unrecognized. On the volar surface of the proximal phalanx, adhesions are more likely to involve the flexor superficialis tendon, where the broad area of Camper's chiasma is in closer contact with the bone than is the flexor profundus tendon. Clinically, extension of the proximal interphalangeal joint will be limited because of the tethering effect of the adhesions between tendon and bone. If the profundus tendon is spared, motions at the distal interphalangeal joint will not be affected.

Treatment for adhesions of the flexor and extensor tendons should therefore be preventative, and early range of motion exercises should be encouraged after any injury. As adhesions become more mature, the use of dynamic splints may be effective. For chronic cases in which adhesions are permanent and refractory to therapy, surgical tendolyses are required. With respect to the dorsal tendon mechanism, adhesions involving the extrinsic tendon component can be released. The patient can then be started on an early program of active and passive exercises. With involvement of one or both lateral bands of the intrinsic component of this mechanism, the band(s) together with its oblique fibers are excised, but the transverse fibers are preserved.

When surgery is required for adhesions involving the flexor system, tendolysis of the flexor superficialis tendon may not be adequate, because the tendon may be too badly damaged to permit its salvage. Excision of the tendon may be warranted in such cases. As with extensor tendon releases, early active range of motion exercises are started immediately after surgery. Flexion exercises against resistance or the use of a forceful dynamic extension splint should be avoided for several weeks if the vinculum longus to the profundus had to be sacrificed during tendolysis or excision of the flexor superficialis because circulation to the profundus would be compromised in such cases and there would be a danger of it rupturing.

Fractures

The treatment of fractures in this area is difficult because of the necessity of restoring alignment and maintaining stability of the bone to facilitate early exercises (Fig. 26-19). Various classifications can be used for proximal phalangeal fractures, including the anatomic region of the bone that is damaged or whether or not the fracture is intraarticular. Regardless of fracture location, it may involve the articular area at either end of the bone. This discussion will group fractures according to location: base, shaft, and neck/head regions.

Base Fractures

Fractures of the base are frequently angulated volarly because of the pull of the intrinsic muscles. The degree of angulation is difficult to visualize by lateral roentgenogram

A

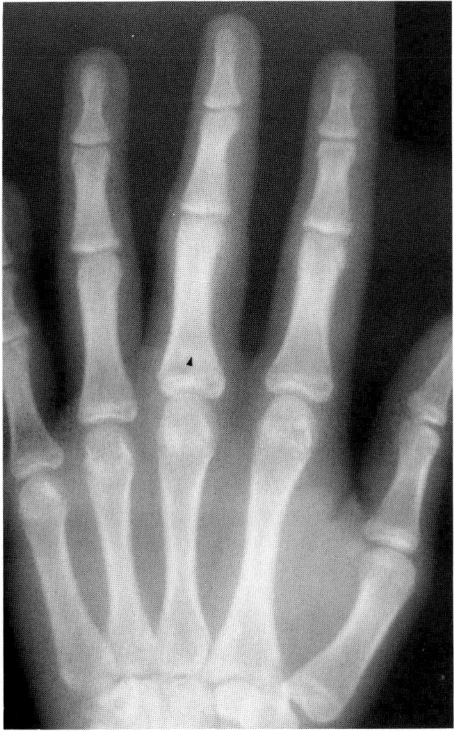

B

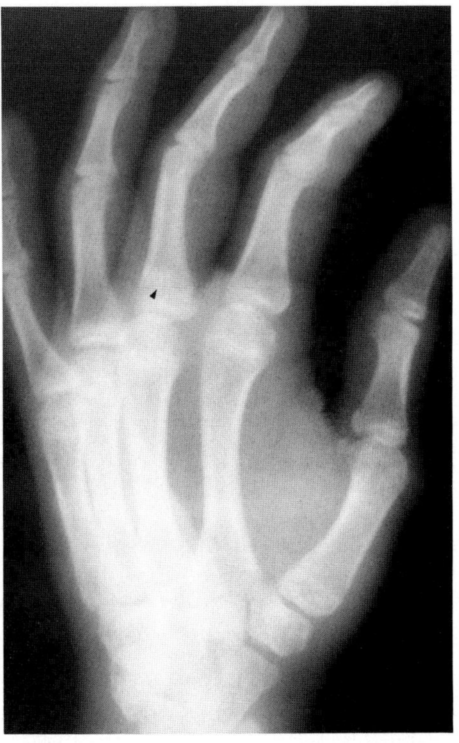

FIG. 26-19 A and **B,** A careful clinical examination of an injured digit is the essential first step in the treatment of any fracture. The oblique fracture at the base of the proximal phalanx of the middle finger appears nondisplaced in these anteroposterior and oblique roentgenograms.

Continued.

C 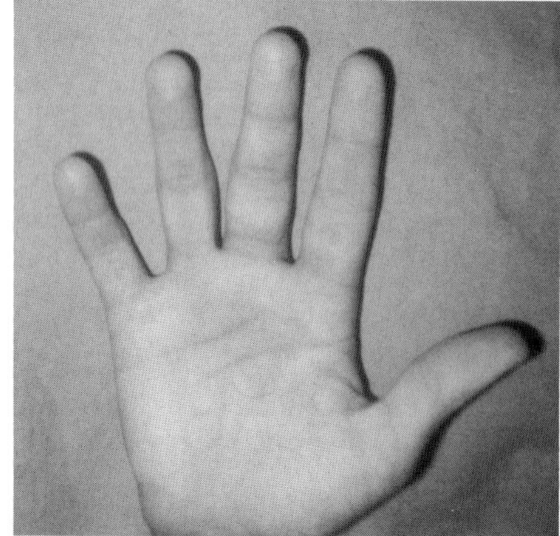

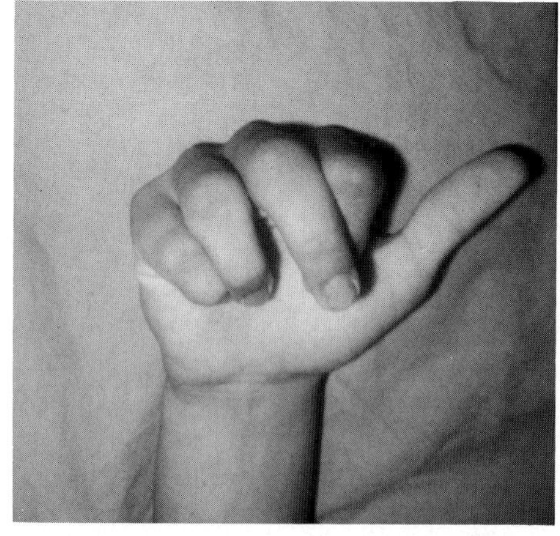 D

FIG. 26-19, cont'd. C and **D,** Clinical examination showed an obvious rotational deformity of the digit, which was corrected by nonoperative measures.

because the proximal phalanges of the uninjured fingers are superimposed on the film. An oblique roentgenogram is helpful, but it also fails to show the true severity of the angulation. Unfortunately, many of these fractures heal in a malunited position, which seriously compromises prehension.[36] Active extension at the proximal interphalangeal joint is diminished because the dorsal tendon mechanism is relaxed, and active flexion may also be affected by the increase in excursion that is required of the flexor tendons as they pass around the volar convexity at the fracture site. Flexion may also become limited at the metacarpophalangeal joint as contractures develop in the collateral ligaments, which are lax due to the angulated portions of the proximal fracture fragment.

Volar angulation of the fracture is often noticed by a depression on the dorsal aspect of the bone, which can be palpated as the examiner's finger moves across the metacarpophalangeal joint and along the dorsal aspect of the phalanx. Reduction of the fracture is achieved by acutely flexing the metacarpophalangeal joint, which relaxes the intrinsics and stabilizes the proximal fragment by tightening the collateral ligaments. The proximal interphalangeal joint is then placed in complete extension to relax the central extensor tendon, thereby further neutralizing any muscle imbalance.[185] The distal fracture fragment is then flexed, correcting the angulation. The digit is immobilized, maintaining the metacarpophalangeal joint in acute flexion and the proximal interphalangeal joint in slight flexion, not exceeding 30 degrees. This position of immobilization is the "safe position," because it reduces the likelihood of contractures at both joint levels. This position should be differentiated from the "position of function," in which the metacarpophalangeal joints are in only slight flexion and the interphalangeal joints in greater flexion. The "position of function" would be appropriate for fusions of these joints, but not suitable for preventing contractures. If the fracture cannot be reduced and stabilized in almost an anatomic position, internal fixation is necessary. Though percutaneous pinning across the flexed interphalangeal joint and down the medullary cavity of the phalanx has been recommended,[9] the technique has the potential of causing scarring in the extensor tendon and/or dorsal hood. Inserting the pins to either side of the central tendon and only into the proximal phalanx is less likely to cause later problems. If percutaneous pinning does not achieve the desired result, the fracture should be opened and pins inserted.

Salter-Harris type II epiphyseal fractures are common injuries in children and usually involve the little finger. If there is lateral deviation at the fracture, reduction is accomplished in the same manner as in adults. A pencil is placed in the web space, which provides leverage for manipulation of the fracture. Rarely is open reduction required. If it is, the use of a single, thin, nonthreaded pin drilled across the epiphyseal plate and removed within 3 weeks is unlikely to cause any growth damage.

With respect to intraarticular fractures at the base of the phalanx, the same method of reduction applies as for nonarticular fractures. However, the likelihood for surgery to restore articular congruity is greater, particularly if the fragment is sizable and associated with joint instability[139] (Fig. 26-20). Intraarticular fractures are also seen in children (Salter-Harris type III) and occur more commonly than those at the base of the middle

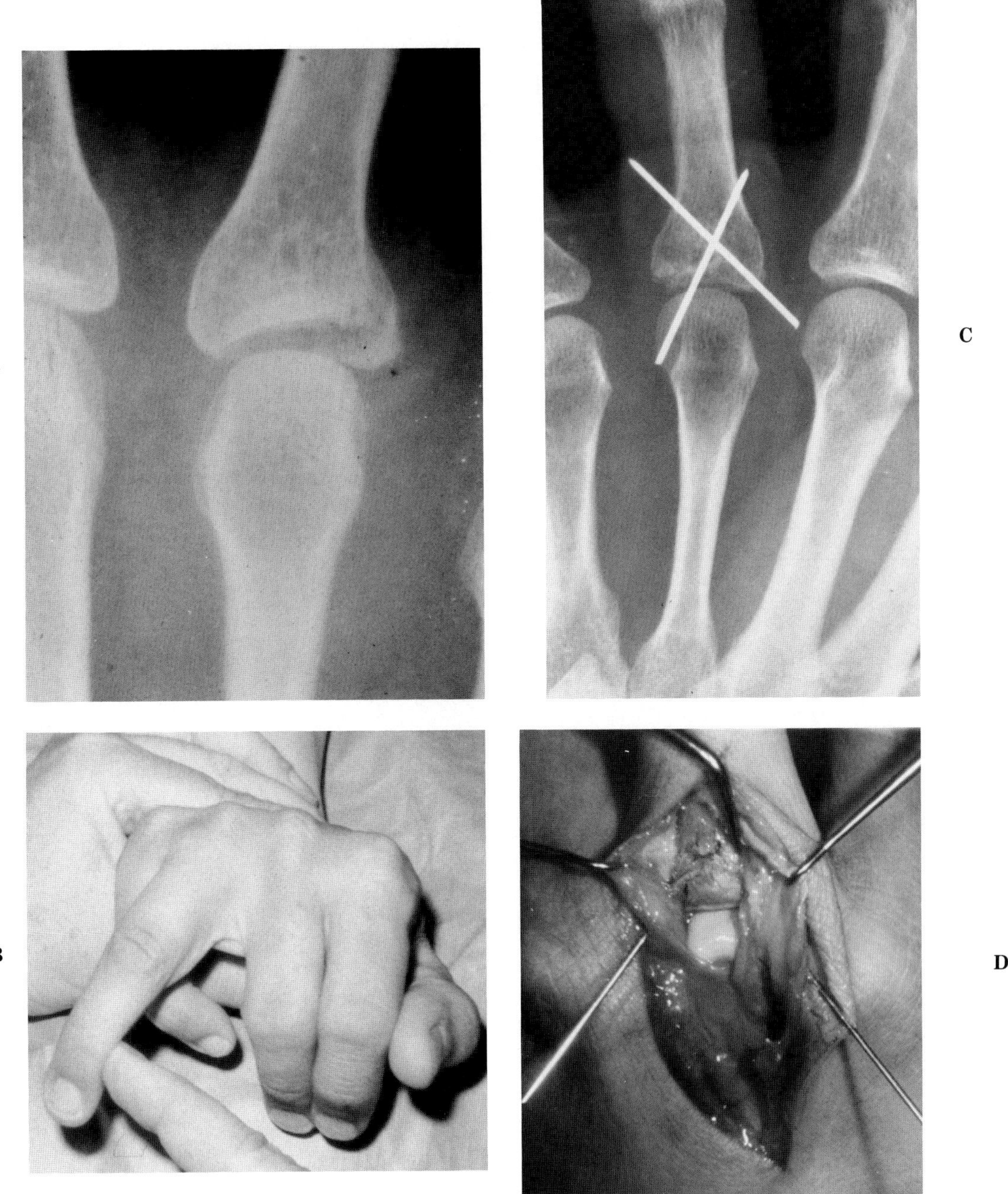

FIG. 26-20. **A** and **B,** This intraarticular fracture of the base of the proximal phalanx resembled a collateral ligament injury with apparent instability of the metacarpophalangeal joint. **C** and **D,** An open reduction and internal fixation of the fracture was necessary. The Kirschner pins were inserted into the sides of the phalanx, avoiding any further damage to the joint.

phalanx as a result of differences in the insertions of the collateral ligaments at these two joint levels. The collateral ligaments for the proximal phalanx insert exclusively into the epiphysis, whereas the insertion of the ligaments at the middle phalanx extend further distally[13] (Fig. 26-21). If surgery is required, it is best carried out through a curved incision to one side of the metacarpophalangeal joint. The transverse and sagittal fibers are incised and the extensor tendon retracted. The underlying capsule is then opened to allow visualization of the fracture site. The bone fragment with its attached collateral ligament is then stabilized using a pin, wire suture, or small screw. The straight dorsal incision,

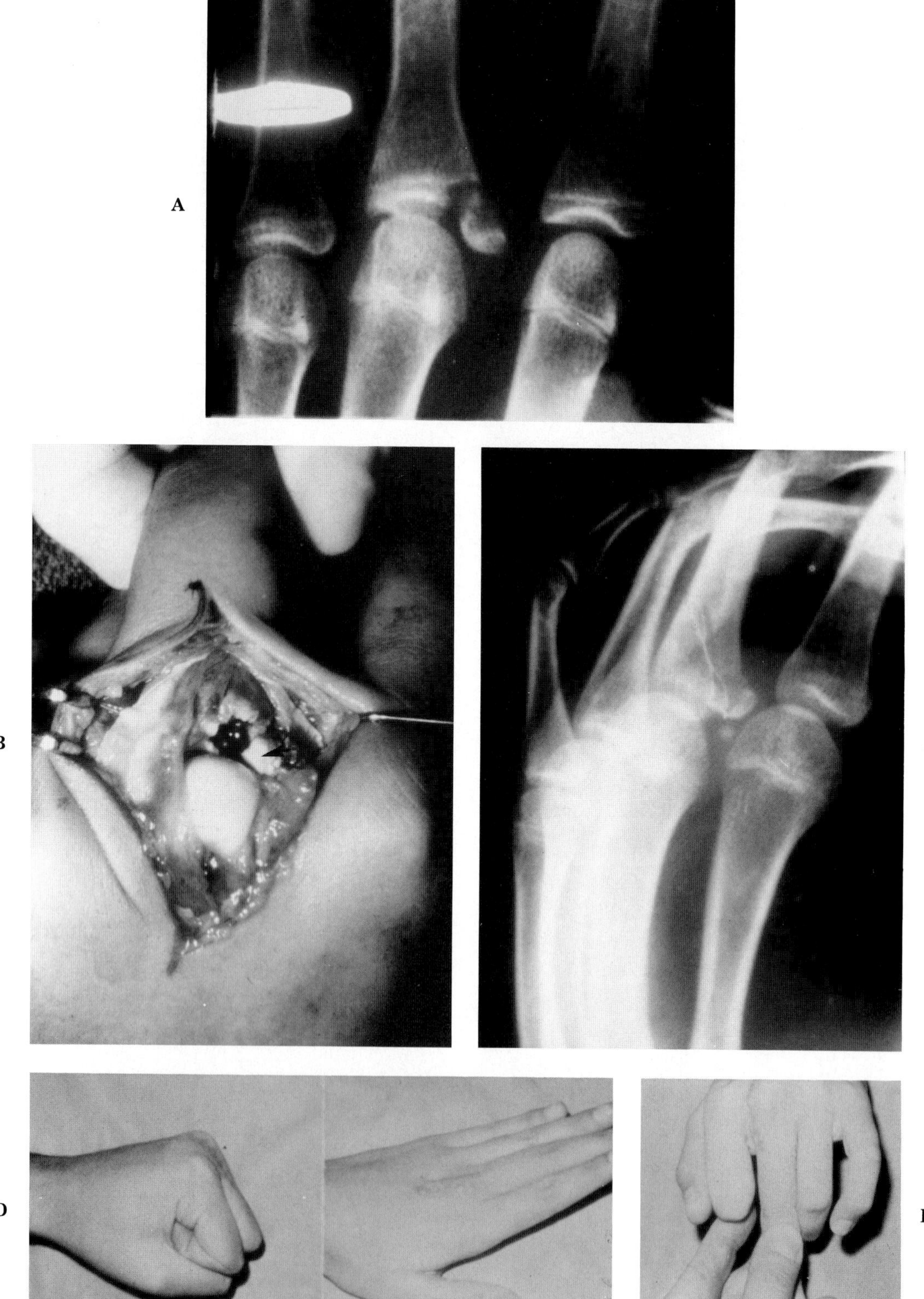

FIG. 26-21. A, An intraarticular fracture sustained in a 16-year-old gymnast. The bone fragment from the epiphysis was displaced and rotated. **B** and **C,** At surgery, the collateral ligament, as anticipated, was attached to the bone fragment *(arrow)*, which was reattached into the phalanx with a wire suture. **D** and **E,** The gymnast regained complete mobility and stability of the finger.

which splits the extensor tendon, should be reserved for operative reduction of displaced T-shaped fractures which cannot be adequately visualized by either a radial or ulnar approach.[55,156] This tendon-splitting incision, though it provides excellent visualization of the entire dorsal and lateral aspects of the phalanx, tends to cause greater scarring and adherence of the extensor mechanism, thereby limiting restoration of mobility. Meticulous closure of the periosteum and tendon as separate layers will reduce but not eliminate the risk of later adhesions.

Shaft Fractures

Shaft fractures may be transverse, oblique, spiral, or comminuted[7]. The spiral type may actually be intraarticular, extending into the proximal interphalangeal joint. If unrecognized and allowed to heal in this position, the fracture spike can block joint flexion. As with any fracture, a complete roentgenographic examination including a direct lateral view is mandatory. Proper roentgenograms at the time of the injury will demonstrate any problem and will often make later, more difficult corrective surgery unnecessary (Fig. 26-22).

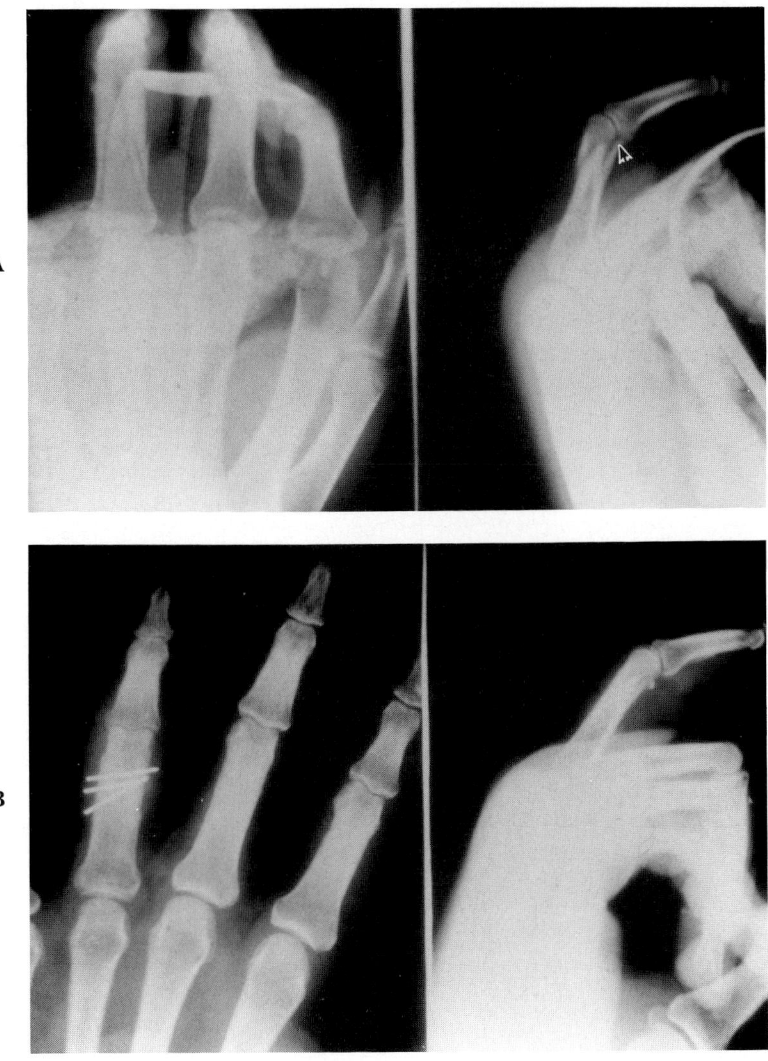

FIG. 26-22. A, A spiral fracture of the proximal phalanx is in good alignment in the posteroanterior roentgenogram. However, the lateral roentgenogram shows displacement with a spike of the proximal fragment *(arrow)* abutting against the base of the middle phalanx. **B,** An anatomic reduction was obtained after surgery, and rigid internal fixation with Kirschner pins permitted early active range of motion exercises.

Most shaft fractures are nondisplaced and can be managed by splint immobilization. Early active range of motion exercises within 3 weeks are important if function is to be restored.[27,181] As the healing progresses, the digit must be protected. Though strapping the injured finger to an adjacent finger ("buddy-taping") is a satisfactory method of protection, it is not a successful method for stabilizing a fracture immediately after the acute injury. Return to full activity should not be permitted until there is roentgenographic evidence of complete healing.

If the fracture cannot be reduced, internal fixation is required. Percutaneous pins enjoy considerable popularity, and various clamps that stabilize the fractures as well as facilitate introduction of the pins have been devised.[11,69,139] However, these methods often fail to achieve a complete reduction, and pin placement may interfere with joint motions.[8] If a fracture is in an unsatisfactory position and reduction and internal fixation are required, the reduction should be anatomic and the fixation precise. This is best achieved by surgery in which an incision is made in the midaxial line on either the radial or ulnar side of the bone. The side of the finger on which the midaxial incision is made matters little for a transverse fracture, and only surgical convenience need be considered. For an oblique fracture, however, it is important to make the incision on the side to which the distal fragment has displaced. In this manner, the unstable distal fragment can be accurately reduced and fixed to the stable proximal fragment. Failure to make the incision on the proper side of the finger will seriously interfere with visualizing the fracture site and make it virtually impossible to achieve a rigid and anatomic reduction unless a second midaxial incision is made on the opposite side of the finger. The extensor tendon mechanism is retracted dorsally, and the bone is subperiosteally exposed. If the proximal portion of the bone must be exposed and the lateral band cannot be adequately retracted dorsally, an incision is made through the oblique and transverse fibers, and the lateral band is retracted in the volar direction. After the fracture is stabilized, the lateral band can be resutured using fine monofilament nylon.

Various techniques for fixation can be used depending on the nature of the fracture, as well as the experience of the surgeon. For oblique and spiral fractures, Kirschner pins are effective. If possible, the pins are inserted in a frontal plane between the flexor and extensor tendons so that the pins will not interfere with the gliding of the tendons. Because fractures may take many weeks and sometimes months to unite, there is no urgency to remove the pins. As a general principle, pins that are left in place for an indefinite period are cut off beneath the skin. Pins that will be removed at a specific time (usually within a few weeks) can be left protruding through the skin. Included in the latter category are pins that transfix joints. Oblique and spiral fractures can also be rigidly fixed using small cortical lag screws, if the length of the fracture is at least twice the width of the bone.[80,127,128]

With transverse fractures, a variety of methods have also been employed, including crossed Kirschner pins, intraosseous wiring combined with a single pin, or tension band fixation on the dorsal or tension side of the bone. The use of a plate and screws, though technically feasible, is rarely necessary. The relative bulk of these devices applied to a small bone with limited soft tissue coverage tends to interfere with tendon gliding.

Neck/Head Fractures

Fractures of the distal end of the phalanx involve either the extraarticular neck portion of the bone or the intraarticular condyles. Phalangeal neck fractures are much more common in children than adults. Displacement of the phalangeal head can be severe, often exceeding 90 degrees. In the anteroposterior roentgenograms, the rotated head presents an ovoid appearance similar to a metacarpal head epiphysis.[40] Because there is no epiphysis at this end of the phalanx, this roentgenographic sign should alert the examiner to a serious problem. The lateral roentgenogram will clearly demonstrate that the phalangeal head is not only displaced dorsally, but also rotated so that its articular surface faces dorsally and its fractured side volarly. An attempt should be made to manipulate the displaced head back into position by applying firm digital pressure to the dorsal aspect of the acutely flexed joint.[139] Because there is no appreciable remodeling at this end of the bone, any residual angulation is unacceptable.[8,112] Surgery for this fracture is difficult because of the small size of the phalangeal head fragment and the limited area available for stabilization. The fracture is exposed through a midaxial incision, and, if possible, crossed Kirschner pins are drilled across the fracture site. The first pin is drilled from the head into the proximal shaft. In young children, the phalangeal head is very small and there may be room for only a single pin. If the thinnest-caliber Kirschner pins are still too wide, straight needles can be substituted. It may be necessary to make a second midaxial incision on the opposite side of the finger to insert a pin from that direction. The problem of fixation is not as difficult in adults, in whom the large bone fragments permit other techniques to be used, including intraosseous wiring.[114]

Condylar fractures can be unicondylar or bicondylar. Unicondylar fractures are common in athletic injuries and, unfortunately, delayed treament is common because good joint mobility often remains.[174] Lateral inclination of the finger soon becomes obvious as the joint tilts toward the side of the displaced condyle. Open reduction and internal fixation of the displaced condyle are necessary using either Kirschner pins or a lag screw[38] (Fig. 26-23). The fracture is exposed either by a midaxial incision and dorsal retraction of the lateral band, or by a curved incision and entering into the joint between the central slip and the lateral band. Care is taken not to disturb the insertion of the central slip or damage the collateral ligament, which provides the blood supply to the condylar fragment.[127,128] Bicondylar fractures present even a greater surgical challenge. The two condyles are first stabilized to each other, then fixed to the shaft of the bone. The surgical approach is, by necessity, an extensive one, and a significant permanent loss of mobility should be anticipated with these fractures.

PROXIMAL INTERPHALANGEAL JOINT AREA

Anatomy

In no other area of the hand is the anatomy as complex and interrelated as at the proximal interphalangeal joint. Though each anatomic structure in this area is important to the function of the others, the extensor tendon system and the joint capsule deserve special attention because of the frequency of injuries to both and the deleterious effect these injuries have on function.

The extensor system is actually a fascial-tendon expansion with both extrinsic and intrinsic components. At the proximal interpha-

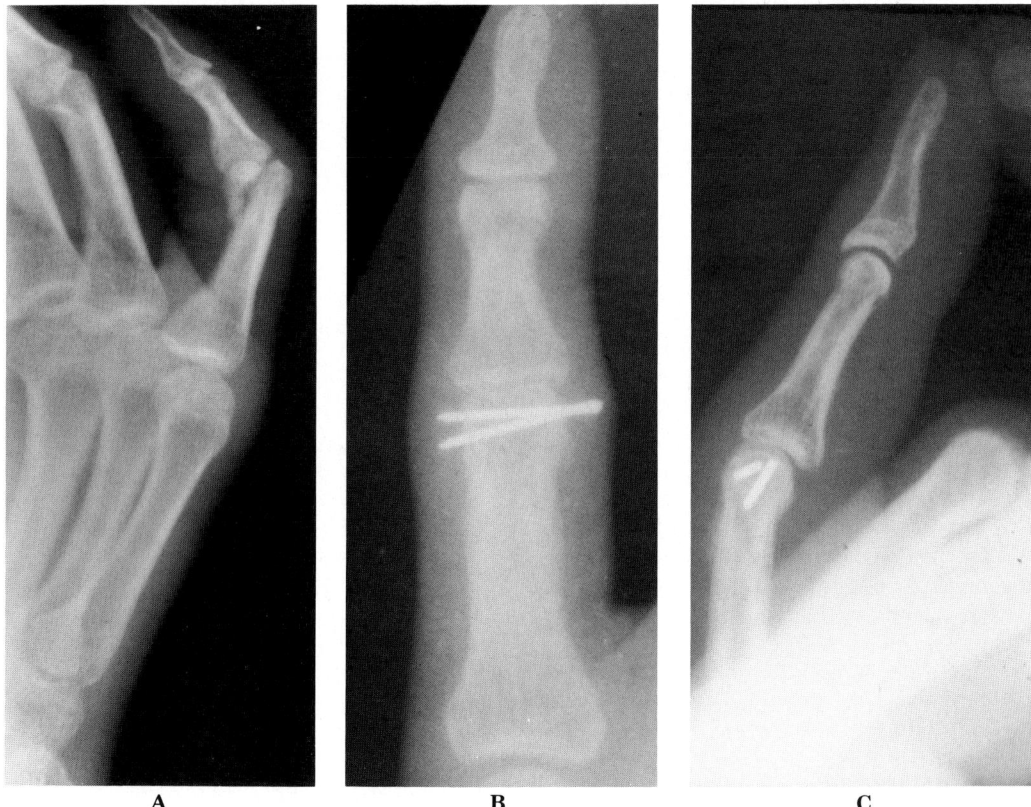

FIG. 26-23. A, An intercondylar fracture of the proximal phalanx, which was untreated for 2 weeks. **B** and **C,** An open reduction and internal fixation was required. During the operation, the collateral ligament to the fracture fragment was not disturbed.

Continued.

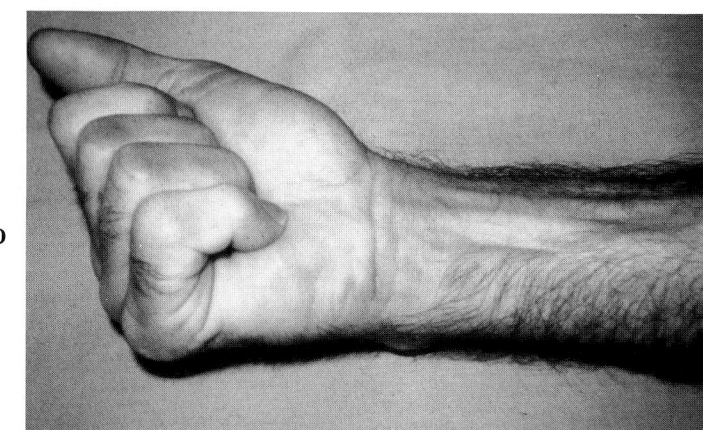

D

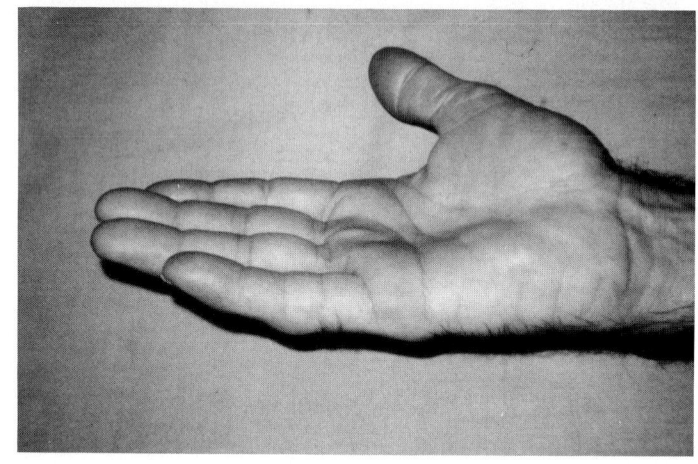

E

FIG. 26-23, cont'd. D and **E,** Post-operative mobility.

langeal joint, the entire expansion lies dorsal to the axis of the joint with its central tendon (extrinsic component) inserting at the base of the middle phalanx and its two lateral tendons, the lateral bands (intrinsic components), continuing distally and joining to form a single tendon. The insertion of this terminal extensor tendon into the base of the distal phalanx is more secure than is the insertion of the central tendon into the middle phalanx. All the tendons that make up the extensor mechanism and their fascial connections have fixed and critical lengths, and only a few millimeters of displacement, shortening, or lengthening will often result in a diminution of their power and deformity of a finger.[26] Because the three joints within each finger are an intercalated linkage system, a deformity at the proximal interphalangeal joint will always produce deformities at the adjacent metacarpophalangeal and distal interphalangeal joints. The limited tolerance for change in the length of any part of the extensor mechanism is not shared by the flexor system, where there is an independent flexor (flexor digitorum superficialis and profundus) for each interphalangeal joint.

The proximal interphalangeal joint itself is a hinge or ginglymus joint, permitting a wide range of motion in a flexion-extension arc ranging from 100 to 110 degrees. The articular surfaces consist of the head of the proximal phalanx, which has two condyles of almost perfect curvature separated by a shallow intercondylar groove.[45] The articular surface of the middle phalanx is broad, and its anatomic features are the reciprocal of the proximal phalanx, consisting of two depressions separated by a median ridge. These two joint surfaces form a tongue-and-groove configuration that facilitates movement in the sagittal plane but resists lateral or rotational stresses. In the transverse diameter, the joint surfaces are about equal, but in the sagittal plane, the base of the middle phalanx covers only one half of the head of the proximal phalanx.[45]

Thus in extension a considerable portion of the condyles protrudes volarly and can easily be palpated.

Laterally, the interphalangeal joint is supported by two layers of soft tissues. The more superficial layer is thin and consists of the transverse and oblique fibers of the retinacular ligaments of Landsmeer and the intermediate bundle of Cleland's ligament.[37] The deeper layer, which is much thicker, consists of collateral ligaments that are quadrangular in shape and arise from small fossae on the sides of the head of the proximal phalanx and insert into the volar one third of the middle phalanx and into the distal margins of the volar plate. The collateral ligaments are 2 to 3 mm in thickness, and their widths at origin and insertion are almost one half of their length.[46] Some of the ligaments fibers run in a more oblique direction and insert into the sides of the volar plate, forming the accessory collateral ligaments. Unlike the ligaments at the metacarpophalangeal joint level, whose tension depends on the position of the joint, the ligament tension at the proximal interphalangeal joints varies little from extension to flexion.

The volar plate, or glenoid fibrocartilage, forms the floor of the joint. Though similar to the plate at the metacarpophalangeal joint, the volar plate has several distinct differences. The distal attachment of its thick cartilaginous portion is only at its lateral margins, where it becomes confluent with the insertion of the collateral and accessory collateral ligaments. These attachments into the lateral volar tubercles of the middle phalanx at the "critical corners" provide the main resistance against hyperextension of the joint.[19,20] The central portion of the distal end of the plate, making up more than three quarters of its width, has no firm insertion into the phalanx, which in this area consists of the volar tubercle of the median ridge. The plate attachment in this area is to the periosteum on the metaphyseal portion of the bone, which gives the plate a meniscoid character. This configuration facilitates movement of the plate away from the base of the middle phalanx during flexion.[19,61] Proximally, the plate thins in its central portion, which allows passage for important capsular vessels.[67] The lateral portions are much thicker. They attach to the ridges just proximal to the condyles inside the tendon sheath, just inside the walls of the distal portion of the second annular (A-2) pulley, and confluent with the origin of the proximal portion of the first cruciate (C-1) pulley.[19] These proximal attachments, referred to as the "lower fibers" of the capsule,[103] or the "check-rein ligaments",[46] produce a swallow-tail configuration at the proximal portion of the plate.[19] Dorsally, the joint capsule is intimately connected with the extensor apparatus, and it is difficult to separate the two. The central tendon not only functions as an active extensor of the joint but also serves as a dorsal ligament.[45]

Tendon Injuries

Acute Boutonnière Deformity

Tendon injuries in the proximal interphalangeal joint area are usually closed and almost always involve the central slip of the extensor tendon mechanism. Aside from injuries to the terminal extensor tendon at the distal interphalangeal joint, which will be discussed in a subsequent section, injuries to the central tendon are the most common closed tendon injuries in athletes.[27,120] They result from direct trauma to the tendon or from sudden forced flexion of the joint. Often the athlete neglects to seek immediate medical attention or, if attention is sought, an accurate diagnosis may not be made. Initially, there may be only a paucity of objective clinical findings. The joint may be only slightly swollen and there may be little or no loss of active extension. The boutonnière deformity, which in France is curiously anglicized and referred to as the "buttonhole deformité," may not be present. However, after a week or two, as the lateral bands slip volarly, the characteristic deformity becomes obvious.

An index of suspicion and a careful physical examination are necessary if an accurate diagnosis is to be made at the time of the injury and prompt, effective treatment is to be instituted. Localization of the area of maximum tenderness is important; it will be over the insertion of the central tendon into the base of the middle phalanx. Though any loss of joint extension is significant, it is not by itself pathognomonic of tendon injury. A more important clue to the injury may be obtained by observing active and passive flexion at the distal interphalangeal joint after first stabilizing the proximal interphalangeal joint in extension. With disruption of the central tendon, even slight volar slippage of the lateral bands will significantly compromise active and passive flexion at the distal joint.[22] Roentgenograms are usually negative except in those rare cases in which the tendon avulses from the dorsal base of the phalanx with a fragment that can be clearly visualized on a lateral roentgenogram. If the roentgenograms are negative, treatment is to splint the proximal interphalangeal joint in full extension, leaving the distal interphalangeal joint free. Active and passive flexion exercises for the distal interphalangeal joint are encouraged to prevent contracture of the retinacular ligaments.[151] Continuous splinting for the proximal interphalangeal joint is maintained for 4 to 5 weeks, followed by periodic splinting for an additional 2 weeks. During this time active

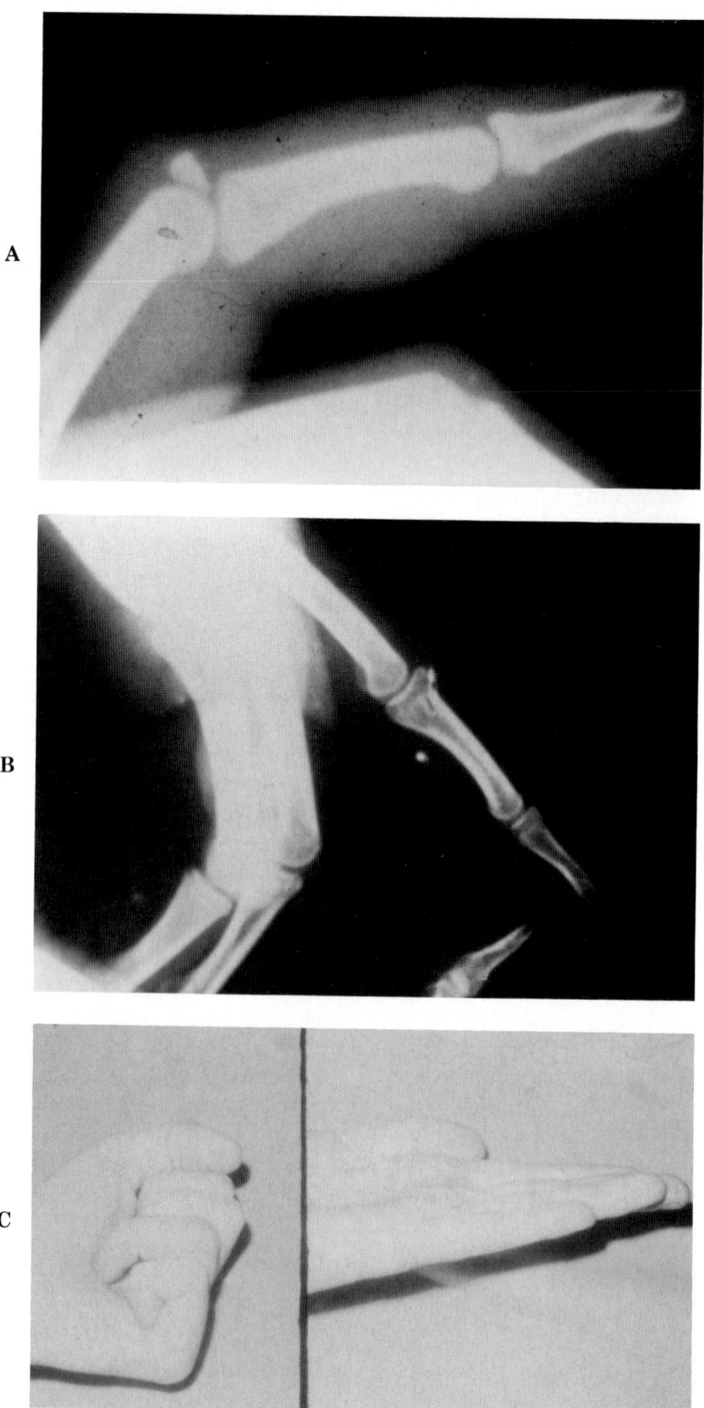

FIG. 26-24. A, The central tendon avulsed with a large fracture fragment from the base of the middle phalanx, resulting in an acute boutonniere deformity. **B,** The fragment was reattached with the cerclage wire. **C,** Postoperative mobility.

range of motion exercises are encouraged for all joints. Only in those rare cases of avulsion fracture is surgery required for the acute injury. If the fragment is large enough, a transverse drill hole is made in it as well as in the phalanx, and the fracture is then reattached using a cerclage 30- to 32-gauge wire (Fig. 26-24). If the fragment is small, the wire suture is passed through the central tendon rather than the fragment and then anchored to the phalanx. The wire suture must be passed deep to the lateral bands before it is threaded through the phalanx to avoid limiting the excursion of the lateral bands.

Subacute Boutonnière Deformity

If the injury is untreated for several weeks, contractures develop at both interphalangeal joints. In this subacute stage, it may be possible to improve passive extension of the proximal interphalangeal joint by the use of serial casts, which are changed weekly, or dynamic splints. After joint extension is achieved, the digit is splinted for several weeks followed by active range of motion exercises. These patients usually regain satisfactory function of the injured finger without surgery, though mobility is rarely completely restored (Fig. 26-25).

Chronic Boutonnière Deformity

When the condition is chronic, the flexion contracture at the proximal interphalangeal joint and extension contracture at the distal interphalangeal joint have become rigid. The chronic boutonnière deformity is among the most difficult and challenging problems to treat. The original injury confined to the central extensor tendon has progressed to volar displacement and fixation of the lateral bands, fibrosis with shortening of the transverse and oblique retinacular ligaments, and contractures of the collateral ligaments at both interphalangeal joints. Essentially there are two problems: an incompetent extensor tendon mechanism and the more serious flexion contracture at the proximal interphalangeal joint. Though it is technically feasible to treat both problems with a single operation, namely a capsulectomy at the proximal interphalangeal joint to restore full passive extension and a reconstruction of the tendon mechanism, the

A

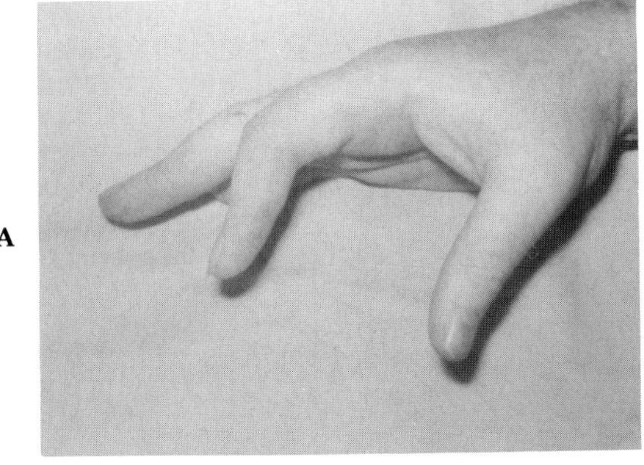

B

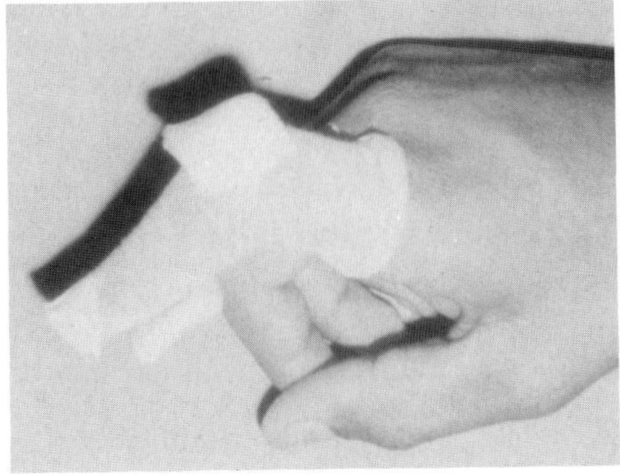

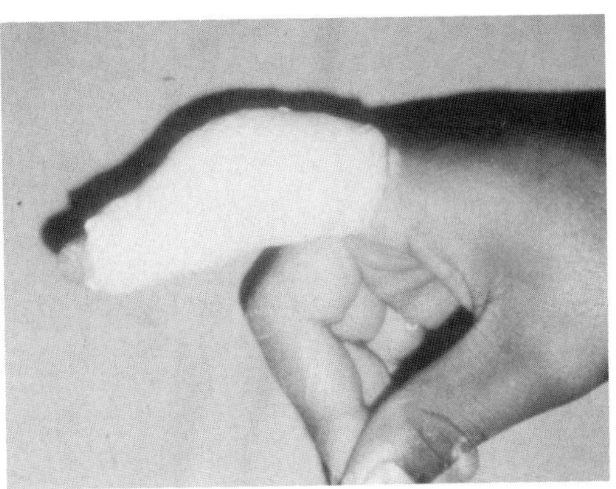

C

FIG. 26-25. A, Closed injury to the extensor tendon at the proximal interphalangeal joint that ocurred 6 weeks earlier. **B** and **C,** Serial plaster casts were applied each week to correct the secondary joint contracture. The casts are applied with padding limited only to the pressure areas over the dorsal aspect of the proximal interphalangeal joint and the volar aspect of the distal interphalangeal joint.
Continued.

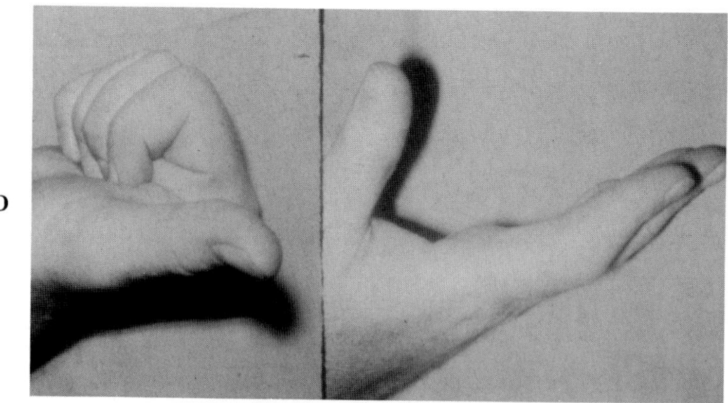

FIG. 26-25, cont'd. D, After four serial casts, the patient regained complete flexion at both interphalangeal joints with only a slight impairment in extension at the proximal interphalangeal joint.

result would be poor. Postoperative care following a capsulectomy, which involves early active and passive exercises, is radically different from that following tendon reconstruction, which requires that the digit be immobilized for several weeks. Capsulectomy and tendon reconstruction carried out together would in all likelihood convert the stiff flexed finger into a stiff extended one.

The primary objective with a chronic boutonnière deformity is to improve passive joint mobility by nonoperative measures. If this can be achieved, then the only problem remaining is the damaged extensor tendon, which then can be improved by surgery. Serial casts followed by dynamic splints are used to treat the joint contractures. Passive extension at the proximal interphalangeal joint must be restored before surgery for the tendon problem can be considered. A variety of surgical techniques are available to reconstruct the tendon, and all have the same goals: to advance the scarred and retracted central extensor tendon to the level of its normal insertion at the base of the middle phalanx, and to relocate the displaced lateral bands to their normal position dorsal to the axis of motion at the proximal interphalangeal joint (Fig. 26-26). The extension or hyperextension at the distal interphalangeal joint can be managed either by passive flexion of the joint and fixation in a more functional flexed position with a Kirschner pin for several weeks; or, if the joint cannot be manipulated, by division of the terminal extensor tendon. A mild flexion contracture at the distal joint is much more functional than a hyperextension contracture.

If the joint contractures do not respond to conservative measures and remain rigid, a two-stage procedure is required. Capsulectomy is the first procedure, and after satisfactory passive mobility is restored, the dorsal tendon mechanism is reconstructed. This two-stage procedure is rarely indicated because of the prolonged period of rehabilitation required, usually a minimum of 6 months. Before this extensive reconstructive program is considered, the boutonnière deformity should be causing a significant disability. Equally important, the patient must have a complete understanding of the complexity of his problem, the limited objectives of the surgical procedures, and the necessity for complete cooperation in the postoperative therapy. In some cases for which two-stage procedure is planned, the function of the extensor mechanism improves after capsulectomy, and a second operation becomes unnecessary.

Pseudoboutonnière Deformity

Pseudoboutonnière deformity is often confused with boutonnière deformity. The two deformities bear a superficial resemblance in that the proximal interphalangeal joint is in a flexed position in both. The difference can be distinguished by observing the distal interphalangeal joint: there is an extension or hyperextension contracture in the boutonnière deformity, but normal mobility in the pseudoboutonnière deformity.[161] The two deformities also differ in their mechanism of injury and the time it takes for joint contractures to appear. Boutonnière deformity results from damage to the central extensor tendon, and joint contractures develop soon after the injury. In contrast, pseudoboutonnière deformity follows a hyperextension injury, which tears the volar capsule of the proximal interphalangeal joint. The flexion contracture develops as a later complication.[120,121,122] Rarely, a severe and chronic pseudoboutonnière deformity can develop into a boutonnière defor-

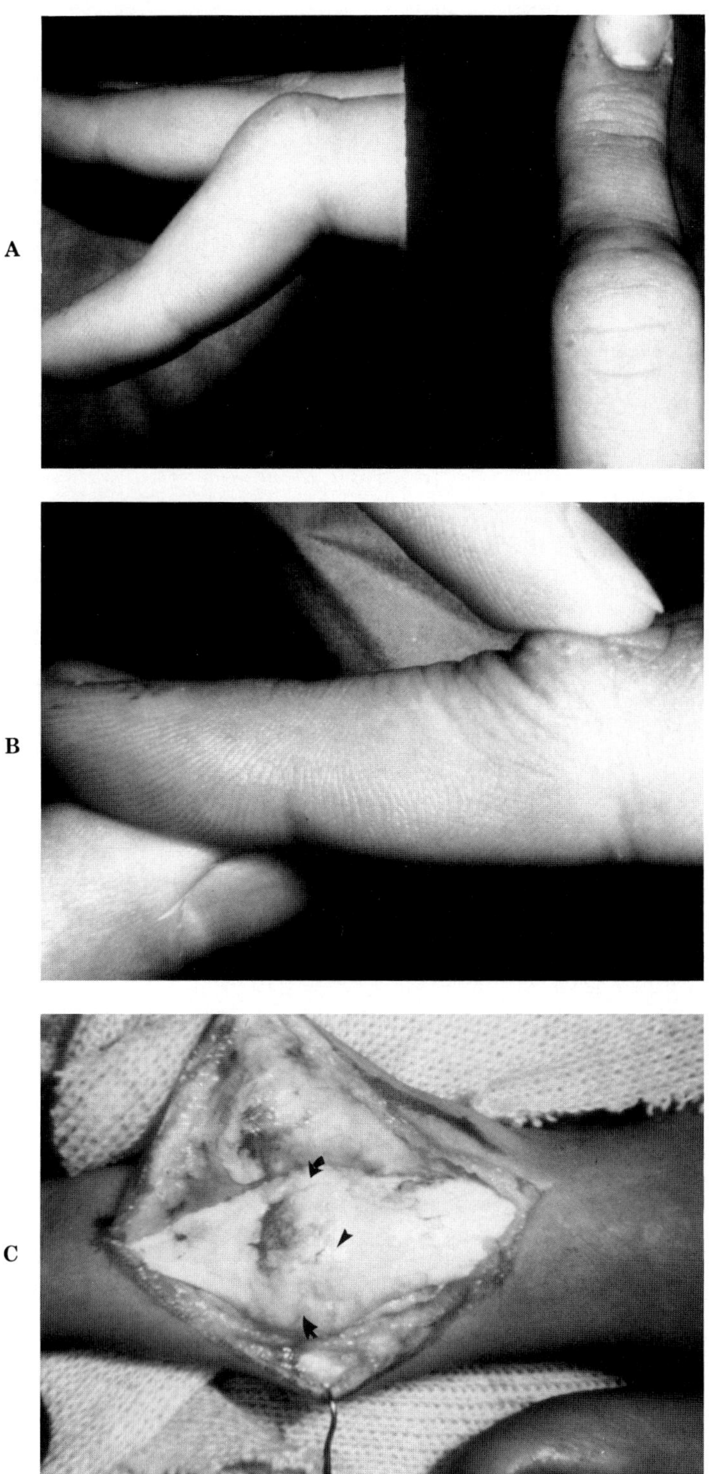

FIG. 26-26. A and **B,** A Chronic boutonnière deformity in a young patient with full passive extension of the proximal interphalangeal joint. This is the ideal situation for reconstructive surgery. **C,** The central tendon was scarred and retracted *(small arrow)* and both lateral bands *(curved arrows)* were subluxed volar to the axis of motion at the joint.

Continued.

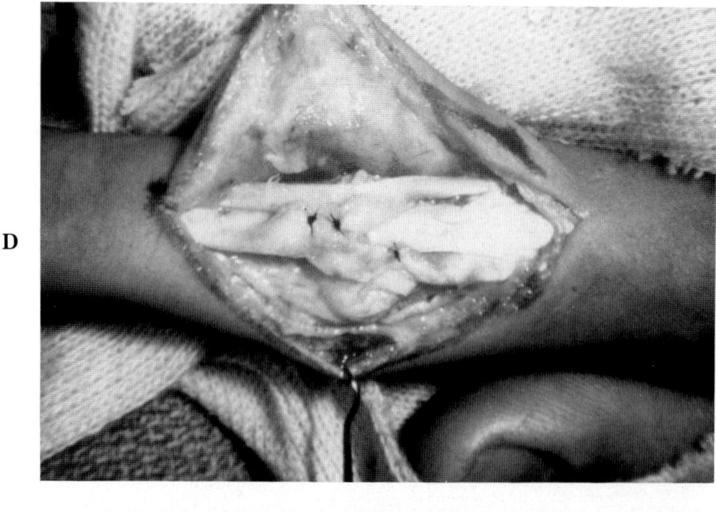

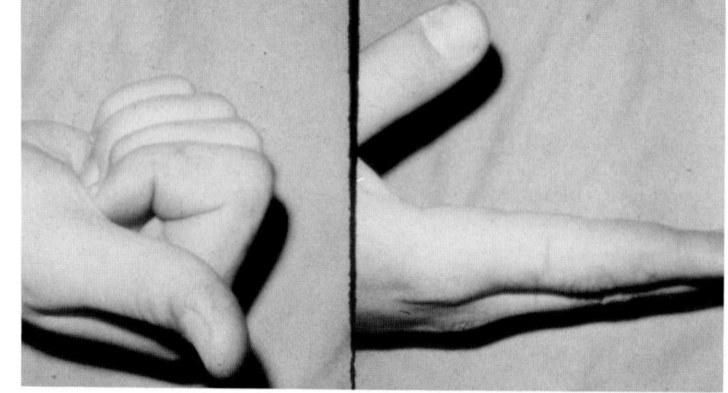

FIG. 26-26, cont'd. D, The lateral bands were replaced dorsally and the central tendon advanced. Sutures were placed in the extensor mechanism distal to the joint level to avoid producing a later extension contracture. **E,** Postoperative mobility.

Boutonnière versus Pseudoboutonnière deformity

Boutonnière deformity
- Etiology
  - Central extensor injury
- Natural history
  - Joint contractures develop easily
- Findings
  - PIP flexed
  - DIP—Hyperextended or extension contraction

Pseudoboutonnière deformity
- Etiology
  - Hypertension injury to PIP joint with volar plate injury
- Natural history
  - Joint contracture develops later
- Findings
  - PIP flexed
  - DIP—normal mobility

mity as the central slip elongates over the flexed proximal interphalangeal joint, which permits the lateral bands to slip volarly. Secondary contractures of the retinacular ligaments then develop, limiting flexion at the distal interphalangeal joint, and the transformation is completed.

Initial treatment for pseudoboutonnière deformity involves active and passive exercises and the use of dynamic extension splints to restore extension at the proximal interphalangeal joint. If the proximal interphalangeal joint contracture is rigid and disabling, surgical release followed by early exercises is necessary. Because there is no damage to the dorsal tendon mechanism in these cases, the prognosis for regaining mobility is better than after surgery for a boutonnière deformity.

Ligament Injuries

Injuries to the ligaments at the proximal interphalangeal joint are among the most common injuries affecting the hand. Their incidence is impossible to establish because medical attention is rarely sought for most of them. Many dislocations spontaneously reduce or are reportedly "snapped back into place" by the injured athlete. Medical attention is usually sought only because the finger remains painful, swollen, and stiff weeks after the injury. These athletes frequently describe their injury as a "jammed finger," which may represent a spectrum of diagnoses ranging from a mild first-degree sprain to a third-degree sprain resulting in instability, subluxation, or dislocation, or even a fracture-dislocation of the joint. Obviously, a delay of weeks in treating an unstable joint or a fracture-dislocation will result in a serious and permanent impairment. Fortunately, most chronic "jammed fingers" represent first- or second-degree sprains, and no appreciable harm is caused by the delay in treatment. The athlete is often concerned by the persistent joint swelling, and he must be informed that it may take up to 18 months for the swelling to reach a point of maximum improvement. With severe injuries, some permanent enlargement of the joint should be anticipated.

Volar Plate

Acute injuries. Injuries to the volar capsule occur most commonly in sports activities, in either the recreational amateur athlete or professional.[67] The volar plate is the primary static restraint limiting joint extension. Experimental studies in fresh anatomic specimens show that when stress is applied slowly to the joint, there is a gradual attenuation of the proximal attachments.[20,21] If this stress is continued, the middle phalanx dislocates dorsally, taking with it the volar plate, which can then be entrapped over the head of the proximal phalanx and block reduction. Because a slow hyperextension force is an unusual mechanism of injury, proximal disruption and entrapment of the plate within the joint is a clinical rarity. When these unusual dislocations do occur, a lateral roentgenogram view will show persistent incongruity of the joint following attempted reduction[73,101] (Fig. 26-27).

With rapid loading of the joint, which is the usual method of injury, the plate fails at its distal insertion. Two types of distal ruptures are encountered, and each may occur with or without avulsion of a bone flake from the metaphyseal area of the middle phalanx.[20,21] In the type I rupture, the damage is confined to the thin center portion of the plate, and its important corner attachments remain intact. Though these injuries may be initially painful and cause swelling and stiffness, there is no instability with stress testing. Overtreatment must be avoided. If immobilization is used it should be for a brief period, not exceeding 1 week. "Buddy taping" for an additional 1 or 2 weeks is all that is required for these injuries. If the hyperextension force on the joint continues, the distal lateral attchments at the plate rupture and the lateral capsule tears between the accessory collateral and collateral ligaments, producing the type II injury. The middle phalanx can then shift dorsally, hinging on the origins of the collateral ligaments. If the split in the lateral capsule is minor, the joint will be hyperextended, sometimes as much as 70 to 80 degrees. However, the articular surfaces remain in contact as the middle phalanx articulates with the dorsal aspect of the head of the proximal phalanx.[43] When the lateral capsular tear is more severe, the middle phalanx actually dislocates dorsally, producing a bayonet alignment with the proximal phalanx. A closed reduction can usually be achieved by simply pushing the displaced middle phalanx over the head of the proximal phalanx. Traction should be avoided, because it could cause entrapment of soft tissues within the joint and prevent reduction.[21] There is rarely any lateral instability after reduction, because the collateral ligaments remain intact.[19,20,21,46,94] Treatment involves the use of a dorsal block splint. This prevents the joint from extending the last 20 to 30 degrees but permits active and even passive flexion exercises. The presence of an avulsion fracture in type II injury may even be considered fortunate, because the patient will usually receive medical treatment. The problem occurs with type II injuries without a chip fracture, because volar instability of the joint often goes unrecognized. Without appropriate dorsal block splinting, the joint may sublux or progress to chronic volar instability.

Occasionally, a compressive force on the joint or an axial force on the partially flexed finger may cause the volar base of the middle phalanx to shear dorsally against the condyles of the proximal phalanx. This results in a fracture-dislocation. These injuries often represent the most complex and difficult-to-treat intraarticular fractures encountered in hand trauma.[85] Except for some swelling, the finger may look normal after the injury. Unfortunately, the athlete often neglects to seek immediate medical attention, which complicates treatment and compromises the ultimate return of joint mobility.

The extent of articular disruption at the base of the middle phalanx determines stability following reduction. Instability is not a

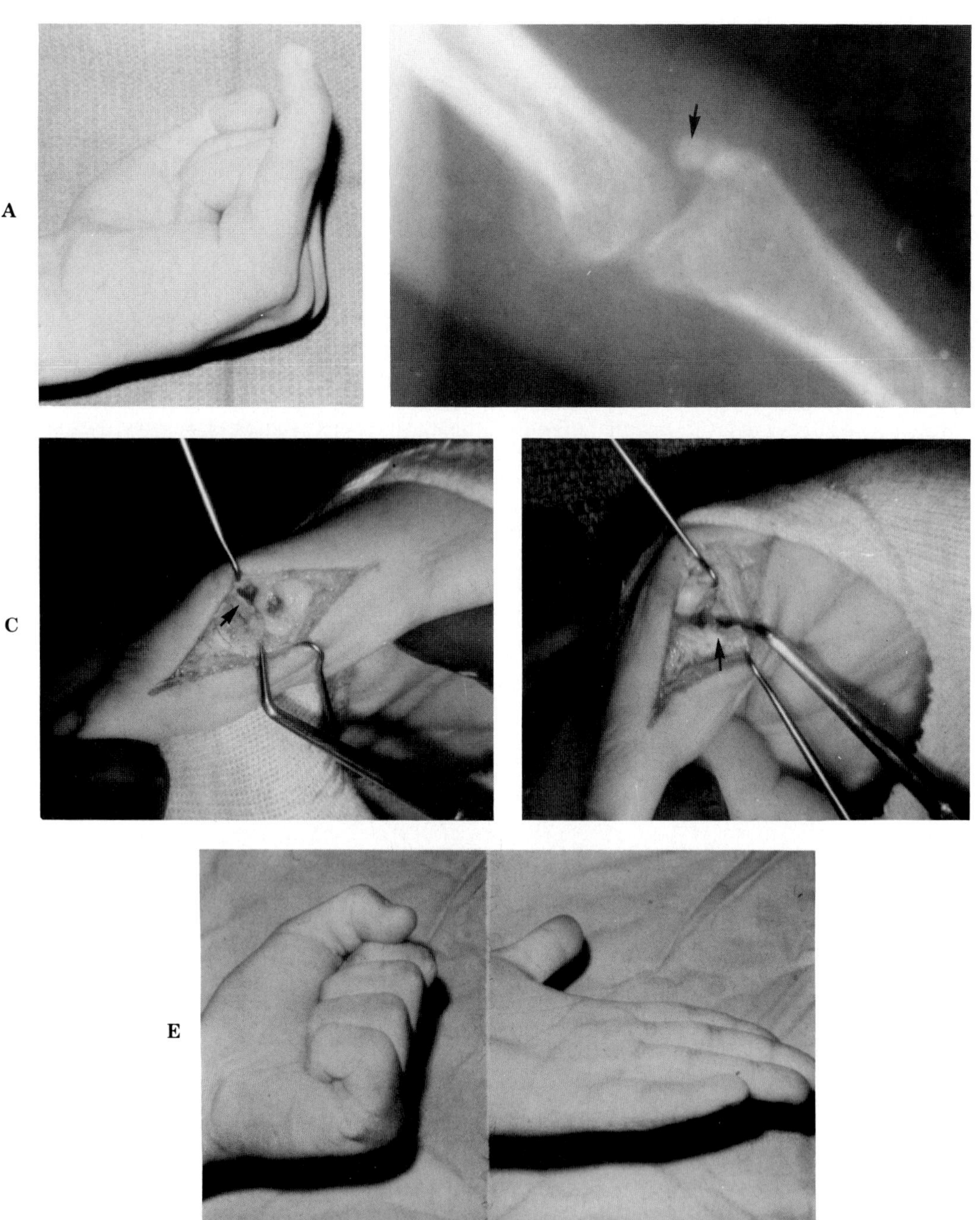

FIG. 26-27. A and **B,** The lateral roentgenogram of an irreducible dorsal dislocation shows incongruity of the joint. The small bone fragment was attached to the volar plate, which had detached proximally and was dorsal to the head of the proximal phalanx. **C** and **D,** At surgery, the plate, which was interposed between the joint, prevented reduction. As soon as it was mobilized *(arrow),* the subluxation was reduced. **E,** Postoperative mobility.

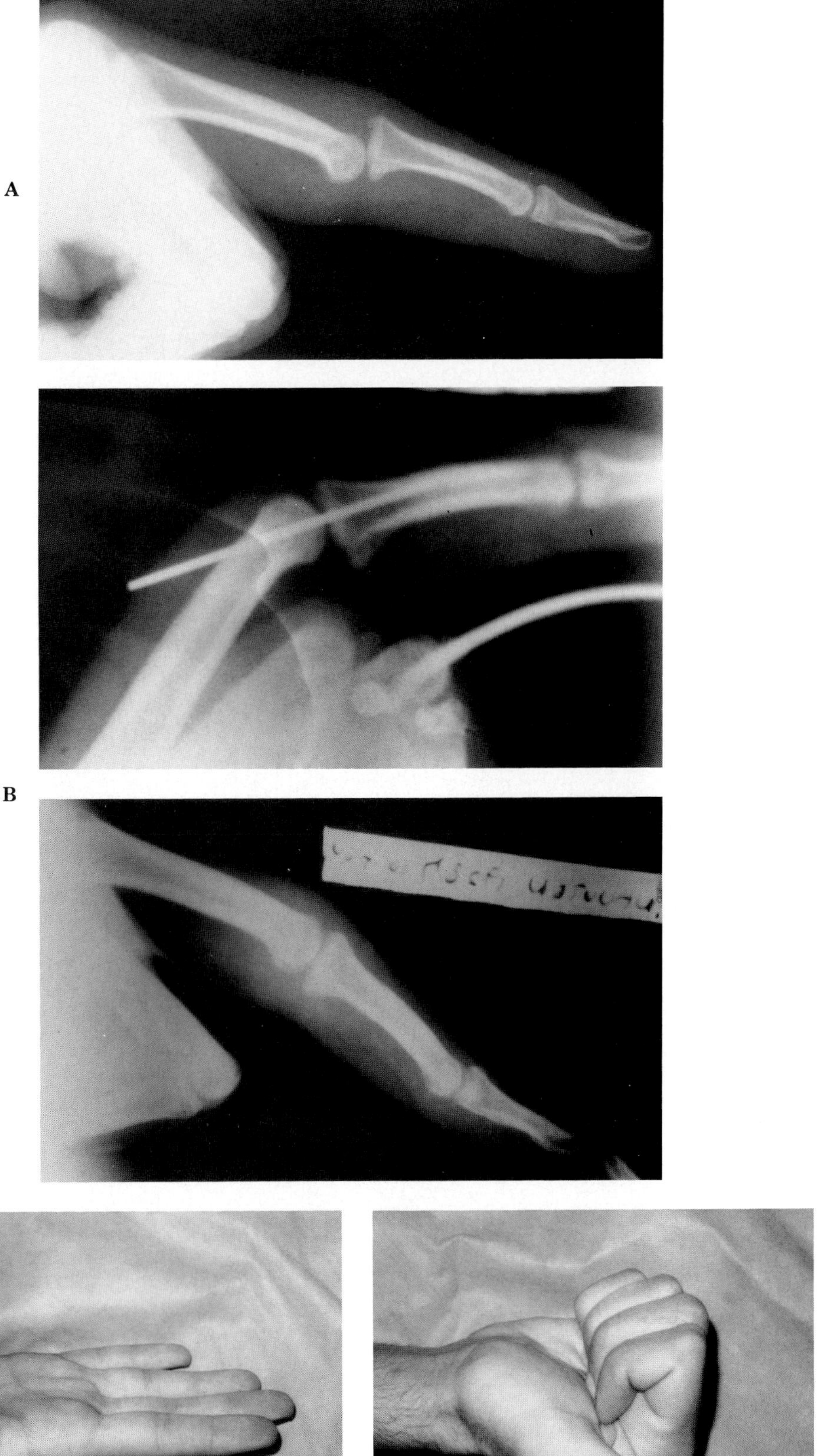

FIG. 26-28. A, A dorsal subluxation of a proximal interphalangeal joint. **B,** The volar fracture fragment was small, and the joint was easily reduced by manipulation and percutaneously pinned for 3 to 4 weeks. **C** and **D,** The joint remained stable. The patient regained complete digital mobility.

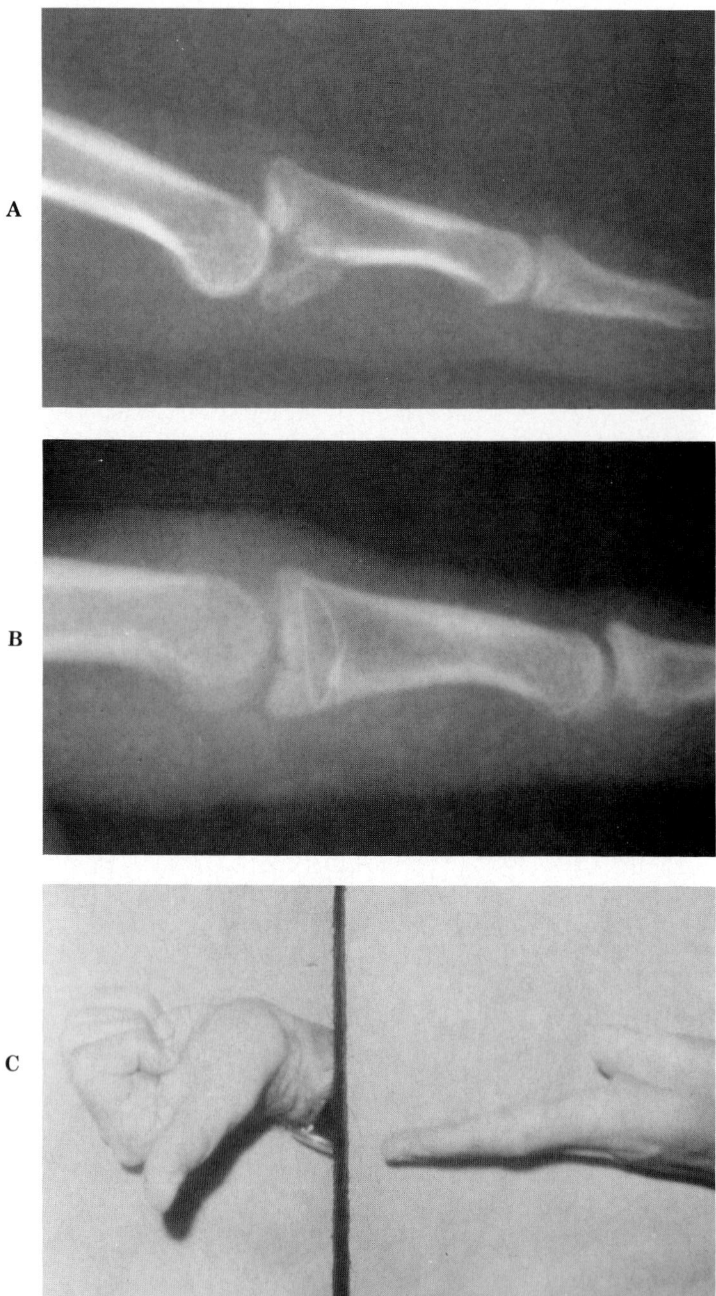

FIG. 26-29. A, Intraarticular fracture of the base of the middle phalanx resulted from a shear force. **B,** Articular congruity was restored by an open reduction and cerclage wire fixation of the fracture fragment. **C,** Postoperative mobility.

problem with small avulsion fractures, because the volar plate and only a small portion of the collateral ligaments have disrupted. However, instability should be anticipated with larger fragments that make up a third or more of the articular surface. This is because most if not all of the collateral ligament insertions into the middle phalanx have been detatched. The restraining forces on the middle phalanx are lost, and the bone subluxes dorsally. Surgery is necessary, and if possible the volar fragment is reattached using a Kirschner pin or, preferably, an interosseous wire suture (Figs. 26-28 and 26-29).

Frequently, the volar fragment is severely comminuted, precluding any reattachment. In these situations, the fragments can be excised and the volar plate advanced into the

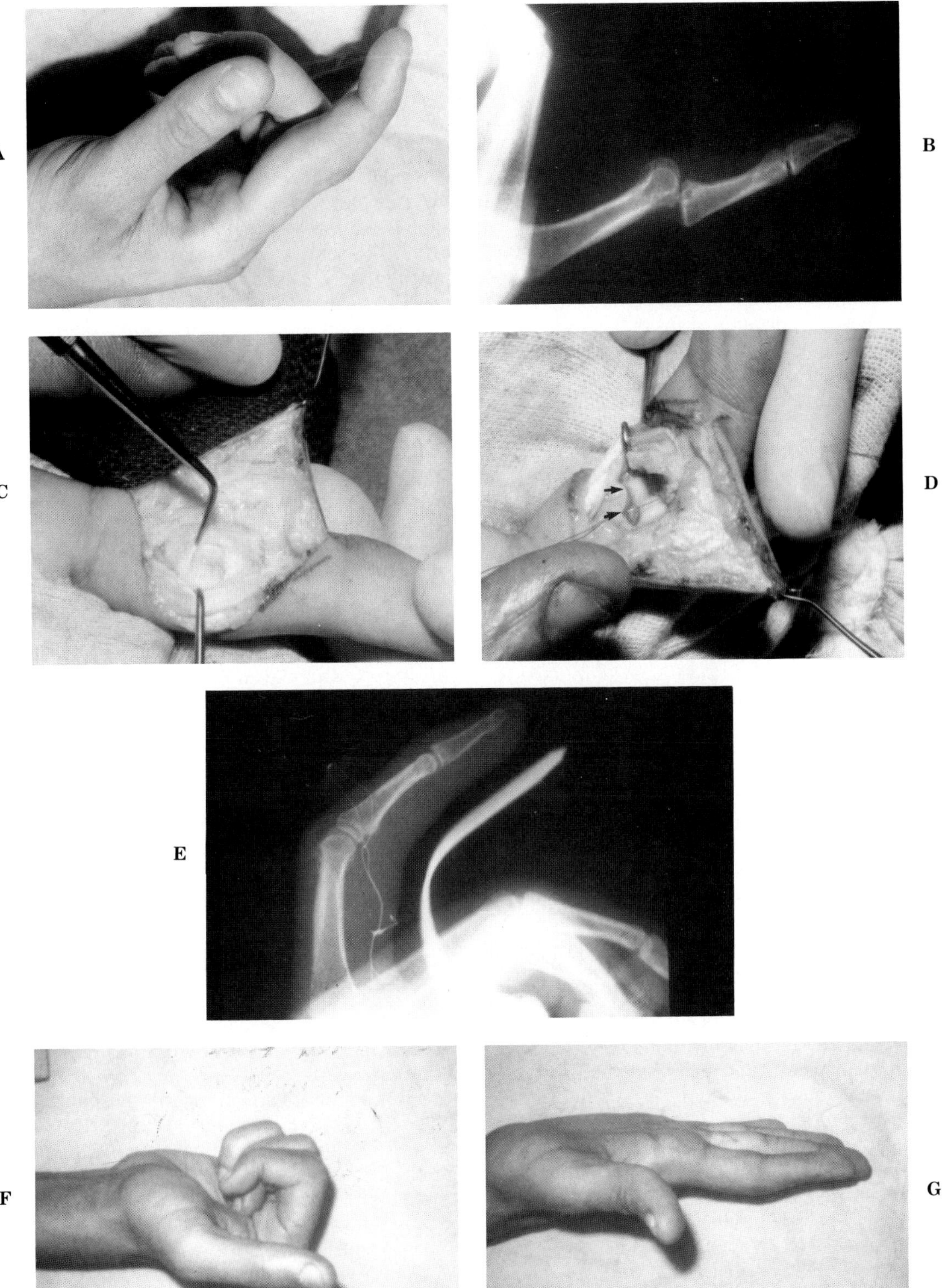

FIG. 26-30. A and **B,** Dorsal dislocation of a proximal interphalangeal joint with compression of the volar one third of the base of the middle phalanx. **C,** Through a volar approach, the joint was explored. With the tendons retracted, the plate was visualized. It had avulsed distally with several small bone fragments and retracted *(probe)*. **D** and **E,** The volar plate was reattached into the middle phalanx using a pull-out wire suture, and the digit was immobilized for 3 to 4 weeks before active range of motion exercises were started. **F** and **G,** Postoperative motions of the digit were satisfactory.

defect of the base of the middle phalanx[46] (Fig. 29-30). A Bruner-type zigzag incision is made on the volar aspect of the digit with the apex of the incision at the midaxial point on either the radial or ulnar side of the proximal interphalangeal flexion crease. A triangular-shaped skin flap is elevated, and both neurovascular bundles are identified and protected. The tendon sheath between the A-2 and A-4 pulleys is then excised to permit retraction of the flexor tendons and inspection of the joint. The volar plate can be retracted proximally and the middle phalanx extended to allow visualization of the defect in its articular surface. Division of any remaining portions of the collateral ligaments to the middle phalanx facilitates the exposure. Small fragments are debrided from the joint as well as from the distal portion of the plate. The joint is then reduced and stabilized in slight flexion (about 30 degrees) using a thin, nonthreaded Kirschner pin. The volar plate is then inserted into the defect in the base of the middle phalanx using a pull-out wire suture. Proper placement of this suture is critical to the procedure. It should first be threaded into the plate with its two ends emerging from the distal corners and then passed into corresponding drill holes that have been made in the lateral margins of the articular defect in the middle phalanx. The wires exit on the dorsal aspect of the bone. Traction on the pins pulls the plate snugly into the defect, thereby restoring volar stability. Postoperatively, the finger is immobilized for 3 weeks. The pin is then removed and active range of motion exercises begun. Passive flexion also should be encouraged, but passive extension should be avoided for several more weeks. If at that time there is an extension deficit greater than 35 degrees, a dynamic extension splint can be used. Though mobility is rarely restored completely, this difficult operation restores stability as well as a satisfactory range of motion to the severely injured joint.

An alternative procedure is to use a skeletal traction device. Its application is based on the fact that a single axis of rotation for flexion/extension is located between the dorsal and palmar bundles of the collateral ligaments at their origin, on the sides of the head of the proximal phalanx. The device maintains reduction; provides distraction, which permits reduction of the fracture fragments by ligamentoaxis; protects the joint surface from compressive loading; and, most importantly, allows for active and passive exercises. The procedure is simpler than an operative repair and will become more widely used for difficult fracture-dislocations when a suitable device becomes commercially available.[79]

Chronic injuries. Chronic injuries to the volar plate involve either an unrecognized fracture-dislocation or volar instability. Treatment for a chronic fracture-dislocation depends on the condition of the joint surfaces. If secondary degenerative arthritic changes have not yet developed, the contracted capsule is released and the volar plate advanced, as for the acute injury. In selected cases, an osteotomy of the malunited fracture at the base of the middle phalanx can be considered to salvage some joint function. Once arthritic changes develop, surgical options are either implant arthroplasty or arthrodesis, with arthrodesis being the preferred treatment for the active athlete.

Chronic volar instability is a rare and interesting condition. There is considerable conjecture why instability develops rather than the more commonly encountered flexion contracture. One theory is that the sparse vascularity at the distal insertion of the plate results in insufficient bleeding to cause scarring after rupture, which would permit adherence of the plate to the bone from which it avulsed.[140] This would explain the tendency for poorer healing when the plate avulses without a fragment from the metaphyseal area of the middle phalanx. The absence of a bone fragment indicates that there was no "fracture bleeding," and without bleeding there is less likelihood for scarring.[21] In addition, if the joint is not immobilized after the acute injury or if there are multiple hyperextension injuries, any small clots that form may be washed away by the flow of the synovial fluid between the joint and flexor tendon sheath. The ruptured plate fails to heal and rounds off, similar to what occurs to the ends of flexor tendons severed within their sheaths.[20,83]

With chronic volar instability, the middle phalanx hyperextends, and its articular surfaces frequently get caught in a position on the dorsal aspect of the head of the proximal phalanx. Slight passive flexion is required to "unlock" the joint before it can be actively flexed. The objective of treatment is to restore a volar restraint to complete joint extension. Various surgical procedures have been described: reattaching the avulsed plate into the middle phalanx,[80,144] shifting a portion of the proximal part of the collateral ligament volarly on the head of the proximal phalanx,[102] or reconstructing a plate substitute using either a free tendon graft[2] or the flexor superficialis tendon in the finger.[97,107,183]

I prefer to use the flexor superficialis ten-

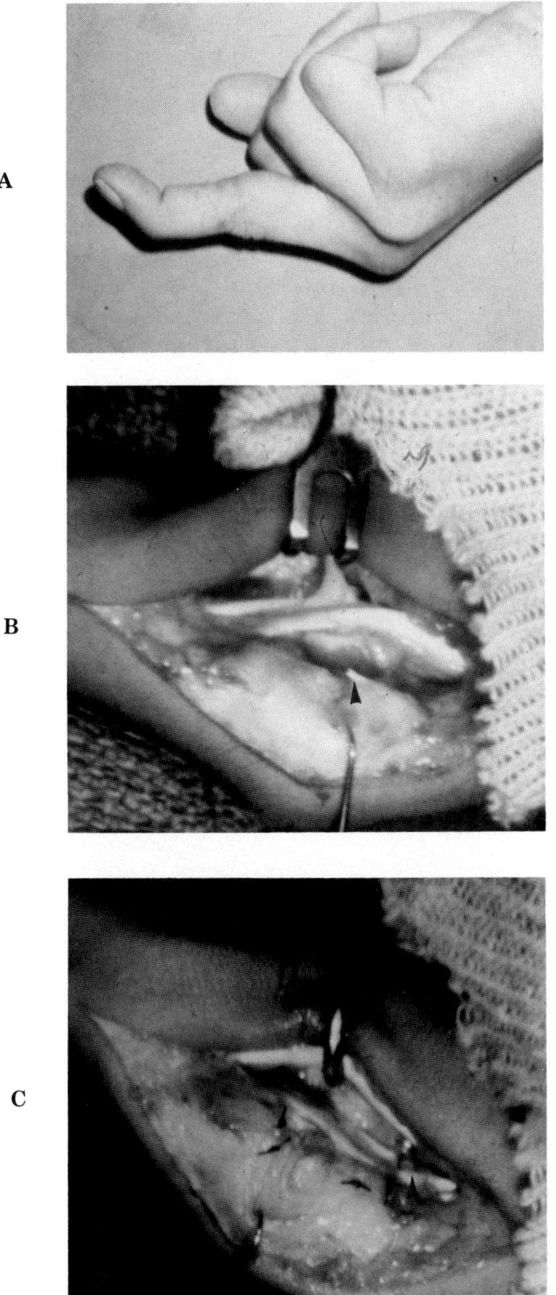

FIG. 26-31. A, Chronic volar instability of the proximal interphalangeal joint in a baseball player. The middle phalanx would frequently get caught in the hyperextended position and the patient would have to passively "unlock" it to permit flexion. **B,** At surgery, the volar plate was torn distally. **C,** The flexor superficialis tendon *(arrow)* was attached into a trough made in the proximal phalanx with the proximal interphalangeal joint in 20 to 30 degrees of flexion. The edge of the tendon was also sutured to the edge of the volar plate. *Continued.*

don because of its strength (Fig. 26-31). A midaxial incision is made along the side of the finger that is most convenient for the surgeon; radial side for the index and middle fingers and ulnar side for the ring and little fingers. The tendon sheath between the A-2 and A-4 pulleys is excised and the flexor tendons retracted, with care taken to avoid damage to their vincula. The ruptured plate will be clearly visible with its smooth distal edge. The joint is then fixed in a slightly flexed position of 20 to 30 degrees with a thin, nonthreaded

D

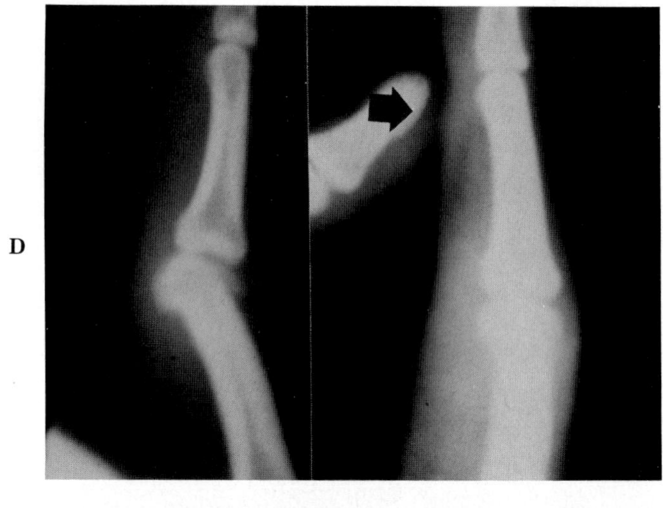

E

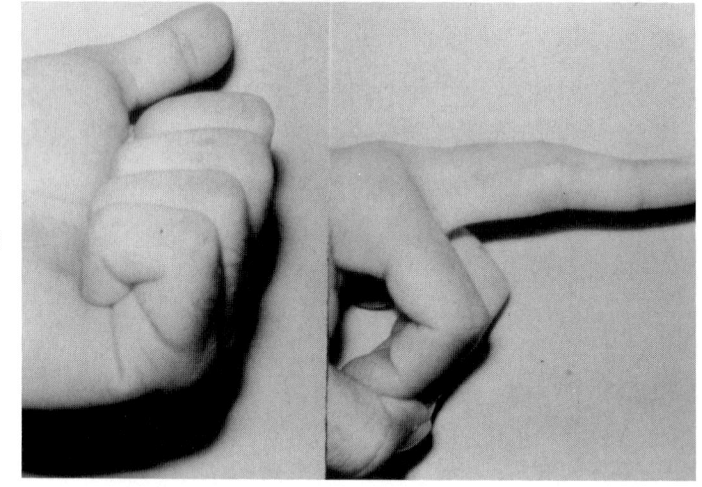

FIG. 26-31, cont'd. D, Comparison of preoperative and postoperative lateral roentgenograms. Preoperatively, the joint was unstable with active extension. Postoperatively, hyperextension was eliminated even to passive forces. (Arrow indicates direction of passive force of examining finger.) The patient regained complete mobility. The 20 degree deficit to full extension was insignificant.

Kirschner pin. A transverse trough is made with a power burr across the diaphyseal portion of the proximal phalanx, and the dorsal surface of the flexor superficialis tendon is roughened. Care is taken not to damage the opposite surface of the tendon, which is in contact with the flexor profundus. Two drill holes are made in the lateral margins of the trough, and the entire flexor superficialis tendon is then sutured into the trough with a pull-out wire suture. The suture in the tendon should be placed in such a way that it will pull the tendon snugly into the trough. There is no danger of pulling the tendon too tightly, because the degree of joint flexion has already been fixed by the transarticular Kirschner pin. The ends of the wire suture are then tied over padding on the dorsal surface of the phalanx to avoid pressure sores on the skin. The edge of the superficialis tendon is sutured to the edge of the volar plate, thereby adding further reinforcement. After 3 weeks, the pin is removed and active exercises including passive flexion are begun. The objective is a joint that has full flexion but is prevented from extending completely by the tenodesis effect of the flexor superficialis tendon.

Collateral Ligaments

Acute injuries. Lateral dislocation of the proximal interphalangeal joint results after a rupture of one collateral ligament, usually the radial, and most if not all of the insertion of the volar plate.[120,158] The joint hinges laterally on the intact collateral ligament. Usually, the dislocation can be easily reduced, and the torn ligament will resume its normal position. Though only one of the collateral ligaments remains intact, the joint is relatively stable because of the congruity of the tongue-and-groove configuration of its articular surfaces and the compressive effect provided by the intact flexor and extensor tendon systems. After reduction, the joint should be immobilized for 2 to 3 weeks in slight flexion. Additional protection can be achieved by "buddy taping" to the finger on the side of the ligament rupture for several additional weeks. In those dislocations which are reduced spontaneously, the joint will appear deceptively normal. However, stress testing will readily demonstrate instability and the need for immobilization. Surgery is indicated in those rare acute cases in which reduction cannot be achieved or if the joint redislocates with active motion.

Chronic injuries. Chronic lateral instability is rare. It is usually seen in athletes who report multiple dislocations or whose previous injuries never received adequate treatment. Clinically, there is slight enlargement of the joint on the side of the damaged ligament, which is most frequently the radial collateral ligament. Stress testing will readily demonstrate the degree of instability and, if it is greater than 20 degrees, it usually indicates a complete disruption of the collateral ligament.[100] In mild cases, "buddy taping" to the adjacent digit during sports activities may suffice. In more severe cases requiring surgery, the procedure depends on the operative findings. If possible, the avulsed collateral ligament is reinserted into the phalanx. This may be feasible even in chronic cases because the ligament rarely ruptures in its midsubstance (Fig. 26-32). Usually, the most volar and proximal fibers of the ligament tear first, followed by the dorsal fibers, because the joint is laterally angulated. If there is no recognizable ligament tissue, a new ligament must be reconstructed using either a portion of the volar plate[53] or the flexor superficialis tendon[107] (Figs. 26-33 and 26-34).

Volar Dislocations

Volar dislocation is far less common than dorsal or lateral dislocation. This is fortunate, because volar dislocation tends to cause residual joint stiffness. The injury results from sudden forceful flexion of the middle phalanx or from violent torsional injury to the joint. When the force is primarily flexion, the head of the proximal phalanx ruptures through the extensor tendon mechanism, tearing the central slip. Reduction can usually be achieved by closed measures and must be confirmed by roentgenograms, particularly a lateral view showing congruity of the joint surfaces. Though some authors recommend surgery to repair the central slip,[127,172] the preferred treatment is the same as for the closed acute boutonnière deformity.

In irreducible cases, the mechanism of injury is primarily a torsional force that results in disruption of one collateral ligament and partial avulsion of the volar plate. As the middle phalanx rotates volarly, the condyle of the proximal phalanx causes a longitudinal tear in the extensor mechanism. Usually, the tear is between the central slip and the ipsilateral lateral band, which slips volar to the condyle and entraps it (Fig. 26-35). In some situations, the tear is between the central slip and the contralateral band, and both the central slip and ipsilateral lateral band become

Text continued on p. 558.

A

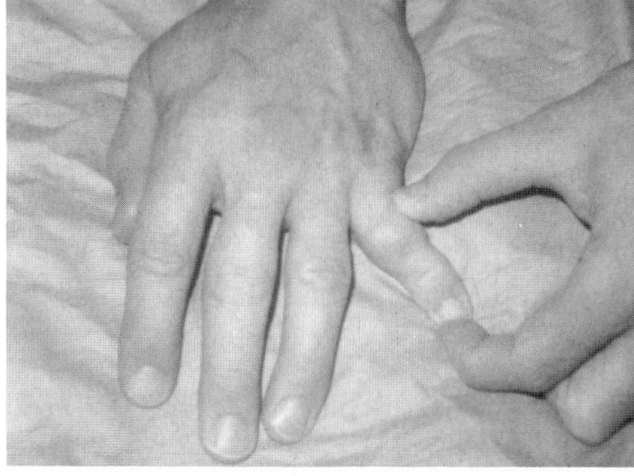

B

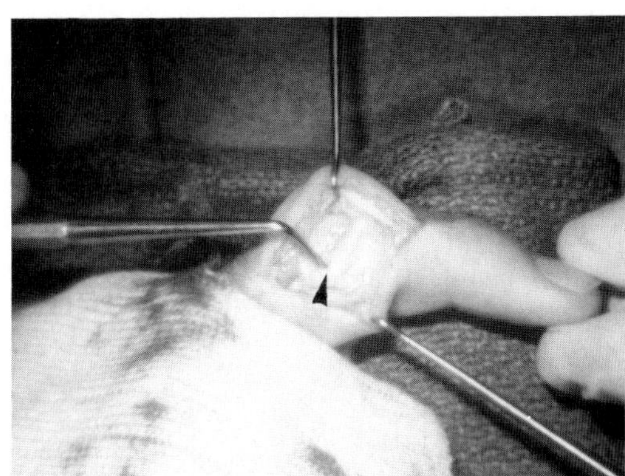

FIG. 26-32. A, Chronic lateral instability of the proximal interphalangeal joint of the little finger in an athlete who reported multiple ulnar dislocations, none of which received any treatment. **B,** The collateral ligament was scarred and attenuated proximally *(probe)*.

Continued.

C

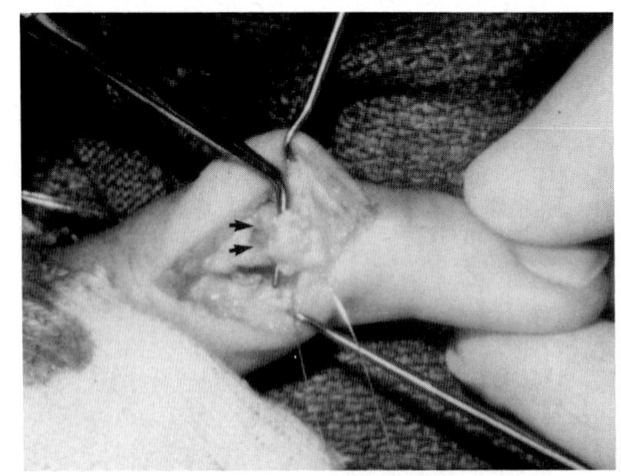

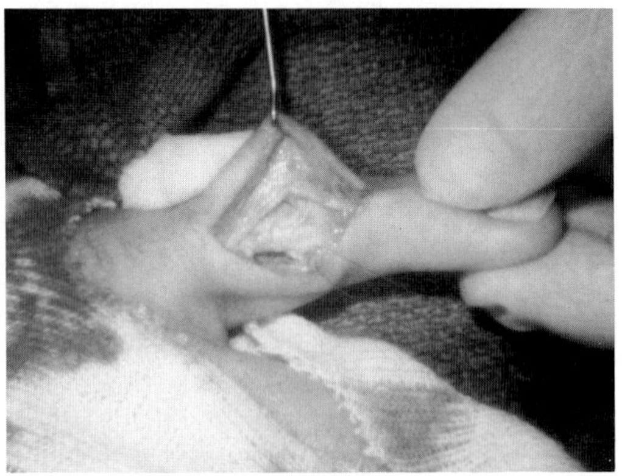

D

E

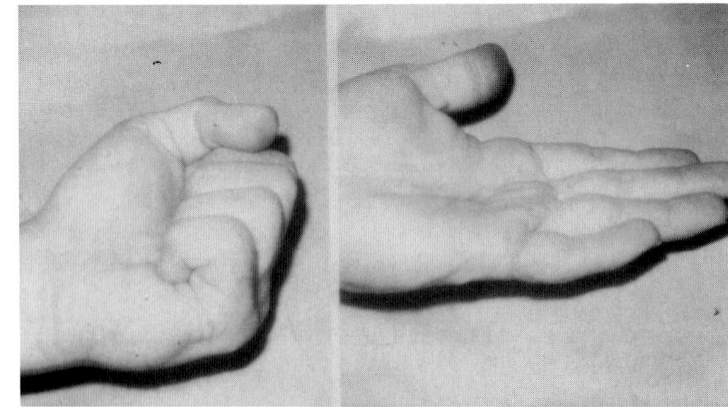

FIG. 26-32, cont'd. C and **D,** A trough was made in the side of the head of the phalanx *(small arrow),* and the normal portion of the ligament was reinserted into the bone. **E,** Postoperatively, stability and mobility were restored .

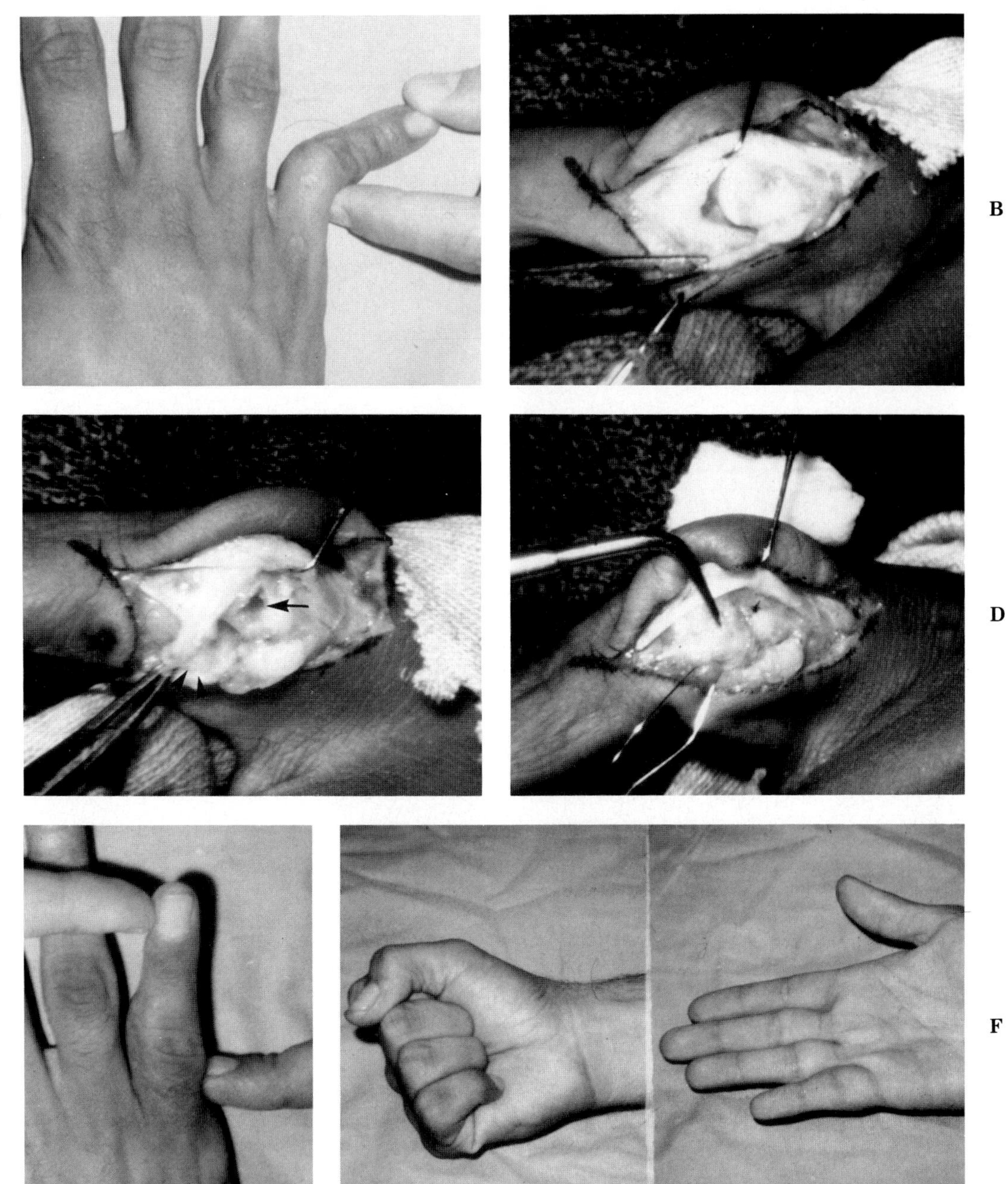

FIG. 26-33. A, Chronic lateral instability. **B,** At surgery, there was no recognizable ligamentous tissue. **C,** A portion of the volar plate *(arrow)* was mobilized, and a trough *(arrow)* was made in the side of the head of the phalanx. **D,** The volar plate (under the probe) was attached into the side of the bone using a pull-out wire suture. **E** and **F,** Postoperatively, mobility and stability were restored.

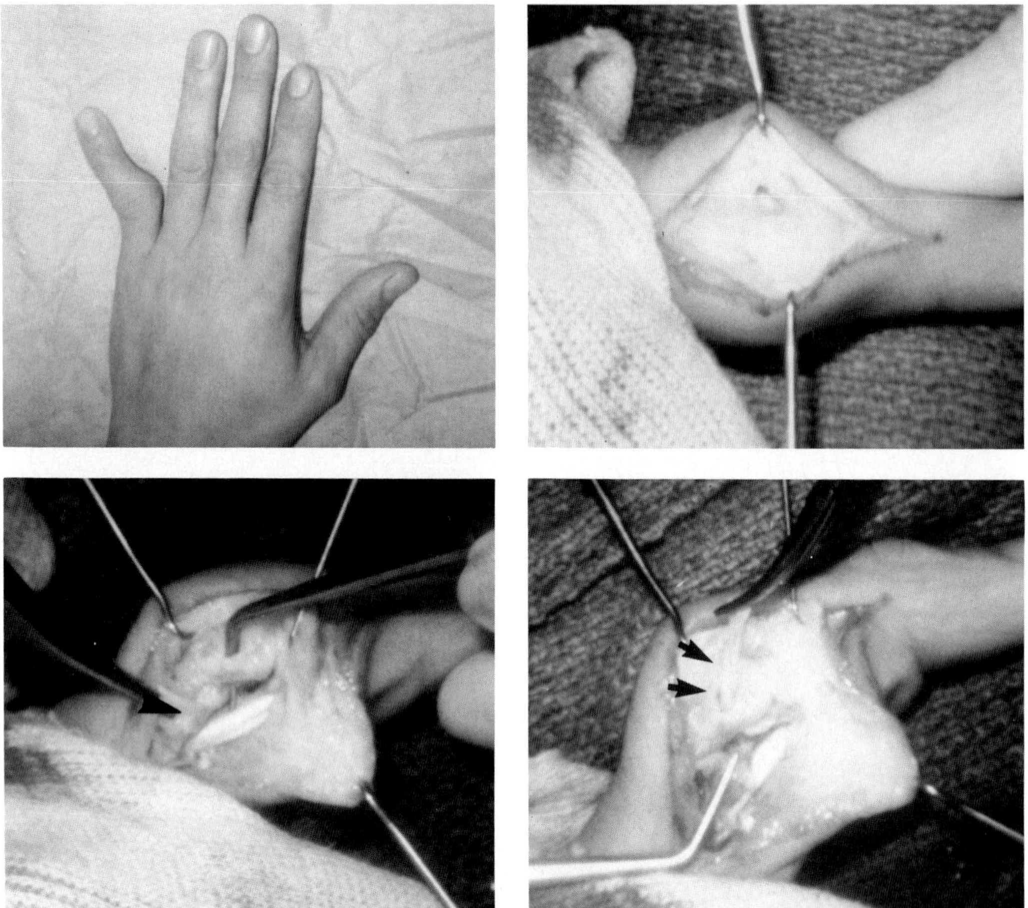

A

B

C

D

FIG. 26-34. A, Chronic lateral instability. **B,** At surgery, there was scarring of both the collateral ligament and volar plate, and neither structure was suitable to reconstruct the ligament. **C,** A hole *(probe)* was drilled in the head of the phalanx, and one slip of the flexor superficialis tendon was detached proximally *(arrow)*. **D,** The tendon was passed through the head of the phalanx and sutured into the side of the middle phalanx.

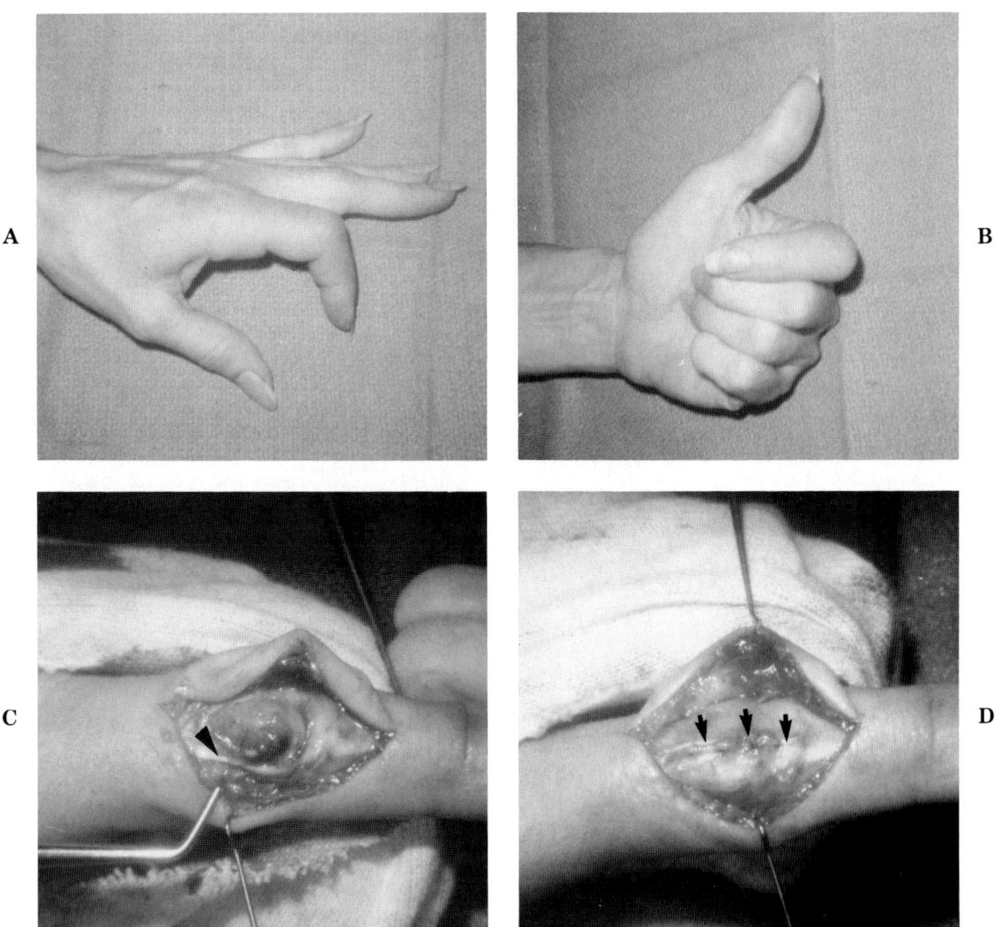

FIG. 26-35. A and **B,** This irreducible volar dislocation followed a twisting injury to the index finger. The finger was obviously malrotated. **C,** The radial collateral ligament was torn, and the radial lateral band was dislocated volar to the radial condyle of the head of the phalanx. **D,** Following reduction, the rent in the dorsal hood was repaired.

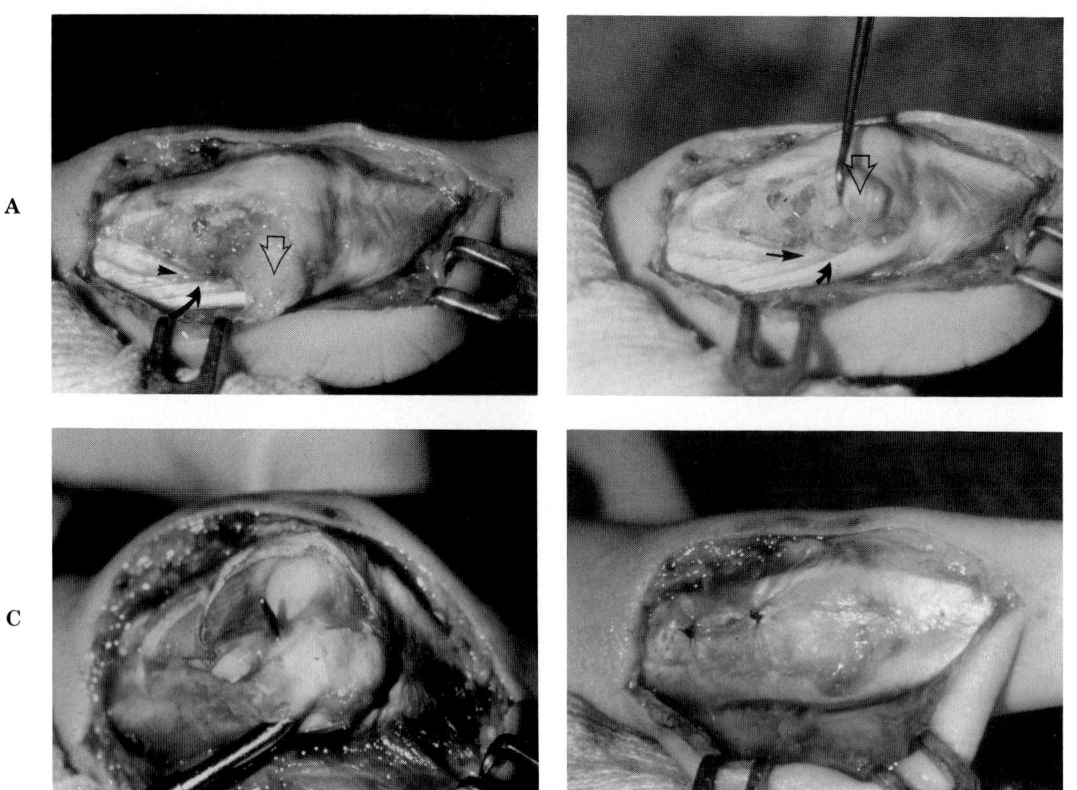

FIG. 26-36. **A** and **B,** An irreducible volar dislocation with both the central slip *(small arrow)* and radial lateral band *(large arrow)* dislocated beneath the condyle at the phalanx. The collateral ligament *(open arrow)* was torn from its insertion into the middle phalanx. **C,** The central tendon (under the probe) remained intact. **D,** After reduction, the tear between the lateral band that was not displaced and the central tendon was a sutured with fine, nonabsorbable sutures.

entrapped[90,133,137,155] (Fig. 26-36). The roentgenograms in these cases may not show a complete dislocation, as in those injuries where the central slip is torn. However, a lateral roentgenogram will show incongruity of the joint, and the proximal and middle phalanges will project differently. One of the phalanges will appear in a lateral projection whereas the other will appear slightly oblique because of the rotational deformity of the joint. Closed reduction should be attempted with the metacarpophalangeal and proximal interphalangeal joints in flexion to relax the displaced lateral band. The joint is then rotated and extended, which may allow the lateral band to slip back into its normal position.[43] If this maneuver is unsuccessful, surgery is necessary. A curved incision is made over the dorsal aspect of the joint with the apex of the incision at the midaxial line on the side where the ligament disrupted. The displaced and entrapped portion of the extensor mechanism, the lateral band, and possibly the central slip are liberated. This can usually be accomplished by use of a blunt instrument such as a dental probe. If the collateral ligament is found to have avulsed cleanly from the bone, it can be resutured. However, this is rarely the situation, and the ligament usually appears frayed. Attempting to reapproximate it with multiple sutures is likely to result in increased scarring and therefore should be avoided. The longitudinal tear in the dorsal tendon mechanism should be sutured with fine 5-0 nonabsorbable nylon sutures. Because the extensor mechanism is intact, active range of motion exercises can be started within 1 week. Paradoxically, the prognosis is far better after an irreducible dislocation that requires surgery than after a reducible volar dislocation, because in the former the extensor mechanism is displaced but not disrupted.

Dorsal Capsular Injuries

Though chronic volar instability can result from injuries to the volar plate and chronic lateral instability can result from injuries to either collateral ligament, chronic dorsal instability never occurs. Though there is a joint capsule dorsally, it is thin and ineffective as a dorsal stabilizer. The central extensor tendon, by virtue of its strength and wide insertion, functions both as the important active extensor of the joint and its dorsal ligament. If the central tendon is damaged as the result of a traumatic avulsion or laceration or if it becomes attenuated, its function as both an active extensor and a dorsal stabilizer is lost, and a boutonnière deformity develops. Dorsal instability is therefore not clinically possible.

MIDDLE PHALANX AREA

Anatomy

The middle phalanx has several distinct anatomic differences from the proximal phalanx. Besides being shorter, its volar surface is not as concave as the proximal phalanx, and its dorsal surface is flatter. The lateral crest in the shaft portion of the bone, where the slips of the flexor digitorum superficialis insert are also thicker, rougher, and wider.[154] The base of the bone is much wider than its shaft, and on its dorsal aspect is a ridge that separates the base from its articular surface. In the middle of the ridge is a prominent tubercle for attachment of the central extensor tendon. The ridge extends volarly to each side, where it ends with tubercles onto which the collateral ligaments insert. The head of the bone is similar to the configuration of the head of the proximal phalanx.

Tendon Injuries

Acute injuries to the extensor tendon mechanism in this area are rare, except for lacerations. Secondary adhesions after blunt trauma or fractures are more common. A similar paucity of closed injuries is encountered in the flexor tendons, though rare avulsions of the flexor superficialis tendon have been reported after hyperextension injuries.[23,65]

Fractures

Fractures of the middle phalanx tend to be more transverse than at the proximal phalanx.[25,139] Most fractures occur distal to the insertion of the flexor superficialis tendon, which results in flexion of the proximal fragment and extension of the distal fragment. If the fragment occurs proximal to the insertion of the superficialis but distal to the insertion of the central extensor slip, the reverse deformity occurs with extension of the proximal fragment and flexion of the distal fragment. With fractures in the middle of the bone, the angulation may be in either direction, and this may be more a result of the direction of the trauma than of the pull of the flexor superficialis tendon.[28,55] Closed reduction for these angulated fractures can usually be accomplished. If the fracture is stable, the digit is immobilized with the metacarpophalangeal joint in acute flexion and the proximal interphalangeal joint in slight flexion. Because the fractures are in the cortical diaphyseal portion of the bone, healing is slow. Though active range of motion exercises can usually be started within 2 to 3 weeks, the digit must be protected until there is roentgenographic evidence of complete healing, which may take 10 to 12 weeks or even longer. For those unstable fractures, internal fixation, usually with Kirschner pins, is required.

DISTAL INTERPHALANGEAL JOINT AREA

Anatomy

A distal interphalangeal joint is a hinge or ginglymus joint whose articular and capsular components are similar to those of a proximal interphalangeal joint, but with certain distinct variations. The head of the middle phalanx is bicondylar and fits snugly into the concave surface of the base of the distal phalanx. The condyles of the middle phalanx in the middle finger are symmetric, and the longitudinal axes for both middle and distal phalanges are in a straight line. In the index, ring, and little fingers, however, the condyles of the middle phalanges are more asymmetric in their widths, anteroposterior dimensions, and projections. The difference in condylar projections accounts for the ulnar deviation of the index finger toward the middle finger and the radial deviation of the ring and little fingers toward the middle finger seen in many individuals. Differences also exist in the extension-flexion arcs between the two interphalangeal joints. Passive hyperextension exists in the distal interphalangeal joint, but not at a proximal interphalangeal joint, and this is reflected in the distance that the cartilage over the head of the middle phalanx extends proximally. A reciprocal situation exists with flexion, which is less at a distal interphalangeal joint. This is consistent with the more limited cartilage over the volar aspect of the head of a middle phalanx as compared to the head of a proximal phalanx.[154]

With respect to the capsular structures, the "check-rein" configuration of the ligaments that tether the volar plate at a proximal interphalangeal joint is not present distally, and this permits passive joint hyperextension. The location of the insertion of the flexor profundus and superficialis tendons may explain the differences in flexion between the interphalangeal joints. The insertion of the flexor superficialis tendon is several millimeters distal to the base of the middle phalanx. When the tendon contracts, the insertion moves away from the proximal interphalangeal joint, increasing its mechanical advantage. The flexor profundus insertion, however, because of its closer proximity to the joint, does not have this advantage.[46] Dorsally, the synovium and joint capsule are in intimate contact with and virtually inseparable from the terminal extensor tendon. The insertion of the tendon is not limited to the dorsal tubercle at the base of the distal phalanx as it is with the insertion of the central tendon into the base of the middle phalanx. Rather, its insertion is over a wide area extending to the nail matrix. The skin around the joint is firmly fixed by Cleland's ligaments.

Tendon Injuries

Extensor Tendons

Acute injuries. Injuries to the terminal extensor tendon are common in athletes, particularly those who catch or hit a ball (i.e., baseball, football, basketball, and volleyball). The usual history is a ball striking the extended finger, forcing the distal interphalangeal joint into acute flexion. The vast majority of these injuries are closed and result in acute stretching or rupture of the terminal extensor tendon or its avulsion from the base of the distal phalanx, often with a small bone fragment. The patient complains of pain, swelling, and tenderness over the dorsal aspect of the joint and notices its flexed position. The deformity is frequently referred to as a "mallet" or "baseball" finger, but both terms are misnomers. The finger does not actually resemble a mallet, and numerous activities besides baseball can be responsible for the problem. A more accurate and descriptive term is "drop" finger.[1] The distal joint is flexed because of the relatively unopposed action of the flexor profundus tendon. The damaged terminal extensor tendon slides proximally, increasing the extension forces at the proximal interphalangeal joint. In loose-jointed patients, a secondary hyperextension deformity may develop at this joint. With the flexed position at the distal joint, the finger assumes a swan-neck appearance.

Treatment for the acute injury is splinting of the distal joint in extension or slight hyperextension for at least 6 weeks. Application of the splint to the dorsal aspect of the joint is usually more comfortable and functional than a splint on the volar aspect because it allows for tactile sensibility at the pulp.[123] Commercial splints are also available, but they tend to cover the volar aspect of the digit tip and may pose more of a functional impairment than a dorsally applied splint. It is important that the joint not be splinted in hyperextension, which causes the dorsal skin to blanch because of the risk of causing an ulcer. This is more likely to occur immediately after the injury, when there may be considerable swelling. It is important that the joint be maintained in extension at *all* times. The patient should be seen periodically to check for any skin irritation. When the splint is changed, the joint is maintained in an extended position. The cooperative and reliable patient can be instructed in the technique of changing the splint without allowing the distal joint to inadvertently flex. The proximal interphalangeal joint is not immobilized and should be exercised to prevent stiffness. After 6 weeks, the splint is removed several times each day for active range of motion exercises and the splint can be discontinued after another 2 to 3 weeks.

Occasionally, it may be an unrealistic burden for a patient to maintain an extension splint for the many weeks necessary for effective treatment, (e.g., a surgeon). In these situations, a Kirschner pin can be drilled across the joint to maintain it in full extension, and the patient can resume most of his activities.[71]

Surgery is reserved for injuries in which there is an open laceration[51,175] or a fracture with the distal phalanx volarly subluxed.[39,191] Subluxations with fractures are likely to occur when the dorsal fragment is large. In these situations, the loss not only involves the dorsal support of the extensor tendon, but also the lateral support provided by both collateral ligaments, which remain attached to the dorsal fragment. Surgery is not indicated solely on the basis of the size of the dorsal fragment or the distance of its displacement; in the absence of any subluxation, surgery should be avoided. The operation is technically difficult and involves potential complications such as scarring of the matrix with nail deformity and joint stiffness. Even displaced avulsion fractures heal with satisfactory remodeling of the articular surface (Fig. 26-37). A dorsal beak may persist in these cases but is rarely symptomatic. With subluxations of the distal phalanx, however, there is no alternative but to reduce the joint and transfix it with a Kirschner pin. If the avulsed fragment is large, it can also be stabilized with a pin.

A "drop" finger can also be caused by a

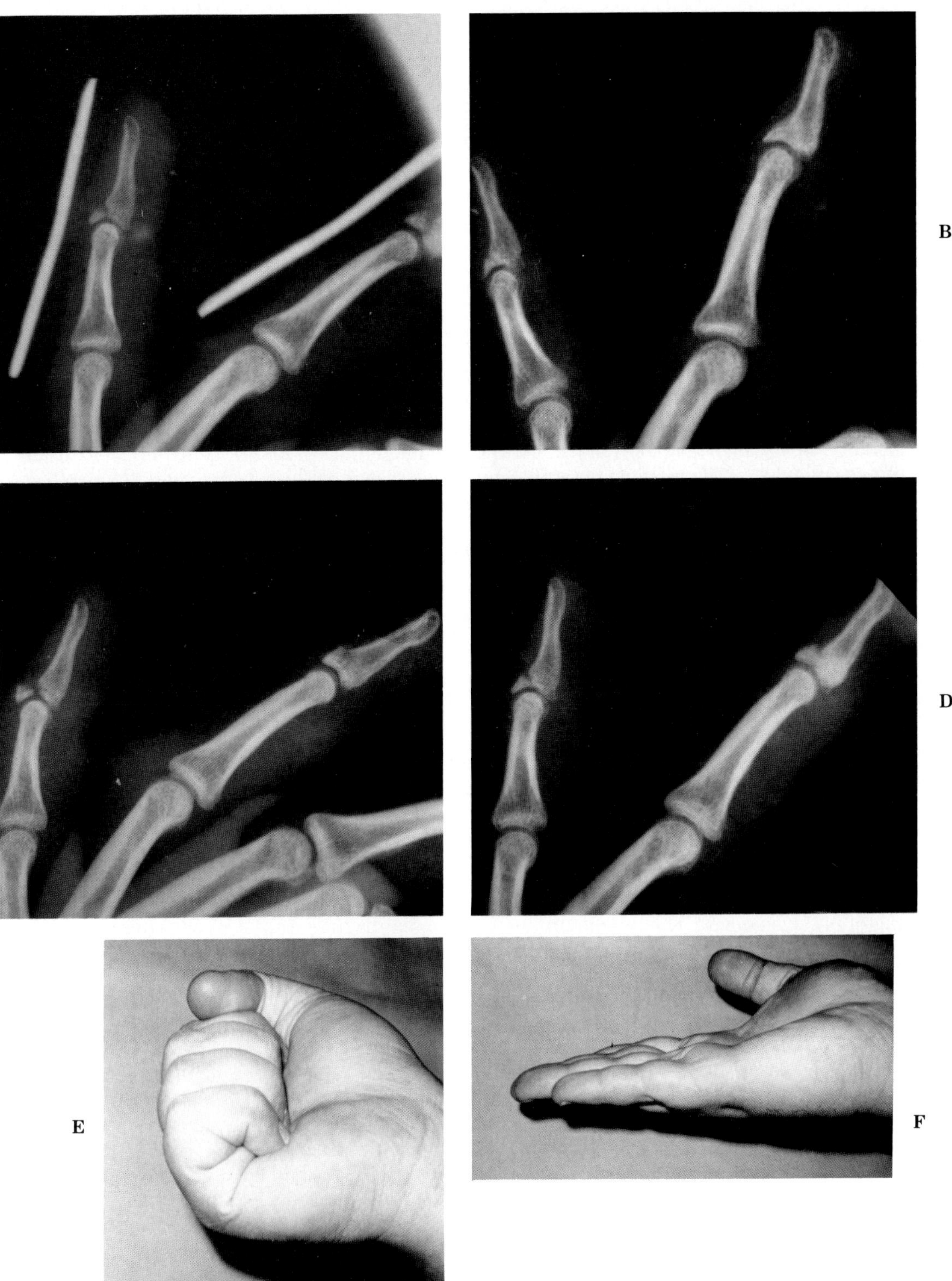

FIG. 26-37. A and **B,** "Drop" ring and little fingers with avulsion fractures of the distal phalanges were treated by dorsal extension splints. Surgery was necessary since neither injured phalanx was volarly subluxed. **C,** At 6 weeks, the fractures were beginning to heal. **D,**The fractures had completely healed at 12 weeks. **E** and **F,** The patient regained complete mobility of both fingers.

forced hyperextension injury to the distal joint that fractures the dorsal base of the distal phalanx. Surgery is often necessary for these rare injuries, because the fracture fragment usually exceeds 50% of the articular surface. More importantly, the intact portion of the bone is often subluxed volarly.[109]

Chronic injuries. Frequently, the patient with an injury to the extensor tendon neglects to seek medical attention for weeks and sometimes months after the injury. If the delay is a few weeks, extension splinting should still be used if there is no joint subluxation. In more chronic cases, extension splinting will be of no benefit. If the deformity does not cause disability, no treatment is necessary. If the deformity interferes with function and passive extension of the joint remains intact, reconstruction of the terminal extensor tendon may be feasible. Tenotomy of the central extensor tendon at the proximal interphalangeal joint has also been recommended, but such a procedure jeopardizes mobility at a joint where mobility is more important than at the originally injured joint.[18,75] If the distal interphalangeal joint is chronically subluxed or arthritic changes have developed, arthrodesis is indicated.

Flexor Tendons

Acute injuries. Avulsion of the flexor profundus tendon is the result of violent overstretching of a tendon whose muscle is contracting against resistance. These injuries typically occur in young adult male athletes who participate in sports such as football and rugby in which there is grabbing and clutching of one's opponent. The athlete, in an attempt to stop his opponent, forcefully grasps the opponent's jersey. As the opponent struggles to free himself, the injured athlete's finger becomes caught in the jersey and is suddenly extended. Though any finger can be injured in this way, the ring finger is most commonly involved. Various theories concerning the propensity for injury to this finger have been proposed and include the limited independent flexion of the ring finger resulting from the common muscle belly of the profundi[76]; the weakness of the insertion of the profundus into the distal phalanx of the ring finger as compared to the middle finger[115]; the arrangement of the interconnections between the extensor tendons, the juncturae tendinae, which limit independent extension of the ring finger[110,111]; and that with grasp the ring finger is "longest" and therefore the most vulnerable to injury.[29] Frequently, the seriousness of the injury is not immediately apparent to the athlete because there is no obvious deformity as in extensor tendon injury. Though there is pain, swelling, and often ecchymoses along the tendon sheath, the athlete is unaware of the loss of flexion at the distal joint. The diagnosis can also be missed by the physician who does not specifically test for function of the flexor profundus tendon. Roentgenograms may show radiopacity if the tendon avulsed with a bone fragment from the base of the distal fragment. The ruptured tendon usually retracts to the level of the proximal interphalangeal flexion crease or even into the palm, where further retraction is prevented by the tethering effect of the lumbrical muscle (Fig. 26-38). If the tendon avulses with a large fragment, it is usually caught at the level of the A-4 pulley, preventing further proximal retraction of the tendon[109] (Fig. 26-39). However, an avulsion associated with a large bone fragment to which the tendon was no longer attached and had retracted to an even more proximal level has been reported.[108] Avulsions associated with fractures of the distal phalanx have also been reported.[168]

Surgery is necessary for all acute ruptures of the flexor profundus tendon. If there is marked swelling and ecchymoses, the operation should be deferred until the soft tissue reaction to the injury subsides. Elevation and warm soaks will hasten the process, and the operation can usually be performed within 1 week. Any further delay should be avoided, because a secondary contracture of the muscle belly will develop, precluding the possibility of reinsertion of the tendon.

Chronic injuries. A profundus avulsion that is not diagnosed until weeks after the injury may still be reinserted depending on its level of retraction. The greater the distance of retraction, the greater the contracture of the muscle belly and the less likelihood of repair. The ideal situation would be a profundus avulsion that remains in proximity to the distal interphalangeal joint, tethered by an intact vinculum breve. This would be unusual, because the vinculum breve usually tears with the profundus and the tendon retracts at least to the level of the proximal interphalangeal joint, where it becomes adherent to the two slips of the flexor superficialis tendon. A tendolysis is necessary to mobilize the profundus and assess the degree of secondary muscle contracture. The tendon end is grasped with a straight clamp and traction is placed on it in an attempt to bring it to the base of the distal phalanx. This test should be carried out with the wrist in neutral position and the digit in extension (Fig. 26-40). If the tendon can-

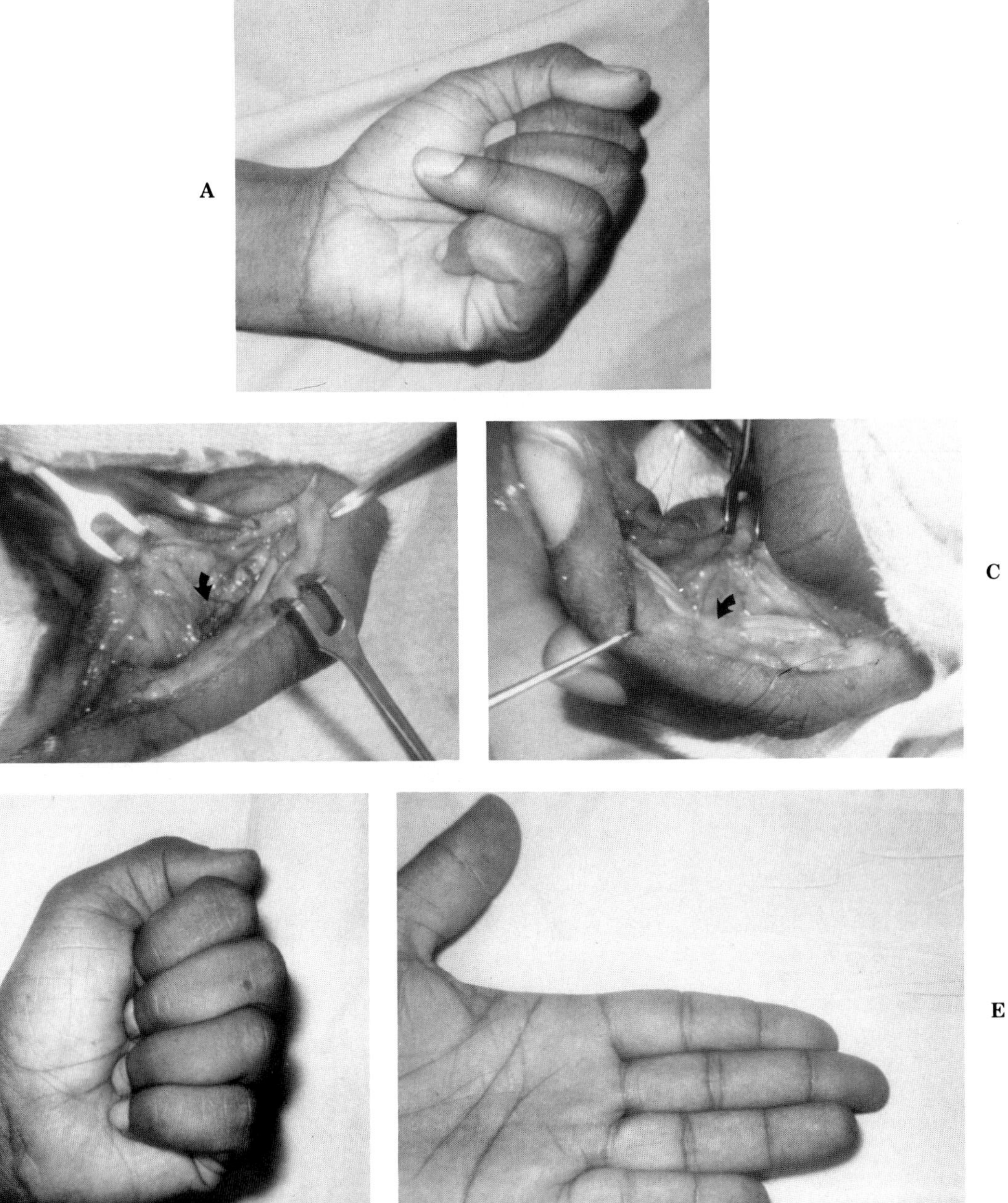

FIG. 26-38. A, Rupture of the flexor profundus tendon in the ring finger of a football player. **B,** The tendon avulsed from its insertion and retracted to the level of the proximal interphalangeal joint *(arrow)*. **C,** The tendon was reinserted into the distal phalanx using a pull-out wire suture. The A-4 pulley *(arrow)* was preserved. **D** and **E,** Postoperative mobility.

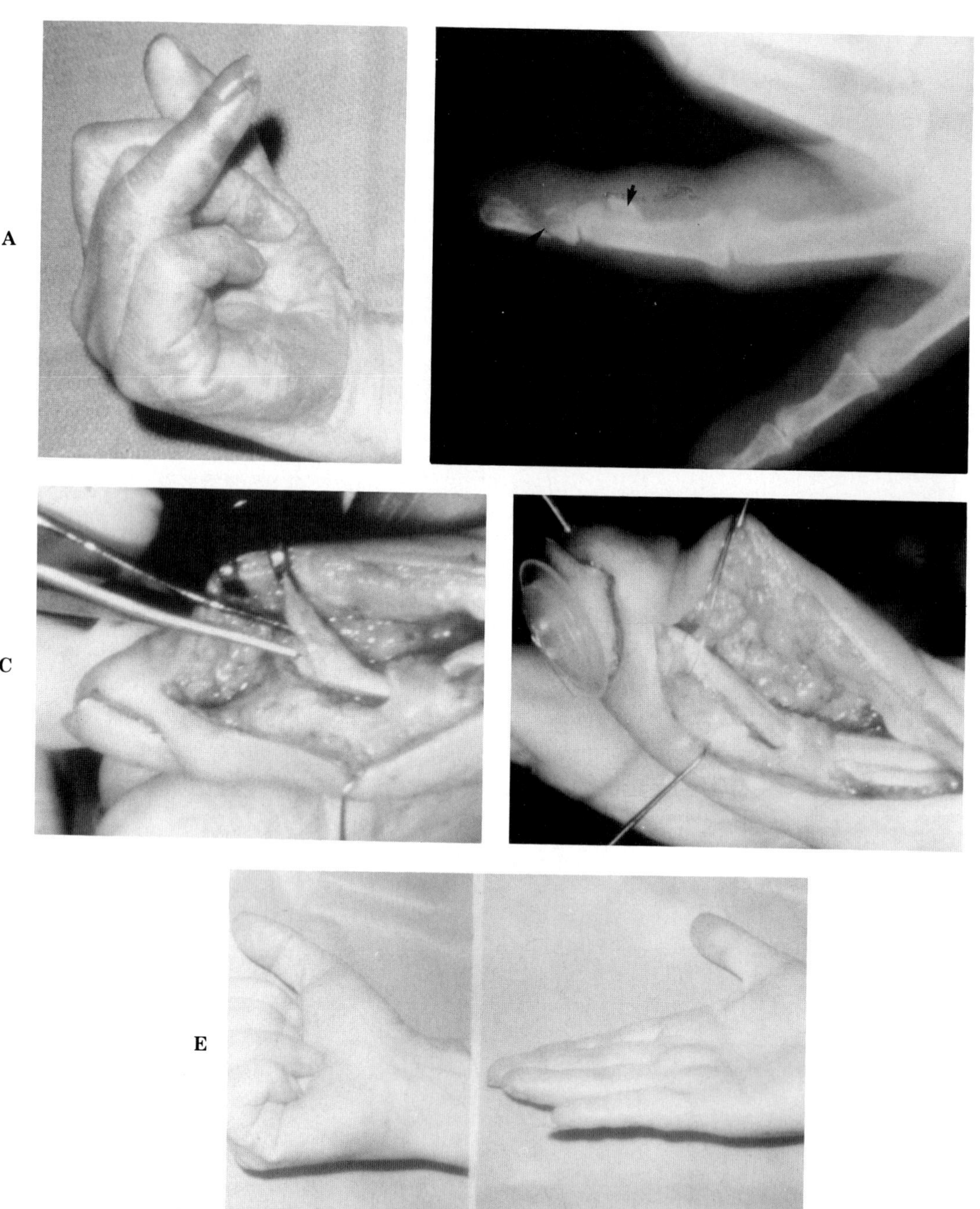

FIG. 26-39. **A,** Avulsion of the flexor profundus tendon, which also limited flexion at the proximal interphalangeal joint. **B,** Roentgenograms showed an avulsion fracture *(small arrow)* as well as a fracture of the distal phalanx *(arrow)*. **C,** At surgery, the forceps is grasping the bone fragment with its attached flexor profundus tendon. **D,** The bone fragment and tendon were reattached with a pull-out wire suture and a Kirschner pin was inserted to stabilize the distal phalanx. **E,** Postoperative mobility.

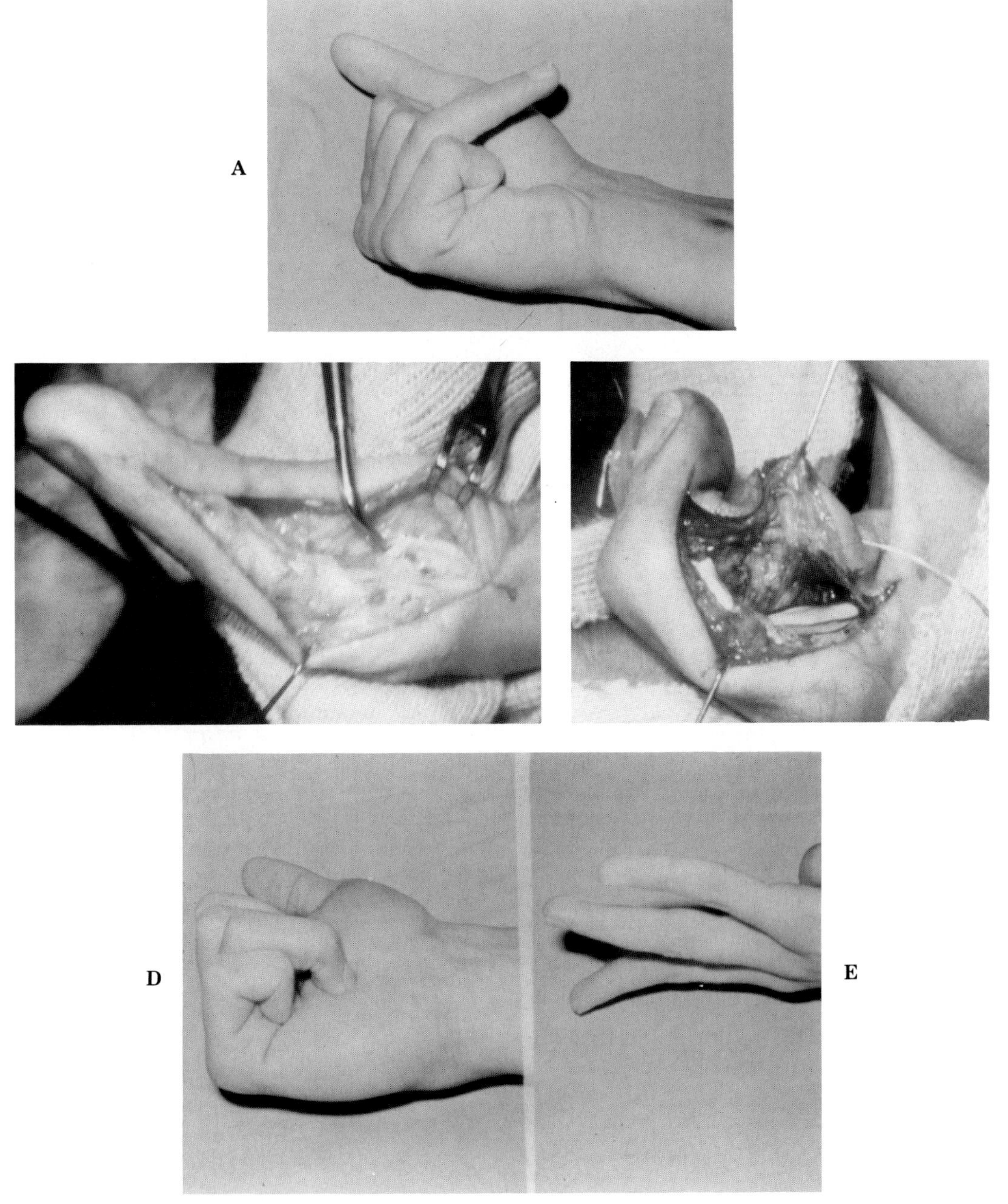

FIG. 26-40. A, A flexor profundus rupture in a 16-year-old. The injury was untreated for 4 weeks. **B,** At surgery, the profundus tendon retracted to the level of the proximal interphalangeal joint *(probe)*. **C,** Some contracture of the muscle had occurred, but because it was not severe and the patient was young, the tendon was reinserted into the distal phalanx. The finger was in considerable flexion after the reattachment. **D,** A dynamic extension splint was required after the eighth postoperative week to correct a flexion contracture. **E,** The patient ultimately regained good mobility.

not be advanced, a contracture of its muscle must be considered. Reinsertion of the tendon under such circumstances might be technically possible by flexing the wrist and fingers enough to relax the muscle-tendon unit; however, this would result in a severe flexion contracture of the digit. If the avulsed profundus has retracted to the base of the digit or into the palm and the injury is of longer standing than a few weeks, a secondary muscle contracture is even more likely. It is difficult to determine the level of tendon retraction before surgery unless the avulsion is accompanied by a bone fragment that is visualized on a lateral roentgenogram.

Treatment for the chronic case in which repair of the avulsed tendon is no longer possible depends on the degree of functional impairment. For the patient who has normal mobility at the proximal interphalangeal joint and is asymptomatic, no treatment is necessary. If, however, there is volar instability of the distal joint or the loss of terminal joint flexion interferes with grasp, surgery is warranted. The most predictable procedure is an arthrodesis. Resection of the retracted profundus may be indicated at the same time if a tender lump representing the end of the tendon persists in the digit or palm. In certain situations, a flexor tendon graft, either as a single[117] or staged procedure[82] can be considered. Tendon graft in the presence of an intact flexor superficialis tendon is a difficult procedure and has the potential to compromise normal mobility at the proximal interphalangeal joint. Therefore the procedure should be reserved for young patients[70,176] or for well-motivated adults, such as musicians, who require active flexion of their distal interphalangeal joint and clearly understand the risks.[110]

Ligament Injuries

Dislocations of the distal interphalangeal joints are far less common than those of the proximal interphalangeal joints. The greater stability at the distal joint is the result of its strong collateral ligaments, the adjacent insertions of the flexor and extensor tendons, and the much shorter lever arm of the distal phalanx.[46] When a dislocation does occur, it is either lateral or dorsal, and it is often compound because of the density of the cutaneous ligaments that firmly anchor the skin to the underlying structures. Reduction can usually be achieved by closed manipulation using digital block anesthesia. If the skin is torn, local debridement, irrigation, and antibiotics are required. Occasionally, when the dislocation is irreducible as a result of entrapment of the volar plate,[143] flexor tendon,[148] or an osteochondral fracture fragment,[182] surgery is required. Following reduction by either closed or open measures, the joint is stable. Immobilization need not exceed 2 weeks. Chronic instability is a rare complication.

Fractures

Fractures of the distal phalanges are common and usually result from crushing injuries. Unless the crush is severe, these fractures are rarely displaced, because there are no tendons spanning the bone to deform it. In addition, the phalanx is normally stabilized by the nail dorsally and the fibrous septa in the pulp tissue volarly.[27] Treatment is primarily directed to the soft tissue component of the injury. A subungual hematoma is often present. If the pain is severe, usually described as "pounding" or "throbbing," it can be quickly relieved by draining the hematoma. The simplest, most effective, and most painless method is using the end of a straightened paper clip, heated by a flame until it is red hot, to burn a hole through the nail. Aseptic technique with preliminary cleansing of the nail is important, because the hole alters any closed fracture of the underlying phalanx into an open one. There may also be hemorrhage into the pulp tissue on the volar aspect of the digit tip. If the swelling is severe it can be partially decompressed with multiple puncture wounds made by a needle. A splint is used primarily for symptomatic relief of pain rather than bone stabilization and therefore can be confined to the distal segment of the finger.

In those rare fractures which are displaced, the nail matrix may become interposed between the fracture fragments, resulting in later deformity of the nail and possibly a nonunion. These complications can be avoided by repairing the nail matrix with fine absorbable sutures. Kirschner pin fixation is required only if the soft tissue support of the bone has been lost.

In the young patient whose epiphyseal plate is still open, acute flexion force on the distal joint is more likely to cause a fracture through the plate than an avulsion of the extensor tendon. Though the injury clinically resembles a "drop" finger deformity, there is a transverse fracture through the base of the distal phalanx. These are compound injuries, because the proximal portion of the nail slips out from under the eponychium and lies superficial to it, preventing reduction. Reduction can usually be accomplished by slightly hyperextending the joint and then replacing the nail under the eponychium.[166,194] In chronic cases, it may be necessary to resect the proximal portion of the nail and use internal fixation.

Thumb

CARPOMETACARPAL (TRAPEZIOMETACARPAL) JOINT AREA

Anatomy

The trapeziometacarpal or basal joint of the thumb has often been referred to as a "saddle" joint because of the configuration of its articular surface, which is concave in its radioulnar dimension and convex in its volar-dorsal dimension.[147] The articular surface of the base of the metacarpal has a reciprocal concave-convex configuration, and together the two joint surfaces resemble opposed saddles.[104] If these two saddles had deep congruous surfaces, the joint would be capable of only flexion, extension, abduction, and adduction, but not rotation. The joint would be similar to a western-type saddle, whose deep seat formed by the horn in front and high cantle in the rear permit the rider to move in essentially two planes, forward and backward and side to side. Rotational movements are prevented by the deep contour of the seat and the rider's intimate contact with it. To rotate, the rider must lift his buttocks off the seat by pressing down with his feet on the stirrups. In the trapeziometacarpal joint, the articular surfaces are neither deep nor perfectly congruous (Fig. 26-41). Rather, they resemble the English-type saddle, whose low contours permit the rider not only to move forward and backward and side to side, but also to rotate.

Rotation at the trapeziometacarpal joint, whether pronation or supination, is facilitated not only by the shallow contours of the articular surfaces, but also by the laxity of the joint capsule[160] (Fig. 26-42). Pronation or opposition occurs as the longitudinal axis of the metacarpal rotates 20 to 30 degrees from the corresponding axis of the fixed trapezium.[48] Though the joint capsule permits mobility, it also provides for stability. The relative importance of its component ligaments for this latter function is controversial. At the base of the metacarpal is a prominent beak which, when the joint is in neutral position, faces the distal portion of the ridge of the trapezium. Anchoring these two bony prominences is a stout ligament referred to by a variety of terms including the "ulnar ligament,"[160] "anterior oblique ligament,"[135] or simply "volar ligament." "Volar ligament" is probably the most appropriate name, because it accurately describes the position of the ligament in its relationship to the thumb. Laterally the joint capsule is thin, but dorsally it thickens into the posterior oblique ligament which, together with the volar ligament, has an important role in joint stability.[77] In flexion and opposition, the volar beak of the metacarpal is in close contact with the trapezium, but in

A

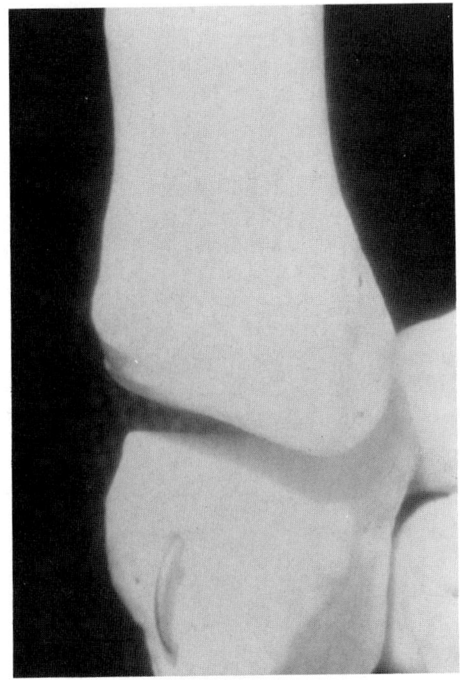

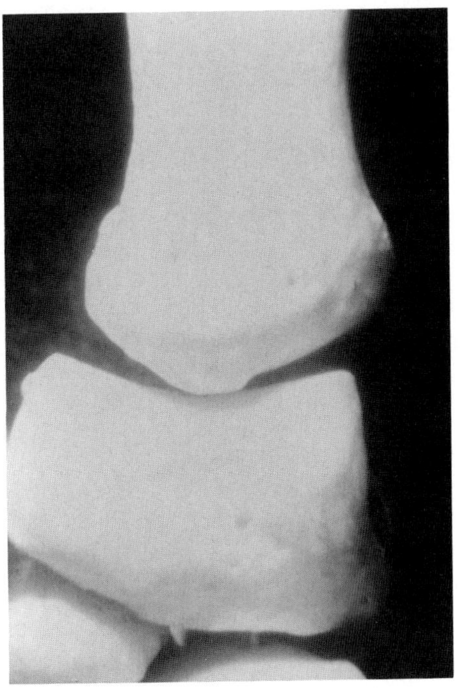

B

FIG. 26-41. Views of a trapeziometacarpal joint. **A,** Volar. **B,** Dorsal.

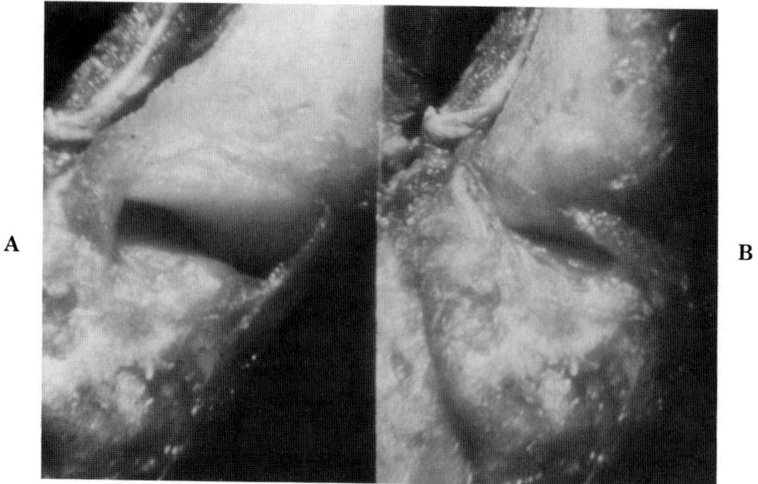

FIG. 26-42. Laxity of the joint capsule permits rotation. **A,** Supination. **B,** Pronation.

abduction and extension it is slightly elevated and pulls away from the trapezium. Further retraction of the metacarpal is prevented by the volar ligament. The importance of these anatomic features will be discussed in the section on treatment for Bennett's fractures.

Muscle-Tendon Injuries

Acute closed injuries to the extrinsic tendons or intrinsic muscles are rare at the level of the trapeziometacarpal joint. A chronic strain resulting in deQuervain's tenosynovitis at the wrist level can also affect the abductor pollicis longus more distally, causing pain, swelling, and tenderness at its insertion into the base of the first metacarpal.

Ligament Injuries

Acute Injuries

Acute traumatic dislocation of a trapeziometacarpal joint is an unusual injury that has been referred to as a "Bennett's fracture without a fracture."[132] This may be inaccurate, because, though a displaced Bennett's fracture is invariably unstable after reduction, a dislocation may be quite stable.[190] Treatment for the dislocation that is stable after reduction is immobilization with a thumb spica cast for several weeks. For dislocations that remain unstable after reduction, there is some controversy concerning the nature of the pathology and treatment. Some believe that the volar ligament is invariably torn,[47] whereas others report that the volar ligament remains intact, but the dorsal capsule is disrupted.[167] Regardless of the particular ligament that is injured, the preferred treatment is reduction followed by stabilization by percutaneous insertion of one or two Kirschner pins. The pins are maintained for a minimum of 6 weeks. The objective of such treatment is for sufficient scarring to develop at the site of the capsular tear to prevent later joint laxity or instability. An indication for surgery for the acute injury is if the base of the metacarpal cannot be anatomically reduced, which would indicate interposition of ligamentous tissue.[43] If surgery is required and the volar ligament is found to have been disrupted, repair is difficult if not impossible because of the short length and relative inaccessibility of the ligament. A new ligament must be reconstructed, and the most predictable technique is to use a strip of the flexor carpi radialis tendon.[49] The trapeziometacarpal joint is visualized through a curved incision extending from the ulnar border of the first metacarpal around the base of the thumb into the thenar crease of the palm. Care must be taken to avoid damaging the sensory branches of the radial and musculocutaneous nerves and the palmar cutaneous branch of the median nerve. The thenar muscles are detached from their origins and mobilized distally. The lateral capsule is incised and the joint surfaces inspected. A drill hole is made in the base of the metacarpal in a dorsal-to-volar direction, with the drill point emerging at the volar beak of the bone. The hole is gradually enlarged using progressively larger-sized drills. The flexor carpi radialis tendon is then exposed through several small transverse incisions along its course in the distal forearm. The tendon is split longitudinally, and one half of its diameter is divided approximately 6 cm proximal to the wrist flexion crease. To mobilize and split the tendon in its more distal portion, the sheath covering its passage under the crest of the trapezium must be divided. Care must be taken in splitting the tendon in this location because its distal insertion must be maintained. This part of the operation is facilitated by adequate surgical exposure and by palmar flexion of the wrist, which relaxes the tendon. The detached half of the tendon is now passed through the hole in the metacarpal in a volar-to-dorsal direction. A suture is placed into the end of the tendon, and the suture is passed through the eye of a large curved needle that was inserted into the hole in a retrograde fashion. As the needle is withdrawn, the suture is carried through the hole as well. Traction on the suture pulls the tendon through the bone. The metacarpal is then reduced and stabilized to the adjacent trapezium with a thin nonthreaded Kirschner pin, avoiding spearing of the tendon that is running through the bone. The tendon that emerges on the dorsal aspect of the metacarpal is then passed deep to the abductor pollicis longus and sutured to the dorsal and lateral portions of the capsule. It can also be passed around the intact portion of the flexor carpi radialis and back up to the metacarpal and sutured to its periosteum. The thenar muscles are reattached and a plaster splint applied, immobilizing the thumb and wrist. After 4 weeks, the pin is removed and active range of motion exercises are started. These exercises are carried out three to four times daily, the splint being worn at all other times. After an additional week, the splint is discontinued and the frequency of exercises is increased. Active resistive exercises to restore extrinsic and intrinsic muscle strength are begun in the sixth or seventh week.

Chronic Injuries

For acute dislocations that remain unstable after closed reduction and immobilization or for cases of chronic laxity with no secondary arthritic changes, reconstruction of a volar ligament by the same technique described in the previous section is required (Fig. 26-43). If arthritis has developed, arthroplasty or arthrodesis would be indicated.

Fractures

Fractures of the first metacarpal have two features that distinguish them from fractures of the other metacarpals: their potential to cause an adduction contracture of the web space and the greater importance of maintaining or restoring stability for the trapeziometacarpal joint as compared to the carpometacarpal joints of the fingers.[185] Two important fractures occur at the base of the first metacarpal, and both are intraarticular: Bennett's fracture and Rolando's fracture.

Bennett's Fracture

In the latter part of the nineteenth century, Edward Bennett described an oblique intraarticular fracture of the first metacarpal.[10] The fracture results in a subluxation or dislocation as the articular surface of the bone splits, separating the main portion of the metacarpal from its volar beak. The beak remains in place by the intact volar ligament, but the metacarpal shaft is displaced radially and dorsally by the pull of the abductor pollicis longus tendon. The dislocation component of the injury is far more important than the size of the volar fragment. If the dislocation is not accurately reduced, malunion with persistent subluxation of the joint will occur, ultimately leading to secondary arthritic changes and significant disability with pain and weakness. A careful roentgenographic examination to determine the presence of any articular incongruity is therefore the first essential step in the treatment of these fractures. Tomograms may also be required if conventional roentgenograms do not adequately visualize the articular surfaces of the metacarpal and trapezium.

A variety of treatments for a Bennett's fracture have been proposed, including closed manipulation and cast immobilization,[142,149] closed reduction, and Kirschner pin fixation between the first and second metacarpals[89] or across the trapeziometacarpal joint. Stabilization of the joint is accomplished by either inserting the pin at the base of the metacarpal[189] or intramedullarly through the head of the metacarpal and across into the trapezium.[193] Transfixion of the fracture fragment itself has also been proposed,[165] as has skeletal traction.[173] In most cases, an accurate reduction can be obtained by manipulation and percutaneous fixation of the joint with one or two Kirschner pins. Transfixion of the small fracture fragment should be avoided because of the risk of causing it to rotate or shift in position as the pin is drilled into the bone. Choosing the proper method of reduction is essential, because the thumb must be held in the position that permits the most accurate alignment of the fracture fragments. As mentioned in the section on anatomy, the volar beak of the metacarpal normally pulls away from its contiguous trapezial articular surface with abduction and extension. Further retraction is prevented by the volar ligament, a restraint that is lost after a Bennett's fracture. Therefore placing the thumb in this position to reduce the fracture has the opposite effect,

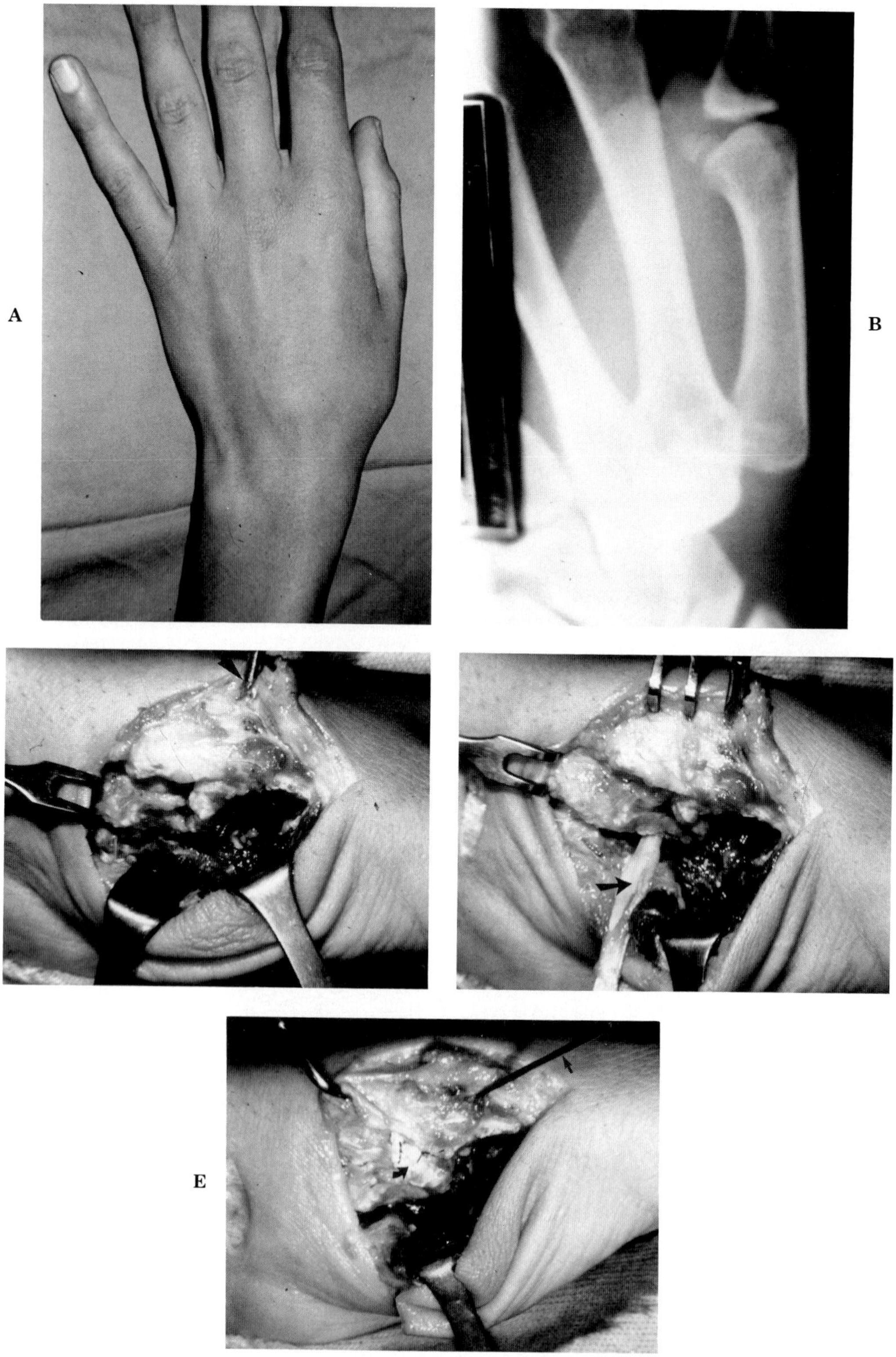

A B C D E

FIG. 26-43. A and **B,** Chronic instability of the trapeziometacarpal joint. The roentgenogram shows radial subluxation of the metacarpal base with irregularity at its volar beak. **C,** A drill hole was made going from dorsal to volar with the drill tip *(arrow)* emerging near the volar beak. **D,** The flexor carpi radialis tendon *(arrow)* was split for a distance of approximately 8 cm, and one half of its diameter was divided proximally. Its distal insertion was maintained. **E,** The tendon *(arrow)* is passed through the hole in the metacarpal going from volar to dorsal and then brought around to be sutured to the capsule. A Kirschner pin *(arrow)* was inserted to stabilize the trapeziometacarpal joint in its reduced postion.

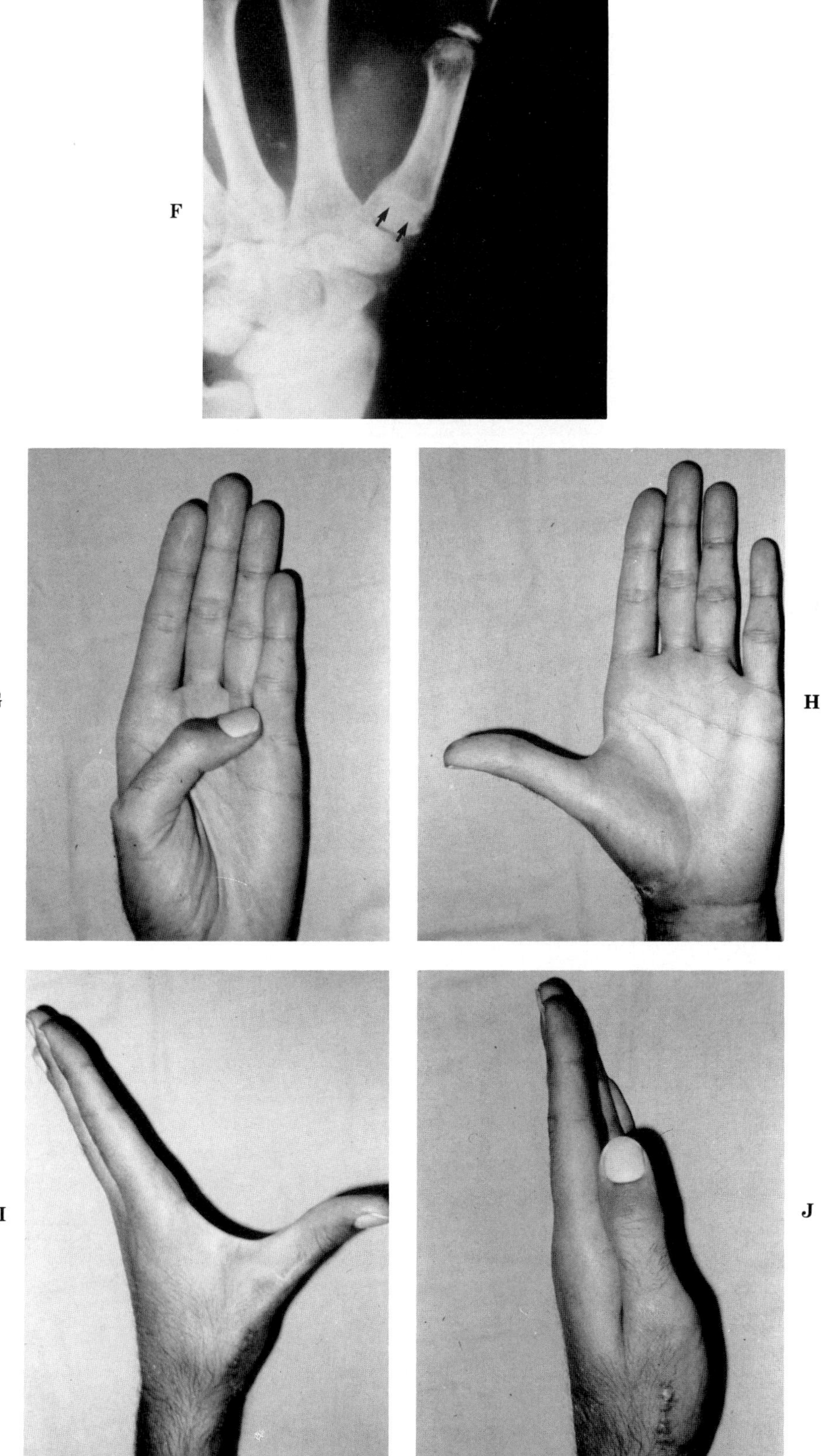

FIG. 26-43, cont'd. F, A postoperative roentgenogram shows the outline of the hole in the base of the metacarpal. **G** to **J,** Stability was restored, and the patient regained complete mobility.

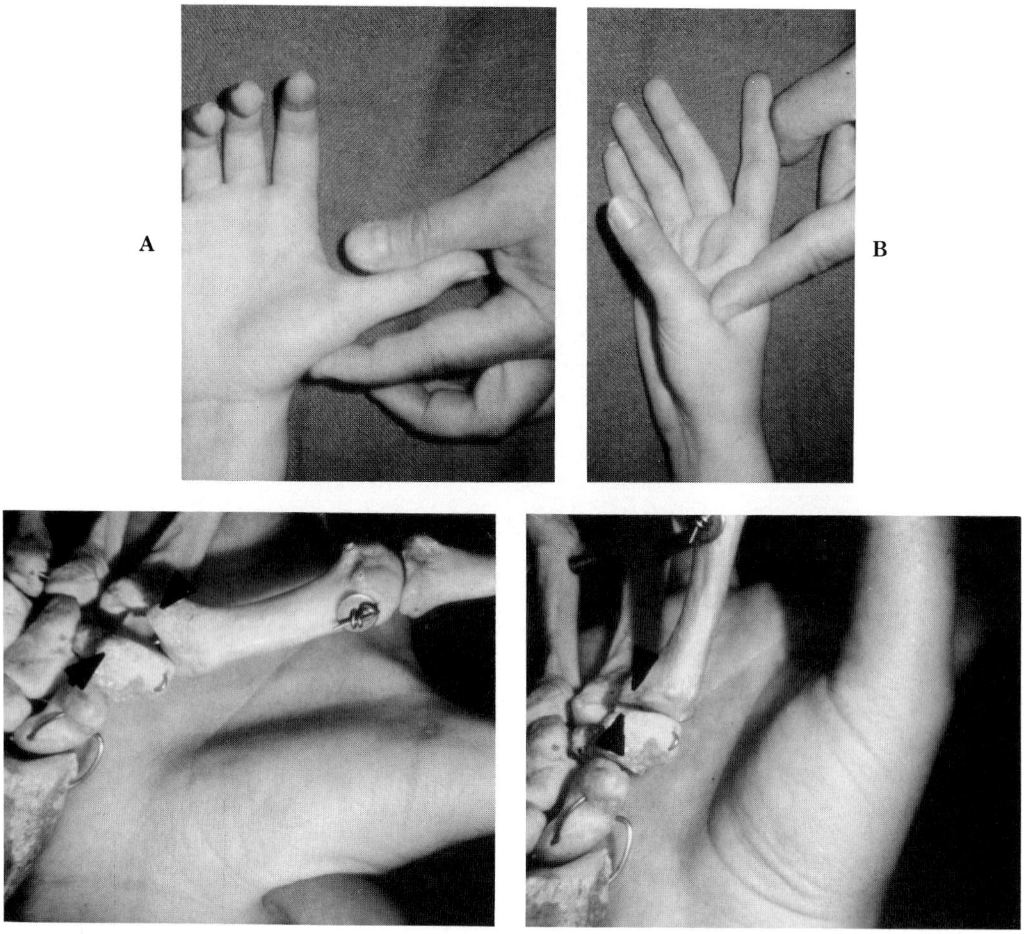

A

B

C

D

FIG. 26-44. Incorrect and correct methods of reducing a Bennett's fracture. **A,** Extension (incorrect). **B,** Pronation (correct). **C,** In extension, the volar beak of the base of the metacarpal is distracted from the trapezium. **D,** In opposition, the articular surfaces of the metacarpal and trapezium are in close contact with each other.

and the tendency is for the fracture to distract even further. The metacarpal must be held in flexion and opposition, because in this position the volar beak of the bone fits snugly into the corresponding surface of the trapezium[160] (Fig. 26-44). If an accurate reduction cannot be obtained and articular incongruity persists, operative reduction is necessary.[62] Internal fixation is usually provided by Kirschner pins, though a small cortical screw can also be used if the fracture fragment is of ample size (Fig. 26-45).

Rolando's Fracture

Rolando's fracture is another type of intra-articular fracture at the base of the metacarpal. In its classic presentation, Rolando's fracture has a T- or Y-shaped configuration. These fractures tend to be more comminuted than Bennett's fractures and are therefore usually more serious. When the comminution is severe, skeletal traction may be the only feasible method of treatment.[63,186] The traction, provided by a single Kirschner pin inserted into the metacarpal in an oblique direction going from distal and ulnar to proximal and radial, exerts two forces of pull on the fracture. One force is longitudinal, which corrects the varus deformity and restores articular congruity. Occasionally, these fractures are impacted, and cancellous bone grafting may be required to restore satisfactory reduction.[92]

METACARPAL AREA

Anatomy

Effective hand function depends to a large measure on the ability of the thumb to oppose. The importance of its capacity to face the other fingers was recognized by Hippocrates, who referred to the thumb as the "anti-hand."[195] The anatomic structures responsible for this function include the trapeziometacar-

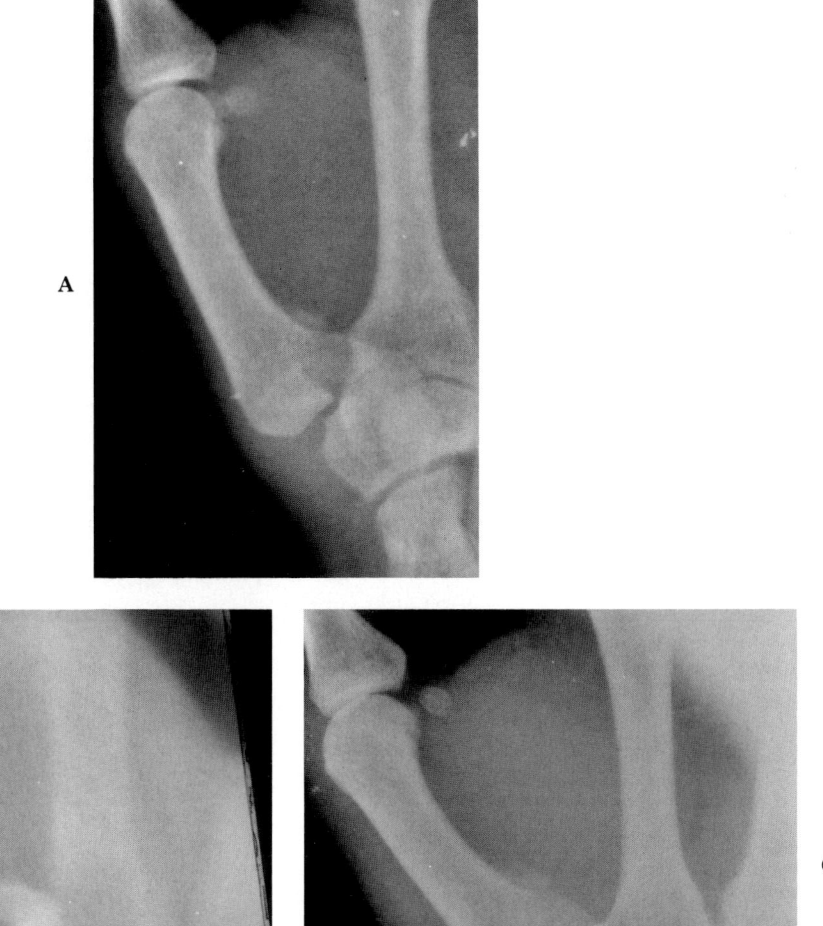

FIG. 26-45. A, A Bennett's fracture that was untreated for 2 weeks. **B,** Tomograms were obtained to more clearly visualize the incongruity at the fracture site. **C,** An open reduction was required, and the fracture was internally fixed with a Kirschner pin.

pal joint, at which the circumduction movement occurs, and the intrinsic muscles that power this movement. These muscles almost totally encircle the first metacarpal and, except for a narrow area along the dorsal aspect of the bone, form a muscular sleeve for it.

Muscle/Tendon Injuries

Muscle strains are commonly thought to be confined to the larger muscles in the arm and forearm. Such injuries are seen in sports requiring lifting, pushing, throwing, or the use of racquets. These same activities can also affect the intrinsic muscles of the hand, most notably the intrinsics of the thumb. As the demand on these muscles exceeds their ability to function effectively, the muscles fatigue. Such problems may be seen in the individual who forcefully grips his racquet without ever relaxing his grip, even when not hitting the ball. It can also occur in the individual who tightly grips a pen while writing for extended periods and in musicians who practice continuously for many hours. An analogous, if exaggerated, situation for the muscles in the lower extremity would be the long-distance runner who attempted to run two marathons within days of each other, a feat that would almost certainly result in severe muscle strains. As with any acute strain, cessation of the activity and rest are the essential first steps in treatment. Application of cold compresses may also help to limit soft tissue swelling. Effective and prompt treatment of the relatively benign acute strain will lessen the risk of a chronic condition, in which recovery is more difficult and disability more prolonged.

Fractures

Fractures of the first metacarpal account for 25% of metacarpal fractures, second only to fractures of the fifth metacarpal.[62,146] The vast majority of thumb metacarpal fractures are intraarticular and the two most important varieties, Bennett's and Rolando's fractures, have already been discussed. Extraarticular fractures are usually less problematic, and when they are at the base of the bone they tend to be transversely oriented. Most are radially angulated with the distal fragment adducted and supinated.[27] If the angulation does not exceed 20%, there is rarely any functional impairment because of the wide range of mobility at the adjacent trapeziometacarpal joint. For more severely angulated fractures, reduction is required. This can usually be accomplished by closed measures involving abduction and pronation of the distal fragment. Occasionally the angulation will have a greater effect on limiting extension of the thumb rather than its abduction. Some individuals compensate for this problem by hyperextending their metacarpophalangeal joint. Extraarticular fractures can also be obliquely oriented where there is a propensity for shortening. The distal shaft fragment may actually impinge on the dorsoradial margin of the trapezium, which requires open reduction and Kirschner pin fixation.[146] In the skeletally immature individual, a fracture can involve the proximal metaphyseal epiphyseal plate. They are usually Salter-Harris type II fractures, which respond well to closed reduction and immobilization.[139]

METACARPOPHALANGEAL JOINT AREA

Anatomy

The metacarpophalangeal joint of the thumb is a condyloid joint, like its counterpart in the fingers, but with important differences. The shape of the head of the first metacarpal is usually less spherical, and its articular surface is wider and flatter with more limited cartilage on its dorsal aspect[91] (Fig. 26-46). There is also greater constancy of the sesamoids in the thumb, which are located in the lateral margins of the volar plate and incorporated into the tendon of the flexor pollicis brevis radially and the adductor pollicis ulnarly. In the fingers, the sesamoids are also within the volar plate, but are not associated with the intrinsic muscles.[72] The insertions of the intrinsic muscles in the thumb form thicker and stronger tendinous and aponeurotic expansions on the sides of the joint than is seen in the fingers.[4] This is particularly evident medially, where the adductor muscle and its aponeurosis provide strong support as they span the interval from the volar plate and medial sesamoid to the border of the extensor pollicis longus tendon. Laterally, the support is not as strong where the insertions of the

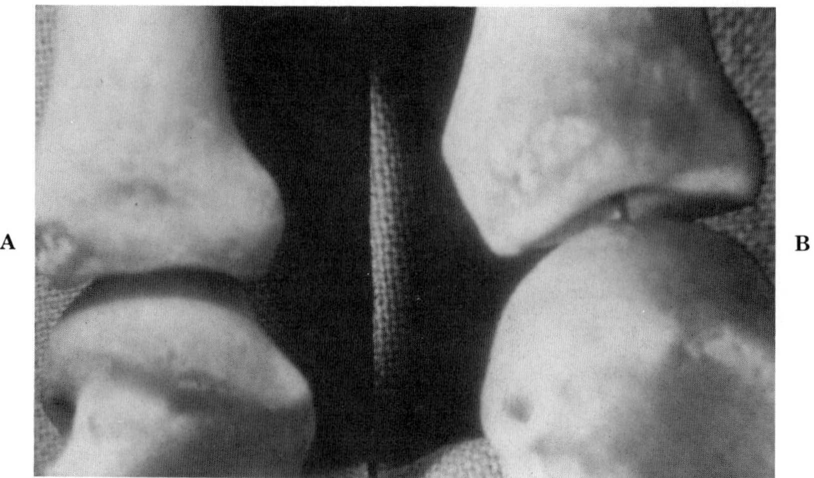

FIG. 26-46. Comparative views of the metacarpophalangeal joints. **A,** Thumb. **B,** Finger.

thenar muscles have three components. The flexor pollicis brevis provides two of these components with a deep head insertion into the volar plate and lateral sesamoid, similar to the insertion of the adductor pollicis, and a more superficial insertion on the volar portion of the side of the proximal phalanx. The third component of this lateral expansion is the abductor pollicis brevis, which makes up the most superficial layer and inserts over a broad area more dorsal and distal to the underlying flexor pollicis brevis. Both the adductor and abductor aponeurotic expansions extend dorsally on both sides of the joint and stabilize the extensor pollicis longus in its midline position. This tendon is also stabilized more proximally by radial and ulnar sagittal bands that attach to the volar plate. The extensor pollicis longus, by virtue of its position, is an important extensor of the metacarpophalangeal joint in addition to its more obvious function as the extensor of the interphalangeal joint. The extensor pollicis brevis, which inserts into the base of the proximal phalanx and dorsal capsule, functions only as an extensor of the metacarpophalangeal joint.

The collateral ligaments have two important functions: they provide lateral stability and dorsal support for the phalanx. Without the dorsal support, the flexors, particularly the intrinsics, no longer function as flexors of the metacarpophalangeal joint. Instead they translocate the phalanx, causing a volar subluxation or dislocation.[169]

The anatomic features of the metacarpophalangeal joint are consistent with its function of a limited hinge. Though the flexion-extension arc varies, including the ability of some individuals to hyperextend the joint, motions are usually more limited than in the metacarpophalangeal joints of the fingers.[35] Abduction and adduction motions are definitely more limited in the metacarpophalangeal joint of the thumb, in which the priority of function is stability rather than mobility.

Tendon Injuries

The most likely tendons to be injured in a closed injury are the extensors. Because the extensor pollicis brevis and extensor pollicis longus are intimately connected with the dorsal capsule and the adductor and abductor aponeurotic expansions, they are usually damaged after a subluxation or dislocation. They will be discussed with subluxation and dislocation injuries in the following section.

Ligament Injuries

Dorsal Capsule

Anterior dislocation of the metacarpophalangeal joint is a rare injury that tears the dorsal capsule and the extensor pollicis brevis at its insertion. A concomitant injury to one of the collateral ligaments is common because, rather than the joint being forced in a purely anterior direction, it is more commonly deviated anteromedially or antero-laterally.[163] Even a pure flexion injury is likely to cause some damage to the collateral ligaments. If there is any tendency for persistent subluxation after a closed reduction, it indicates that the dorsal portions of the collateral ligaments have been torn. Surgery is necessary to repair the dorsal capsule. Temporary Kirschner pin fixation of the joint is recommended to protect the repair, because the flexor forces on the joint are more powerful than the extensor forces (Fig. 26-47). If there is also lateral instability as the result of rupture of a collateral ligament, repair of the ligament is also required.

Volar Plate

Acute injuries. Dorsal dislocations are at least ten times more common than volar dislocations. They result from a hyperextension injury to the joint that tears the volar plate, usually at its proximal attachment.[163] The head of the metacarpal herniates between the intrinsic muscles, which insert into both the radial and ulnar sesamoids. The dislocation is clearly seen on a lateral roentgenogram which also aids in determining the location of the tear in the volar plate. If the sesamoids remain close to the dislocated phalanx, the plate must be intact distally but torn proximally. Unlike a volar dislocation, a dorsal dislocation may not be readily reducible by closed measures, because the volar plate may be interposed between the dislocated phalanx and the dorsal surface of the metacarpal head. A closed reduction should be attempted and may be successful if carried out properly. Pressure is applied in a distal direction on the base of the dislocated phalanx while the metacarpal is maintained in a flexed and adducted position to relax the intrinsic muscles. If closed reduction is unsuccessful, surgery is necessary to release the entrapped plate. After either closed or operative reduction, a dorsal splint is applied to the digit to prevent complete metacarpophalangeal joint extension but allow for active flexion exercises.

Chronic injuries. Hyperextension at the metacarpophalangeal joint is normally opposed passively by the volar plate and actively by the intrinsic muscles. The flexor pollicis brevis is the most effective intrinsic muscle limiting active hyperextension because of its advantageous line of pull.[178] A distinction must be made between a joint that can actively hyperextend and one that is volarly unstable. The ability to actively hyperextend the metacarpophalangeal joint is not a pathologic condition and can be observed in many individuals. With pressure of the thumb tip against the fingertips or against an object, the hyperextension in a normal thumb disappears, and the joint is stable in slight flexion. With volar instability, however, the joint fails to stabilize during prehension and continues to hyperextend. This is a pathologic condition that may produce a significant disability. Conservative treatment should be tried, including the use of a small dorsal splint to block metacarpophalangeal joint extension and active resistive exercises to strengthen the intrinsic muscles. If these measures fail and the disability is significant, surgery should be considered. An effective procedure is to advance the conjoined tendon of the insertion of the abductor pollicis brevis and the important flexor pollicis brevis. This technique increases the flexion forces of the muscles on the joint,

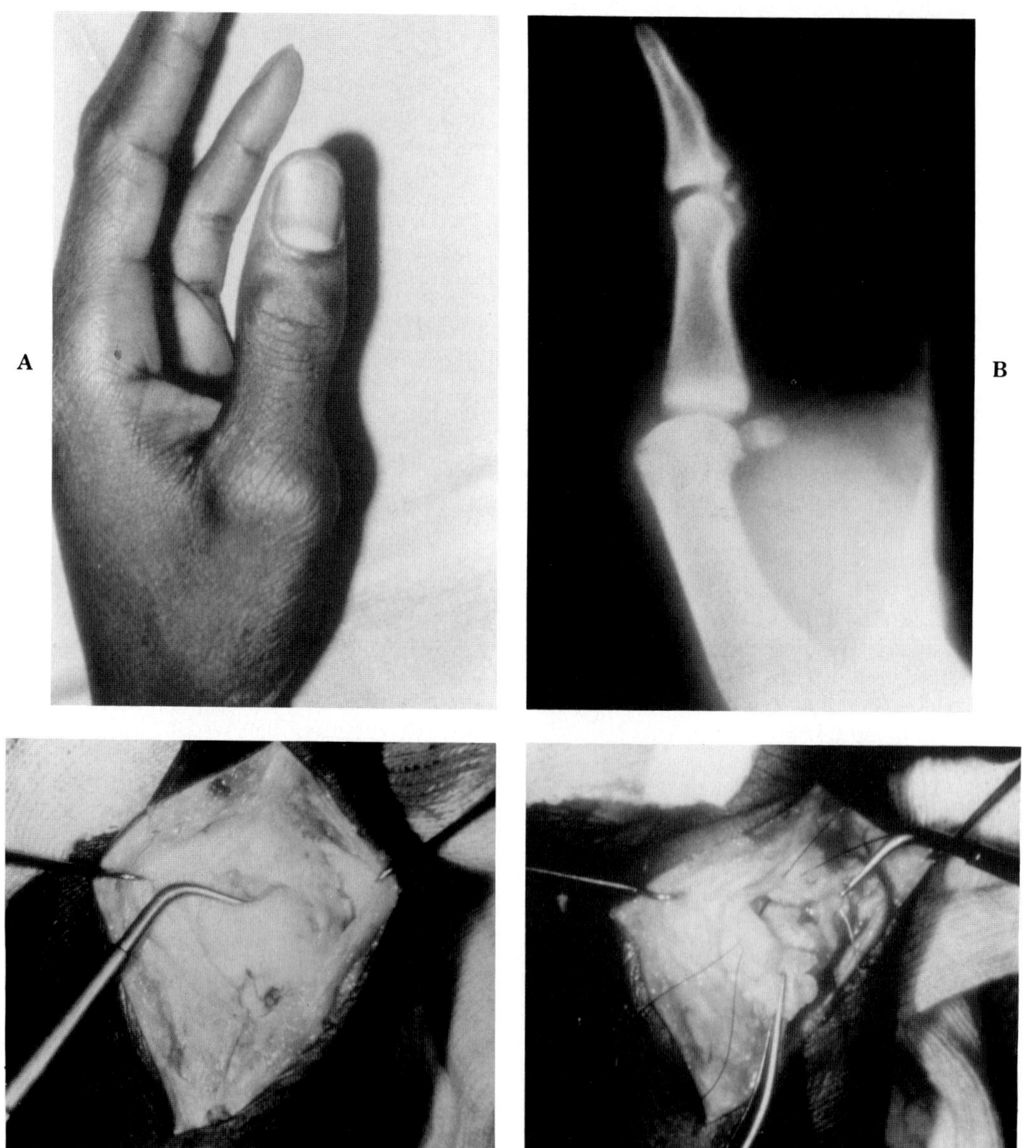

FIG. 26-47. A and **B,** This boxer had chronic pain in the metacarpophalangeal joint of his thumb, which was volarly subluxed. **C** and **D,** At surgery, the dorsal capsule *(probe)* was torn and repaired with nonabsorbable sutures.

thereby eliminating the volar instability[152] (Fig. 26-48).

Ulnar Collateral Ligament Injuries

Acute injuries. Instability following an injury to the ulnar collateral ligament is common, resulting in a condition often referred to as a "gamekeeper's thumb." The term does not refer to an acute injury but to a chronic occupational condition that was observed in Scottish gamekeepers.[31] These workers killed hares by placing their thumbs and index fingers on the animals' heads and hyperextending their necks. The abduction force that this repetitive activity placed on the gamekeeper's thumb gradually weakened the ulnar collateral ligament, resulting in progressive joint instability. By common usage and tradition, "gamekeeper's thumb" has been used to indicate an acute as well as a chronic injury to the ligament. A more appropriate term for the acute injury would be "skier's thumb" because skiing is responsible for most such injuries. It is estimated that between 15% to 25% of all skiing injuries involve the thumb. In 90% of these injuries the damage is to the

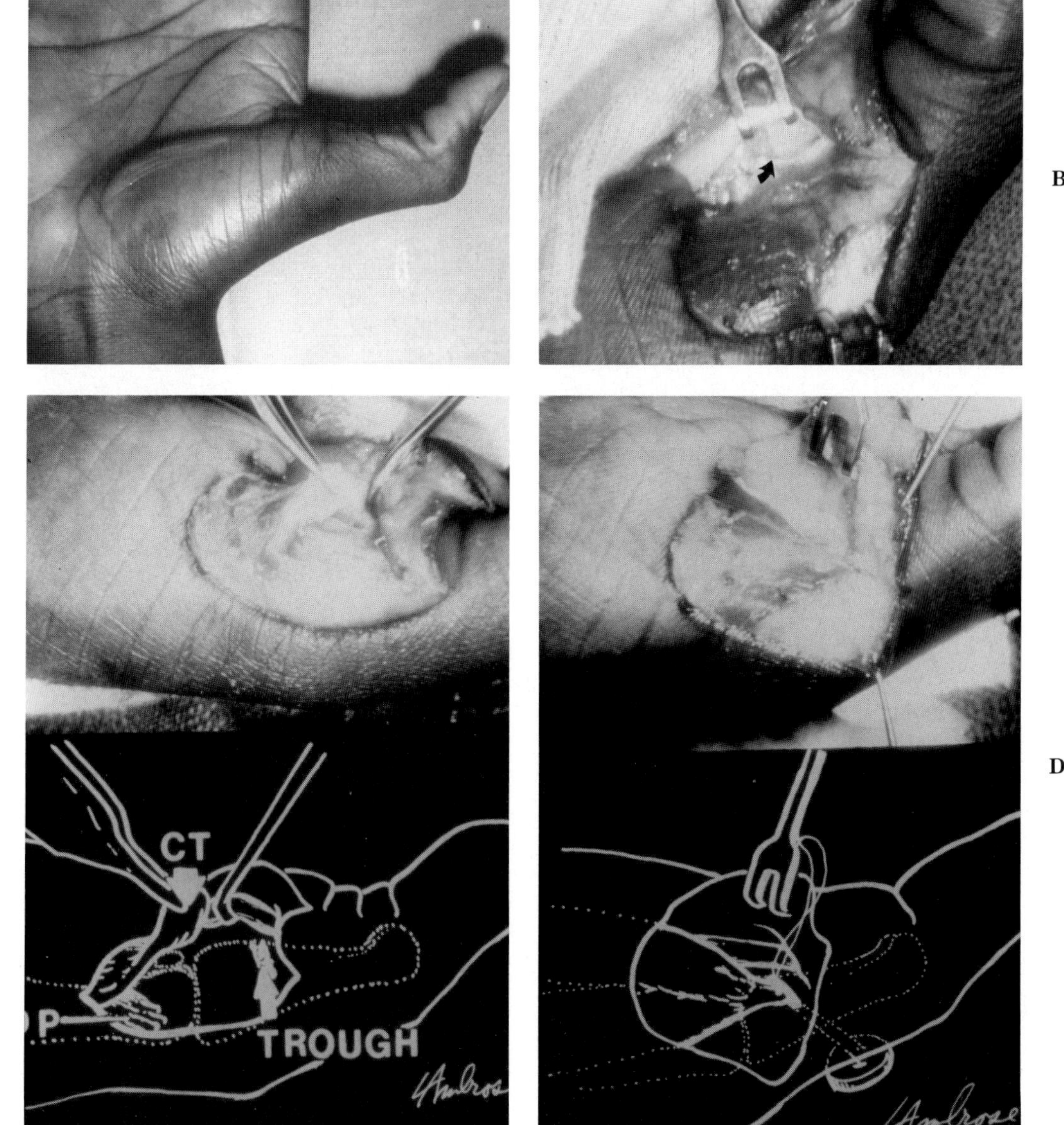

FIG. 26-48. A, Chronic volar instability of the metacarpophalangeal joint in a thumb. **B,** The volar plate is usually intact in these problems, though it is often attenuated. **C,** The conjoined tendon of the abductor pollicis and flexor pollicis brevis is removed, and a trough is made at a more distal level on the phalanx. **D,** The tendon is advanced into the trough.

Continued.

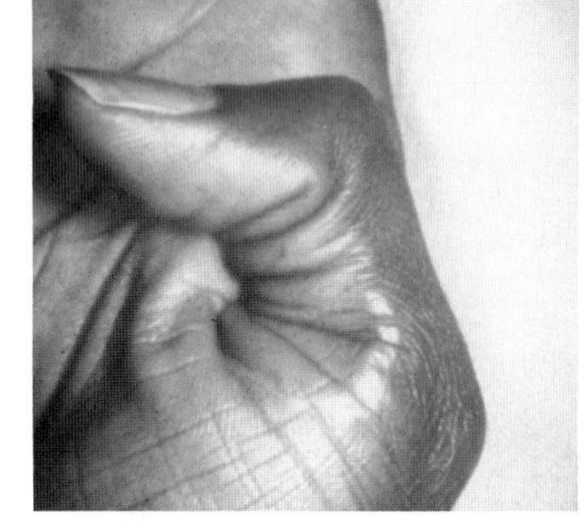

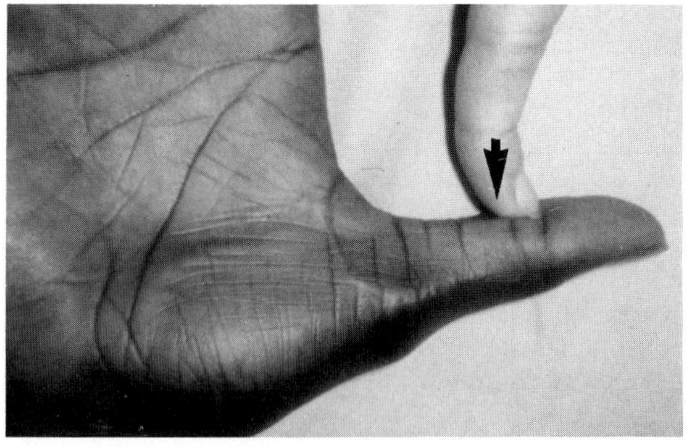

FIG. 26-48, cont'd. E and **F,** Postoperatively, flexion was not impaired, and the previous dorsal instability was corrected.

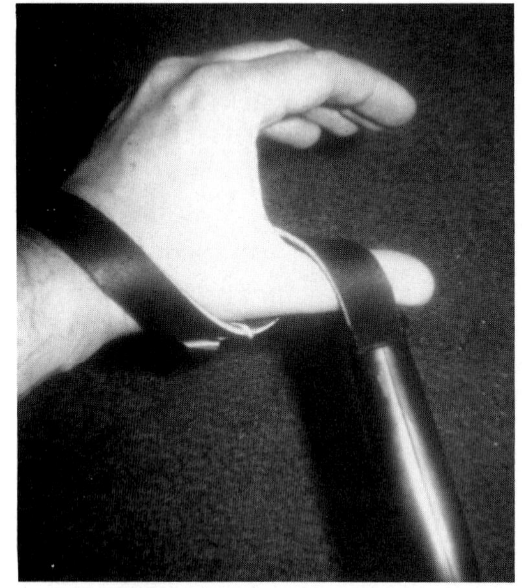

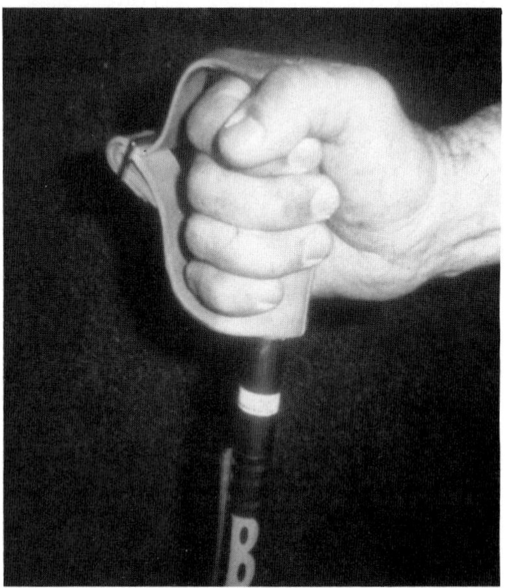

FIG. 26-49. A, The strap on a ski pole may catch around the skier's thumb, pulling it into abduction. **B,** Ski pole with a sword-type grip.

ulnar collateral ligament of the metacarpophalangeal joint.[52,131] The straps on ski poles have been incriminated as the major cause of these ligament injuries.[136,169] As the skier falls, the far end of the pole gets caught in the snow. The strap, which lies across the palm, pulls the thumb into radial deviation. Poles with sword grips, in which the retention strap is across the dorsum of the hand, should reduce the incidence of these injuries (Fig. 26-49). Unfortunately, this has not proved to be the situation; ulnar collateral ligament injuries occur with even greater frequency in skiers using sword grip poles.[131] Apparently, as the palm of the hand strikes the snow, the pole remains wedged in the first web space, resulting in forced abduction of the thumb. The safest poles are those without any grip restraints, because these poles are more likely to fly away from the falling skier. Ulnar collateral ligament injuries will still occur, but their incidence will be significantly reduced.

The diagnosis and proper classification of the type of ligament sprain depends on a careful examination. The purpose of the examination is to differentiate between the partial injury, in which joint stability has not been compromised, and the third-degree or complete ligament disruption, which results in instability and requires surgery. Marked swelling and particularly ecchymoses should alert the examiner to the possibility of a severe ligament injury. The resting attitude of the thumb should be observed and any radial angulation of the joint noted. The area of maximum tenderness should also be determined: whether it is at the insertion of the ligament into the proximal phalanx, where it most commonly fails; or whether it is proximal, at the origin of the ligament on the side of the metacarpal head. Joint stability is best evaluated by stress testing but should always be preceded by conventional roentgenograms. These roentgenograms are necessary to determine if there is a large, undisplaced intraarticular fracture or an undisplaced epiphyseal injury in the young patient who has not reached skeletal maturity. To avoid altering an undisplaced fracture into a displaced one, stress testing should obviously be avoided.

A common roentgenographic finding, best visualized on the posteroanterior view, is a small fracture fragment. It is usually seen at the base of the proximal phalanx. A rarer roentgenographic finding best seen on a lateral view is volar subluxation of the proximal phalanx. When this occurs, there must be a concomitant tear of the dorsal capsule and insertion of the extensor pollicis brevis in addition to a possible tear of one of the collateral ligaments. The fracture fragment usually results from an avulsion injury as the ligament pulls from the bone. If the fragment is attached to the collateral ligament, the distance of its displacement from the phalanx or metacarpal indicates the distance of displacement of the collateral ligament. If the fragment is displaced, the joint is usually unstable, and surgery is required. Occasionally, the fragment may be only minimally displaced, but because it makes up a significant portion of the articular surface, surgery will also be necessary.

Though a displaced fragment is almost always associated with an unstable joint, a nondisplaced fragment does not necessarily indicate joint stability. It is possible for a ligament to be completely avulsed and displaced from its insertion and yet for an undisplaced fracture fragment to be seen on roentgenogram. The fragment in such a case is not the result of the avulsion force but rather of a violent shear force as the phalanx came in contact with the metacarpal head.[178] Therefore the presence of an undisplaced fragment does not necessarily indicate that the ligament is nondisplaced and the joint is stable.

Special roentgenographic procedures including stress roentgenograms,[84,127] arthrography,[66,159,179] and stress arthrography[17] have been recommended as useful tests in determining the severity of ligament damage and the necessity for surgery. Though these examinations undoubtedly provide documentation for obvious pathologic findings, they are by no means infallible and may even be misleading. They should never be used as the sole criterion for surgery. The decision for such treatment depends on the findings of a properly performed stress test.

The technique of carrying out a stress test and interpreting its results are controversial. Opinions vary as to the position in which the metacarpophalangeal joint should be held during the examination. These positions vary from full extension,[136,169] to slight flexion,[127,131] to complete flexion,[145] or even a combination of extension and flexion.[43,47,177] The rationale for holding the joint in full flexion is that the collateral ligaments are maximally tight in this position; therefore any instability indicates a disruption.[21] A practical problem with testing the joint in full flexion is that it may show what appears to be angulation of the joint but is actually axial rotation of the metacarpal at its trapeziometacarpal joint. This occurs because the metacarpal is "locked" by both collateral ligaments when the metacarpophalangeal joint is in full flexion. Stressing the joint in this position may simply rotate the entire metacarpal. Even if the metacarpal is firmly stabilized and prevented from rotating, rotation can still occur at the metacarpophalangeal joint. This is likely to occur in individuals who have a large flexion arc at their metacarpophalangeal joint because of a lax dorsal capsule. Again, the joint may appear to be angulating, giving a false positive impression of collateral ligament instability (Fig. 26-50).

The preferred method of stress testing is with the joint in full extension. Unlike the metacarpophalangeal joints of fingers, the metacarpophalangeal joint of a thumb must be functionally stable in extension, and it is important to evaluate stability in this position. A possible objection to this method of examination is that a third-degree collateral ligament injury may go unrecognized if the accessory collateral ligament, which is taut in extension, is uninjured. This has not proved to be a problem, and a joint that is unstable in extension yet stable in flexion has not been observed. Testing the joint in full extension eliminates rotation of the metacarpal at its trapeziometacarpal joint and rotation of the proximal phalanx at its metacarpophalangeal joint. The examiner stabilizes the metacarpal

A
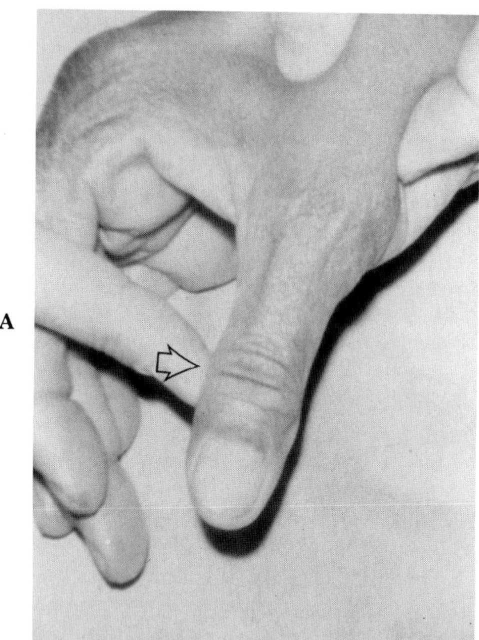

B
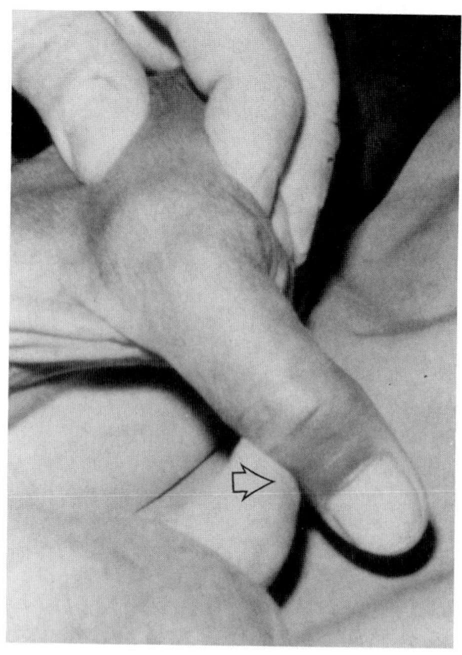

FIG. 26-50. A and **B,** Testing stability of the ulnar collateral ligament in the thumb of a normal individual. In extension, the thumb was stable, but in flexion it appeared to be unstable. This was caused by the laxity of the dorsal capsule at the metacarpophalangeal joint.

with the thumb and index finger of one hand and, with the thumb and index finger of the other hand, grasps the interphalangeal joint, applying force in a radial direction. If there is instability, the joint will angulate. The degree of angulation should be documented. The examiner stresses the joint with one hand and measures the angulation using a goniometer with the other hand. This is done by placing the index finger (right index finger when testing stability of a right thumb) on the radial side of the metacarpal head and stressing the joint with this thumb on the ulnar side of the distal segment. With the other hand, the examiner places a goniometer on the top of the patient's thumb or along its ulnar border to measure the degree of joint angulation. Angulation greater than 30 to 35 degrees, or 15 to 20 degrees greater than the angulation in the uninjured joint, is considered significant and requires surgery.

Occasionally, the adductor aponeurosis becomes interposed between the avulsed ligament and its insertion, thereby precluding any possibility of healing with immobilization of the joint as the sole method of treatment. Described by Stener, the lesion that commonly bears his name is the result of a violent abduction injury.[177] The degree of radial angulation of the joint at the time of the trauma must exceed 60 degrees for the proximal edge of the adductor aponeurosis to move distal to the site of the ligament avulsion. When the joint spontaneously realigns itself, the ligament lies external to the aponeurosis. These lesions are usually found in injured thumbs in which there is marked instability and in which there may be angulation in the resting position (Fig. 26-51).

The treatment for a partial first- or second-degree ligament injury in which there is no instability is immobilization for 4 to 5 weeks. If there is severe swelling after the injury, a molded volar gutter splint may be used for the first week until the swelling subsides. This is followed by a thumb spica cast for an additional 3 to 4 weeks. Conservative treatment has also been recommended for the acute injury in which there is obvious joint instability. Proponents of conservative treatment reserve surgery only for cases in which there is later disability or in which the diagnosis of instability is delayed for weeks after injury.[35,136] The rationale for delaying surgery is that not all acutely unstable thumbs will remain painful after a period of immobilization, and that if a later problem develops successful surgery is still possible. However, most physicians do not share this rationale and favor early surgery for the unstable joint. The predictability of early surgery to restore stability and reduce the likelihood of later pain, weakness, and secondary

A

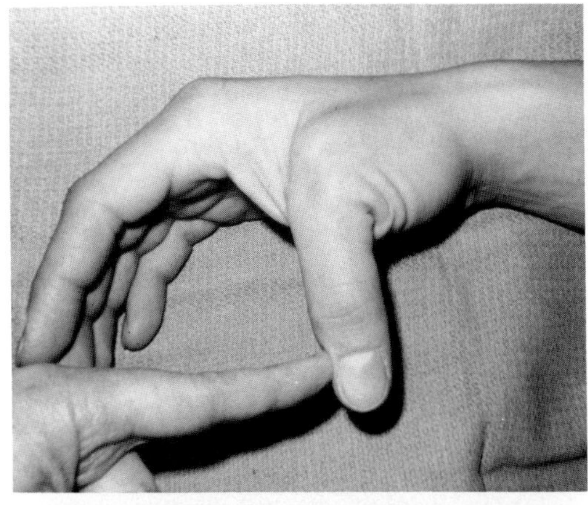

B

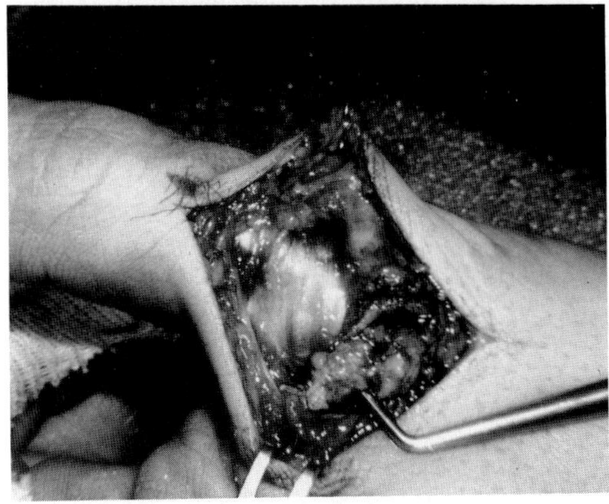

FIG. 26-51. A, Complete instability of the metacarpophalangeal joint with radial stress. **B,** At surgery, the distal end of the collateral ligament *(probe)* was external to the abductor aponeurosis. This is a classic Stener lesion.

arthritis is far greater than when immobilization is used as the primary treatment.*

Because a chronically unstable joint can be successfully treated by surgery and insertion of an avulsed ligament is often possible weeks or even months after the injury, one may question the necessity of operating on the acutely unstable thumb. The rationale is simply that it is preferable to repair a ligament than to reconstruct one. Late ligament repair is possible if the ruptured end remains close to its bony insertion. However, if the ligament retracts or folds on itself after injury, the scarring that develops within weeks precludes repair. Late ligament repair would also be impossible for the Stener lesion. Because it is difficult to determine before surgery if the ligament has ruptured in a fashion which would make later repair possible, it is preferable to operate for the acute injury. The operation is carried out as soon as the patient's general medical condition and the local wound condition permit. If the thumb is markedly swollen and ecchymotic, it is preferable to delay the operation for several days.

At surgery, a curved incision is made on the ulnar side of the thumb with the apex of the incision at the midaxial line of the metacarpophalangeal joint. Skin flaps are elevated. Care must be taken to identify and protect the sensory branches of the radial nerve. Placement of a retractor around these branches should be avoided, because prolonged retraction during the operation can lead to permanent numbness and dysesthesias. If a Stener lesion is present, the normally well-defined edge of the aponeurosis will be obscured by a mass, which represents the retracted and displaced end of the collateral ligament. An incision is made in the aponeurosis along the ulnar edge of the extensor pollicis longus tendon. This permits retraction of the hood further radially, exposing the entire dorsal capsule, which is often torn transversely. The ulnar aspect of the hood is mobilized volarly to visualize the collateral ligament. There is usually some bleeding at the site of the capsular injury or within the joint. An incision is then made along the dorsal edge of the collateral ligament and the dorsal capsule is reflected. The incision should be along the entire length of the ligament, especially to the bony edge of the phalanx. At this point an infolding of the synovial lining, forming a type of meniscal cushion, may be noted. The collateral ligament can now be carefully inspected and the precise location of the damage determined. Intraarticular visualization of the ligament is sometimes necessary, because few changes may be seen on its outside, though its deeper fibers are ruptured. Usually, the ligament is ruptured at its insertion into the phalanx, but it may also be ruptured proximally or even within its substance. If the ligament has folded back on itself, it will appear as a ball of tissue against the metacarpal head. If so, sharp dissection is necessary to unfold it. Freeing the recess between the metacarpal head and the retracted ligament may also be necessary to restore the length of the ligament before reinsertion. The ligament can be mobilized even further by incising the accessory collateral ligament.

The most secure method of fixation is to reinsert the ligament directly into the bone. This is accomplished by making a slot on the ulnar side of the phalanx if it is ruptured distally or on the side of the metacarpal head if

*References 46, 57, 64, 81, 119, 131, 177.

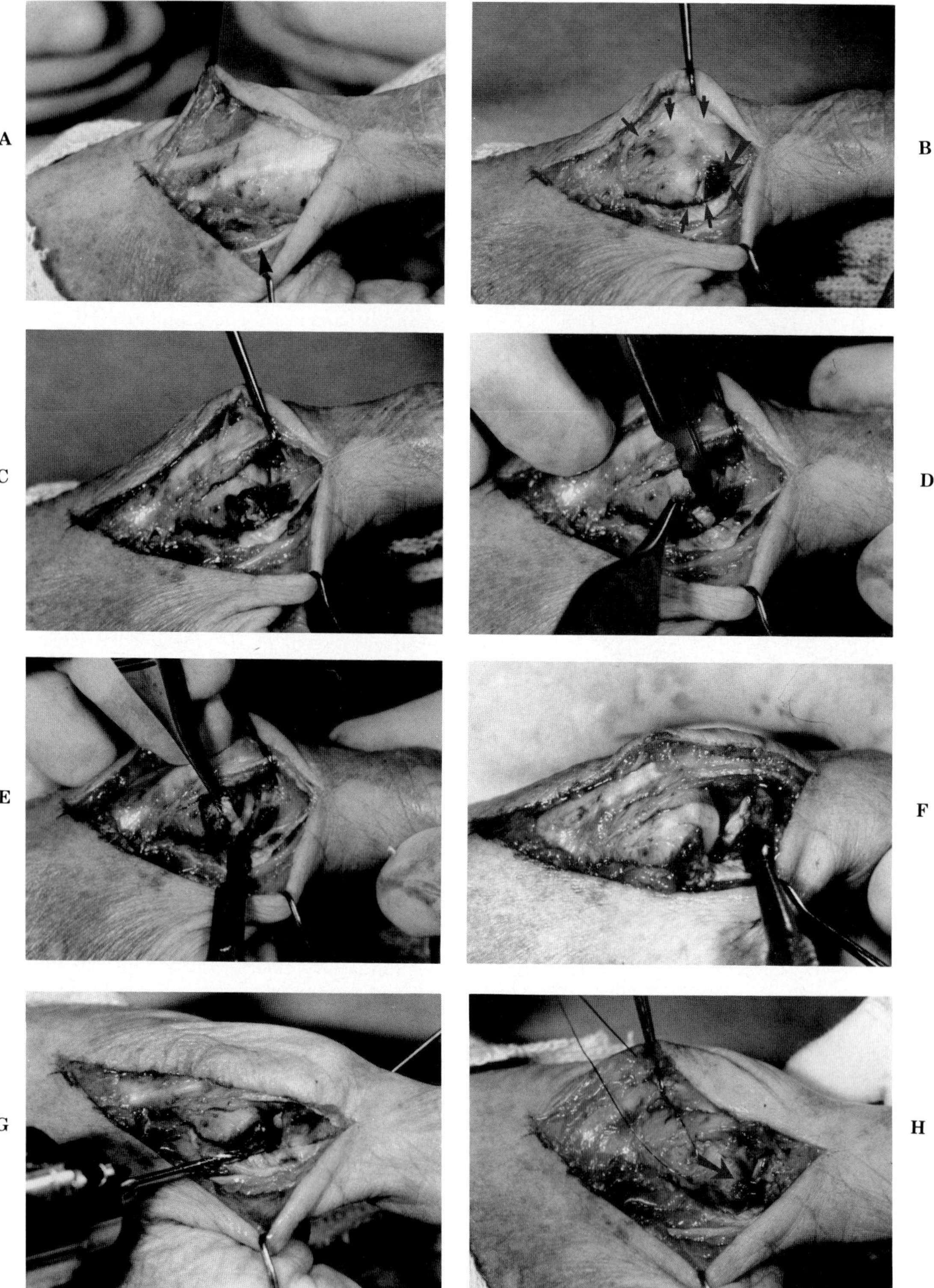

FIG. 26-52. A, A curved incision is made on the ulnar side of the joint, and care must be taken to identify and protect the sensory branches of the radial nerve *(arrow)*. **B,** The hood is incised *(arrow)* to the volar aspect of the extensor tendon. Hemorrhage was noted at the site of the ligament insertion into the phalanx *(large arrow)*. **C,** An incision is made along the dorsal edge of the ligament, retracting the dorsal capsule (under hook). **D** and **E,** Freeing the interval between the ligament and the metacarpal head and releasing the accessory fibers of the collateral ligament may facilitate advancement and reattachment of the ligament. **F,** A dorsal-volar transverse trough is made in the base of the proximal phalanx. **G,** A drill hole is made in the trough, and a Keith needle is inserted.

it is ruptured proximally. A dental chisel is used for this purpose. The slot must be deep and broad enough to accommodate the ligament. Care must be taken while levering the chisel into the bone not to cause a fracture of the articular surface. This can be avoided by starting the slot several millimeters distal to the joint surface. If a fracture fragment accompanies the ruptured ligament, it can be excised before insertion. If the fragment makes up more than 15% of the articular surface, it should be reinserted with the ligament.[43] A pull-out wire suture is used. Padding should always be placed beneath the button on the radial side of the thumb to prevent any pressure irritation on the skin. One or two 4-0 nylon mattress sutures are used to reinforce the ligament repair. If the dorsal capsule is torn, it too is repaired. The incision made in the capsule along the dorsal edge of the ligament is now closed. If there is any tendency for the metacarpophalangeal joint to remain flexed, the sutures between the dorsal capsule and collateral ligament are inserted obliquely to pull the capsule proximally. The joint is now gently stressed to test the efficacy of the repair. The incision in the adductor aponeurosis is also closed with 4-0 nylon mattress sutures. It is unnecessary to transfix the joint with a Kirschner pin routinely. This should be reserved for cases in which there is a concomitant volar subluxation. Postoperatively, a volar plaster splint is applied to immobilize the thumb and wrist (Fig. 26-52). After 5 to 6

I

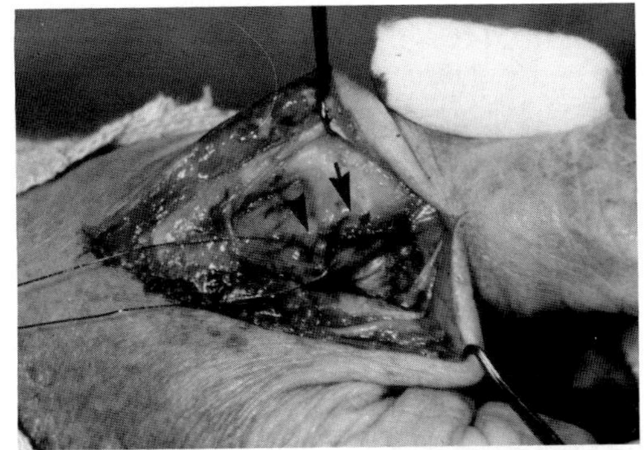

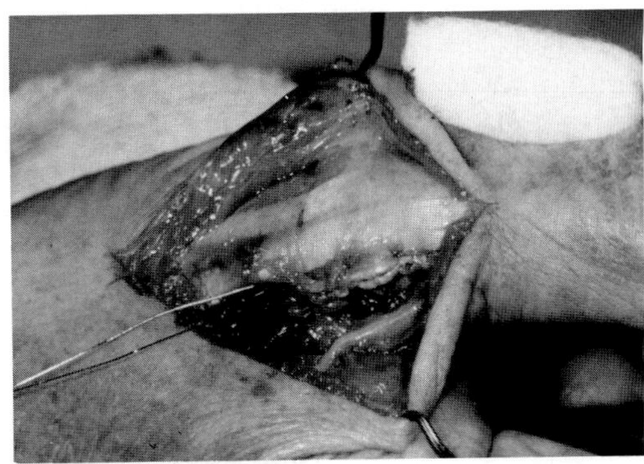

J

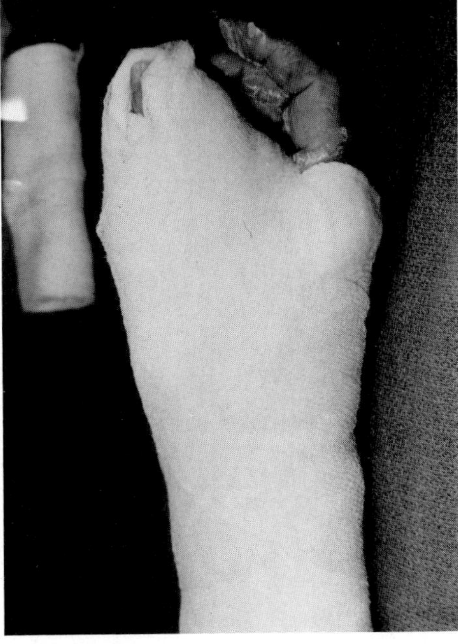

K

FIG. 26-52, cont'd. H and **I,** The ligament is reinserted using a pull-out wire suture, and padding is placed beneath the button on the radial side of the thumb. **J,** The dorsal capsule is sutured to the dorsal edge of the repaired ligament. **K,** The dorsal hood is repaired. Postoperatively, the thumb and wrist are immobilized. A properly applied volar plaster splint is preferable to a thumb spica cast, because it is more comfortable for the patient and facilitates changing the bandages.

weeks, the splint is removed several times daily for active range of motion exercises. After an additional week, the splint is removed, and the exercises are increased to an hourly frequency. Ideally, all activities that place the thumb at risk of reinjury should be avoided for another 6 weeks. This delay may be unreasonable for the professional or serious amateur athlete. If situations warrant, the thumb can be protected by the use of an orthosis. For the athlete who wears a glove, such as the skier or hockey player, a small dorsal gutter splint can be fabricated to fit inside the glove (Fig. 26-53).

Chronic injury. Chronic instability, the true "gamekeeper's thumb," is common. It occurs when athletes dismiss their acute injury as trivial and neglect to seek prompt medical attention. Only as their pain persists and they remain unable to grasp effectively do they seek medical attention. As with the acute thumb injury, conventional roentgenograms are an important part of the examination. If secondary arthritic changes have developed, arthrodesis is the preferred operation. Arthrodesis may also be indicated for the chronically painful thumb, which may not be unstable. This situation is usually encountered in the athlete who reports multiple injuries, none of which was severe enough alone to rupture the ligament but whose cumulative effect has resulted in a diffusely painful joint.

In addition to lateral instability, the extensor pollicis longus tendon may be displaced in a chronic injury because of stretching of the adductor dorsal aponeurotic expansion. The tendon displacement causes increased force on the distal phalanx, resulting in hyperextension of the interphalangeal joint. This condition is analogous to the common thumb deformity seen in patients with rheumatoid arthritis.[169]

For unstable joints in which roentgenograms show no appreciable arthritis, surgical repair of the ligament or some type of soft tissue reconstruction is warranted. As previously stated, a ligament ruptured at either its insertion or origin can often be reinserted into the bone weeks or even months after injury. If reinsertion is possible, it is preferred. If, however, the ligament is found to be irreparable at surgery, joint stability must be restored by another method. Techniques fitting into two categories have been proposed: transferring a tendon to the ulnar side of the metacarpophalangeal joint or reconstructing a new ligament using a tendon graft.[3,177,180] Tendon transfers have included using the extensor in-

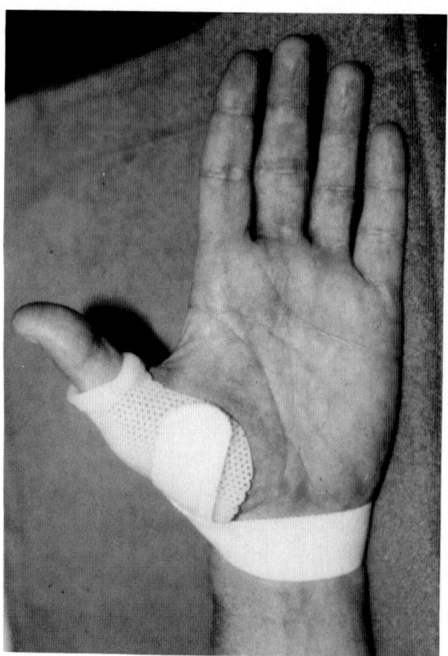
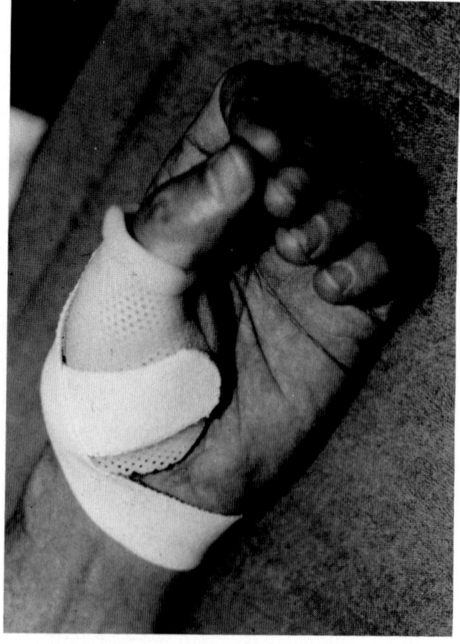

FIG. 26-53. Molded splints fabricated from lightweight thermoplastic materials provide protection for the joint following a first- or second-degree sprain or for the third-degree sprain recovering from surgery. These splints can often be worn while the athlete continues participating in his or her sport, whether it be basketball, gymnastics, hockey, or skiing. In sports such as hockey in which a glove is worn, the splint can be worn underneath.

dicis proprius,[96] a portion of the abductor pollicis longus,[60] the adductor pollicis,[136] and the extensor pollicis brevis.[162] Proponents for each of these procedures report generally favorable results.

The other surgical option is to reconstruct a new ligament using a tendon graft. This option will restore stability, and the technique to be described satisfies the primary objective of any surgical procedure—it is easily replicable and the predictability of success is high. The surgical approach is identical to that used for the acute injury. The dissection, however, is more difficult because of secondary scarring. This is particularly evident when one is trying to separate the adductor aponeurosis from the underlying dorsal capsule and what remains of the collateral ligament. The dissection should begin distally, where the aponeurosis is usually unscarred and easily separable from the underlying phalanx. As the dissection proceeds proximally, there is usually no longer a distinct plane between the hood and joint capsule, and separating the two can be difficult. After separation is accomplished, the condition of the ligament is evaluated. If scant ligamentous tissue remains, a new ligament should be reconstructed. The plamaris longus tendon is the preferred donor, but in its absence the plantaris tendon, a toe extensor, or on rare occasions the extensor indicis proprius can be substituted. A drill home is made in the metacarpal at its head-neck junction, going in a dorsal-to-volar direction. The drill hole, which is to the ulnar side of the bone, is gradually widened with successively larger drill bits. A deep transverse slot is then made on the ulnar side of the base of the phalanx, as used when an avulsed ligament is reinserted. The tendon graft is passed through the hole in the metacarpal. This is accomplished by first passing the suture through one end of the graft, then passing the suture into the eye of a heavy needle that is introduced in a retrograde fashion into the volar hole in the metacarpal. The needle is withdrawn, pulling the suture through the hole. Traction on the suture then pulls the tendon through as well. If the tendon is thin, as may be the case when a plantaris tendon is used, it should be folded on itself before being passed through the metacarpal. The tendon emerging from the volar hole is then anchored into the medullary cavity of the proximal phalanx using a pull-out wire suture. The other end of the graft, emerging from the dorsal hole in the metacarpal, is sutured to its other end and to the periosteum on the side of the phalanx with several 4-0 nylon mattress sutures. Proper placement of the initial suture is important, because if joint stability is not restored the subsequent sutures will be as ineffective as the first. The role of the assistant is important in stabilizing the joint while the sutures are inserted. With one hand, the assistant retracts a heavy skin hook that is hooked into the ulnar side of the metacarpal head. Meanwhile the other hand, grasping the distal segment of the thumb, deviates the metacarpophalangeal joint into a correct position. Care must be taken not to overcorrect the joint and deviate it ulnarly, which is possible in loose-jointed individuals. The limbs of the tendon graft emerging from the volar and dorsal aspects of the metacarpal and converging to the sides of the phalanx form a horizontal letter V. This approximates the configuration of a normal collateral ligament (Fig. 26-54). The two limbs of the V are then sutured together, which tightens the reconstructed ligament and adds further stability to the joint. If any doubt remains concerning stability, the remaining length of the ligament can be folded back and anchored to the remnant of the collateral ligament on the side of the metacarpal head. Proximal advancement of the dorsal capsule is usually required, because chronically unstable joints tend to be flexed or, in some situations, volarly subluxed. Finally, the adductor aponeurosis is closed. If lax, it should be imbricated to add further reinforcement to the reconstructed ligament. Postoperatively, treatment is the same as for the primarily repaired ligament.

Radial Collateral Ligament Injuries

Acute injuries. The radial collateral ligament is injured approximately one third as frequently as the ulnar collateral ligament.[30,57,169] The injuries result from adduction force on the joint, usually after a fall or sudden ulnar deviation of the thumb. As with injuries to the ulnar collateral ligament, stress testing is necessary to determine if there is significant joint instability. If there is instability, surgery is necessary. The operative findings may vary from those of ulnar collateral ligament rupture. Stener lesion never occurs with rupture of a radial collateral ligament. The location of the ligament damage is not as predictable as with ulnar collateral ligament ruptures, which almost always fail at their distal insertions. A radial collateral ligament may tear with equal frequency at either end, where it can be associated with an avulsion fracture, or it may tear in its midsubstance. Repair and postop-

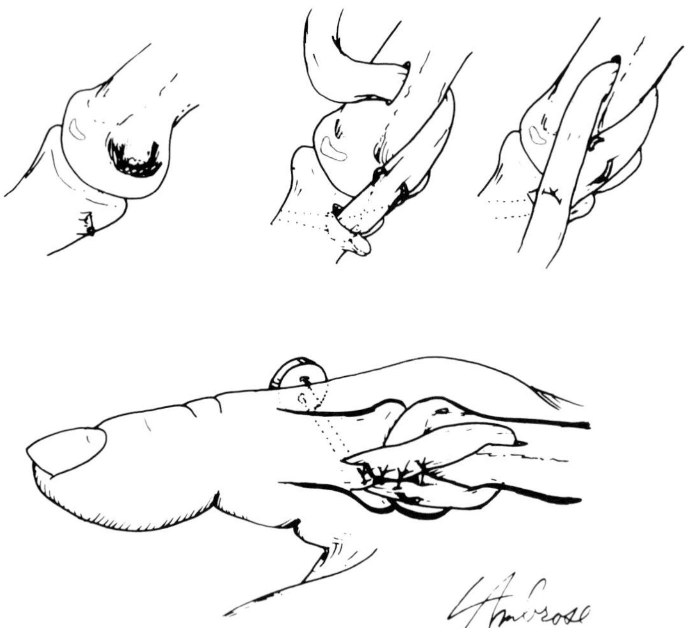

FIG. 26-54. Diagrammatic sequence of reconstruction of a collateral ligament using a tendon graft.

erative treatment are the same as for the ulnar injury.

Chronic injuries. It is probably more likely that a radial collateral ligament rupture will go unrecognized and become a chronic problem than it is that a similar injury to the ulnar collateral ligament will become chronic. With radial collateral ligament rupture, pinch and grip strength are not adversely affected, because the ulnar collateral ligament, essential for these activities, remains intact. Therefore the athlete rarely seeks medical attention at the time of the injury. However, as acute pain and swelling subside, the athlete notes that the radial side of the metacarpal head remains prominent and tender. In severe cases, the proximal phalanx is slightly ulnarly deviated. More importantly, the athlete experiences pain whenever pressure is applied to the radial side of the thumb, as when he pushes open doors, pushes the buttons on some types of door handles, opens lids on large jars, or does push-ups. Chronic radial collateral ligament injuries can be as disabling as chronic ulnar collateral ligament injuries.

If secondary arthritic changes have developed, arthrodesis is recommended. If no such changes exist, the preferred procedure is reinsertion of the ligament into the bone from which it avulsed. If the ligament cannot be salvaged, a new ligament is reconstructed. A tendon graft is used as in the method described for ulnar collateral ligament reconstruction. The abductor aponeurosis is closed and, if lax, is imbricated. The tendon of the abductor pollicis brevis, which is partially detached early in the procedure to allow inspection of the ligament damage can be advanced to add additional lateral support to the joint.

PROXIMAL PHALANGEAL AREA

Anatomy

The anatomic features of the proximal phalangeal area are analogous to the proximal phalangeal area of a finger, where the bone is almost totally ensheathed by the extrinsic and intrinsic muscle systems. The insertions of the intrinsic muscles on both sides of the proximal phalanx in the thumb and their contributions to the adductor and abductor aponeuroses have been described previously.

Tendon Injuries

The problems associated with closed tendon injuries, particularly as they pertain to the dorsal extension expansions, are similar to those encountered in fingers. However, these problems do not have the same deleterious effects on function. Though tendon adherence over the dorsum of the proximal phalanx in a finger will limit proximal interphalangeal joint flexion and seriously impair the function of the finger, similar tendon adherence in a thumb, which limits interphalangeal joint flexion, will have only a negligible effect on overall function. Effective pinch and prehension in the thumb will not be compromised if the interphalangeal joint is not fixed in extension or hyperextension. This occurs because the mobility of the trapeziometacarpal joint, which is essential to thumb function, remains intact.

Nerve Injuries

Neuropathies of the digital nerves in this area can result from any activity that causes local compression. Similar neuropathies can occur in the fingers, but they are not as common as in the thumb, where the ulnar digital nerve is usually affected. This nerve, which lies in a thin layer of subcutaneous tissue, is particularly vulnerable because of its anatomic position superficial to the ulnar sesamoid. With repetitive local trauma, scarring develops. Mobility of the nerve, which is normally limited by the tethering effect of its branches to the overlying skin, becomes even more limited. Continued repetitive compression causes increasing damage to the nerve. The condition is most commonly encountered in bowlers. It is caused by the constant friction between the thumb and grip hole in the ball.[41] Symptoms include pain, local tenderness, and numbness. On examination, a tender mass can usually be palpated as the digital nerve is rolled under the examiner's finger. Percussion over the mass produces distal paresthesias along the side of the thumb. There is usually

A

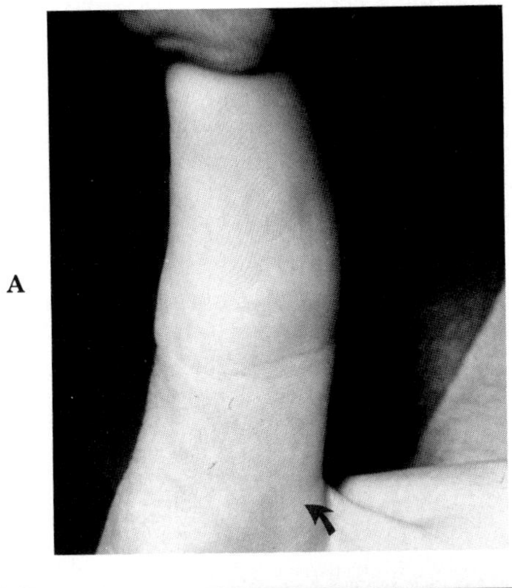

B

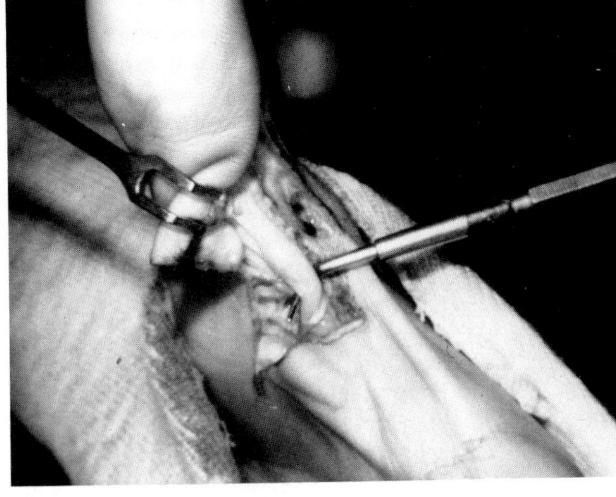

FIG. 26-55. A, Chronic pain and numbness along the ulnar side of a bowler's thumb. The neurovascular bundle at the base of the digit *(arrow)* could be rolled under the examiner's digit. **B,** At surgery, there was marked thickening of the ulnar digital nerve *(over probe)*. An epineurectomy was carried out.

a slight sensory deficit in this area as well. In severe and chronic cases, two-point discrimination may be impaired. Treatment consists of cessation of the activity. In mild cases, the symptoms will disappear within several weeks. If the athlete decides to continue bowling, several changes should be considered, both in delivery technique and in the ball itself, to reduce the risk of recurrence. The bowler should experiment with a three-quarter grip technique, which does not require the entire thumb to be inserted into the ball. If this is unsatisfactory, the hole in the ball can be altered so that the thumb is in greater abduction/extension, which will lessen the pressure between the edge of the hole and the ulnar base of the thumb. Contouring the hole may also be of some benefit. In some cases, the condition remains resistant to all conservative measures, and tenderness and numbness persist. If the disability becomes unacceptable, surgery is warranted. On exploration the digital nerve appears enlarged and resembles a traumatic neuroma. Unlike neuroma caused by laceration, it should not be excised. Rather neurolysis with excision of the thickened epineurium is carried out (Fig. 26-55). The results of such treatment are satisfactory, though some permanent sensory deficit may persist in severe and chronic cases.

Fractures

Fractures of the proximal phalanx are similar to those encountered in the fingers. At the distal end of the bone they can be intraarticular, involving one or both condyles, or extraarticular, through the neck of the phalanx. At the proximal end of the phalanx, fractures are also categorized as either intraarticular or extraarticular. Transverse extraarticular fractures are commonly volarly angulated as a result of the pull of the intrinsic muscles. Treatment for any of these fractures is identical to those of a finger.

INTERPHALANGEAL JOINT AREA

Anatomy

The interphalangeal joint is a hinged joint with a wide range of movement in the flexion-extension arc. Not only is flexion in the range of 90 degrees, but there is also hyperextension to 35 degrees or more. This exceeds the hyperextension seen in any interphalangeal joint of a finger. Structurally, the condyles of the proximal phalanx in the thumb are asymmetric with the ulnar condyle being more prominent, wider, and longer in the anteroposterior plate than the radial condyle. The movements of the joint are therefore not through a single axis of rotation; rather, they change, causing the joint to rotate as it flexes. The rotation is toward pronation, which is in concert with the movements of the other joint of the thumb during opposition.[93]

Tendon Injuries

Closed tendon injuries are far less common at the interphalangeal joint of the thumb than at the distal interphalangeal joints of fingers. When they do occur, they usually involve the extensor tendon. As with a "mallet" or "drop" finger deformity, treatment is conservative and involves extension splinting for 6 weeks. Surgery is reserved for the rare chronic case in which the extension lag is so severe that it presents a significant disability.

Ligament Injuries

Though dislocations at the distal interphalangeal joints of fingers may be either dorsal or lateral, dislocations of the interphalangeal joints of the thumbs are almost always dorsal. Lateral dislocations in thumbs are infrequent because of the wider transverse diameter of the condyles of its proximal phalanx, as compared to the transverse diameter of the condyles of the middle phalanx in a finger. In addition, the greater overall mobility of a thumb tends to dissipate a lateral force on its interphalangeal joint, thereby further reducing the likelihood of lateral dislocation.[47]

Dorsal dislocations in thumbs may be compound, as in fingers. The soft tissue over the distal phalanx is firmly anchored by strong, dense skin ligaments and may tear. The result is a compound injury as the distal phalanx dislocates. Careful wound lavage is important before reduction of the dislocation. Antibiotic prophylaxis is advisable. Occasionally, the volar plate, which remains attached to the distal phalanx, may block the attempted reduction. Surgery may then be necessary. The joint is always stable after reduction, and a dorsal extension block splint is all that is required for several weeks (Fig. 26-56). Chronic instability has not been noted following effective treatment for the acute dislocation.

Fractures

Intraarticular fractures involving the base of the distal phalanx are similar to those encountered in fingers. Treatment is similar as well. One difference in treatment may involve longitudinal fractures, which may be more se-

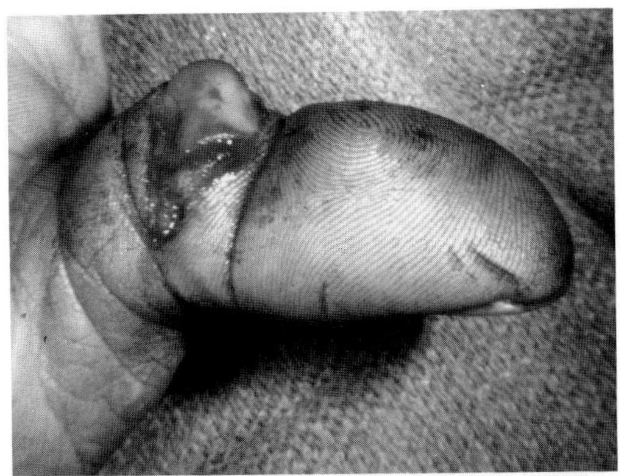

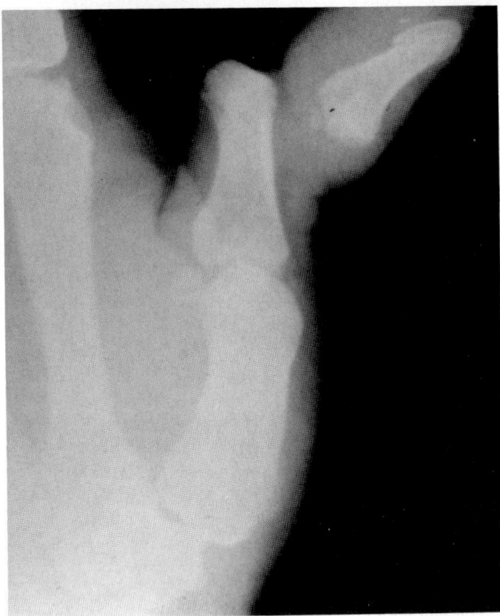

FIG. 26-56. Compound dislocation of the interphalangeal joint of a thumb.

vere in the thumb. The distal phalanx of a thumb is one third wider than the distal phalanx of a finger, because the pulp stability of the thumb is important for prehension. Because the distal phalanx provides for this stability, widely split or displaced longitudinal fractures may require open reduction and internal fixation.[139]

REFERENCES

1. Abouna JM, and Brown H: The treatment of mallet finger: the results on a series of 148 consecutive cases and a review of the literature, Brit J Surg 55:653, 1968.
2. Adams JP: Correction of chronic dorsal subluxation of the proximal interphalangeal joint by means of a criss-cross volar graft, J Bone Joint Surg 41A:111, 1959.
3. Alldred, AJ: Rupture of the collateral ligament of the metacarpophalangeal joint of the thumb, J Bone Joint Surg 37B:443, 1955.
4. Aubriot, JH: The metacarpophalangeal joint of the thumb. In Tubiana R, editor: The hand, vol 1, Philadelphia, 1981, WB Saunders, p 184.
5. Baldwin, LW, et al: Metacarpophalangeal joint dislocations of the fingers: a comparison of the pathological anatomy of the index and little finger, J Bone Joint Surg 49A:1587, 1967.
6. Barenfeld PA, and Weseley MS: Dorsal dislocation of the metacarpophalangeal joint of the index finger treated by late open reduction: a case report, J Bone Joint Surg 54A:1311, 1972.
7. Barton NJ: Fractures of the shafts of the phalanges of the hand, Hand 11:119, 1979.
8. Barton NJ: Fractures of the phalanges of the hand in children, Hand 11:134, 1979.
9. Belsky MR, Easton RG, and Lane LB: Closed reduction and internal fixation of proximal phalangeal fractures, J Hand Surg 9A:725, 1984.
10. Bennett EH: On fractures of the metacarpal bone of the thumb, Br Med J 2:12, 1986.
11. Blalock HS, et al: An instrument designed to help reduce and percutaneously pin fractured phalanges, J Bone Joint Surg 57A:792, 1975.

12. Bloem JJAM: The treatment and prognosis of uncomplicated dislocated fractures of the metacarpals and phalanges, Arch Chir Neerl 23:55, 1971.
13. Bogumill GP: A morphologic study of the relationship of collateral ligaments to growth plates on the digits, J Hand Surg 8:74, 1983.
14. Bohart PG, et al: Complex dislocation of the metacarpophalangeal joint: operative reduction by Farabeuf's dorsal incision, Clin Orthop 164:208, 1982.
15. Bora JW, and Didizian NH: The treatment of injuries to the carpometacarpal joint of the little finger, J Bone Joint Surg 56A:1459, 1974.
16. Bosworth DM: Internal splinting of fractures of the fifth metacarpal, J Bone Joint Surg 19:826, 1937.
17. Bowers WH, and Hurst LC: Gamekeeper's thumb: evaluation by arthrography and stress roentgenography, J Bone Joint Surg 59A:519, 1977.
18. Bowers WH, and Hurst LC: Chronic mallet finger: the use of Fowler's central slip release, J Hand Surg 3:373, 1978.
19. Bowers WH, et al: The proximal interphalangeal joint volar plate. I. An anatomical and biomechanical study, J Hand Surg 5:79, 1980.
20. Bowers WH: The proximal interphalangeal joint. II. A clinical study of hyperextension, J Hand Surg 6:77, 1981.
21. Bowers WH: Sprains and joint injuries in the hand, Hand Clin 2:93, 1986.
22. Boyes JH: Bunnell's surgery of the hand, ed 5, Philadelphia, 1970, JB Lippincott, p 439.
23. Boyes JH, Wilson JN, and Smith JW: Flexor tendon ruptures in the forearm and hand, J Bone Joint Surg 42:637, 1960.
24. Brewerton DA: A tangential radiographic projection for demonstrating involvement of metacarpal heads in rheumatoid arthritis, Br J Radiol 40:233, 1967.
25. Brunet ME, and Haddad RJ: Fractures and dislocations of the metacarpals and phalanges, Clin Sports Med 5:773, 1986.
26. Burton RI: Extensor tendon: late reconstruction. In Green DP, editor: Operative hand surgery, ed 2, New York, 1988, Churchill Livingston, p 2073.
27. Burton RI, and Eaton RG: Common hand injuries in the athlete, Orthop Clin North Am 4:809, 1973.
28. Butt WD: Fractures of the hand: treatment and results, Can Med Assoc J 86:815, 1962.
29. Bynum DK, and Gilbert JA: Avulsion of the flexor digitorum profundus: anatomic and biomechanical considerations, J Hand Surg 13A:222, 1988.
30. Camp RA, Weatherway RJ, and Miller EB: Chronic posttraumatic radial instability of the thumb metacarpophalangeal joint, J Hand Surg 5:221, 1980.
31. Campbell CS: Gamekeeper's thumb, J Bone Joint Surg 37B:148, 1955.
32. Carroll C, Moore JR, and Weiland AJ: Posttraumatic ulnar subluxation of the extnesor tendons: a reconstructive technique, J Hand Surg 12A: 227, 1987.
33. Carroll RE, Sinton W, and Garcia A: Acute calcium deposits in the hand, JAMA 157:422, 1955.
34. Clifford RH: Intra-medullary wire fixation of hand fractures, Plast Reconstr Surg 11:366, 1953.
35. Coonrad RW, and Goldner JL: A study of the pathological findings and treatment in soft tissue injury of the thumb metacarpophalangeal joint, J Bone Joint Surg 50A:439, 1968.
36. Coonrad RW, and Pholman MH: Impacted fractures in the proximal portion of the proximal phalanx of the finger, J Bone Joint Surg 51A:1291, 1969.
37. Cozzi EP: The proximal interphalangeal joints: a study of the para-articular fibrous structures. In Tubiana, R, editor: The hand, vol 2, Philadelphia, 1985, WB Saunders, p 869.
38. Crawford GP: Screw fixation of the phalanges and metacarpals, J Bone Joint Surg 58A:487, 1978.
39. Crawford GP: The molded polyethelene splint for mallet finger deformities, J Hand Surg 9A:231, 1984.
40. Dixon GL, and Moon NF: Rotational supracondylar fractures of the proximal phalanx in children, Clin Orthop 83:151, 1972.
41. Dobyns JH, et al: Bowler's thumb: diagnosis and treatment. A review of seventeen cases, J Bone Joint Surg 54A:751, 1972.
42. Doyle JR: Extensor tendons: acute injuries. In Green DP, editor: Operative hand surgery, ed 2, New York, 1988, Churchill Livingstone, p 2045.
43. Dray GJ, and Eaton RG: Dislocations and ligament injuries in the digits. In Green DP, editor: Operative hand surgery, ed 2, New York, 1988, Churchill Livingston, p 777.
44. Dray G, Millender LH, and Nalebuff EA: Rupture of the radial collateral ligament of a metacarpophalangeal joint to one of the ulnar three fingers, J Hand Surg 4:346, 1979.
45. Dubousset JF: The digital joints. In Tubiana R, editor: The hand, vol 1, Philadelphia, 1981, WB Saunders, p 191.
46. Eaton RG: Joint injuries of the hand, Springfield, Ill, 1971, Charles C Thomas, p 15.
47. Eaton RG: Acute and chronic ligamentous injuries of the fingers and thumb. In Tubiana R, editor: The hand, vol 2, Philadelphia, 1985, WB Saunders, p 877.
48. Eaton RG, and Littler JW: A study of the basal joint of the thumb: treatment of its disabilities by fusion, J Bone Joint Surg 51A:661, 1969.
49. Eaton RG, and Littler JW: Ligament reconstruction for the painful thumb carpometacarpal joint, J Bone Joint Surg 55A:1655, 1973.
50. El-Bacha A: The carpometacarpal joints. In Tubiana R, editor: The hand, vol 1, Philadelphia, 1981, WB Saunders, p 158.
51. Elliott RA: Intrinsics to the extensor mechanism of the hand, Orthop Clin North Am 1:335, 1970.
52. Engkvist O, Balkfors B, and Lindsjo U: Thumb injuries in downhill skiing, Int J Sports Med 3:50, 1982.
53. Faithfull DK: Treatment of chronic instability of the digital joints using a strip of volar plate, Hand 13:36, 1981.
54. Flatt AE: The care of the rheumatoid hand, St Louis, 1963, The CV Mosby Co.
55. Flatt AE: Fractures: Care of minor hand injuries, ed 3, St Louis, 1972, The CV Mosby Co.
56. Frank G: Injuries of the hand. In Donoghue DH, editor: Treatment of injuries to athletes, ed 4, Philadelphia, 1984, WB Saunders, p 298.
57. Frank WE, and Dobyns JH: Surgical pathology of collateral ligamentous injuries of the thumb, Clin Orthop 83:102, 1972.

58. Freeland AE, Jabaley ME, and Hughes JE: Stable fixation of the hand and wrist, New York, 1986, Springer-Verlag.
59. Froimson AI: Tenosynovitis and tennis elbow. In Green DP, editor: Operative hand surgery, ed 2, New York, 1988, Churchill Livingstone, p 2117.
60. Frykman G, and Johansson O: Surgical repair of rupture of the ulnar collateral ligament of the metacarpophalangeal joint of the thumb, Acta Orthop Scand 112:58, 1956.
61. Gad P: The anatomy of the volar part of the capsules of the finger joints, J Bone Joint Surg 49B:362, 1967.
62. Gedda KO: Studies on Bennett's fracture: anatomy, roentgenology and therapy, Acta Chir Scand Suppl 193, 1954.
63. Gelberman RH, Vance RM, and Zakaib GS: Fractures at the base of the thumb:
64. Gerber C, Senn E, and Matter P: Skier's thumb: surgical treatment of recent injuries to the ulnar collateral ligament of the thumb's metacarpophalangeal joint, Am J Sports Med 9:171, 1981.
65. Gibson CT, and Manske PR: Isolated avulsion of a flexor digitorum superficialis tendon, J Hand Surg 12A:601, 1987.
66. Gilbert A, and Busy F: The contribution of arthrography to the diagnosis of lesions of the digital ligaments. In Tubiana R, editor: The hand, vol 2, Philadelphia, 1985, WB Saunders, p 904.
67. Gilbert A, et al: Lesions of the volar plates. In Tubiana R, editor: The hand, vol 2, Philadelphia, 1985, WB Saunders Co, p 904.
68. Gingrass RP, Fehring B, and Matloub H: Intraosseous wiring of complex hand fractures, Plast Reconstr Surg 66:383, 1980.
69. Glasgow M, and Lloyd GJ: The use of modified AO reduction forceps in percutaneous fracture fixation, Hand 13:214, 1981.
70. Goldner JL, and Coonrad RW: Tendon grafting of the flexor profundus in the presence of a completely or partially intact flexor sublimis, J Bone Joint Surg 51A:527, 1969.
71. Green DP, and Rowland SA: Fractures and dislocations in the hand, In Rockwood CA, and Green DP, editors: Fractures, Philadelphia, 1975, JB Lippincott.
72. Green DP, and Terry GC: Complex dislocation of the metacarpophalangeal joint: corrective pathological anatomy, J Bone Joint Surg 55A:1480, 1973.
73. Green S, and Posner MA: Irreducible dorsal dislocation of the proximal interphalangeal joint, J Hand Surg 10A:85, 1985.
74. Gropper PT, and Bowen V: Cerclage wiring of metacarpal fractures, Clin Orthop 188:203, 1984.
75. Grundberg AB, and Reagan DS: Central slip tenotomy for chronic mallet finger deformity, J Hand Surg 12A:545, 1987.
76. Gunter GS: Traumatic avulsion of the insertion of the flexor digitorum profundus, Aust NZ J Surg 30:1, 1960.
77. Harvey FJ, and Bye WD: Bennett's fracture, Hand 8:48, 1976.
78. Harvey FJ, and Hume KF: Spontaneous recurrent ulnar dislocation of the long extensor tendons of the fingers, J Hand Surg 5:492, 1980.
79. Hastings H: Complex articular fractures of the base of the middle phalanx: treatment by hinged external fixation, Paper presented at the 42nd Annual Meeting of the ASSH, San Antonio, 1987.
80. Heim V, and Pfeiffer KM: Small fragment set manual. Technique recommended by the ASIF group (ewiss association for the study of internal fixation), ed 2, New York, 1982, Springer-Verlag.
81. Helm RH: Hand function after injuries to the collateral ligaments of the metacarpophalangeal joint of the thumb, J Hand Surg 12B:252, 1987.
82. Honner R: The late management of the isolated lesion of the flexor digitorum profundus tendon, Hand 7:171, 1975.
83. Howard LD: Treatment of posttraumatic recurvatum deformities of the proximal interphalangeal joint with occasional locking, but with otherwise free joint mobility. In Cramer LM, and Chase RA, editors: Symposium on the hand, vol 3, St Louis, 1971, The CV Mosby Co, p 33.
84. Isani A: Small joint injuries requiring surgical treatment, Orthop Clin North Am 17:407, 1986.
85. Isani A, and Melone CP: Ligamentous injuries of the hand in athletes, Clin Sports Med 5:757, 1986.
86. Ishizuki M: Injury to the collateral ligament of the metacarpophalangeal joint of a finger, J Hand Surg 13A:444, 1988.
87. Jahss SA: Fractures of the metacarpals: a new method of reduction and immobilization, J Bone Joint Surg 20:178, 1938.
88. James JIP: Fractures of the proximal and middle phalanges of the finger, Acta Orthop Scand 32:401, 1962.
89. Johnson EC: Fractures of the base of the thumb: a new method of fixation, JAMA 126:27, 1944.
90. Johnson FG, and Green MH: Another cause of the irreducible dislocation of the proximal interphalangeal joint of a finger: a case report, J Bone Joint Surg 48A:542, 1966.
91. Joseph J: Further studies of the metacarpophalangeal and interphalangeal joints of the thumb, J Anat 85:221, 1951.
92. Jupiter JB, and Silver MA: Fractures of the metacarpals and phalanges. In Chapman MW, editor: Operative orthopaedics, vol 2, Philadelphia, 1988, JB Lippincott, p 1235.
93. Kapandji IA: Biomechanics of the interphalangeal joint of the thumb. In Tubiana R, editor: The hand, vol 1, Philadelphia, 1981, WB Saunders, p 188.
94. Kaplan EB: Extension deformities of the proximal interphalangeal joints of the finger: an anatomical study, J Bone Joint Surg 18:781, 1939.
95. Kaplan EB: Dorsal dislocation of the metacarpophalangeal joint of the index finger, J Bone Joint Surg 39A:1081, 1957.
96. Kaplan EB: The pathology and treatment of radial subluxation of the thumb with ulnar displacement of the head of the first metacarpal, J Bone Joint Surg 43A:541, 1961.
97. Karthaus RP, and van der Werf GJIM: Operative correction of posttraumatic and congenital swan-neck deformity: a new technique, J Hand Surg 239, 1986.
98. Kelsey JL, et al: Upper extremity disorders: a survey of their frequency and cost in the United States, St Louis, 1980, The CV Mosby Co.
99. Kettelkamp DB, Flatt AE, and Moulds R: Traumatic dislocation of the long finger extensor: a clinical, anatomical, and biomechanical study, J Bone Joint Surg 53A:229, 1971.
100. Kiefhaber TR, Stern PJ, and Grood ES: Lateral stability of the proximal interphalangeal joint, J Hand Surg 11A:661, 1986.

101. Kjeldal I: Irreducible compound dorsal dislocation of the proximal interphalangeal joint of a finger, J Hand Surg 11B:49, 1986.
102. Kleinert HE, and Kasdan ML: Reconstruction of chronically subluxated proximal interphalangeal finger joint, J Bone Joint Surg 47A:958, 1965.
103. Kuczynski K: The proximal interphalangeal joint: anatomy and causes of stiffness in the fingers, J Bone Joint Surg 50B:656, 1968.
104. Kuczynski K: The thumb and the saddle, Hand 7:120, 1975.
105. Landsmeer JMF: Anatomical and functional investigation of the articulations of the human finger, Acta Anat 25, 1955.
106. Lane CS: Detecting occult fractures of the metacarpal head: the Brewerton view, J Hand Surg 2:131, 1977.
107. Lane CS: Reconstruction of the unstable proximal interphalangeal joint: the double superficialis tenodesis, J Hand Surg 3:368, 1978.
108. Langa V, and Posner MA: Unusual rupture of a flexor profundus tendon, J Hand Surg 11A:227, 1986.
109. Lange RH, and Engber WD: Hyperextension mallet finger, Ortho 6:1426, 1983.
110. Leddy JP: Flexor tendon: acute injuries. In Green DP, editor: Operative hand surgery, ed 2, New York, 1988, Churchill Livingston, p 1955.
111. Leddy JP, and Packer JT: Avulsion of the profundus insertion in athletes, J Hand Surg 2:66, 1977.
112. Leonard MH, and Dubracik P: Management of fractured fingers in the child, Clin Orthop 73:160, 1970.
113. Lipscomb PR: Management of fractures of the hand, Am Surg 29:277, 1963.
114. Lister G: Intraosseous wiring of the digital skeleton, J Hand Surg 3:427, 1978.
115. Manske PR, and Lesker PA: Avulsion of the ring finger flexor digitorum profundus: an experimental study, Hand 10:52, 1978.
116. Massengill MD, et al: Mechanical analysis of Kirschner wire fixation in a phalangeal model, J Hand Surg 4:351, 1979.
117. McClinton MA, Curtis RM, and Wilgis EFS: One hundred tendon grafts for isolated flexor digitorum profundus injuries, J Hand Surg 7:224, 1982.
118. McCoy PJ, and Winsky AJ: Limbrical loop operation for luxation of the extensor tendons of the hand, Plast Reconstr Surg 44:142, 1969.
119. McCue FC, et al: Ulnar collateral ligament injuries of the thumb in athletes, J Sports Med 2:70, 1974.
120. McCue FC, Honner R, Johnson MC, and Geick JH: Athletic injuries of the proximal interphalangeal joint requiring surgical treatment, J Bone Joint Surg 52A:937, 1970.
121. McCue FC: The elbow, wrist and hand. In Kulund D, editor: The injured athlete, Philadelphia, 1982, JB Lippincott, p 295.
122. McCue FC, et al: A pseudo-boutonniere deformity, Hand 7:166, 1975.
123. McCue FC, and Wooten SL: Closed tendon injuries of the hand in athletes, Clin Sports Med 4:741, 1986.
124. McElfresh EC, and Dobyns JH: Intra-articular metacarpal head fractures, J Hand Surg 8:383, 1983.
125. McLaughlin HL: Complex "locked" dislocation of the metacarpophalangeal joints, J Trauma 5:683, 1965.
126. McMaster PE: Tendon and muscle ruptures: clinical and experimental studies on the causes and location of subcutaneous ruptures, J Bone Joint Surg 15:705, 1983.
127. Melone CP: Joint injuries of the fingers and thumb, Emerg Med Clin North Am 3:319, 1985.
128. Melone CP: Rigid fixation of phalangeal and metacarpal fractures, Orthop Clin North Am 17:424, 1986.
129. Milch H, and Green HH: Calcification about the flexor carpi ulnaris tendon, Arch Surg 36:600, 1938.
130. Milford L: The Hand, St. Louis, 1982, The CV Mosby Co.
131. Miller RJ: Dislocation and fracture dislocations of the metacarpophalangeal joint of the thumb, Hand Clin 4:45, 1988.
132. Moberg E, and Stener B: Injuries to the ligaments of the thumb and fingers: diagnosis, treatment and prognosis, Acta Chir Scand 106:166, 1953.
133. Murakam Y: Irreducible volar dislocation of the proximal interphalangeal joint of the finger, Hand 6:87, 1974.
134. Murphy AF, and Stark HH: Closed dislocations of the metacarpophalangeal joint of the index finger, J Bone Joint Surg 49A:1579, 1967.
135. Napier JR: The form and function of the carpometacarpal joint of the thumb, J Anat 89:362, 1955.
136. Neviaser RJ, Wilson JN, and Lievano A: Rupture of the ulnar collateral ligament of the thumb (gamekeeper's thumb): correction by dynamic repair, J Bone Joint Surg 53A:1357, 1971.
137. Neviaser RJ, and Wilson JN: Interposition of the extensor tendon resulting in persistent subluxation of the proximal interphalangeal joint of the finger, Clin Orthop 8:118, 1972.
138. Nutter PD: Interposition of sesamoids into metacarpophalangeal dislocations, J Bone Joint Surg 22:730, 1940.
139. O'Brien ET: Fractures of the metacarpals and phalanges. In Green DP, editor: Operative hand surgery, ed 2, New York, 1988, Churchill Livingston, p 709.
140. Ochiai N, et al: Vascular anatomy of flexor tendons. I. Vascular system and blood supply of the profundus tendon in the digital sheath, J Hand Surg 4:321, 1979.
141. O'Donoghue DH: Treatment of injuries to athletes, Philadelphia, 1970, WB Saunders Co.
142. Opgrande JD, and Westphal SA: Fractures of the hand, Orthop Clin North Am 14:779, 1983.
143. Palmar AK, and Linscheid RL: Irreducible dorsal dislocation of the distal interphalangeal joint of the finger, J Hand Surg 2:406, 1977.
144. Palmar AK, and Linscheid RL: Chronic recurrent dislocation of the proximal interphalangeal joint of the finger, J Hand Surg 3:95, 1978.
145. Palmar AK, and Louis DS: Assessing ulnar instability of the metacarpophalangeal joint of the thumb, J Hand Surg 3:542, 1978.
146. Pellegrini UD: Fractures of the base of the thumb, Hand Clin 4:87, 1988.
147. Pieron AP: The first carpometacarpal joint. In Tubiana R, editor: The hand, vol 1, Philadelphia, 1981, WB Saunders Co, p 169.
148. Pohl AL: Irreducible dislocation of a distal interphalangeal joint, Br J Plast Surg 29:227, 1976.
149. Pollen AG: The conservative treatment of Bennett's fracture: subluxation of the thumb metacarpal, J Bone Joint Surg 50B:91, 1968.

150. Posner MA: Injuries to the hand and wrist in athletes, Orthop Clin North Am 8:593, 1977.
151. Posner MA: Hand and digit injuries. In Scott NW, Nissonson B, and Nicholas JA, editors: Principles of sports medicine, Baltimore, 1984, Williams & Wilkins, p 178.
152. Posner MA, and Ambrose L: Intrinsic muscle advancement to treat chronic palmar instability of the metacarpophalangeal joint of the thumb, J Hand Surg 13A:110, 1988.
153. Posner MA, and Ambrose L: The boxer's knuckle; dorsal capsule rupture of the metacarpophalangeal joint of a finger, J Hand Surg 14A:229, 1989.
154. Posner MA, and Kaplan EB: Osseous and ligamentous structures. In Spinner M, editor: Kaplan's functional and surgical anatomy of the hand, Philadelphia, 1984, JB Lippincott Co, p 23-51.
155. Posner MA, and Wilenski M: Irreducible volar dislocation of the proximal interphalangeal joint of a finger caused by interposition of an intact central slip: a case report, J Bone Joint Surg 60A:133, 1978.
156. Pratt DR: Exposing fractures of the proximal phalanx of the finger longitudinally through the dorsal extensor apparatus, Clin Orthop 15:22, 1959.
157. Pulvertaft RG: Operative treatment of the injuries of the phalanges and metacarpal bones and their joints. In Fullong R, editor: Operative surgery, ed 2, Philadelphia, 1969, JB Lippincott.
158. Redler I, and Williams JT: Rupture of a collateral ligament of the proximal interphalangeal joint of the finger: analysis of 18 cases, J Bone Joint Surg 49A:322, 1967.
159. Resnick D, and Danzig LA: Orthopaedic evaluation of injuries of the first metacarpophalangeal joint: gamekeeper's thumb, AJR 126:1046, 1976.
160. Riordan DC, and Kaplan EB: The thumb. In Spinner M, editor: Kaplan's functional and surgical anatomy of the hand, Philadelphia, 1984, JB Lippincott Co, p 113.
161. Ruby LK: Common hand injuries in the athlete, Orthop Clin North Am 33:819, 1980.
162. Sakellarides HT, and DeWeese JW: Instability of the metacarpophalangeal joint of the thumb: reconstruction of the collateral ligaments using the extensor pollicis brevis tendon, J Bone Joint Surg 58A:106, 1976.
163. Sedel L: Dislocation of the metacarpophalangeal joint. In Tubiana R, editor: The hand, vol 2, Philadelphia, 1985, WB Saunders, p 915.
164. Sedel L: Dislocation of the carpometacarpal joints. In Tubiana R, editor: The hand, vol 2, Philadelphia, 1985, WB Saunders Co, p 926.
165. Segmuller G, and Schoneuberger F: Fractures of the hand. In Weber BG, Bruner C, and Freuler F, editors: Treatment of fractures in children and adolescents, New York, 1980, Springer-Verlag.
166. Seymour N: Juxta-epiphyseal fracture of the terminal phalanx of the finger, J Bone Joint Surg 48B:347, 1966.
167. Shah J, and Patel M: Dislocation of the carpometacarpal joint of the thumb: a report of four cases, Clin Orthop 175:166, 1973.
168. Smith JH: Avulsion of a profundus tendon with simultaneous intraarticular fracture of the distal phalanx: case report, J Hand Surg 6:600, 1981.
169. Smith RJ: Post-traumatic instability of the metacarpophalangeal joint of the thumb, J Bone Joint Surg 59A:14, 1977.
170. Smith RJ, and Kaplan EB: Rheumatoid deformities at the metacarpophalangeal joints of the fingers, J Bone Joint Surg 49A:31, 1967.
171. Smith RJ, and Peimer CA: Injuries to the metacarpal bones and joints, Adv Surg 2:341, 1977.
172. Spinner M, and Choi BY: Anterior dislocation of the proximal interphalangeal joint: a case of rupture of the central slip of the extensor mechanism, J Bone Joint Surg 52A:1329, 1970.
173. Sponberg O, and Thoren L: Bennett's fracture: a new method of treatment with oblique traction, J Bone Joint Surg 45B:732, 1963.
174. Stark HH: Troublesome fractures and dislocations of the hand: American Academy of Orthopedic Surgeons instructional course lectures, vol 19, St Louis, 1970, The CV Mosby Co.
175. Stark HH, Boyes JH, and Wilson JN: Mallet finger, J Bone Joint Surg 44A:1061, 1962.
176. Stark HH, et al: Flexor tendon graft through intact superficialis tendon, J Hand Surg 2:456, 1977.
177. Stener B: Displacement of the ruptured ulnar collateral ligament of the metacarpophalangeal joint of the thumb: a clinical and anatomical study, J Bone Joint Surg 44B:869, 1962.
178. Stener B: Acute injuries to the metacarpophalangeal joint of the thumb. In Tubiana R, editor: The hand, vol 2, Philadelphia, 1985, WB Saunders Co, p. 895.
179. Stothard J, and Caird DM: Experience with arthrography of the first metacarpophalangeal joint, Hand 13:257, 1981.
180. Strandell G: Total rupture of the ulnar collateral ligament of the metacarpophalangeal joint of the thumb, Acta Chir Scand 118:72, 1959.
181. Strickland JW, et al: In Strickland JW, and Steichen JB, editors: Difficult problems in hand surgery, St Louis, 1982, The CV Mosby Co, p 126.
182. Stripling WD: Displaced intra-articular osteochondral fracture: cause for irreducible dislocation of the distal interphalangeal joint, J Hand Surg 7:77, 1982.
183. Swanson AB: Surgery of the hand in cerebral palsy and the swan neck deformity, J Bone Joint Surg 42A:951, 1960.
184. Sweterlitsch PR, Torg JS, and Pollack H: Entrapment of a sesamoid on the index metacarpophalangeal joint: report of two cases, J Bone Joint Surg 51A:995, 1969.
185. Thiomine JM: The management of recent fractures of the phalanges and metacarpals. In Tubiana R, editor: The hand, vol 2, Philadelphia, 1985, WB Saunders Co, p 763.
186. Thoren L: A new method of extension treatment in Bennett's fracture, Acta Chir Scand 110:485, 1956.
187. Vanik RK, et al: The comparative strengths of internal fixation techniques, J Hand Surg 9A:216, 1984.
188. Vom Saal FH: Intramedullary fixation in fractures of the hand and fingers, J Bone Joint Surg 35A:5, 1953.
189. Wagner CJ: Methods of treatment of Bennett's fracture-dislocations, Am J Surg 80:230, 1950.
190. Watt N, and Cooper G: Dislocation of the trapeziometacarpal joint, J Hand Surg 12B:242, 1987.
191. Webbe MA, and Schneider LH: Mallet fractures, J Bone Joint Surg 66A:658, 1984.
192. Wheeldon FT: Recurrent dislocation of extensor tendons, J Bone Joint Surg 36B:612, 1954.

193. Wiggins H, Bundens W, and Park B: A method of treatment of fracture-dislocations of the first metacarpal bone, J Bone Joint Surg 36A:810, 1954.
194. Wood UE: Fractures of the hand in children, Orthop Clin North Am 7:527, 1976.
195. Zancolli E: Movements of the thumb: opposition mechanics. Structural and dynamic bases of hand surgery, ed 2, Philadelphia, 1979, JB Lippincott Co, p 105.

CHAPTER 27 Tendon Injuries of the Hand

Lawrence H. Schneider

The athlete's hand, active in sporting activities, is at risk for specific tendon injuries.[6,35,40] These include injury at both the flexor and extensor insertions at the base of the distal phalanx, as well as the closed extensor injury at the proximal interphalangeal (PIP) joint, which will later develop into the boutonnière deformity. These will often appear trivial at the time of injury and yet may produce considerable impairment to the athlete's hand. In order to avoid a misdiagnosis, which would lead to inadequate treatment, it is necessary to be aware of these lesions.

FLEXOR PROFUNDUS RUPTURE

Avulsion of the profundus flexor from the base of the distal phalanx is a relatively frequent sports injury.* While football is the sport that seems to produce the majority of these problems, avulsion can occur in almost any sporting activity.[6] The condition will often be initially seen as a "jamming" injury with swelling and pain at the distal interphalangeal joint. These findings will overshadow the fact that distal joint flexion has been lost. At times with proximal migration of the tendon end, the symptoms may be at the PIP joint. This condition will therefore frequently be missed if the trainer or physician is unaware of the usual presentation. Because early and direct repair is generally the best treatment, it is important that the condition is recognized. When missed, and the period for direct repair has been passed, other treatment options are available for the treating surgeon.

Pertinent Anatomy

The flexor digitorum profundus proceeds through the superficialis decussation and finally broadens into a flat tendon that inserts into the proximal third of the palmar aspect

*References 2, 5, 8, 11, 12, 16, 41.

of the distal phalanx (Fig. 27-1). The blood vessel containing vinculum breve runs from the dorsal surface of the distal end of the tendon to the distal joint capsule and for a variable distance on to the palmar aspect of the middle phalanx. The profundus tendon is the only flexor of the distal interphalangeal joint.[44]

Mechanism of Injury

The injury is most often a closed avulsion of the tendon; it occurs when the patient is strongly flexing his or her finger and a sudden extension force is applied to that finger. This happens classically when a tackler in football grasps the jersey of an opponent who pulls forcefully away.[56] While the ring finger is most commonly involved, the reason for this is not entirely clear, and several theories have been advanced. Gunter[20] thought that the ring finger was most frequently involved because of this finger's lack of independent action. He pointed out that the long flexor of the ring finger offers the most resistance to extension when the hand is in a fist position, and therefore it is most likely to rupture at the insertion. Others have supported this belief.[28,29] Wenger[56] had a similar explanation to Gunter, stating that the most logical explanation is the lack of independent extension of the ring finger when the other digits are tightly flexed. He explained this with photographs. Manske and Lasker[31] tested the breaking strength of the profundus tendon insertion at its attachment to bone. They found that the ring finger profundus insertion was weaker than the insertion of the profundus in adjacent fingers. However, this relative weakness at the attachment is not of a great magnitude and so this theory may only offer a partial explanation.

Examination

The lesion may be a pure avulsion of the flexor tendon from its insertion at the distal phalanx or the tendon can bring along a piece of bone from the distal phalanx.[7] Examination will reveal loss of terminal joint flexion and tenderness along the flexor sheath. One can sometimes feel the torn distal end of the tendon and thereby localize it. When the tendon retracts to the palm a mass will be palpable.

The flexor digitorum profundus is the only flexor of the distal interphalangeal joint and its avulsion will be obvious when the tip is tested for flexion power. The patient may have proximal swelling at the PIP joint if the tendon has migrated there, or tenderness may be present in the palm in those cases where the proximal end of the tendon has pulled into that area.

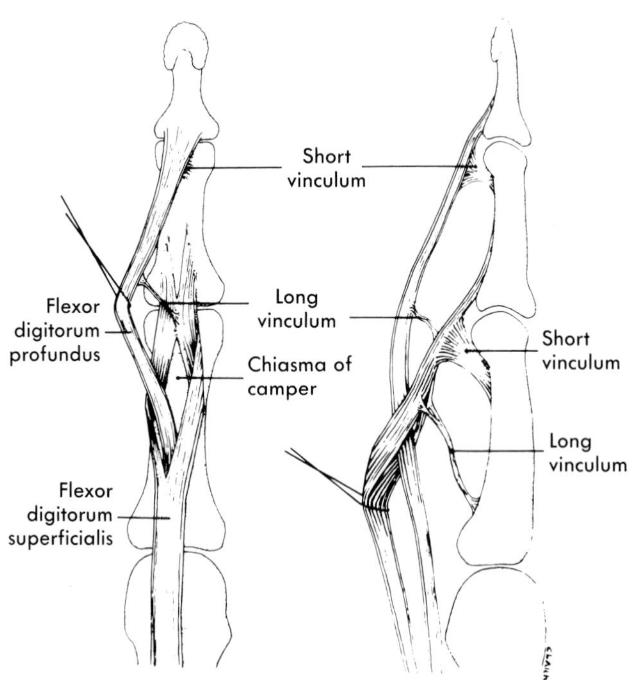

FIG. 27-1. Anatomy of the flexor system. The flexor digitorum profundus (FDP) passes through the tails of the flexor digitorum superficialis (FDS) on its way to its insertion on the distal phalanx. At this insertion it is susceptible to avulsion in forceful hyperextension injuries at the distal joint.

Roentgenographs

Roentgenographic studies are needed to show whether or not bone is involved. The significance of these injuries will sometimes confuse the unwary examiner. The roentgenogram may show that a significant segment of bone from the base of the distal phalanx has been avulsed, and this may distract from the nature of the tendon injury. On other occasions, when just a small fragment of bone from the distal phalanx has been avulsed by the tendon, this small piece of bone seen at the level of the PIP joint in the lateral view may lead the examiner to think that this is a minor chip fracture of the PIP joint.

Classification

Early recognition is beneficial, because prompt restitution of the flexor profundus system carries a better prognosis in terms of distal joint flexion[54]. Leddy and Packer[29] presented a classification of these injuries based on the location of the distal end of the tendon.

Leddy and Packer Classification of Avulsion Injuries of the Flexor Digitorum Profundus (FDP)

TYPE 1

The tendon end is located in the palm with both vincula ruptured. This type, in my experience, is not often associated with a fracture. Early reattachment of the FDP is recommended, preferably within the first 2 weeks of injury (Fig. 27-2).

A

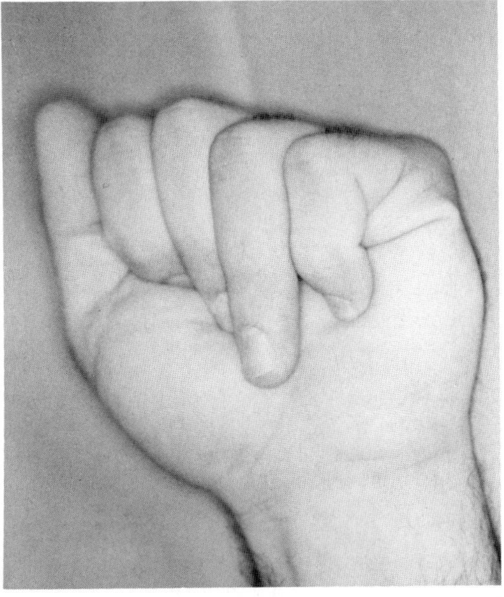

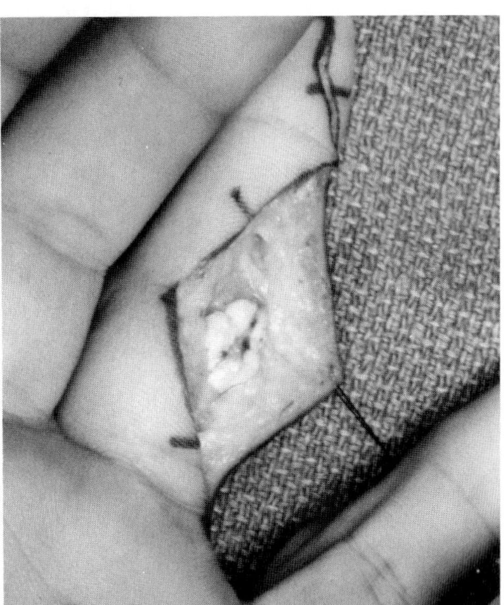

B

C

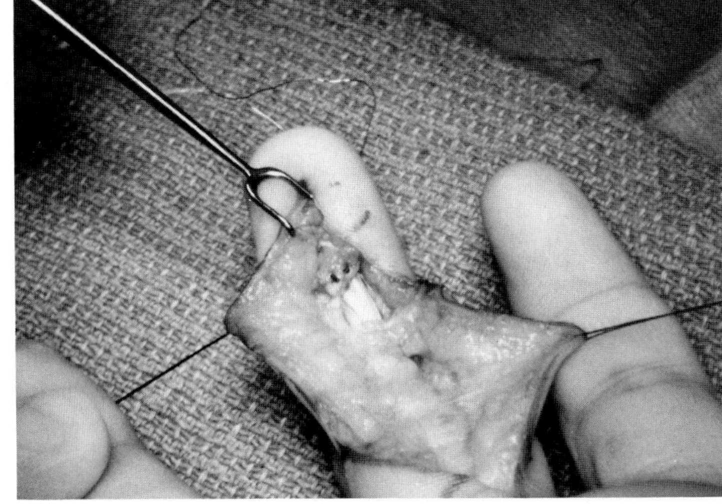

FIG. 27-2. Rupture of the ring finger profundus in a rugby player. **A,** Loss of active flexion is seen at the ring finger 3 days after injury. **B,** the tendon was avulsed from the distal phalanx and was retrievable from the palm—a type 1 injury. **C,** Reattachment to the distal phalanx was done using the Bunnell technique.

Continued.

D

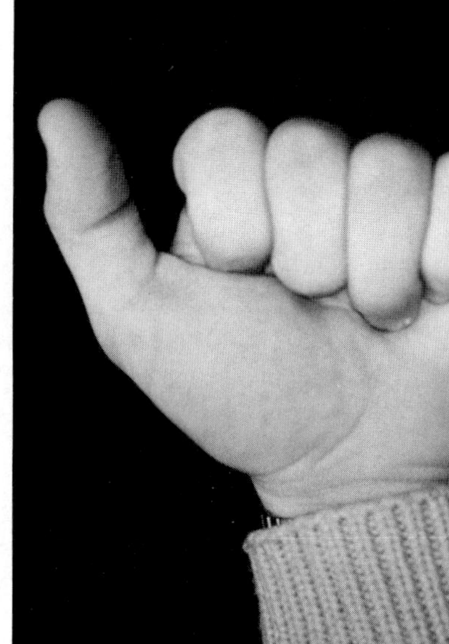

E

FIG. 27-2, cont'd. **D,** and **E,** Range of motion was achieved at 6 months.

A

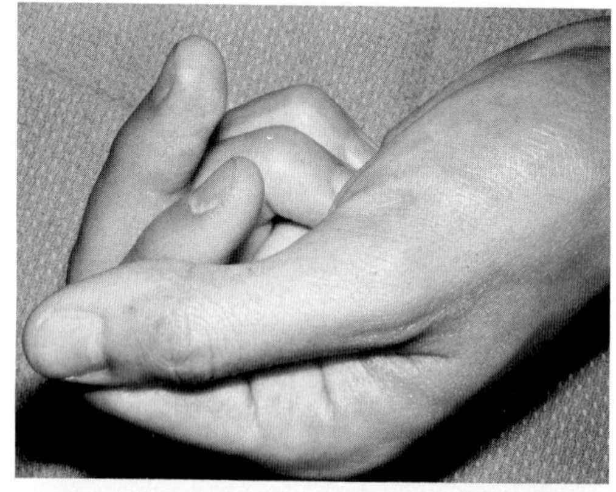

B

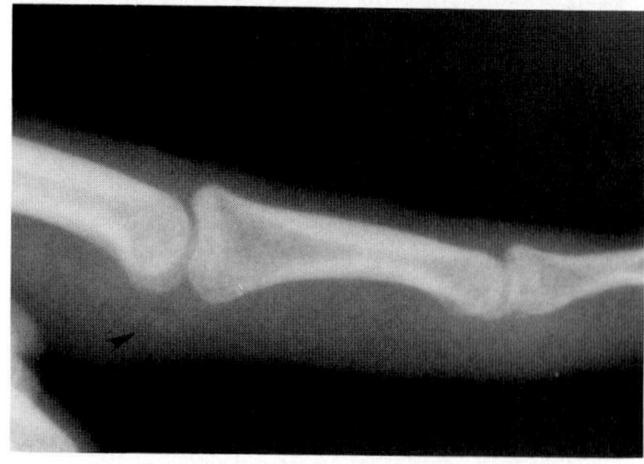

FIG. 27-3. Rupture of the flexor digitorum profundus along with a small bone fragment. **A,** Loss of flexion at the distal joint of the long finger. **B,** Roentgenogram showed a small bone fragment that was present at the level of the proximal interphalangeal joint—a type 2 injury.

Continued.

TYPE 2

In these cases the tendon along with the small bone fragment from the distal phalanx retracts to the level of the PIP joint. The long vinculum remains intact. In these cases a small fragment of bone is seen in the lateral view at the proximal interphalangeal joint, and this gives a clue as to the location of the flexor digitorum profundus (Fig. 27-3). Certainly, early reattachment is indicated, but this lesion is not as emergent a problem as the type 1 injury; reattachment can be done up to 4 weeks after injury, with certain reservations as noted below, but rarely beyond that time.

TYPE 3

This lesion is associated with a large bony fragment. In this instance the fragment, being large, hangs up on the A-4 pulley just proximal to the distal interphalangeal joint, keeping the tendon out in the finger. Treatment is open reduction and internal fixation, which serves to restore the continuity of the tendon system (Fig. 27-4).

Robins and Dobyns,[42] Smith,[48] and Langa and Posner[26] have recognized a variant of the type 3 lesion in which not only is the bone fractured but, in addition, the tendon is avulsed from the bony fragment. It would be impossible preoperatively to identify this lesion, which demands both restoration of the joint by open reduction and internal fixation and also a tendon repair. This is a rare injury, and my experience includes just one case in

C

D

E

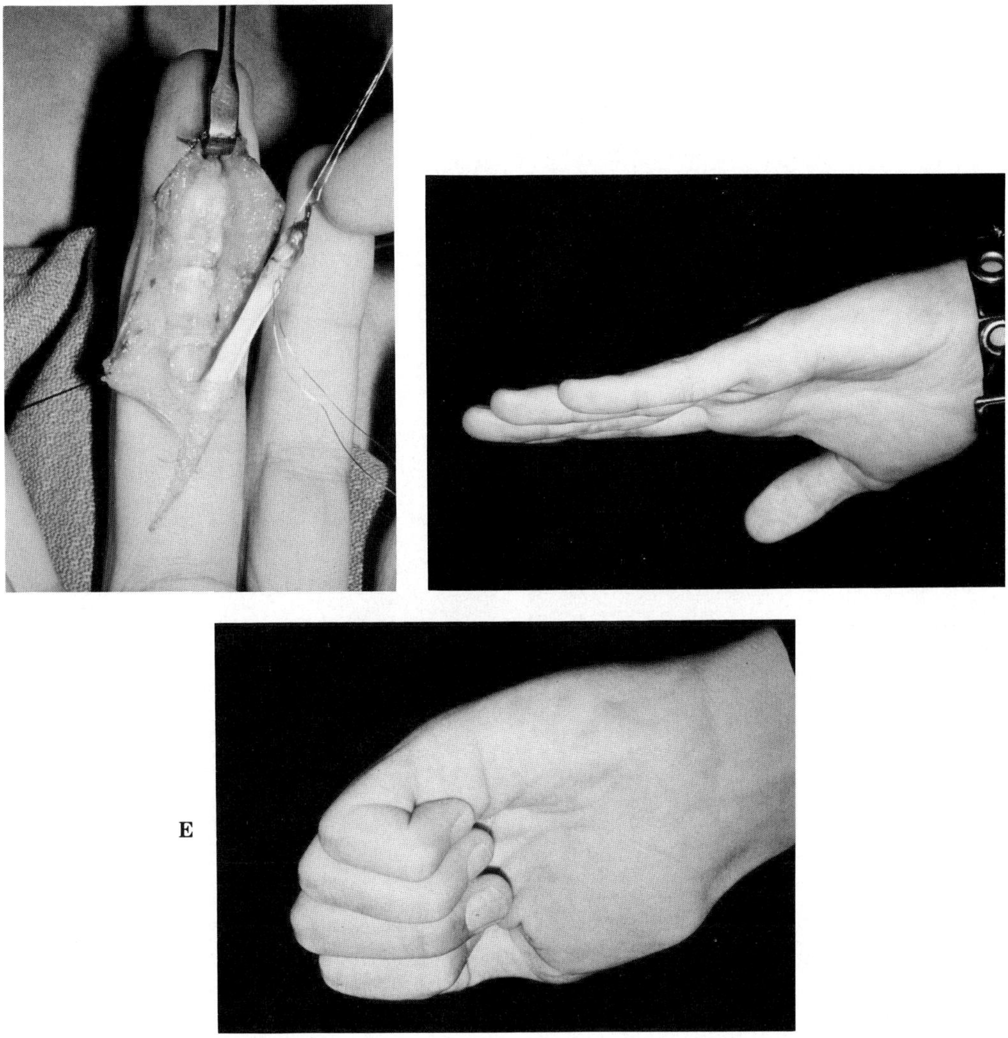

FIG. 27-3, cont'd. C, The tendon is retrieved and is going to be replaced at the distal joint using a Bunnell pull-out technique. **D,** and **E,** Range of motion is excellent at 3 months.

A

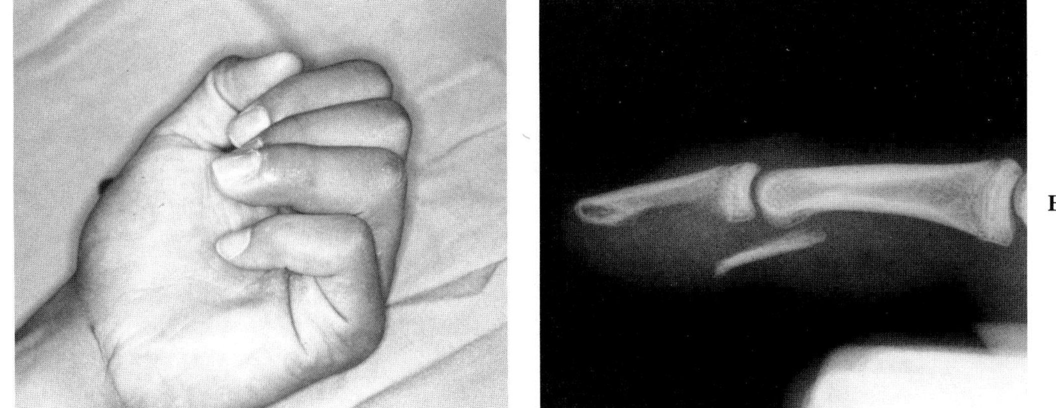

B

FIG. 27-4. Rupture of the flexor profundus with a large bone fragment—type 3 lesion. **A,** Painful swelling is seen at the distal joint. This overshadows the loss of distal joint flexion. **B,** Roentgenograph shows a large fragment that is hung up on the A-4 pulley. There is also a fracture across the base of the phalanx.

Continued.

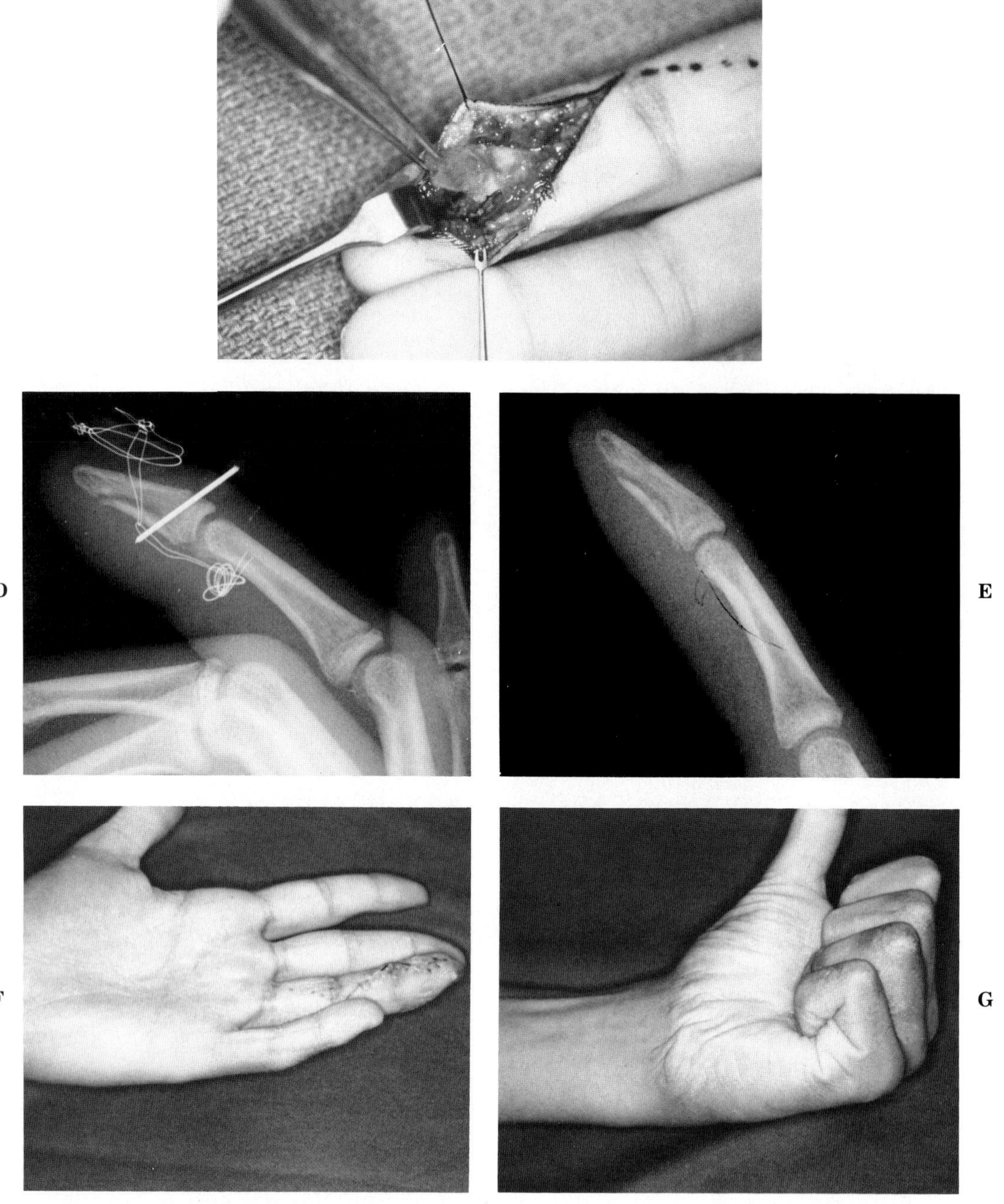

FIG. 27-4, cont'd. C, The tendon is seen to be attached to the fragment from the distal phalanx. **D,** Reattachment is carried out using a pull-out wire and a Kirschner wire. **E,** After healing, the fragment is held in place by fibrous union. **F,** and **G,** Early range of motion at 4 weeks.

which I used both Kirschner wires and the pull-out wire technique (Fig. 27-5).

Treatment

Acute Lesions

There is no nonoperative treatment for acute lesions. Splinting the finger for comfort is not unreasonable, but plans should be made for early operative reattachment of the tendon.[39] When recognized early, the reattachment of the tendon end gives the best chance for a good result in terms of distal joint function.

Type 1 lesions. In type 1 lesions the tendon is retrieved as atraumatically as possible and threaded up the flexor sheath (preserving as much sheath as possible), doing as little damage to that structure as possible. At the distal

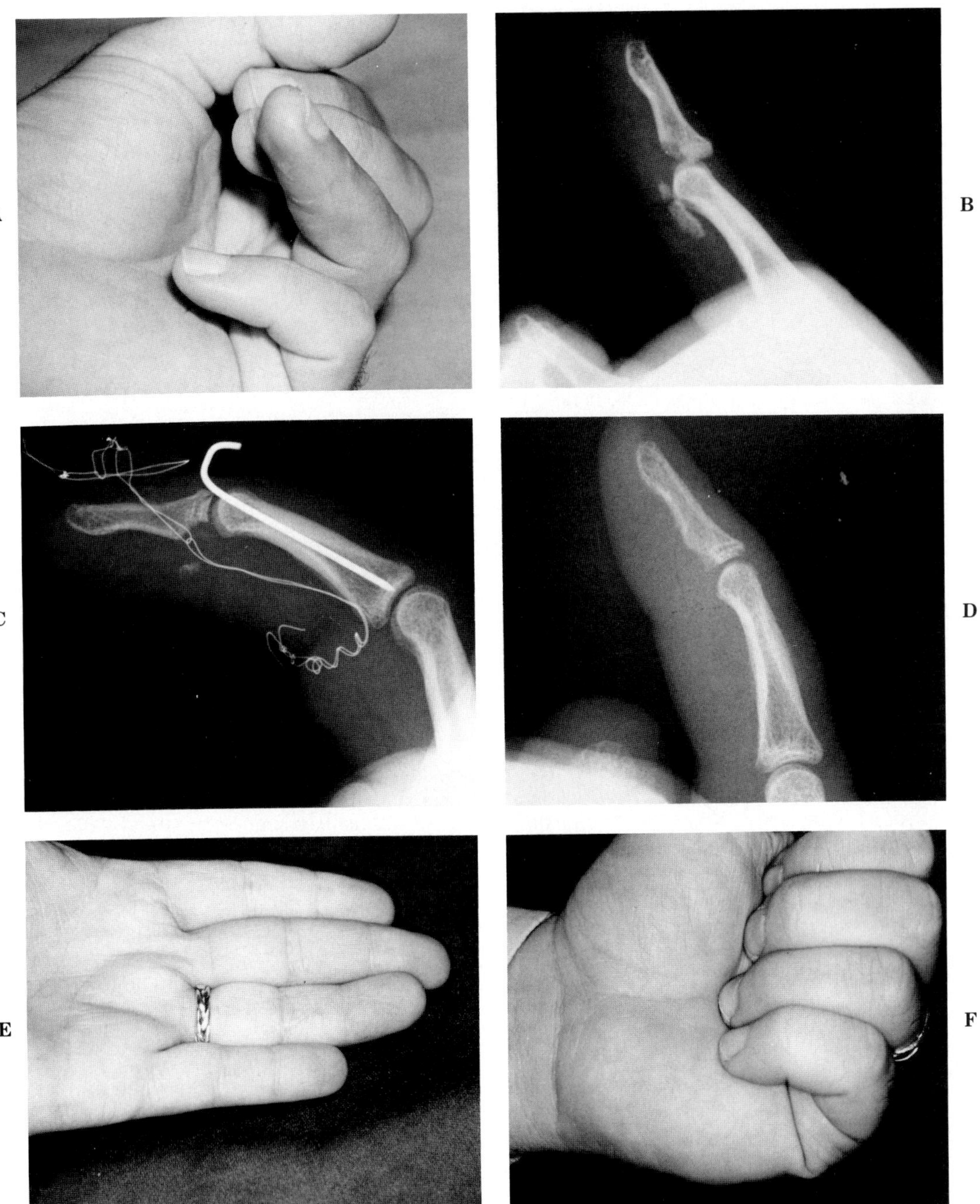

FIG. 27-5. Fracture of the distal phalanx with, in addition, separation of the profundus tendon from the fragment. This finger sustained an avulsive force when caught in the reins of his horse. **A,** Loss of flexion with pain at the distal joint. **B,** The roentgenograph showed bony avulsion from the base of the distal phalanx and dorsal displacement of the distal phalanx. **C,** On exploration, the tendon was found to be separated from the bone fragment. The joint was reduced and stabilized with a Kirschner wire, the bone fragments were discarded, and the tendon was attached directly to the distal phalanx by a pull-out wire. **D,** Roentgenographic appearance 6 years later. **E,** and **F,** Range of motion at the ring finger at 6 years.

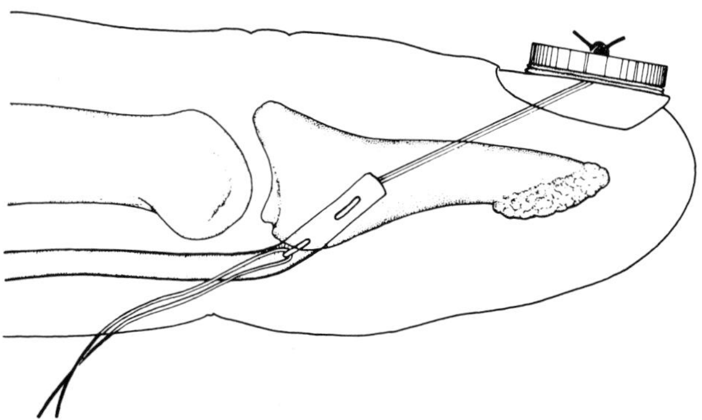

FIG. 27-6. Bunnell technique for reattachment of the flexor profundus to the distal phalanx. (From Schneider LH: Flexor tendon injuries, Boston, 1985, Little, Brown & Co. Used with permission.)

phalanx the tendon is reattached to bone. The Bunnel tendon-to-bone juncture is best.[44] This should be done early, preferably before 2 weeks have elapsed. If done later, the profundus muscle may contract and shorten. With reattachment the surgeon may find that the finger will be placed in excessive flexion when it is on the operating table. This will be recognized by placing the hand flat on the table with the wrist in the neutral position. There will be a break in the normal cascade of the fingers. It is a mistake to accept this posture. The surgeon should be prepared preoperatively to abandon the direct repair and either accept the situation or go to tendon grafting or fusion of the joint.

Type 2 lesions. In this lesion the tendon does not pull as proximally as in type 1 but stays in the finger, so it is not as emergent a procedure. I have reattached these successfully at a later time, again using the Bunnell technique. The pull-out wire in the tendon can incorporate the fracture fragment and be used to pull the fragment into its bed in the distal phalanx.

The reattachment to bone is done using the Bunnell pull-out wire technique (Fig. 27-6). The patient is mobilized early, as in the protected mobilization program.[44] This procedure in these lesions in which the tendon has pulled into the palm is usually performable up to approximately 2 weeks. I have treated a patient in whom the short vinculum of the profundus remained intact and the tendon end had migrated only to the level just proximal to the distal interphalangeal (DIP) joint. A patient such as this could probably be treated quite late. Obviously this could not have been predicted before exploration, so the exact time that one can successfully carry out a reattachment is not fixed, and exploration may be needed to make a definitive determination.

Late Lesions

There are patients in whom the initial diagnosis was missed or, as is not uncommon, athletes who will elect to defer their treatment when seen at the time of injury. Not infrequently we see an athlete with this lesion past the time that direct repair can be accomplished. Typical is the football player who comes in after the season with loss of distal joint flexion. When passive motion at the DIP joint has been maintained, the choices for treatment include the following.[23,39]

1. *Accepting the lesion as it stands.* This is particularly pertinent for patients who have a fully functional flexor superficialis to motor the PIP joint. Most of the useful arc of motion of the finger has been maintained when the superficialis is fully functional. There is considerable risk to this function, if while the tendon graft is being passed through or around the superficialis decussation, damage is done to this complex area, resulting in adhesion formation and an overall reduction in function. In fingers that are not particularly soft or supple but that show good FDS function, it may be justifiable to again offer no treatment. This is particularly true when the distal joint is not hyperextensible.

2. *Stabilization of the tip by fusion or tenodesis.* If the distal joint is unstable, particularly if it tends to hyperextension, fusion can be offered. If damage at the PIP joint results in a flexion contracture at that level, tenolysis and joint release at that joint can be combined with a distal joint fusion without going into more complex procedures. This salvage in which proximal joint function is restored or preserved with stabilization of the distal joint has been referred to as the "superficialis finger."[44] At the same sitting one might excise the proximal portion of the FDP if it is coiled up in the palm and causing a troublesome mass at that location. If at the time of tenolysis

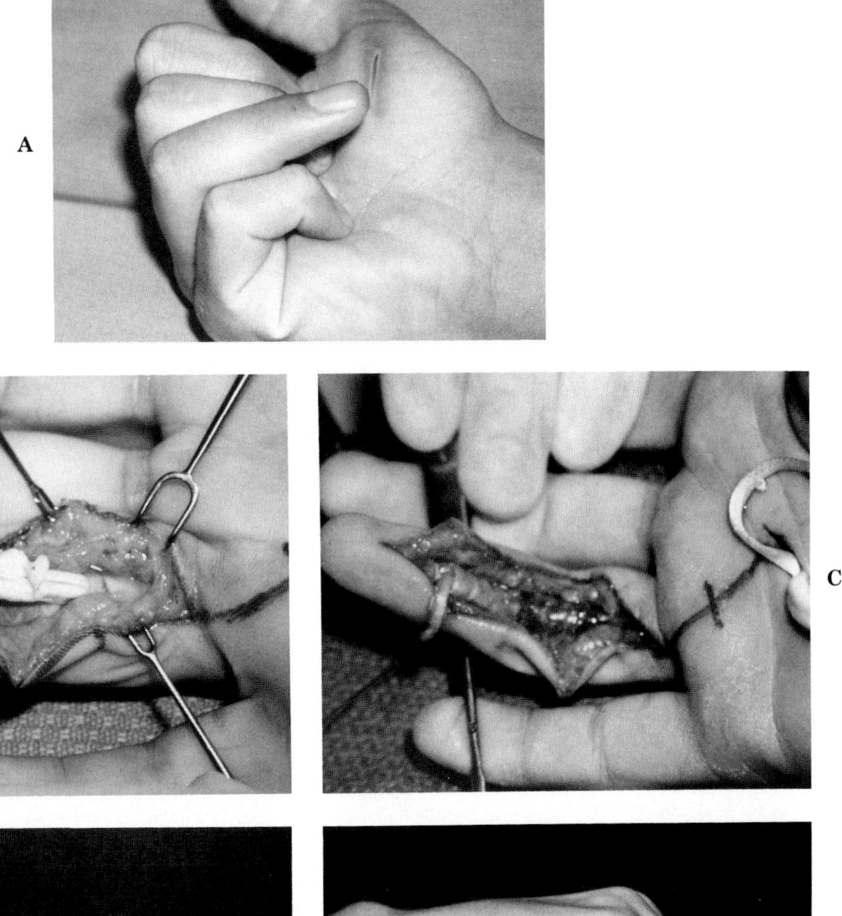

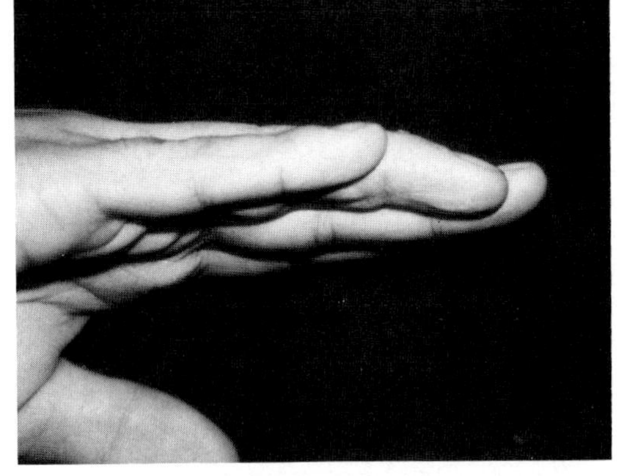

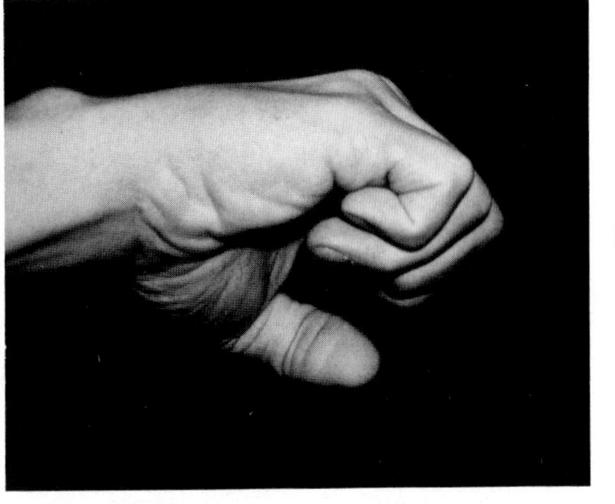

FIG. 27-7. Closed rupture of the flexor digitorum profundus in a 17-year-old football player who reports for treatment 4 months after injury. **A,** Posture of the finger in attempted flexion of the ring finger. **B,** The tendon has been retrieved but is not advanceable to the distal phalanx. **C,** A tendon graft from the palmaris longus is placed within the flexor retinaculum. **D,** and **E,** Range of motion returned to the distal interphalangeal joint after 6 months.

of the intact but adherent flexor superficialis a graft for distal joint function has been elected, the staged technique is used.[44]

3. *Tendon graft through the intact flexor superficialis in one or two stages*. This last technique is the only way that motion can be returned to the distal phalanx. Contrary to other opinions, this reconstructive procedure is even better indicated in those in whom the PIP is not normal. It is noted that this procedure is done at considerable risk to the function of the finger, and both patient and surgeon should consider the risks when offering this procedure. The patient may opt for one of the more predictable procedures. In my opinion the tendon graft is better indicated in the young and on the ulnar side of the hand (Fig. 27-7). In my experience, which includes

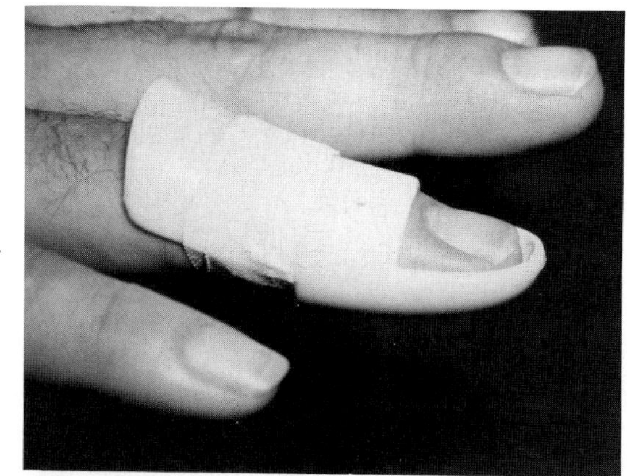

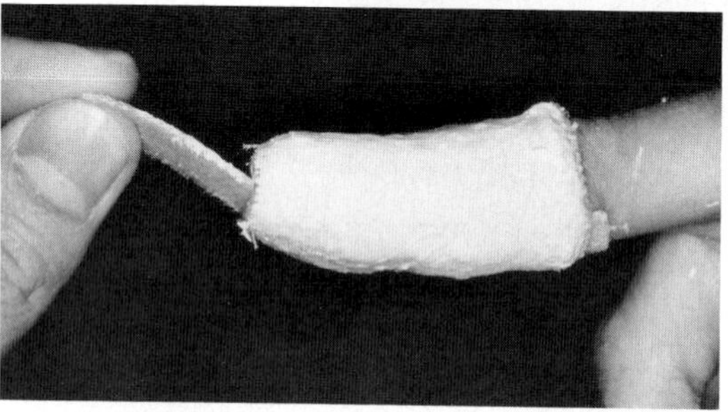

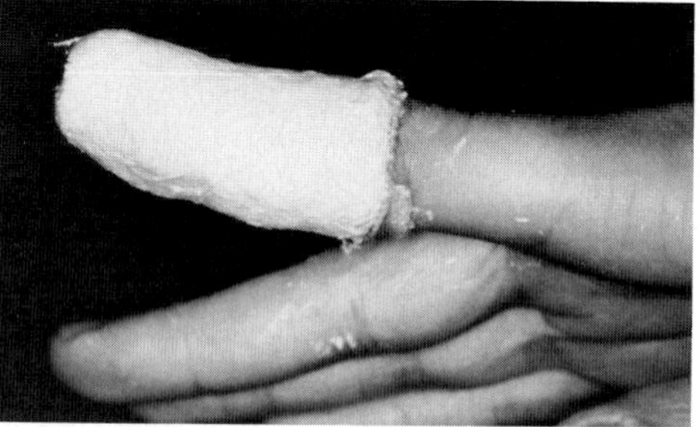

FIG. 27-8. Immobilization devices for mallet fingers. **A,** Plastic splint is comfortable and allows for proximal interphalangeal joint motion. It can additionally be wrapped with tape when the patient is participating in sports. **B,** and **C,** Finger cast applied over adherent tape is a reliable form of immobilization.

22 palm-to-fingertip one-stage tendon grafts, flexor tenolysis was carried out as a secondary procedure in approximately 50% of cases.[45] Where heavy scarring is found or in those patients who need joint release or tenolysis of the superficialis, then the two-staged tendon reconstruction is indicated.[44]

MALLET FINGER INJURY

Mechanism of Injury

Disruption of the terminal extensor mechanism at the distal interphalangeal joint will produce an extensor lag at that joint.[21,52] This lesion, the mallet finger, which has also been referred to as a baseball finger, is incurred when an object, often a ball, strikes the tip of the extended finger, forcing it suddenly into flexion. This activity tears the extensor mechanism from the base of the distal phalanx. The tendon may be just stretched or attenuated, or torn completely from the bone, resulting in a soft tissue mallet finger. If the deformity is associated with a fracture in which a fragment of bone comes off from the dorsum of the distal phalanx with the tendon, a mallet fracture is present.

Types of mallet injuries

- Soft tissue mallet finger—
  tendon is stretched, attenuated, or avulsed
- Mallet fracture—
  tendon is detached with a portion of distal phalanx

Pertinent Anatomy

The distal extensor tendon, formed from contributions from the lateral bands over the middle phalanx, terminates in a central tendon that inserts into the base of the distal phalanx.[53] Some of the fibers of the oblique retinacular ligament also blend into the central tendon and contribute to the extension at the distal interphalangeal joint. Interruption of this extensor mechanism will lead to varying degrees of drooping of the distal phalanx (an extensor lag). In patients with hyperextensile PIP joints, the PIP joint tends to adopt a hyperextension posture. This is because with proximal migration of the extensor force more power into extension is placed on the PIP joint. This will lead to stretching of the volar supportive structures at the PIP joint. With attempts at extension this problem worsens. The flexor profundus exaggerates the deformity at the DIP with more tension placed

A

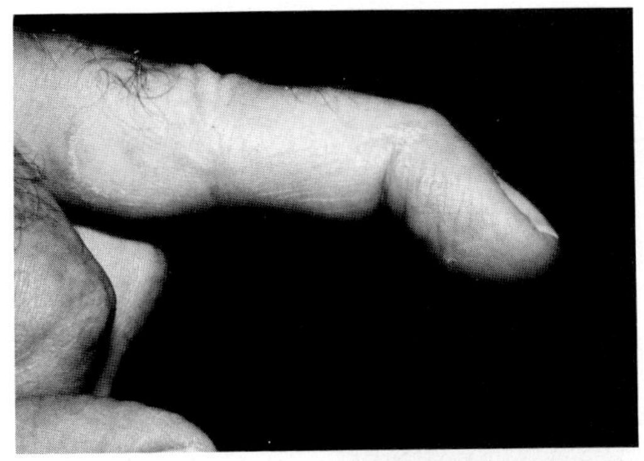

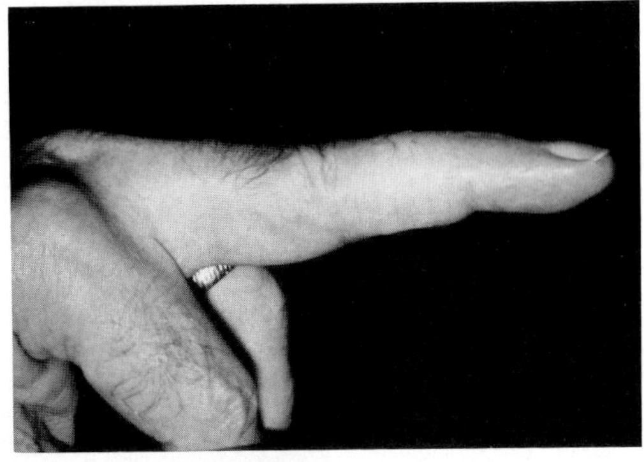

B

C

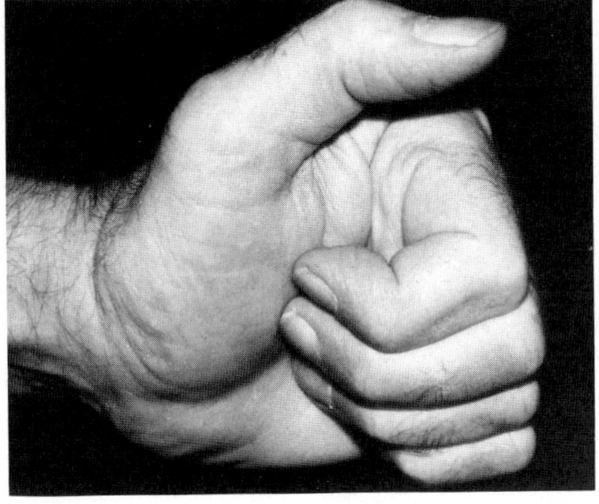

FIG. 27-9. Mallet finger. **A,** A 60-year-old man who stubbed his finger playing catch with his grandchild. He had a 45-degree extensor lag at the distal joint. He was treated in a splint, as seen in Fig. 27-8, A, for 8 weeks. **B,** and **C,** Range of motion achieved at 4 months.

in it by the hyperextension at the PIP. With time a swan-neck deformity (hyperextension at the PIP joint and flexion at the DIP joint) may result.

Examination

The patient usually recognizes and points out to the examiner that he or she has lost terminal joint extension. There may be erythema over the dorsum of the joint and some pain with the injury, but there can be remarkably few symptoms. Inability to actively extend the distal phalanx will be present to a varying degree. The exact amount of extension loss can be better estimated when compared with an adjacent normal finger, because many patients normally hyperextend at the distal interphalangeal joint.

Roentgenographs

Roentgenographs should be taken to rule out fracture.

Treatment

Acute Soft Tissue Mallet Injuries

Acute soft tissue mallet injuries can be treated by well-proven nonoperative methods.[1]

Splints. Many kinds of splints have been recommended; these are applied with the distal joint in extension (Fig. 27-8). One should not force the joint into hyperextension because this risks sloughing of skin on the dorsum of the joint. This treatment requires 6 to 8 weeks of uninterrupted immobilization in extension at the DIP joint. The important point with this treatment is educating the patient to avoid removing the splint to test for healing. If the splint is to be changed, the joint must be kept in full extension. In the past the PIP joint would be included, but this is now known not to be necessary. Inclusion of the more proximal joint may be helpful in the more active or uncooperative patient.

Circular finger castings. The splinting program is difficult to apply in many active athletes and circular finger casting may be a more predictable method of immobilization. In very active or uncooperative patients, inclusion of the PIP joint in 45 degrees of flexion in the finger cast will, in addition, help keep the splint from slipping off (Fig. 27-9). The immobilization should not be placed in excessive extension to avoid skin sloughs on the dorsum of the distal joint.

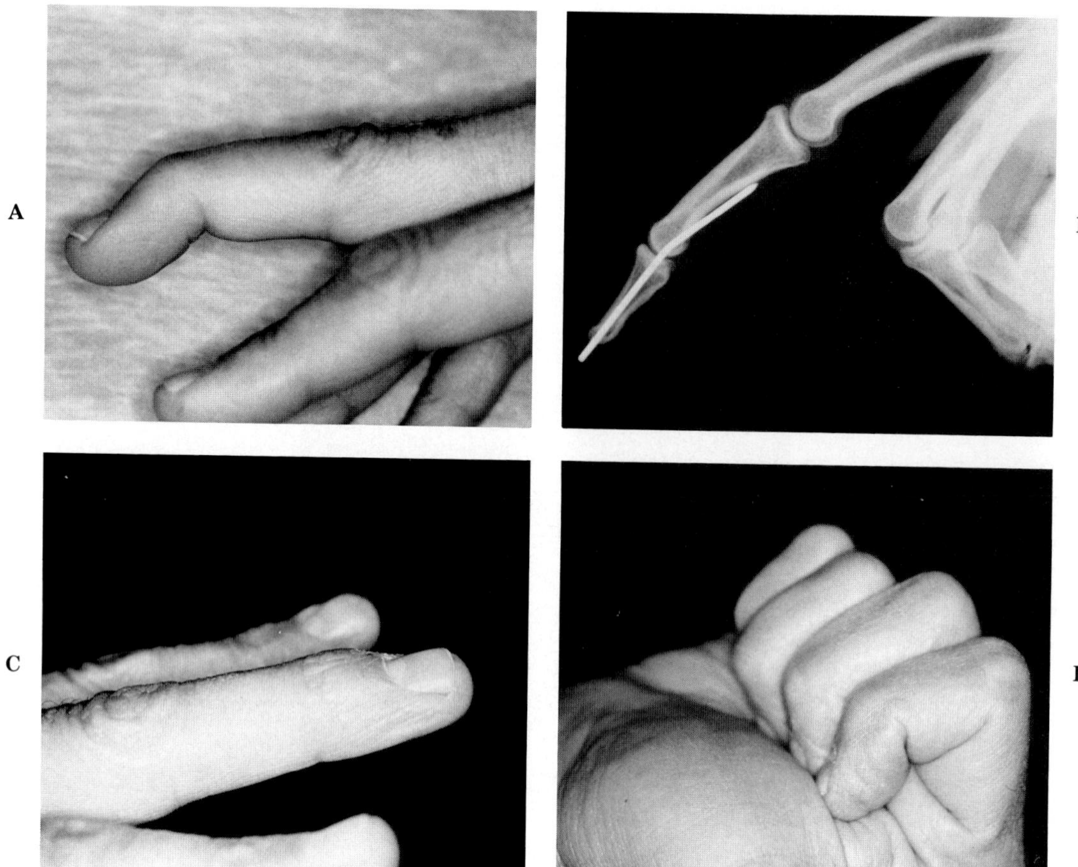

FIG. 27-10. Mallet finger treated by percutaneous Kirschner wire fixation of the distal joint. **A,** Mallet finger in a 50-year-old surgeon. **B,** A 0.62 Kirshner wire was used to transfix the distal interphalangeal joint in extension. The pin was cut off subcutaneously and he resumed activities. It is noted that he inadvertently bent the pin. **C,** and **D,** Extension and flexion at 2 years.

Percutaneous wire fixation. Operative repair is rarely indicated in the acute closed mallet finger. One form of operative treatment is the use of a percutaneous Kirschner wire to fix the DIP joint in extension.[9,10] This is done under metacarpal block of the digital nerves with a single 0.045 Kirschner wire. In the active patient the pin can be cut off beneath the skin and activity allowed (Fig. 27-10). In risk situations the finger should be additionally protected with an external splint.

Open operative repair. Authors have used open operative treatment for the acute soft tissue mallet finger injury. In my experience these are rarely indicated. Hillman recommended immobilizing the distal joint with a suture placed percutaneously.[22] I would see little indication for this procedure.

Chronic Soft Tissue Mallet Injuries

Not infrequently the mallet injury soft tissue goes untreated and the patient presents himself for treatment later. This is usually because the significance of the injury was missed or underestimated. Selection of a treatment method is determined on an individual basis based on the significance of symptoms and amount of dysfunction present. An array of procedures are available. Judgment is required in their selection, and in fact many of these chronic mallet fingers have little functional impairment and are better left untreated. (A famous professional baseball catcher is said to have had eight untreated mallet fingers and to have done well.)

When treatment is elected there are various options.

Splint application, as in the acute case. It is known that splints may be adequate treatment even for a late mallet finger. A recent paper showed good results in patients who were treated by late splinting 4 to 18 weeks after injury.[38] In fact it is not really known what the outside time period is in which splinting will still effectively correct the problem. The disadvantage of late splinting is the

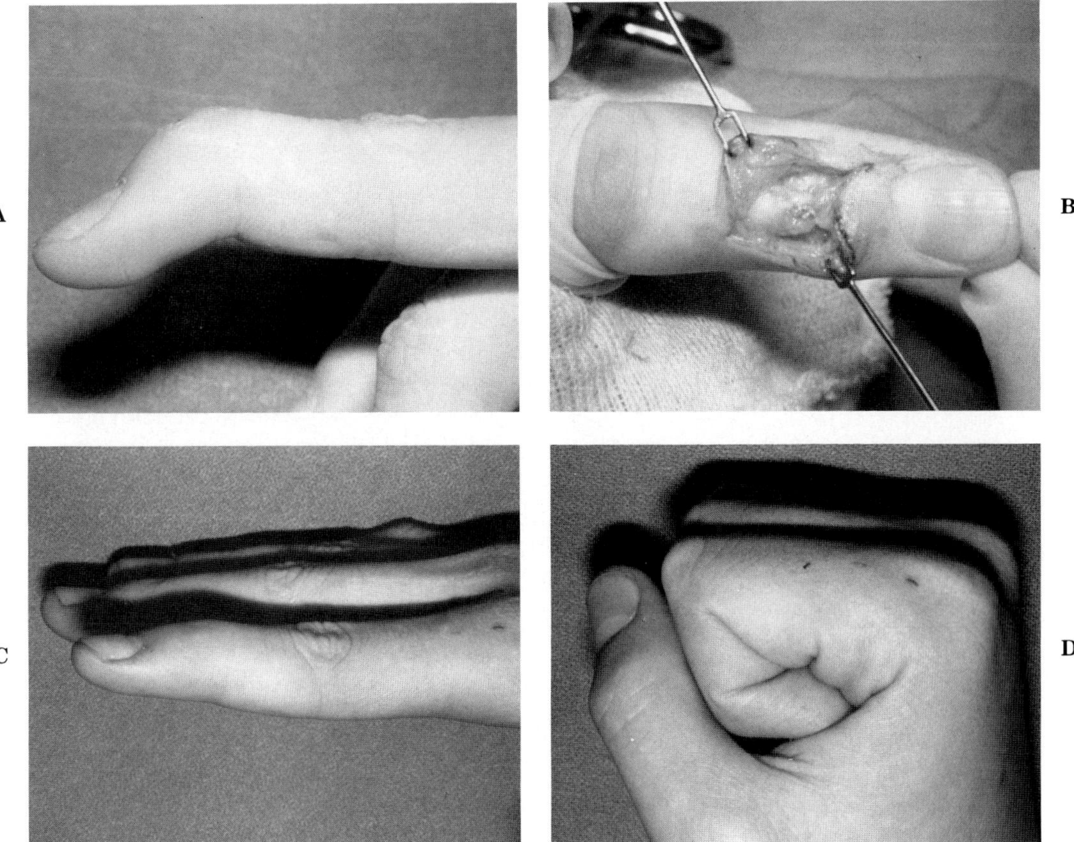

FIG. 27-11. Chronic mallet finger of the index finger in a 16-year-old boy. **A,** This lesion was 5 months old with chronic swelling seen at the dorsum of the joint. **B,** The tendon showed scarring and granulation tissue at the area of disruption. This scarring was excised and the tendon ends were sutured. A Kirschner wire was used to transfix the joint for 6 weeks. **C,** and **D,** Excellent recovery at 6 months is seen in these photos.

unpredictability of this technique. The advantages of the use of nonoperative treatment in a prolonged long program must be weighed with the fact that many of the operative reconstructive techniques used are also unpredictable.

Surgical reattachment or shortening of the extensor tendon will usually recover extension in most cases.[15] The joint needs to be kept extended full time for 6 to 8 weeks and a Kirschner wire is left in place for most of this time. The problem is that most of these, if protected long enough, will restore extension at the price of some flexion loss at the distal joint. In young cooperative patients this can be a reasonable procedure (Fig. 27-11).

Fowler's technique is a procedure in which the central slip is released at the PIP joint, which allows the extensor system to more strongly pull distally at the DIP joint, thereby improving extension at that joint.[4,17] This procedure risks the development of a boutonnière deformity.

Tenodermodesis. For late untreated mallet fingers, Iselin has described a procedure in which the skin and extensor mechanism are excised over the DIP joint in an elliptical fashion.[24] The skin-tendon edges are then reapproximated by three or four nonabsorbable sutures. The aftercare includes splinting for 5 weeks full time and at night for an additional 4 weeks.

Oblique retinacular ligament reconstruction. In this procedure a free tendon graft is inserted along the course of the oblique retinacular ligament from the flexor sheath overlying the proximal phalanx and is distally attached to the terminal extensor tendon. This procedure was described by Thompson et al and is technically rather complex.[51] It is said to have been simplified by Kleinman and Petersen.[25] I have no experience with this technique.

Fusion. This reliable, predictable procedure is indicated in the patient with painful arthrosis of the joint after failed treatment.

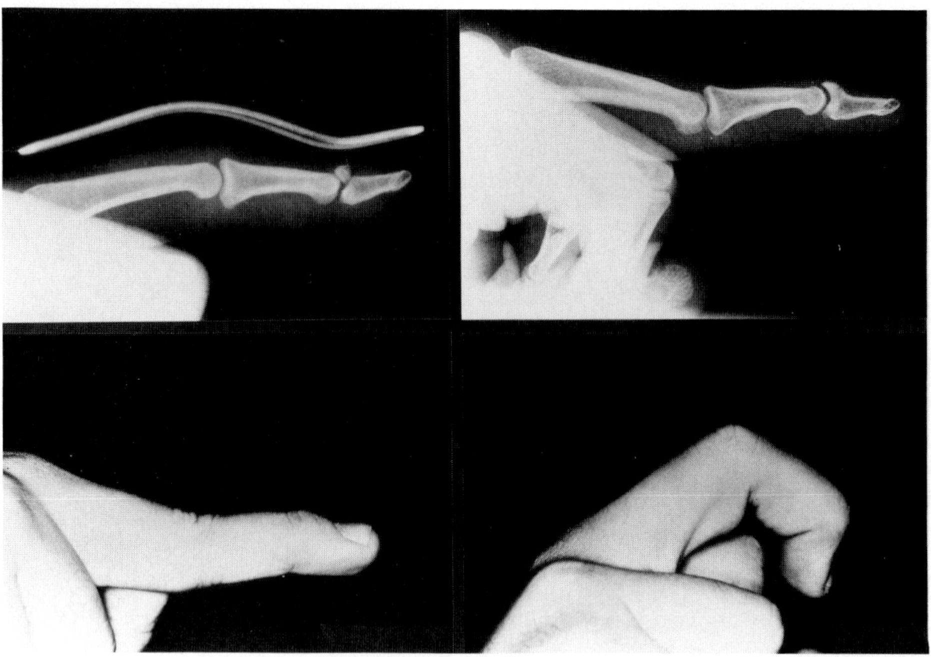

FIG. 27-12. Mallet fracture. A significant fracture of the base of the distal phalanx with articular surface disruption is seen at the *upper left*. Dorsal splinting was shortened to distal to the proximal interphalangeal joint at 2 weeks. The joint was kept in extension uninterrupted for 6 weeks. The range of motion achieved at 2 years is seen *below right and left* and the roentgenogram at that time is seen in the photo, *upper right*. The patient was asymptomatic. This joint has a remarkable ability to remodel, obviating the need for operative treatment. (From Wehbe MA, and Schneider LH: Mallet fractures, J Bone and Joint Surg 66A:658-669, 1984. Used with permission.)

Acute Mallet Fractures

It should be noted that mallet fractures, an injury not infrequently associated with sports, is caused by avulsion of the terminal extensor tendon with a portion of the base of the distal phalanx. Many treatments have been advocated but virtually all of these injuries can be treated by well-proven nonoperative techniques.[46,55] This means uninterrupted splinting of the DIP joint in zero degrees of extension for 6 to 8 weeks. This joint has been seen to remodel despite significant involvement of the articular surface and even with displacement (Fig. 27-12).

Chronic Mallet Fractures

The use of a splint for a patient who is initially seen with this lesion at a late date can still be tried. The cut off time for splint treatment for untreated injuries is not known at this time.

The chronic untreated mallet fracture can often be accepted by the patient if symptoms are not severe. On one occasion I excised the dorsal bump and reset (shortened) the extensor tendon with some improvement. Fusion of the joint for painful arthrosis is reasonable in symptomatic patients.

Hyperextension Variant of the Mallet Injury

Mention should be made of the hyperextension variant of the mallet injury. Lange and Engber[27] brought our attention to this injury, which was recognized by Bohler.[3] Bohler stated that all mallet fractures did not occur in flexion injuries by avulsion of the bone by the tendon. In the hyperextension variant, the base of the distal phalanx is jammed against the head of the middle phalanx, resulting in a major fracture fragment at the dorsal base of the distal phalanx. Lange and Engber reported that we should be careful not to hyperextend these injuries in splints because this leads to displacement and possible palmar subluxation of the joint.[27] I believe that this lesion can be treated in the same manner as the usual mallet fracture. Care is taken to splint in minimal flexion or the straight position, but treatment is not really different from that for the mallet fracture sustained in the usual way.

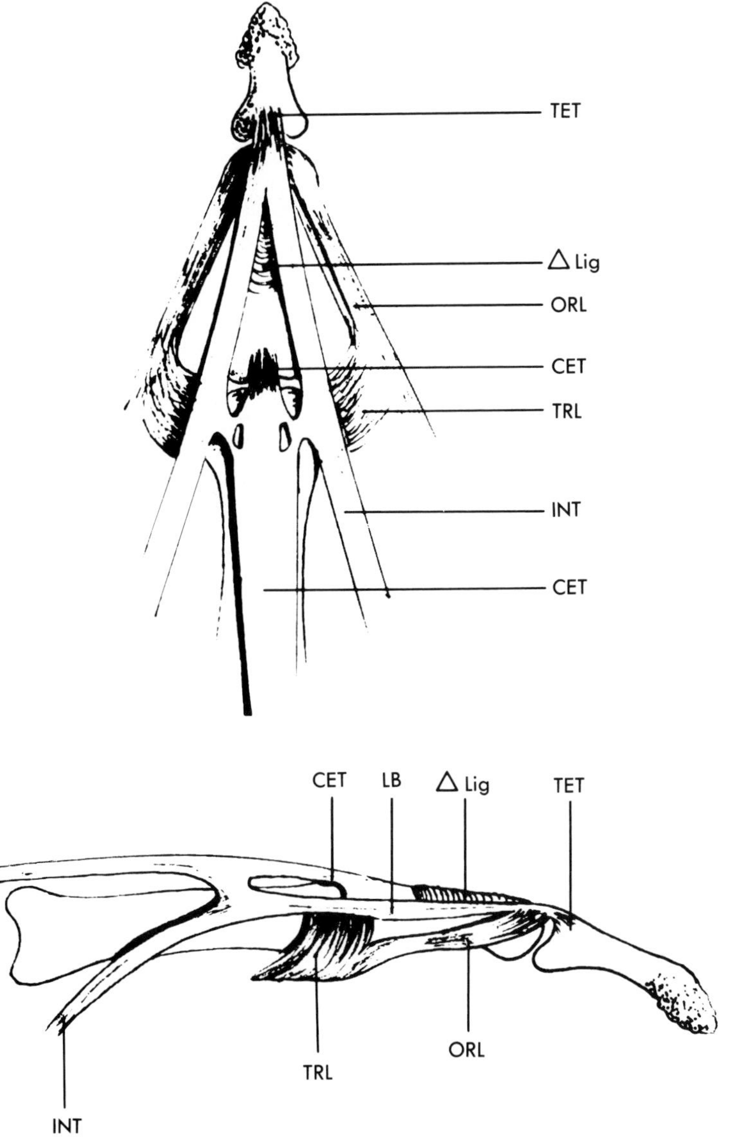

FIG. 27-13. Extensor anatomy. *CET*, central extensor tendon; *LB*, lateral band; Δ, Lig triangular ligament; *TET*, terminal extensor tendon; *INT*, intrinsic tendon; *TRL*, transverse retinacualar ligament; *ORL*, oblique retinacular ligament. (From Schneider LH, and Smith KL: Boutonniere deformity. In Hunter JM, Schneider LH, and Mackin EJ, editors: Tendon surgery in the hand, St. Louis, 1987, The CV Mosby Co. Used with permission.)

BOUTONNIÈRE DEFORMITY

Disruption of the extensor mechanism at the dorsum of the proximal interphalangeal joint level can lead to a boutonnière (buttonhole) deformity in which there is loss of active extension at the proximal interphalangeal joint and secondary hyperextension at the distal interphalangeal joint. This deformity can be very disabling to the athlete, and once established, it is difficult to treat. The lesion can be caused by an open injury (laceration) to the extensor mechanism at the proximal interphalangeal joint but in the athlete will more often be associated with a closed "jamming" injury, which forcibly flexes the PIP joint while it is in the extended position.[53]

Pertinent Anatomy (Fig. 27-13)

The extensor hood, also referred to as the extensor or dorsal apparatus, is formed at the metacarpophalangeal (MP) joint level by contributions from both the extrinsic extensor systems and the intrinsic tendons.[52] As the extensor tendon system progresses distally from the hood mechanism, a central slip forms that inserts into the base of the middle phalanx. The extrinsic extensor also contributes two lateral slips that merge with contributions from the intrinsic tendons to form the lateral bands. The major portions of the intrinsic tendons make up these lateral bands while a lesser part goes to the central slip. The lateral bands progress distally and become more dorsal over the middle phalanx and ultimately join each other to insert as the terminal extensor tendon at the base of the distal phalanx. An important ligament over the middle phalanx, the triangular ligament, bridges the two lateral bands and holds these bands in a dorsolateral position. This ligament limits the palmar displacement of these lateral bands in flexion.

Also of importance is the retinacular ligament system. There are two identifiable retinacular ligaments: transverse and oblique. The transverse retinacular ligaments, which insert on the lateral aspect of the lateral bands, serve to prevent the lateral bands from coming dorsally to the midline in extension. The oblique retinacular ligaments run from a palmar position at the proximal phalanx and the flexor sheath and progress dorsally alongside the middle phalanx and finally insert into the distal phalanx alongside the terminal tendon. The retinacular ligaments serve to coordinate movement at the proximal and distal interphalangeal joints. When the finger normally flexes at the distal joint, the oblique retinacular ligament tightens and tends to flex the proximal joint. The passive extension of the proximal joint also causes extension at the distal joint through these oblique retinacular fibers.

Mechanism of Injury

The mechanism of formation of the boutonnière deformity begins with damage to the central tendon mechanism at the PIP joint by a flexion force that is applied while the joint is being extended.[57] The deformity itself will often be delayed in appearance especially in the closed athletic injury. At first the patient may be able to actively extend the PIP joint using the lateral bands. With ongoing attempts at function, active flexion of the joint will force the head of the proximal phalanx to "buttonhole" through a defect in the torn or stretched central slip (Fig. 27-14). This will subsequently cause stretching or tearing of the triangular ligament and will push the lateral bands more laterally and palmward. When the lateral bands arrive at a point palmar to the axis of motion of the PIP joint, they become flexors of the joint and are the cause of the deformity. The resulting increased tension in the lateral bands causes increased ex-

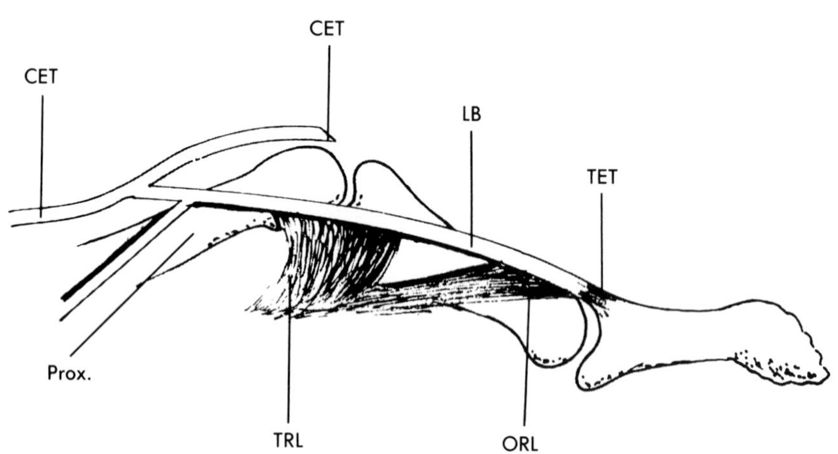

FIG. 27-14. The boutonnière deformity. Rupture of the central tendon at the proximal interphalangeal joint starts the process that leads to the boutinnière deformity. *CET,* central extensor tendon; *LB,* lateral band; *Prox,* Proximal phalanx; *TET,* terminal extensor tendon; *INT,* intrinsic tendon; *TRL,* transverse retinacular ligament; *ORL,* oblique retinacular ligament; (From Schneider LH, and Smith KL: Boutonnière deformity. In Hunter JM, Schneider LH, and Mackin EJ: Tendon surgery in the hand, St. Louis, 1987, The CV Mosby Co. Used with permission.)

tensor force to act at the distal interphalangeal joint, forcing that joint into the extended position. At first the problem is flexible, but with time the transverse retinacular ligaments tighten, holding the now shortened lateral bands below the axis of the proximal interphalangeal joint, and the deformity becomes fixed. Further, the oblique retinacular ligament, with contracture, accentuates the extended position at the distal joint.

Examination

The boutonnière deformity is missed frequently in the acute phase because of its delayed development. The examiner must therefore be alert to the existence and possibility of this lesion. A swollen, painful PIP joint after a "sprain or jam" should raise suspicion, especially when the swelling and tenderness are noted to be predominantly dorsal at the PIP joint. This joint will adopt a position of slight flexion with the DIP joint tending toward extension.[15] The presence of a volar dislocation at the PIP joint should also alert the physician to the boutonnière injury and after reduction appropriate splinting in the extended position is maintained.

Roentgenographs

Roentgenographic examination is done to rule out a fracture and may help in the diagnosis of a boutonnière injury if there is a small bone fragment avulsed from the dorsum of the middle phalanx (rare).

Treatment

Acute Boutonniére Deformity

When this injury is recognized, splinting in the extended position at the PIP joint with the DIP joint left free is indicated.[50] The immobilization of the PIP joint in extension should be maintained uninterrupted for 6 to 8 weeks. When the splint is changed, the patient should resist the temptation to "test the healing." While the patient is wearing the splint,

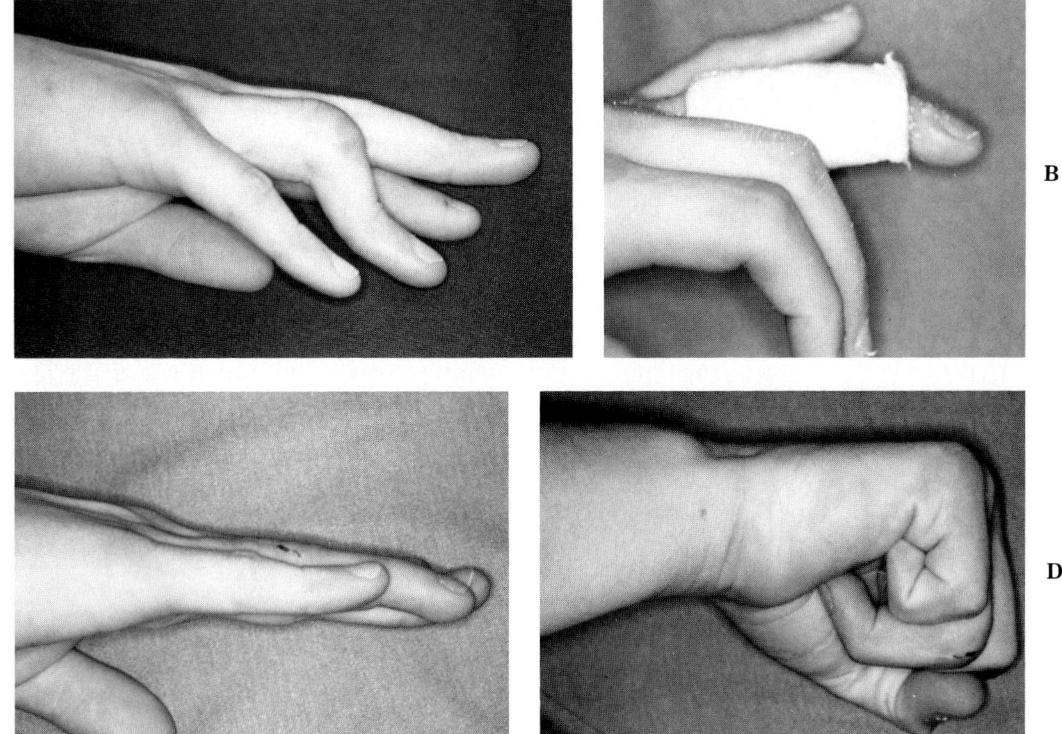

FIG. 27-15. Acute boutonnière deformity in a 15-year-old. The finger is still supple. **A,** The deformity with flexion at the proximal joint and hyperextension at the distal joint. **B,** A finger cast has been applied and the finger will remain in extension at the proximal joint for 6 weeks. The patient is encouraged to flex the distal joint while in the cast. **C,** and **D,** Range of motion at 3 months. (From Schneider LH: Injuries to tendons. In Bora FW, editor: The pediatric upper extremity, Philadelphia, 1986, WB Saunders Co. Used with permission).

active and passive flexion of the DIP joint is carried out. This maintains mobility in the distal joint and is felt to help keep the lateral bands up in their dorsolateral position at the middle phalanx. While all types of dorsal and palmar splints have been used for immobilization of the PIP joint in this problem, I have preferred the use of a plaster cylinder cast for the active age-group. This is applied in the extended position at the PIP joint. If, because of swelling, full extension could not be achieved, then the cast is changed weekly until this position is obtained. Six weeks of casting is recommended and then the patient is protected in the extended position for an additional 2 weeks. In athletic activities an additional 4 to 6 weeks of intermittent splinting is recommended (Fig. 27-15).

While the majority of acute boutonnière injuries can be treated by nonoperative means, a displaced fracture fragment avulsed from the base of the middle phalanx is an indication for open treatment. This would be treated by open reduction and internal fixation by Kirschner wires or fine screws if the fragment cannot be reduced by closed means.[53]

Treatment of acute boutonnière injury

- Splint PIP in extension
- Leave DIP free
- Maintain immobilization full time for 6-8 weeks
- Protect with splint during athletic activities for an additional 4-6 weeks
- ORIF large displaced fracture of middle phalanx base

Under certain conditions where splinting is difficult to use, the application of a transarticular Kirschner wire is indicated for immobilization in the fresh boutonnière deformity. This 0.045 of an inch pin is driven obliquely across the joint and left in place for 4 to 5 weeks and then splint protection is maintained for an additional 1 to 2 weeks. While the pin is strong it has been my policy to add a splint for extra protection to the finger for athletic activities.

While early treatment is recommended for this lesion when it is recognized in the acute stage, the point when closed treatment will not work is really unknown. It is at least 2 months but may even be longer.

Chronic Boutonnière Deformity

Not infrequently these patients present with the deformity at a late date. Treatment differs between those problems that are supple with full range of passive motion and those fixed deformities.

Supple deformities

Nonoperative treatment. Casting is a reasonable method of treatment within 8 weeks of the time of the injury in the supple deformity. Once applied, casting is continued for 8 weeks. Protective splinting is used after this while the patient is being mobilized. Actually the maximal period after injury during which nonoperative treatment could be applied is not known. Souter[50] stated that the 6-week cutoff in his study of Pulvertaft's cases was arbitrary and that closed treatment could probably be initiated even later. This treatment could be applied by either the various splint devices or even a transarticular Kirschner wire.

Operative treatment. It is to be noted that not all patients with this problem need to be treated. A mild deformity that is not worsening (is stable) can often be accepted, since the risks of operative treatment are significant. The problem in treatment here is that extension is relatively easy to regain by surgical treatment but flexion may be difficult to recover postoperatively. An untreated finger with a slight flexion deformity at the PIP joint that flexes fully is more desirable than an operated finger, which is stiff in the extension range. Therefore when an examiner chooses operative repair, the deformity should be significant.

There are many techniques described in the literature. These take widely different approaches but when considering what is known, the reader should view with suspicion those procedures that are based on the tight fixation of the lateral bands over the dorsum of the proximal interphalangeal joint, because these will prevent the free flexion of that joint and therefore not be successful.

Techniques available include the following:

1. Redistribution of forces at the joints (Littler and Eaton[30])
2. Use of a tendon graft (Nichols[36])
3. Reconstruction using the lateral bands (Matev[32] and Salvi[43])
4. Direct anatomical repair of the central slip (Souter,[44] Elliott,[15] Grundberg,[19] Pardini,[37] Smith,[49] Urbaniak,[54] and Zancolli.[57])

I prefer the last technique, in which the central slip is reattached to the middle phalanx. Elliot[15] describes this in detail (Fig. 27-16). The lateral bands are mobilized by transection of the transverse retinacular liga-

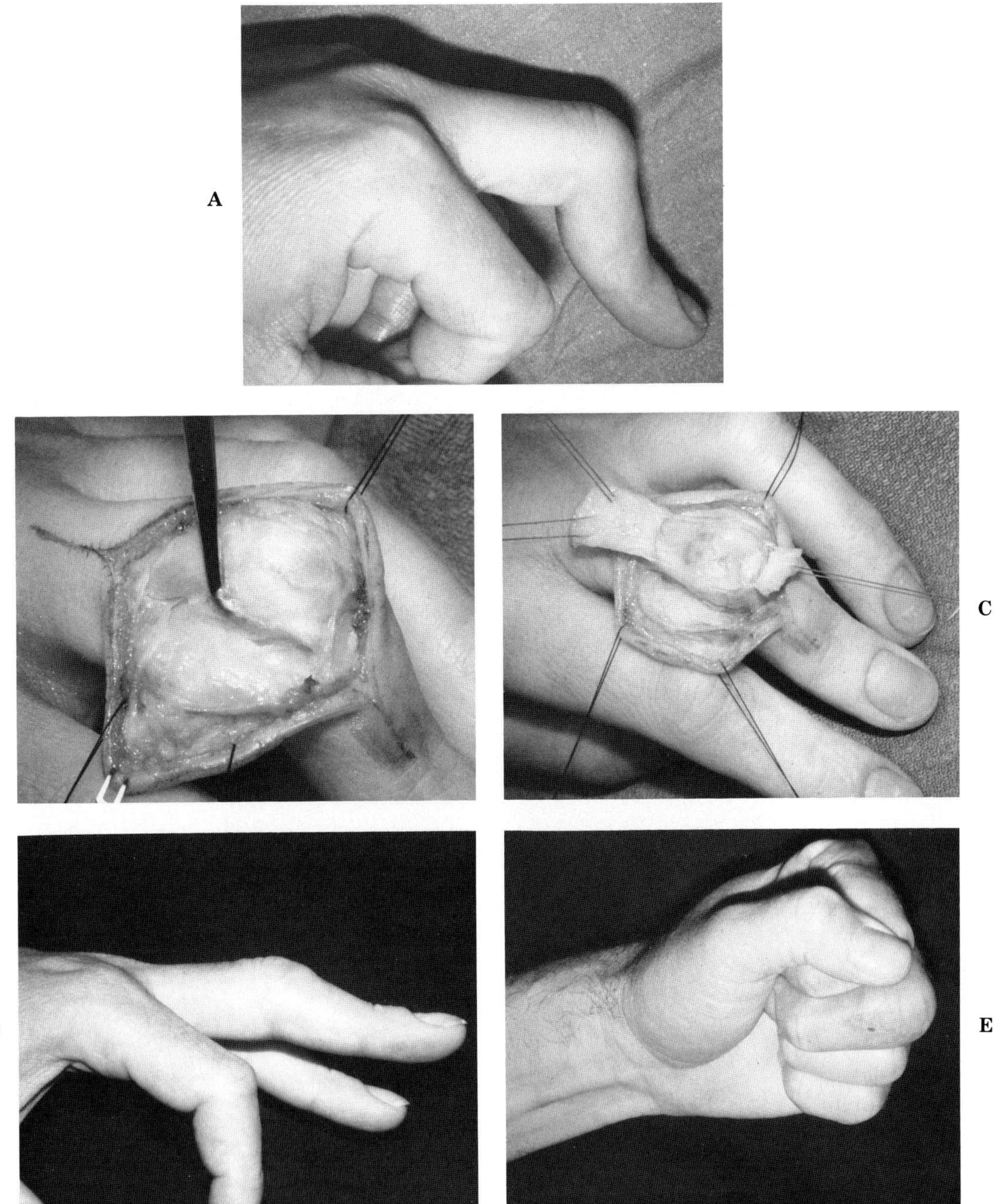

FIG. 27-16. Boutonnière deformity—surgical treatment. **A,** The deformity failed to respond to nonoperative care. **B,** The scarred extensor mechanism at the PIP joint. The probe is showing the transverse retinacular ligament, which is contracted and holding the lateral bands volar to the axis of the joint. These bands are released. **C,** The central tendon is mobilized and will be shortened and reattached to the middle phalanx. **D,** and **E,** The range of motion at 8 months.

ments and the central slip is mobilized, advanced, and repaired. In the chronic case it is noted that the central slip defect will have been filled in with scar tissue, which the surgeon will excise before reattachment to the base of the middle phalanx. The amount of central slip to be removed is very little and it is beneficial to perform this surgery with the patient under local anesthesia so as to better estimate the tension in the repair. The joint is pinned in the extended position to protect the repair. Postoperatively the finger is kept in extension for 6 weeks; 4 with pin protection and 2 more in an extension splint. The recovery period then stresses the recovery of flexion while trying not to lose the regained extension at the PIP joint.

Fixed deformity. When patients have this condition, an attempt can be made to increase joint motion by hand therapy, including range of motion exercises, dynamic splinting, and serial plasters. When these are unsuccessful in recovering passive extension at the PIP joint, this motion will have to be achieved with a surgical procedure that releases the transverse and oblique retinacular ligaments as part of the mobilization of the lateral bands. This will often be sufficient to allow full extension and then the surgeon can proceed to repair the extensor mechanism at the central slip as noted above. It may be necessary, however, in severely fixed cases, to also release the accessory portion of the collateral ligaments or even the volar plate. In advanced articular stiffness, especially where there has been intraarticular damage, it may be nec-

A

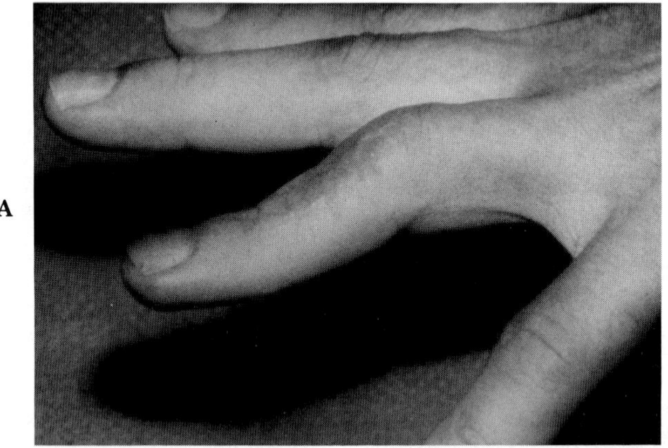

B

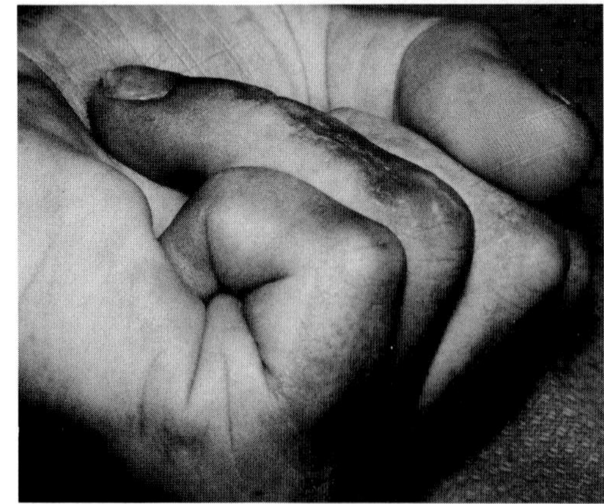

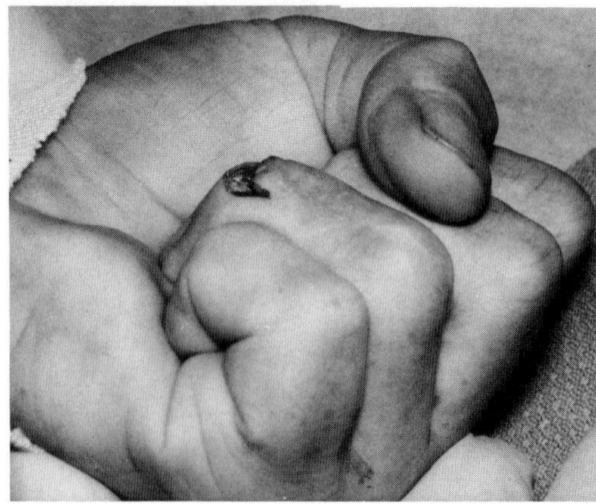

C

FIG. 27-17. Salvage of the chronic boutonnière deformity. The extensor release at the distal joint (Dolphin). **A,** Surgery had been attempted for this deformity. **B,** The patient was most troubled by loss of flexion at the distal joint at his ring finger. This interfered with his power grip. **C,** Transection of the terminal extensor tendon is done with the patient under local anesthesia. It is seen on the operating table that distal joint flexion is immediately increased.

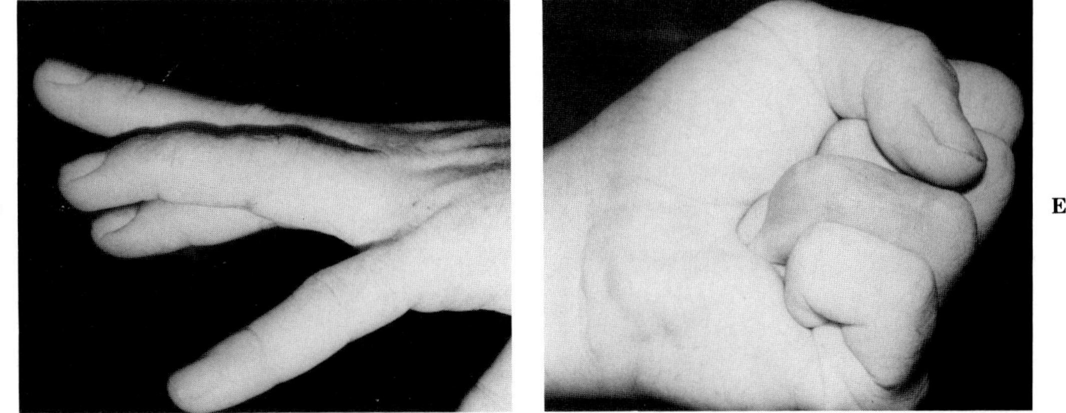

FIG. 27-17, cont'd. D, Posture of the finger in extension at 3 months is improved. **E,** Flexion at 3 months. The finger can now grip.

FIG. 27-18. Tendonitis in a karate player. **A** to **C,** Nodularity seen at the metacarpal phalangeal joint level from frequent punching activity. These masses were asymptomatic.

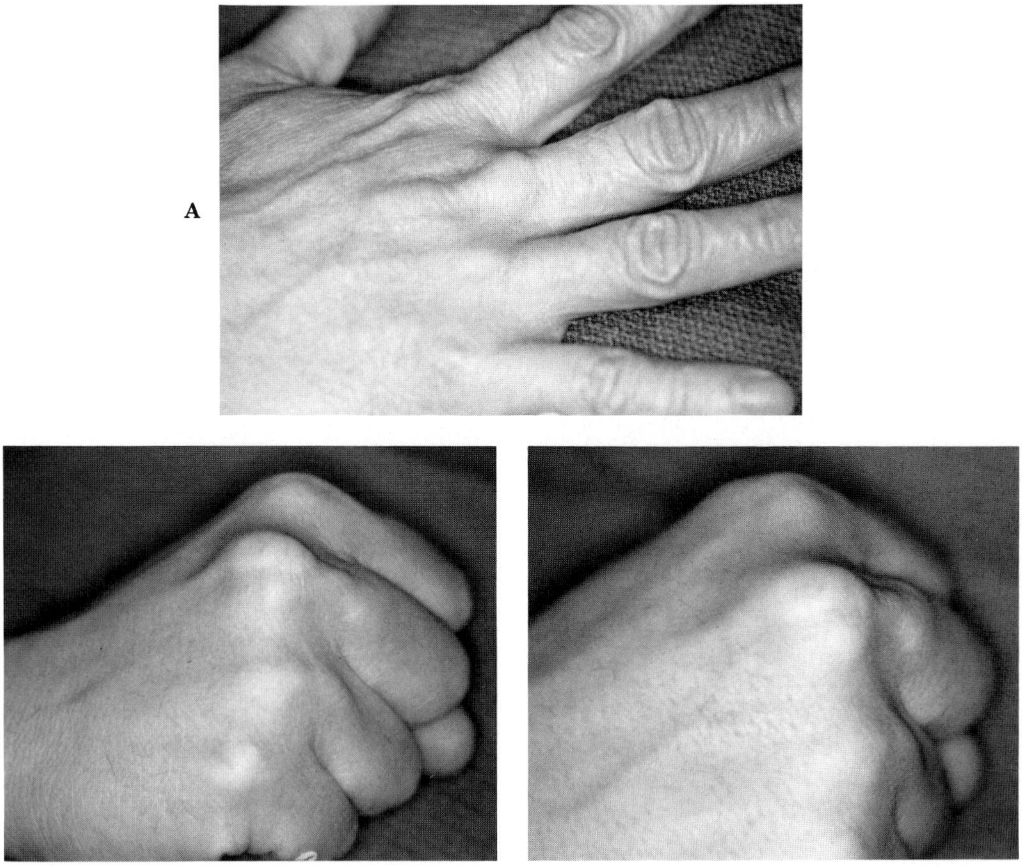

essary to reconstruct the joint using a Swanson implant arthroplasty technique[47] or even to fuse the joint in a useful position. A patient with an implant arthroplasty would be protected by buddy-taping the finger to an adjacent finger for athletic activities.

A procedure that has proved useful in the salvage of the finger with a chronic boutonnière deformity, especially in patients who have difficulty grasping because of the fixed hyperextension at the DIP joint, is the transection of the terminal extensor tendon at the distal joint. The operation has been credited to Fowler[17] and described by Dolphin.[14] This immediately improves distal joint flexion, and therefore grasp improves, although extension, provided by the oblique retinacular ligament, may be floppy. This procedure is best indicated at the ulnar border of the hand (ring and little fingers) where power grip is important (Fig. 27-17).

Curtis et al[13] have presented a step-by-step approach to the management of the chronic boutonnière deformity. When surgery is needed it is done in steps modified as the procedure progresses. This approach is very reasonable and should be reviewed by all who treat these lesions.

Pseudoboutonnière Deformity

McCue and colleagues[33,34] have pointed out that some volar plate injuries at the PIP joint that are seen late present with flexion deformities at the PIP joint and an extension posture at the DIP joint that resembles the boutonniere deformity.[33,34] It is important to differentiate these lesions from the true boutonnière because the problem is quite different and treatment, by necessity, is different. It is noted, when diagnosing this condition, that the DIP extension deformity is not severe and active and passive flexion motion at the DIP is possible. Another clue was the roentgenographic appearance of calcification and spurring proximal to the PIP joint at the proximal phalanx. This represents the palmar plate injury and a spontaneous repair reaction. This pseudoboutonnière is a joint lesion and is treatable by operations aimed at release of the palmar plate contracture.

Pseudoboutonnière deformity

- Results from volar plate injury, not extensor injury
- Flexion deformity at PIP joint like true boutonnière
- Milder DIP extension deformity in pseudoboutonnière
- Acute and passive DIP motion possible in pseudoboutonnière
- Calcification and osteophyte formation may occur at volar aspect of distal portion of proximal phalanx

Summary of Boutonnière Treatment

Overall, those experienced in the treatment of the boutonnière deformity will agree that a nonoperative approach is generally preferred in the treatment of this lesion. In mild deformities that persist after conservative therapy, one may elect to accept the problem, since there is considerable risk of increasing the impairment if surgery is unsuccessful. When surgery is elected there should be careful consideration for the indications and the pathologic condition here. Surgery with the patient under local anesthesia is helpful to evaluate both the problem and the effects of treatment during the procedure. This, combined with aftercare that is closely supervised, is critical if one is to obtain better results with this difficult entity.

HYPERTROPHY OF THE EXTENSOR MECHANISM AT THE METACARPOPHALANGEAL (MP) JOINT IN THE KARATE HAND

This condition is seen at the metacarpophalangeal joint level of karate practitioners and presents as a mass that moves with the extensor apparatus. There is a history of repeated striking of the fist against a post as part of the practice routine. The mass represents hypertrophy of the extensor mechanism in response to this trauma and has been called hypertrophic infiltrative tendonitis, the "HIT" syndrome, by Gardner.[18] Unlike his case, in which surgery was performed, my two patients with this condition were asymptomatic and no treatment was necessary (Fig. 27-18).

REFERENCES

1. Abouna JM, and Brown H: The treatment of mallet finger, Br J Surg 55:653, 1968.
2. Blazina ME, and Lane C: Rupture of the insertion of the flexor digitorum profundus in student athletes, J Am Coll Health Assoc 14:248, 1966.
3. Bohler L: Finger fractures. In Bohler L: The treatment of fractures, New York, 1956, Grune & Stratton, p. 976.
4. Bowers WH, and Hurst LC: Chronic mallet finger: the use of Fowler's central slip release, J Hand Surg 3:373, 1978.
5. Boyes JH, Wilson JN, and Smith JW: Flexor tendon ruptures in the forearm and hand, J Bone Joint Surg 42A:637, 1960.

6. Burton R, and Eaton R: Common hand injuries in the athlete, Orthop Clin North Am 4:808, 1973.
7. Buscemi MJ, and Page BJ: Flexor digitorum profundus avulsions with associated distal phalanx fractures, Am J Sports Med 15:366, 1987.
8. Carroll RE, and Match RM: Avulsion of the flexor profundus tendon insertion, J Trauma 10:1109, 1979.
9. Casscells SW, and Strange TB: Intramedullary wire fixation of mallet-finger, J Bone Joint Surg 39A:521, 1957.
10. Casscells SW, and Strange TB: Intramedullary-wire fixation of mallet finger, J Bone Joint Surg 51A:1018, 1969.
11. Chang WH, Thoms OJ, and White WL: Avulsion injury of the long flexor tendons, Plast Reconstr Surg 50:260, 1972.
12. Culver JE et al: Avulsions of the profundus and superficialis tendons of the ring finger, Am J Sports Med 9:184, 1981.
13. Curtis RM, Reis RL, and Provost JM: A stage technique for the repair of the traumatic boutonnière deformity, J Hand Surg 8:167, 1983.
14. Dolphin JA: Extensor tenotomy for chronic boutonnière deformity of the finger, J Bone Joint Surg 47A:161, 1965.
15. Elliott RA: Injuries to the extensor mechanism of the hand, Orthop Clin North Am 1:335, 1970.
16. Fomar RC, Nelson CL, and Phalen GS: Ruptures of the flexor tendons in the hands of non-rheumatoid patients, J Bone Joint Surg 54A:579, 1972.
17. Fowler SB: Extensor apparatus of the digits, J Bone Joint Surg 31B:477, 1949.
18. Gardner RC: Hypertrophic infiltrative tendinitis (Hit syndrome) of the long extensor: the abused Karate hand, JAMA 211:1009, 1970.
19. Grundberg AB: Anatomic repair of boutonnière deformity, Clin Orthop Rel Res 153:226, 1980.
20. Gunter GS: Traumatic avulsion injuries of the insertion of the flexor digitorum profundus, Aust N Z J Surg 30:1, 1960.
21. Hallberg D, and Lindholm A: Subcutaneous rupture of the extensor tendon of the distal phalanx of the finger: "Mallet finger," Acta Chir Scand 119:260, 1960.
22. Hillman FE: New technique for treatment of mallet fingers and fractures of distal phalanx, JAMA 161:1135, 1956.
23. Honner R: The late management of isolated lesion of the flexor digitorum profundus tendon, Hand 7:171, 1975.
24. Iselin F, Levame J, and Godoy J: A simplified technique for treating mallet fingers: tenodermodesis, J Hand Surg 2:118, 1977.
25. Kleinman WB, and Petersen DP: Oblique retinacular ligament reconstruction for chronic mallet finger deformity, J Hand Surg 9A:399, 1984.
26. Langa V, and Posner MA: Unusual rupture of a flexor profundus tendon, J Hand Surg 11A:227, 1986.
27. Lange RH, and Engber WD: Hyperextension mallet finger, Orthopedics 6:1426, 1983.
28. Leddy JP: Avulsions of the flexor digitorum profundus, Hand Clin North Am 1:77, 1985.
29. Leddy JP, and Packer JW: Avulsion of the profundus tendon insertion in athletes, J Hand Surg 2:66, 1977.
30. Littler JW, and Eaton RG: Redistribution of the forces in the correction of boutonnière deformity, J Bone Joint Surg 49-A:1267, 1967.
31. Manske PR, and Lesker PA: Avulsion of the ring finger flexor digitorum profundus tendon: an experimental study, Hand 10:52, 1978.
32. Matev I: Transposition of the lateral bands of the aponeurosis of longstanding "boutonnièrre deformity" of the fingers, Br J Plast Surg 17:281, 1964.
33. McCue FC, and Garroway RY: Sports injuries to the hand and wrist. In Schneider RC, Kennedy JC, and Plant ML, editors: Sports injuries, Baltimore, 1985, Williams & Wilkins, p.743.
34. McCue FM et al: Athletic injuries of the proximal interphalangeal joint requiring surgical treatment, J Bone Joint Surg 52A:937, 1970.
35. Mosher JF: Flexor and extensor tendon injuries. In Pettrone FA, editor: AAOS symposium on upper extremity injuries in athletes, St Louis, 1986, The CV Mosby Co.
36. Nichols HN: Repair of the extensor tendon insertions in the fingers, J Bone Joint Surg 33A:836, 1951.
37. Pardini AG, Sosta RD, and Morais MS: Surgical repair of the boutonnièrre deformity of the fingers, Hand 11:87, 1979.
38. Patel MR, Desai SS, and Bassini-Lipson, L: Conservative management of chronic mallet finger, J Hand Surg 11A:570, 1986.
39. Posch JL, Walker PJ, and Miller H: Treatment of ruptured tendons of the hand and wrist, Am J Surg 91:669, 1956.
40. Posner MA: Injuries to the hand and wrist in athletes, Orthop Clin North Am 8:593, 1977.
41. Reef TC: Avulsions of the flexor digitorum profundus: an athletic injury, Am J Sports Med 5:281, 1977.
42. Robins PR, and Dobyns JH: Avulsion of the insertion of the flexor digitorum profundus tendon associated with fracture of the distal phalanx. In Symposium on tendon surgery in the hand, St Louis, 1975, The CV Mosby Co.
43. Salvi V: Technique for the boutonnière deformity, Hand 1:96, 1969.
44. Schneider LH: Flexor tendon injuries, Boston, 1985, Little, Brown & Co Inc.
45. Schneider LH: Treatment of isolated flexor digitorum profundus injuries by tendon grafting. In Hunter JM, Schneider LH, and Mackin EJ editors: Tendon surgery in the hand, St. Louis, 1987, The CV Mosby Co, p.307.
46. Schneider LH: Fractures of the distal phalanx, Hand Clin North Am 4:537-547, 1988.
47. Schneider LH, and Smith KL: Boutonnière deformity. In Hunter JM, Schneider LH, and Mackin EJ, editors: Tendon surgery in the hand, St Louis, 1987, The CV Mosby Co, p.349.
48. Smith JH: Avulsion of the profundus tendon with simultaneous intraarticular fracture of the distal phalanx, J Hand Surg 6:600, 1981.
49. Smith RJ: Boutonnière deformity of the fingers Bull Hosp Joint Dis 27:27, 1966.
50. Souter WA: The problem of the boutonnière deformity, Clin Orthop Rel Res 104:116, 1974.
51. Thompson JS, Littler JW, and Upton J: The spiral oblique retinacular ligament, J Hand Surg 3:482, 1978.
52. Tubiana R, and Valentin P: The anatomy or the extensor apparatus of the fingers, Surg Clin North Am 44:897, 1964.
53. Tubiana R, and Valentin P: The physiology of the extension of the fingers, Surg Clin North Am 44:907, 1964.

54. Urbaniak JR, and Hayes MG: Chronic boutonnière deformity-an anatomical reconstruction, J Hand Surg 6:379, 1981.
55. Wehbe MA, and Schneider LH: Mallet fractures, J Bone Joint Surg 66A:658, 1984.
56. Wenger DR: Avulsion of the profundus tendon insertion in football players, Arch Surg 106:145, 1973.
57. Zancolli E: Structural and dynamic bases of hand surgery, ed 2, Philadelphia, 1979, JB Lippincott Co.

CHAPTER 28 Rehabilitation and Protection of the Hand and Wrist

Vi A. Mayer
Frank C. McCue III

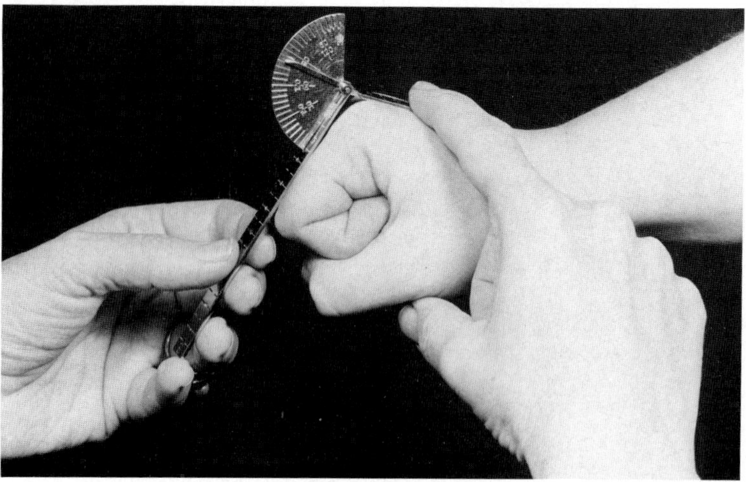

FIG. 28-1. Goniometer designed to measure small joints of the hand.

The hand and wrist are vulnerable to injury in almost every sport. Mismanagement from either a medical or a rehabilitation standpoint can result in significant disability and limitation in function. Functional use of hands requires adequate mobility, stability, and sensibility as well as freedom from pain.

All athletic injuries of the hand and wrist should be evaluated by an orthopaedist in a timely manner. To help the athlete avoid a functional residual deficit, we must provide him or her with an early diagnosis, accurate treatment, proper rehabilitation, and protection from reinjury.

Most hand and wrist injuries sustained during athletics are closed injuries involving ligaments, bones, tendons, and neurovascular structures, and these injuries can be treated conservatively. However, when surgical intervention is indicated, it is important that the surgeon be trained in the techniques of hand surgery. Close follow-up is of paramount importance, especially when dealing with young athletes who are impatient about restrictions that may be imposed on them. Their immaturity does not allow them to see the wisdom of compliance. It is helpful to communicate with parents or coaches for support in gaining their cooperation.

CLINICAL EXAMINATION

Clinical examination of the hand is a skill that requires an understanding of functional anatomy of the hand as well as a complete history of the mechanism of injury. A systematic examination should include evaluation of deformity, instability, tenderness, active and passive motion, and edema, as well as nerve and tendon function. Accurate documentation of findings is of great importance. Whenever possible, standardized means of measurements should be used. The **American Society for Surgery of the Hand** (ASSH)[2] and the **American Society of Hand Therapists** (ASHT)[24] have both established guidelines for clinical assessment of the hand. Patient treatment is based on the results of a thorough clinical examination as well as on accurate documented measurements.

Hand evaluation

- Deformity
- Instability
- Tenderness
- Motion (active and passive)
- Edema
- Neural function
- Tendon function

Goniometry

A standardized method of measuring and recording joint motion was established by the American Academy of Orthopaedic Surgeons in 1965[1] (Fig. 28-1). Both active motion (tendon excursion) and passive motion (joint mo-

Tendinous causes of limited active motion

- Lack of continuity
- Inflammation
- Adherence
- Attenuation
- Sheath constriction

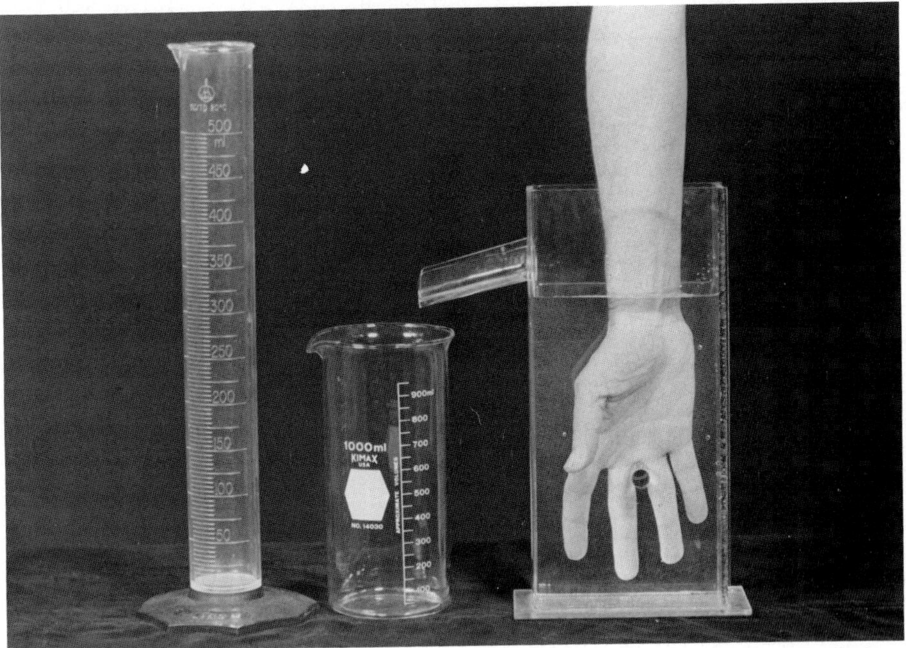

FIG. 28-2. The hand is lowered into the volumeter until the web space between the middle and ring finger is resting on the dowel. The wrist is held in neutral, then the forearm is aligned with the hand. When used according to instructions, accuracy should be within 10 ml.

bility) of flexion and extension should be measured and documented. Limitation of passive motion may be indicative of problems either within the joint itself or of the capsular structures surrounding it. Limitation of active motion may have several causes involving tendons. Causes may include lack of continuity, inflammation, adherence, attenuation, and constriction of sheath.

Frequent goniometric assessments are helpful in monitoring the effectiveness of a therapeutic program. One should be especially responsive to substantial discrepancies that exist between active and passive motion.

Hand Volume Assessment

Edema is most easily detected on the dorsum of the hand. Bony prominences appear rounded off and there are diminished lines over the joints. Edema on the palmar surface is not as easily detected but is most obvious when flexion exercises are performed. Often, complete motion will not be possible because edema is present. Subtle edema may be best observed by doing a comparative examination of the contralateral extremity.

Evaluating volume changes in the hand is necessary to evaluate the effectiveness of methods of edema control that are being used. Hand volume may be assessed by several methods. **Circumferential measurements** of the wrist, palm, and fingers are acceptable if they are measured and recorded in a consistent manner using identical bony markings or joint creases. Results should be recorded in centimeters. A more accurate means of assessing edema is possible with the use of a **hand volumeter*** (Fig. 28-2). Its use is based on Archimedes' principle of water displacement.[14] The displaced water is measured in a beaker. Often, it is helpful on initial examination to measure the contralateral hand to establish norms for each patient. A comparative study is appropriate only in the absence of appreciable deformity.

Hand volume assessment

- Circumferential measurements
- Hand volumeter

Manual Muscle Testing

Manual muscle testing is an effective way of determining the strength of individual mus-

*Available from Volumeters Unlimited, Idyllwild, CA, 92349.

TABLE 28-1 Manual muscle testing

Muscle Grade	Range of Motion (ROM)
5 = Normal	Complete ROM against gravity with full resistance
4 = Good	Complete ROM against gravity with some resistance
3 = Fair	Complete ROM against gravity with no resistance
2 = Poor	Complete ROM with gravity elminated
1 = Trace	Slight contractility with no joint motion
0 = Zero	No evidence of contractility

From Seddon H: Surgical disorders of peripheral nerves, ed 2, New York, 1975, Churchill Livingstone.

grading systems exist for evaluating muscle strength. The most frequently used system is a numerical system devised by Seddon, which grades muscles from 0 to 5 (Table 28-1).[54] Testing should occur only when there is no fear of aggravating the injury. Muscle strength should then be compared to the contralateral extremity.

Criteria for grading muscle strength have recently improved. However, there continues to be some degree of subjective interpretation by the examiner.

Sensibility Testing

Despite the fact that without sensation hand function is tremendously impaired, research into the mechanisms of sensibility has lagged enormously behind research into motor function. Aspects of sensory rehabilitation are often excluded from texts. Seddon and Bowden[11] were among the first to distinguish between "academic and functional sensibility" recovery in evaluating regeneration. **Academic recovery** is judged in terms of motor and sensory recovery, such as ability to perceive pin-prick, touch, and temperature changes, while **functional recovery** is judged in terms of the patient's ability to use the hand for functional activities. Tests performed by physicians to evaluate spinal tracts and central nervous system pathways do not correlate with the hand's ability to function[21] (Fig. 28-3). The credit for bringing this differentiation to worldwide attention belongs to Moberg,[43,44] who also spent several decades researching and publishing material on the importance of functional sensory testing.

Because of the vast number of clinical methods available for testing sensibility and the complexity of many tests, a tendency exists to exclude formal testing for sensibility from evaluations of the upper extremity. It is the challenge of the therapist or trainer to choose tests that are practical as well as appropriate to assess patients in the clinical setting. Tests should be administered in a standard manner to eliminate as many variables as possible, thereby allowing follow-up evaluations to be reliably compared.

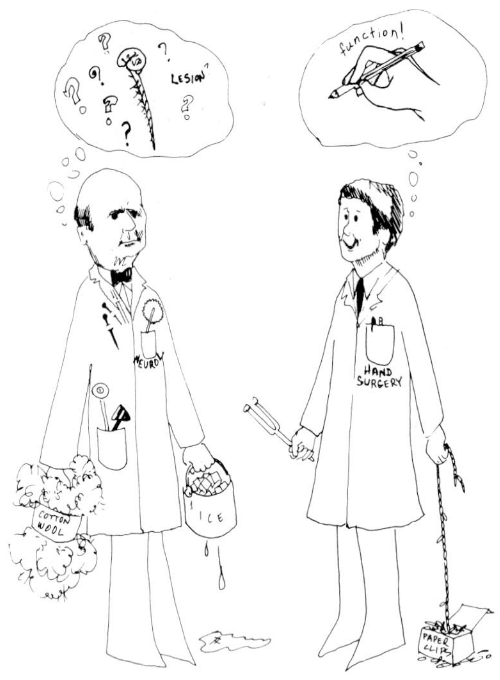

FIG. 28-3. Academic recovery does not equal functional recovery. (From Dellon AL: Evaluation of sensibility and re-education of sensation in the hand, Baltimore, 1981, Williams & Wilkins Co.)

Weber Two-Point Discrimination

In 1853 Weber described a sensibility test that would provide qualifiable results. He described the use of calipers whose points were held against the skin at different distances apart until the patient was unable to distinguish between one or two points of contact on the skin, with vision occluded.[21]

Moberg recognized several limitations of the Weber test and further refined its use to include the following [43,44]:

1. Quiet environment
2. Positioning of the tested area to prevent movement

3. Use of a blunt rather than a sharp-tipped instrument
4. Application of least possible pressure, trying not to make the skin blanch

Two-point discrimination is usually measured only in the fingertips. Tables vary from author to author. The American Society for Surgery of the Hand has accepted the following classification: less than 6 mm is normal, 6 to 10 mm is fair, 11 to 15 mm is poor. Rather than referring to charts or tables for normal values, it is advisable to test areas of normal sensation as well as areas thought to have diminished sensation. The results should then be compared to establish normal values for each patient. A review of the literature reveals that the Weber two-point test results leave considerable room for interpretation of normal functional results.

Moving Two-Point Discrimination

Moving two-point discrimination as described by Dellon[20] adds the variable of motion to the test. Dellon thought that moving two-point discrimination would measure the recovery status of quickly adapting receptors. As a result of his studies, he noted that the improvements in moving two-point discrimination coincided with improvements in patients' functional abilities more frequently than did static two-point discrimination. Moving two-point discrimination is performed similarly to the two-point discrimination test; however, the stimulus is moved longitudinally rather than merely placed on the skin.

Grip and Pinch Testing

Grip

Various injuries to the hand and wrist can interfere with the athlete's ability to perform activities requiring grip. Grip depends on skeletal mobility, joint integrity, and a combination of contraction and relaxation of the intrinsic and the extrinsic muscle groups. Grip consists of three stages—opening of the hand, closing of the digits to grasp an object, and regulating the force of pressure.[56] Napier divided grip into two types: power and precision.[45]

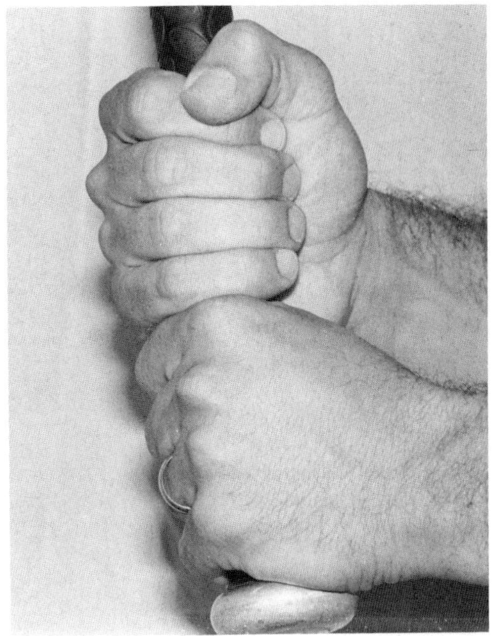

FIG. 28-4. Power grip.

During **power grip,** the wrist is held in dorsiflexion, allowing the long flexors to press the object against the palm. The thumb may be either clasped over the flexed fingers or held tightly against a handle in adduction. Swinging a baseball bat is an example of power grip (Fig. 28-4).

Problems that may interfere with maximal power grip include lack of mobility or weakness of the fourth and fifth rays. Limited mobility as well as pain in the carpals and wrist may also play a role in decreased functional grip.

In performing **precision grip,** the athlete may hold the wrist in volar flexion or dorsiflexion, and the thumb is opposed to semiflexed fingers. The intrinsic muscles play an important role in required finger motion. Precision grip is required in grasping a baseball (Fig. 28-5).

The Jamar hydraulic dynamometer provides an accurate and reliable method of measuring grip strength[6] (Fig. 28-6). The adjustable handle allows an accurate evaluation of overall hand strength. Grip strength is altered by the size of the object being grasped, and therefore readings should be taken in all five grip spans. To measure grip strength the

Grip

Requirements
- Skeletal mobility
- Joint integrity
- Muscle coordination

Stages
- Hand opening
- Closing digits
- Regulating forces

Types
- Power
- Precision

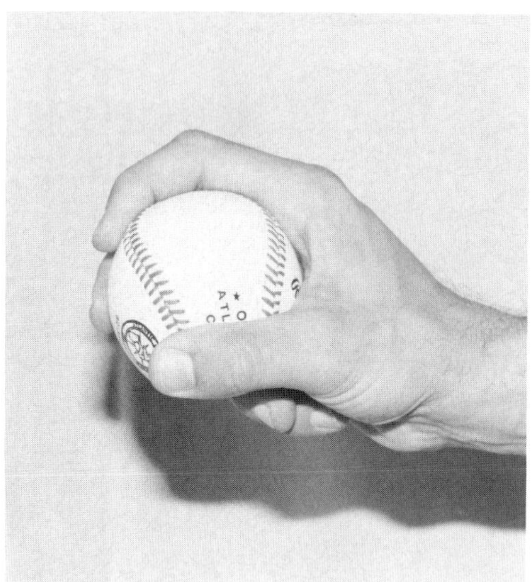

FIG. 28-5. Precision grip.

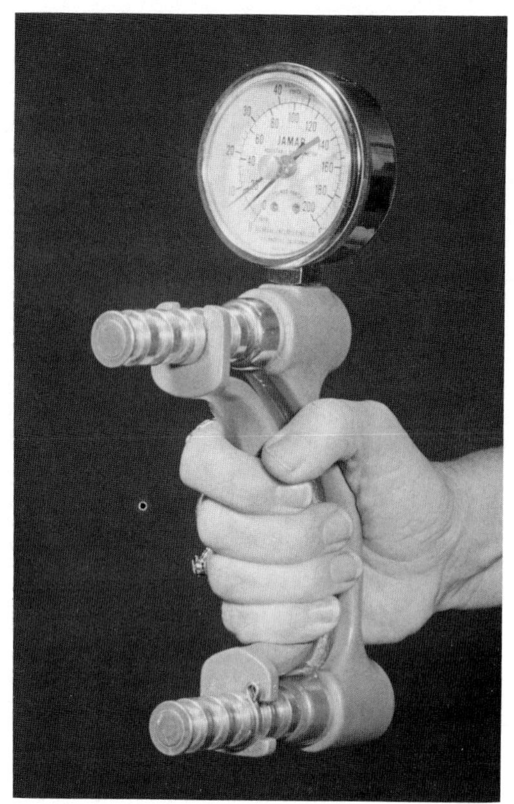

FIG. 28-6. Jamar hydraulic dynamometer.

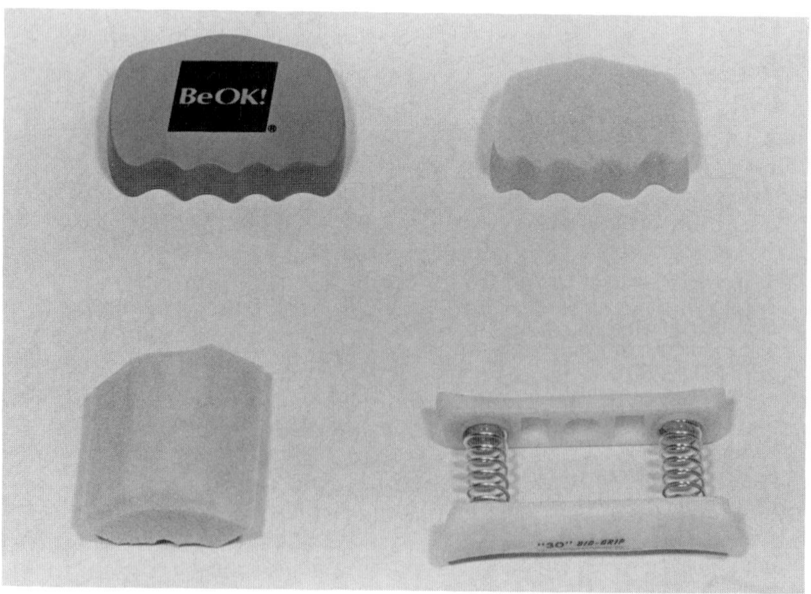

FIG. 28-7. Grippers of variable resistance.

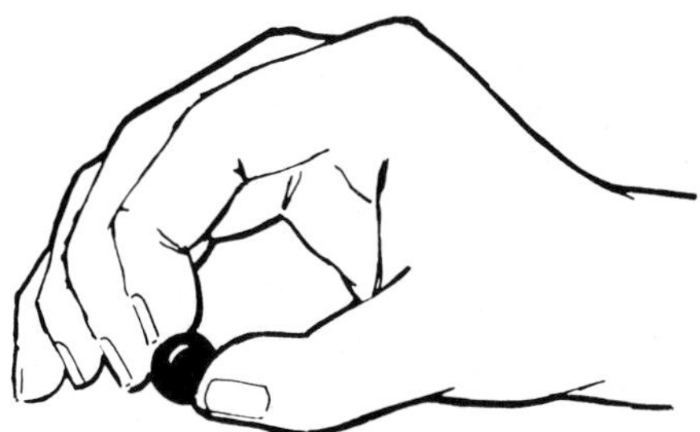

FIG. 28-8. Opposition occurs between the thumb and index finger and is used for picking up small objects. (From Malick MH: Manual on static hand splinting, Pittsburgh, 1972, Harmarville Rehabilitation Center.)

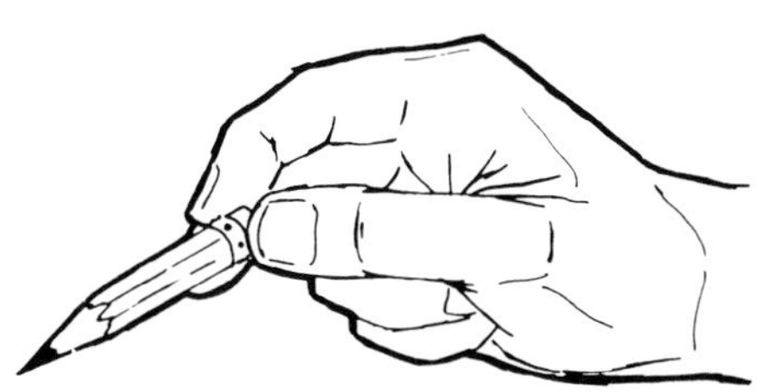

FIG. 28-9. Three-point prehension used to grasp and stabilize large objects, most commonly used during functional activity. (From Malick MH: Manual on static hand splinting, Pittsburgh, 1972, Harmarville Rehabilitation Center.)

arm should be held at the side. The elbow should be flexed at 90 degrees, with the wrist held in neutral. The athlete should be instructed to apply maximal effort in grasping the dynamometer. He should be observed so that substitute patterns are not used. Initially, the right and left hand should be tested alternately. The noninvolved extremity may be used for comparison. Most individuals demonstrate a 5% to 10% difference between their dominant and nondominant extremities.[6] Adequate norms for grip strength are not available, although Schmidt and Toews[53] reported that correlations existed between grip strength and height, weight, and age.

Grip strengthening exercises should not be painful. Adequate finger motion should be present before strengthening is initiated. Often it is necessary to start with gentle isometric exercises, gradually increasing effort until pain is no longer a factor. Then the patient progresses to gentle resistance that is gradually increased in graded increments (Fig. 28-7).

Pinch

Opposing the index and middle finger to the thumb is called "three-point prehension"

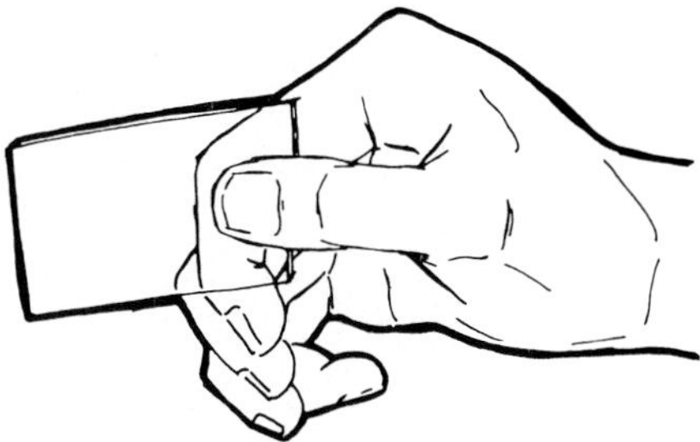

FIG. 28-10. Lateral or key pinch. The most powerful form of pinch. (With permission from Malick, Maude H: Manual on static hand splinting, Pittsburgh, 1972, Harmarville Rehabilitation Center.)

and is considered to be a weak form of precision grip[15] (Figs. 28-8 and 28-9). Strength and stability are equally important in performing pinch. Adequate thumb function is vital to athletes who perform competitively.

Pressing the thumb against the lateral border of the index finger is termed "key" or "lateral pinch" and is considered to be a form of power grip (Fig. 28-10).

Pinch may be measured with the use of a commercial pinch gauge (Fig. 28-11). Strengthening exercises to improve pinch may include the use of therapeutic putty, which is available in various graded resistances.

PATHOLOGIC CONDITIONS

Wrist Injuries

The wrist is a complex joint, consisting of 21 separate articulations and a network of ligaments. Nowhere else in the body are so many nerves, tendons, vessels, bones, and ligaments concentrated in such a small area. When a person falls, a great deal of force is absorbed by the wrist, resulting in severe compression.

The frequency of wrist injuries, together with the various possible mechanisms of injury and multiple roentgenographic views available, make diagnosis of traumatic wrist injuries difficult (see Chapter 24). To further complicate the problem, obtaining a careful history and physical examination is not always helpful. Memory for the mechanism of injury may be vague or lost in the excitement of the game. Clinical examination may show generalized tenderness and swelling with pain, as well as limitation of motion in various positions. Despite a lack of a definitive diagnosis, protection should continue as long as symptoms persist (Fig. 28-12). If roentgenographic studies continue to be normal, symptomatic

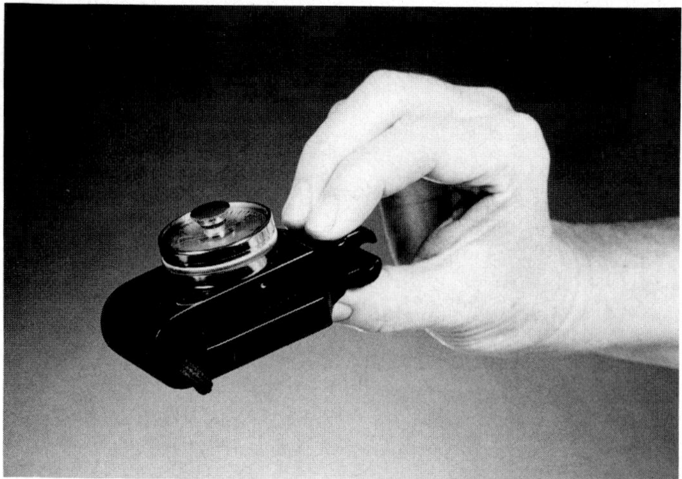

FIG. 28-11. Commercial pinch gauge.

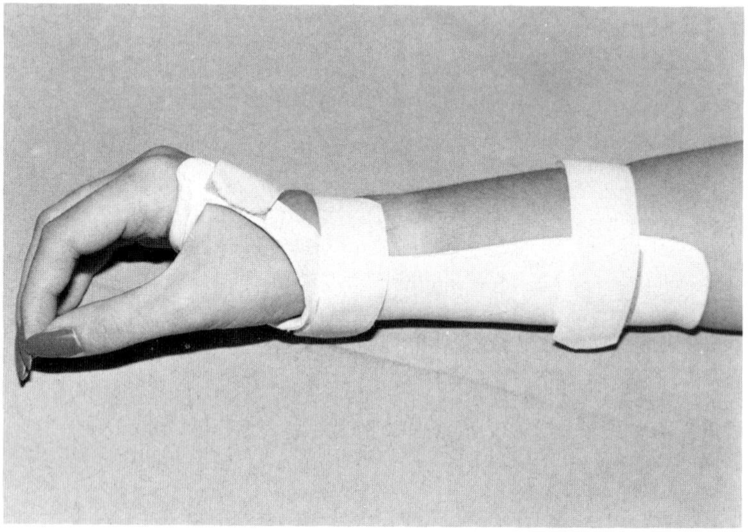

FIG. 28-12. Wrist support splint.

treatment should occur. If serious problems are passed off as minor and treated inadequately, progressive damage to the joint will occur. Medical treatment and rehabilitation become not only more difficult, but prolonged as well. Return to competition may be delayed or, in some situations, impossible.

Restoring Mobility

The wrist will show some degree of limitation of motion after being immobilized for a few weeks. The degree of stiffness present increases with age as well as with severity of the injury. Active exercises of the wrist should be started as soon as adequate healing has occurred. In some situations, it may be possible to remove the splint only for early active exercises. The protective splint is replaced after exercises. This method of early motion is helpful in preventing further stiffness from occurring in spite of incomplete healing. Limitations in pronation and supination are often overlooked after wrist immobilization. Active forearm exercises should be initiated.

When progress plateaus with the use of active exercises, active assistive exercises should be initiated. Pain should also be a factor in determining when to begin active assistive exercises.

Because of the many articulations present in the wrist, joint mobilization is an effective means of overcoming appreciable limitations of motion. Mobilization refers to any procedure that increases mobility of soft tissue or joints.[32,42,47] Mennell, Kaltenborn, and Paris have well-established instruction programs for joint mobilization, which is considered a special area of study. It is recommended that therapists and trainers attend a specialized course to become proficient in one of the aforementioned methods.

Before returning to competition unprotected, a program of progressive resistive exercise should have been a part of the rehabilitation program. Timing of resistive exercise is important. The injury should be well healed, edema should be controlled, and active motion should be substantial and pain free. Providing resistive exercises before adequate healing has occurred will only serve to create tissue reaction and ultimately delay return to competition.

Restoring wrist mobility

- Active exercises
- Active assisted exercises
- Joint mobilization
- Progressive resistance exercises

Restoring Strength

Strength can also be attained by returning the athlete to functional activity. It is psychologically and physically beneficial to allow an athlete to practice partial activity for brief periods as soon as he or she is able to perform comfortably. This is especially helpful in ball handlers. Patients should be monitored carefully for symptoms of overuse. Often they are anxious to return to activity and will overexert if they are not carefully supervised.

Modalities

The wrist is particularly responsive to the use of various modalities. Application of heat before exercise, followed by ice after exercise, is often useful to control tissue reaction brought about by exercise.

Hamate Hook Fractures

Hamate hook fractures most often occur in athletes who participate in baseball, golf, tennis, racquetball, and squash.[38,48] The injury usually occurs when the athlete loses control of the handle of the equipment and the handle strikes the hypothenar area. The fracture occurs with less frequency from direct trauma, such as that which results from a fall.

Resultant patient complaints include a poor grip and wrist pain that is increased by both passive and active dorsiflexion. Symptoms of ulnar nerve impingement or tendonitis of the flexor digitorum profundus of the little finger may also occur. On clinical examination, deep pressure produces discomfort over the hook itself.

In an acute nondisplaced fracture, conservative methods of treatment include a short gauntlet cast for mobilization and a silicone cast for use during competition when reaction has subsided. Forces on the muscular attachment to the fracture often result in nonunions. If symptoms persist, the displaced hook may be surgically removed (see Fig. 23-16). Postoperative therapy consists of application of modalities to improve scar tone and massage to provide desensitization, as well as to improve soft tissue mobility. During the early phase of treatment, protecting the area with either padded gloves or equipment is helpful, because it allows the athlete to continue sports activities.

Thumb Injuries

The thumb may be considered to have three different functional units: (1) flexion and extension of the metacarpophalangeal (MCP) and interphalangeal (IP) joints, (2) abduction and adduction, and (3) opposition.

Loss of thumb function is said to result in loss of 50% of total hand function. Injuries sustained to the thumb during athletics may include Rolando's fracture, Bennett's fracture-dislocation, metacarpal dislocations and fractures, and collateral ligament sprains.

The remarkable mobility of the thumb is said to result from the function of the carpometacarpal joint.

The MCP joint of the thumb owes its stability to a complex arrangement of ligamentous, capsular, and musculotendinous supporting structures. It is the joint in the hand that is most affected by ligamentous instability. Injury to the ulnar collateral ligament is quite common in skiers and in ball handlers. Injury to the radial collateral ligament occurs much less frequently. Laxity of the ulnar collateral ligament results in weakness of grasp and pinch, but the radial side of the joint does not receive such stress. Consequently, the functional residual is much less debilitating.

Ligamentous injuries to the thumb usually do not respond well to conservative treatment. Inadequate treatment, especially in complete tears, jeopardizes the most important function of the hand, namely the ability to pinch.

General principles of hand therapy should be followed in restoring thumb mobility.

TABLE 28-2 Positioning guidelines for PIP joint injuries

Injury	Joint Position	Splint Surface
Articular fractures	30 degrees flexion	Volar
Fracture-dislocations	Block at 25 degrees flexion; allow full flexion	Dorsal
Boutonnière deformity	Full extension	Volar
Pseudoboutonnière deformity	Full extension	Volar
Collateral ligament injuries		
Mild strain	Functional position	Volar
Incomplete tear	30 degress flexion	Volar
Volar plate injuries	25-30 degrees flexion	Volar or dorsal

From Gieck JH, and Mayer V: Clinics in sports medicine, Philadelphia, 1986, WB Saunders Co.

Splinting may be indicated to restore thumb web space. Joint mobilization may be indicated to restore flexion to the MCP and IP joints.

Proximal Interphalangeal (PIP) Joint Injuries

In no instance are early diagnosis, proper medical treatment, and quality rehabilitation more important in preventing residual deformity than in the proximal interphalangeal (PIP) joint. Inadequate long-term protection during practice and competition can lead to reinjury and permanent disability.

The exact number of injuries to PIP joints that occur during athletic activity is unknown. Dislocations are often reduced on the sidelines by the coach or trainer and taped to an adjacent finger. Several weeks later, when the joint remains stiff, swollen, and painful and a contracture begins to ensue, medical attention is usually sought. Occasionally, incorrect diagnosis will be made by an inexperienced practitioner. If the condition does not improve or deteriorates in spite of adequate conservative treatment, reexamination or a second medical opinion is advisable.

Common injuries to PIP joints that occur during athletic activity may include articular fractures, fracture dislocations, boutonnière deformities, pseudoboutonnière deformities, and collateral ligament and volar plate injuries. Splinting guidelines are provided in Table 28-2. Confusion exists between the boutonnière deformity and the pseudoboutonnière deformity. The classical **boutonnière deformity** consists of hyperextension of the MP joint, flexion of the PIP joint, and hyperextension of the distal interphalangeal (DIP) joint. The boutonnière deformity is the result of disruption of the central slip of the extensor digitorum communis tendon over the PIP joint. The **pseudoboutonnière deformity** resembles a classic boutonnière deformity, but is caused by disruption of the volar plate at its proximal membranous portion without disruption of the central slip. The pseudoboutonnière consists of a flexion contracture of the PIP joint, which is more resistant to correction by passive extension than the classic boutonnière; slight hyperextension of the DIP joint; and roentgenographic evidence of calcification at the proximal attachment of the volar plate.[39] Many commercial splints exist for mobilization of PIP injuries (Fig. 28-13).

PIP joint injuries

- Articular fractures
- Fracture dislocations
- Boutonnière deformities
- Pseudoboutonnière deformities
- Collateral ligament sprains
- Volar plate injuries

Treatment

When the deformities are treated conservatively, therapeutic measures should consist of dynamic and/or static splinting exercises, as well as modalities to control pain and edema. Splints should be fabricated so as not to restrict motion of the MCP and DIP joints. How early an athlete with PIP joint injury can safely return to play with proper protection is a medical decision. In most instances splints can be fabricated to allow an athlete to return to competition. Buddy tapes do *not* allow adequate protection for painful, swollen joints. Adequate protective splinting should continue until motion is complete and pain free.

Proper management of injuries to the PIP joint can significantly reduce the deformity often seen in athletes who do not receive

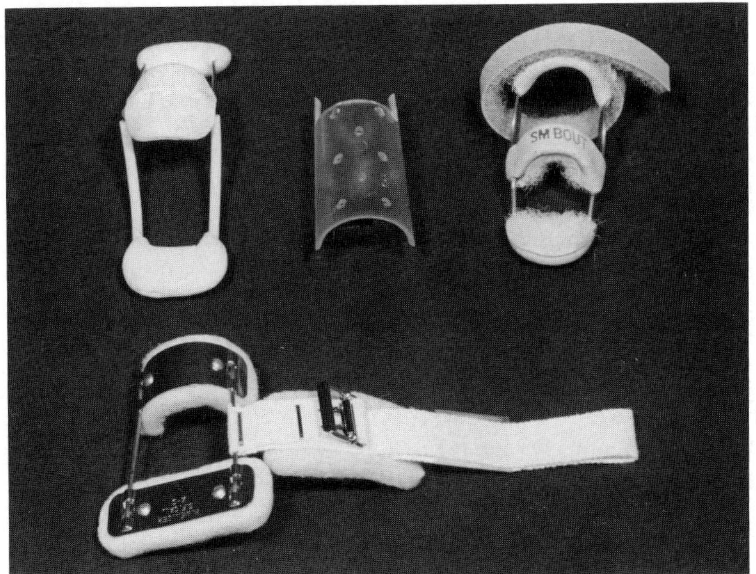

FIG. 28-13. Splints available for treatment of PIP injuries.

proper medical care, rehabilitation, or protective splinting.

Distal Interphalangeal (DIP) Joint Injuries

Injury to the extensor mechanism is one of the most common hand injuries sustained by athletes. The injury occurs when a force, such as a hard thrown ball, strikes the extended fingertip and forces the distal phalanx into flexion while the extensor mechanism is actively contracting. The distal joint may be passively, but not actively, extended.[38]

The most common rupture of the extensor tendon occurs at the insertion into the base of the distal phalanx and is called a **mallet finger.** Most mallet fingers can be treated by conservative methods. Surgical repair of the extensor tendon in the area of the DIP joint is difficult because of a poor blood supply.[38] When the DIP joint is immobilized to treat acute mallet finger, the distal phalanx may be positioned in neutral or slight hyperextension. The degree of hyperextension should not exceed the position at which the dorsal skin begins to blanch. Studies have shown that the degree of hyperextension at which skin begins to blanch is widely variable.[51] Crawford obtained satisfactory results in 151 patients with mallet finger with the use of premolded polythene stack splints, which maintain the joint in a neutral position[19] (Fig. 28-14). Metal splints may be placed on the dorsal or volar surface of the digit. Splints should be removed

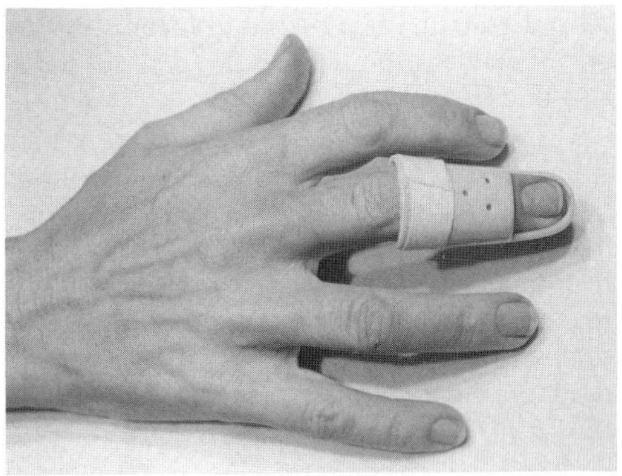

FIG. 28-14. Stack mallet finger splint.

for hand care. When removing the splint, the athlete should be instructed not to allow the distal phalanx to drop into flexion. This may be accomplished by gradually removing the splint while supporting the distal phalanx with the thumb. Splinting should continue for at least 8 weeks, at which time exercises may be initiated to restore mobility. If DIP extension decreases at this time, splinting may be renewed on a full- or part-time basis. Protection during athletic activity should continue until gains in motion have reached a plateau and the joint is no longer sore.

Overuse Syndromes

Repetitive microtrauma or overuse injuries were once thought to occur only in unfit adult weekend athletes. We now know that such injuries can occur in anyone who does repetitive movements. Overuse injuries occur when too much activity is done over too short a period with inadequate conditioning or improper techniques. Injuries can occur in the workplace, as well as in competitive or recreational sports, and may involve individuals of all ages. Early conservative treatment of overuse injuries is best. Treatment should consist of rest and protection to reduce inflammation and pain, and the athlete should cease performing the activity that contributed to the problem. The athlete's period of inactivity should be minimized by closely monitoring rehabilitation and supervising activity, thereby preventing consequential recurrence.

Carpal Tunnel Syndrome

Carpal tunnel syndrome may occur from the repetitive motion or long periods of gripping, throwing, bicycling, and performing repetitive motion with the wrist held in flexion.[18] Classic symptoms include wrist pain, which may radiate up the arm and intensify at night, and episodic numbness of the thumb, index, and middle fingers.

Conservative treatment should consist of splinting the wrist in 10 degrees of dorsiflexion, administering nonsteroidal antiinflammatory medications and therapeutic modalities, and ceasing the activity that created the reaction. Treatment should continue until motion is complete and pain free.

If conservative treatment is not successful, the athlete should be referred for medical evaluation. Decompression has been reported to be necessary in several young athletes.[25]

de Quervain's Disease

de Quervain's disease is the result of stenosing tenosynovitis of the abductor pollicis longus and extensor pollicis brevis. The disease creates pain in the area of the first dorsal compartment and the radial styloid. It has a much higher incidence in women. The disease does not often occur in athletes. Splinting is not always helpful, but judicious use of injections is acceptable.

Tendon Injuries

Extensor tenosynovitis. Extensor tenosynovitis, or tendonitis, involves the dorsal extensor retinaculum and the individual extensor dorsal compartments. The condition frequently occurs in lifting and throwing sports. Generally, the condition is treatable through rest, therapeutic modalities, the use of antiinflammatory drugs, and protective splinting or sufficient padding to prevent a reoccurrence of the condition.

Trigger finger. Trigger fingers result from repetitive trauma along the pulley system at the base of the fingers. Handball players, baseball catchers, gymnasts, and weightlifters may be prone to the condition. Incidence of trigger finger may be decreased by the use of gloves or padding applied to the palmar aspect of the hand. Treatment may include rest, therapeutic modalities, antiinflammatory medications, and corticosteroid injections. Alleviation of the conditions that contribute to the problem may include reviewing handgear worn by the athlete. If symptoms persist in spite of conservative treatment, release of the A1 pulley is indicated.

Rehabilitation

Therapeutic heat and cold reduce pain and inflammation and must be applied before an exercise program is initiated. The main goal of rehabilitation is to enable the athlete to resume normal activity when healing is taking place, rather than to allow complete healing before exercise is resumed.[26] Although early motion is important, exercises should only be done in a pain-free range. The longer the immobilization period, the greater the impact disuse atrophy and limited mobility will exhibit. After a therapeutic modality is used, passive exercise consisting of a slow, steady stretch should be initiated for 30 to 60 seconds and repeated several times.

The next progression during the acute stage of overuse injury is strengthening or isometric exercises, which are most effective in the acute stage of treatment. Isometric exercise involves contraction of the muscle, allowing no joint motion. The athlete should only exert force that is comfortable. As healing occurs, the force can be increased. The exercises should be performed with the joint held in various positions for 6 to 10 seconds. The athlete may then progress to using free weights. Progression of the exercise program should be monitored carefully. Resistive exercises in the acute stage of healing will aggravate the symptoms. As normal strength returns, exercises to improve endurance are added. The athletic activity that contributed to the injury may be initiated at this time.

An important activity of the practitioner is to review techniques the athlete uses while performing the activity that created the injury. Unless corrected, the injury is apt to reoccur.

Pitfalls in the rehabilitation of overuse injuries include inadequate rehabilitation time and the return to activity before adequate healing has occurred.

Digital Nerve Injuries

Direct repetitive trauma over the palm and digits, such as is required in many sports, makes digital nerve injuries in the hand a common occurrence. Digital neuromas may also result.

Symptoms may be so severe as to interfere with the athlete's functional ability. Neuromas usually respond to conservative treatment, such as transcutaneous electrical nerve stimulation (TENS) and desensitization programs. Evaluating the athlete's equipment is also recommended, since padding or glove use may help to reduce stress to the painful area.

Bowler's thumb involves the ulnar digital sensory nerve of the thumb and may be so painful as to incapacitate the bowler. Contributing factors to neuroma formation among bowlers may include use of a ball that is too heavy or oversized. Improper bore spread, as well as poor bowling technique, may also contribute to the injury.

Evaluation of the bowler's ball and technique should be provided. If conservative treatment is unsuccessful, referral for surgical consideration is indicated. Best results require early treatment, with either conservative or surgical intervention.[22]

Vascular Injuries

Ischemia of the hand and fingers secondary to repetitive blunt trauma has been labeled the **hypothenar hammer syndrome.**[3,16] Constant trauma to the hypothenar area may cause spasms of the ulnar artery, thromboses, and aneurysms of the hand.[29] The condition has been reported to occur in baseball, karate, rugby, handball, lacrosse, and volleyball. Any athlete who participates in a sport that involves repetitive trauma against the palmar surface of the hand is at risk of developing vascular injuries.[2]

Signs and symptoms of athletes with impending vascular injury include coolness, numbness, cyanosis, paleness, and a positive response to the Allen test.[55] The Allen test can be carried out on a single digit by expressing the blood out of it, occluding both digital arteries, and then releasing the radial digital artery and noting the filling of the digit. The same procedure is carried out on the ulnar digital artery. This procedure independently evaluates the patency of each digital vessel. Athletic trainers can be helpful by providing conservative therapy, reviewing the athlete's techniques, evaluating equipment, and supplying additional protection. Often the use of a glove or application of padding to relieve stress in vulnerable areas is helpful.

An obvious need exists for improvement of the protective gear offered to athletes who perform activities traumatic to the palm and hypothenar area. Studies have reported a correlation between the repetitive trauma to the fingers from catching a ball and the number of years played, frequency of practice, and position played.[2]

Neuromas

Neuromas occur after axonal injury with mechanical disruption of the endoneural myelin barrier. A neuroma of some degree is always produced at the point of injury to a nerve. Not all neuromas are painful. If a neuroma is painful, however, initial treatment should be directed toward conservative methods of desensitization rather than toward operative procedures.

Conservative Treatment

Neuromas may be treated with local anesthetic injections. Although results have not been published, TENS has been used for desensitization of painful neuromas for many years. Desensitization techniques used in the treatment of painful neuromas and hyperesthetic scars are similar. Although some neuromas may respond to a program of manual desensitization alone, TENS appears to speed up the process. In the treatment of painful neuroma and hyperesthetic scars, conventional TENS should be used. Electrode placement should be in continuity with the involved nerve, with the distal electrode placed as near the painful site as possible. As the site becomes less painful, the electrode should be placed closer to the neuroma. If conservative treatment is successful, ultimately it should be possible to place the electrode over the neuroma site.

Application of TENS should be followed by a program of manual desensitization. A protocol for manual desensitization developed at the Curtis Hand Center of Baltimore, Maryland, includes a regimented program of various graded stimuli (textures) that progresses from moving touch to constant touch, and ends with percussive stimulation. Each stimulus is performed in a proximal to distal direction, then progresses horizontally from left to right, from right to left, and finally from a distal to a proximal direction. When stimulation in all directions is tolerated, the stimulus or texture is upgraded and training begins at step 1—proximal to distal—and progresses through the various directions and textures as tolerated. The next step of manual desensitization is constant touch, which is reeducated by applying various pressures to the area. The eraser of a pencil or a fingertip may be used as the stimulus. The final stage of desensitization is percussion, which may begin with gentle tapping of a fingertip or the eraser of a pencil.

The staff of the Downey Hand Center of Downey, California, have developed a sensitivity test and kit that is commercially available for testing and treatment of hyperesthesia.[59]

It is important to note that the gradual progression of stimulation is important to the treatment of painful neuromas. Often athletes with hyperesthetic areas are only instructed to perform a percussive type of stimulation. Obviously, compliance to this request is not possible. A successful desensitization program is dependent on a thorough evaluation, as well as a manual desensitization program that is nonpainful. TENS and injections may also be helpful, though the importance of the physiologic and psychologic bases for manual desensitization cannot be overstressed. Stimulation through functional use is also an important aspect of reeducation.

Painful neuromas that do not respond to conservative treatment should be referred for evaluation for surgical intervention.

Reflex Sympathetic Dystrophy

Reflex sympathetic dystrophy (RSD) is a vasomotor dysfunction that is characterized by hyperesthesia, burning pain, edema, discoloration, and stiffness in an extremity. It occurs after a variety of injuries such as fractures, lacerations, surgical incisions, and soft tissue injury. Involvement may be limited to one or two digits, or it may be so severe as to involve the entire extremity. The mechanism of injury can be so trivial that the patient may have difficulty recalling the incident that directly precipitated the complaints. There is no known correlation between the severity of the injury and the intensity of the symptoms of RSD, unless one suffers a related peripheral nerve injury. The latter patients would most appropriately be diagnosed as having **causalgia,** and because of the associated nerve damage, the syndrome may result in more retractable pain, neurologic deficit and dysfunction, and less successful resolution of symptoms, even with maximal treatment. The pathologic consequences occur in the skin, muscle, blood vessels, and bones of the extremity and can significantly affect its function. Symptoms of the condition occur in various degrees and may go through changes that can persist for several years if untreated.[33] These include:

1. Edema. Edematous changes may begin as a pitting type of edema, which eventually becomes brawny and ultimately results in a periarticular thickening of the joints.
2. Discoloration. Initial appearance may be pale or cyanotic or a combination of both. Eventually a redness develops, especially over the dorsum of MCP and IP joints, and may progress to include the flexor creases of the hand.
3. Hyperhidrosis. Although present in early stages, hyperhidrosis decreases with time. Unusual dryness occurs in later stages.
4. Paresthesia. Initially, paresthesia occurs in response to light touch. Ultimately, skin takes on a tight, glossy appearance. Subcutaneous tissue atrophies and progresses until fingertips become very thin.

There is no neurologic deficit in RSD, per se, that results from nerve damage. Rather, the patient complains of a vague, yet severe, nondermatomal burning pain in the extremity. There is no specific diagnostic laboratory test for RSD, but any test that reflects a change in blood flow in the extremity may support the diagnosis.[55]

Sympathetic Blocks

Since the likelihood of spontaneous resolution of the symptoms is low, RSD requires treatment. Traditional management involved temporary or permanent blockade of the sympathetic nervous system of the affected extremity with local anesthetics or phenol or alcohol, respectively. Although several regional anesthetic techniques result in sympathectomy, a series of five to seven stellate ganglion blocks is usually performed (one block every 1 to 3 days) for the upper extremity. The same number of lumbar sympathetic blocks is completed for the lower extremity. These techniques result in only sympathetic block (there is no numbness, weakness, or paralysis), and they significantly decrease the hypersensitivity to even gentle stimuli and the burning pain of the extremity. Restoration of comfort without comprehensive hand therapy to decrease edema and restore mobility is inadequate treatment. The patient must be involved in rehabilitation concurrent with and after the nerve blocks. Some cases of RSD require only gentle hand therapy at first, but then therapy becomes progressively more intense, frequent, and extensive. A few patients with intractable symptoms and good, albeit temporary, improvement with nerve block therapy will require surgical sympathectomy.[52]

Treatment of RSD

- Stellate ganglion blocks
- Hand rehabilitation
- TENS
- Medication

Transcutaneous Electrical Nerve Stimulation

Transcutaneous electrical nerve stimulation (TENS) as an adjunct has also been shown to be beneficial when the electrodes are placed over the vascular supply to the affected extremity.[52] In this location, the stimulation affects sympathetic tone, a change not generally produced by traditional dermatomal stimulation. Maximal therapy would be TENS for 60 minutes, then having the unit in place (if the patient so desires) but turned off for a similar amount of time during waking hours. TENS may be useful in patients with a low tolerance for nerve blocks or as an initial treatment in mild cases. Selected patients are capable of increasing blood flow to the affected extremity on command after learning hypnosis.

Medical Management

Most of the common analgesic medications are of little benefit to the patient with RSD, because the primary pain is sympathetically mediated. Even nonsteroidal antiinflammatory drugs (NSAIDs) may have little effect because the edema associated with the RSD is the result of the alteration in blood flow, not a peripheral inflammatory mechanism. Some use is made of α- and β-adrenergic blocking drugs (i.e., phenoxybenzamine 10 to 40 mg four times a day or propranolol 10 to 40 mg four times a day, respectively) in attempts to manipulate the peripheral circulation and relieve the intense vasoconstriction. Calcium channel blocking drugs (i.e., nifedipine 10 to 20 mg t.i.d.) have also been used, since they produce some vasodilitation and may interrupt painful discharges from the injured extremity that serve only to retrigger the exaggerated response in sympathetic tone that results in the clinical syndrome of RSD.[52]

Restoration of comfort without a comprehensive rehabilitation program to restore mobility and decrease edema is inadequate treatment.

Rehabilitation

Nowhere in hand rehabilitation is the expression "no pain, no gain" more *inappropriate* than in the treatment of patients with reflex sympathetic dystrophy. A vigorous exercise program is definitely *not* what the doctor should order. Overly zealous, passive exercises performed to the point of pain will surely increase the symptoms of dystrophy. Active exercises stopping short of the point of pain are indicated. Short exercise periods of several minutes performed throughout the day are more effective than longer exercise periods performed less frequently. Patients should be informed of the symptoms of overuse to better monitor their exercise program and their level of activity. In selected postoperative cases, controlled joint manipulation may be indicated immediately after successful administration of regional blocks. This procedure may be necessary to reduce tendon and soft tissue adherence, thereby allowing active motion to occur.

As treatment progresses, a custom-made static thermoplastic splint may be fabricated in a position of comfort to promote relaxation. The splint should gradually be altered until the functional position is obtained. If contractures are present, it may be necessary to ultimately adjust the splint to an intrinsic plus position. The splint should be removed periodically for exercise periods. As hand function improves, wearing time should be decreased. Use of dynamic splints is contraindicated in the acute stage of the condition. They should not be used until edema has subsided and their use does not produce discomfort or an exacerbation of symptoms.

As clinicians, it is important that we be aware of the early symptoms of reflex sympathetic dystrophy. It is prudent to refer athletes to the team physician for review if their symptoms appear to be out of proportion to their injury, or if they do not appear to be improving in spite of therapeutic efforts. Early recognition and proper management of the condition produce the best results.

EDEMA

Prevention Of Edema

If left untreated, edema can be responsible for delaying healing and causing pain, as well as limiting mobility with subsequent compromised functional use. The prevention and treatment of edema present a constant challenge to trainers and therapists. We are doing the athlete a disservice if we do not promptly alleviate factors that contribute to the formation of edema immediately after injury oc-

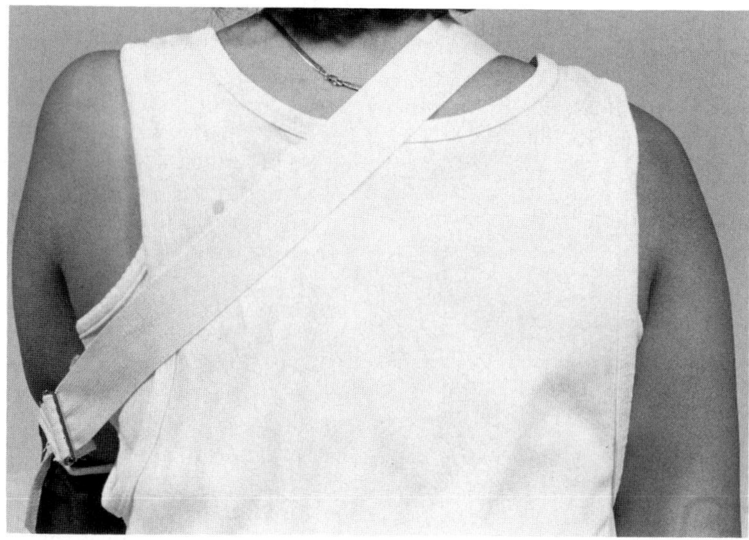

FIG. 28-15. Proper position of sling strap.

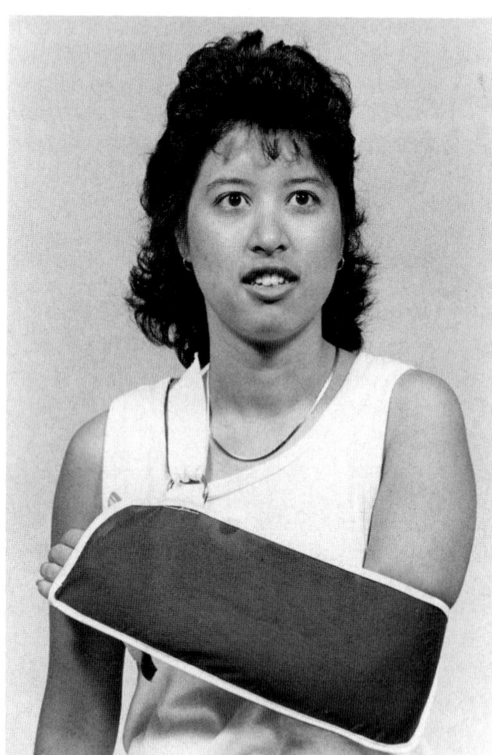

FIG. 28-16. Properly fitted sling.

curs. Several factors may contribute to the formation of edema:

1. The hand may be immobilized in a dependent position such as that which occurs from an ill-fitting sling.
2. Painful wrists that are not splinted in dorsiflexion usually drop into palmar flexion.
3. If left unsupported, hands assume a guarded position. The wrist will drop into palmar flexion while the MCPs and PIPs will assume an extended position. As edema forms, the longitudinal and the transverse arch are eventually lost because of pressure that is created on the dorsum of the hand. Injured hands should be splinted in a functional position.
4. Attempts to hold the extremity in an elevated position for long periods of time without the use of slings or splints. Sling use should be alternated with elevation and active exercises to all uninvolved joints of the extremity.
5. The exercise program for adjacent uninvolved structures may be inadequate.

Elevation

When slings are used, wearing time and proper application should be discussed. The back strap is diagonally positioned so that the weight of the extremity is supported on the opposite shoulder (Fig. 28-15). The elbow and forearm should rest directly on the trough of the sling. The wrist and the midportion of the hand should be supported by the trough of the sling (Fig. 28-16). Allowing the wrist to take on a position of ulnar deviation and palmar flexion will contribute to the formation of edema (Fig. 28-17).

If a sling is used for extended periods of time, the athlete should be instructed to periodically remove the sling and perform active exercises to all uninvolved joints that the sling is immobilizing. Constant use of a sling can result in a shoulder adduction internal rotation deformity that may eventually develop into a frozen shoulder or shoulder-hand syndrome.

Instruction for elevation while in a supine position should also be provided. Placing the hand anywhere over the trunk while lying down is considered elevation. To increase comfort, it is helpful to support the arm with pillows and therefore promote relaxation. It is best to support the extremity in a comfortable position using pillows of various sizes for support (Fig. 28-18). Providing instruction for awkward positions or asking the athlete to hold the extremity in a specific position while at rest should be avoided.

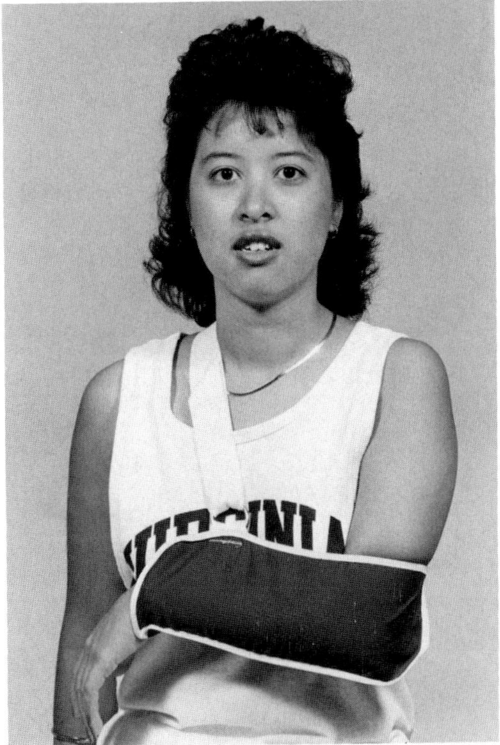

FIG. 28-17. Ill-fitted sling.

Splints

Static splints are indicated to provide support, thereby preventing strain of a severely edematous or painful hand and wrist. The splints should be molded in either a functional or intrinsic plus position, depending on diagnosis and clinical examination. When splinting is used for edema control, the use of straps should be discouraged. Use of Coban* or an Ace wrap distributes the pressure over a larger area, thereby providing compression to further reduce edema.

Continuous static splinting of an edematous hand can result in joint stiffness. The effects of immobilization may be counteracted by instructing the athlete to remove his splint often during the day to perform active exercises.

Exercise

Short exercise periods performed often are most effective in preventing edema formation. Having the athlete elevate the extremity while

*Available from Medical Products Division, 3M Company, St. Paul, Minn.

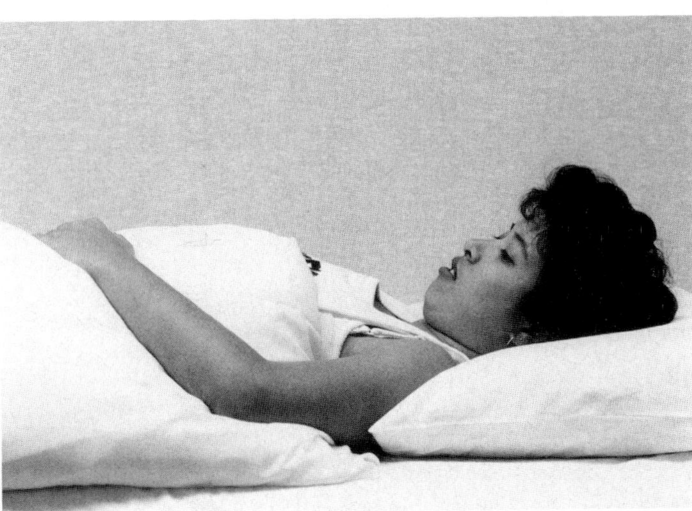

FIG. 28-18. Elevated position while at rest.

performing active "pumping" types of exercise will further enhance edema reduction.

During active movement, the blood flow is directly related to the degree of activity in the muscle. Firm fist-making exercise with the extremity elevated should be encouraged periodically throughout the day. Shortened rapid attempts at finger flexion are ineffective. Passive movement produces very little change in blood flow to the limb, though it is helpful in preventing adhesions and maintaining joint mobility. In summary, the only exercise program that is of any consequence in reducing edema is one of *firm, active motion* that takes the digits through as large an arc of motion as comfort allows, performed while the limb is elevated (Fig. 28-19).

Reduction of Edema

One or more of the following techniques may be used to facilitate venous flow, thereby reducing edema in the upper extremity. Instruction provided should be explicit. The athlete should be informed of the consequences of inadequate or total noncompliance. When properly executed, these techniques can do much to reduce edema; however, when carried out poorly they may contribute to an increase in edema.

Constant or Intermittent Compression

Intermittent and constant devices provide an added dimension to rehabilitation of the hand and wrist when they are used for edema control.[28,57] Gentle pressure applied to the digits is effective in improving mobility in extension. One can also observe an appreciable improvement in flexion after compression because of decreased volume throughout the hand.

Constant compression devices such as the Jobst air splint may be used in the following manner (Fig. 28-20).

Preparation. Place stockinette on the portion of the extremity to be placed in the splint.

Position. Position the hand in the air splint so that compression will occur at the fingertips.

Support. Support the extremity on an elevated or inclined surface.

Inflation. Using the airbulb, inflate the splint to tolerance. Initially, it may be necessary to start with gentle pressure and gradually increase it as tolerance increases. The pressure

A

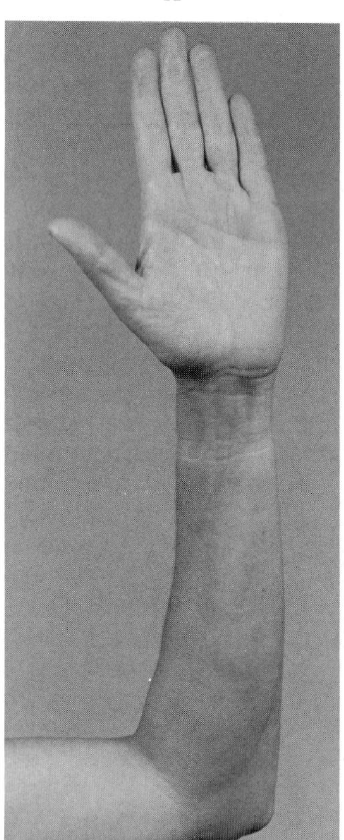

B

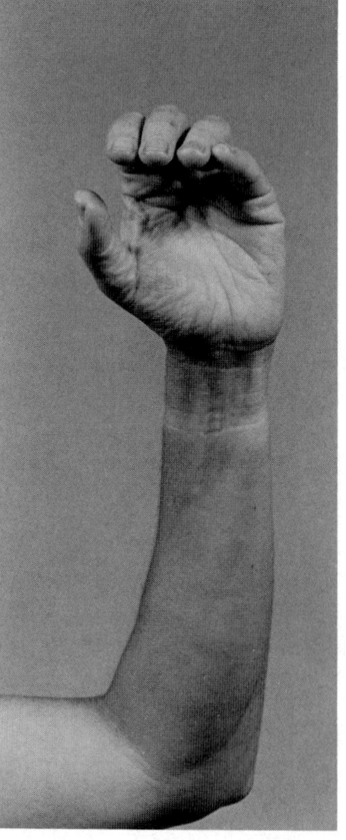

C

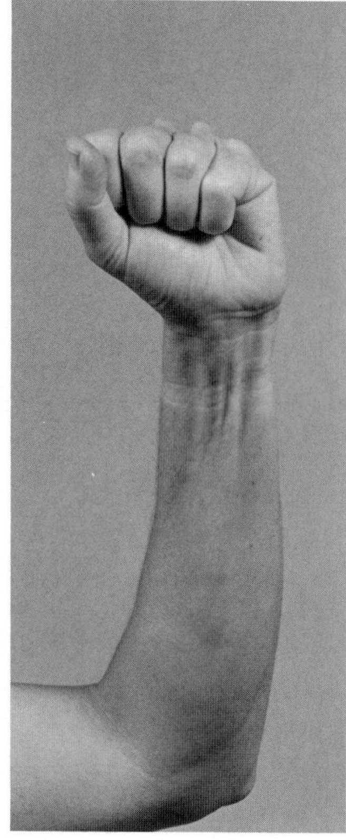

FIG. 28-19. A to **C,** Pumping exercises used for edema reduction.

should not be so great as to create throbbing, tingling, or numbness.

Adaptations. If IP flexion contractures are present, it may be necessary to place light padding in the palm, thereby reducing painful stress that may occur from forcing the fingers into extension. To increase mobility in finger flexion, the fingers may be loosely taped to encourage composite flexion before being placed in the splint.

Utilization. When the splint for edema control is used with the digits held in extension, it may be left in place for 20 minutes. However when the splint is used to increase mobility and the fingers are taped in flexion, it must be removed after 10 minutes.

This method of edema control is particularly helpful for use with athletes who are experiencing a moderate degree of edema and do not have access to a training room or clinic on a regular basis. Static compression may also be used as an adjunct to intermittent compression as part of a home program in situations where edema is persistent.

Intermittent compression is provided with the use of a compression pump and a pneumatic sleeve. To reduce edema in acute injuries, the external intermittent pressure device increases interstitial pressure, thereby forcing lymphatic fluids back into the venous system. The arm should be elevated on an inclined surface or positioned on pillows at approximately a 30- to 45-degree angle to take advantage of gravity. It is not necessary to check the athlete's blood pressure before compression. Pneumatic sleeves are available for the hand and wrist, as well as for the full arm. In treating injuries of the hand and wrist, the shorter pneumatic sleeve is generally adequate. In treating the upper extremity, 30 to 40 mm Hg provides adequate pressure. The pressure applied should not elicit sensations of throbbing, tingling, or numbness. Various alterations in treatment may be employed when treating acute hand injuries. Small open wounds are not a contraindication to its use; however, these wounds should be covered with a sterile dressing. Felt or foam padding may be used to protect pin sites that are painful to pressure. Padding may also be used to support the palmar surface of the hand if pressure applied to the extended fingers is painful.

Contrary to the belief that more pressure is better, it is not necesary to continually increase the pressure as tolerance improves. Increasing the pressure beyond 40 mm Hg may lead to an increase rather than a reduction in hand volume. After edema is reduced through the use of intermittent compression, the volume loss may be maintained by the use of compression gloves or Coban bandage. Air splints may also be used for maintaining losses as part of a home program.

Massage

Retrograde massage is an important aspect of edema reduction programs involving the hand and wrist. The force of the massage stroke should begin distally and progress proximally. It is beneficial to support the hand on an inclined surface when performing mas-

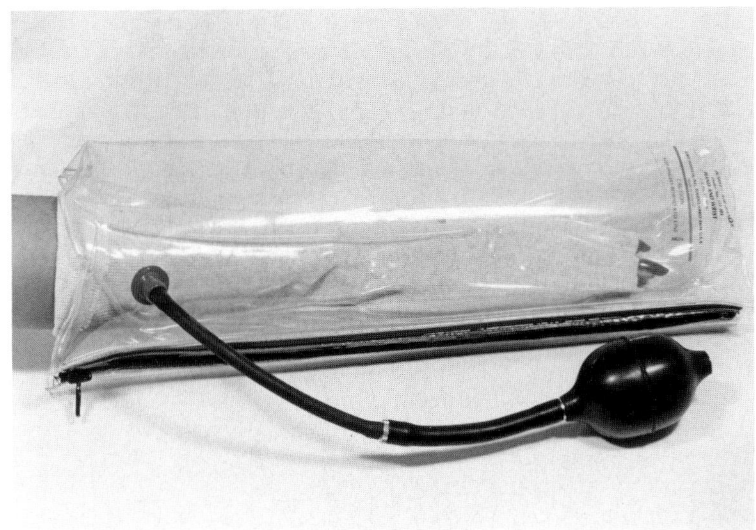

FIG. 28-20. Jobst air splint.

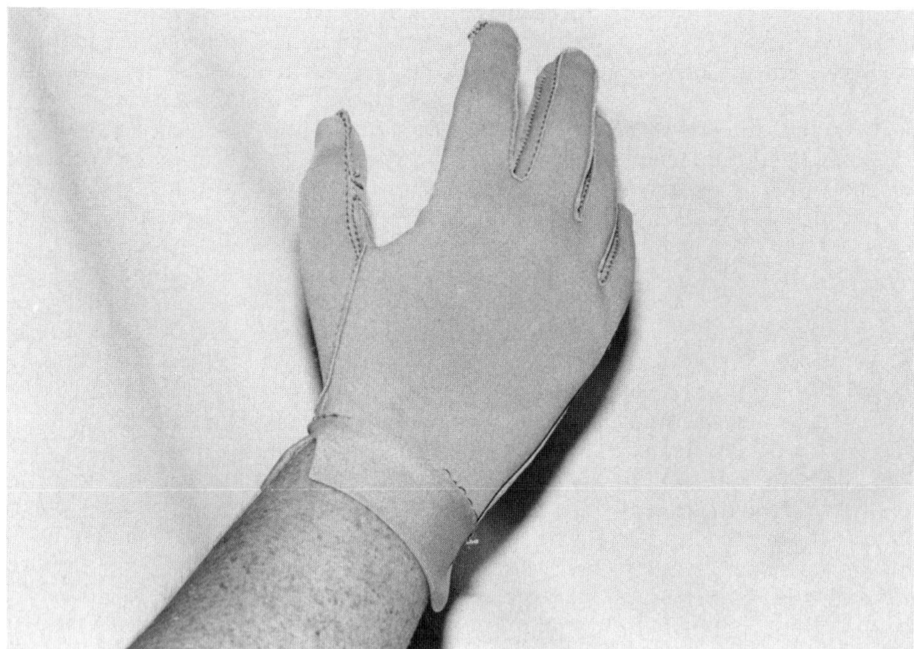

FIG. 28-21. Compression glove.

sage. The athlete should be instructed in techniques of retrograde massage so that it may be incorporated into the home program.

Coban is an effective means of reducing edema in the hand. One layer is wrapped proximally to the palm starting at the distal end of the digit. All involved fingers and the palm should be wrapped proximally to the edematous area. The pressure applied should provide adequate compression, but care should be taken to avoid creating a sensation of throbbing, tingling, or numbness.

Two-inch Coban is appropriate for wrapping the palm and forearm; however, the one-inch width is most practical for wrapping digits. An important feature of Coban is that is does not limit mobility. Coban is also effective when used to secure static finger or hand splints in place. Its use is particularly advantageous in that the use of strapping or circumferential taping may result in increased edema.

Compression Gloves

Compression gloves provide external pressure that is helpful in maintaining volume loss after treatment (Fig. 28-21). After wearing the gloves, patients often report a decrease in discomfort and increase in functional use of the hand. Many varieties of compression gloves are commercially available. Aris Gloves* sells gloves in department stores. One size fits all, and they are available for both men and women. Jobst† produces compression gloves that are available in several sizes. They also make custom-made edema control garments on request.

Therapeutic Cold

Use of therapeutic heat is contraindicated in treatment of extremities where edema is present. A local effect of therapeutic cold is pain suppression. Cold creates vasoconstriction and is also believed to elevate the pain threshold of sensory nerve fibers, thereby decreasing the degree of pain that is perceived. As a consequence, patients usually experience less pain and guarding and therefore are better able to perform active movement.

A direct application of an ice pack for a 5-minute interval is usually all that a patient will tolerate.

EXERCISE

Exercises may be classified in four categories: (1) active, (2) active assistive, (3) passive, and (4) resistive.

Active exercise is the only modality of hand

*Aris Gloves, New York, N.Y., 10016.

†Jobst Institute, Inc., Toledo, Ohio, 43694.

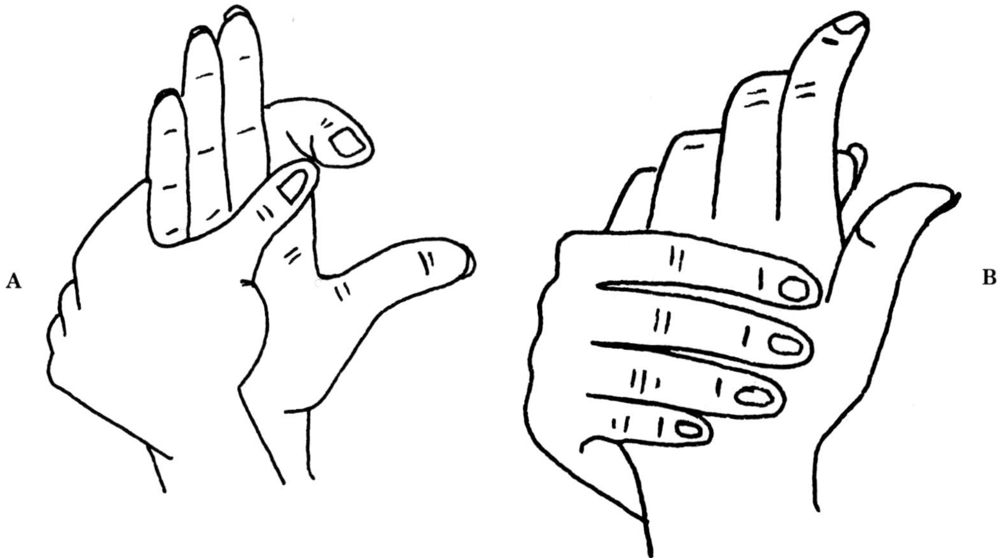

FIG. 28-22. Isolation of active PIP joint motion. **A,** Volar view. **B,** Dorsal view.

therapy ever shown to be of lasting benefit in the rehabilitation of athletically related hand injuries. Its role, therefore, cannot be overemphasized.[5] Active exercises should be initiated as soon as pain subsides and adequate healing of soft tissue and fractures has occurred. Through active motion, it is possible to preserve anatomic structure and tissue nutrition, as well as to prevent adhesions and permit lymphatic drainage.

Active motion must be within pain tolerance. Exercises should be performed gently to avoid tissue reaction but frequently to increase mobility. Tendon adhesions can be avoided with early continuous active exercises aimed at full tendon excursion in both directions.[58] Because active motion plays a primary role in hand therapy, it may be difficult for the practitioner to determine when other types of exercises are indicated.

If passive motion does not exceed active motion, it is necessary to upgrade the exercise program to overcome restriction of joint range. This can be accomplished by several means.

Less tissue reaction occurs when patients are taught to perform active assistive exercises by applying gentle force for short periods several times during the day. When performing active assistive exercises, patients are more likely to respond to pain and will not incite tissue reactions. As healing occurs, patients should be taught to distinguish between discomfort and pain. Discomfort created by a properly applied force is tolerable and beneficial; *pain is not*. The degree of force and number of repetitions should be altered until no tissue reaction occurs. As further healing occurs, intensity should be increased while tissue reaction is continually monitored.

Purely passive exercises play a small role in hand therapy. Effective alternatives to passive motion, besides active assistive exercise, include joint mobilization and static and dynamic splinting.

If passive motion exceeds active motion in spite of what appears to be an adequate active exercise program, it may be necessary to initiate gentle resistive exercises using a light rubber band to overcome weakness or adherence of tendons. It is important that tension applied is gentle enough to allow motion of the joint.

Active Exercise

Isolated-Blocking Exercise

Because active exercises play a substantial role in preventing tendon adherence, teaching the athlete to perform active isolated or blocking exercises to the flexor digitorum profundus or flexor digitorum sublimus in a timely manner is of utmost importance. The athlete should be instructed to stabilize the joint proximal to the one that is being exercised, using the opposite hand to provide better mechanical advantage (Fig. 28-22). Flexion exercises should be done gently and sustained for 10 seconds, with maximal power stopping just short of pain. Many individuals require additional assistance to learn the tech-

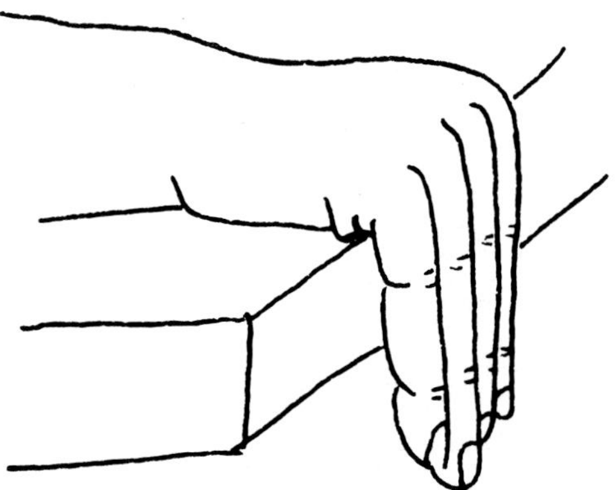

FIG. 28-23. Supporting forearm and wrist on a stationary surface allows for easier active MCP joint isolation.

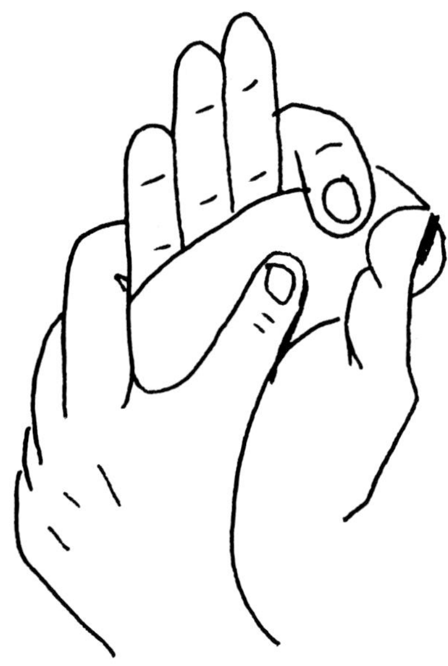

FIG. 28-24. Exercise aids may be necessary to accomplish proper execution of blocking exercises.

nique. Initially, it is helpful to explain that isolated motion is a mental rather than a physical process. By applying effort that is too forceful, they simultaneously contract the flexor and extensor muscles, producing a paradoxic type of motion. Much time and effort can be spent in helping patients to overcome this habit.

Various methods of instruction that implement methods of proprioceptive neuromuscular facilitation (PNF) or biofeedback may be used. Possible methods include practicing isolation of an uninvolved DIP joint, flexing all PIP joints simultaneously, or performing bilateral MCP flexion exercises over the edge of a table top (Fig. 28-23). Many commercial exercise aids are available to assist the therapist. To be effective, devices should support the bone proximal to the joint being exercised to obtain the best mechanical advantage. Devices should also conform to the architecture of the hand by not forcing it into awkward or painful positions (Fig. 28-24).

Passive Exercise

Clinical experience shows that the benefits of passive motion in the hand are transient at best.[5] Passive motion should be included in a hand therapy program only when active motion is not possible. When passive motion is indicated, the athlete should be instructed to perform the exercises himself. Since pain deters athletes from stressing joints, they are less likely to increase symptoms by overexercising.

Passive exercises have been widely used in the past by physical therapists and have been responsible, in part, for alienating the relationship between physical therapists and the early hand surgeons. Surgeons observed that after physical therapy, their patients often appeared to experience increased swelling and decreased mobility, which they attributed to overzealous passive exercises performed by the therapist. Bunnell thought that applying vigorous passive exercises to joints was equivalent to spraining them on a regular basis. He thought the rationale for use of passive motion was unscientific and must be based on comparisons to inanimate objects, such as rusty hinges.[12] As a result of their philosophic differences, early hand surgeons abandoned the use of therapists and personally supervised their patients' rehabilitation. This practice continued until the middle 1970s. By this time, many hand surgeons had trained therapists in what they thought were proper atraumatic techniques of hand rehabilitation. As a result of the physicians' efforts, the American Society of Hand Therapists was founded in 1978.

Many alternative methods of improving passive motion in the hand and wrist exist. They include gentle active assistive exercises, static splinting, and slow, deliberate stretch-

Techniques to improve passive range of motion

- Gentle active assisted exercises
- Static splinting
- Dynamic splinting
- Joint mobilization

ing such as that provided by dynamic splints and joint mobilization.

Resistive Exercise

Resistive exercises should only be initiated in the face of pain-free motion. The patient begins with light resistive materials and gradually increases resistance. The therapist continues to monitor for symptoms of tissue reaction as resistance is upgraded.

Monitoring Exercise Program

Exercises do not have to be painful to be effective. Pain is not gain; it is also not the enemy. Brand describes pain as being the patient's own living cells indicating the limits of the exercise.[13]

Therapists are taught to respect pain. In turn, they must teach patients its significance. Therapists must upgrade rehabilitation programs adequately to make therapeutic gains, but not so rapidly as to create tissue reaction.

As tissues heal, they are able to tolerate stresses that produce discomfort. During this phase, it is necessary to help the athlete differentiate between discomfort and pain.

Tissue reactions should be carefully monitored. If increased edema or pain occurs, the therapeutic program should be reviewed and altered accordingly. This is especially important in dealing with individuals who are unable to differentiate between pain and discomfort.

Experience has taught us that compliance with a consistent therapeutic program is superior to an overzealous exercise program performed in a haphazard or inconsistent manner. In the evaluation of a therapeutic program, an apparent lack of progress may be the result of too much rather than too little exercise.

Composite Flexion

Attaining composite flexion, or "making a fist," is often the only general clinical impression used in evaluating successful rehabilitation of hand injuries.

However simplistic it may appear, careful attention should be paid to restoring composite finger flexion. Unless contraindicated, all initial home programs should consist of exercises for composite motion as well as isolated joint or blocking motion of the digit. The therapist or trainer should provide instruction to flex digits actively around a cylindric object that is almost within current grasp. When patients are able to grasp the object comfortably, therapists or trainers should instruct them to progress gradually to grasping smaller cylindric objects. This exercise is an excellent means of improving motion, because individuals often relate to grasping the object as an activity rather than as an exercise, and they are generally more spontaneous in their performance. Initially, it may be necessary to instruct the patient to grasp rather than squeeze the object. Patients are often tempted to squeeze before adequate healing has occurred to allow their efforts to be therapeutic.

It may be necessary to augment an active exercise program for obtaining composite finger flexion with the use of a static serial splint. Dynamic splints and flexor gloves are suitable alternatives to splinting.

Intrinsic Versus Capsular Tightness

The test for intrinsic tightness is to place the intrinsics on a stretch by extending the MCP joints while passively flexing the PIPs. Then the patient relaxes the intrinsics by flexing the MCPs several degrees while passively flexing the PIP joints. If the PIP joints demonstrate greater passive flexion when the intrinsics are relaxed (flexed MCPs), intrinsic tightness is present. If the degree of passive PIP flexion is unchanged by altering the position of the MCP joints, a joint contracture is present[30] (Fig. 28-25).

Routine therapeutic efforts to improve composite finger flexion are generally not effective in overcoming intrinsic tightness.

Methods of overcoming intrinsic tightness consist of applying a slow, steady force to the middle phalanges while supporting the MCPs in extension. This is best accomplished by the use of dynamic splinting. A volar base is fabricated on the forearm and wrist, extending distally to support the MCP joints in extension. Individual finger cuffs are attached to the proximal phalanx of each digit. Tension is directed toward the outrigger, which is attached to the base of the splint. The outrigger and cuffs should be altered to maintain a continuous 90-degree angle on the digits as improvement occurs. An alternate method of overcoming intrinsic tightness is to use progressive static splinting.

Overcoming intrinsic contracture

- Dynamic splinting
- Serial static splints

Maintaining or Restoring PIP Extension

Maintaining or restoring PIP extension is one of the greatest challenges of rehabilita-

A

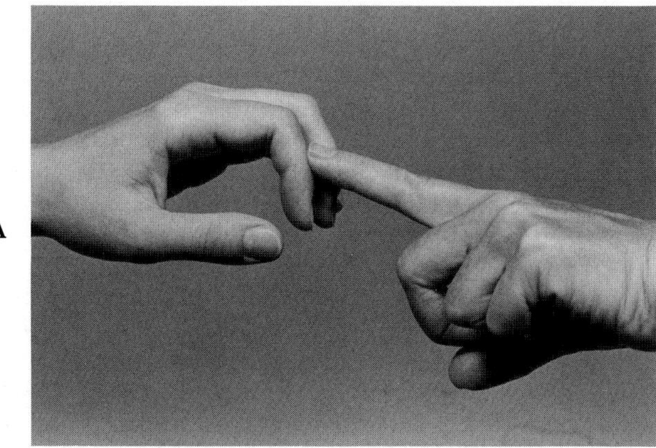

B

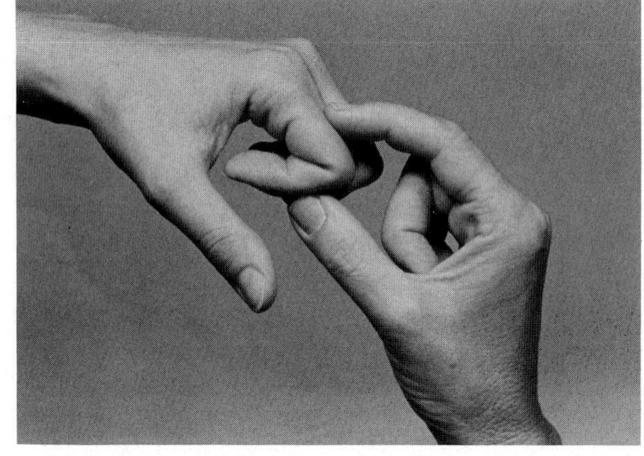

FIG. 28-25. A and **B,** Testing intrinsic tightness.

tion. The challenge becomes even greater if measures to preserve extension are not initiated early in the treatment program.

The flexor muscles in the hand are four times stronger than the extensor muscles.[12] Very few activities require resistive finger extension. The primary function of the extensor muscles is to move the fingers out of the palm. The functional or working position of the hand involves finger flexion.

It is crucial to the therapy program that extension be evaluated often so that mobility is maintained. Loss of PIP extension may occur if splinting is discontinued before adequate soft tissue healing has occurred. It may further be decreased when either substantial gains in flexion are attained or there is increased functional use of the hand.

Isolated PIP extension exercises should be a part of all exercise programs involving digits. To perform active isolated PIP extension exercises, the patient positions the wrist in a neutral position and stabilizes the MCPs in maximal flexion by supporting them with the opposite hand. The athlete should be instructed to actively extend the PIP joints (Fig. 28-26).

To further counteract the imbalance, it is often necessary to statically splint the PIP joints in extension. Splints may be worn at night to avoid interfering with functional use and therapeutic programs designed to improve mobility.

MODALITIES

Therapeutic Heat

Therapeutic heat decreases pain and muscle spasms, reduces joint stiffness, and increases collagen extensibility.

Hydrocollator

Hydrocollators (hot packs) apply moist heat directly to the skin surfaces and have the advantage of being applied while the hand is held in elevation. However, any compromise of peripheral circulation or presence of insensitive digits contraindicates the use of hydrocollators.

Patients should be checked often during

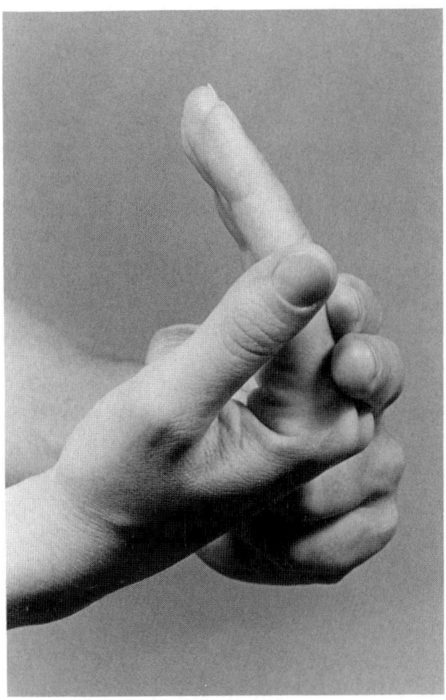

FIG. 28-26. Active isolated PIP extension.

treatment to ensure that the intense heat is well tolerated. It is especially important to observe bony prominences or contracted joints for indications of intolerance. Placing weights on hot packs in an attempt to improve finger extension should be discouraged, especially if significant contractures are present.

Hot packs are especially effective when used before wrist exercises.

Whirlpool

Despite the popularity of the whirlpool, it is often used unnecessarily and indiscriminately. Improper use of the whirlpool may not only provide an ineffective modality in some situations, but also the temperature of the water, together with the dependent position of the extremity, often results in increased edema. This technique, used in previous years, has given the whirlpool a bad name. Hand surgery literature is filled with the perils created by the improper use of the whirlpool. Bell and Horton state: "Probably no device deserves more credit for perpetuating hand disability than the whirlpool."[7] The whirlpool can be used in the treatment of hand and wrist injuries if indications, contraindications, and precautions as to its use are employed.

The dependent position can be eliminated by slightly abducting the shoulder and flexing the elbow so that the water level just covers the hand during treatment. One can avoid compromising the vascularity of an injured extremity or damaging an insensitive area with extremes of hot or cold temperatures. A wide variety of treatment temperatures are cited in the literature.[3,7,25,31] Recommended temperatures for providing general whirlpool range from 95° to 105° F for heat, and from 55° to 65° F for cold whirlpool. It is important to note that these statistics are not provided for the treatment of upper extremities. To determine desirable or appropriate water temperatures, it is important to review all information obtained through clinical examination and the available medical information. Hand volume should be observed before and after whirlpool treatment, and water temperature decreased if volume increases. Active exercises are also effective in combating edema if they are performed during whirlpool treatment.

Whirlpool therapy

Proper whirlpool use
- Hand is elevated
- Appropriate temperature

Improper whirlpool use
- Hand is dependent
- Inappropriate temperature

Recommended whirlpool temperatures
- Heat: 95°-105° F
- Cold: 55°-65° F

In the treatment of open wounds, a disinfectant added to the whirlpool water, together with a clean whirlpool has been shown to reduce the local bacteria count.[8,45] Following treatment, the tank should be drained and thoroughly cleaned. Carefully followed cleaning procedures and periodic cultures are necessary. If cleaning and culturing procedures are not carefully followed, open wounds should not be treated in the whirlpool.

In the absence of open wounds, paraffin or hydrocollator pads along with elevation may be a better method of providing heat before exercise. Whirlpool is not effective when heat is the only desired objective.

Paraffin

The paraffin bath is particularly effective in the rehabilitation of hand and wrist injuries. The advantage of paraffin is that it contours and heats all surfaces, thereby providing an even heating effect. The presence of oil provides lubrication to dry skin and improves elasticity, making it especially effective as a precursor to massage. Joints can be positioned on a stretch, providing maximal benefit from the heat that is applied to contracting structures. The temperature of 126° F can create skin problems in the face of vascular compromise, neurologic deficits, or early reflex sympathetic dystrophy. Paraffin treatment is also not indicated in individuals with open wounds or exposed internal hardware.

Directions for paraffin application

- Elevate if edema is present.
- Remove all jewelry, and wash and dry hand well.
- With fingers slightly abducted, dip hand and wrist into the bath. Remove quickly and allow to cool. Having started the treatment, maintain constant position of the fingers to maintain heat longer.
- When the paraffin has cooled enough to be comfortable, resume dipping. Continue dipping until you have built up approximately 10 layers of paraffin.
- Cover the hand with clear plastic wrap or a plastic bag. Wrap tightly in a towel to maintain heat.
- Leave the paraffin in place for 20 minutes or as long as the effect of heat is appreciated.
- It is best to dispose of used paraffin.

Fluidotherapy

Fluidotherapy* was introduced as a form of therapeutic heat in 1974.[9] Fluidotherapy is based on the discovery that in certain hydrodynamic conditions, solid particles can be suspended in air. Essentially, the mixture is similar to a dry whirlpool, which provides massage action and carries heat to body tissues in an effective manner. Because the heat generated is dry (115° to 120° F), temperatures are generally comfortably tolerated. Borrell and his associates have stated that under these conditions, heat absorbed by the body is four to six times as great as in other forms of hydrotherapy or paraffin treatments.[10] Advantages to this treatment include a decrease in manpower and utilities, in that plumbing usage and filling and emptying the apparatus between uses is not indicated. Elevation and active exercises are possible during its use.

Therapeutic Ultrasound

Therapeutic ultrasound is widely used in sports medicine clinics. Through the years, various claims have been made concerning the effects of ultrasound. Although its thermal effects have been well documented in the literature,[49] research concerning its nonthermal effects has not been conclusive. Contraindications to ultrasound treatment include areas that are insensate, since pain sensation is one of the best indicators of overdosage. Acutely injured or edematous extremities should also not be treated with ultrasound. It has been determined that within therapeutic dosage, ultrasound is safe to use over epiphyseal growth areas.[3]

Contraindications to ultrasound use

- Insensate regions
- Open wounds
- Edema

Ultrasound treatments to the hand and wrist should always be provided under water. Both the extremity and ultrasound head should be submerged. The head should be placed approximately 2.5 cm from the surface to be treated. The dose varies according to the depth of tissue treated and state of the injury, for example, acute versus subacute.

Therapeutic Cold

Therapeutic cold may also be used to decrease pain, muscle spasm, and inflammation. It increases joint stiffness, however, and causes vasoconstriction. Cold is most effective when used immediately after injury and during the acute stage of healing to reduce the effects of edema.

Cold may be used both before and after exercise to reduce resultant edema. Cold is often required after treatment in rehabilitating wrist injuries.

Duration of cold treatments is dependent on patient tolerance. Icing may be done for 5 to 10 minutes, while cool whirlpool is usually provided for 10 to 20 minutes.

In overuse syndromes, cold treatments should be continued until the joint is pain-free throughout its range and edema is no longer present. In other diagnoses, it is appropriate to progress to the use of heat when edema subsides or when cold is no longer effective as a preexercise modality.

Contrast Therapy

Contrast therapy may be indicated between acute and subacute phases of rehabilitation. In progressing from the use of cold to the use of heat, it may be necessary to bridge the gap between using cold or heat as a precursor to

*Fluidotherapy Corporation, 7001 Mullins St., Suite A, Houston, TX 77081.

exercise. Contrast therapy consists of alternately submerging the extremity in warm water (102° F) for 2 minutes followed by submergence in cool water (55° to 65° F) for 2 minutes. Beginning with heat, five sessions should take place, always ending in cold.

Transcutaneous Electrical Nerve Stimulation

Transcutaneous electrical nerve stimulation (TENS) has gained wide acceptance as a method of reducing pain in athletes with both acute and chronic problems. TENS offers different forms of stimulation that are achieved by adjustment of the amplitude, pulse rate, and pulse width of the pulsed wave form. They are classified as conventional, brief intense, and low frequency.

TENS techniques

- Conventional
- Low-frequency
- Brief intense

Conventional

Conventional TENS is based on the Melzack and Walls gate control theory of pain.[41] Parameters for conventional TENS require a high rate, low width wave form, with amplitude adjustment until the patient is able to perceive a tingling sensation in the extremity. Onset of pain relief may occur relatively quickly. Conventional TENS is the most commonly used and is the recommended choice for postoperative pain and treatment of reflex sympathetic dystrophy.

Low-Frequency

The effect of low-frequency TENS is attributed to the release of a naturally occurring morphinelike substance called endorphins.[27] Parameters for low-frequency TENS require low pulse rate, high pulse width, and an increase in amplitude until a visible muscle contraction is present. Not all models of TENS units can be adjusted adequately for low rate stimulation because they are manufactured with a preset width. Low-frequency TENS may be provided in a bursting mode or pulsed train, which has been described as more comfortable by patients with upper extremity problems. Because it creates a muscle contraction, low-frequency TENS should not be performed on athletes who have not been given medical clearance for active exercises.

Brief Intense

Clinical applications for brief intense TENS are not numerous. Parameters for brief intense TENS require high rate and high pulse width and increased amplitude until a strong muscle contraction occurs. Brief intense TENS is beneficial in controlling pain before suture removal or debridement. Stimulation time should be brief, because muscle fatigue occurs rapidly.

Postoperative

Conventional TENS is used for postoperative pain. Sterile electrodes may be applied in the operating room. Best results are obtained when the TENS functions before the patient awakes from anesthesia or before an anesthetic block wears off. Whenever possible, patients should be familiarized with the unit before surgery. Postoperative TENS is particularly beneficial in situations where early motion is desirable. Indications for postoperative TENS may include tenolysis, neurolysis, a previous history of pain problems, or reflex sympathetic dystrophy. When TENS is used, postoperative exercise programs should be structured and monitored to guard against excessive activity.

TENS is an invaluable tool in rehabilitation of the upper extremity. It can play an impressive role in the treatment of crush injuries, painful swollen hands, sensitive scars, painful neuromas, overuse syndrome, and any situation in which adequate healing has occurred, but active motion is inhibited by the pain.

Electrodes

Although standard carbon electrodes are most economical, they must be covered evenly with conducting gel to be effective. Preparation and application are often difficult for patients with hand involvement. Self-adherent electrodes, although more expensive, are often indicated to allow independent application. Skin reaction is not a common problem, though the skin under electrodes should be checked for any indications of adverse reaction. The electrodes should not be placed over open or irritated areas.

Electrodes are available in various sizes. In treatment of the hand and wrist, electrodes may either be too large or too inflexible to allow adequate skin contact. One should investigate the various types and sizes of electrodes available before using TENS. In some situations, it is necessary to trim overly large electrodes. When reducing the size of one electrode on a given channel, it is important not to exceed a 2:1 ratio of electrode sizes.

This will prevent burning under the smaller electrode.

Electrodes are usually placed over the painful site (neuroma), though they can also be placed over dermatomes, myotomes, trigger or acupuncture points, peripheral nerve pathways, vascular channels (reflex sympathetic dystrophy), or proximal and distal to a painful scar. The numerous waveforms available are confusing, because none has proved more effective than others.[17] When purchasing units for a clinic, it is important to become acquainted with several units. The therapist should choose those with two channels that will best suit the needs of the patients. When choosing units to be used in home programs, simplicity in operation is advantageous. It is also wise to choose units that can be operated and maintained by individuals with hand impairment.

Contraindications

Contraindications to TENS rarely occur in the athletic population. TENS should not be used during pregnancy, over the carotid sinus, over the chest in the presence of cardiac problems, over the eyes or mucosal membranes, after cerebrovascular accidents, or with individuals who rely on pacemakers.[36]

Electrical Stimulation

The High-voltage galvanic stimulator (HVGS) is an excellent modality used in sports medicine because of its multiple benefits and simplicity of use. The HVGS can be used for edema and pain control, the treatment of acute injuries, and muscle stimulation. Its effectiveness in promoting wound healing has been substantiated in the literature. Electrodes for the HVGS unit are too large to be practical for muscle stimulation of the hand.

Galvanism is a continuous, waveless, unidirectional current that is referred to commercially as direct current. Galvanic current is chemical in action; as it passes through the body, it breaks up some of the molecules encountered into their component atoms or ions. Ions have either a positive or negative electric charge, and they either attract or repel each other. The most important feature of the galvanic current is polarity. Each has distinctive attributes and produces different therapeutic effects.

The box below outlines the effects produced at the respective poles. The various effects are produced at the site of the active electrode.

The effect of muscle stimulation includes a decrease in muscle spasm. The current causes intermittent tetanic contraction, which in turn results in muscle relaxation. HVGS is usually more effective than low voltage because it can provide a stronger contraction. It is also capable of providing contraction of deeper muscles.

The use of electrical stimulation to produce contraction of muscles of the hand and wrist is better achieved by stimulators other than HVG units. The size of the electrodes is more compatible for stimulation of muscles of the hand and wrist. A smaller pulse width is more effective when stimulating smaller muscles.

To be effective for use as a muscle stimulator, muscles must be innervated when using HVGS.

SENSORY REEDUCATION

Before 1971 poor sensibility following nerve repair was thought to be the result of the surgical procedure. When clinicians observed patients who demonstrated different levels of functional recovery with identical levels of injury and measured clinical sensation (academic recovery), they attributed the variation to motivational factors and persistent use of the extremity.

Dellon and colleagues[21] postulated that the failure of patients to achieve full recovery of functional sensation in the hand following peripheral nerve injury was related to failure by the patient to achieve his full sensory potential.

Their study presented evidence to support the premise that following nerve injury, pa-

HVGS effects

Positive pole
- Attracts acid
- Repels alkali
- Hardens tissue
- Relieves pain
- Reduces edema
- Facilitates tissue granulation

Negative pole
- Attracts alkali
- Repels acid
- Softens tissue (including scar tissue)
- Has antibacterial effect

tients could be reeducated to correctly interpret, with the cerebral cortex, the profiles of impulses that occur in response to a known peripheral stimulus. A formal sensory reeducation program is based on learning principals of attention, reenforcement, feedback, and memory to improve hand function. The patient can learn to decipher altered messages that are being sent to the brain by nerve fibers that are less populated, smaller, and disorganized when compared to their preinjury state.

Dellon and his associates' study demonstrated that the usual pattern of sensation of functional recovery in the hand occurs in the following sequence[21] (Fig. 28-27):

1. Pain (no longer tested)
2. Vibration of 30 cps (hertz)
3. Moving touch
4. Constant touch
5. Vibration of 256 cps (hertz)

A pain-free hand is necessary before sensory reeducation is undertaken. Painful neuromas, paresthesias, and other painful situations discovered in the initial evaluation should be treated before beginning training. Their specific treatment has been discussed earlier in this chapter.

Dellon has outlined detailed techniques involved in the early and late phase of sensory reeducation.[21]

SPLINTS

It is not possible to provide optimal hand rehabilitation without using static or dynamic splints. Splints may be protective, supportive, and/or corrective in design.

Faulty positioning of a limb during either rest or activity could cause deformity if impairment of nerves, muscles, or joints is present. To successfully prevent the development of deformity, we must understand the basic pathologic condition, recognize factors that lead to deformity, and provide appropriate treatment.

Position for static immobilization

- Wrist—30 degrees dorsiflexion
- MCPs—70 degrees flexion
- PIPs—10-20 degrees flexion
- Thumb—Full abduction

Static Splints

When static splinting of the entire extremity is indicated, the hand and wrist should be placed in an intrinsic plus, clam digger, or antideformity position (Fig. 28-28). This preferred position of immobilization preserves the functional length of tissues. The wrist should be placed in approximately 30 degrees of dorsiflexion. The thumb should be placed in full abduction. MCPs should be positioned in 70 degrees of flexion. PIPs should be positioned in 10 to 20 degrees of flexion. During periods of immobilization, it is important to preserve the arches of the hand. Volar splints are best and should be fabricated to support the proximal and distal transverse arches, as well as the longitudinal arches.

The intrinsic plus position maintains liga-

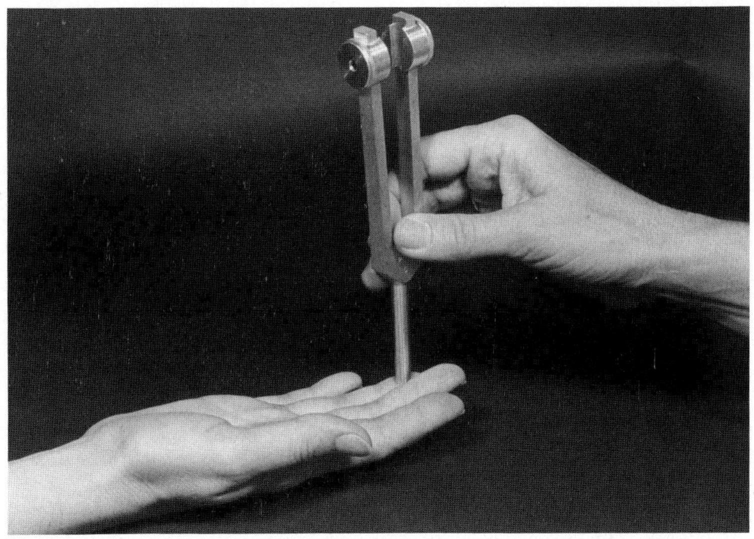

FIG. 28-27. Tuning fork used to test vibratory sense.

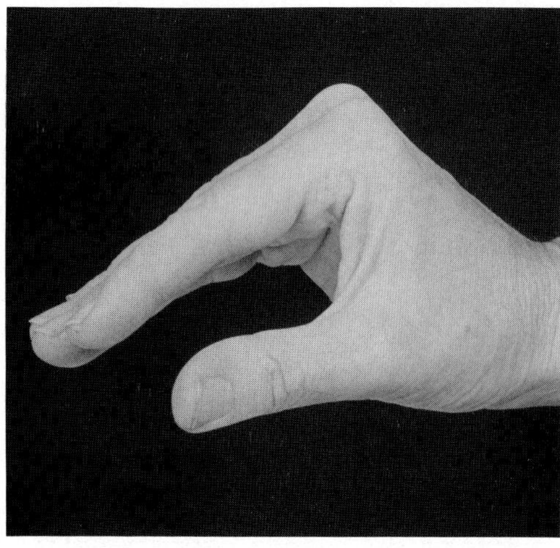

FIG. 28-28. Intrinsic plus—clam digger or antideformity position.

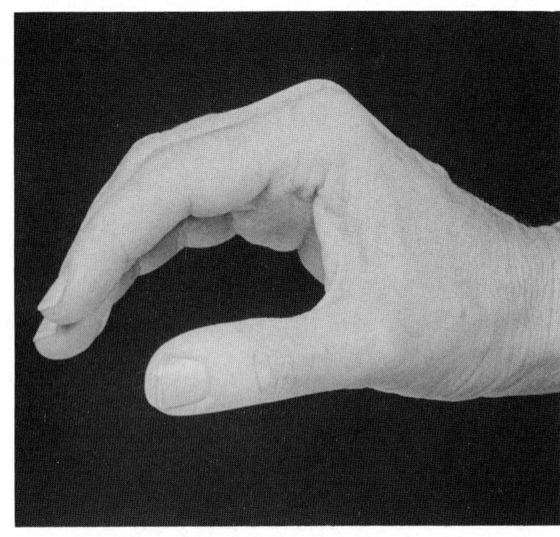

FIG. 28-30. Functional position.

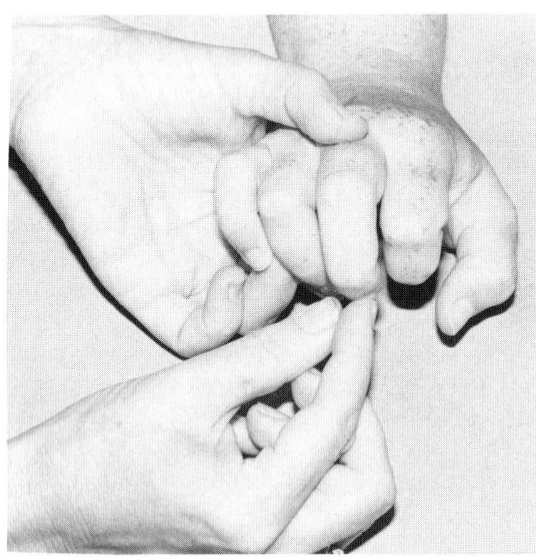

FIG. 28-29. Exercise effective in counteracting tight intrinsic muscles that may result from prolonged immobilization.

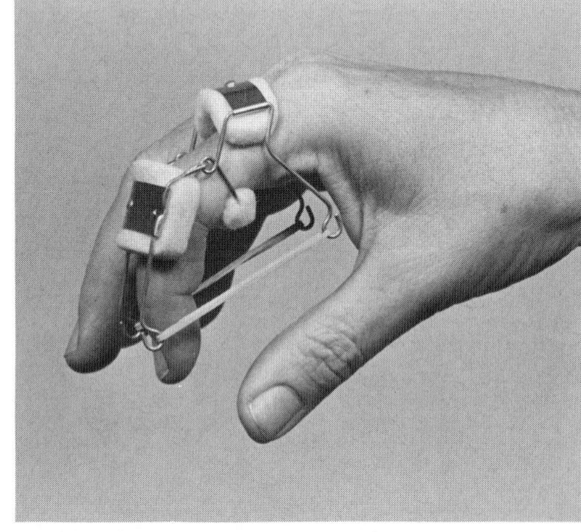

FIG. 28-31. Finger bender splint designed to increase PIP flexion.

ments of the digital joints under maximal tension, thereby preventing joint contractures. The position also encourages intrinsic tightness; however, tightness can be combated by initiating intrinsic stretching exercises. To stretch intrinsic muscles passively, the MP joints are placed in extension while the PIPs and DIPs are flexed (Fig. 28-29).

An alternate position for splinting the hand is in a functional position (Fig. 28-30). The wrist is placed in 30 degrees of dorsiflexion. The MPs are flexed in approximately 45 degrees of flexion, while the PIP joints are in 10 to 20 degrees of flexion. The thumb may be placed in opposition or adduction depending on its involvement. Care should be taken to preserve the web space. The functional position is preferred when splinting is indicated to promote relaxation.

Dynamic Splints

Dynamic splints employ traction devices such as rubber bands or springs to alter passive motion of a joint (Fig. 28-31). They may be helpful in accomplishing the following objectives:

1. Prevention or correction of deformities of the hand or wrist
2. Prevention of joint stiffness by maintaining mobility

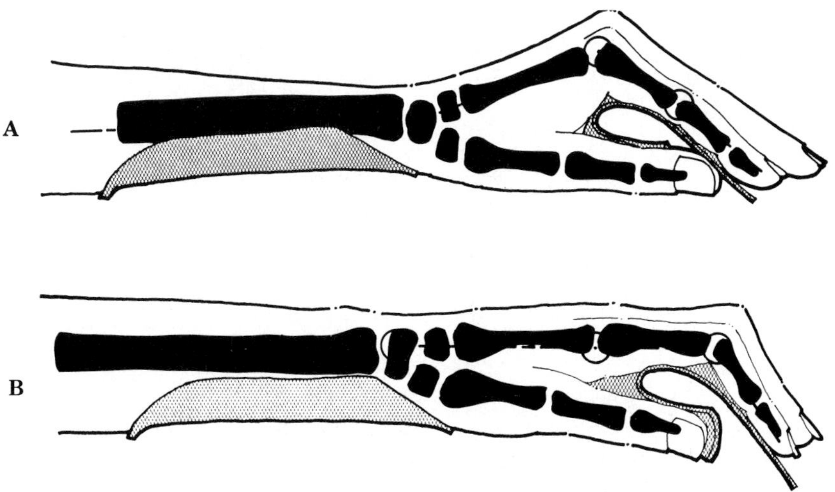

FIG. 28-32. A, Properly applied splint. **B,** Improperly applied splint. (From Malick MH: Manual on dynamic hand splinting with thermoplastic materials, Pittsburgh, 1974, Harmarville Rehabilitation Center.)

3. Strengthening of weak muscles by encouraging proper positioning and assistance
4. Increasing functional capacity of the hand by stabilizing it in a better position for function, in order to provide mechanical assistance

The philosophy of dynamic splinting is based on the theory of prolonged stretching of tissues, similar to that which is used by orthodontists in the bracing of teeth. The bone proximal to the joint being moved must be stabilized, and the line of pull should be at right angles to the axis of the bone being affected.[50] The line of pull must be adjusted frequently to maintain the correct direction of pull (90 degrees) as joint motion increases.

Splints should provide adequate stretch without being painful. Patients should be aware of a pulling sensation but not of pain. Rather than prescribing a structured routine, the therapist should instruct the patient to wear the splint until reaching maximal tolerance, at which time the splint should be removed. Wearing time may be relatively short at first but should quickly increase. If wearing time does not progress, the splint should be checked. Lack of effectiveness may be caused by an ill-fitting splint, excessive tension applied to the bands, or in inadequate healing that does not allow tolerance of the forces exerted by the splint. Splinting programs should be supplemented with an exercise program and encouragement of functional use of the extremity.

Dynamic splints provided to improve mobility should not be used for exercising, as pulling against the bands strengthens the opposite motion the splint was designed to improve.

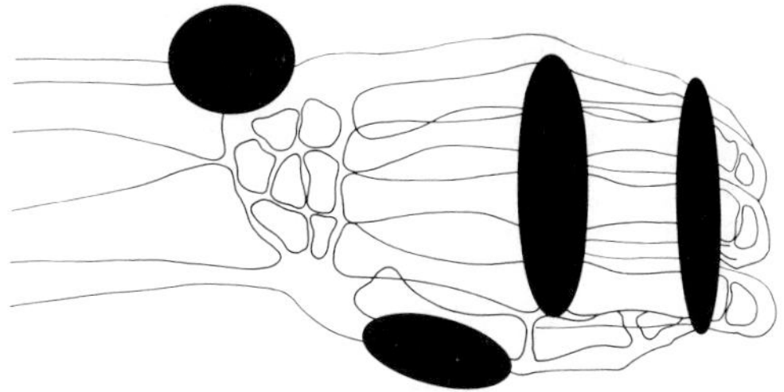

FIG. 28-33. Dorsal view of pressure areas to consider when fabricating splints. (From Malick MH: Manual on dynamic hand splinting with thermoplastic materials, Pittsburgh, 1974, Harmarville Rehabilitation Center.)

Precautions

Splints should be checked often. Ill-fitting splints can contribute to rather than prevent deformity (Fig. 28-32). Changes in hand volume and improvement in motion necessitate splint alteration. Caution should be taken to avoid creating irritation over bony prominances caused by friction.[35,36] This is especially important when fabricating splints that will be worn during functional use of the extremity. In the hand, pressure areas may occur over the heads of the metacarpals, the pisiform, and the base of the first metacarpal (Fig. 28-33). In the forearm, the radial and styloid processes may create similar problems

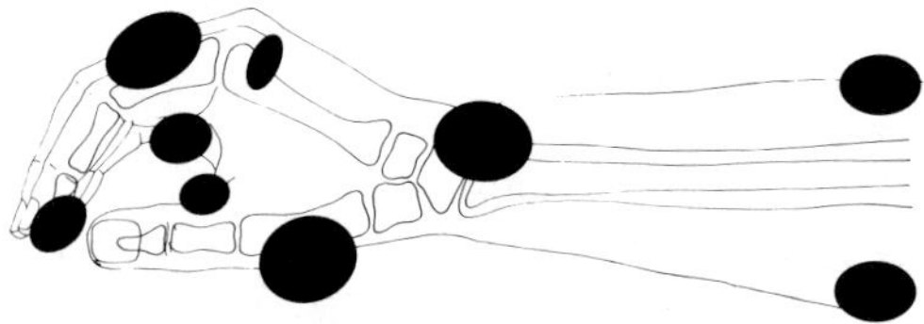

FIG. 28-34. Radial view of pressure areas to consider when fabricating splints. (From Malick MH: Manual on dynamic hand splinting with thermoplastic materials, Pittsburgh, 1974, Harmarville Rehabilitation Center.)

(Fig. 28-34). Eliminating pressure over bony prominances may be done in several ways. Avoiding the area, dispersing pressure over a larger area, or padding are all acceptable means of avoidance. Padding is most often used when protective splints are fabricated for use during athletic activity.

Techniques to eliminate pressure on bony prominences

- Padding
- Avoiding the area
- Dispensing pressure over greater area

Materials

Many low temperature plastic splinting materials are available on the market today. Thickness and rigidity of splinting materials should be considered. Bulky material will interfere with dexterity, while thin material may not be strong enough to withstand the pressure placed on them during athletic activity. The use of perforated rather than nonperforated splinting material should not be considered in the fabrication of certain types of protective athletic splints. In the author's experience, several splints made from perforated materials have broken in areas of high stress, making their use inadvisable for protection in sports that require heavy repetitive activity.

Protective

When fabricating splints to be used for protection during activity, the therapist must have basic knowledge of anatomy and kinesiology of the hand, as well as familiarity with the level of skill required of each athlete.

While at rest, the transverse metacarpal arch takes on a concave appearance (Fig. 28-35). When the hand is engaged in functional activities, the arch becomes even more pronounced (Fig. 28-36). The second and third metacarpals are immobile, while the first,

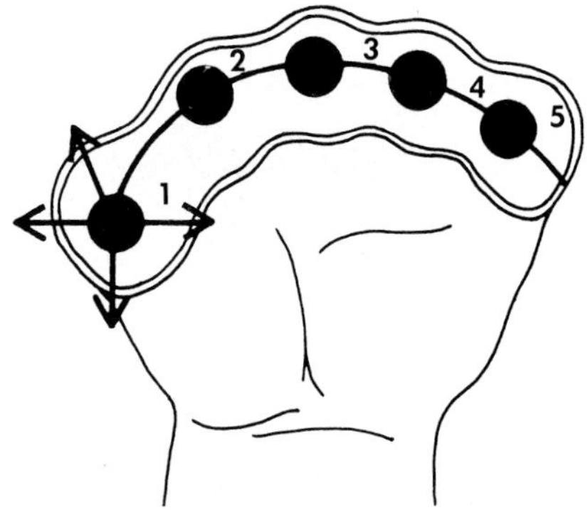

FIG. 28-35. Transverse metacarpal arch at rest. (From Malick MH: Manual on dynamic hand splinting with thermoplastic materials, Pittsburgh, 1974, Harmarville Rehabilitation Center.)

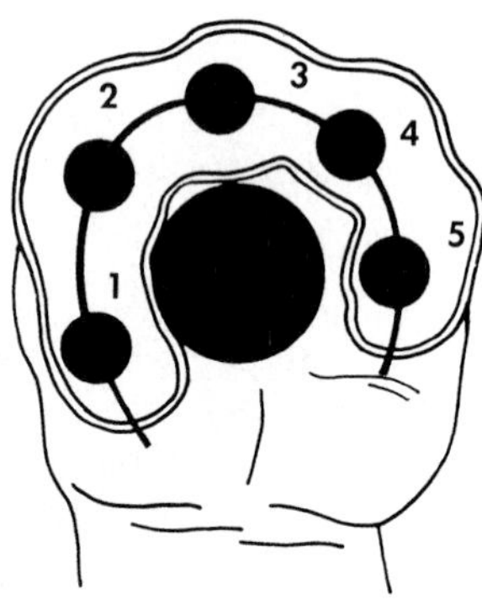

FIG. 28-36. Transverse metacarpal arch during function. (From Malick MH: Manual on dynamic hand splinting with thermoplastic materials, Pittsburgh, 1974, Harmarville Rehabilitation Center.)

fourth, and fifth metacarpals are mobile. Failure to accommodate the transverse metacarpal arch into splints, casts, or protective gear will result in decreased dexterity and need for further joint mobilization when splinting is discontinued (Fig. 28-37).

The longitudinal arch consists of MCP, PIP, and DIP flexion. Positioning of the longitudinal arch during splinting is dictated by the medical condition. Possible positions include intrinsic plus, functional position, or optimal position for athletic participation.

Having access to athletic equipment in the clinic or training room allows a better functional position for immobilization, thereby permitting the athlete to perform all aspects of activity; for example, a baseball player should be able to grasp and release a bat. Having equipment available will allow the thera-

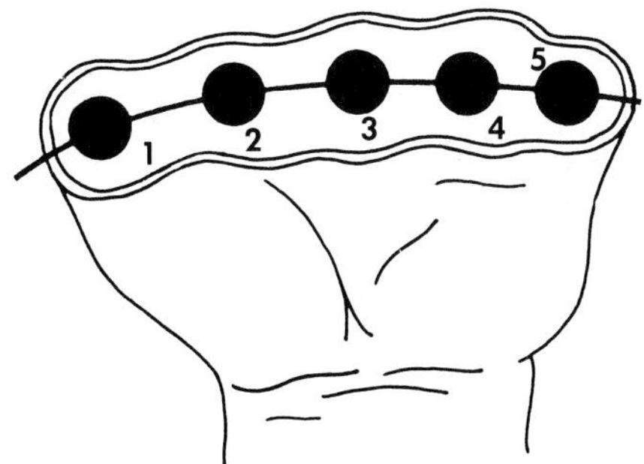

FIG. 28-37. Transverse metacarpal arch, nonfunctional position. (From Malick MH: Manual on dynamic hand splinting with thermoplastic materials, Pittsburgh, 1974, Harmarville Rehabilitation Center.)

pist to immobilize the patient's finger in a compromised position that will permit adequate mobility to perform all aspects of the sport (Fig. 28-38).

When fabricating splints, as much length as possible should be maintained for mechanical leverage (Fig. 28-39). Care should be taken not to restrict motion of uninvolved joints. Skin creases created by joints are helpful landmarks to use in designing finger splints (Fig. 28-40).

Metacarpophalangeal Joint and Wrist

Safe support for the wrist or MCP should be circumferential. Fiberglass or silicone casts provide an excellent means of protec-

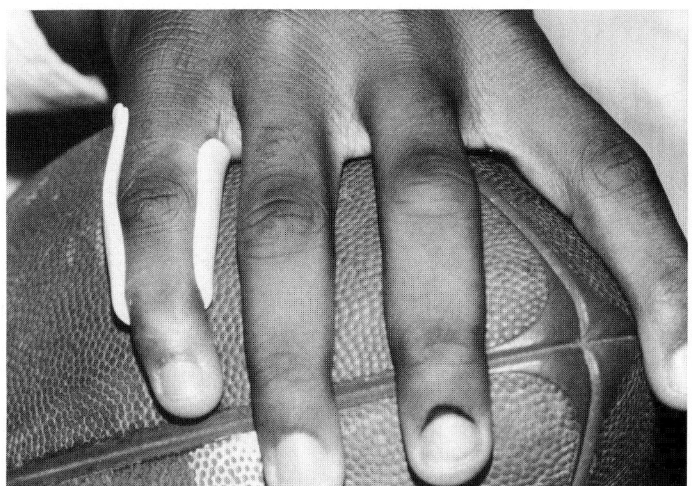

FIG. 28-38. Protective device molded to allow maximal function.

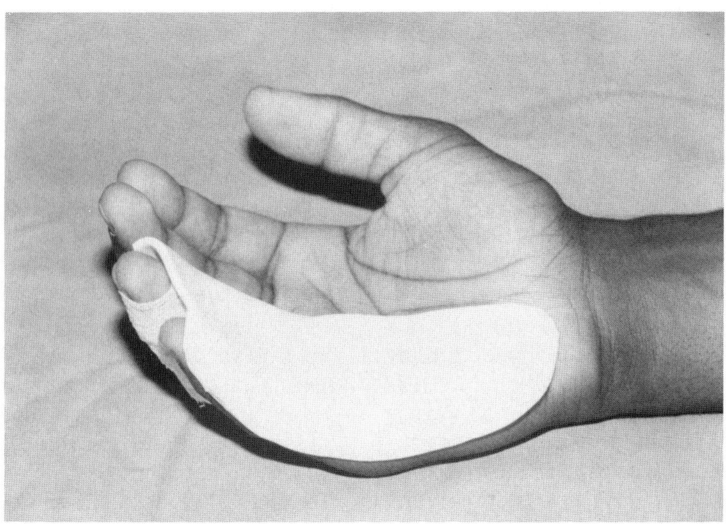

FIG. 28-39. Protection should be of adequate length but should not limit mobility of uninvolved joints.

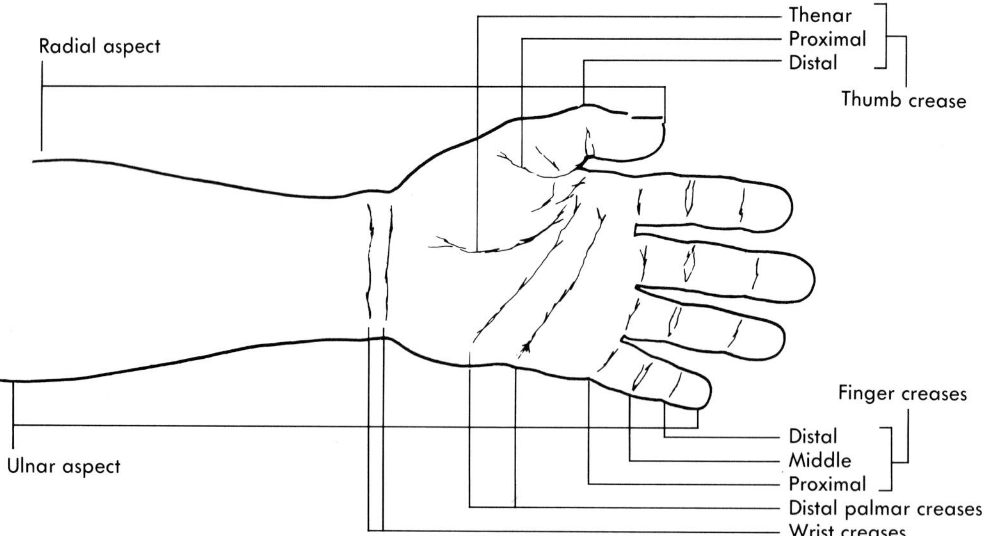

FIG. 28-40. Skin creases on volar surface of the hand created by joints. (From Malick MH: Manual on static hand splinting, Pittsburgh, 1972, Harmarville Rehabilitation Center.)

tion. Rules regarding acceptable protective splints vary between states, as well as between professional, college, and high school teams.

If adequately padded, fiberglass or regular casts are allowed. This method provides excellent protection and eliminates the need for changing casts. Another means of protection is the soft or silicone rubber cast. Initially introduced in the 1970s, soft casts are widely used today in both sports medicine and hand clinics.[4]

RTV silicone is available in quantities of 1 pound or 12 pound containers. Since not all casts require one pound of silicone, much material is wasted. Buying the larger quantity and dividing it into 4 ounce portions may be a reasonable and economical solution to the problem of wasted material.

Storage

RTV may be stored in the refrigerator. Larger quantities may be stored in the freezer, which seems to increase its shelf life.

Thumb

When adequate healing has occurred, safe-effective protection should be provided to allow the athlete to return to participation. In designing thumb protection, it is important to consider the diagnosis and the position the athlete plays. Stability is always more important than mobility. The proper position of protection is essential, because protection in an improper position may cause reinjury. When positioning the thumb from ulna collateral ligament (UCL) injuries, the carpometacarpal (CMC) joint should be slightly flexed and adducted. Protection should prevent extension and abduction, the mechanism that created the initial injury (Fig. 28-41).

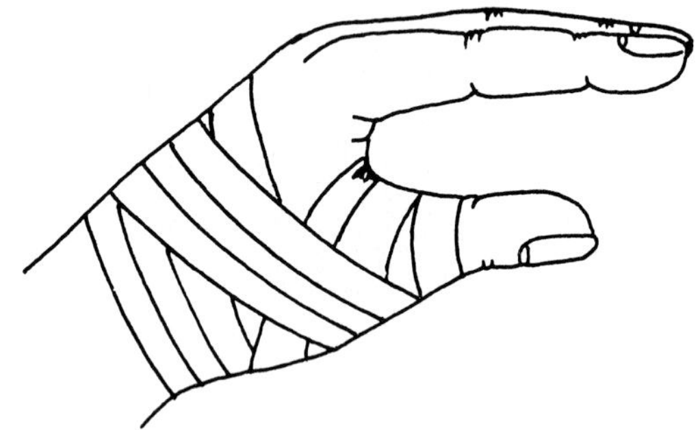

FIG. 28-41. Protected thumb position for UCL injury. (From Gieck JH and Mayer V: Protective splinting for the hand and wrist. In McCue FC, editor: Clinics in sports medicine, Philadelphia, 1986, WB Saunders Co.)

Methods of thumb protection may be provided by various means: using low temperature plastic (Fig. 28-42); taping the index finger to the thumb to provide a buddy type of anchor (Fig. 28-43); or taping the thumb to the hand for stability (Fig. 28-44). Obviously, this method of protection is not suitable for ball handlers.

Soft cast: instructions for fabricating silicone rubber casts [23,38]

Supplies needed

Tongue blades
Vaseline
4 rolls of Kling* a silicone compound
Scissors
One 2 or 3-inch Ace wrap
Talcum powder
Approximately 1 lb RTV 11 silicone and catalyst
1-inch adhesive tape
Paper towels
Topper sponge gauze strip or 1/16-inch polyform strip
Plastic covering for work surface

Method of fabrication

Divide 1 lb of silicone into four 4 oz containers.
Add 20 drops of catalyst per 4 oz (only mix when needed).
Tape area to be protected.
Cover area of the hand, wrist, and forearm to be supported within the rubber cast with vaseline to prevent silicone from adhering to skin tape.
Loosely wrap the hand-forearm with enough Kling for 2 layers, then apply prepared silicone with the tongue blade. (Smooth out and cover well).
Loosely wrap another two layers of Kling and apply more silicone. It is at this point that internal support is added. We use a strip of polyform to add additional support to the fracture site, but ½ × 2 inch strips of topper also work well. Impregnate the topper sponge, then put into position.
Continue to wrap Kling—three layers before applying silicone thereafter. Prepare additional silicone as needed. Most splints require from 12 to 16 oz of silicone. We suggest using all of the kling and silicone. Wipe away excess with a paper towel.
After the rubber cast is completed, wrap loosely with a plastic wrap, then the 2 or 3 inch Ace wrap. Do not press or squeeze rubber cast while it is curing.
Curing time is approximately 3 hours.
To remove, cut along ulnar border with bandage scissors.
Trim splint and check fit.
Remove tape, wipe vaseline off arm with paper towels, then wash with soap and water.
Silicone casts are nonporous and should only be worn during practice and games. The hand and forearm should be dusted with powder before wearing the rubber cast. The cast is held in place with adhesive tape. If worn for more than several hours at a time, the skin may become macerated. Fiberglass or regular hard casts should be worn during the day as well as during practice.

*Johnson and Johnson, New Brunswick, New Jersey, 08903.

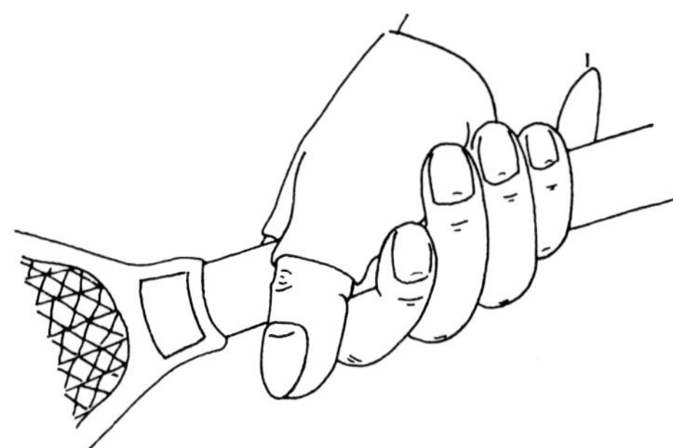

FIG. 28-42. MCP protection. (From Gieck JH and Mayer V: Protective splinting for the hand and wrist. In McCue FC, editor: Clinics in sports medicine, Philadelphia, 1986, WB Saunders Co.)

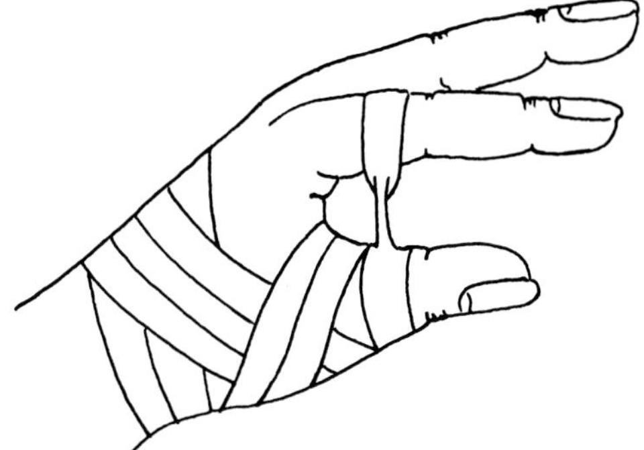

FIG. 28-43. Buddy taping. (From Gieck JH and Mayer V: Protective splinting for the hand and wrist. In McCue FC, editor: Clinics in sports medicine, Philadelphia, 1986, WB Saunders Co.)

ADAPTED EQUIPMENT

Many types of commercial gloves are available to protect athletes' hand from injury. Such protection should be used whenever it is available. Lacrosse gloves are well designed since they allow adequate function while providing protection. Most hand injuries in lacrosse players today occur because the player alters or cuts away some of the glove's protection to afford better mobility.

Baseball catchers may add additional padding to the palms of their mitts to reduce shock and consequently decrease the possibility of developing thromboses or aneurysms of the radial or ulnar arteries.

Skiers should not wear short gloves. Long gloves can protect a skier's wrists from injuries such as cuts, which may occur from the edge of a ski.[36] Children's ski gloves should be checked to ensure that they are long enough to be protective.

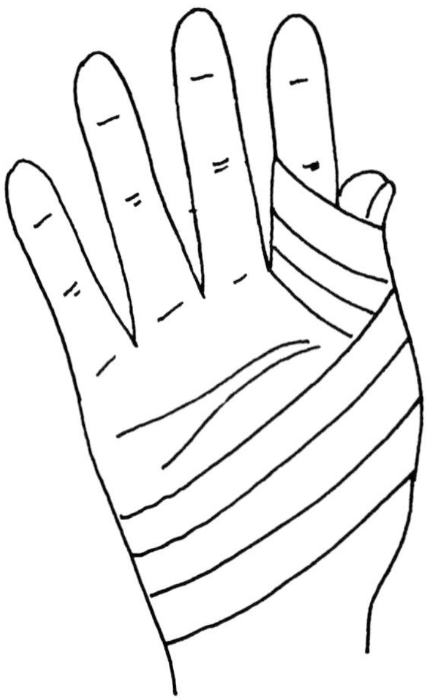

FIG. 28-44. Maximal thumb stability. (From Gieck, JH and Mayer V: Protective splinting for the hand and wrist. In McCue FC, editor: Clinics in sports medicine, Philadelphia, 1986, WB Saunders Co.)

It is recommended that long distance cyclists wear padded gloves. Extra padding in the hypothenar region helps to decrease prolonged pressure from handle bars. Pressure in this area can cause compressure of the ulnar nerve through Guyon's canal. Adaptations may be provided to the athlete's glove or sports equipment to allow practice of skills before having adequate mobility to compete (Fig. 28-45).

HOME PROGRAM

The home program is often considered the most important aspect of hand rehabilitation. Nowhere is its importance greater than in the treatment of athletic injuries.

Injuries sustained by athletes are usually produced by circumstances inherent to their respective sport. When allowed to return to competition, they are exposed to similar recurrent trauma, making reinjury more likely. In the rehabilitation of athletes, our goal is to obtain normal function to the greatest degree possible in the shortest possible time.

Therapists or trainers should provide athletes with adequate instruction so that they are able to carry out all aspects of their programs at home on a daily basis. Instruction should include the use of modalities, exercise aids, splints, and therapeutic exercise. Oral, written, and visual instruction are often required. The symptoms of overuse should also be provided so that athletes are able to monitor an appropriate level of activity.

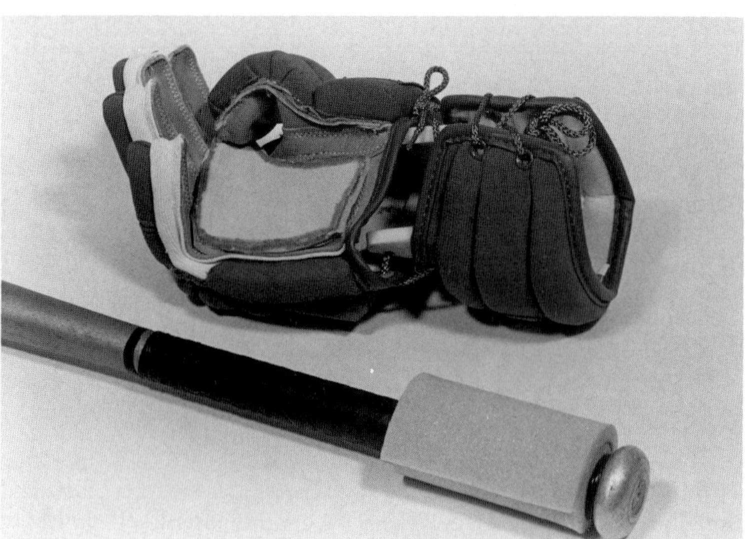

FIG. 28-45. Padding may be applied to the palmar aspect of a la-crosse glove to compensate for limited grasp. A padded bat would better suit a similar need in a baseball player. (From Gieck JH and Mayer V: Protecive splinting for the hand and wrist. In McCue FC, editor: Clinics in sports medicine, Philadelphia, 1986, WB Saunders Co.)

Trainers or therapists should review the home program frequently to assure that athletes are using proper techniques and to upgrade and/or alter the program according to findings in the most recent evaluation.

REFERENCES

1. American Academy of Orthopaedic Surgeons: Joint motion: method of measuring and recording, Chicago, 1965, The Academy.
2. American Society for Surgery of the Hand: The hand—examination and diagnosis, Aurora, Ill, 1978, The Society.
3. Arnheim DD: Modern principles of athletic training, ed 7, St Louis, 1989, The CV Mosby Co.
4. Basset FH, Malone T, and Gilchrist R: A protective splint of silicone rubber, Am J Sports Med 7:358, 1970.
5. Beasley R: Rehabilitation of the hand. In Hunter J et al, editors: Rehabilitation of the hand, St Louis, 1978, The CV Mosby Co, p 97.
6. Bechtol CO: Grip test: the use of a dynamometer with adjustable handle spacings, J Bone Joint Surg 36A:820, 1954.
7. Bell AT and Horton PG: The use and abuse of hydrotherapy in athletics: a review, Athl Train 22(2):115, 1987.
8. Bohannon RW: Whirlpool versus whirlpool and rinse for removal of bacteria from a venous stasis ulcer, Phys Ther 62(3):304, 1982.
9. Borrell RM et al: Fluidotherapy: evaluation of a new heat modality, Arch Phys Med Rehab 58:69, 1977.
10. Borrell RM et al: Comparison of in vivo temperatures produced by hydrotherapy, paraffin wax treatment, and fluidotherapy, Phys Ther 69:1273, 1980.
11. Bowden REM: Factors influencing functional recovery. In Seddon HJ, editor: Peripheral nerve injuries, London, 1954, Her Majesty's Stationery Printing Office, p. 298.
12. Boyes JH: Bunnell's surgery of the hand, ed 5, Philadelphia, 1970, JB Lippincott Co.
13. Brand PW: Clinical mechanics of the hand, St Louis, 1985, The CV Mosby Co.
14. Brand P and Wood H: Hand volumeter instruction sheet, Carville, La 1973, U.S. Public Health Service Hospital.
15. Brunet ME and Haddad RJ: Fractures and dislocations of the metacarpals and phalanges, Clin Sports Med 5(4):773, 1986.
16. Buchout BC and Warner MA: Digital perfusion of handball players: effects of repeated ball impact on the structures of the hand, Am J Sports Med 8(3):206, 1980.
17. Burke ER: Ulnar neuropathy in bicyclists, Phys Sports Med 9(4):53, 1981.
18. Cabrera JM and McCue FC: Nonosseous athletic injuries of the elbow, forearm and hand. Clin Sports Med 5(4):681, 1986.
19. Crawford GP: The molded polythene splint for mallet finger deformities, J Hand Surg 9A:231, 1984.
20. Dellon AL: The moving 2 point discrimination test: clinical evaluation of the quickly-adapting fiber receptor system, J Hand Surg 3:474, 1978.
21. Dellon AL: Evaluation of sensibility and re-education of sensation in the hand, Baltimore, 1981, Williams & Wilkins Co.
22. Dobyns JH, et al: Bowler's thumb: diagnosis and treatment; a review of seventeen cases, J Bone Joint Surg 54A:751, 1972.
23. Duncan R: Personal communication, 1987.
24. Fess E and Moran C: Clinical assessment recommendations, Indianapolis, 1981, American Society of Hand Therapists.
25. Gibson CT and Manske PR: Carpal tunnel syndrome in the adolescent, J Hand Surg 12A(2):279, 1987.
26. Gieck JH and Saliba EN: Application of modalities in overuse syndrome, Clin Sports Med 6(2):427, 1987.
27. Goldstein A: Opioid peptides cendorphins in pituitary and brain, Science 193:1081, 1976.
28. Greenberg S and Braun R: Therapeutic uses of the air bag splint for the injured hand Am J Occup Ther 31:38 1977.
29. Ho PK, Dellon AL, and Wilgis EFS: True aneurysms of the hand resulting from athletic injury: report of two cases, Am J Sports Med 13(2):136, 1985.
30. Hoppenfeld S: Physical examination of the spine and extremities, Norwalk, Conn., 1976, Appleton-Century-Crofts.
31. Hunter J et al, editors: Rehabilitation of the hand, ed 2, St Louis, 1984 The CV Mosby Co.
32. Kaltenborn F: Manual therapy for the extremity joints: specialized techniques, tests and joint-mobilization, ed 2, Oslo, 1976, Olaf Norlis Bokhandel.
33. Lankford, LL: Reflex sympathetic dystrophy. In Green D, editor: Operative hand surgery, Vol 1, New York, 1982, Churchill-Livingstone, Inc.
34. Malick M: Manual on static hand splinting. Pittsburgh, 1970, Harmarville Rehabilitation Center.
35. Malick M: Manual on dynamic hand splinting with thermoplastic materials, Pittsburgh, 1974, Harmarville Rehabilitation Center.
36. Mannheimer JS and Lampe GN: Transcutaneous electrical nerve stimulation, Philadelphia, 1984, FA Davis Co.
37. Match RM: Laceration of the median nerve from skiing, Am J Sports Med 6:22, 1978.
38. McCue FC and Garroway RY: Sports injuries: mechanisms, prevention and treatment, Baltimore, 1985, Williams & Wilkins.
39. McCue FC et al: A pseudoboutonniere deformity, J Br Soc Surg Hand 7:166, 1975.
40. McCue FC et al: Hand and wrist injuries in the athlete, Am J Sports Med 7:257, 1978.
41. Melzak R and Wall PD: Pain mechanism: a new theory, Science 150:971, 1965.
42. Mennell J: Joint pain: diagnosis and treatment using manipulative techniques, Boston, 1964, Little Brown & Co.
43. Moberg E: Objective methods for determining the functional value of sensibility of the hand, J Bone Joint Surg 40B:454, 1958.
44. Moberg E: Criticism and study of methods of examining sensibility in the hand, Neurology 12:8, 1962.
45. Napier J: The prehensile movements of the human hand, J Bone Joint Surg, 38B:902, 1956.
46. Nieder H et al: Reduction of skin bacterial load with use of the therapeutic whirlpool, Phys Ther 55(5):482, 1975.
47. Paris S: Extremity dysfunction and mobilization, Prepublication edition, St Augustine, Fla, 1980, Institute Press Inc.
48. Parker RD et al: Hook of the hamate fractures in athletes, Am J Sports Med 14(6):517, 1986.
49. Payton O, Lamb BR, and Kasey M: Effects of therapeutic ultrasound on bone marrow in dogs, Am J Phys Ther Assoc 55:20, 1975.
50. Pearson S: Dynamic splinting. In Hunter J et al, editors: Rehabilitation of the hand, St Louis, 1978, The CV Mosby Co, p. 621.

51. Rayan GM and Mullins PT: Skin necrosis complicating mallet finger splinting and vascularity of the distal interphalangeal joint overlying skin, J Hand Surg 12A(4):548, 1987.
52. Rowlingson J: Personal communication, 1987.
53. Schmidt TT and Toews JV: Grip strength as measured by the Jamar dynamometer, Arch Phys Med Rehab 51(6):321, 1970.
54. Seddon H: Surgical disorders of peripheral nerves, ed 2, New York, 1975, Churchill-Livingstone, Inc.
55. Sugawara M et al: Digital ischemia in baseball players, Am J Sports Med 14(4):329, 334, 1986.
56. Tubiana R: Architecture and functions of the hand. In Tubiana R, editor: The hand, Philadelphia, 1978, WB Saunders Co, p. 19.
57. Vasudevan SV and Melvin JL: Upper extremity edema control: rationale of the techniques, Am J Occup Ther 33(8):520, 1979.
58. Wilson RL and Carter MS: Management of hand fractures. In Hunter JM et al, editors: Rehabilitation of the hand, ed 2, St Louis, 1984, The CV Mosby Co.
59. Yerxa EJ et al: Development of a hand test for use in desensitization of the hypersensitive hand , Am J Occup Ther 37(3):176, 1983.

ADDITIONAL READINGS

Barr N: The hand: principles and techniques of simple splintmaking in rehabilitation, London, 1975, Butterworth.

Baugher WH and McCue FC: Anterior fracture-dislocation of the proximal interphalangeal joint: a case report, J Bone Joint Surg 61A(5):779, 1979.

Beasley R: Rehabilitation of the hand. Hunter J et al, editors: Rehabilitation of the hand, St Louis, 1984, The CV Mosby Co, p. 154.

Bergfeld JA et al: Soft playing splint for protection of significant hand and wrist injuries in sports, Am J Sports Med, 10:293, 1982.

Birrer RB: Sports medicine for the primary care physician, Norwalk, Conn. 1984, Appleton-Century-Crofts.

Black SH: Blisters and torn hands disrupt gymast's training, First Aider 48(6):10, 1979.

Blazina ME and Lane C: Rupture of the inserter of the flexor digitorum profundus tendon in student athletes, J Am Coll Health Assoc 14:248, 1966.

Borrell RM and Henley EJ: Fluidotherapy in a hand clinic, Arch Phys Med Rehab 60:536, 1979.

Buck-Gramcko D, Hoffman R, and Neumann R: Hand trauma: a practical guide, Stuttgart, 1986, Thieme Inc.

Campbell Reid DA, and McGrouther DA: Surgery of the thumb, London, 1986, Butterworth & Co.

Cannon N: Manual of hand splinting, New York, 1985, Churchill-Livingstone, Inc.

Carroll RE and Match RM: Avulsion of the profundus tendon insertion, J Trauma 10:1109, 1970.

Chang WH, Thoms OJ, and White WL: Avulsion injury of the long flexor tendons, Plast Reconstr Surg 50:260, 1972.

Cohn BT and Froimson AI: Case report of a rare mallet finger injury, Orthopedics 9(4):529, 1986.

Commandre F and Viani JL: The football keeper's thumb, J Sports Med Phys Fitness 16(2):121, 1976.

Conn J, Bergan JJ, and Bell JL: Hypothenar hammer syndrome post-traumatic digital ischemia, Surgery 68:1122, 1970.

Cooney WP: Sports injuries to the upper extremity. How to recognize and deal with some common problems, Postgrad Med 76(4):45, 1984.

Culver JE: Instabilities of the wrist, Clin Sports Med 5(4):725, 1986.

Culver JE et al: Avulsion of the profundus and superficialis tendons of the ring finger, Am J Sports Med 9(3):184, 1981.

Dawson WJ and Pullos N: Baseball injuries to the hand, Ann Emerg Med 10(6):302, 1981.

Dellon AL and Jabaley ME: Reeducation of sensation in the hand following nerve suture, Clin Orthop Rel Res 162:75, 1982.

Dobyns JH, Sim FH, and Linscheid RL: Sports stress syndromes of the hand and wrist, Am J Sports Med 6(5):236, 1978.

Doran GA: Towards preventing reinjury in contact sport, J Sports Med Phys Fitness 24(2):90, 1984.

Dunham W et al: Bowler's thumb, Clin Orthop 83:99, 1972.

Eckman PB et al: Ulnar neuropathy in bicycle riders, Arch Neurol 32:130, 1975.

Editorial, Br Med J 2(6103):1622, 1977.

Ellsasser JC and Stein AH: Management of hand injuries in a professional football team, Am J Sports Med 7(3):178, 1979.

Fess E, Gettle K, and Strickland J: Hand splinting: principles and methods, St Louis, 1981, The CV Mosby Co.

Fess E and Phillips C: Hand splinting: principles and methods, ed 2, St Louis, 1987, The CV Mosby Co.

Flatt A: The care of minor hand injuries, ed 4, St Louis, 1979, The CV Mosby Co.

Folmar RC, Nelson CL, and Phalen GS: Ruptures of the flexor tendons in hands of non-rheumatoid patients, J Bone Joint Surg 54A:579, 1972.

Ganel A, Aharonson Z, and Engel J: Gamekeeper's thumb: injuries of the ulnar collateral ligament of the metacarpophalangeal joint, Br J Sports Med 14(2/3):92, 1980.

Garrett WE: Strains and sprains in athletes, Postgrad Med 73(3):200, 1983.

Gerber C, Senn E, and Matter F: Skier's thumb: surgical treatment of recent injuries to the ulnar collateral ligament of the thumb's metacarpophalangeal joint, Am J Sports Med 9(3):171, 1981.

Gieck J and Buxton BP: Reflex sympathetic dystrophy, Athl Train 22(2):120, 1987.

Gieck JH and Mayer V: Protective splinting of the hand and wrist, Clin Sports Med 5(4):795, 1986.

Gieck J and McCue F: Conservative treatment and rehabilitation of athletic injuries to soft tissue of the hand, J Natl Athl Train Assoc 318:56, 1971.

Gray RE, Freeland AE, and Harrison RB: Rotatory subluxation of the scaphoid, J Miss State Med Assoc 26(2):39, 1985.

Green DP, editor: Operative hand surgery, vol 1, New York, 1982, Churchill-Livingstone, Inc.

Green DP, editor: Operative hand surgery, vol 2, New York, 1982, Churchill-Livingston, Inc.

Gunter GS: Traumatic avulsion of the insertion of flexor digitorum profundus, Aust NZ J Surg 30(1):2, 1960.

Hollis LI: Hand rehabilitation. In Hopkins H, and Smith H, editors: Willard and Spackman's occupational therapy, ed 5, Philadelphia, 1978, JB Lippincott Co.

Hopkins H and Smith H, editors: Willard and Spackman's occupational therapy, ed 5, Philadelphia, 1978, JB Lippincott Co.

Hunter J et al, editors: Rehabilitation of the hand, St Louis, 1978, The CV Mosby Co.

Isanti A and Malone CP: Ligamentous injuries of the hand in athletes, Clin Sports Med 5(4):757, 1986.

Jabaley ME and Freeland AE: Rigid internal fixation in the hand: 104 cases, Plast Reconstr Surg 77(2):288, 1986.

Johnson RP: The acutely injured wrist and its residuals, Clin Orthop Rel Res 149:33, 1980.
Kalenak A et al: Athletic injuries of the hand, Am Fam Phys 14(5):136, 1976.
Kauer JMG: Functional anatomy of the wrist, Clin Orthop Rel Res 149:9, 1980.
Kettelkamp DB, Flatt AE, and Moulds R: Traumatic dislocation of the long finger extensor tendon: a clinical, anatomical, and biomechanical study, J Bone Joint Surg 53A:229, 1971.
Kiel JH: Basic hand splinting: a pattern designing approach, Boston, 1983, Little Brown & Co.
Knight KL: Taping a mallet finger, Phys Sports Med 133(11):140, 1985.
Kulund DN: The injured athlete, Philadelphia, 1982, JB Lippincott Co, p. 314.
Lampe GN: TENS technology and physiology, Randolph, Me 1984, Codman & Shurtleff.
Leach RE: The prevention and rehabilitation of soft tissue injuries, Int J Sports Med 3:18, 1982.
Leddy JP and Coyle MP, Jr: Injuries of the flexor and extensor tendons, Prim Care 7(2):259, 1980.
Leddy JP and Packer JW: Avulsion of the profundus insertion in athletes, J Hand Surg 2:66, 1977.
Linscheid RL and Dobyns JH: Athletic injuries of the wrist, Clin Orthop Rel Res 198:141, 1985.
Linscheid RL et al: Traumatic instability of the wrist, J Bone Joint Surg 54:1612, 1972.
Lister G: The hand: diagnosis and indications, ed 2, New York, 1984, Churchill-Livingstone, Inc.
Loosli A and Garrick JG: The functional treatment of a third proximal phalanx fracture, Am J Sports Med 15(1):94, 1987.
Lowrey CW et al: Digital vessels trauma from repetitive impact in baseball catchers, J Hand Surg 1(3):236, 1976.
Lunn PG and Lamb DW: "Rugby finger"—avulsion of profundus of ring finger, J Hand Surg 9(1):69, 1984.
Malick M and Carr JA: Flexible elastomer molds in burn scar control, Am J Occup Ther 34(9):603, 1980.
Mallach JD: Palmar arch thrombosis, Br Med J 2:28, 1962.
Mannheimer JS: Electrode placement for transcutaneous electrical nerve stimulation, Am J Phys Ther 58:1455, 1978.
Manske PR and Lesker PA: Avulsion of the ring finger flexor digitorum profundus tendon: an experimental study, Hand 10:52, 1978.
Martin AF: Ulnar artery thrombosis in the palm, J Bone Joint Surg 36B:438, 1954.
Mayer V and Gieck JH: Rehabilitation of hand injuries in athletes, Clin Sports Med 5(4):783, 1986.
Mayfield JK: Mechanism of carpal injuries, Clin Orthop Rel Res 149:45, 1980.
Mayfield JK: Wrist ligamentous anatomy and pathogenesis of carpal instability, Orthop Clin North Am 15:209, 1984.
Mayfield JK, Johnson RP, and Kilcoyne R: Carpal dislocations: pathomechanics and progressive perilunar instability, J Hand Surg 5:226, 1980.
McCue FC: The elbow, wrist and hand. In Kulund D, editor: The injured athlete, Philadelphia, 1982, JB Lippincott Co.
McCue FC and Abbott JL: The treatment of mallet finger and boutonniere deformities, Va Med Mon 94:623, 1966.
McCue FC and Wooten SL: Closed tendon injuries of the hand in athletes, Clin Sports Med 5(4):741, 1986.
McCue FC et al: Athletic injuries of the proximal interphalangeal joint requiring surgical treatment, J Bone Joint Surg 52A:937, 1970.
McCue FC et al: The coach's finger, J Sports Med 2:270, 1974.
McCue FC et al: Ulnar collateral ligament injuries of the thumb in athletes, J Sports Med 2:70, 1974.
McCue FC et al: Hand injuries in athletes, Surg Rounds, 1:8, December 1978.
McElfresh EC and Dobyns JH: Intra-articular metacarpal head fractures, J Hand Surg 8A(4):383, 1983.
Micheli LJ: Pediatric and adolescent sports medicine, Boston, 1984, Little, Brown & Co.
Millander LH, Nalebuff EA, and Kadson E: Aneurysms and thrombosis of the ulnar artery in the hand, Arch Surg 105:686, 1972.
Moberg E: Splinting in hand therapy, New York, 1984, Thieme-Stratton.
Mosher JF: Current concepts in the diagnosis and treatment of hand and wrist injuries in sports, Med Sci Sports Exerc 17(1):48, 1985.
O'Donoghue DH: Treatment of injuries to athletes, Philadelphia, 1984, WB Saunders Co.
Palmar AK, Dobyns JH, and Linscheid RL: Management of posttraumatic instability of the wrist, secondary to ligament rupture, J Hand Surg 3:507, 1978.
Peimer CA, Sullivan DJ, and Wild DR: Palmar dislocation of the proximal interphalangeal joint, J Hand Surg 9A(1):39, 1984.
Peppard A: Thumb taping, Phys Sports Med 10(4):139, 1982.
Posch JL, Walker PJ, and Miller H: Treatment of ruptured tendons of the hand and wrist, Am J Surg 91:669, 1956.
Primiano GA: Skier's thumb injuries associated with flared ski pole handles, Am J Sports Med 13(6):425, 1985.
Primiano GA: Functional cast immobilization of thumb metacarpophalangeal joint injuries, Am J Sports Med 14(4):335, 1986.
Reef TC: Avulsion of the flexor digitorum profundus: an athletic injury, Am J Sports Med 5(6):281, 1977.
Rothwell AG: The pseudo-boutonniere deformity, NZ Med J 89(628):51, 1979.
Roy S and Irvin R: Sports medicine prevention, evaluation, management, and rehabilitation, Englewood Cliffs, NJ, 1983, Prentice-Hall, Inc.
Ruby LK: Common hand injuries in the athlete, Orthop Clin N Am 11(4):819, 1980.
Ryan JR: Fracture and dislocation about the carpal lunate, Ann Emerg Med 9(3):158, 1980.
Sakellarides HT: Treatment of recent and old injuries of the ulnar collateral ligament of the MP joint of the thumb, Am J Sports Med 6(5): 255, 1978.
Schneider RC, Kennedy JC, and Plant ML, editors: Sports injuries: mechanisms, prevention, and treatment, Baltimore, 1985, Williams & Wilkins.
Smith JH: Avulsion of the profundus tendon with simultaneous intraarticular fracture of the distal phalanx: case report, J Hand Surg 6:600, 1981.
Spinner M: Kaplan's functional and surgical anatomy of the hand, ed 3, Philadelphia, 1984, JB Lippincott Co.
Stark HH et al: Fracture of the hook of the hamate in athletes, J Bone Joint Surg 59A(5):575, 1977.
Stokes HM: The seriously uninjured hand—weakness of grip, J Occup Med 25(9):683, 1983.
Toews JV: A grip-strength study among steelworkers, Arch Phys Med Rehab 45(8):413, 1964.

Torres J: Little finger splint, Am J Occup Ther 29(4):230, 1975.

Trombly C, editor: Occupational therapy for physical dysfunction, ed 2, Baltimore, 1983, Williams & Wilkins.

Tubiana R: Injuries to the extensor apparatus on the dorsum of the fingers. In Verdan C, editor: Tendon surgery of the hand, New York, 1979, Churchill Livingstone, Inc. p. 119.

Tubiana R: Examination of the hand and upper limb, Philadelphia, 1984, WB Saunders.

Tubiana R, editor: The hand, vol 1, Philadelphia, 1981, WB Saunders Co.

Tubiana R, editor: The hand, vol 2, Philadelphia, 1985, WB Saunders Co.

Valenza J et al: A clinical study of a new heat modality, J Am Pod Assoc 69(7):440, 1979

Volz RG, Lieb M, and Benjamin J: Biomechanics of the Wrist, Clin Orthop Rel Res 149:112, 1980.

Watson FM: Simultaneous interphalangeal dislocation in one finger, J Trauma 23(1):65, 1983.

Wenger DR: Avulsion of the profundus tendon insertion in football players, Arch Surg 106:145, 1973.

Wood, MB and Dobyns JH: Sports-related extraarticular wrist syndromes, Clin Orthop 202:93, 1986.

Wray RC, Young VL, and Holtman B: Proximal interphalangeal joint sprains, Plast Reconstr Surg 74(1):101, 1984.

Wynn-Parry CB: Rehabilitation of the hand, ed 3, London, 1973, Butterworth & Co.

Zemel NP and Stark HH: Fractures and dislocations of the carpal bones, Clin Sports Med 5(4):709, 1986.

CHAPTER 29 Athletic Taping and Protective Equipment

Robert C. Reese, Jr.
T. Pepper Burruss
Joseph Patten

Soft tissue injuries to the wrist and hand can be protected with a variety of wrist-taping techniques. Taping is most often used after a mild hyperextension (dorsiflexion) injury. Less commonly, palmar flexion injuries are the basis for a wrist-taping technique. In both instances, taping is used to limit motion and protect the damaged structures.

WRIST TAPING

Hyperextension Wrist Injury

Wrist extension taping is designed to limit the extension of the wrist and thus protect structures that may be injured after a forced dorsiflexion injury. The goal is to limit wrist extension to a range of motion that is comfortable for the athlete and will allow effective participation in sports.

Technique

It is best to apply this taping technique with the athlete standing facing the person taping. The athlete's fingers can rest on the taper's chest to provide secure support for the hand and wrist while the tape is being applied. The wrist is held in a neutral to slight dorsiflexion position (Fig. 29-1).

In general, no shaving is required for this technique if underwrap is applied. Occasionally, the area on the forearm at which the anchor strips are placed is shaved to allow better fixation of the anchor strips to the skin. If no underwrap is available and repeated taping is necessary, shaving from the forearm to the hand is indicated. Either way, tape adhesive spray is used.

Underwrap is applied circumferentially from the hand (just proximal to the metacarpophalangeal joints of the fingers) to the midforearm (Fig. 29-2). Anchor strips are applied at the midforearm, over the wrist, and around the hand, just proximal to the metacarpal heads. When the anchor strips are applied along the hand, it is very important to have the athlete hold the fingers abducted as far as possible (Fig. 29-3). This prevents tape application with the transverse metacarpal arch in a compressed position. If taping is done with the fingers in a resting or adducted position, pain often occurs during activity in the region of the interosseous muscles between the metacarpals.

Check reins are most often prepared by cre-

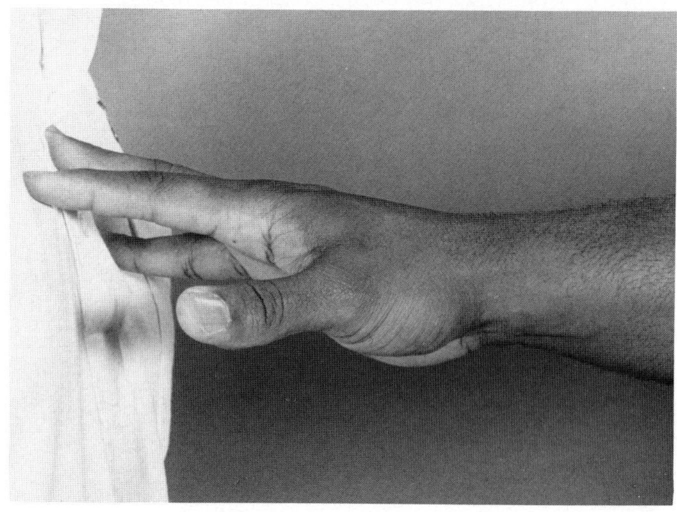

FIG. 29-1. Position for wrist taping. Both athlete and taper should be comfortable.

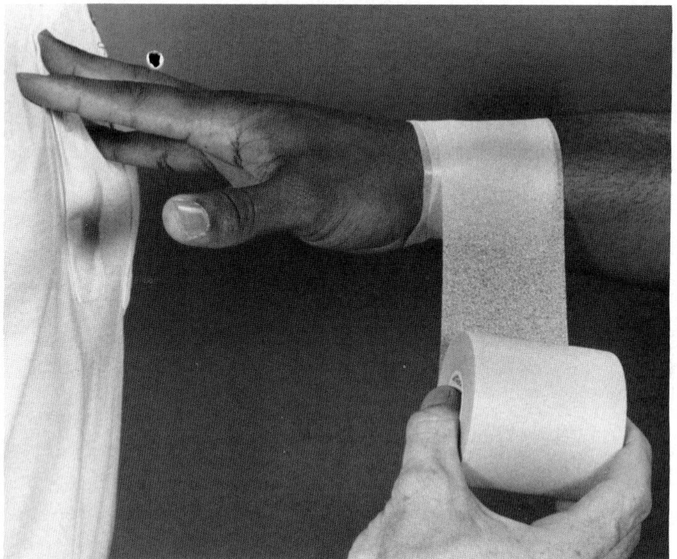

FIG. 29-2. Application of underwrap.

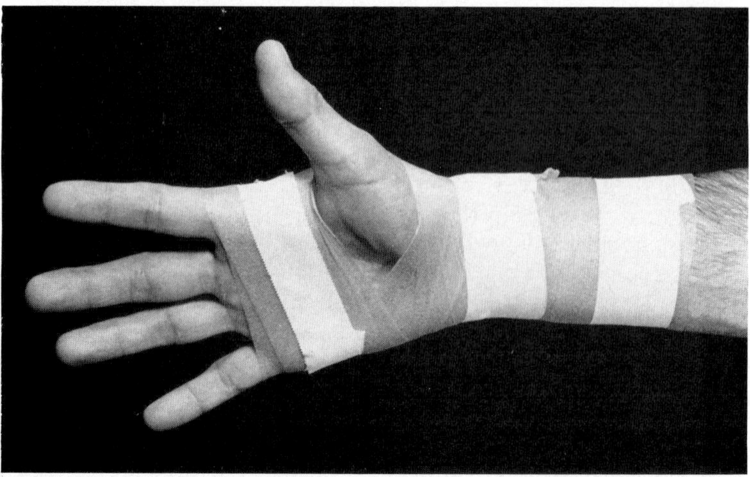

FIG. 29-3. Anchor strips are applied to midforearm, wrist, and hand. Athlete holds fingers wide apart while hand anchor strip is placed.

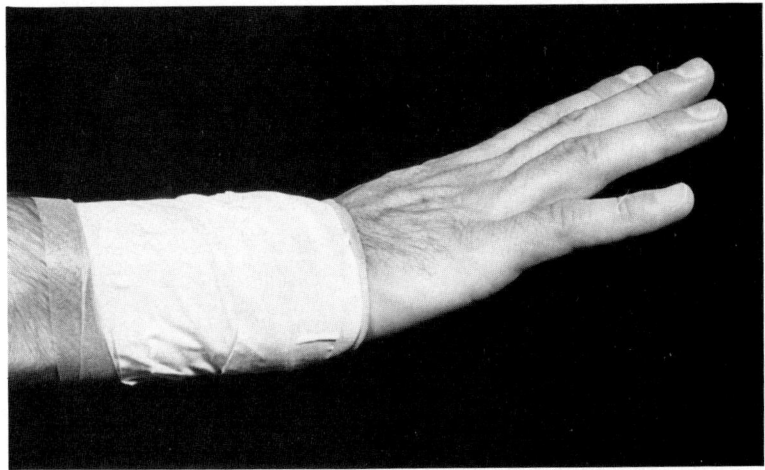

FIG. 29-7. "Bulk" technique uses repeated circles of tape around the wrist.

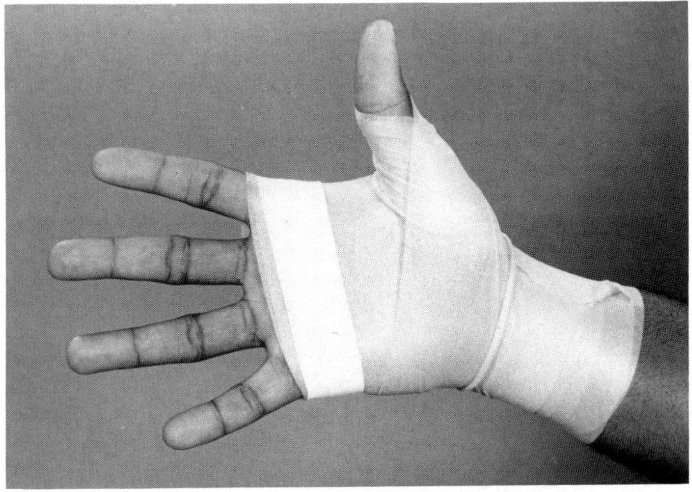

FIG. 29-8. Anchor strips around the metacarpal heads for thumb spica technique.

However, this position can be varied and the position selected should depend on the examination of the injured region and an appropriate plan to limit specific motions. The position can vary in both the flexion/extension plane and in the abduction/adduction plane. After the thumb has been positioned as indicated, underwrap is applied to the thumb.

Anchor strips of cloth adhesive tape are placed around the metacarpal heads (Fig. 29-8). Figure eight check reins are next applied around the thumb and continued over the wrist in a circumferential pattern (Fig. 29-9). These check reins are varied by reversing the tape direction with each application. The tape direction is dictated by the motion being restricted. The check reins are anchored with tape extending from the wrist to the thumb, the strip beginning at the forearm and continuing longitudinally to the interphalangeal joint of the thumb (Fig. 29-10). Circumferential loops of tape are applied in a continuous strip to anchor and solidify the tape job. The taping is completed with a figure eight piece of tape that incorporates the thumb, hand, and wrist.

Variations

A somewhat less bulky form of spica immobilization can be created by initially applying figure eights around the thumb only.

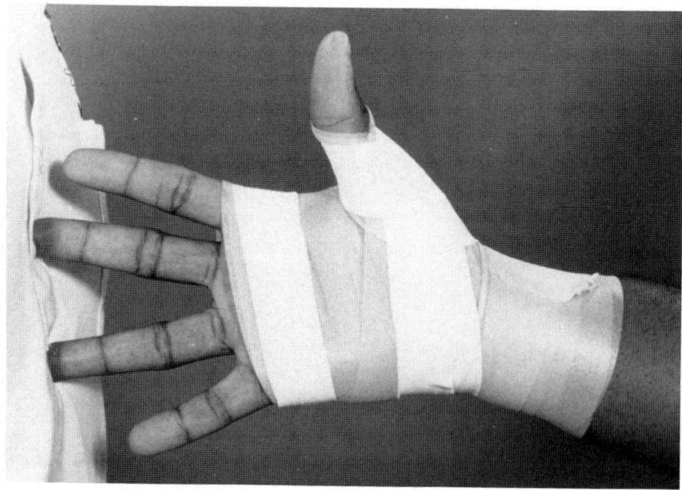

FIG. 29-9. Figure eight check reins around the thumb.

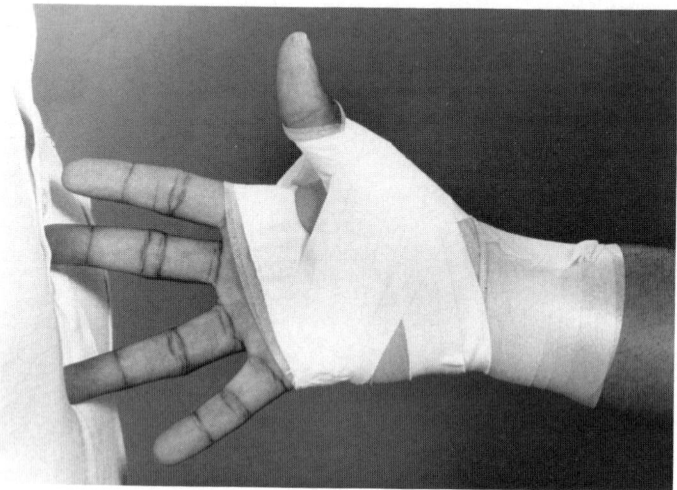

FIG. 29-10. Longitudinal check reins from wrist to thumb.

This will reduce the amount of tape material around the wrist and hand and is appropriate for athletes who require unencumbered thumb movement. However, because of the lack of bulk, the restriction gained and protection afforded are less optimal than with the full tape spica technique. If the wrist needs to be free, then more tape can be applied to the thumb in the figure eight pattern (see Fig. 29-9). These extra layers provide bulk to limit motion. When this extra tape is added, it must be borne in mind that tight is not right, but rather it is the bulk that does the job.

Abbreviated Thumb Taping

Athletes who use equipment in their hands, as do football quarterbacks or hockey players, may require a tape application that can limit thumb extension yet allow the wrist to remain mobile. The abbreviated thumb technique is designed for that purpose. Interestingly, it was created by Pinky Newell of Purdue University for use by Bob Griese in a Rose Bowl game.

Technique

Tape adhesive spray and underwrap are applied around the forearm, wrist, and hand.

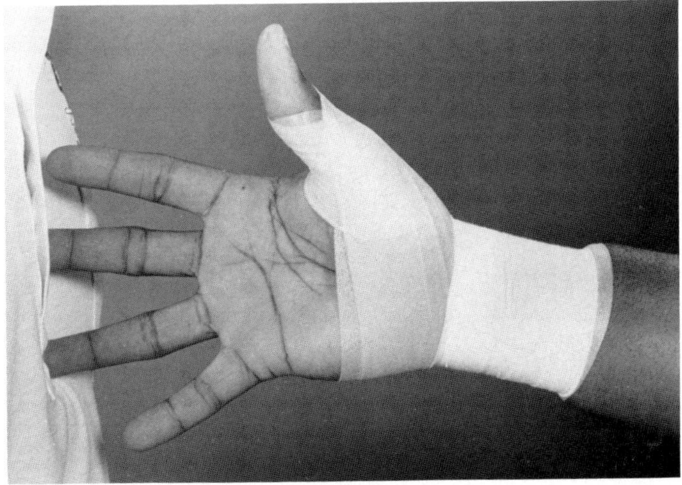

FIG. 29-11. Abbreviated thumb taping technique. Note proximal position of anchor strips.

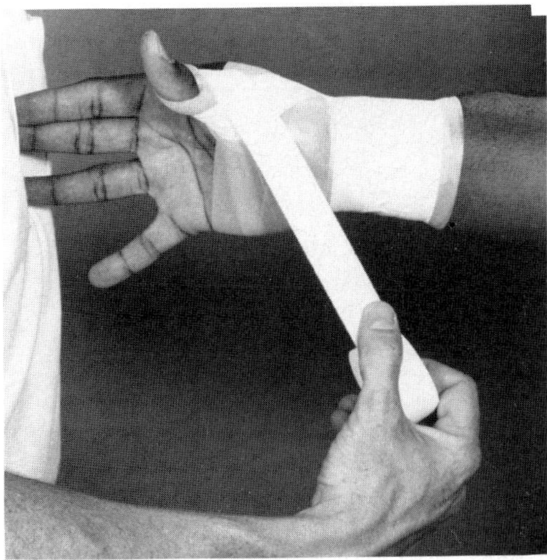

FIG. 29-12. Figure eight application for abbreviated technique.

Using 1-inch adhesive cloth tape, a series of two figure eights are applied in opposite directions from the thumb to the wrist. However, the point of application at the wrist is made more proximal than in the usual thumb spica application (Fig. 29-11). This permits greater wrist motion than in the standard thumb spica technique.

Next, a series of abbreviated figure eights are applied, with the thumb positioned just short of the maximum extension desired. This continuous strip should begin on the anchor strip on the wrist, angle up toward the base of the thumb (metacarpophalangeal joint) as if another figure eight were going to be applied. Instead of encircling the thumb, however, the tape is pressed down and redirected to the opposite side of the hand, distal to proximal and around the wrist (Fig. 29-12). The distal point of the tape should be pinched at the redirected angle, so that it adheres to itself, and laid over itself as the next continuous abbreviated figure eight is brought up, overlapping approximately half the width of tape. This should be continued until the proximal point of the interphalangeal joint of the thumb has been reached. To complete the technique, one final figure eight is laid on, designated more as an anchor strip rather than for support.

By use of this method, in effect, a series of check reigns preventing extension has been achieved, flexion has not been limited, and he palm of the hand is free for grasping (Fig. 29-13).

FINGER TAPING

Injuries to the fingers are quite common in contact sports. A variety of taping techniques are available to support and protect fingers during athletic participation.

Buddy Taping

Buddy taping is used when support of a finger is required but restriction of motion is undesirable. The support for the injured finger is supplied by an adjacent finger, which acts as a splint. In general, buddy taping is indicated in uncomplicated PIP joint injuries and stable, healing fractures of the proximal

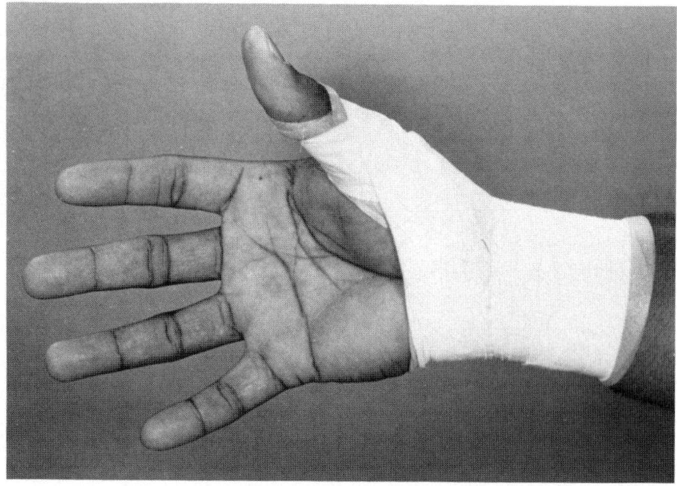

FIG. 29-13. Completed abbreviated tape technique for thumb; palm of hand is left free for grasping.

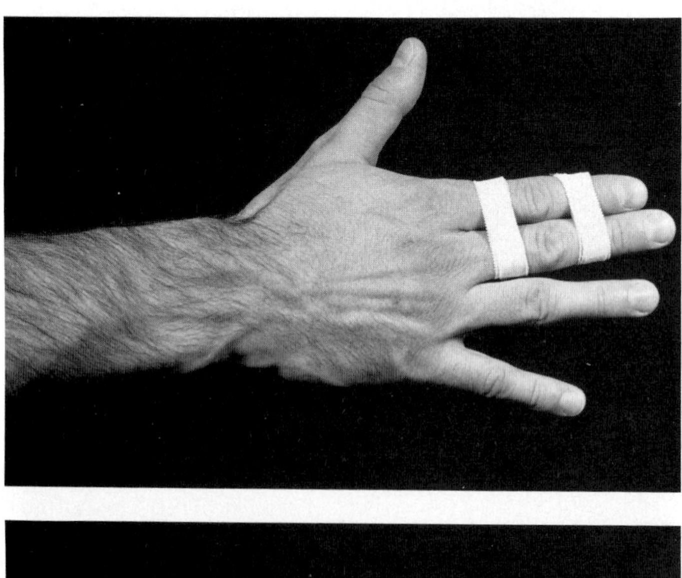

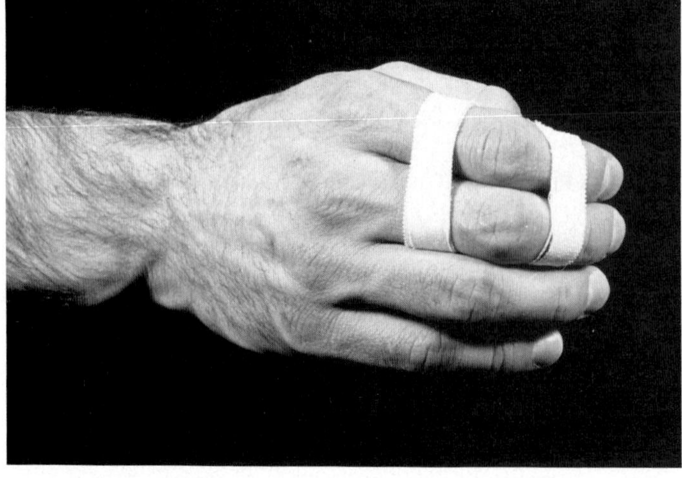

FIG. 29-14. Buddy taping. Taping over joints is avoided.

and middle phalanx. Buddy taping can be done with any two fingers and is easiest to apply when the index, middle, or ring fingers are injured.

Technique

The technique is quite simple; the injured finger and its adjacent support finger are taped together with circumferential strips centered over the proximal and middle phalanxes (Fig. 29-14). If necessary, the distal phalanxes can be taped together, but occasionally, this is not achievable because of disparities in finger lengths. In this regard, buddy taping of the little and ring fingers is also difficult to fashion because the PIP and DIP joints are at different levels. With care, however, a satisfactory buddy taping technique can be carried out between any two fingers. Finally, in some instances, thin foam rubber can be applied between the two fingers for added comfort, if necessary.

Compression Taping for Swelling

After interphalangeal joint injury, such as a sprain or dislocation, soft tissue swelling often ensues and further adds to soft tissue injury, delaying healing and impairing performance. A useful taping technique has been devised to limit swelling and allow continued athletic participation with relatively minimal impedance of the involved finger. This taping technique is used after the injury has been fully evaluated clinically and radiographically, to ascertain that no other more appropriate form of intervention is indicated.

Technique

A layer of underwrap is applied across the injured joint. Circumferential layers of elastic tape are then placed over the injured joint (Fig. 29-15). The elastic tape is applied firmly, but not too tightly. A single layer of cloth tape is used over the elastic tape to solidify the tape. The injured finger and an adjacent finger are

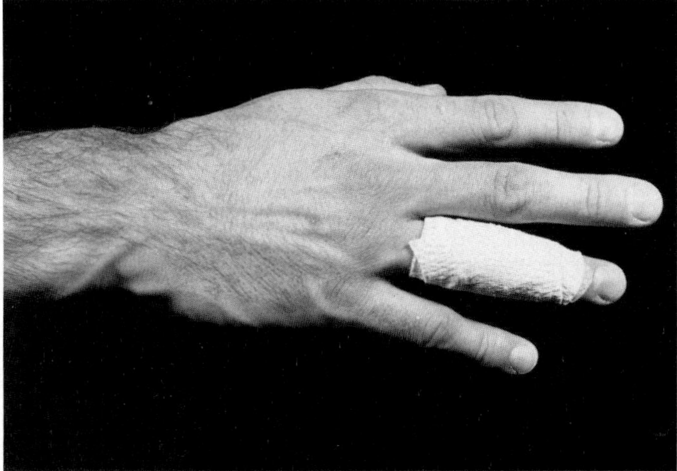

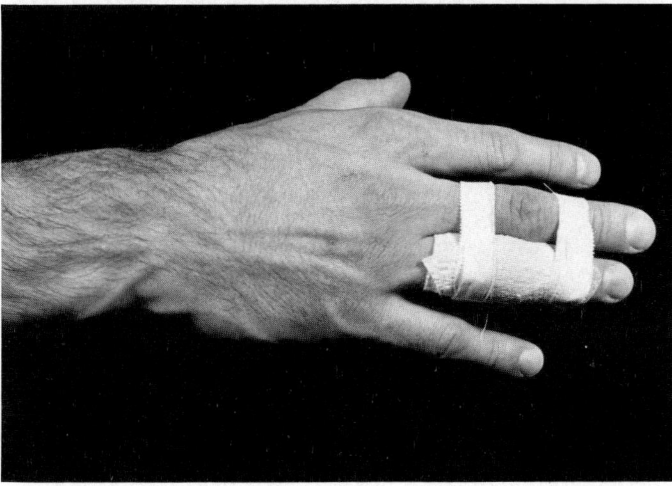

FIG. 29-15. Compression taping for swelling with elastic tape.

buddy taped together to provide splinting. At all times, the neurovascular function is checked to assure that compromise is not occurring. A self-adhering compression wrap, such as Coban and cotton wading, such as Webril, can be substituted for the underwrap and elastic tape, then secured with cloth adhesive tape.

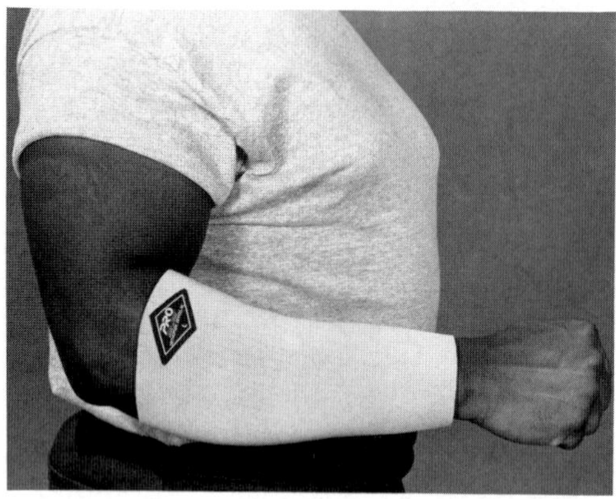

FIG. 29-16. Neoprene sleeves for forearm protection.

PROTECTIVE EQUIPMENT

Forearm

The forearm is subject to both contusions and abrasions in sports, and several types of equipment are available to protect the athlete from these injuries. Neoprene sleeves are quite popular and serve well as protection for the forearm (Fig. 29-16). Other commercially available pads are generally made from elasticized cloth, incorporating some foam rubber (Fig. 29-17).

Occasionally, a hard shell is desired, as in recovery from a forearm fracture. These can be custom made from thermomoldable plastic and created to protect the appropriate anatomic location desired. It is important the outside of the hard shell be adequately padded to protect opposing athletes from injury (Fig. 29-18).

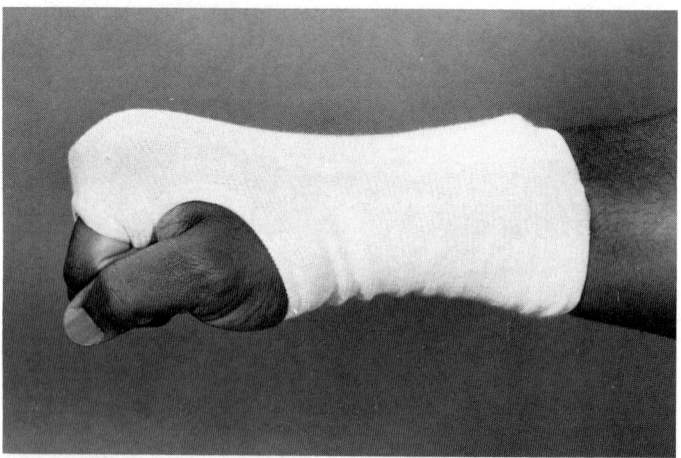

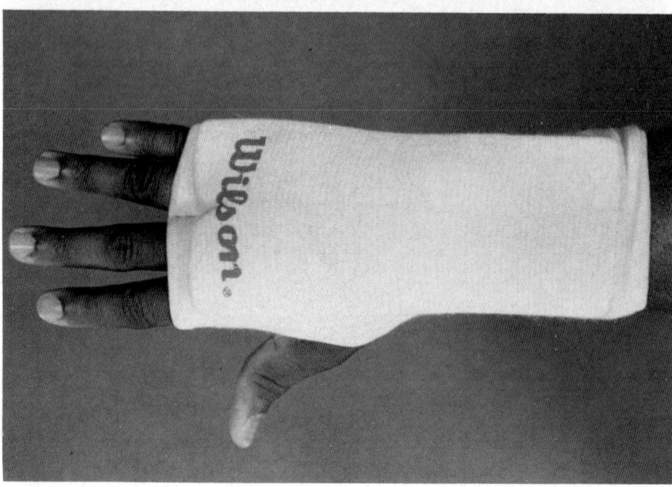

FIG. 29-17. Foam and cloth forearm padding.

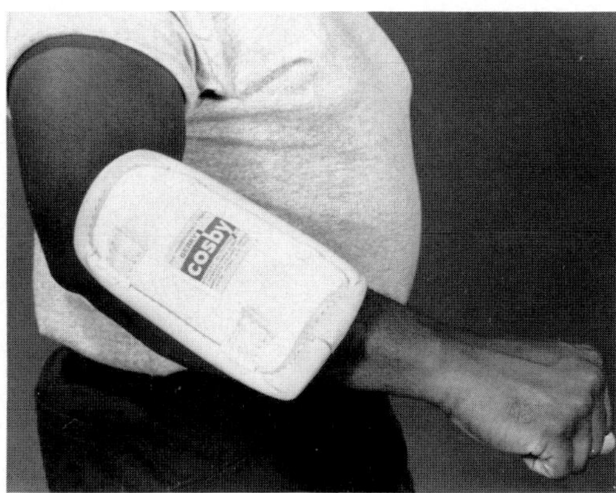

FIG. 29-18. A hard shell can be fabricated for additional forearm protection.

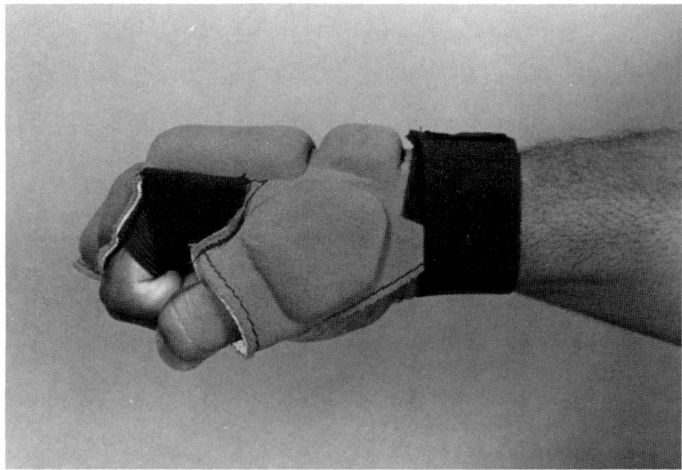

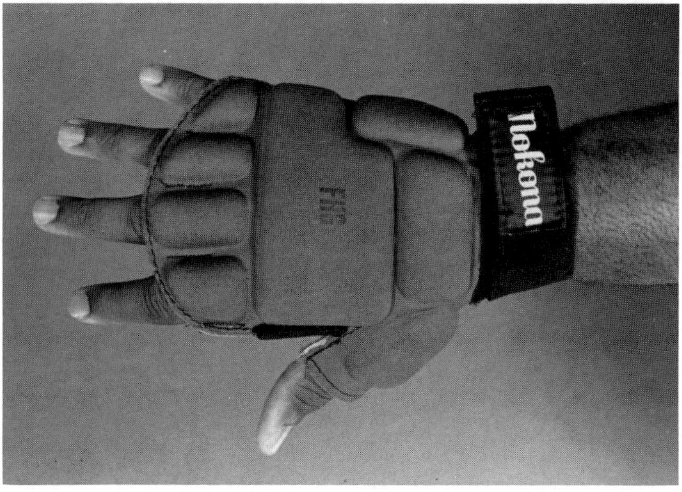

FIG. 29-19. Padded gloves, like these used by football offensive linemen, are designed to provide protection to dorsum of the hand and metacarpophalangeal region.

Continued.

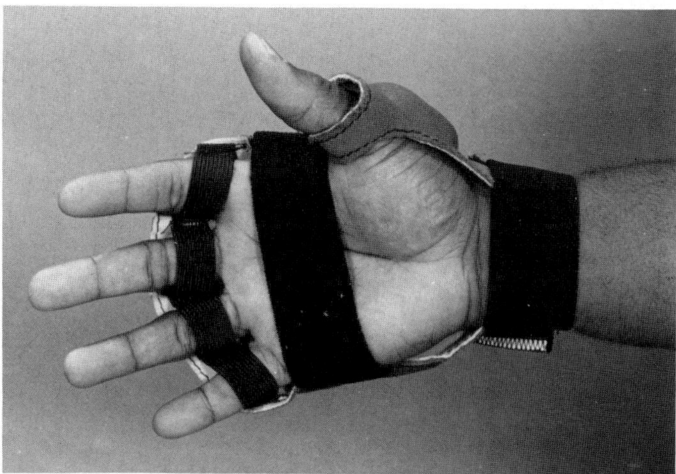

FIG. 29-19, cont'd. Padded gloves, like these used by football offensive linemen, are designed to provide protection to dorsum of the hand and metacarpophalangeal region.

Wrist and Hand

Hand protection is generally obtained with the use of specialized gloves. These gloves incorporate special padding, as dictated by the need of the athlete. For example, in football, offensive linemen use gloves with padding in the dorsum of the glove, which protects the metacarpophalangeal joints (Fig. 29-19).

Occasionally, a cast can be used to protect an injured area of the wrist or hand during athletic participation. These casts are usually made from synthetic cast material, such as fiberglass, and often extend to completely enclose the hand. Adequate padding is required outside the hard shell to protect other athletic participants from injury.

For an additional discussion of specialized equipment used in the rehabilitation of wrist and hand injuries, see Chapter 28.

PART V Skeletally Immature Athletes

CHAPTER 30 Upper Extremity Injuries in the Skeletally Immature Athlete

Jack T. Andrish

Part of the uniqueness of the skeletally immature athlete is the presence of open growth plates (Fig. 30-1). This cartilaginous structure is the vehicle for longitudinal growth via endochondral ossification. Injury to the growth plate carries with it not only reality of consistent and expeditious healing but also the potential for early or late growth disturbance.

Trauma to the growth plate may be acute or chronic. Acute injury is well recognized and described. Salter and Harris,[54] and more recently Ogden,[42] have written on the subject and have provided classifications for acute growth plate fractures (Fig. 30-2). These injuries, of course, do happen to young athletes, but a more unusual injury is the chronic **stress-related growth plate reaction** that is seen as a result of athletic abuse.[52,66] The growth plate may be required to withstand several different types and combinations of stress (i.e., tension, compression, shear, and torsion). Within certain physiologic limits, tension or compression may stimulate growth. However, forces beyond these limits will retard or stop growth[42] (Fig. 30-3).

The periosteum plays a vital biomechanical role in stabilizing the growth plate. The insertion into the epiphysis is strong, and the periosteum itself is a relatively thick and tough structure. Furthermore, the undulations of the growth plate are thought to help resist displacement by shear stresses. The growth plate is most resistant to tension and least resistant to torsion.[42] Over the metaphysis and diaphysis of long bones, the periosteum is loosely attached. This becomes more firmly attached to the growth plate at the perichondrium and, as noted, the epiphysis. Tendons and ligaments tend to insert at the area of the perichondrium. This allows tensile stress to be received by a tensile-responsive structure (i.e., the growth plate). Muscles, on the other hand, tend to originate from the periosteum directly over the metaphysis and diaphysis. This is a loose arrangement with few areas of direct connection to the bone, whereas the tendon insertion into perichondrium carries on into the physeal and epiphyseal cartilage (Fig. 30-4).

Although fractures may occur across the growth plate, more typically at least some

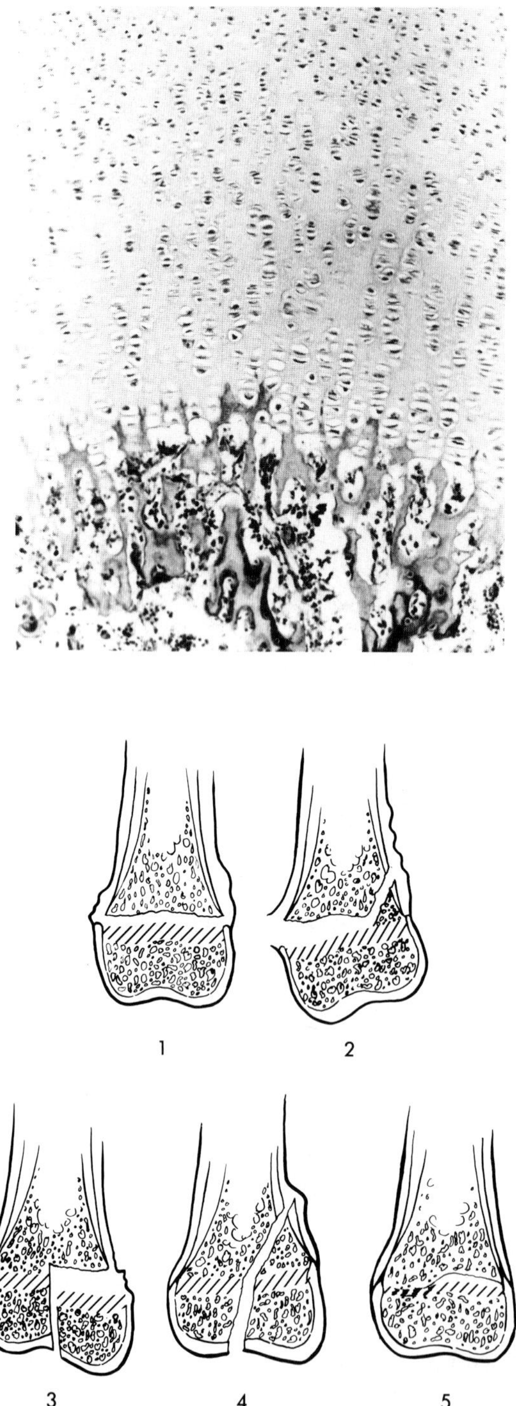

FIG. 30-1. The histology of the growth plate is well recognized. This includes the typical columnar orientation of cells with progressive cellular hypertrophy, provisional calcification, and finally endochondral ossification.

FIG. 30-2. Although other fracture classifications exist, the Salter-Harris classification remains as a practical and popular standard.

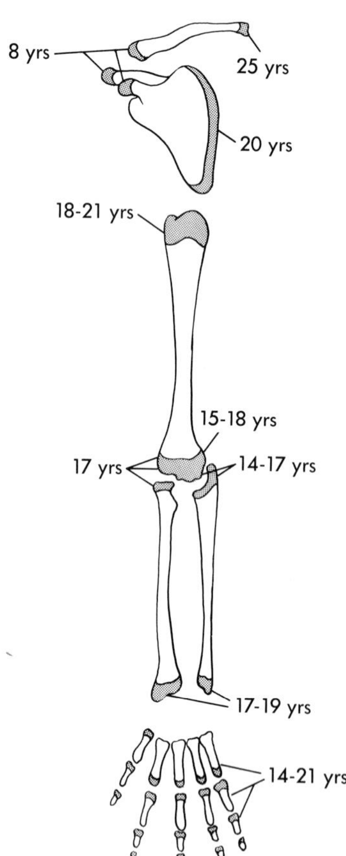

FIG. 30-3. Although significant variations exist in the exact time of growth plate closure, the sequence of closure is generally consistent. (Modified from Ogden JA: Skeletal injury in the child, Philadelphia, 1982, Lea & Febiger.)

component of the injury will be transverse through it. The zone of hypertrophy and the zone of provisional calcification have been most often implicated as the anatomic site of growth plate fractures[54] (see Fig. 30-1).

There are other differences between the musculoskeletal systems of immature and mature athletes. First of all, the plasticity of young bone is greater. Bone tends to get stiffer and more brittle with age. Immature epiphyses are also softer than mature calcified bone. This feature also makes the cartilagi-

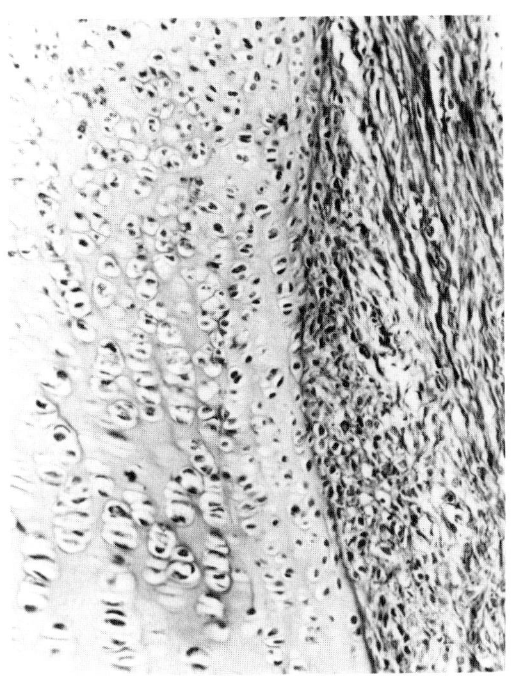

FIG. 30-4. The perichondrium not only provides a physical restraint to the growth plate, but also serves in the transition of tendinous and periosteal attachments extending into the physeal and epiphyseal cartilage.

nous epiphysis susceptible to stress in a different way from the bony epiphysis of the adult. Many of the so-called osteochondroses have their origins in chronic, repetitive trauma to the cartilaginous epiphysis.

Because of the increased plastic behavior of young bone, greenstick fractures are common. Permanent deformation may occur (angular), although most often this deformity is small and fully remodeled during further growth of the bone. Large, angular deformities of long bones may not fully correct themselves, and certainly rotational deformities do not correct themselves with further growth and development (Fig. 30-5).

Just as the epiphyseal ends of growing long bones have special anatomic features related to the cartilage model, secondary ossification, and joint formation, the apophyses also have different features. These growth plates are frequently found on irregularly shaped bone, such as the pelvis, or on metaphyseal areas, such as the tibial tubercle. Although these growth areas generally do not contribute to longitudinal growth, they do contribute to form and usually serve as attachment sites for tendons and ligaments. As in the lower extremities, repetitive traction stress, such as is

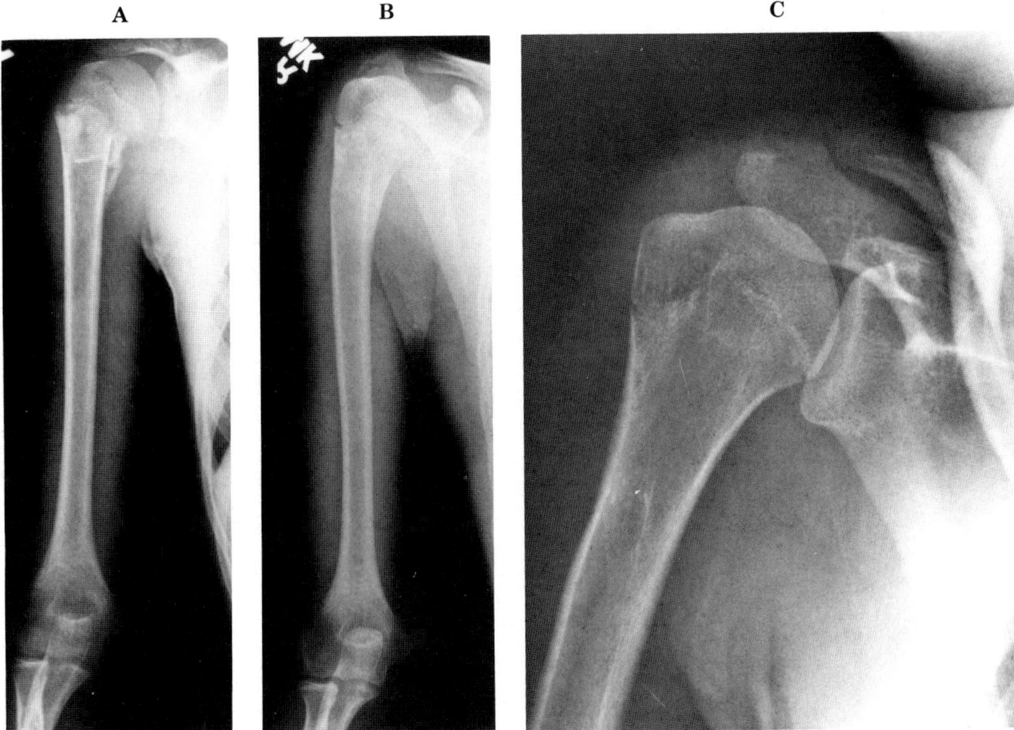

FIG. 30-5. A, This 12-year-old skier sustained a proximal humeral fracture with moderate displacement. **B,** Managed with a sling and swath for 3 weeks, uneventful healing occurred. **C,** Five years later, the bony contour is normal.

encountered in organized youth sports, can lead to bony changes resulting from stress-induced apophyseal growth disturbances.[66]

EPIDEMIOLOGY

During a 10-year period from January 1977 to December 1986, there were 17,384 new sport-related injuries registered in our Section of Sports Medicine at the Cleveland Clinic Foundation. Of these, 3387 (19.5%) were in young people aged 15 and under; 502 (14.8%) of these injuries to young athletes involved the upper extremity. Of course, these figures do not reflect the true incidence or prevalence of upper extremity injuries in youth sports, which surely must be higher.[6,11,13,18] They do, however, represent the frequency with which they are encountered in a general sports medicine clinic.

A further breakdown of injury prevalence is shown in Table 30-1. From this we can see that the region most commonly injured is the shoulder (44.6%), with the elbow (21.3%) and the hand (16.1%) following.

CLINICAL EVALUATION

In a discussion of specific injuries of the upper extremities, one must always keep in mind that all is not necessarily what it seems to be when evaluating the skeletally immature athlete. The presence of open growth plates provides additional mechanisms to consider as causes of clinical instability or deformity (acute or chronic). Further, pliable cartilaginous epiphyses provide the opportunity for the development of osteochondroses that may cause joint pain or swelling. Accordingly, roentgenographic examination of the injured part is mandatory to arrive at a definitive diagnosis. Even then, the roentgenograph may be misleading. Acute growth plate fractures, nondisplaced, may have roentgenographs that are initially interpreted as normal, only to demonstrate evidence of fracture 10 to 14 days later when periosteal reaction becomes apparent. Loose bodies may be cartilaginous and radiolucent, later to become calcified and apparent. Osteochondritis dissecans may be purely cystic and easily missed, only to become sclerotic and fragmented at a later time.

The moral to this is that the skeletal system in the child is evolving and undergoing continual change and remodeling. In the diagnosis and management of injuries to children, we must always keep this concept of dynamics in mind. Especially in children, the longitudinal evaluation of injuries over time is necessary not only to be able to make the precise diagnosis, but also to better predict the outcome.

SHOULDER

Anatomy

Fig. 30-3 depicts the various epiphyseal centers about the shoulder and their approximate ages at closure. One can see that these closures are relatively late; thus many school-aged athletes will be subject to the peculiarities of injuries to the growth plate. For instance, the medial clavicular physis may remain open until age 25, the proximal humerus until ages 18 to 21. As one would expect, the firm periosteal attachments to the epiphysis play a major role during the generation of injuries. At the proximal humerus, the periosteum has been shown to be thick and tough posteriorly, thus preventing posterior displacement of physeal fracture fragments.[10] Additionally, the rotator cuff attachments onto the physis extend medially onto the metaphysis, further contributing to the characteristic type II fractures seen in children (Fig. 30-6).

TABLE 30-1 Prevalence of upper extremity injuries in athletes aged 15 and under

Area of Injury	Percentage (N = 17,384)
Shoulder	36.5
Acromioclavicular-sternoclavicular	8.1
Upper arm	3.8
Elbow	21.3
Forearm	4.4
Wrist	9.8
Hand	16.1

Data from Cleveland Clinic Foundation, Section of Sports Medicine, 1977 to 1986.

TABLE 30-2 Prevalance of injury to the shoulder

Area of Injury	Percentage (N = 224)
Instability	
Subluxable	19.6
Dislocatable	11.2
	30.8
Impingement syndrome	15.6
Rotator cuff strain	13.4
	29.0
Fractures	13.0
Nerve pinch	6.7

Data from Cleveland Clinic Foundation, Section of Sports Medicine, 1977 to 1986.

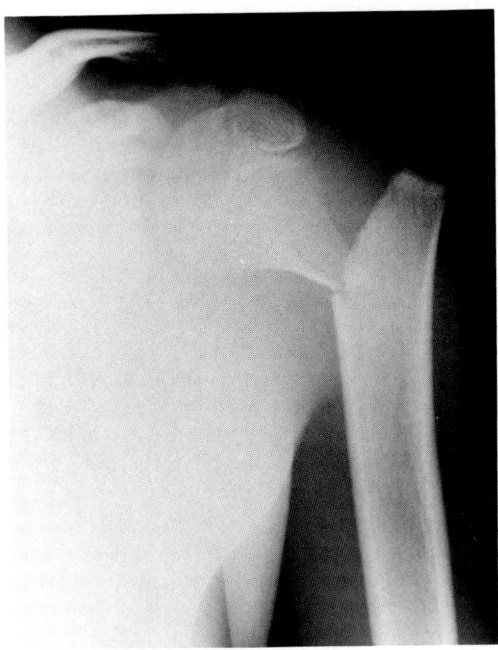

FIG. 30-6. The large metaphyseal component to this type II growth plate injury is apparent in this 12-year-old boy.

Injury Statistics

In our series, 44.6% of injuries to the upper extremity involve the shoulder; we consider the acromioclavicular joint, the clavicle and the sternoclavicular joint to be part of the shoulder complex as well as the traditional inclusion of the glenohumeral joint. Table 30-2 depicts the most frequent, specific injuries to this area. As can be seen, even in this young age-group, shoulder instability accounted for the most frequent diagnoses (30.8%), followed closely by problems of the rotator cuff (impingement and/or strain) (29%).

Instability Problems

As with adults, most typically the young athlete with shoulder instability will have anterior dislocations or subluxations. The reported incidence of recurrence of symptomatic instability is high. Despite recent reports of success with initial immobilization for 3 to 6 weeks and subsequent rehabilitation, the topic is still controversial.[26] Our approach has been to offer 3 to 4 weeks of sling and swath immobilization after the initial reduction, followed by a rehabilitation program that emphasizes rotator cuff strengthening. However, the first recurrence of dislocation is usually a bad sign and should signal an alert to consider surgical repair. Because of open growth plates, young bones, and inconsistent compliance with postoperative regimens, we prefer an operative approach that does not leave metal behind. A standard anterior capsulorrhaphy, such as in the Putti-Platt or the Bankhart type of repair, should achieve a 95% success rate as measured by prevention of recurrent dislocations.*

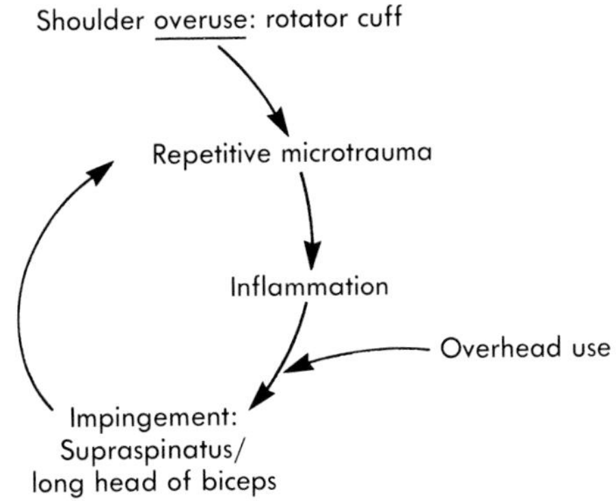

FIG. 30-7. Overuse can result in impingement syndrome. Successful treatment and management are directed toward each phase.

The management of subluxation has been similar to that of dislocation except for the initial period of immobilization. It has been our experience that this injury is often more insidious in its presentation and not amenable to this early detection and treatment. However, we have had an equally effective (or ineffective) response to rehabilitation programs. Surgical repair may offer generally better results.

Impingement Syndrome

Problems related to inflammation of the rotator cuff are common in the young athlete. This is especially true in the competitive swimmer, in whom this is seen most frequently.[22] Neer[39] has alerted the orthopedic community to the pathoanatomy of shoulder impingement, and Jobe[31] has defined the relationship of this entity to repetitive microtrauma. This symptom complex of shoulder pain (usually anterior but frequently poorly localized) begins as an inflammatory response of the rotator cuff (and at times the long head of the biceps tendon) to overuse. The accompanying swelling of peritendinous and bursal tissue then becomes subject to impingement with overhead activities.[41] The supraspinatus and the biceps tendon are most often involved with impingement by the coracoacromial arch. With impingement of inflamed structures, continuation of overhead activities, such as in swimming, will cause self-perpetuation of the cycle (Fig. 30-7).

Our treatment for this condition is as de-

*References 5, 9, 28, 29, 40, 43, 51, 55, 65.

scribed by others.[22,31,39,61] As with most overuse syndromes, successful treatment is usually nonoperative and includes activity modification (relative rest), oral antiinflammatory medications, and cryotherapy.

The subsequent management and rehabilitation include a rehabilitation program emphasizing flexibility and strengthening of the rotator cuff and also a gradual return to the sport activity (see Chapter 5).

We have had variable success with operative treatment of the impingement syndrome. For the young person with refractory shoulder pain, subacromial decompression is advocated.[61] Resection of the coracoacromial ligament alone can be effective in the athlete under age 25.[30] Over this age, acromioplasty is also required. With the development of arthroscopic techniques of subacromial decompression, we now can debride the subacromial bursa and release the coracoacromial ligament without violating the deltoid attachment on the acromion. This has significant implications for rehabilitation. If needed, an arthroscopic acromioplasty can be added. At this time, comparative studies of arthroscopic subacromial decompression and open procedures are incomplete. Our impression, however, is that the arthroscopic technique offers distinct advantages. Not all recurrent and refractory shoulder pain in the young athlete results from the impingement syndrome; occult shoulder instability can also mimic the symptoms of impingement.[20,50] This must be kept in mind during the formulation of the diagnosis, and at the time of arthroscopy both adequate physical examination of the shoulder and a direct look within the glenohumeral joint should be included.[8,63] Subacromial injection of a local anesthetic agent at the time the patient is seen in the office can also be helpful in establishing the diagnosis of impingement.

Acromioclavicular Injuries and Fractures

Acromioclavicular separations are uncommon in the skeletally immature athlete.[16] When seen, their management is usually no different from that required for the older athlete.[14,19,45,58] An injury unique to the young athlete involves a fracture of the distal clavicle (Fig. 30-8). In effect, this injury is analogous to the metaphyseal fracture seen with growth plate injuries. Usually the coracoclavicular ligaments remain intact and attached to the distal clavicle. Occasionally this deformity may necessitate open reduction and internal fixation with pins placed across the acromioclavicular joint and fracture. However, since considerable remodeling potential exists in children with this injury, some authors advocate nonoperative management regardless of deformity.[16]

Little League Shoulder and Elbow

It is, of course, difficult to discuss upper extremity injuries in the skeletally immature

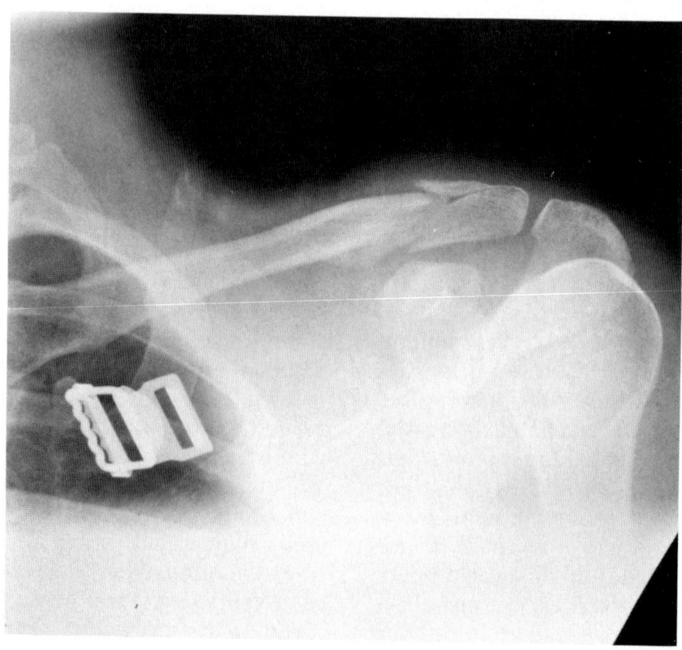

FIG. 30-8. Although skeletally mature, this young athlete sustained a metaphyseal fracture of the distal clavicle, lateral to the coracoclavicular ligaments. Closed management with a Kenny-Howard sling resulted in successful union and prevention of deformity.

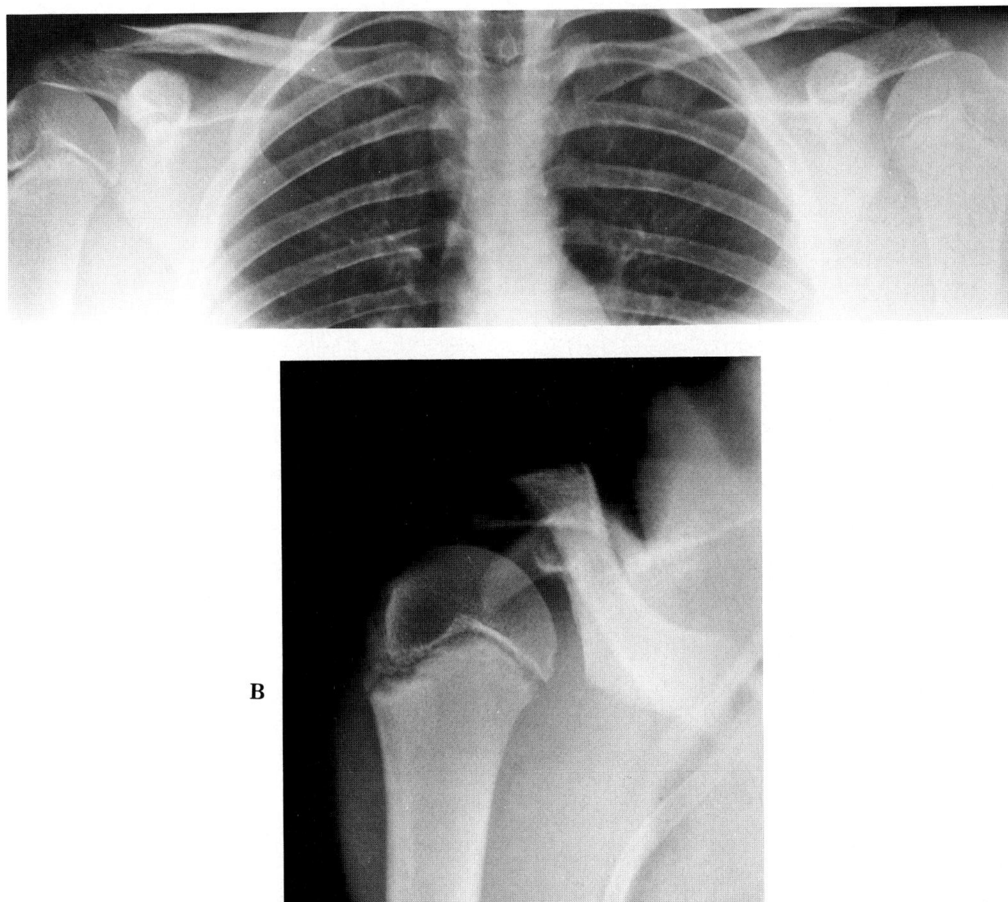

FIG. 30-9. This 13-year-old right-handed pitcher experienced three weeks of right shoulder pain midway through his baseball season. Roentgenographs of both shoulders **(A)** demonstrate asymmetry of the proximal humeral growth plates. An isolated roentgenograph of the right proximal humerus **(B)** clearly demonstrates growth plate widening and irregularity.

athlete without mentioning the entities referred to as little league shoulder or little league elbow. Adams brought attention to this in 1965 with his study of little league baseball pitchers in California.[1] Several studies since then have confirmed its existence, but emphasized the lower frequency.[21,24,34,62] Little league shoulder is characterized by pain occurring in a dominant shoulder of a skeletally immature throwing athlete. Radiographs easily demonstrate a widening of the proximal humeral growth plate. This is considered to be either a stress-related change or a subacute type I growth plate fracture (Fig. 30-9). In either case the treatment is easy: the athlete simply stops throwing for 4 to 6 weeks. Complete healing occurs uniformly and no adverse sequelae result.

ELBOW

Anatomy

Types of injury patterns about the elbow seen in skeletally immature athletes are heavily influenced by age. The distal humerus of the newborn has a single cartilaginous model of the epiphysis. However, by as early as 3 months, the ossification center of the capitellum appears (Fig. 30-10). Table 30-3 depicts the sequential times of appearance for

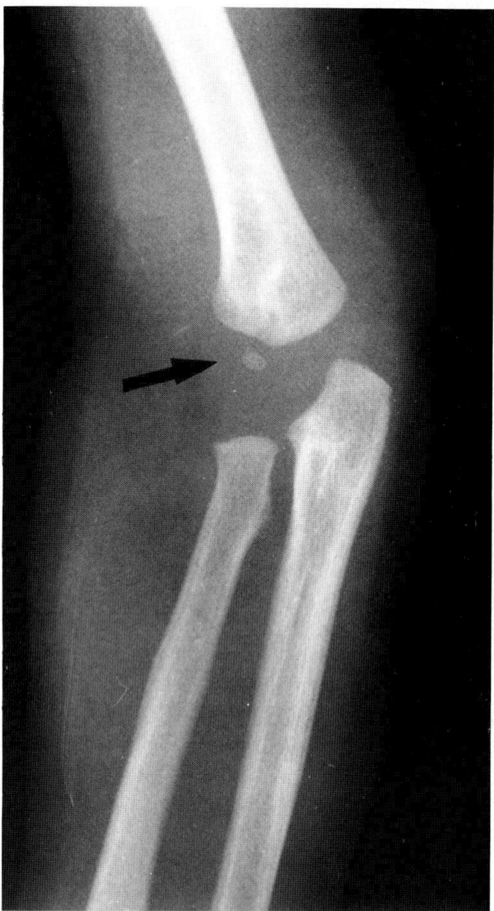

FIG. 30-10. At 12 months of age, the secondary center of ossification for the capitellum is apparent. At this age, however, much of the elbow can still be a roentgenographic mystery.

TABLE 30-3 Age of appearance for secondary ossification centers: elbow

	Males	Females
Capitellum	1-2 months	1-6 months
Radial head	3-6 years	3-6 years
Medial epicondyle	5-7 years	3-6 years
Trochlea	8-10 years	7-9 years
Olecranon	8-10 years	8-10 years
Lateral epicondyle	12 years	11 years

Modified from Ogden JA: Skeletal injury in the child, Philadelphia, 1982, Lea & Feibiger.

the secondary ossification centers about the elbow.[1] It is not unusual for any of these centers of ossification to appear first as two or more foci that later coalesce to become a single bony centrum. The trochlea commonly develops in this manner. Furthermore, this fragmented appearance and development of ossification centers need not be symmetrical. Table 30-4 indicates the time of fusion of these ossification centers. Although the sequence of appearance and closure of these ossification centers is consistent, the actual ages involved are variable, and most figures quoted in the literature are recognized as being approximations.

TABLE 30-4 Age of fusion for secondary ossification center: elbow

	Males (Years)	Females (Years)
Capitellum	14.5	13
Radial head	16	14
Medial epicondyle	17	14
Trochlea	13	11.5
Olecranon	16	14
Lateral epicondyle	15	12.5

Modified from Pappas AM: Elbow problems associated with baseball during childhood and adolescence, Clin Orthop 164:30-41, 1982.

TABLE 30-5 Prevalence of injury to the elbow

Injury	Percentage (N = 107)
Tendonitis	21.5
Fracture	15.0
Strain	12.2
Osteochondritis dissecans	7.5

Data from Cleveland Clinic Foundation, Section of Sports Medicine, 1977 to 1986.

Injury Statistics

Of the injuries to the upper extremity that we encountered in the skeletally immature athlete, 21.3% involved the elbow. As expected, the most frequent types of injury were related to overuse (Table 30-5). Fractures accounted for 15% and osteochondritis dissecans 7.5% of elbow complaints seen in our clinic.

Pappas has provided an excellent review of elbow problems developing in young pitchers.[44] From his experience, injury patterns were distinct and related to stages of development. In childhood, which he defined as terminating with the appearance of all secondary centers of ossification, most problems are related to the secondary ossification centers. Radiographs may demonstrate irregularly shaped or fragmented osseous development. At this stage, the problems are usually self-limited if the offending repetitive stress is avoided. Adolescence ends when all ossifica-

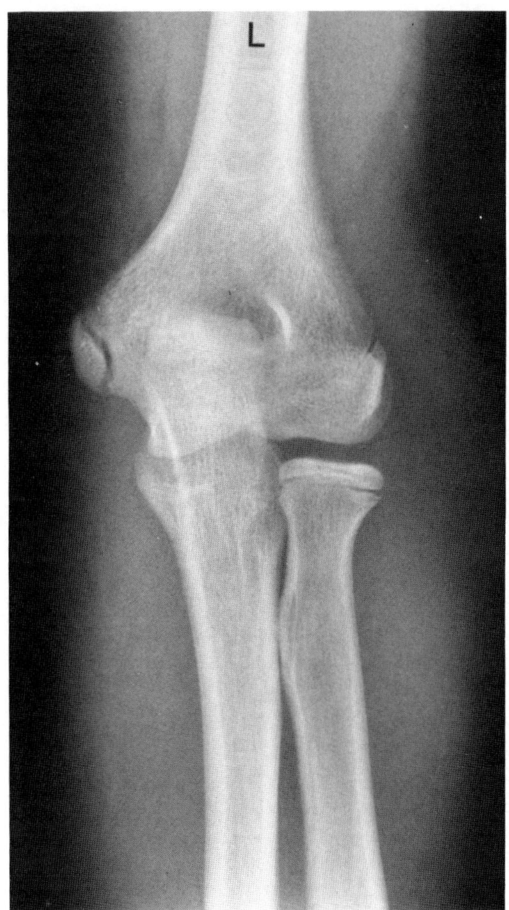

FIG. 30-11. Although hypertrophy of the medial humeral epicondyle can be a normal variant of the dominant upper extremity, widening of the apophysis combined with clinical pain and tenderness can be one characteristic feature of little league elbow.

tion centers have fused; problems characteristic of this adolescent period include avulsions, physeal separations, and avascular necrosis.

Little League Elbow

By far the most widely recognized elbow injuries occurring in youth sports are related to throwing—the little league elbow. Numerous studies have analyzed and discussed the pathologic forces generated about the elbow during throwing.[3,12,44] The throwing mechanism consists of three phases: the wind-up or cocking phase, the forward motion or acceleration phase, and the follow-through.[44] Each of these phases will place unique force patterns about the elbow.[12,44,64] During the late cocking phase, distraction forces are produced medially, compressive forces are applied laterally, and translational forces exist across the articulation between the olecranon and humerus. These forces neutralize during the acceleration phase. The follow-through produces excessive forces posteriorly throughout the triceps contraction, and compressive and shear forces across the radial capitellar joint with the rapid pronation of the forearm.

Clinical features that have been described in association with the little league elbow[24,34] include flexion contractures and increased valgus carrying angle. Radiographically, hypertrophy of the medial epicondyle is present but probably represents a normal variant of a dominant extremity. Fragmentation of the trochlea, olecranon and medial epicondyle can exist, as well as widening of the distance between the medial epicondyle and the humeral metaphysis (Fig. 30-11).

Clinical findings in little league elbow

- Flexion contracture
- Increased valgus carrying angle

Roentgenographic findings in little league elbow

- Medial epicondyle hypertrophy or fragmentation
- Trochlear fragmentation
- Olecranon fragmentation
- Widening of distance between medial epicondyle and humeral metaphysis

Avascular necrosis of the capitellum or of the radial head is also well recognized in the syndrome of elbow pain occurring in young pitchers. Except for the problems related to avascular necrosis or osteochondritis dissecans (see the next section), most of the features of little league elbow are either self-limiting, responding to a simple reprieve from throwing, or are normal anatomic variations of no clinical significance.

Osteochondritis Dissecans

The exception to the relatively benign course of well-treated little league elbow is the presence of osteochondritis dissecans of the capitellum, radial head, or both. By no means limited to pitchers, it may be seen in young gymnasts, basketball players, and virtually any active child.[46] Of the theories that exist to explain the cause,* most relate to avascular necrosis produced on a susceptible epiphysis

*References 2, 7, 32, 33, 35, 38, 44, 56.

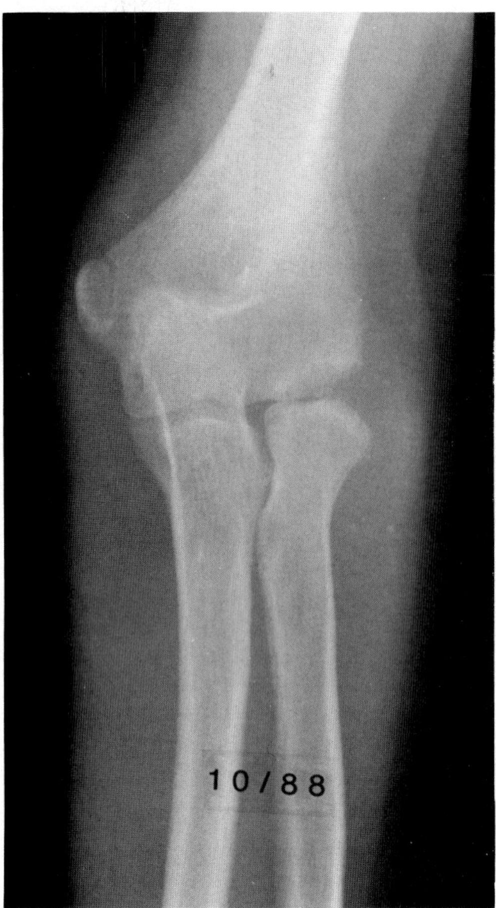

FIG. 30-12. The excessive valgus stress that occurs at the elbow during the act of throwing generates extreme compressive forces across the radial-capitellar joint. This young pitcher with chronic elbow pain illustrates the typical radiographic features of osteochondritis dissecans. This includes not only cystic and sclerotic changes of the capitellum, but also deformity of the radial head.

that receives repetitive compression or shearing forces. Typically the capitellum may show cystic changes or a radiographic pattern of sclerosis and loose body formation. The radial head may be deformed (Fig. 30-12). Intraarticular findings include softening and fissuring of the articular surfaces of the radiocapitellar joint; at times there may be subchondral collapse and bony eburnation. Intraarticular loose bodies are common. They may be osteocartilaginous, as seen in osteochondritis dissecans, or they may be purely cartilaginous, representing by-products of articular surface degeneration.

Treatment of osteochondritis dissecans varies. There is no doubt that some lesions in skeletally immature elbows will heal if provided with the proper environment. This treatment includes a strict avoidance of any throwing, as well as impact loading activities as seen in gymnastics. Pain, tenderness, contracture, and radiographic changes provide objective parameters to judge activity of the disease. Once loose-body formation has occurred, or healing has been incomplete (as is usually the case) and symptoms persist, surgical intervention will be required.[36] Traditionally, this has consisted of an arthrotomy with joint debridement (Fig. 30-13). Drilling of the osteochondritis dissecans lesion to stimulate either healing of the loose body within the lesion or fibrocartilaginous filling of a defect has been advocated.[36] This approach can provide relief of pain and mechanical symptoms, but usually does not result in much improvement in reducing contracture. More recently, arthroscopy has been applied to the management of this problem. Although the technique of arthroscopy of the elbow is more demanding and certainly has greater potential risk of injuries to neurovascular structures, with attention to detail the procedure is reasonable and the clinical effectiveness of arthroscopic joint debridement and loose-body removal make it rewarding for surgeon and young patient alike. It has become our preferred method of surgical management of osteochondritis dissecans of the elbow.

Flexion Contractures

Perhaps no entity involving the young elbow has been more frustrating to manage than the significant flexion contracture. Repetitive hyperextension, as occurs with throwing, can lead to traction injury of the anterior joint capsule, fibrosis, and contracture. Although some degree of flexion contracture may exist in 10%[24,34] of little league pitchers, most contractures are of less than 15 degrees and of little functional significance. Simple rest (i.e., avoiding hard throwing) will effect a cure in most instances. However, persistent abuse or the association of osteochondritis dissecans or remote elbow fracture can result in significant contractures of 30 degrees or more. Treatment initially consists of active range of motion and active assisted range of motion exercises. Throwing is prohibited, as are impact loading activities. Three months usually provide a reasonable measure of time to judge effectiveness of this rehabilitation program.

An adjunct worth using in refractory cases is the dynamic splinting program, as seen with the Dynasplint.[27] This device applies an extension moment to the elbow, with tension adjusted to avoid increasing elbow pain and

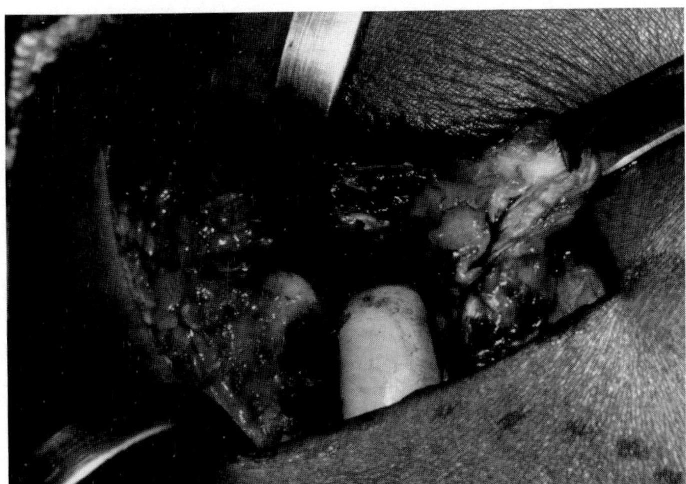

FIG. 30-13. Large osteochondral fragments of the capitellum frequently require debridement. The traditional arthrotomy with removal of loose osteochondral fragments and curettage and drilling of the subchondral bone is frequently required. However, arthroscopic debridement has less morbidity and comparable clinical results.

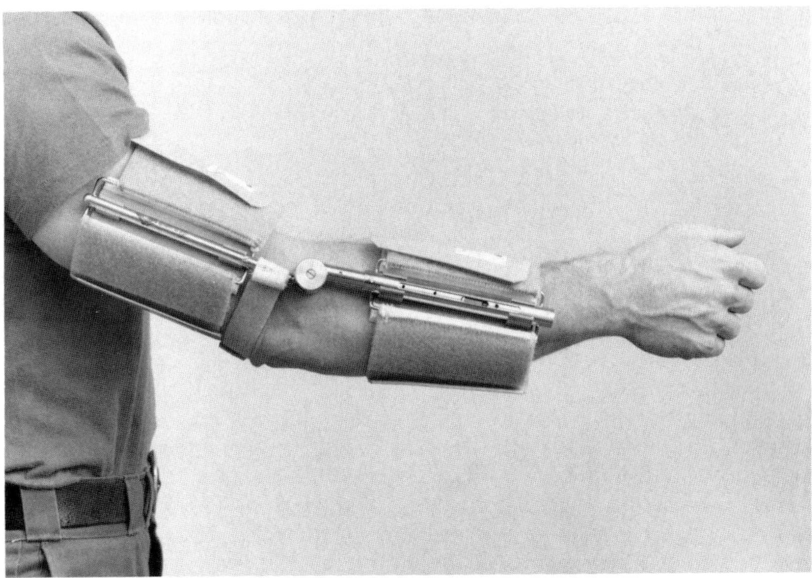

FIG. 30-14. Surprisingly good results with recalcitrant flexion contractures can be achieved with a part-time regimen of dynamic splinting. Application of the Dynasplint is shown.

soreness. It is worn as a nighttime orthosis, as tolerance permits, usually 12 hours per day. Our experience has been that these dynamic orthoses can generally reduce the contractures by half of their initial amount over a 3-month period.

Surgical treatment of flexion contractures about the elbow yields unpredictable results. Even young elbows, however, can have osteophytic formation on the olecranon as well as within the olecranon fossa. Loose bodies may also reside in the posterior recess and with this scenario, surgical debridement (open or arthroscopic) of osteophytes and removal of loose bodies can have a significant influence in regaining motion. A postoperative regimen with a continuous passive motion machine as well as dynamic splints will further improve results (Fig. 30-14).

Fractures and Dislocations

The most common elbow fracture seen in the young athlete is the **fracture/separation of the medial epicondyle** (Fig. 30-15).

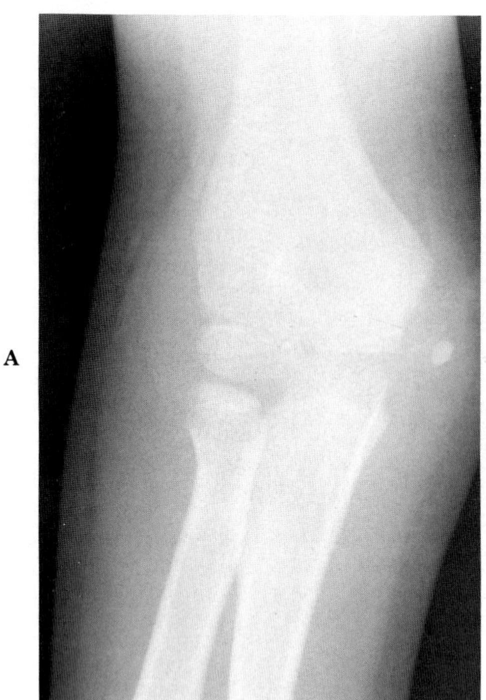

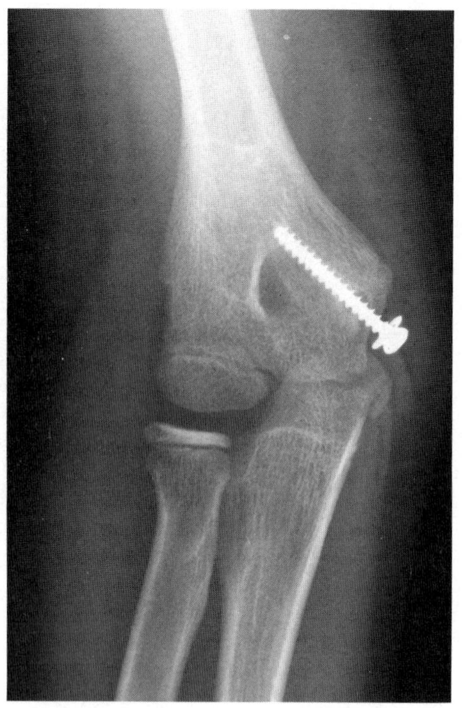

FIG. 30-15. Progressive displacement of the medial epicondyle occurred in this 11-year-old boy despite cast immobilization. **A,** Open reduction was required, and although crossed K-wire fixation is usually adequate, **B,** a screw with a spiked plastic washer was required in this instance.

This injury is frequently the childhood counterpart of the adult elbow dislocation.[46,59] However, the mechanism need not be a product of violent hyperextension and valgus stress but may also represent an avulsion fracture, as can be seen with throwing.[25] Treatment depends on the amount of displacement and the degree of associated elbow instability. Displacement greater than 5 mm, especially if combined with elbow instability, should direct the surgeon toward open reduction and internal fixation with crossed pins. Surgical exploration should include identifying the ulnar nerve, because this structure can be intimately involved with and even within the fracture. After the nerve has been identified and protected, the epicondyle is reduced and pinned. Postoperatively, the elbow is immobilized for 3 weeks. In epicondyle fractures that are minimally displaced (less than 5 mm), closed treatment is preferred, that is, a long arm cast for 3 weeks. However, radiographic checks should be made at some point during the first week, because the pull of the flexor/pronator musculature can lead to further displacement despite external immobilization. Finally, the same valgus stress combined with hyperextension that injures medial structures can injure lateral structures as well. Most typically, this is to the radial neck in the young athlete but may be to the radial head in the teenager or beyond. The **radial neck fracture** usually does well and is associated with little morbidity. In fact, a good deal of angulation can be accepted before reduction is even necessary[47] (Fig. 30-16). If the child is under 10 years of age, angulation of up to 30 or 40 degrees may be compatible with adequate remodeling and good function. In the child over 10 years of age, less remodeling potential exists and no more than 15 degrees of angulation should be accepted.[42] Immobilization is carried out for 3 to 4 weeks in angulated radial neck fractures, especially in those requiring open or closed reduction. For minimally angulated fractures, motion may be initiated as soon as comfort allows.

Radial head fractures can be troublesome. Although displacement may be minimal, loss of motion can be significant. If the clinical examination demonstrates good motion, including pronation and supination, closed treatment should be used. A simple sling or posterior splint for 7 to 10 days, followed by active range of motion activities, is all that is necessary. Further immobilization

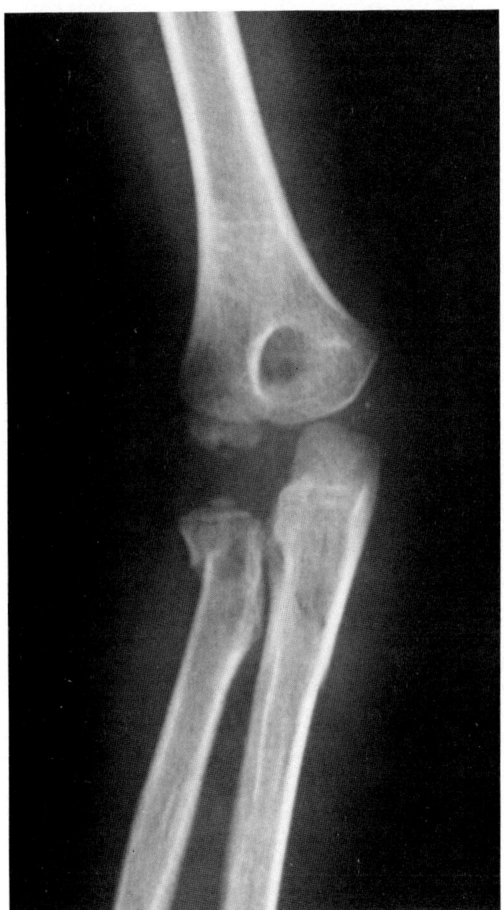

FIG. 30-16. Moderate displacement and angulation, as depicted in this child, is easily remodeled. Angulation of 30 to 40 degrees may be compatible with adequate remodeling and good function.

can lead to excessive stiffness and contracture. However, if the initial displacement is greater than 3 mm or if pronation and supination is limited, open reduction should be performed. Internal fixation with K-wires or small fragment screws is advocated.

WRIST AND FOREARM

As one might expect, athletic injuries about the wrist unique to the skeletally immature athlete are those involving the growth plate. The distal radius undergoes spontaneous closure of its physis by 17 years in the female and 19 years in the male.[23] As shown in Table 30-1, in our experience 9.8% of injuries to the young upper extremity were to the wrist.

Fractures

Most of the wrist fractures in our study consisted of routine **distal radial fractures,** either metaphyseal, epiphyseal, or both. The common types of tendonitis do occur, but in the skeletally immature athlete an occult underlying stress reaction of bone or growth plate may masquerade as tendonitis. Bone scans are not as routinely helpful here because of the normally increased uptake about the growth plates. However, we still obtain bone scans if our index of suspicion suggests an "atypical" tendonitis pattern.

Stress-Related Injuries

Several authors have described stress-related injuries of the skeletally immature wrist. These have for the most part involved young gymnasts and consisted of radiographic changes compatible with stress-induced changes of the distal radial or distal ulnar growth plates. These radiographic patterns include widening, irregularity, cystic changes, or haziness of the growth plate.[52,56] Actual growth plate slippage or fractures of the distal epiphyses have been described.[48]

Roentgenographic changes in stress-related wrist injuries

- Widening and irregularity of physis
- Cystic changes
- Haziness of the physis
- Growth plate displacement

The mechanism of injury behind these stress-related growth plate changes relates to repetitive hyperextension and rotation, as exemplified by the gymnast practicing a twisting vault technique.[48] This technique causes the wrist on the side of the twist to go into hyperextension and ulnar deviation (Fig. 30-17). Other activities in gymnastics have been implicated. In particular, the dowel grip used by gymnasts to increase their hook-grip strength has been associated with painful stress-related changes of the distal radial and ulnar growth plates. It is theorized that dependence on this device allows increased tensile forces to be generated across the distal radial and ulnar growth plates, eventually leading to stress injury.[66] As with other overuse injuries in young people, they are self-limiting if allowed time to rest properly.

HAND

Although adult types of hand injuries, including sprains and dislocations, can occur in the young athlete, fractures are the most common event that brings them to the physician's office (Table 30-6). And, as one would expect,

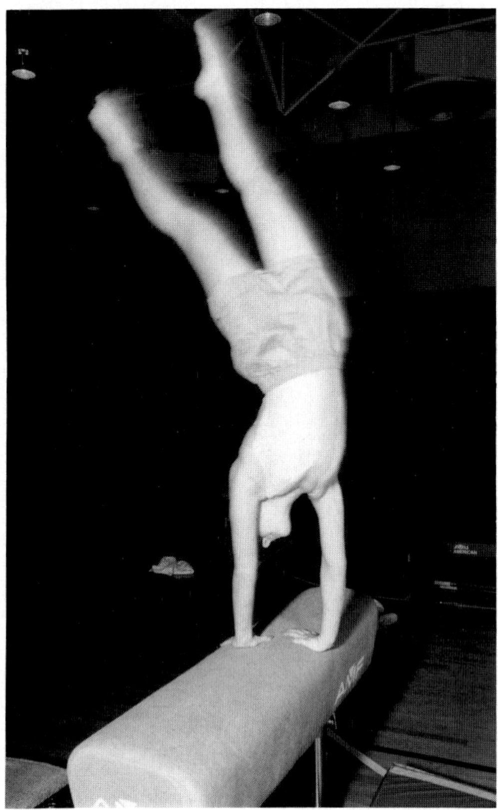

FIG. 30-17. Repetitive impact loading on the extended upper extremity, often combined with rotational forces, have been associated with stress-related growth plate changes of the distal radius and ulna.

these fractures are usually epiphyseal growth plate fractures, which tend to heal rapidly and well with closed reduction and external immobilization alone.[15,53] Remodeling of angular deformity of fractures within the plane of motion of the adjacent joint helps further. However, as with adults, rotational deformity does not correct itself and can be especially troublesome in the hand. Finally, since most of these fractures involve the growth plate, the possibility of late deformity caused by premature or asymmetrical growth arrest must be kept in mind when arranging adequate clinical follow up.

TABLE 30-6 Prevalence of injury to the hand

Injury	Percentage (N = 81)
Fracture	
Phalangeal	40.7
Metacarpal	16.1
	56.8
Sprain	24.7
Contusion	14.8

Data from Cleveland Clinic Foundation, Section of Sports Medicine, 1977 to 1986.

SUMMARY

The upper extremity is a marvel of engineering design and neuromuscular control, performing a multitude of precise and intricate movements throughout a wide range of motion, yet often sustaining large externally and internally generated forces—a tribute to our evolution. On the other hand, sport tends to push us to our limits of physiologic tolerance, and the young athlete is no exception.[4,17,49,57] Although adult patterns of injury virtually without exception can and do occur in the young, the majority of injury patterns in the young upper extremity are influenced by the existence of a growth plate.[37,60] This structure often represents the weak link in the musculoskeletal system and sustains injury (either chronic or acute) preferentially over ligaments, tendons, or bones. The good news is that the vast majority of these childhood sport trauma injuries will heal well, without sequelae, with relatively simple closed methods of treatment. There are exceptions, however, and we must forever be aware of and alert to these mischievous and at times vicious injury patterns.

Our attention should further be directed not only at the treatment of injury, but also, especially in dealing with youth, on prevention. Careful analysis of the mechanisms of injury and the athletic environments associated with the production of injury patterns has provided and will continue to provide the knowledge necessary to formulate rational guidelines for the prevention of athletic abuse.

REFERENCES

1. Adams JE: Injury to the throwing arm in the elbow joints of boy baseball players, Calif Med 102:127-132, 1965.
2. Aichroth P: Osteochondral fractures and their relationship to osteochondritis dissecans of the knee: an experimental study in animals, J Bone Joint Surg 53B(3):448, 1971.
3. Albright JA et al: Clinical study of baseball pitchers: correlation of injury to the throwing arm with method of delivery, Am J Sports Med 6(1):15, 1978.
4. Allen ME: Stress fracture of the humerus: a case study, Am J Sports Med 12(3):244, 1984.
5. Arenon JG and Regan K: Decreasing the incidence of recurrence of first time anterior shoulder dislocations with rehabilitation, Am J Sports Med 12(4):283, 1984.
6. Blitzer CM et al: Downhill skiing injuries in children, Am J Sports Med 12(2):142, 1984.
7. Campbell CJ and Ranawat CS: Osteochondritis dissecans: the question of etiology, J Trauma 6(2):201, 1966.

8. Cofield RH and Irving JF: Evaluation and classification of shoulder instability with special reference to examination under anesthesia, Clin Orthop 223:32, 1987.
9. Cofield RH, Kavanagh BF, and Frassica FJ: Anterior shoulder instability, Instr Course Lect 34:210, 1985.
10. Dameron TB and Reibel DB: Fractures involving the proximal humeral epiphyseal plate, J Bone Joint Surg 51A(2):289, 1969.
11. DeHaven KE: Elbow problems in the adolescent athlete, Cleve Clin Q 42(2):297, 1985.
12. DeHaven KE and Evarts CM: Throwing injuries of the elbow in athletes, Orthop Clin North Am 4(3):801, 1973.
13. Devereaux MD and Lachman SM: Athletes attending a sports injury clinic—a review, Br J Sports Med 17(4):137, 1983.
14. Dias JJ et al: The conservative treatment of acromioclavicular dislocation: review after five years, J Bone Joint Surg 69B(5):719, 1987.
15. Eaton RG: The dangerous chip fracture in athletes, Instr Course Lect 34:314, 1985.
16. Eidman DK, Siff SJ, and Tullos HS: Acromioclavicular lesions in children, Am J Sports Med 9(3):150, 1981.
17. Emans JB: Upper extremity injuries in sports. In Pediatric adolescent sports medicine, Boston, 1984, Little & Brown.
18. Estwanik JJ et al: Injuries in interscholastic wrestling, Phys Sports Med 8(3):111, 1980.
19. Galpin RD, Hawkins RJ, and Grainger RW: A comparative analysis of operative versus nonoperative treatment of grade III acromioclavicular separations, Clin Orthop 193:150, 1985.
20. Garth WP, Allman FL, and Armstrong WS: Occult anterior subluxations of the shoulder in noncontact sports, Am J Sports Med 15(6):579, 1987.
21. Grana WA and Rashking A: Pitcher's elbow in adolescents, Am J Sports Med 8(5):333, 1980.
22. Greipp JF: Swimmer's shoulder: the influence of flexibility and weight training, Phys Sports Med 13(8):92, 1985.
23. Greulich WW and Pyle SI: Radiographic atlas of skeletal development of the wrist and hand, Stanford, Calif, and Oxford, England, 1950, Stanford University Press and Oxford University Press.
24. Gugenheim JJ et al: Little league survey: the Houston study, Am J Sports Med 4(5):189, 1976.
25. Haw DWM: Avulsion fracture of the medial epicondyle of the elbow in a young javelin thrower: case report, Br J Sports Med 15(1):47, 1981.
26. Henry JH and Genung JA: Natural history of glenohumeral dislocation revisited, Am J Sports Med 10(3):135, 1982.
27. Hepburn GR and Crivelli KJ: Use of elbow Dynasplint for reduction of elbow flexion contractures: a case study, J Orthop Sports Med Phys Ther 5(5):269, 1984.
28. Hovelius L: Anterior dislocation of the shoulder in teen-agers and young adults: five year prognosis, J Bone Joint Surg 69A(3):393, 1987.
29. Hovelius L et al: Recurrences after initial dislocation of the shoulder: results of a prospective study of treatment, J Bone Joint Surg 65A(3):343, 1983.
30. Jackson DW: Chronic rotator cuff impingement in the throwing athlete, Am J Sports Med 4(6):231, 1976.
31. Jobe FW and Jobe CM: Painful athletic injuries in the shoulder, Clin Orthop 173:117, 1983.
32. Langenskiold A: Can osteochondritis dissecans arise as a sequel of cartilage fracture in early childhood? An experimental study, Acta Chir Scand 109:204, 1955.
33. Langer F and Percy EC: Osteochondritis dissecans and anomalous centres of ossification: a review of 80 lesions in 61 patients, Can J Surg 14:208, 1971.
34. Larson RL et al: Little league survey: the Eugene study, Am J Sports Med 4(5):201, 1976.
35. Linden B and Telhag H: Osteochondritis dissecans: a histologic and autoradiographic study in man, Acta Orthop Scand 48:682, 1977.
36. McManama GB et al: The surgical treatment of osteochondritis of the capitellum, Am J Sports Med 13(1):11, 1985.
37. Micheli LJ: Overuse injuries in children's sports: the growth factor, Orthop Clin North Am 14(2): 337, 1983.
38. Nagura S: The so-called osteochondritis dissecans of Konig, Clin Orthop 18:100, 1960.
39. Neer CS: Anterior acromioplasty for the chronic impingement syndrome in the shoulder, J Bone Joint Surg 54A(1):41, 1972.
40. Nielsen AB and Nielsen K: The modified Bristow procedure for recurrent anterior dislocation of the shoulder, Acta Orthop Scand 53:229, 1982.
41. Norwood LA et al: Anterior shoulder pain in baseball pitchers, Am J Sports Med 6(3):103, 1978.
42. Ogden JA: Skeletal injury in the child, Philadelphia, 1982, Lea & Febiger.
43. Paavolainen P et al: Recurrent anterior dislocation of the shoulder: results of Eden-Hybbinette and Putti-Platt operations, Acta Orthop Scand 55:556, 1984.
44. Pappas AM: Elbow problems associated with baseball during childhood and adolescence, Clin Orthop 164:30, 1982.
45. Post M: Current concepts in the diagnosis and management of acromioclavicular dislocations, Clin Orthop 200:234, 1985.
46. Priest JD and Weise DJ: Elbow injury in women's gymnastics, Am J Sports Med 9(5):288, 1981.
47. Rang M: Children's fractures, Philadelphia, 1974, JB Lippincott Co.
48. Read MTF: Stress fractures of the distal radius in adolescent gymnasts, Br J Sports Med 15(4):272, 1981.
49. Rettig AC and Beltz HF: Stress fracture in the humerus in an adolescent tennis tournament player, Am J Sports Med 13(1):55, 1985.
50. Rowe CR: Recurrent transient anterior subluxation of the shoulder: the "dead arm" syndrome, Clin Orthop 223:11, 1987.
51. Rowe CR, Zarins B, and Ciullo JV: Recurrent anterior dislocation of the shoulder after surgical repair: apparent causes of failure and treatment, J Bone Joint Surg 66A(2):159, 1984.
52. Roy S, Caine D, and Singer KM: Stress changes of the distal radial epiphysis in young gymnasts: a report of twenty-one cases and a review of the literature, Am J Sports Med 13(5):301, 1985.
53. Ruby LK: Common hand injuries in the athlete, Clin Sports Med 2(3):609, 1983.
54. Salter RB and Harris WR: Injuries involving the epiphyseal plate, J Bone Joint Surg 45A(3):587, 1963.
55. Simonet WT and Cofield RH: Prognosis in anterior shoulder dislocation, Am J Sports Med 12(1):19, 1984.

56. Smith AD: Osteochondritis of the knee joint: a report of three cases in one family and a discussion of the etiology and treatment, J Bone Joint Surg 42A(2):289, 1960.
57. Sullivan JA: Recurring pain in the pediatric athlete, Pediatr Clin North Am 31(5):1097, 1984.
58. Taft TN et al: Dislocation of the acromioclavicular joint: an end-result study, J Bone Joint Surg 69A(7):1045, 1987.
59. Teitz CC: Sports medicine concerns in dance and gymnastics, Pediatr Clin North Am 29(6):1399, 1982.
60. Tibone JE: Shoulder problems of adolescents: how they differ from those of adults, Clin Sports Med 2(2):423, 1983.
61. Tibone JE et al: Shoulder impingement syndrome in athletes treated by an anterior acromioplasty, Clin Orthop 198:134, 1985.
62. Torg JS, Pollack H, and Sweterlitsch P: The effect of competitive pitching on the shoulders and elbows of preadolescent baseball players, Pediatrics 49(2):267, 1972.
63. Tulos HS, Bennett JB, and Braly WG: Acute shoulder dislocations: factors influencing diagnosis and treatment, Instr Course Lect 33:364, 1984.
64. Tulos HS and King JW: Lesions of the pitching arm in adolescents, Clin Orthop 200:264, 1972.
65. Wagner KT and Lyne ED: Adolescent traumatic dislocations of the shoulder with open epiphyses, J Pediatr Orthop 3(1):61, 1983.
66. Yong-Hing K, Wedge JG, and Bowen CVA: Chronic injury to the distal ulnar and radial growth plates in an adolescent gymnast, J Bone Joint Surg 70A(7):1087, 1988.

PART VI Neurologic and Vascular Problems

CHAPTER 31 Neurovascular Injuries

George Pianka
Elliott B. Hershman

The spectrum of athletic injuries that involve the upper extremity include both acute injuries to and chronic conditions of the neurovascular structures. These problems can be difficult to diagnose at times and often are considered only after other, more common, athletic injuries are eliminated from diagnostic consideration. Injury to the neurovascular structures, however, should always be considered in the differential diagnosis of an athletic injury. Neurovascular problems can be the primary problem, as in "bowler's thumb,"[10,55,83] or secondary to other ongoing processes, as with ulnar neuritis[27,31] resulting from chronic valgus instability of the elbow. Whether primary or secondary in nature, the neurovascular condition must be addressed to permit safe return to athletics.

Injury to the neurologic system can occur in numerous anatomic locations and create symptoms in the upper extremity. In particular, cervical spine trauma often leads to either peripheral nerve injury at the root level or spinal cord injury in the cervical region.[2] Neck injury must always be considered when athletes describe neurologic symptoms in the upper extremity.[4] The diagnostic approach to differentiating these problems is discussed at length in Chapter 1.

Neurologic problems can arise from injury to the major nerves, as in brachial plexus trauma, or to smaller peripheral nerves, as occurs in carpal tunnel syndrome. The level of injury can often be localized from the results of a detailed physical examination. Other diagnostic modalities can be used to confirm or refute the clinician's diagnostic impression. These techniques include nerve conduction studies, electromyography, and spinal cord or cortical evolved potentials.

Like neurologic injury, vascular problems can arise in a multitude of sites in the upper extremity. Both arterial and venous injuries can occur, and problems range from injury to the large subclavian vessels to involvement of the significantly smaller ulnar artery. In chronic vascular problems, the roentgenographic evaluation (arteriography or venography) often is an important diagnostic modality because the physical examination can be quite unrevealing. This is in contrast to acute vascular occlusion, which often manifests dramatic physical findings.

In any of these injuries, it is important the pertinent anatomy be understood so the physical examination is precise and informative. Once an exact diagnosis is reached, appropriate treatment and counseling can be offered.

ANATOMY

Brachial Plexus

The neurologic elements of the upper extremity originate from the cervical portion of the spinal cord. Cervical roots 5,6,7, and 8, as well as thoracic root 1, contribute to the innervation of the upper extremity.

The brachial plexus is formed by the junctions of the ventral rami of the C5, C6, C7, C8, and T1 spinal nerve roots. Occasionally, there may be a contribution from C4, designated as a prefixed plexus, or less frequently from T2, designated a postfixed plexus. Although observed anatomically, these variations have little clinical significance in most instances. These rami are formed from a dorsal root, which is sensory, and a ventral root, which is motor. The ventral rami lie between the anterior and middle scalene muscles where they share space with the subclavian artery. The plexus continues distally over the first rib and deep to the sternocleidomastoid muscle in the posterior cervical triangle, a region bordered by the trapezius muscle, sternocleidomastoid muscle, and superior border of the clavicle.

The five ventral rami unite just above the clavicle to form three trunks: the upper trunk, consisting of roots C5 and C6; the middle trunk, consisting of root C7; and lower trunk, consisting of roots C8 and T1 (Fig. 31-1). Just below the level of the clavicle, each trunk divides into an anterior and posterior division. These divisions contribute to the formation of three cords.

The posterior divisions from each trunk form the posterior cord, which has contributions from C5, C6, C7, C8, and slightly from T1. The anterior divisions of the upper and middle trunks form the lateral cord, which has contributions from C5, C6, and C7. The anterior division of the lower trunk forms the medial cord, which has contributions from C8 and T1. The three cords, lateral, posterior, and medial, are named in reference to their posi-

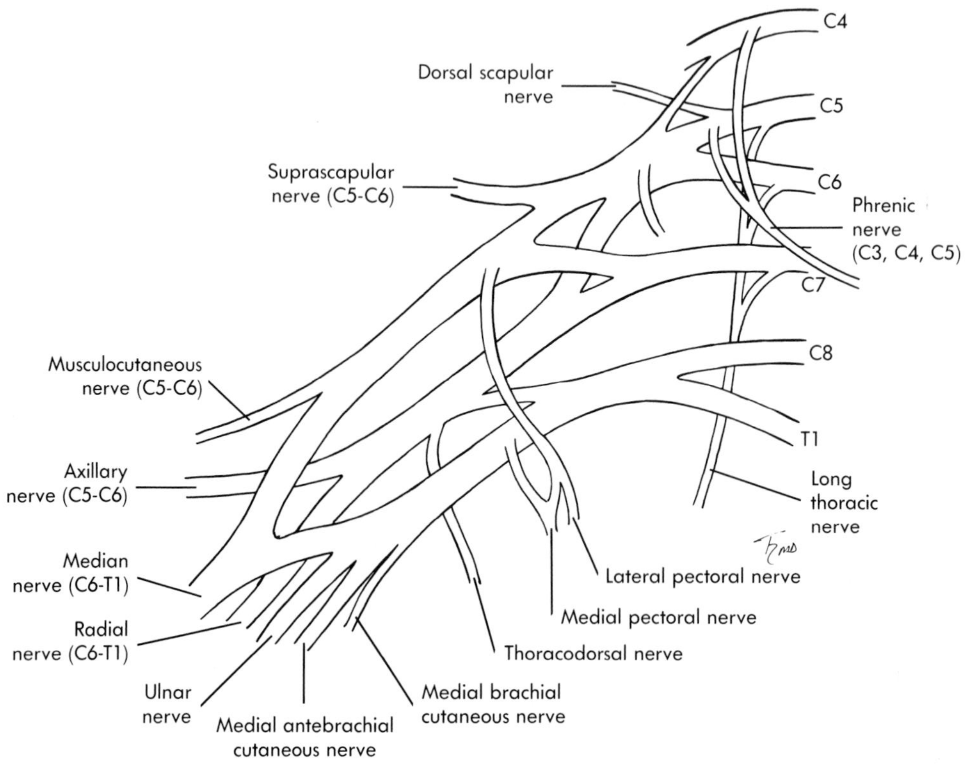

FIG. 31-1. The brachial plexus.

TABLE 31-1 Major branches of the brachial plexus

Peripheral Nerve	Root Composition	Origin
Long thoracic	C5, C6, C7	Cervical roots
Dorsal scapula	C5	Cervical root
Suprascapular	C5, C6	Upper trunk
Upper subscapular	C5	Posterior cord
Lower subscapular	C5, C6	Posterior cord
Thoracodorsal	C7, C8	Posterior cord
Lateral pectoral	C5, C6, C7	Lateral cord
Medial pectoral	C8, T1	Medial cord
Medial brachial cutaneous	C8, T1	Medial cord
Medial antebrachial cutaneous	C8, T1	Medial cord
Axillary	C5, C6	Posterior cord
Radial	C6, C7, C8	Posterior cord
Median	C5, C6, C7, C8, T1	Medial and lateral cords
Musculocutaneous	C5, C6	Lateral cord
Ulnar	C8, T1	Medial cord

tion relative the axillary artery, running just below the pectoralis minor muscle.

The three cords divide to give five terminal branches to the upper extremity, whereas other branches arise more proximally, either from the cords, trunks, or roots, to supply the shoulder girdle musculature. These branches are summarized in Table 31-1.

The radial nerve is the terminal branch of the posterior cord, the middle trunk, and the C7 ventral ramus. It receives contributions from the upper and lower trunks. The axillary nerve is a branch from the posterior cord, which originates proximal to the radial nerve. Other direct branches from the posterior cord are the thoracodorsal nerve and the upper and lower subscapular nerves.

The ulnar nerve is the terminal branch of the medial cord and lower trunk, arising from the C8 and T1 ventral rami. The medial pectoral nerve and the medial brachial and antebrachial cutaneous branches are also terminal divisions of the medial cord.

The median nerve is formed from continuing portions of the medial and lateral cords. The lateral cord, which arose from the upper and middle trunks, contributes mainly sensory fibers from the ventral rami of C5, C6, and C7. These fibers join with the primarily motor contribution from a branch of the medial cord, originating at the C8 and T1 ventral rami.

The suprascapular nerve is a branch arising from the upper trunk, consisting of the C5 and C6 ventral rami. The C5 ventral ramus sends contributions to the phrenic nerve and provides another branch to form the dorsal scapular nerve. The long thoracic nerve is formed from contributions of the ventral rami of C5, C6, and C7 nerve roots.

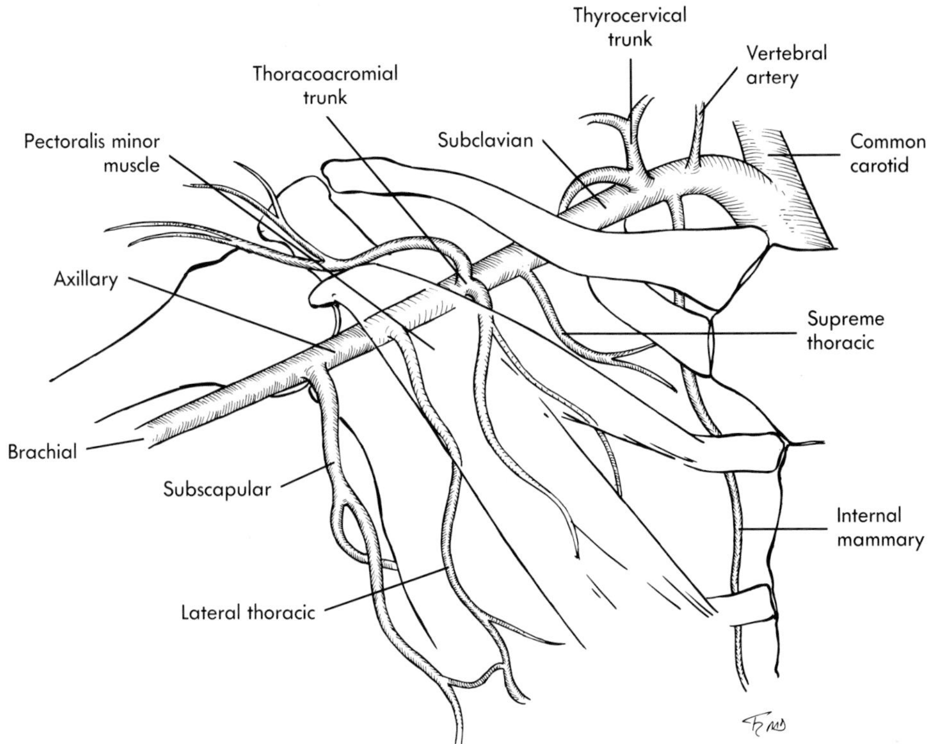

FIG. 31-2. Arterial anatomy of the shoulder region.

Axillary artery branches

- Supreme thoracic
- Thoracoacromial
- Lateral thoracic
- Subscapular
- Anterior humeral circumflex
- Posterior humeral circumflex

Axillary Vessels

The subclavian vessels arise from the aortic arch on the left side and from the innominate (brachiocephalic) artery on the right. The subclavian artery has the transverse scapular artery as a branch and becomes the axillary artery as it crosses the upper border of the first rib. The axillary veins tend to follow the artery and its branches. The brachial plexus is located around the artery. The axillary artery, axillary vein, and brachial plexus travel through the axilla enclosed within the axillary sheath, a fibrous tunnel that is a continuation of the fascia of the neck.

The axillary artery is often described by its relationship to the pectoralis minor: the first segment lies proximal to the pectoralis minor, the second directly behind it, and the third, distal to it. There are six main branches arising from the axillary artery — supreme thoracic, thoracoacromial, lateral thoracic, subscapular, anterior humeral circumflex, and posterior humeral circumflex (Fig. 31-2). The axillary artery becomes the brachial artery as it crosses the lower border of the teres major.

Arm

The brachial artery continues down the arm along the medial aspect of the biceps. It passes into the elbow region beneath the biceps aponeurosis (lacertus fibrosis).

In the upper arm, the radial nerve lies behind the artery, the ulnar nerve is medial to the artery, and the median nerve can be found anterolateral to the artery. The radial nerve continues posterior, winds around the humerus, and continues along the lateral border of the distal humerus. The ulna nerve becomes more medial as it courses distally, passing through the intermuscular septum to lie posteriorly near the point it crosses the elbow, behind the medial epicondyle.

In the arm, the musculocutaneous nerve supplies innervation to the biceps brachii, coracobrachialis, and brachialis muscles. Posteriorly, the triceps are innervated by the radial nerve. In addition, the radial nerve provides innervation to the anconeus and brachioradialis muscles. The ulna and median nerves have no motor branches in the arm, but rather contribute to the forearm, wrist, hand, and fingers with both motor and sensory fibers.

Forearm

The terminal branches of the medial, ulnar, and radial nerves provide all of the motor innervation to the muscles of the forearm and hand. The sensory innervation of the forearm and hand is also supplied by these nerves, with the exception of the medial aspect of the proximal forearm (medial antebrachial cutaneous nerve) and varying portions of the mid- to distal lateral forearm (cutaneous portion of the musculocutaneous nerve).

The median nerve lies medial to the brachial artery on the anterior surface of the brachialis at the elbow. It passes with the brachial artery beneath the lacertus fibrosus, then continues between the two heads of the pronator teres. It provides motor control to the pronator teres, flexor carpi radialis, palmaris longus, and flexor digitorum superficialis. The nerve runs between the heads of the flexor digitorum superficialis and continues to the wrist, deep to the flexor digitorum superficialis muscle. An important branch of the median nerve arises about 5 cm below the medial epicondyle. This branch, the anterior interosseous nerve, continues down the forearm on the interosseous membrane and gives motor innervation to the flexor digitorum profundus (index and middle fingers), flexor pollicis longus, and pronator quadratus. The various tissues the median nerve passes through account in large part for the entrapment syndromes that can occur.

The ulnar nerve passes into the forearm between the heads of the flexor carpi ulnaris and continues to the wrist under the cover of this muscle tendon unit. The nerve supplies motor innervation to the flexor carpi ulnaris and the ulnar portion of the flexor digitorum profundus (ring and little fingers).

The radial nerve supplies all the innervation to the extensor aspect of the forearm. After winding posteriorly around the humerus, the nerve comes to lie on the lateral side of the arm. In the region of the elbow, the nerve divides into motor (posterior interosseous) and sensory (superficial radial) branches. The location of this bifurcation is variable and can occur proximal or distal to the elbow.

The majority of the motor supply on the extensor aspect is afforded by the posterior interosseous nerve. This nerve provides innervation to the muscles listed in the accompanying box. The radial nerve or superficial branch generally provides innervation to the

Posterior interosseous nerve–innervated muscles

- Supinator
- Extensor digitorum
- Extensor digiti minimi
- Extensor carpi ulnaris
- Abductor pollicis longus
- Extensor pollicis brevis
- Extensor pollicis longus
- Extensor indicis

extensor carpi radialis longus and/or brevis, but the innervation is variable.

The brachial artery divides into two branches, the radial and ulnar arteries. The radial artery passes through the forearm, between the brachioradialis and the flexor carpi radialis. The ulnar artery travels with the ulnar nerve, between the flexor carpi ulnaris and the flexor digitorum profundus.

Wrist and Hand

The median nerve passes through the wrist in the carpal tunnel. Here it lies beneath the transverse carpal ligament (flexor retinaculum). Proximally in the carpal tunnel, it is found on the radial side of the superficial flexor tendons, but distally it comes to lie directly beneath the transverse carpal ligament. It gives off the important motor branch to the thenar muscles then continues to branch, providing motor innervation to the first and second lumbricals and sensory innervation to the palmar aspect of the thumb, index finger, middle finger, and radial aspect of the ring finger.

The ulnar nerve passes under the volar carpal ligament in Guyon's canal. It generally divides at about the level of the distal pisiform into its terminal superficial and deep branches. The superficial branch provides sensory innervation to the palmar aspect of the little finger and ulnar aspect of the little finger and ring finger. The deep branch provides motor innervation to the hypothenar muscles, the interosseous muscles, the third and fourth lumbricals, the adductor pollicis, and the deep head of the flexor pollicis brevis.

The superficial radial nerve provides sensory innervation to the dorsum of the hand and radial digits (thumb, index, and middle). Often the dorsum of the ulna digits has sensory innervation from branches of the dorsal branch of the ulnar nerve.

The radial artery and ulnar artery each branch to form a deep and superficial component. These branches go on to form the deep and superficial palmar arches. The completeness of these vascular arches is variable, but the deep is more constant than the superficial.

For the reader interested in further discussion of the anatomy of wrist and hand, see Chapter 21 for additional information.

PHYSICAL EXAMINATION

The physical examination with respect to neurovascular injuries should be part of every routine physical examination. A number of specific features of the neurologic and vascular examinations are important to discuss.

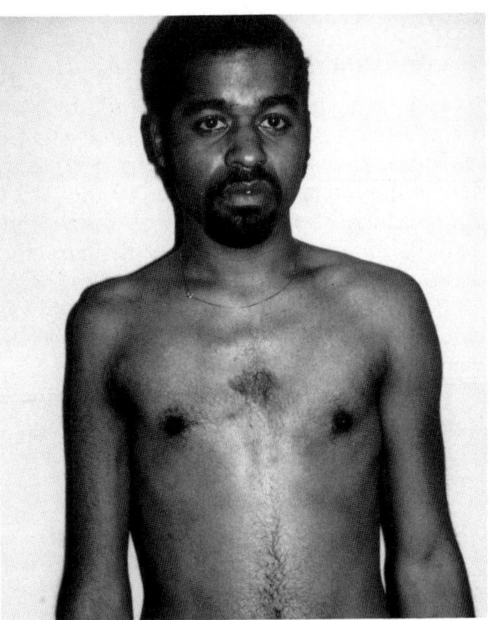
A

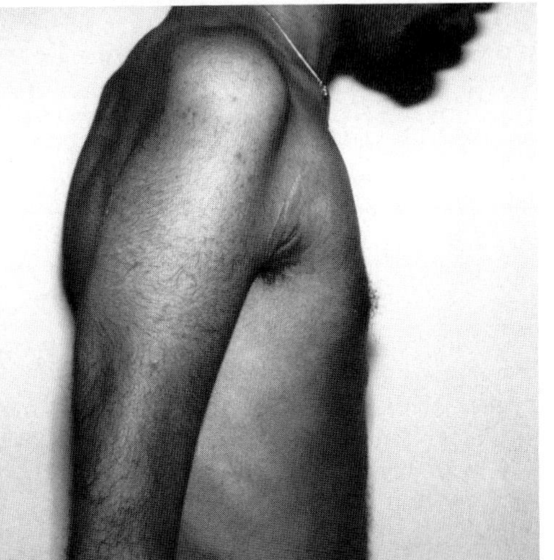
B

FIG. 31-3. A and **B,** Atrophy can often be used to delineate the region of nerve injury. This lesion has led to atrophy of the right deltoid and biceps, easily noted with careful observation.

Observation

The patient should be observed carefully, with the trunk and upper extremities disrobed. Subtle areas of atrophy or deformity can be observed in this manner (Fig. 31-3). Discoloration, swelling, and general skin color should be noted because abnormalities may arise in these characteristics with both venous and arterial problems. Any skeletal deformity should be documented.

Joint Evaluation

The active and passive range of motion of the neck, shoulders, elbows, wrists, and hands should be measured. Stability of joints should be evaluated because recurrent instability can result in neurovascular problems.

Motor Examination

The motor evaluation is one of the most important components of the neurologic evaluation. A thorough motor examination can often define the site of lesion. It is important to differentiate between root level injuries and peripheral nerve injuries, and this can often be done on the basis of the motor examination. The various innervation patterns that can be identified by careful motor examination are outlined in Table 31-2.

When motor function is graded in athletes, it is important to recall the classic muscle grading system.[99] In this system, strength is graded as follows:

Grade		Findings
5	**Normal (N)**	**Able to withstand full resistance**
4	**Good (G)**	**Able to withstand some resistance**
3	**Fair (F)**	**Able to move against gravity**
2	**Poor (P)**	**Able to move with gravity eliminated**
1	**Trace (T)**	**Able to contract without movement**
0	**Zero**	**No evidence of contraction**

In athletes, however, strength measurement by manual muscle testing may be difficult because of the tremendous strength of many athletes. Often the examiner cannot overcome an athlete's strength in the injured extremity because of the great strength of the athlete. In this setting, quantifiable strength measurement may be of value. This can be done by using dynamometers, such as Cybex isokinetic equipment, or by using hand-held measuring devices such as the NISMAT—Nicholas Manual Muscle Tester. It must be remembered that strength testing, in general, has limitations resulting from pain and test-subject efforts, so results must be judged in their clinical setting.

Reflex Examination

The reflexes of the upper extremity are listed in Table 31-3. Reflexes should be judged in terms of their quality, not just their presence or absence, in order to evaluate for subtle reflex abnormalities.

Sensory Evaluation

Sensory disturbances can occur in either a dermatomal (root) distribution or in the distribution of peripheral nerves. These are illustrated in Fig. 31-4. If spinal cord lesions are suspected, it is important to evaluate all sensory functions, including light touch, temperature, vibration, position sense, and pain (pin prick).

Vascular Evaluation

Pulses can be evaluated at the wrist for both the radial and ulna arteries. The Allen test should be performed if vascular injuries are suspected at the wrist. In this test, both the radial and ulnar arteries are occluded by the examiner. The patient opens and closes the hand until the hand is blanched. The examiner then releases the pressure on the radial artery and notes the filling of the hand from radial to ulnar. The procedure is then repeated with the examiner releasing the ulnar artery initially. Comparisons are made in the patterns of vascular refill.

The brachial artery is easily palpated at the elbow, just medial to the lacertus fibrosus. Obliteration of the pulse implies a vascular problem proximally in the axillary or subclavian region.

Venous tone and patterns should be observed. In axillary vein thrombosis, the venous pattern of the involved extremity is increased and the dorsal hand veins do not collapse when raised to the level of the heart (Fig. 31-5).

Adson's test may be helpful in the diagnosis of thoracic outlet syndrome. It is performed by extending the arm and locating the radial pulse. The head is turned to the side being tested. A positive test occurs when the radial pulse is obliterated by the turned head. A modification of this test has the patient turn his or her head to the opposite side.[107]

In an examination for a neurologic injury, Tinel's sign should be sought. To elicit Tinel's sign, percussion is performed over a nerve

TABLE 31-2 Patterns of motor innervation

Root Innervation (predominant)

C5	*C6*	*C7*	*C8*	*T1*
Deltoid Biceps Rhomboids Supraspinatus Infraspinatus	Wrist extensors	Triceps Wrist flexors Finger extensors	Finger flexors Hand intrinsics	Hand intrinsics

Peripheral Nerve Innervation

Dorsal scapula	***Long thoracic***	***Suprascapular***
Rhomboids	Serratus anterior	Infraspinatus Supraspinatus
Thoracodorsal	***Subscapular***	***Lower subscapular***
Latissimus dorsi	Subscapularis	Subscapularis Teres major
Medial pectoral	***Lateral pectoral***	***Musculocutaneous***
Pectoralis major Pectoralis minor	Pectoralis major	Coracobrachialis Biceps Brachialis
Median	***Anterior interosseous***	***Axillary***
Pronator teres Flexor carpi radialis Palmaris longus Flexor digitorum superficialis Abductor pollicis brevis Opponens pollicis Flexor pollicis brevis (superficial) Radial two lumbricals	Flexor digitorum profundus (radial half) Flexor pollicis longus Pronator quadratus	Deltoid Teres minor
Radial	***Posterior interosseous***	***Ulnar***
Triceps Anconeous Brachioradialis Extensor carpi radialis longus and brevis	Supinator Extensor digitorum Extensor digiti minimi Extensor carpi ulnaris Abductor pollicis longus Extensor pollicis brevis Extensor pollicis longus Extensor indicis	Flexor carpi ulnaris Flexor digitorum profundus (ulnar half) Flexor pollicis brevis (deep) Hypothenar muscles Adductor pollicis Interossei Ulnar two lumbricals

TABLE 31-3 Upper extremity reflexes

Muscle	Root (predominant)
Biceps	C5
Brachioradialis	C6
Triceps	C7

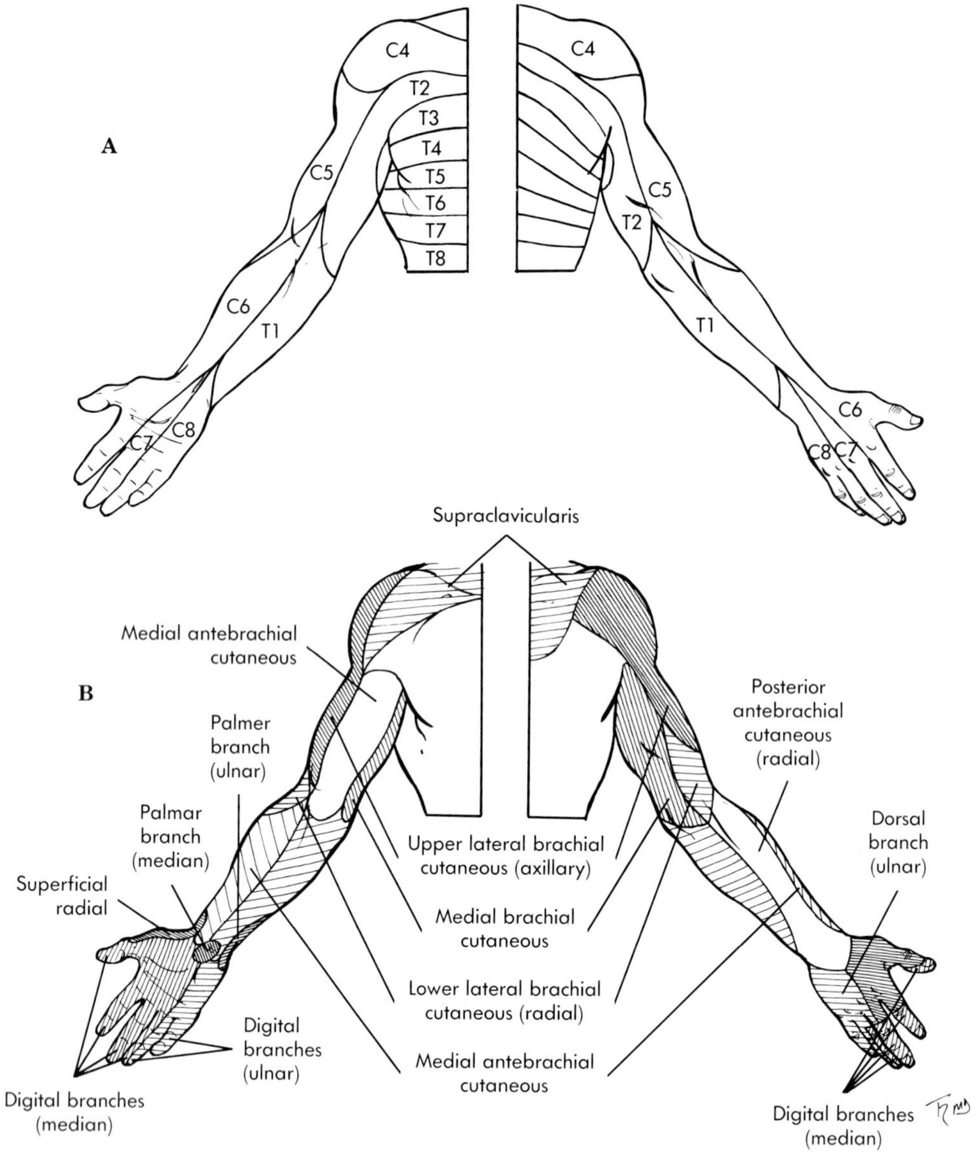

FIG. 31-4. Sensory distribution. **A,** Root dermatomes. **B,** Peripheral nerve distribution.

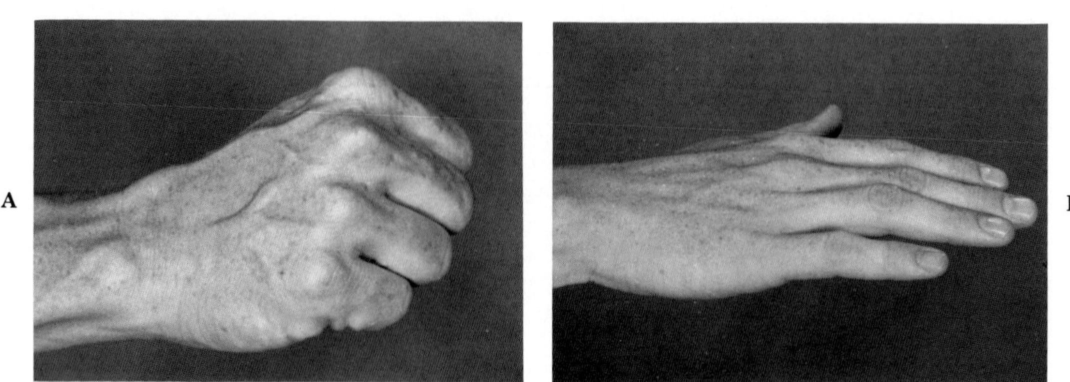

FIG. 31-5. Evaluation of axillary vein patency. **A,** Hand at side, normal prominent venous tone. **B,** Hand at heart level, veins collapse when axillary vein is patent. If appearance of hand is similar to **A,** axillary vein thrombosis is suspected.

from distal to proximal. The point of maximal pain may represent an entrapment lesion.

ADJUNCTIVE TESTS

The most commonly performed test for evaluation of neurologic injury is electrophysiologic examination. This includes two components—an electromyogram (EMG) and a nerve conduction study (NCS).

An EMG is performed by placing small needles into the muscle being evaluated and observing the nature of the electrical activity in the muscle. Complete denervation leads to absense of total electrical activity. Partial (acute) denervation, indicative of a lesion that has structural integrity of the nerve but functional loss, will present a pattern of fibrillations on the EMG evaluation. These patterns of injury will not generally appear until 2½ to 3 weeks after a neural injury. As healing occurs, these fibrillation potentials will disappear, often leaving a pattern of large motor units demonstrated by increased duration and amplitude of the motor units' potentials. This represents sprouting of the intact motor nerves to take over "orphaned" muscle cells. These large units can be found permanently in the EMG after significant injury, if repair occurs.

The NCS represents direct measurement of nerve conduction throughout the extremity. The measurements are obtained by direct stimulation of the nerve proximally in the extremity and measurement of the time until the impulse reaches a point more distal in the extremity. The standard nerve conduction velocities have been published and are readily available. In addition, the time of conduction across certain regions is also evaluated and compared with the opposite extremity, if uninvolved.

These measurements are known as latency and are typically calculated for the areas across the cubital tunnel (ulnar nerve), carpal tunnel (median nerve), and Guyon's canal (ulnar nerve). Prolonged latency implies a block in nerve conduction in the anatomic region being studied.

For vascular problems, invasive testing may be required. Arterial problems are often evaluated with arteriography. If a proximal lesion is suspected, a catheter can be inserted into the femoral artery and advanced to the aortic arch or subclavian artery. Here, contrast injection will define lesions at the subclavian, axillary, and brachial level. Distal lesions can be evaluated similarly or by a brachial contrast injection technique.

On the venous side, venography performed by contrast injection into the hand is indicated if venous occlusion is seriously suspected.

Other more elaborate tests of vascular function include Doppler ultrasound, impedance plethysmography, and vascular phase technetium scanning. These techniques are best used in conjunction with vascular surgeons as part of a comprehensive evaluation.

CLASSIFICATION OF TRAUMATIC NERVE INJURIES

In 1943, Seddon described a classification for traumatic nerve injuries. This classification is useful in describing the degree of injury and the potential for recovery.[91,99] The three classes are as follows:

Neuropraxia—a minimal nerve injury that leads to a temporary, fully reversible nerve conduction block.

Axonotmesis—a moderate injury in which there is interruption of the axons and their myelin sheaths. The endoneural tubes, however, remain intact to guide regeneration.

Neurotmesis—a severe injury in which a nerve is severed completely or destroyed and regeneration cannot occur spontaneously.

Most sports injuries result in either neuropraxia or axonotmesis. However, in moderate athletic trauma, nerves can be injured in such a way that a component of the nerve has a neurotmesis injury, but the majority of injury is usually axonotmesis.[106] Differentiation may be difficult clinically and electrophysiologically.

CRANIAL NERVE INJURIES

Spinal Accessory Nerve

The spinal accessory nerve (eleventh cranial nerve) is the sole motor nerve to the trapezius muscle. The superficial course of this nerve makes it susceptible to injury. The nerve lies in the subcutaneous tissue on the floor of the posterior cervical triangle in its course to innervate the trapezius muscle.[96] Blunt trauma and surgery in the posterior cervical triangle are the two predominant causes of injury to this nerve, resulting in paralysis of the trapezius muscle. This lesion, although uncommon, is painful, deforming, and disabling.

A direct, forceful blow to the neck in the area of the posterior cervical triangle can cause a crushing injury to the nerve where it passes under the upper border of the trapezius

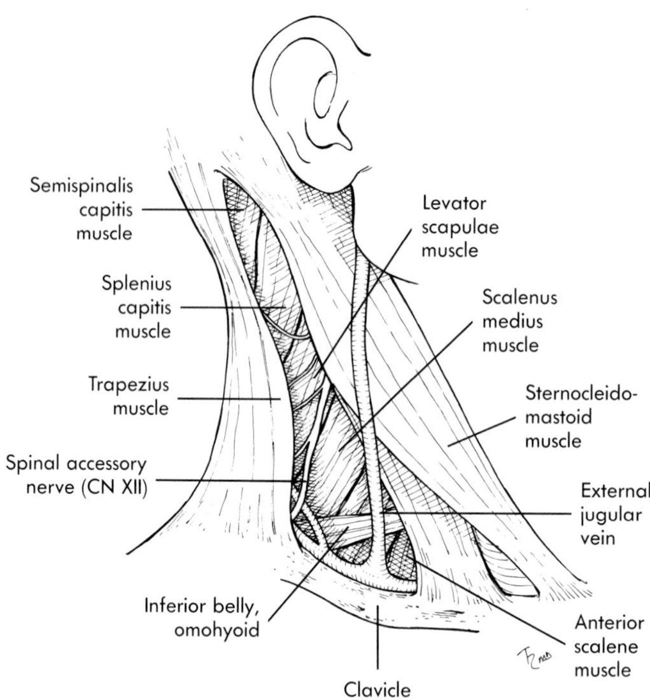

FIG. 31-6. Injury to the spinal accessory nerve can occur from blunt trauma in the region where the nerve crosses the border of the trapezius in the posterior cervical triangle.

(Fig. 31-6). This can be the result of contact between athletes or contact between an athlete and a piece of equipment. Another mechanism is an injury that depresses the shoulder while the head is forced in the opposite direction, resulting in a traction injury to the nerve.[110] Football, lacrosse, and hockey are some of the sports in which this type of injury has occurred.[53,108]

Manifestations of this injury include a dull ache or pain, with drooping of the shoulder and noticeable weakness in arm elevation and abduction. On examination, the patient is unable to shrug his or her shoulders and shows winging of the scapula when viewed from behind. The scapula is rotated downward and displaced laterally as a result of the lack of the suspensory action of the trapezius. This is because of the paralysis of the upper and central portion of the muscle that attaches to the acromion and normally pulls the shoulder upward and inward. The scapula is stabilized on the chest wall by the lower portion of the muscle, and this normal function, which prevents rotation and translation, is lost. The trapezius not only helps suspend the shoulder, but provides a firm base from which the deltoid muscle acts in elevating the arm. The pain is thought to be caused by overuse of the levator scapulae and rhomboid muscles and from brachial radiculitis caused by stretching of the brachial plexus.[13]

Initial treatment is conservative. The arm is put into a sling and physical therapy for active and passive exercise is provided to avoid contractures in the arm and shoulder. Paralysis may persist for 3 to 12 months in closed injuries. The function of the trapezius is so vital that even strengthening adjacent muscle groups is inadequate to compensate for the extensive lost functions.

For lesions caused by open trauma or iatrogenic injury, neurolysis and nerve grafting have given variable results, but are generally more successful when performed within 6 months. After 1 year, reconstructive procedures, using muscle transfers, are performed to improve shoulder function in isolated injuries,[13] whereas stabilization procedures are preferred for more widespread weakness and neuromuscular disorders.

Dynamic procedures that involve muscle transfers have consisted of transferring the levator scapulae and rhomboid muscles, the Eden-Lange procedure.[13,63] Static fixation of the scapula to the spinous processes has been done using fascia lata grafts.[28]

If the lesion is mild and reversible, athletic participation can be attempted when healing has occurred and dynamic stabilization of the scapula has been achieved through muscle rehabilitation and reeducation. For severe lesions, with little or no functional return, athletic participation will be restricted insofar as the involved extremity is concerned.

BRACHIAL PLEXUS PROBLEMS

The brachial plexus is formed by the ventral rami of cervical spinal nerves (C5 through 8 and T1). The nerves then emerge between the anterior and middle scalene muscles traveling below the sternocleidomastoid muscle and under the clavicle to the axilla. The ventral rami of the fifth and sixth spinal nerves interconnect to form the upper trunk, C7 continues as the middle trunk, and C8 and T1 combine to form the lower trunk. After decussation and reassembly, lateral, posterior, and medial cords are formed from which the terminal nerves to the arm are derived. Knowledge of the brachial plexus and its innervations is essential to proper diagnosis of injuries to this area, in addition to prognostic implications.

Acute Traumatic Injury

Because of its superficial location, surrounding bony structures, and the mobility of the neck and shoulders, the brachial plexus is vulnerable to injury. Traction injuries are found in various contact sports, such as football and wrestling.[3] The majority of information on brachial plexus injuries has come from cases of high-velocity trauma, such as motorcycle accidents.[66,89] Fracture-dislocations of the shoulder may also injure the brachial plexus, whereas dislocations without associated fractures usually injure the axillary nerve more than the brachial plexus. Clavicle fractures and their active callus or hematoma may also cause injury to the brachial plexus or chronic compression. Another example of brachial plexus compression occurs during hiking with heavy backpacks, when the brachial plexus is compressed between the clavicle and first rib by the weight of the pack and the shoulder straps (Fig. 31-7). Damage to the brachial plexus may also occur as root avulsions (Fig. 31-8). Cervical nerve root avulsion has a consistently poor prognosis because the nerve cannot be repaired and does not regenerate. Careful evaluation of brachial plexus injuries is essential in order to render appropriate treatment and prognosis.

Supraclavicular traction injuries of the brachial plexus have notoriously bad prognoses, probably because of the frequency of root avulsions.[89] In addition to a thorough examination, electromyography is a helpful adjunct in localizing injuries of the brachial plexus because the paraspinal muscles can be tested and will indicate the severity of nerve damage. Myelography can be used to show root avulsions by demonstrating pseudomeningoceles. Histamine skin testing helps to determine whether the sensory lesion is pre- or postganglionic. An absent flare response indicates a postganglionic injury and therefore a more favorable prognosis. Infraclavicular lesions have a relatively good prognosis with a return of motor function in the injured cord or terminal branch.[66,89] Lesions of the upper trunk are more common and have better prognoses than lesions of the lower trunk.[89] Persistent pain in the presence of a brachial plexus injury, regardless of its location, indicates a poor prognosis. The presence of Horner's syndrome is usually a bad prognostic sign in a brachial plexus injury as well.

Knowing the location of the injury (i.e., neuropraxia, axonotmesis, or neurotmesis and involvement of the cervical spinal roots), one can better anticipate the likelihood of spontaneous improvement or the need for surgery. In closed injuries, without a gross disruption in the brachial plexus, early institution of physical therapy is recommended to prevent contractures. Neuropraxic injuries

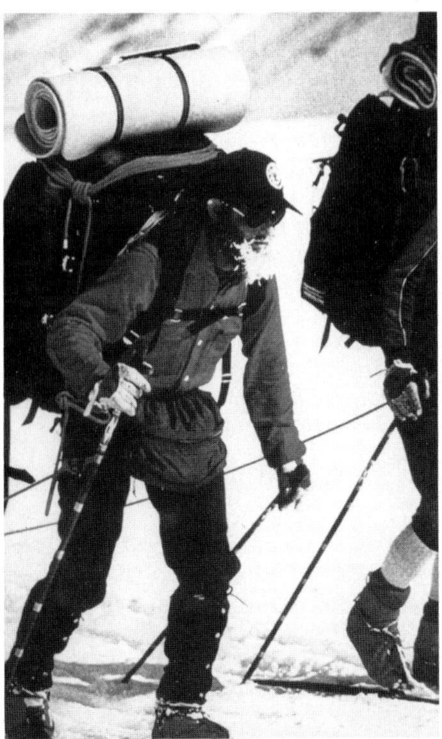

FIG. 31-7. Long periods of direct pressure by the axillary straps of heavy back pack can lead to plexus injury.

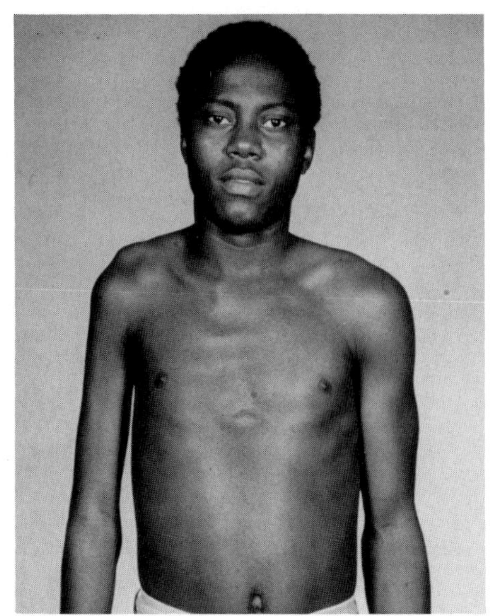

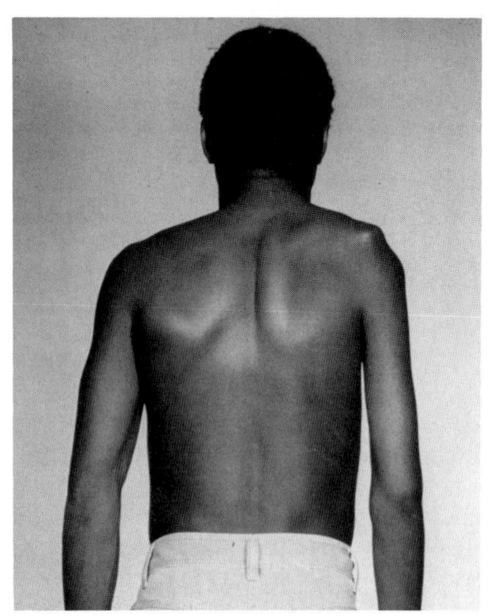

FIG. 31-8. A&B Sandlot football player with C5 C6 root avulsions. Injury occurred when shoulder struck ground and neck was driven to opposite side. Gross atrophy of deltoid biceps and spinati is present. Scapula is winging.

may take 3 to 4 months to show improvement. The majority of brachial plexus injuries in sports are low-velocity injuries, such as shoulder dislocations, with good prognoses for recovery because the nerves are in continuity and the lesion is either a neuropraxia or a axonotmesis. After 4 months of observation with no improvement, and electrophysiologic studies showing continued axonal degeneration, surgery may be indicated to either repair the disruption in the plexus or use cable nerve grafts. Emphasis is placed on restoring the nerve supply to proximal muscles because effective regeneration of nerves to muscles in the hand rarely occurs in adults. Approximately 2 years are required to obtain the axonal regeneration and return of function. At the end of this period, tendon transfers may be considered to improve the residual muscle function in the arm and shoulder.

The "Burner" Syndrome

The "burner" syndrome is a term used to describe a specific upper-trunk brachial plexus injury that occurs in contact sports.[11] It is most commonly seen in football and has also been termed upper trunk brachial plexopathy or the stinger syndrome.[85]

The brachial plexus consists of contributions of ventral rami of the fifth, sixth, seventh, and eighth cervical roots and the first thoracic root. Classically, burners involve the C5 and C6 components of the brachial plexus. The injury usually results from a player making head, neck, and/or shoulder contact with an opposing player.[85] The entire shoulder girdle is depressed in its relation to the neck. This mechanism is similar to the mechanism of an acromioclavicular sprain; however, the point of contact is somewhat different (Fig. 31-9). The player immediately feels a sharp burning pain in the shoulder, radiating into the arm and hand (Fig. 31-10). The pain is described as burning in nature, hence the origin of the descriptive name of this syndrome. The burning is accompanied by weakness of the biceps, spinati, and/or deltoid muscles, causing weakness in shoulder abduction, external rotation, and elbow flexion. The symptoms usually last for a few minutes, but may persist for 2 weeks or longer. Persistent pain and weakness beyond 2 weeks indicates a more severe injury to the brachial plexus. Clancy et al[21] have classified these lesions by their clinical features (Table 31-4). Some players experience repeated episodes of burners. Although permanent neurologic deficits are rare, they nevertheless have been reported.

It is important to repeatedly examine athletes who sustain a burner. Often weakness develops in the days or weeks following the injury. Repeated examination will identify those athletes in whom weakness develops in the postinjury period.

There is still some controversy with regard to the exact site and nature of the injury. It

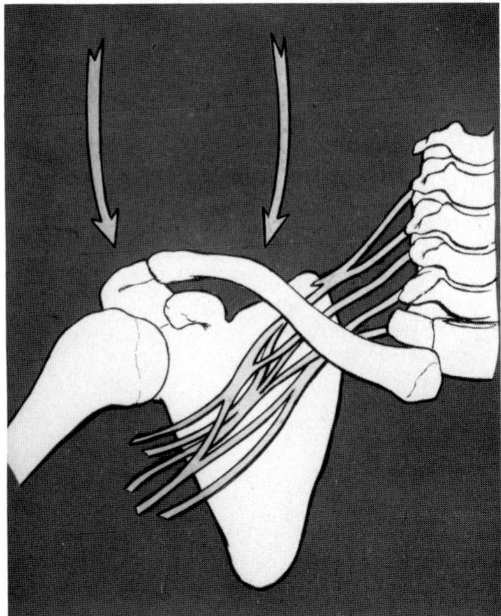

FIG. 31-9. Point of conduct is A-C joint injuries is over acromion (*left arrow*). In burner syndrome impact occurs more medially (right arrow).

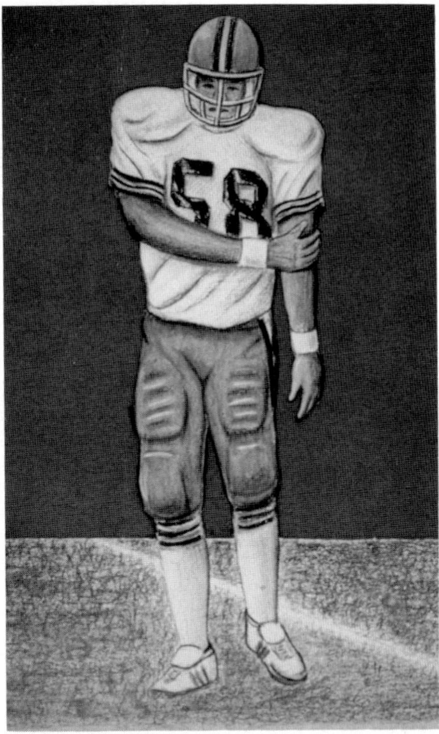

FIG. 31-10. Burner syndrome causes sharp burning pain in shoulder, arm and hand. The athlete may hold the affected arm as they leave field.

TABLE 31-4 Clinical classification of brachial plexus injuries

Grade	Findings
I	Transitory motor/sensory loss; may last minutes to hours; complete recovery within 2 weeks.
II	Significant motor weakness/sensory loss; neurologic examination abnormal at least 2 weeks.
III	Motor and sensory loss at least 1 year's duration.

From Clancy WG, Brand RL, and Bergfeld, JA: Am J Sports Med, 5:209, 1977.

is uncertain whether the injury is at the cervical root level,[20] ventral rami, or in the brachial plexus.[80] Many authors, however, believe the lesion in the true burner syndrome is at the upper trunk level.[11,21,85] Burners most often are a transitory physiologic block of some or all axons in the involved nerve and would be classified as a neuropraxia by Seddon's classification of nerve injury. Axonotmesis probably does occur in more severe injuries and would coincide with prolonged symptoms weeks from the time of injury. Electromyography can be helpful in defining the site and extent of the lesion after a period of 3 weeks from the time of the injury. The electromyographic findings compatible with a brachial plexopathy in a player with burners are fibrillation potentials demonstrated in the upper-trunk–innervated shoulder girdle musculature (deltoid, biceps, supraspinatus, and infraspinatus) and normal activity in the cervical paraspinal musculature. Often the lesion is mild electrophysiologically, and the site of injury may be difficult to determine.[106] Other studies have found fibrillation potentials in the neck muscles of players with burners consistent with cervical radiculopathy.

Cervical spine fracture or dislocation may evoke symptoms much like those seen with burners and central cervical spinal cord syndrome.[2,71] Therefore a player with an acute burner symptom should be treated as an unstable cervical spine injury because of the similarity in presentation. Roentgenographs and cervical cord evaluation will be negative in the burner syndrome.

Once the diagnosis has been made, the athlete with weakness should be restricted from competition and reexamined on a regular basis. When shoulder strength has returned to normal, participation in athletics can be resumed. Athletes will often use neck rolls; special pads, and extra high shoulder pads to help limit neck motion when they return to football

A

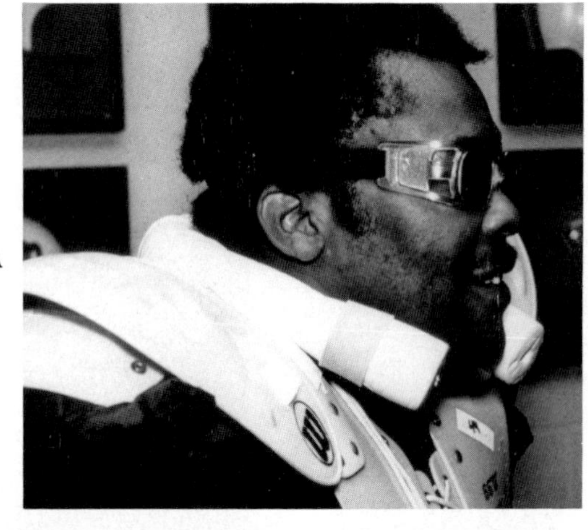

B

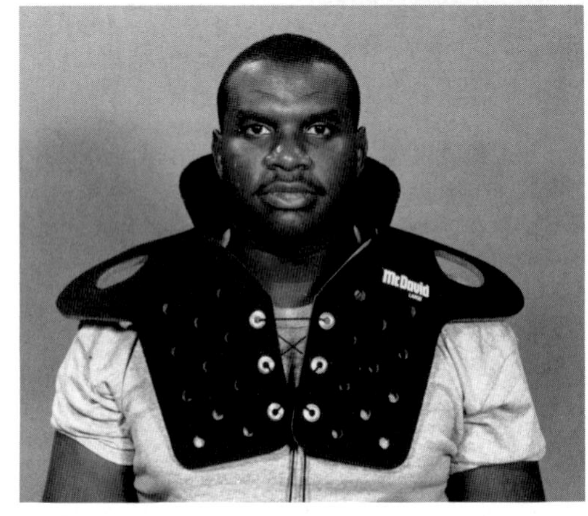

C

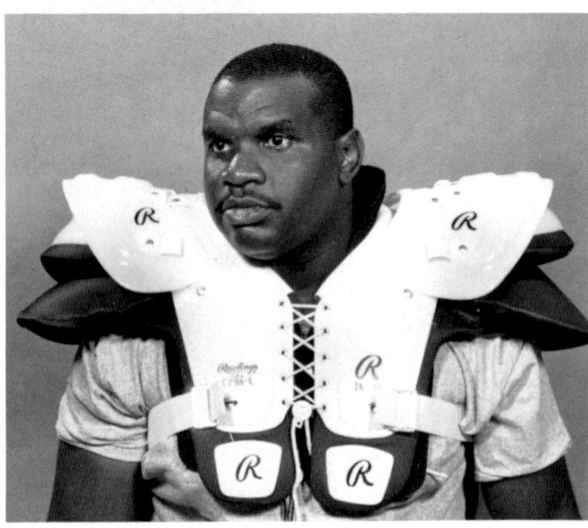

FIG. 31-11. Neck rolls. **A,** Under shoulder pad devices. **B,** High shoulder pads. **C,** Both pads somewhat limit neck mobility.

(Fig. 31-11). The efficacy of these pads is undetermined. All athletes should however participate in a neck, shoulder, and upper trunk strengthening program.

The EMG may remain abnormal for years, with large motor unit potentials commonly appearing, so repeat electromyography is not often indicated to determine the time for athletic return.[11] Rather, the return to normal strength should be the factor relied on in most situations.

Acute Brachial Neuropathy

Acute brachial neuropathy (ABN) is an uncommon cause of shoulder pain and disability. It can, however, present in association with athletic activity and must therefore be included in the differential diagnosis of athletes with shoulder pain.[51]

ABN is a clinical entity of unknown cause, characterized by the acute or subacute onset of shoulder pain associated with weakness and sometimes with wasting of various forequarter muscles.[102] Involvement is most common in the shoulder and proximal arm. This syndrome can develop in athletes during or following their athletic activity, but the onset cannot usually be related to a specific traumatic event.[51] Characteristically, pain is severe and continues despite cessation of activity. Physical examination often reveals scapular winging, weakness (deltoid, supraspinatus, infraspinatus, biceps, and/or triceps most commonly), and occasional sensory deficit. Electromyography usually reveals diffuse plexus involvement.

Once the entity is diagnosed, treatment consists of two phases.[51] In phase 1, support for the affected extremity, rest, and analgesics are indicated. Gentle range of motion exercises are important to maintain joint mobility. Once the severe pain has resolved, the athlete enters phase 2, or the rehabilitative phase. The entire extremity and upper body requires rehabilitation to regain strength in damaged motor units. The need for rehabilitation of all muscles in the upper body must be emphasized because subclinical muscle involvement is common in this entity. Likewise, the trunk-scapula relationship must be considered because serratus anterior and rhomboid involvement frequently occurs.

The issue of returning to sports is difficult to address because the number of athletes reported with this condition is small. Return to participation can generally be considered on a case by case basis when individuals have reached a plateau in their strength development. Athletes should be told at the outset that scapula winging may persist because improvement is generally not observed in this aspect of ABN.[51]

Neurologic Thoracic Outlet Syndrome

Thoracic outlet compression syndrome refers to an uncommon condition in which nerves or vessels or both are compressed in the root of the neck or axilla. Two clearly defined forms of this condition have been described.[25,30,33] One is a neurologic syndrome that involves the lower trunk of the brachial plexus and is caused by abnormal nerve stretch and/or compression.[25] Another is a vascular form that involves the subclavian artery and vein and is more common in men than in women.[30,33] Although there are no reports of specific sports causing this problem, athletic activities that involve the use of the upper limbs will exacerbate the symptoms.[82] Depending upon the mechanism and level of compression, several disorders are included under the title of thoracic outlet syndrome: cervical rib syndrome, scalenus-anticus syndrome, Wright's hyperabduction syndromes (including pectoralis minor syndrome), and costoclavicular syndrome.*

The neurologic form of thoracic outlet syndrome often occurs in women of slim build and drooping shoulders. Presenting symptoms include aching pain in the side or back of the neck that extends across the shoulder and down the arm along the inner aspect of the arm and parasthesias in the ulnar aspect of the hand. The sensory findings extend more proximally than an ulnar nerve lesion, whereas the motor findings include thenar and intrinsic muscle weakness and wasting.[25,65,82,88]

Anatomically, an elongated transverse process of C7 and a cervical rib may be found. A fibrous band often extends from the cervical rib to the first thoracic rib, and the lower brachial trunk is stretched and angulated over this band.[88,107] Damage to the C8 and T1 spinal nerves from other causes must be ruled out, such as Pancoast tumor, neurofibromas, cervical spondylosis, cervical disk herniation, carpal tunnel syndrome, and cubital tunnel syndrome.

Symptoms of neurologic thoracic outlet syndrome

- Aching neck pain
- Radiation into arm, forearm (ulnar side)
- Parasthesias, ulnar aspect of hand
- Intrinsic muscle weakness

Evaluation should include cervical spine and chest roentgenographs. At times, electrophysiologic studies can be useful, and reduced ulnar sensory nerve action potentials (SNAP) can be recorded.[107] To rule out other diseases that can cause C8 and T1 spinal nerve root pathologic conditions, myelography and CAT scans can also be indicated as part of the workup.

Once the diagnosis of a neurologic thoracic outlet syndrome is made, every effort should be made to manage the patient conservatively.[65] Shoulder muscle exercises are often prescribed, along with local heat and a cervical collar. Surgery should be reserved for persistent symptoms for up to 3 or 4 months unless there is intractable pain, vascular compromise, or neurologic loss.[87] Supraclavicular exploration with division of the fibrous band, if present, is the recommended approach, whereas the transaxillary approach is used for first rib resection.[33,45] While relief of pain is consistent, muscle weakness and wasting do not usually resolve significantly.

AXILLARY VESSEL INJURY

Vascular Thoracic Outlet Syndrome

The vascular form of thoracic outlet syndrome (TOS) is uncommon. It is characterized by a well-developed cervical rib producing stenosis and poststenotic dilation of the subclavian artery.[30] The subclavian artery is angulated over the cervical rib and further compressed by the scalenus anterior muscle anterior to it.[33] The initial symptoms may vary from intermittent blanching of the hand and fingers as a result of embolization from a thrombus in the subclavian artery to a sudden catastrophic occlusion.

Evaluation should include examination and auscultation of the supraclavicular fossa for the presence of a mass and a bruit. The pulses in the arm may be absent or diminished. The Adson test can be used to reproduce the symptoms by abducting and externally rotating the arm and raising the hand above the head. If

*References 15, 30, 45, 66, 103, 107, 109.

the radial pulse disappears, then a lesion of the subclavian artery should be suspected. Unfortunately, this maneuver is of questionable value because up to 80% of healthy people will demonstrate a positive test.[107] Another provocative test is to have the patient raise both arms overhead and rapidly open and close his or her hand; this will cause cramping very quickly if vascular TOS is present.[107]

The diagnosis is confirmed by angiography, and the treatment is usually first rib resection.[30,87,103] If acute occlusion of the subclavian artery has occurred, then immediate surgery is indicated with first rib resection, removal of the thrombus, and embolectomy. Axillary artery injury has been reported in shoulder dislocation, scapular neck fracture, humeral neck fracture, and clavicle fracture. Examination will show a diminished pulse in the involved extremity; the color and temperature may or may not be decreased, depending on the extent of injury. A difference in the blood pressure between the two limbs can be measured. If a major vascular injury is suspected, an angiogram is mandatory. Vascular repair is performed along with stabilization of an unstable fracture, if present.

Subclavian Vein Thrombosis

"Effort" thrombosis is a term used to describe a subclavian and axillary vein thrombosis caused by direct or indirect injury to the vein as a result of physical activity.[1] This is a form of thoracic outlet syndrome that accounts for less than 2% of all reported incidents of deep-vein thrombosis. This entity has been reported in competitive swimmers[105] and hockey players.[18] Effort thrombosis has important short-term ramifications, such as severe disability and pulmonary embolism, that have been reported to occur in 12% of patients with subclavian vein thrombosis.[6]

The symptoms and disability may persist for a prolonged period of time in 68% to 75% of cases. Although the majority of cases result from trauma or use of cervical venous catheters, a small portion of the cases are related to various activities that require shoulder abduction.

The clinical presentation of effort thrombosis varies dramatically from intermittent, nonspecific symptoms that consist of a generalized aching of the arm, with a degree of fullness and swelling, to a dramatically swollen, painful arm with dependent rubor. Typically, this occurs in males 15 to 40 years of age, often after a particular physical activity. The symptoms may appear immediately or up to 2 weeks later. The most common symptom noted with time is increased swelling of the arm, which responds to elevation. Swelling may be accompanied by abnormal subcutaneous vein distention, which worsens if the arm is exercised.

A venogram will demonstrate occlusion of the axillary and subclavian veins, although the study itself may result in extension of the thrombosis. Doppler studies have been useful in distinguishing intermittent compression from thrombosis.

The recommended treatment of effort-induced thrombosis is usually conservative. A strict regimen of arm elevation is begun, and the patient is anticoagulated with heparin for 10 days.[70] At that time, conversion to warfarin is done to achieve therapeutic levels that prevent extension of the clot and promote recanalization of the vein.

Some of the chronic symptoms noted by patients who have had this entity include easy fatigability of the arm, recurrent swelling, and tightness in the arm. Surgical intervention with thrombectomy may be indicated if a localized thrombus is present in order to avoid the high risk of chronic symptoms. Surgery is not indicated if an extensive thrombus is present. Chronic symptoms have been reported in 75% of patients treated conservatively. Early clot dissolution with intravenous streptokinase has been achieved with success, provided the clot is less than 2 weeks old.[9]

Other procedures attempted have included decompression of the costoclavicular space and removal of the clavicle or anterior scalene muscle and local fibrinolytic therapy and first rib resection when the clot has resolved.

PERIPHERAL NERVE LESIONS

Shoulder Region

Long Thoracic Nerve

Isolated paralysis of the serratus anterior muscle has been described in a wide variety of sports, including tennis, golf, gymnastics, soccer, bowling, weight lifting, ice hockey, wrestling, archery, basketball, and football.[46] The long thoracic nerve originates from the ventral rami of C5, C6, and C7 cervical nerves and travels beneath the brachial plexus and clavicle over the first rib. The nerve then travels along the lateral aspect of the chest wall to innervate the serratus anterior muscle (Fig. 31-12). Its superficial course and length make it especially vulnerable to injury. Damage to the nerve may be caused by blows to either the shoulder or lateral thoracic wall. Excessive use of the shoulder or prolonged traction,

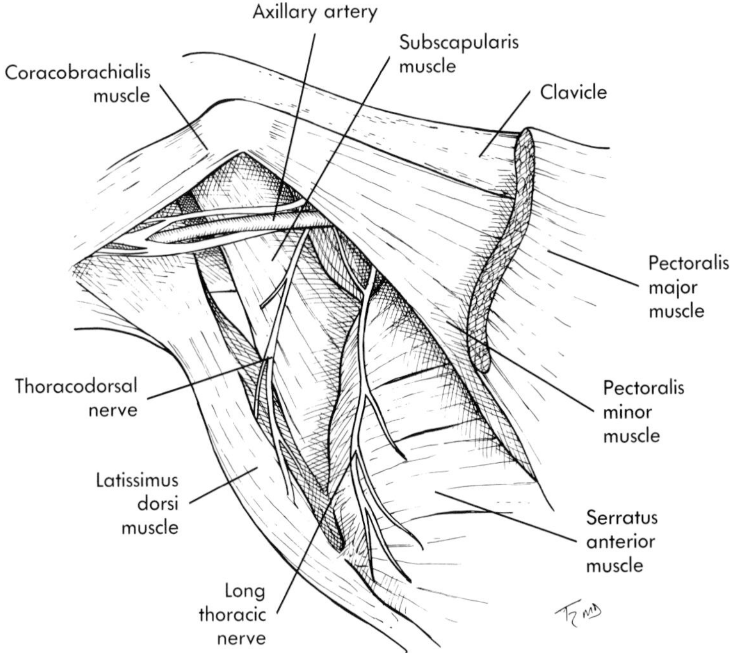

FIG. 31-12. Course of the long thoracic nerve.

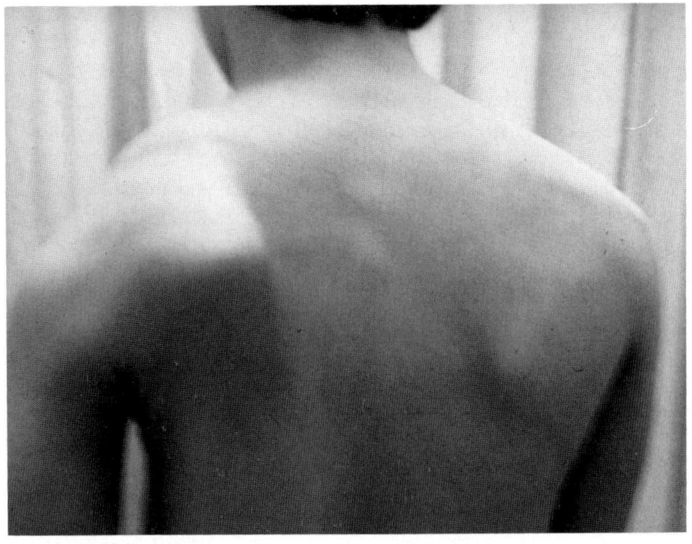

FIG. 31-13. Winging of the left scapula in a weight lifter with injury to the long thoracic nerve.

such as in cycling, have been found to cause this nerve injury.

The clinical features include dull ache or pain around the shoulder girdle, a winged scapula, and decreased active shoulder motion.[37,58] Pain may be increased when the head is tilted to the contralateral side or when the ipsilateral arm is raised above the head. Often, painless winging of the scapula may be the clinical presentation of someone involved in any of the sports mentioned above. Winging of the scapula is especially prominent during forward pushing, as in push-ups (Fig. 31-13). More severe pain is usually indicative of an acute brachial plexus neuropathy with involvement of other muscles of the arm and shoulder.[51] An idiopathic form of serratus anterior paralysis has been identified. The term "neuralgic amyotrophy" was coined by Parsonage and Turner in 1948 to describe the shoulder girdle syndrome or paralytic brachial neuritis that occasionally may affect only the long thoracic nerve.[76]

The serratus anterior stabilizes the scapula on the posterior thoracic wall, thereby providing a firm point for muscles arising from the scapula to move the arm. The serratus anterior, together with the trapezius and levator scapulae, act to upwardly rotate the scapula and thus allow greater glenohumeral motion.

Other conditions, such as polymyositis, muscular dystrophy, and cervical spondylosis, must be ruled out.[58] Electromyographic findings of denervation have proved valuable in the diagnosis and prognosis of this injury.

There is no consensus on treatment of this condition, but generally, conservative measures, such as rest from the associated sport and physical therapy, are advised. The prognosis for serratus anterior paralysis is generally good, with recovery occurring up to 2 years after injury.[44]

Return to sports can be considered when the shoulder girdles have symmetric strength parity. The likelihood of complete resolution of scapula winging is low and should not be used as a criterion for return to athletics.

Suprascapular Nerve

The suprascapular nerve originates from the upper trunk of the brachial plexus and consists of contributions from the fifth and sixth cervical roots. The nerve runs in the posterior triangle of the neck, passing under the body of the omohyoid muscle and anterior border of the trapezius muscle to the scapular notch, where it is firmly fixed in a fibroosseous tunnel. The nerve runs through the scapular notch, which is covered by the transverse scapular ligament, to innervate the supraspinatus muscle, and gives off sensory fibers to the capsular and ligamentous structures of the shoulder and acromioclavicular joint (Fig. 31-14). The majority of entrapment neuropathies of the suprascapular nerve reported have been in the area involving the transverse scapular ligament.[22,47] The nerve then continues around the lateral border of the spine of the scapula, through the spinoglenoid notch, to innervate the infraspinatus muscle. Entrapment here would give symptoms of infraspinatus muscle involvement.

Entrapment of the suprascapular nerve has been associated with traction injuries to the shoulder and with repetitive use of the shoulder.[38] Direct trauma to the shoulder, including shoulder dislocation or fracture, is the most common cause of suprascapular nerve injury.[111]

Activities such as weight lifting, volleyball,[36] and backpacking have been found to cause this rare nerve entrapment syndrome, with trauma from cross-body adduction being implicated in a neuropraxia type of injury to the nerve.[35] Asymptomatic isolated infraspinatus muscle paralysis has been found in volleyball players as a result of cocking of the arm and follow-through while serving.[36]

Clinical findings include atrophy of the supraspinatus and/or infraspinatus muscles (Fig. 31-15) and poorly localized pain in the posterolateral aspect of the scapula. There is often a loss of strength in abduction and external rotation of the arm.[97] Rotator cuff patho-

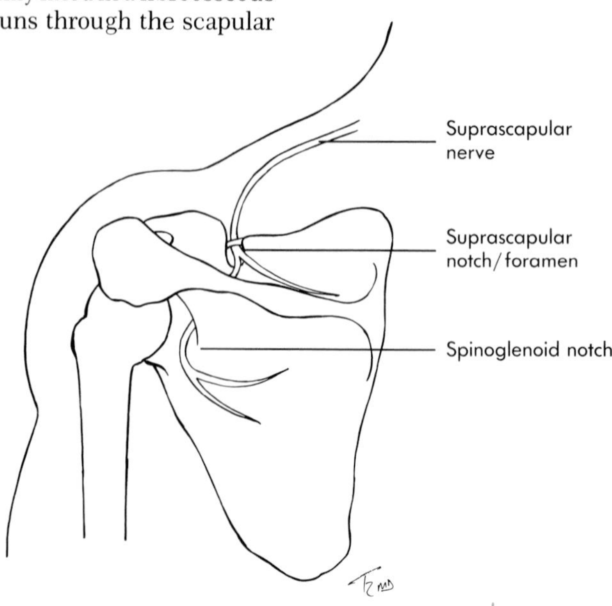

FIG. 31-14. Course of the suprascapular nerve. Entrapment can occur at the suprascapular notch or spinoglenoid notch.

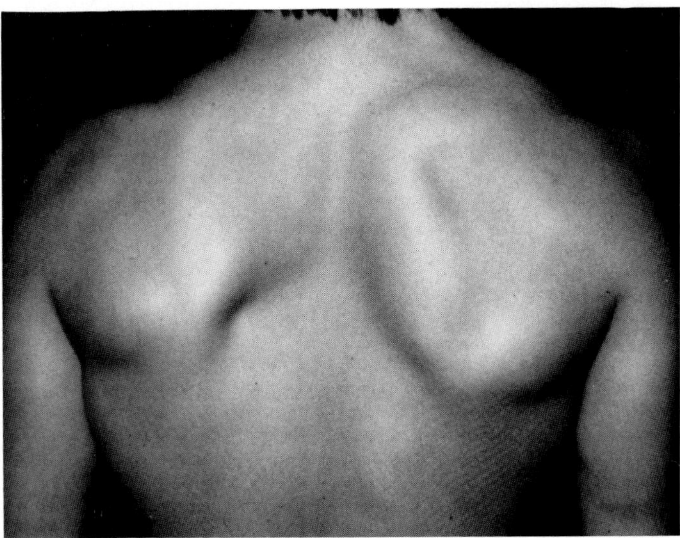

FIG. 31-15. Wrestler with suprascapular nerve injury at suprascapular notch. Observe atrophy of infraspinatus notch and supraspinatus fossa.

logic conditions must be considered in the differential diagnosis in addition to cervical radiculopathy, myopathy, and brachial plexus neuropathy.

Often, roentgenographic, electromyographic, and nerve conduction studies confirm the clinical picture of suprascapular nerve entrapment at the suprascapular or spinoglenoid notch. Conservative therapy with rest, antiinflammatory medication, and physical therapy may be unsuccessful in relieving the symptoms, and surgical decompression may be necessary.[47,100] Explorations of the suprascapular nerve have revealed hypertrophy of the transverse scapular ligament and anomalies of the suprascapular notch. Compression of the spinoglenoid notch has also been identified.

The surgical procedures have ranged from excision of the transverse scapular ligament or spinoglenoid ligament to deepening the suprascapular notch.[39,81] Ganglion cysts often have been found to compress the suprascapular nerve at the notch of the scapula.[54,74,101] The clinical response to decompression of the nerve has varied from no improvement to full restoration of muscle bulk and power and resolution of pain.[47,104]

If return of supraspinatus and infraspinatus function occurs, resumption of participation in athletics can occur. However, since the infraspinatus supplies 90% of the external rotation power of the shoulder and the supraspinatus stabilizes the humeral head in the genoid during elevation, residual weakness will often preclude a safe return to athletics, as the deficits make safe participation difficult to achieve.

Axillary Nerve

The axillary nerve branches from the posterior cord of the brachial plexus and contains fibers from the C5 and C6 nerve roots. The nerve then travels laterally and downward, passing just below the shoulder joint and into the quadrilateral space. The axillary nerve next curves around the posterior and lateral portion of the proximal humerus, divides into anterior and posterior branches, and innervates the deltoid and teres minor muscles (Fig. 31-16). A cutaneous sensory branch of the nerve supplies the lateral aspect of the upper arm.

The usual mechanism of injury to the axillary nerve is trauma, either a direct blow to the shoulder,[12] fracture of the proximal humerus,[14] or a shoulder dislocation, all of which cause stretching of the nerve. Axillary nerve injuries occur in many sports, such as football, wrestling, gymnastics, mountain climbing, or rugby.[8] When the arm is displaced away from the trunk, tension is placed on the nerves. This tension or stretch is most severe for the nerves with the shortest distance from the brachial plexus to their muscle insertion. This would help explain the frequent involvement of the axillary nerve in injuries to the shoulder.

The degree of injury to the axillary nerve can vary. The initial presentation may be weakness in elevation and abduction of the arm, with or without numbness along the lateral aspect of the upper arm. Weakness in abduction may not be readily apparent because the supraspinatus alone may effectively abduct the arm. Wasting of the deltoid muscle subsequently develops (Fig. 31-17). When-

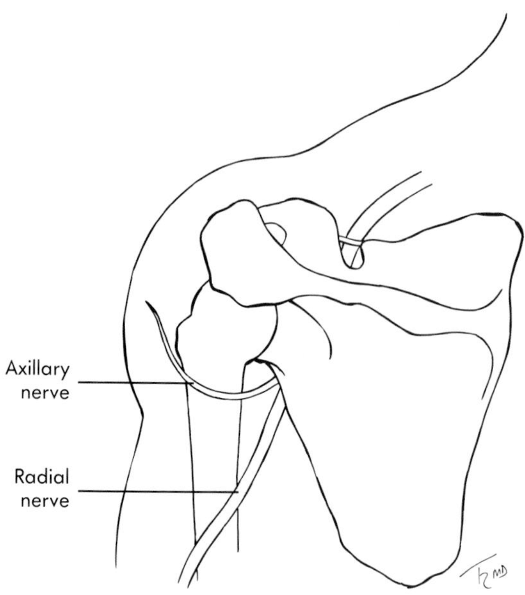

FIG. 31-16. Course of the axillary nerve as it travels posterior to the proximal humerus.

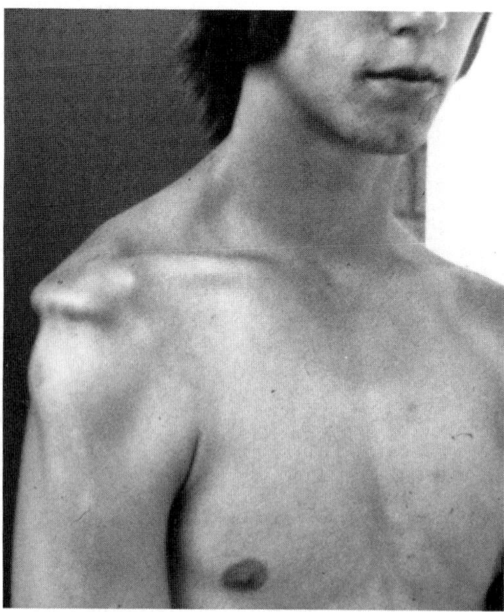

FIG. 31-17. Wasting of the deltoid from isolated axillary nerve injury.

ever an axillary nerve injury is considered, one must rule out a posterior cord injury by testing the latissimus dorsi muscle, the nerve of which branches proximal to the axillary nerve, and by testing the muscles innervated by the radial nerve.

Electrophysiologic testing can be used to determine whether there has been a partial or complete axillary nerve injury. If the injury is partial, the treatment is rest, physical therapy, and a sling. Because of the short course of the axillary nerve, some degree of recovery should be expected within 3 months. Surgical intervention is recommended if there is no sign of improvement by 3 to 4 months. Exploration and neurolysis or nerve grafting often give good results.[77] With any form of treatment, participation in athletics can be resumed when strength parity has been achieved.

Quadrilateral Space Syndrome

The quadilateral space syndrome involves compression of the posterior humeral circumflex artery and axillary nerve. The quadilateral space is on the posterior aspect of the shoulder and its boundaries are: the teres minor superiorly, teres major inferiorly, humeral shaft laterally, and the long head of the triceps muscle medially. The axillary nerve and posterior humeral circumflex artery pierce the internervous plane between the teres minor and teres major, supplying the teres minor and deltoid muscles.[19] A sensory branch innervates the skin on the lateral aspect of the upper arm.

Although it is an uncommon syndrome it has been reported in young people of both sexes.[19] The atypical distribution of pain and paresthesias often result in a delay in diagnosis. The pain is usually intermittant and poorly localized to the anterior aspect of the shoulder. There may be tenderness in the shoulder anteriorly and laterally, often with point tenderness at the insertion of the teres minor. The paresthesias have a nondermatomal distribution in the arm, forearm, and hand. Abduction, elevation, and external rotation of the humerus reproduce or exacerbate the symptoms. There may be a diminished radial pulse with this maneuver which may lead to an erroneous diagnosis of thoracic outlet syndrome. There is no muscle atrophy or neurologic deficit although associated nerve compression syndromes such as carpal tunnel syndrome have been reported.[19] Electrophysiologic testing of the deltoid muscle is normal. Cervical spine and other shoulder diseases such as rotator cuff disease must be differentiated since the pain may awaken the patient at night.

A subclavian arteriogram is used to confirm the diagnosis of quadrilateral space syndrome. The anteriogram is performed with the arm at the side initially and in abduction and external rotation of the arm. The dye is followed laterally to the posterior humeral circumflex artery which will be patent when the arm is at the side and may occlude with the arm in 60 degrees or more of abduction and some external rotation. Bilateral anteriograms are

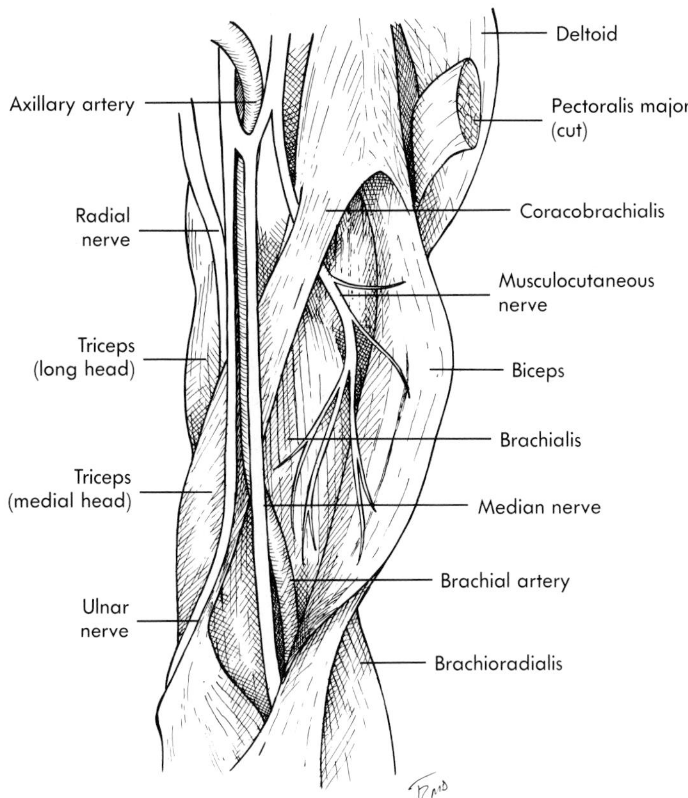

FIG. 31-18. Course of the musculocutaneous nerve in the cutaneous branch of the arm (not shown) continues distally to forearm.

not indicated. About 70% of patients with arteriograms showing occlusion of the posterior humeral circumflex artery do not have symptoms severe enough to undergo surgical decompression and live with their discomfort which may persist.

Surgical decompression of the quadilateral space is performed by detaching the insertion of the teres minor to the humerus and reflecting it medially, thus removing the superior obstruction of the quadrilateral space. Often one finds tethering fibrous bands overlying the neurovascular bundle. After division of these bands, the arm is brought into 110 degrees abduction and 45 degrees external rotation and the pulse should be palpable in the posterior humeral circumflex vessel. The patient is begun an early active range of motion and then muscle strengthening exercises at three weeks.

Elbow Region

Musculocutaneous Nerve

The musculocutaneous nerve is a mixed motor and sensory peripheral nerve that arises from the lateral cord of the brachial plexus and contains fibers from the C5, C6, and C7 nerve roots. The nerve pierces the coracobrachialis muscle below the coracoid process and travels down the arm between the biceps and brachialis muscles, which it also supplies (Fig. 31-18). The sensory component then continues lateral to the biceps and becomes superficial anterolaterally as it penetrates the deep brachial fascia above the elbow. At this point it becomes the lateral cutaneous nerve of the forearm. In its superficial course, the nerve travels through the antecubital fossa between the median cubital vein and cephalic vein. The anterior division of the nerve supplies sensation to the radial half of the volar aspect of the forearm, while the posterior branch supplies the radial third of the dorsal aspect of the forearm.

The presentation of musculocutaneous nerve compression varies according to the site of the lesion.[62] In addition to shoulder dislocations, injury to the nerve proximal to its innervation of the coracobrachialis muscle has been reported to occur in an athlete after throwing a football. The findings in such a case consisted of weakness in elbow flexion, atrophy of the brachialis and biceps brachii, a dull ache in the distal forearm with dysesthesias, and absence of reflex in the biceps. Electrophysiologic studies confirmed the location of the lesion. After 4 months, the neuropraxia resolved with resolution of the symptoms.

Weight lifting has also been associated with musculocutaneous neuropathy below the level of the coracobrachialis muscle that manifested painless weakness and atrophy of biceps muscle and dysesthesia in the volar radial forearm. Strenuous exercise was thought to cause either repetitive injury to the nerve by the coracobrachialis muscle or chronic compression as a result of muscle hypertrophy.[16] Cessation of weight lifting resulted in resolution of the symptoms up to 2 months later.

Positioning the arm in abduction, external rotation, and extension while the patient is under general anesthesia has also resulted in musculocutaneous nerve injury.

This syndrome may be confused with a C5 or C6 radioculopathy, brachial plexus injury (especially one involving the lateral cord), and rupture of the biceps tendon. Differentiation is based on careful clinical examination of other muscle groups innervated by the C5 and C6 nerve roots, sensory examination, and electrophysiologic testing.

A compression syndrome of the lateral cutaneous branch of the musculocutaneous nerve has also been described.[7,35] Symptoms include pain, paresthesias, dysesthesias, and numbness in the distal volar and dorsal forearm. Pain and tenderness are experienced over the nerve in the anterolateral aspect of the elbow or over the lateral humeral epicondyle and may be caused by compression of the nerve between the biceps aponeurosis and tendon against the fascia of the brachialis muscle. The nerve is relatively fixed in this area and injury can result from entrapment and compression.

Vigorous exercise consisting of elbow extension and forearm pronation or resisted elbow flexion has been associated with this compression syndrome.[7] Repeated elbow hyperextension, as occurs in backhanding the ball in racquetball and tennis or carrying heavy packages, is also associated with this sensory neuropathy. Occasionally, repeated pronation and supination of the forearm exacerbates the symptoms. Handbag paresthesia is a condition reported to have occurred because of nerve compression caused by the strap of a heavy bag over the antecubital fossa.[48]

Lateral epicondylitis, cervical radiculopathy, brachial plexopathy, median nerve compression, and ruptured biceps brachii should be differentiated on physical examination and electrophysiologic testing.

Initial treatment of compression of the musculocutaneous nerve at the elbow is nonoperative, consisting of rest, restriction of activities, oral antiinflammatory drugs, and the use of slings and posterior splints to prevent full elbow extension and pronation. If symptoms persist beyond 6 to 12 weeks, then injection of steroids and local anesthetic into the musculocutaneous tunnel at the elbow may be attempted.

After approximately 12 weeks of nonoperative therapy, surgical decompression at the elbow is advised. Unlike proximal musculocutaneous nerve compression, which often resolves spontaneously, compression at the elbow persisted in 7 of 11 cases reported by Bassett and Nunley.[7] All of the patients recovered fully after surgical decompression. A triangular wedge of biceps tendon was excised at the level of the lacertus fibrosus, where the tendon was noted to compress the musculocutaneous nerve against the fascia of the brachialis muscle.

Median Nerve

The median nerve is formed by fibers from C5 to C7 spinal nerves from the lateral cord and C8 and T1 fibers from the medial cord. The nerve runs near the brachial artery, toward the elbow on the medial side (Fig. 31-19).

The nerve passes medial to the biceps tendon and brachial artery at the elbow and courses between the superficial and deep head of the pronator teres, where it is often compressed. Another area of compression is under the tendinous insertion of the flexor digitorum superficialis, an area called the sublimis arch. At this level, a posterior branch of the median nerve arises—the anterior interosseous nerve. This nerve travels under the sublimis bridge and continues distally between the anterior interosseous membrane and the flexor digitorum profundus muscle.

Pronator teres syndrome in athletes is uncommon but has been reported in baseball players.[5] With today's training programs for development of muscle strength, it is surprising that athletes do not more frequently manifest entrapment from repetitive trauma to the nerves.

Four sites have been identified with entrapment of the median nerve in the elbow region[49,50,59,93,94]:

1. Medial supracondylar process and the ligament of Struthers
2. Lacertus fibrosis
3. Between the two heads of the pronator teres muscle
4. Arch of the flexor digitorum superficialis

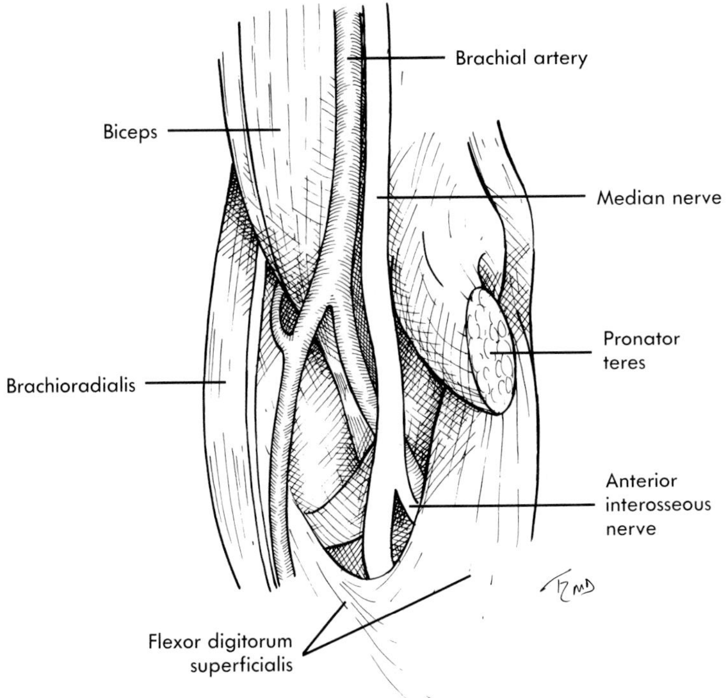

FIG. 31-19. Medial nerve lying medial to the brachial artery. It courses between the heads of the pronator teres and beneath the flexor digitorum superficalis arch—two areas of potential compression.

The median nerve at these levels carries both motor and sensory fibers to the volar forearm flexors (except for the flexor carpi ulnaris), the medial half of the flexor digitorum profundis, and the median-innervated intrinsics. Therefore both sensory and motor findings may be found. Usually there is an aching pain in the volar forearm over the pronator muscle. The pain is worsened by activity, especially repeated pronation movements with the elbow in extension. Altered sensation is found in the medial innervated thumb and digits. Weakness in finger flexion is uncommon, but, if present, is not limited to interphalangeal joint weakness of the thumb and distal interphalangeal joint weakness of the index finger, as in anterior interosseous syndrome. Often the symptoms can be elicited by resistance to forearm pronation and wrist flexion. Tinel's sign may be positive over the pronator muscle. Electrophysiologic studies may or may not be positive. A positive Phalen wrist flexion test may be positive, and this can cloud the diagnosis.

Pronator syndrome

- Volar proximal forearm pain
- Pain worsened with activity
- Abnormal sensibility in volar thumb, index, and middle fingers
- Finger flexor weakness (variable)
- Tinel's sign over pronator teres

On the basis of clinical findings, a 6-month course of conservative treatment is recommended, provided there are minimal or no motor deficits, once the diagnosis of pronator teres syndrome is made. Cessation of repeated pronation is especially advised.

Exploration of the median nerve at the elbow requires extensive surgery to decompress the four possible sites of compression described above.[59,93,94]

Adequate decompression usually affords relief of symptoms in recalcitrant cases. In resistant cases, transfer of the superficial head of the pronator teres posterior to the median nerve may be necessary.

Anterior Interosseous Nerve

The anterior interosseous nerve is a motor branch of the median nerve that arises at or just above the level of the flexor digitorum superficialis arch. It courses distally to innervate the flexor pollicis longus, flexor digitorum profundus (index and sometimes long finger), and pronator quadratus.

A compression neuropathy is often manifested by proximal forearm pain that is made worse with exercise. There is no sensory disturbance in the forearm or hand. The key clinical findings are weakness or paralysis of the anterior interosseous-nerve–innervated muscles.[52] A typical abnormal pinch attitude can be elicited, consisting of extension of the distal interphalangeal joint of the index finger and interphalangeal joint of the thumb, resulting from weakness of the flexor pollicis longus and flexor digitorum profundus to the index finger.[91]

In about 15% of patients, there may be a Martin-Gruber connection, which transports ulnar fibers in the median nerve to the ulnar nerve in the forearm.[95] If present, entrapment of the anterior interosseous nerve will then cause intrinsic muscle paralysis in the hand.

A wide variety of clinical problems can create anterior interosseous nerve syndrome.[34,92,94] Variations in attachment of muscle tendon units, enlarged bursae, thrombosed ulnar collateral blood vessels, tumors, or anomalous passage of the radial artery can be the initiating problem. More commonly, fascial bands on the deep head of the pronator teres or a portion of the tendinous origin of the flexor superficialis are responsible for the compression.[92] Careful electrophysiologic testing often can ascertain the site and extent of neural compression.

There are several reports of anterior interosseous neuropathy occurring after excessive forearm exercise, presumably as a result of compression by the muscles through which the nerve travels.[52] Symptoms resolve quickly when the exercise is stopped. A patient with acute shoulder and arm pain who displays signs of an anterior interosseous neuropathy may have an acute brachial plexus neuropathy with involvement of the fascicles going to the anterior interosseous nerve.[84]

Exploration of the anterior interosseous nerve is recommended if spontaneous improvement is not noted in 6 to 8 weeks.

Radial Nerve

The radial nerve consists of nerve fibers from C5 to T1 spinal nerve roots that travel in the posterior cord of the brachial plexus after giving off the thoracodorsal and axillary branches. The nerve travels down the upper arm in the radial groove of the humerus, pierces the lateral intermuscular septum, and enters the anterior compartment of the arm. Above the elbow, the nerve innervates the triceps, extensor carpi radialis longus and brevis, and brachioradialis. At the elbow, the nerve divides into a motor branch or posterior interosseous nerve and a superficial sensory branch.

Compression syndromes of the radial nerve above the elbow have been reported with sudden forceful contraction of the triceps muscle.[69] The most common cause of high radial nerve palsy is a humeral fracture.[75] Compression of the nerve against the medial side of the humerus occurs in "Saturday night palsy," caused by pressure directly over the nerve on the upper arm.[98]

High radial nerve palsies have been described in various sports, including judo, kendo, baseball, mountain climbing, and skiing.[53] Humeral fractures are often associated with many of the palsies. Chronic compression, as that caused by carrying a heavy backpack, has also caused radial nerve palsies.

Clinical examination is essential to localize the area of injury or compression. In a high radial nerve injury, both motor and sensory deficits are found. The patient is unable to extend the wrist or metacarpophalangeal joints of the hand and has decreased sensation in the first dorsal web space. The triceps are involved only if the injury is proximal to their innervation. On examination a differentiation can be made between radial nerve palsy and posterior interosseous nerve syndrome by noting both radial deviation of the wrist during active wrist dorsiflexion and the lack of sensory findings seen in posterior interosseous nerve syndrome.[93] Proximal lesions, such as in the C7 nerve root or posterior cord of the brachial plexus, can be differentiated by a sensory deficit in the palmar aspect of the third digit and motor abnormalities in the flexor carpi radialis, pronator teres, flexor digitorum superficialis, and flexor pollicis longus. Posterior cord involvement can be demonstrated by deltoid and latissimus dorsi muscle weakness.

Electromyographic and nerve conduction studies can help isolate lesions of the radial nerve.

Prolonged external compression may cause neuronal degeneration requiring several months for recovery.[98] Patients with sleep palsies have almost an 87% chance for full recovery. Radial nerve injuries associated with humeral fractures have a 75% chance of recovering spontaneously, whereas the oblique distal third humeral fracture (Holstein-Lewis) is more controversial, with evidence supporting early exploration because of nerve entrapment in the fracture site.[75]

If the palsy develops after a closed reduction or open reduction and internal fixation, then exploration is often indicated. If no recovery is seen in 8 to 10 weeks, then exploration is performed to repair or release the nerve. Tendon transfers may be needed after a year of observation and maintenance of passive motion.

Posterior Interosseous Nerve

The radial nerve divides 3 cm above or below the elbow into a motor branch (posterior interosseous nerve) and a sensory branch (superficial radial nerve). The motor branch lies 1 cm lateral to the biceps tendon over the anterior capsule of the radiohumeral joint and dorsolateral over the radial neck.

The sensory branch usually arises before the motor branch enters the extensor compartment at the radial tunnel, a space lined by the extensor compartment muscles. The posterior interosseous nerve passes through the supinator muscle at an opening called the arcade of Frohse[68] (Fig. 31-20). This arcade is formed by the proximal superficial head of the supinator and has been shown to have a thickened tendinous edge in 30% of patients, thus creating nerve compression.[73]

Four sites of posterior interosseus nerve compression have been identified (Fig. 31-12): (1) fibrous edge of the extensor carpi radialis brevis, (2) arcade of Frohse, (3) fibrous bands attaching the nerve to the radiohumeral joint, and (4) radial recurrent vessels.[94]

Radial tunnel syndrome was first described by Roles and Maudsley in 1972,[86] and it has often been called resistant tennis elbow because inadequate treatment was often rendered as a result of inaccurate diagnosis.[86]

Most patients with posterior interosseous nerve syndrome are not players of racquet sports, but manual workers.[17] Often tennis elbow or lateral epicondylitis may be present along with radial tunnel syndrome.

Compression of the posterior interosseous nerve in the area of the head of the radius manifests itself as an aching pain in the forearm associated with activity.[23] This is due to the presence of some sensory fibers from the joint, muscle, and skin. The pain is usually well localized in the extensor mass below the elbow and may radiate into the dorsal aspect of the wrist.[61] Repetitive wrist flexion and pronation often exacerbate the symptoms. Hand grip may be weak because of the pain of wrist dorsiflexion.

On examination, tenderness is found over the nerve at the radial neck. No tenderness in the lateral epicondyle of the distal humerus is present; this differentiates it from tennis

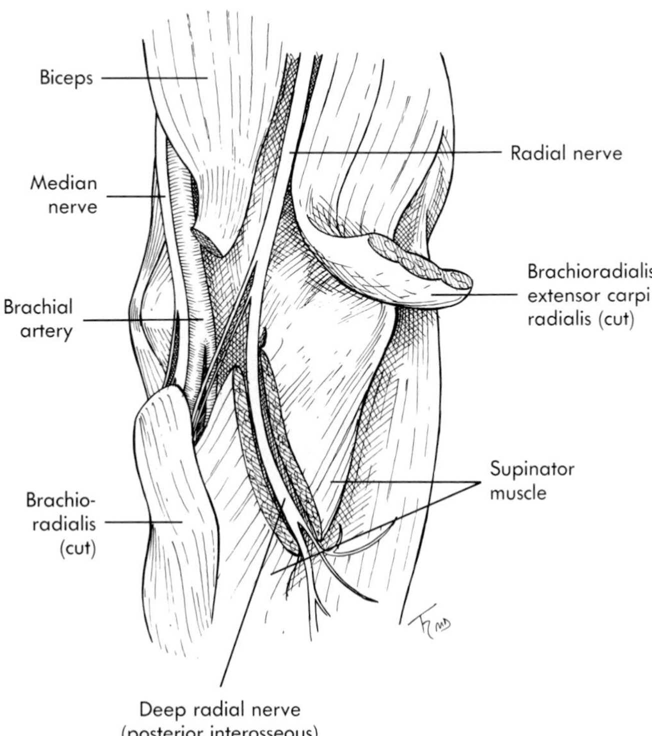

FIG. 31-20. Posterior interosseous nerve travels through the supinator muscle. Compression can occur at the proximal edge of this muscle. (Arcade of Frohese).

elbow. Resistance to middle-finger extension may elicit pain, but this may also be true with tennis elbow. Also, resistance to supination usually elicits the pain. Motor examination is often normal, but some weakness of thumb and finger extension may be found. True paresis has been reported with trauma, such as in Monteggia's fractures, rheumatoid arthritis, or tumors.[67]

Results of electrodiagnostic studies are useful in confirming the lesion, but may prove normal, perhaps because of the intermittent nature of the compression. Other sources of pain in the lateral aspect of the arm include tendonitis, stenosis of the orbicular ligament, tears in the common extensor tendon origin, cervical spine disorders, and radial head pathology.

Treatment of spontaneous posterior interosseus nerve palsy is conservative.[23,61,94] The patient is advised to temporarily change activity, use a resting splint, and try a nonsteroidal antiinflammatory drug. If a mass has been detected or the symptoms persist after 6 months of conservative treatment, surgery may be warranted. Weakness is an indication of severe nerve compression, and surgical decompression should be carried out. Results of surgical decompression have been uniformly good, with success rates above 90%.

Ulnar Nerve

The ulnar nerve is the terminal branch of the medial cord of the brachial plexus after the medial cord sends a contribution to the median nerve. In the humerus, the nerve lies medial to the axillary artery and brachial artery. At the distal third of the humerus, the nerve pierces the medial intermuscular septum and runs along the medial triceps muscle to the groove between the olecranon and medial epicondyle of the humerus. The cubital tunnel lies just behind the medial epicondyle and consists of the ulnar groove, fascial aponeurosis joining the two heads of the flexor carpi ulnaris, and the muscle bellies of these two heads. The nerve courses through the forearm between the flexor digitorum profundis and flexor carpi ulnaris (Fig. 31-21).

The causes of ulnar nerve entrapment in the elbow include the arcade of Struthers, the medial head of the triceps, an anconeus epitrochlearis muscle, the aponeurosis of the flexor carpi ulnaris, osteophytes of the tunnel, ganglia, lipomata, or subluxation of the ulnar nerve. Ulnar nerve entrapment syndrome is a well-documented neuropathy in baseball players, particularly in pitchers.[27,43] Repetitive valgus stress of the elbow is thought to play a key role in the development of this neuropathy. Symptoms include pain in the medial aspect of the proximal forearm that may radiate proximally or distally. Paresthesias, dysesthesias, or anesthesia is usually found in the ulnar half of the ring finger and the little finger. If compression is longstanding, findings may include clumsiness and weakness, with wasting of the intrinsic muscles of the hand. Occasionally, weakness in the flexor profundi to the ring and little finger may be

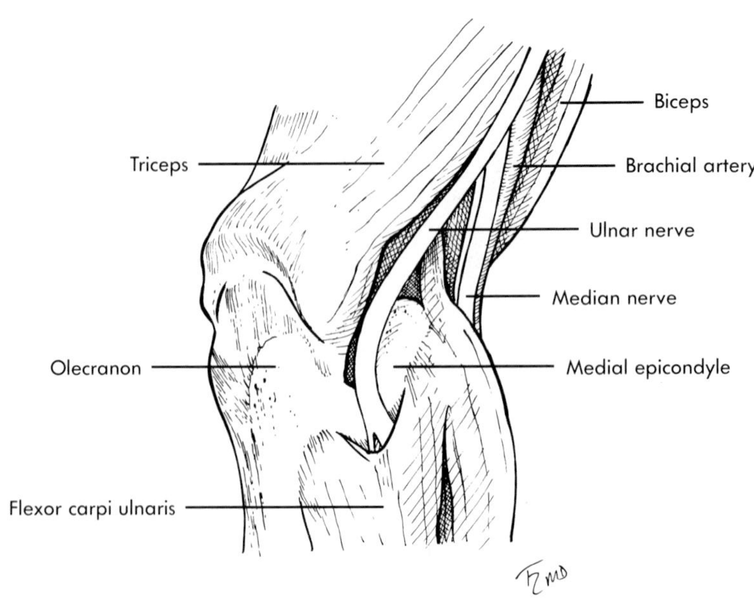

FIG. 31-21. Ulnar nerve entrapment can occur behind medial epicondyle in cubital tunnel.

detected, although this is more common with ulnar nerve injuries above the elbow. A positive Tinel's sign in the cubital tunnel is a frequent finding, with tingling or "shocky" sensations traveling proximally and distally. The elbow flexion test, which consists of full elbow flexion for 5 minutes, often elicits the symptoms. Electrophysiologic studies generally confirm and localize the site of ulnar nerve entrapment. One must carefully exclude disorders of the cervical spinal cord, nerve root, and brachial plexus, such as neurologic thoracic outlet syndrome, which closely resembles ulnar nerve entrapment at the elbow.

Early surgical decompression and submuscular transposition of the ulnar nerve is recommended for baseball players.[26,27] Common associated findings at operation include tearing or calcification of the medial collateral ligament. Players often have scarring over the nerve in the ulnar groove. Surgical decompression of the nerve in this group of patients should not be delayed to wait for EMG changes. Injections into the area of the irritated nerve are not recommended. Approximately 60% of the players in one series returned to their preoperative level of play.[27] During the decompression, the proximal dissection includes resection of the medial intermuscular septum and division of the arcade of Struthers, if one is present.[64] Other procedures used are medial epicondylectomy, decompression, and subcutaneous transposition with a loose fascial sling to prevent a position change of the transposed nerve.[31] Attention must be paid to the relase of the flexor carpi ulnaris aponeurosis, which is thought to play a key role in idiopathic cubital tunnel syndrome.

Wrist

Carpal Tunnel Syndrome

The median nerve enters the hand through the carpal tunnel, which is bordered by the transverse carpal ligament volarly and the wrist bones dorsally. The transverse carpal ligament attaches to the scaphoid and trapezium radially and pisiform and hamate ulnarly. The median nerve shares this space with nine flexor tendons, including the flexor pollicis longus, the flexor digitorum superficialis,[4] and flexor digitorum profundus tendons,[4] all lined by a synovial sheath (Fig. 31-22). The median nerve at this level contains sensory palmar digital branches that innervate the radial three and one-half digits; a motor branch to the thenar eminence, which innervates the abductor pollicis brevis; opponens pollicis and superficial head of the flexor pollicis brevis; and motor branches to the first and second lumbricals.

Clinical features of carpal tunnel syndrome include paresthesias and pain in the wrist, hand, and radial three and one-half digits, especially during sleep. The aching pain may radiate to the elbow or shoulder. With progression of the disease, symptoms occur during the day and can become constant. Patients frequently report stiffness of the fingers in the morning, perhaps caused by swelling around the flexor tendons in the carpal tunnel. Atrophy of the thenar muscles is a late finding in severe carpal tunnel syndrome, but abductor

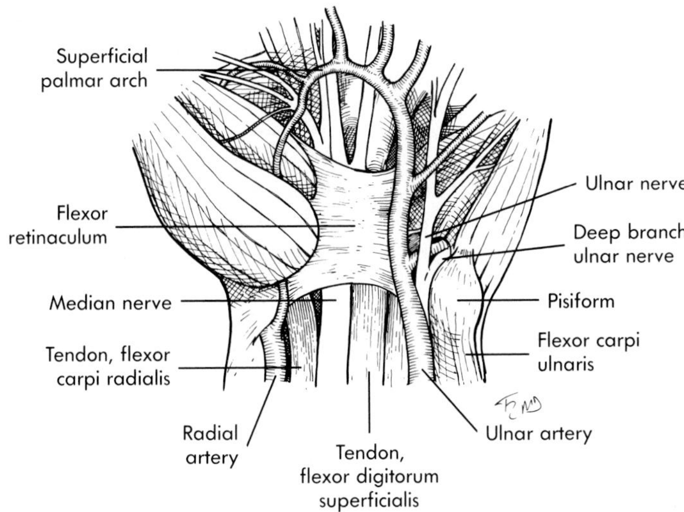

FIG. 31-22. The transverse carpal ligament lies over the median nerve at the carpal tunnel and requires surgical division to relieve symptoms of median nerve compression.

pollicis brevis weakness can often be elicited.[57]

The Phalen wrist flexion test is a sensitive test for carpal tunnel syndrome, but it may be negative.[78,79] A positive Tinel's sign at the wrist may be elicited in approximately 45% of patients with carpal tunnel syndrome. Two-point discrimination may be abnormal, but vibratory sensory testing is more sensitive in detecting early disease. Electromyographic and nerve conduction studies are important in confirming the diagnosis, although they may be negative in 25% of patients with carpal tunnel syndrome. If a patient describes characteristic paresthesias and demonstrates the appropriate signs, such as a positive Phalen test, then there is an 85% certainty of the diagnosis.

Careful clinical examination and electrophysiologic testing can exclude brachial plexus pathology, which is one of the problems in the differential diagnosis of carpal tunnel syndrome. Conditions that may be associated with carpal tunnel syndrome include rheumatoid arthritis; thyroid myxedema; acromegaly; multiple myeloma; amyloidosis; diabetes mellitus; pregnancy; local wrist trauma; hemophilia; alcoholism; tumors, such as ganglia; lipomas; gout; anomalous muscles in the carpal tunnel, such as palmaris profundus; or thrombosis of a persistent median artery.[42]

Local trauma to the wrist has been found to cause carpal tunnel syndrome in cyclists, throwers, and tennis players. Repeated microtrauma to the contents of the carpal tunnel or prolonged wrist extension in these and other sports may produce mechanical irritation or ischemia in the median nerve, resulting in classic symptoms. Carpal tunnel syndrome has also been known to develop in manual workers, such as jackhammer operators. Flexor tenosynovitis resulting from overuse may be a common cause of median nerve compression in the wrist.

Nonsurgical treatment of carpal tunnel syndrome consists of avoidance of activities that produce symptoms, using a wrist splint in 20 to 25 degrees of dorsiflexion, nonsteroidal antiflammatory medication, and sometimes a cortisone injection into the carpal tunnel.[40] The injection is given 1 cm proximal to the distal wrist flexion crease, between the palmaris longus and flexor carpi radialis tendons. Intratendinous injection may weaken the tendon, causing rupture. Intraneural injection may injure the median nerve irreparably. The majority of patients with carpal tunnel syndrome resulting from repetitive trauma will respond to conservative measures.[42] In cases with prolonged symptoms, atrophy, or sensory loss, surgery may be necessary if conservative measures are unsuccessful after 8 to 12 weeks of trial. Division of the transverse carpal ligament has given 90% to 95% of patients good long-term results.[24] There is no consensus as to whether tenosynovectomy and internal neurolysis improve results. Complications include failure to fully divide the transverse carpal ligament and injury to the palmar cutaneous branch of the median nerve.

Ulnar Nerve

The ulnar nerve at the wrist passes between the pisiform bone and the hook of the hamate through Guyon's canal, the floor of which is the transverse carpal ligament and pisohamate ligament, and the roof of which is the palmar fascia and palmaris brevis muscle (Fig. 31-23). Through the canal pass the superficial terminal branch, supplying sensation to the ulnar palm, little finger, and ulnar half of the ring finger, and the deep terminal branch, which supplies the hypothenar muscles, interossei, third and fourth lumbricals, adductor pollicus brevis, first dorsal interosseous, and a portion of the flexor pollicis brevis.

Compression syndromes at Guyon's canal have been reported as a result of chronic repeated external pressure, ganglia, lipoma, rheumatoid synovial cysts, tumors, anomalous muscles, ununited fractures of the hamate, and ulnar artery aneurysms.[72,90] The most common form of compression occurs at the deep terminal branch distal to the branches supplying the hypothenar muscles, caused by compression between the fibrous origin of the abductor and flexor of the fifth finger and the pisohamate ligament against the hook of the hamate.[90] Symptoms include weakness of all ulnar-innervated muscles of the hand except the hypothenar muscles.[57] This form is found in persons who use tools that press into the palm of their hand and in long-distance cyclists, who experience constant pressure from handlebars, and results in motor weakness and wasting of intrinsic muscles.[32,56]

The second most common site of involvement is the main trunk, both sensory and motor, just proximal to or within Guyon's canal. A less common form of compression can occur more distally, at the superficial terminal branch. This results in a sensory loss only and has been reported with an ununited fracture of the hook of the hamate and an ulnar artery aneurysm caused by trauma.[60]

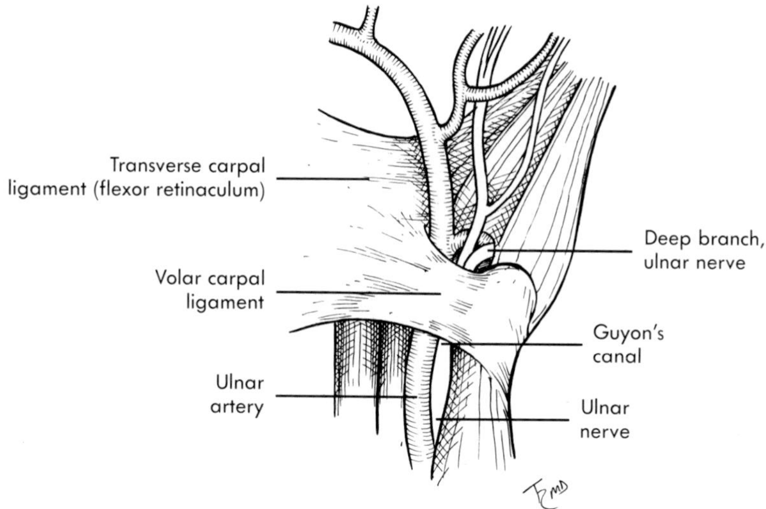

FIG. 31-23. Anatomy of Guyon's canal.

Investigation should consist of a careful history of work habits, hobbies, and previous injuries, and a careful examination of the wrist and hand should follow.

Electrophysiologic studies help localize the neuropathy to the wrist or hand. Careful examination of the dorsal cutaneous branch of the ulnar nerve can help differentiate between a compression at the level of the wrist or proximally.

Occupational causes for the neuropathy have been found to resolve upon discontinuation of the activity in a large portion of patients. Occasionally, surgical decompression is necessary when no improvement is noted or the symptoms worsen. Touring cyclists often achieve relief of their symptoms by wearing cycling gloves and applying proper padding to the handlebars.[32,56]

Hypothenar Hammer Syndrome

The unlar artery travels through Guyon's Canal which is bounded by the hook of the hamate laterally, the pisiform bone medially, the transverse carpal ligament dorsally, and the volar carpal ligament on the palmar aspect. The two centimeter segment of the ulnar artery distal to Guyon's canal is very susceptible to trauma since it is relatively superficial, being covered by a thin layer of subcutaneous tissue, palmaris brevis muscle, and skin. Repetitive trauma to the hypothenar portion of the hand may result in signs and symptoms associated with ischemia to the hand and fingers; often exacerbated by exposure to cold (Raynaud's phenomenon). Spasm, thrombosis, or aneurysm formation of the ulnar artery have been found primarily in male laborers who use hammerlike handles, turning valves or using their palms as hammers, hence the term Hypothenar Hammer Syndrome. A history of trauma; acute, chronic, or repetitive has been reported in all cases.

Patients may present with unilateral numbness in the ulnar innervated digits, ischemic pain with pallor, cold intolerance or sensitivity, and a mass in the hypothenar portion of the hand. Signs include a positive Allen test if the ulnar artery is thrombosed, intrinsic muscle cramping during rapid repetitive movement, and a palapable aneurysm if present. Doppler ultrasonography may help make the diagnosis, while angiography is seldom needed.

A fracture of the hook of the hamate may be associated with thrombosis of the ulnar artery. Raynaud's disease is differentiated by its bilateral involvement, no history of trauma, and higher incidence in women. Other systemic inflammatory and collagen vascular diseases may be excluded by history, physical examination, and diagnostic testing.

Although sympathetic blocks and sympathectomies have been used, surgical excision of the lesion is the most common and effective form of treatment. Direct ulnar artery repairs and vein graft repairs have been done with about a 50% potency rate but excellent clinical improvement.

Hand

Bowler's Thumb

Bowler's thumb is a digital neuropathy of the palmar-ulnar digital nerve that has been described in bowlers and baseball players[10] (Fig. 31-24). The entity is caused by a perineural fibrosis of the ulnar digital nerve of the

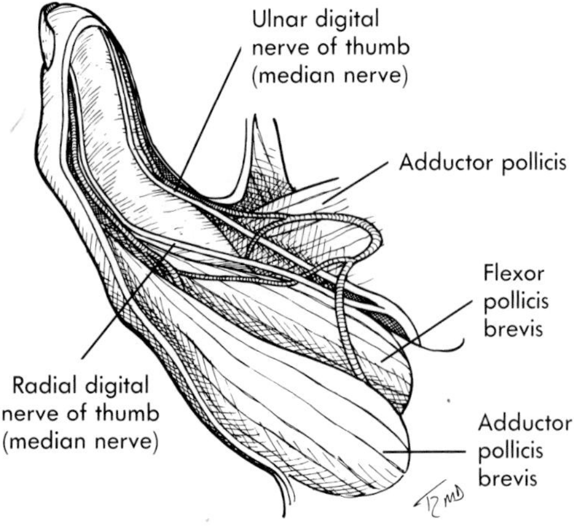

FIG. 31-24. Anatomy of digital nerve of thumbs.

thumb at the metacarpophalangeal crease as a result of chronic compression and repeated trauma to the nerve from the corner of the thumb hole in the bowling ball.[55]

Often the patient reports a tender nodule at the ulnar metacarpophalangeal crease. A Tinel's sign can usually be elicited.[29] There may also be paresthesias and sensory loss in the distribution of the nerve.

Other causes for compression of the nerve include cysts and tumors from the tendon sheath of the thumb, osteophytes, mucinous cysts, rheumatoid tenosynovitis, schwannomas, or digital neuropathies associated with diabetes mellitus and vascular disorders. Even though the digital nerves are superficial, compression neuropathies are quite rare.[83]

Upon recognition of an occupation or sports-related neuropathy, protective measures are instituted.[29] A change in the position of the thumb hole may help, or a splint will help resolve the symptoms. Otherwise, cessation of bowling may be necessary. Surgery is rarely indicated, but in the case of unrelieved symptoms, there has been a report that transposing the nerve posterior to the adductor pollicis tendon yields a good result.[10]

REFERENCES

1. Adams JT and Deweese JA: Effort thrombosis of the axillary and subclavian veins, J Trauma 11:923, 1971.
2. Albright JP et al: Nonfatal cervical spine injuries in interscholastic football, JAMA 236:1243, 1976.
3. Albright JP et al: Head and neck injuries in college football: an eight-year analysis, Am J Sports Med 13:147, 1985.
4. Andrich J, Bergfeld JA, and Ramo RA: A method for the management of cervical injuries in football: a preliminary report, Am J Sports Med 5:89, 1977.
5. Barnes DA and Tullos HS: An analysis of 100 symptomatic baseball players, Am J Sports Med 6:62, March-April, 1978.
6. Barrett T and Levitt LM: Effort thrombosis of the axillary vein with pulmonary embolism, JAMA 146:1412, 1951.
7. Bassett FH and Nunley JA: Compression of the musculocutaneous nerve at the elbow, J Bone Joint Surg 64A:1050, 1982.
8. Bateman JE: Nerve injuries about the shoulder in sports, J Bone Joint Surg 49A:785, 1967.
9. Becker GJ and Holden RW: Local thrombolytic therapy for subclavian and axillary vein thrombosis, Radiology 149:419, 1983.
10. Belsky MR and Millender LH: Bowler's thumb in a baseball player: a case report, Orthopedics 3:122, 1980.
11. Bergfeld JA, Hershman EB, and Wilbourn AJ: Brachial plexus injury in sports: a five-year followup, Orthop Trans 12:743, 1988.
12. Berry H and Bril V: Axillary nerve palsy following blunt trauma to the shoulder region: a clinical and electrophysiological review, J Neurol Neurosurg Psychiatry 45:1027, 1982.
13. Bigliani LU, Perez-Sanz JR, Wolfe IN: Treatment of trapezius paralysis, J Bone Joint Surg G7A:871, 1985.
14. Blom S and Dahlback LO: Nerve injuries in dislocations of the shoulder joint and fractures of the neck and humerus, Acta Chir Scand 136: 461, 1970.
15. Bonney G: The scalenus medius band: a contribution to the study of the thoracic outlet syndrome, J Bone Joint Surg 47B:268, 1965.
16. Braddom RL and Wolfe C: Musculocutaneous nerve injury after heavy exercise, Arch Phys Med Rehabil 59:290, 1978.
17. Bryan FS, Miller LS, and Panijayanond P: Spontaneous paralysis of the posterior interosseous nerve: a case report and reviews of the literature, Clin Orthop 80:9, 1971.
18. Butsch JL: Subclavian thrombosis following hockey injuries, Am J Sports Med 11:448, 1983.
19. Cahill BR and Palmar PE: Quadrilateral space syndrome, J Hand Surg 8:65, 1983.
20. Chrisman OD et al: Lateral flexion neck injuries in athletic competition, JAMA 192(7):613, 1965.
21. Clancy WG, Brand RL, and Bergfeld JA: Upper trunk brachial plexus injuries in contact sports, Am J Sports Med 5:209, 1977.
22. Clein LJ: Supracapsular entrapment neuropathy, J Neurosurg 43:337, 1975.
23. Coonrad RW and Hooper WR: Tennis elbow: its cause, natural history, conversative and surgical management, J Bone Joint Surg 55A:1177, 1973.
24. Cseuz KA et al: Longterm results of operation for carpal tunnel syndrome, Mayo Clin Proc 41:232, 1966.
25. Dale WA: Thoracic outlet compression syndrome: critique in 1982, Arch Surg 117:1437, 1982.
26. Dellan AL: Operative technique for submuscular transposition of the ulnar nerve, Contemp Orthop 4:17, 1988.
27. DelPizzo W, Jobe FW, and Norwood L: Ulnar nerve entrapment syndrome in baseball players, Am J Sports Med 5:182, 1977.
28. Dewar FP and Harris RI: Restoration of function of the shoulder following paralysis of the trapezius by fascial sling fixation and transplantation of the levator scapulae, Ann Surg 132:1111, 1950.

29. Dobyns JH et al: Bowler's thumb: diagnosis and treatment, J Bone Joint Surg 54A:751, 1972.
30. Eastcott HHG: Reconstruction of the subclavian artery for complications of cervical rib and thoracic outlet syndrome, Lancet 2:1243, 1962.
31. Eaton RG, Crowe JF, and Parkes JC: Anterior transposition of the ulnar nerve using a noncompressing fasciodermal sling, J Bone Joint Surg 62A:820, 1980.
32. Eckman PB, Perlstein G, and Altrocchi PH: Ulnar neuropathy in bicycle riders, Arch Neurol 32:130, 1975.
33. Falconer MA and Weddell G: Costoclavicular compression to the subclavian artery and vein: relation to the scalenus anticus syndrome, Lancet 2:539, 1943.
34. Farber JS and Bryan RS: The anterior interosseous nerve syndrome, J Bone Joint Surg 50A:521, 1968.
35. Felsenthal G et al: Forearm pain secondary to compression syndrome of the lateral cutaneous nerve of the forearm, Arch Phys Med Rehabil 65:139, 1984.
36. Ferretti A et al: Suprascapular neuropathy in volleyball players, J Bone Joint Surg 69:260, 1987.
37. Foo CL and Swann M: Isolated paralysis of the serratus anterior, J Bone Joint Surg 65B:552, 1983.
38. Ganzhorn RW et al: Suprascapular nerve entrapment, J Bone Surg 63:492, 1981.
39. Garcia G and McQueen D: Bilateral suprascapular nerve entrapment syndrome, J Bone Joint Surg 63A:491, 1981.
40. Gelberman RH, Aronson D, and Weisman MH: Carpal tunnel syndrome—results of a prospective trial of steroid injection and splinting, J Bone Joint Surg 62A:1181, 1980.
41. Gelberman RH et al: The carpal tunnel syndrome, J Bone Joint Surg 63A:380, 1981.
42. Gerstner DL and Omer GE: Peripheral entrapment neuropathies in the upper extremity, J Musculoskeletal Med 3:14, 1988.
43. Godshell RW: Traumatic ulnar neuropathy in adolscent baseball pitchers, J Bone Joint Surg 53A:359, 1971.
44. Goodman CE, Kenrick MM, and Blum MV: Long thoracic nerve palsy: a follow-up study, Arch Phys Med Rehabil 56:352, 1975.
45. Graham GC and Lincoln BM: Anterior resection of the first rib for thoracic outlet syndrome, Am J Surg 126:803, 1973.
46. Gregg JR, Labosky D, and Harty M: Serratus anterior paralysis in the young athlete, J Bone Joint Surg 61A:825, 1979.
47. Hadley MN: Suprascapular nerve entrapment, J Neurosurg 64:843, 1986.
48. Hale BR: Hand bag paresthesia, Lancet 2:470, 1976.
49. Hantz CR et al: The pronator teres syndrome: compressive neuropathy of the median nerve, J Bone Joint Surg 63A:885, 1981.
50. Herring S and Nilson K: Introduction to overuse injuries, Clin Sports Med 6:225, 1987.
51. Hershman EB, Wilbourn AJ, and Bergfeld JA: Acute brachial neuropathy in athletes, Am J Sports Med (in press).
52. Hill NA, Howard FM, and Huffer BR: The incomplete anterior interosseous nerve syndrome, J Hand Surg 10A:4, 1985.
53. Hirasawa Y and Sakakida K: Sports and peripheral nerve injury, Am J Sports Med 11:420, 1983.
54. Hirayama T and Takemitsu Y: Compression of the suprascapular nerve by ganglion at the suprascapular notch, Clin Orthop 155:95, 1981.
55. Howell AE and Leach RE: Bowler's thumb: perineural fibrosis of the digital nerve, J Bone Joint Surg 52A:379, 1970.
56. Hoyt CS: Ulnar neuropathy in bicycle riders, Arch Neurol 33:372, 1976.
57. Hunt JR: The thenar and hypothenar types of neural atrophy of the hand, Am J Med Sci 141:224, 1911.
58. Johnson JTH and Kendall HO: Isolated paralysis of the serratus anterior muscle, J Bone Joint Surg 37A:567, 1955.
59. Johnson RK, Spinner M, and Shrewsbury MM: Median entrapment syndrome in the proximal forearm, J Hand Surg 4:48, 1979.
60. Kalisman M, Laborde K, and Wolff TW: Ulnar nerve compression secondary to ulnar artery false aneurysm at Guyon's canal, J Hand Surg 7:137, 1982.
61. Kaplan PE: Posterior interosseous neuropathies: natural history, Arch Phys Med Rehab 65:339, 1984.
62. Kim SM and Goodrich JA: Isolated proximal musculocutaneous nerve palsy: case report, Arch Phys Med Rehabil 65:735, 1984.
63. Langenskiold A and Ryoppy S: Treatment of paralysis of the trapezius muscles by the Eden-Lange operation, Acta Orthop Scand 44:383, 1973.
64. Learmonth JR: Technique for transplantation of the ulnar nerve, Surg Gynecol Obstet 75:792, 1942.
65. Leffert RD: Thoracic outlet syndrome. In Omer GE and Spinner M, editors: Management of peripheral nerve problems, Philadelphia, 1980, WB Saunders Co.
66. Leffert RD and Seddon H: Infraclavicular brachial plexus inujuries, J Bone Joint Surg 47B:9, 1965.
67. Lichter RL and Jacobson T: Tardy palsy of the posterior interosseous nerve with a Monteggia fracture, J Bone Joint Surg 57A:124, 1975.
68. Lister GD et al: The radial tunnel syndrome, J Hand Surg 4:52, 1979.
69. Lotem M et al: Radial palsy following muscular effort: a nerve compression syndrome possibly related to a fibrous arch of the lateral head of the triceps, J Bone Joint Surg 53B:500, 1971.
70. Marks J: Anticoagulation therapy in idiopathic occlusion of the axillary vein, Br Med J 1:11, 1956.
71. Maroon JC: "Burning hands" in football, spinal cord injuries, JAMA 238:2049, 1977.
72. McCarroll HR: Nerve injuries associated with wrist trauma, Orthop Clin North Am 15:279, 1984.
73. Nielsen HO: Posterior interosseous nerve paralysis caused by fibrous band compression at the supinator muscle; a report of 4 cases, Acta Orthop Scand 47:304, 1976.
74. Neviaser TJ et al: Suprascapular nerve denervation secondary to attenuation by a ganglionic cyst, J Bone Joint Surg 68A:4:627, 1986.
75. Packer JW et al: The humeral fracture with radial nerve palsy: is exploration warranted? Clin Orthop 88:34, 1972.
76. Parsonage MJ and Turner JWA: Neuralgic amyotrophy: the shoulder girdle syndrome, Lancet 1:973, 1948.
77. Petrucci FS, Morelli A, and Raimohdi PL: Axillary nerve injuries: 21 cases treated by nerve

graft and neurolysis, J Hand Surg 7:271, 1982.
78. Phalen GS: The carpal tunnel syndrome, J Bone Joint Surg 48A:211, 1966.
79. Phalen GS and Kendrick JI: Compression neuropathy of the median nerve in the carpal tunnel, JAMA 16:524, 1957.
80. Poindexter DP and Johnson EW: Football shoulder and neck injury: a study of the stinger, Arch Phys Med Rehabil 65:601, 1984.
81. Rask MR: Suprascapular nerve entrapment: a report of two cases treated by suprascapular notch resection, Clin Orthop 134:266, 1978.
82. Rayan GM: Lower trunk brachial plexus compression neuropathy due to cervical rib in young athletes, Am J Sports Med 16:77, 1988.
83. Rayan GM and O'Donoghue DH: Ulnar digital compression neuropathy of the thumb caused by splinting, Clin Orthop 175:170, 1983.
84. Rennels GD and Ochoa J: Neurologic amyotrophy manifesting as anterior interosseus nerve palsy, Muscle Nerve 3:160, 1980.
85. Robertson WC, Eichman PL, and Clancy WG: Upper trunk brachial plexopathy in football players, JAMA 241:1480, 1979.
86. Roles NC and Maudsley RH: Radial tunnel syndrome: resistant tennis elbow as a nerve entrapment, J Bone Joint Surg, 54B:499, 1972.
87. Roos DB: Experience with first rib resection for thoracic outlet syndrome, Ann Surg 173:429, 1971.
88. Roos DB: Congenital anomalies associated with thoracic outlet syndrome: anatomy, symptoms, diagnosis, and treatment, Am J Surg 132:771, 1976.
89. Rorabeck CH and Harris WR: Factors affecting the prognosis of brachial plexus injuries, J Bone Surg 63B:404, 1981.
90. Shea JD and McClain EJ: Ulnar nerve compression syndromes at and below the wrist, J Bone Joint Surg 51A:1095, 1969.
91. Spinner M: The functional attitude of the hand afflicted with an anterior interosseous nerve paralysis, Bull Hosp Joint Dis 30:21, 1969.
92. Spinner M: The anterior interosseous nerve syndrome with special attention to its variation, J Bone Joint Surg 52A:84, 1970.
93. Spinner M: Injuries to the major branches of the peripheral nerves of the forearm, Philadelphia, 1978, WB Saunders Co.
94. Spinner M and Spencer RS: Nerve compression lesions of the upper extremity, Clin Orthop 104:46, 1974.
95. Stern PJ and Kutz JE: An unusual variant of the anterior interosseous nerve syndrome, J Hand Surg 5:32, 1980.
96. Stewart JD: The brachial plexus. In: Stewart JD, editor: Focal peripheral neuropathies, New York, 1987, Elsevier.
97. Strohm BR, Brand, and Colachis SC Jr: Shoulder joint dysfunction following injury to the suprascapular nerve, Phys Ther 45:106, 1965.
98. Sunderland S: Traumatic injuries of peripheral nerves: simple compression injuries of the radial nerve, Brain 68:5, 1945.
99. Sunderland S: Nerves and nerve injuries, ed 2, Edinburgh, 1978, Churchill Livingstone.
100. Swafford AR and Lichtman DH: Suprascapular nerve entrapment—case report, J Hand Surg 7:57, 1982.
101. Thompson RC Jr, Schneider W, and Kennedy T: Entrapment neuropathy of the inferior branch of the suprascapular nerve by ganglia, Clin Orthop 166:185, 1982.
102. Tsairis P, Dyck PJ, and Mulder DW: Natural history of brachial plexus neuropathy: report of 99 patients, Arch Neurol 27:109, 1972.
103. Urschel HC and Razzuk MA: Management of the thoracic outlet syndrome, N Engl J Med 286:1140, 1972.
104. Vastamaki M: Suprascapular nerve entrapment. AAOS 54th Annual Meeting, Scientific Program, Paper no. 192, 1987.
105. Vogel CM and Jensen JE: "Effort" thrombosis of the subclavian vein in a competitive swimmer, Am J Sports Med 13:269, 1985.
106. Wilbourn AJ, Hershman EB, and Bergfeld JA: Brachial plexopathies in athletes: the EMG findings, Muscle Nerve 9:254, 1986.
107. Wood VE, Twito R, and Verska JM: Thoracic outlet syndrome, Orthop Clin North Am 19:131, 1988.
108. Woodhead AB: Paralysis of the serratus anterior in a world class marksman, Amer J Sports Med 13:359, 1985.
109. Wright IS: The neurovascular syndrome produced by hyperabduction of the arms, Am Heart J 29:1, 1945.
110. Wright YA: Accessory spinal nerve injury, Clin Orthop 108:15, 1975.
111. Zoltan JD: Injury to the suprascapular nerve associated with anterior dislocation of the shoulder: case report and review of the literature, J Trauma 19:203, 1979.

PART VII Sport-Specific Injuries

CHAPTER 32 Biomechanics of Throwing

Jacquelin Perry
Ronald Glousman

The shoulder and elbow provide highly mobile, dynamic, and forceful coordinated motion. While daily activities depend on the upper extremity for lifting and positioning, athletic endeavors require specific and precise motions with propulsive activity. Interaction between static restraints and the dynamic muscle unit allow for the versatile motion and power that is required in competitive performance.

The extent and directions of motion available at any joint are determined by its bony contours and axes of rotation. Mobility is limited by ligamentous restraints. Both the shoulder and elbow use a two-joint complex to expand the mobility provided.

THE SHOULDER JOINT

Shoulder Motion

Vast three-dimensional mobility is provided by the skeletal characteristics of the shoulder (Fig. 32-1). The humeral articular surface is a superiomedially oriented hemisphere (diameter 35 to 55 mm).[32,42] Opposing this is the small, shallow glenoid fossa of the scapula, which has half the contour and one third the surface area.[29] Glenoid area and depth are enlarged by a fibrocartilaginous labrum. This increases the humeral contact areas to 75% vertically and 56% transversely.[47] The effect is enhanced joint stability without impeded mobility from hard bony edges. As a result, the humerus has a wide range of motion in all three planes. Supplementing this is the gliding of the scapula on the thorax as it rotates with the clavicle about the sternal point of origin. The dominance of mobility over stability is even evident in the arm's resting posture.

Shoulder motion patterns

- Elevation
- Rotation—internal/external
- Horizontal flexion and extension

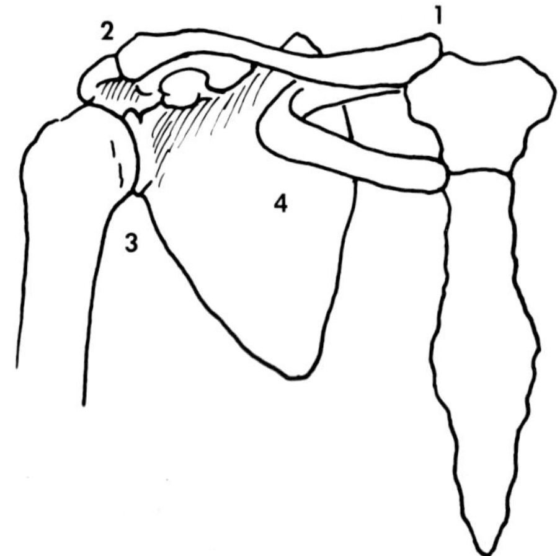

FIG. 32-1. Sites of motion within the shoulder complex. **A,** sternoclavicular joint, **B,** acromioclavicular joint, **C,** glenohumeral joint, **D,** scapulothoracic interface. (From Rowe CR: The shoulder, New York, 1988, Churchill Livingstone, Inc.)

Shoulder mobility is classified by three patterns of motion: elevation, internal/external rotation, and horizontal flexion and extension.

Arm Elevation

Raising the arm from the side of the body to its peak overhead position is a theoretical 180-degree arc. Few men (4%) and less than one third of women (28%) actually attain this range. The men's mean range was 167 degrees and the women's 171 degrees.[13,15] These values still display the shoulder as the most mobile joint in the body. Posterior elevation or extension is about 60 degrees.[33]

Arm elevation is a complex action that is best analyzed as three functional modes: planes of motion, scapulohumeral rhythm, and centers of rotation.

Planes of motion. Neutral elevation of the arm occurs in the plane of the scapula (Fig. 32-2). This is angled approximately 30 degrees anterior to the body's coronal plane.[57] Exact alignment is determined by the contour of the thoracic wall on which the scapula rests.

This alignment of the glenoid fossa is matched by 30 degrees retroversion of the head of the humerus on its shaft (measured in relationship to the intercondylar line at the elbow) (Fig. 32-3). Hence, the glenohumeral joint is designed to follow the plane of the

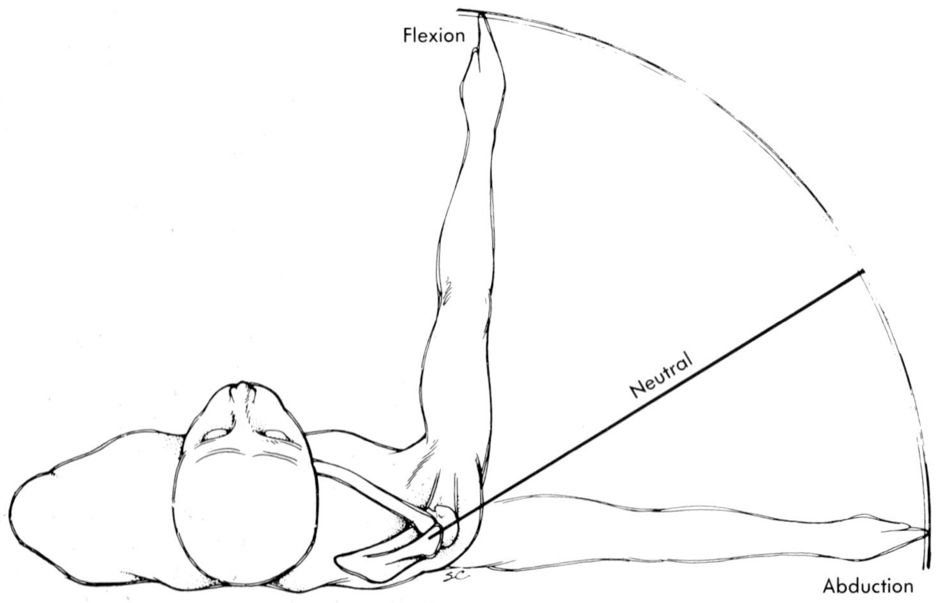

FIG. 32-2. Planes of arm elevation: neutral, flexion, and abduction. (From Rowe CR: The shoulder, New York, 1988, Churchill Livingstone, Inc.)

scapula. As the arm is raised in the scapular plane, the path of the humerus is perpendicular to the face of the glenoid; the joint is in neutral alignment. Johnston noted that the inferior capsule remained without torsion only when the humerus was raised in the scapular plane.[27]

Flexion is sagittal plane elevation (see Fig. 32-2). Placing the arm in this plane includes significant horizontal flexion. Hence the path of the humerus is oblique to the face of the scapula. The inferior joint capsule twists to accommodate this path of arm elevation.[27]

Abduction raises the arm in the coronal plane (see Fig. 32-2). This introduces two limitations. An element of horizontal extension is included in the elevation motion. More significant is the potential for impingement of the greater tuberosity against the acromion, since normal clearance is so minimal that there is no space for tendon thickening. This can be avoided by adding external rotation to the abduction motion.

Differences in the two ranges of motion have necessitated dual testing, because there have been no guidelines for selecting one over the other. The scapular plane represents neutral joint alignment. Clinical experience indicates that it is the simplest path of motion. Patients with limited strength spontaneously choose the scapular plane when asked to raise their arm overhead. Because of such anatomic and clinical findings, it is recommended that the scapular plane be used for basic testing of arm elevation capability.

Scapulohumeral rhythm. Total arm elevation is the sum of motion at two areas: the glenohumeral joint and the gliding of the scapula on the thorax[10] (Fig. 32-4).

Components of arm elevation

- Glenohumeral motion
- Scapulothoracic motion

At the onset of arm elevation, scapular participation has proved to be highly variable. It may be absent, minimal, or even reversed.[22] This lag in scapular motion persisted through the first 60 degrees of flexion and 30 degrees abduction. Once the scapula started to participate, both segments (humerus and scapula) moved continuously and synchronously. Relative humeral and scapular motion was identified by Inman et al. as a 2:1 ratio.[22] Other investigators have found both higher and lower ratios (2.5:1 to 1.25:1).[13,15,42,47] The average among all studies is 1.5:1.[56] Hence, there are approximately 3 degrees of glenohumeral motion for each 2 degrees occurring at the scapula.[13,15,47]

Glenohumeral-scapulothoracic rhythm

- 3 degrees of glenohumeral motion for each 2 degrees of scapulothoracic motion

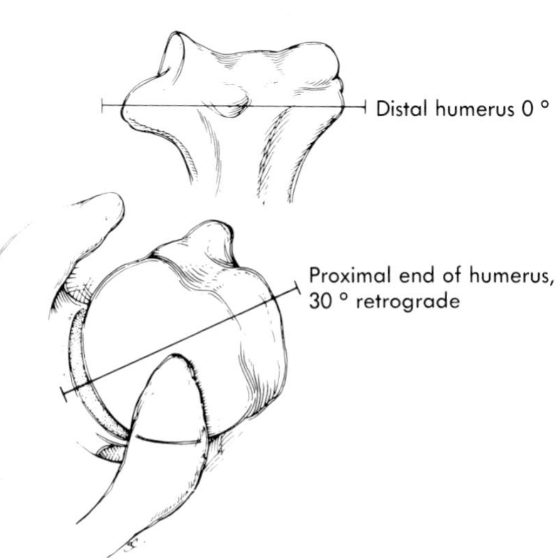

FIG. 32-3. Humeral head retroversion is 30 degrees compared to transverse axis of the elbow. (From Rowe CR: The shoulder, New York, 1988, Churchill Livingstone, Inc.)

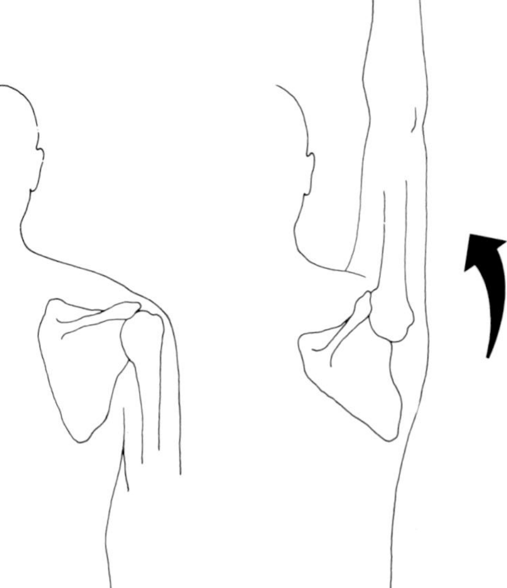

FIG. 32-4. Arm elevation is a combination of scapular and humeral rotation. (From Rowe CR: The shoulder, New York, 1988, Churchill Livingstone, Inc.)

Instant centers of shoulder motion. Each joint has its own pattern of motion. This is defined by its path of instant centers.

Excursion of the humeral head on the glenoid has been described as both gliding and rolling. Direct roentgenologic analysis of the glenohumeral joint demonstrated intraarticular displacement to be minimal. At the onset of arm elevation (zero degrees to 30 degrees) Walker[57] found a 3 mm upward shift. This action appears to be correction of arm sag from its dependent position. During the rest of the elevation range, the point of glenohumeral contact remained within 1 mm of the center of the fossa. Hence rolling is not a significant element of shoulder motion.[14,47] Instead, an intact labrum combined with dynamic control keeps the humeral head centered, making gliding of the humeral surface on that of the glenoid fossa the dominant type of motion within the joint.

Assessment of persons with a painful shoulder showed half of them to have abnormal mechanics.[42] Both humeral head excursion and instant center displacement were increased, with the greater change occurring in excursion.

The scapula was found to follow a more complex path of motion. During its initial setting stage (the first 60 degrees), either there was no motion or the scapula joggled around a center of rotation in the lower part of the blade. Subsequent scapular rotation was grossly centered to the base of the scapular spine until the arm reached 120 degrees. During the final arc, the center of rotation shifted to a point near the base of the glenoid. This marked change in instant center location can be related to scapula motion arising first in the sternoclavicular (SC) and then the acromioclavicular (AC) joints. Clinically, surgeons have found good arm function can be restored despite some compromise in clavicular rotation.[33] Conversely, the clavicle is not an indispensable bone, but its presence adds stability for heavy, overhead arm use.[23]

Scapular rotation also is reflected by the path of the coracoid, while the acromion remains relatively fixed.[57]

Axial Rotation

Internal and external rotation of the arm is a function of the glenohumeral joints. Because of change in relative capsule length, the range varies with arm position (Fig. 32-5). Maximal rotation of approximately 180 degrees is present with the arm at the side of the body (adducted).[7] The larger portion of that range (108 degrees or 60%) is external rotation.[8] Abduction of the arm to 90 degrees reduces the total arc to 120 degrees. Within this range there is more internal than external rotation.[7] At peak elevation (by either flexion or abduction), no more than a jog of rotation is possible.

Horizontal Flexion/Extension

These motions also have been called horizontal adduction/abduction. Within the normal 180 degrees arc, only 45 degrees or 24% is horizontal extension behind the coronal plane.[8] Most of the motion is glenohumeral. As was true in the scapular plane, the humeral head remains centrally located in the glenoid

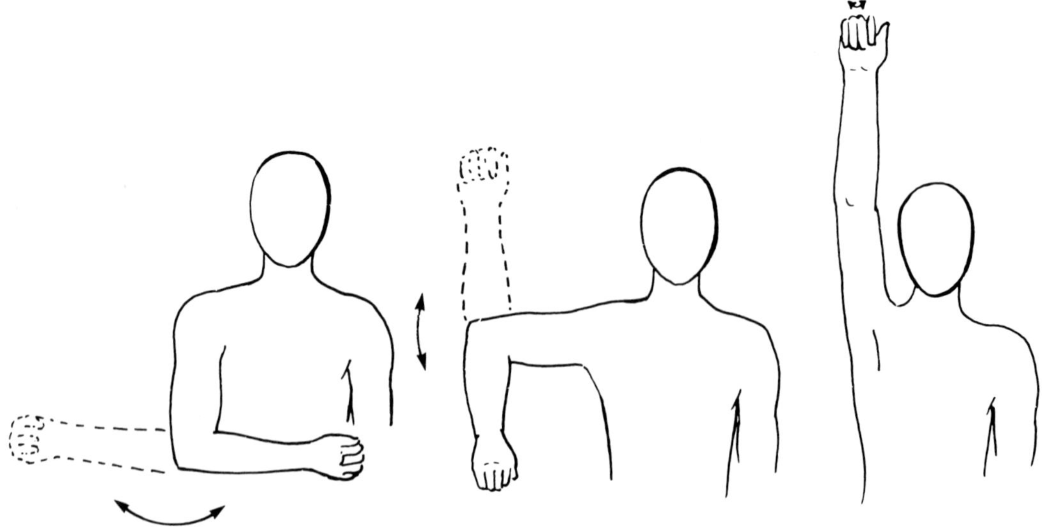

FIG. 32-5. Arm external/internal rotation ranges available with shoulder at zero degrees, 90 degrees, and full elevation. (From Rowe CR: The shoulder, New York, 1988, Churchill Livingstone, Inc.)

fossa. The limitation of this motion is the edge of the humeral articular surface. Further effort leads to impingement between the posterior rims of the glenoid fossa and humeral head as wedging replaces gliding.

Shoulder Muscular Control

Raising the arm from its resting position is the basic shoulder motion. Versatility in hand placement or the path of dynamic arm propulsion is accomplished by varying the plane of arm elevation and supplementing the action with horizontal and rotatory motion. This represents a vast number of possible movement combinations. A simple personal experiment demonstrated that normal selective control is so precise that the arm can be repositioned within 1 degree of the first position. Applying this level of control to the average ranges of shoulder motion indicates that the normal person has the potential to place the hand selectively in 16,000 positions.[40] The fine artist or champion athlete very probably has more precise control and hence a greater number of options available. To allow interpretation of the patterns of muscle control, however, the basic motion patterns will be considered separately.

Elevation

Two sources of control are used to raise the arm: the superficial muscle group and the underlying supraspinatus. Within the superficial musculature, the deltoid is dominant. Its action is supplemented anteriorly by the clavicular head of the pectoralis major, the coracobrachialis and the long head of the biceps brachii. The exact pattern of muscle action varies with the plane of motion selected.

Deltoid. While the deltoid is a continuous muscular sheet wrapped around the shoulder, it functions as three distinct muscles: anterior, middle, and posterior.

The middle deltoid is dominant: it participates in all arm elevation activities.[38,52] Supplementing its action are the anterior and posterior heads. They may act synergistically to add an abductor force or assume primary responsibility for arm elevation in their direction (flexion or extension). Hence the pattern of deltoid action varies with the plane of motion used.

Shoulder flexion

Primary motor
- Anterior deltoid

Secondary motors
- Middle deltoid
- Pectoralis major (clavicular head)
- Coracobrachialis
- Biceps brachii

Scapular plane elevation is provided by combined action of the middle and anterior deltoids[38,52] (Fig. 32-6). Studies using electromyography (EMG) have confirmed the simultaneous action of the anterior and middle deltoids throughout arm elevation.[28,38] Improved leverage of the anterior deltoid improves its contribution as the arm is raised.

Participation of the posterior deltoid in scapular plane elevation is less consistent. By roentgenologic analysis an abduction lever was not identified until the arm reached the 90-degree position.[43]

For flexion, the anterior deltoid is the primary muscle. It is assisted by the clavicular pectoralis major, coracobrachialis, and biceps brachii, as well as the middle deltoid (Fig. 32-7). While only the EMG activity of the cla-

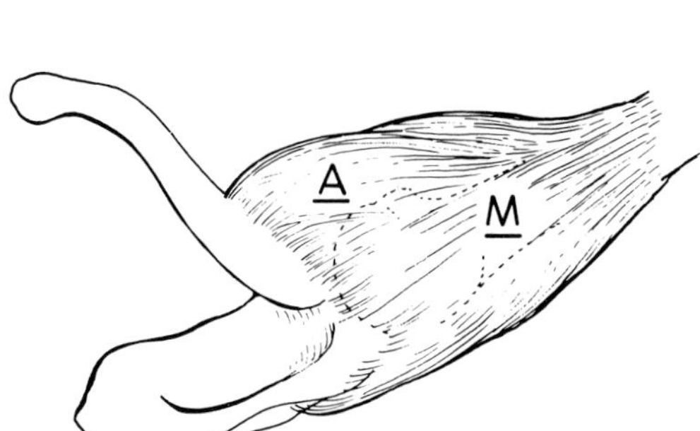

FIG. 32-6. Muscles providing neutral arm elevation (scapular plane). *A*, anterior deltoid; *M*, middle deltoid. (From Rowe CR: The shoulder, New York, 1988, Churchill Livingstone, Inc.)

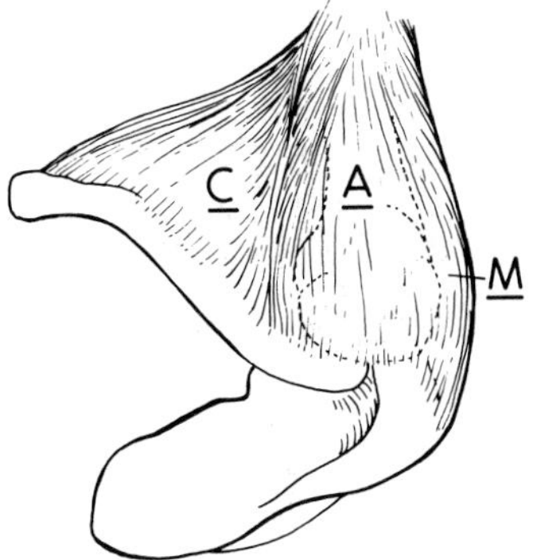

FIG. 32-7. Muscles providing arm flexion (sagittal plane elevation). *C*, clavicular head of the major: *A*, anterior deltoid; *M*, middle deltoid. (From Rowe CR: The shoulder, New York, 1988, Churchill Livingstone, Inc.)

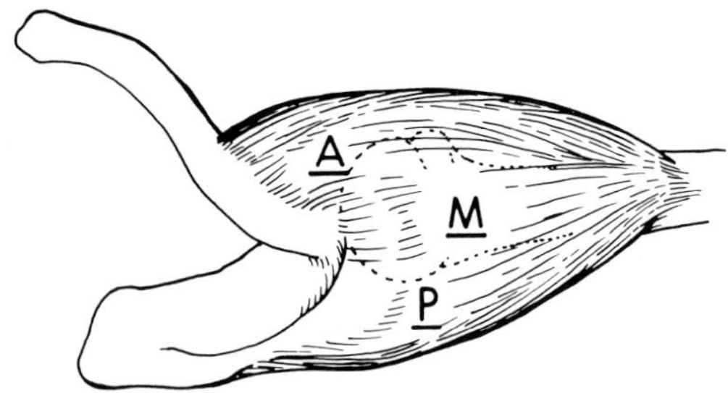

FIG. 32-8. Muscle providing arm abduction (coronal plane elevation). *A*, anterior deltoid; *M*, middle deltoid; *P*, posterior deltoid. (From Rowe CR: The shoulder, New York, 1988, Churchill Livingstone, Inc.)

vicular pectoralis major (CPM) has been studied in detail,[22,49,52] participation by the other muscles has been confirmed. Relative EMG activity of the CPM and deltoid indicated that these superficial muscles provided about 30 percent of the arm elevation effort.

Abduction in the coronal plane adds significant posterior deltoid action to that of the anterior and middle components[38,49] (Fig. 32-8). Conversely, participation of the anterior deltoid is less. This difference is particularly apparent in the arc of motion below 90 degrees.

Hyperextension, or posterior elevation, is dominated by the posterior deltoid. There also is strong participation by the middle deltoid but the anterior muscle is silent.[52]

Effectiveness of the deltoid muscles depends on their functional fiber length. It is greatest with the arm in the dependent rest period and shortest with full glenohumeral elevation. Anatomically, this represents a 33% reduction in the length of the muscle.[30] Functionally, the muscle becomes weaker. Such loss of deltoid strength is avoided by scapular rotation.

The deltoid is anatomically capable of initiating, as well as completing, arm elevation independently because of its mass, even though the leverage at 30 degrees is very low. A strenuous effect (about 54% of maximal) would be required, however, with a corresponding limit in endurance.

Biceps brachii. Between its origin on the superior rim of the glenoid and passage through the bicipital groove on the humeral shaft, the long head of the biceps lies across the top of the humeral head. Contraction of the biceps muscle would thus appear to be a useful humeral head depressor. Limitations to its effectiveness result from its distal attachment to the radius; hence it is an elbow muscle. EMG analysis of pitching confirmed that the need for elbow control was the stimulus for biceps action, not humeral elevation. Also, peak activity of the biceps was only 36% of its maximal capacity with a 9 cm^2 cross section and only half of the muscle related to the long head. The humeral force is small. The stabilizing force at the glenohumeral joint is therefore limited.

Supraspinatus. This muscle is active in all patterns of arm elevation.[22,38,52] Its short leverage (2.2 cm) and modest size (6 cm^2) limit the torque that can be produced, however. Maximal effort (calculated as 98%) could accomplish arm elevation to 30 degrees but not higher. Because this intensity of action would leave no endurance for a second effort, assistance, not initiation of abduction, is its role. A recent anatomic study identified greater strength capability of the supraspinatus. The authors used the shortness and obliquity of the fibers to calculate a larger functional cross section than has been reported previously. The failure to identify independent supraspinatus action leaves this interpretation in doubt, however.

Deltoid-supraspinatus relationships. Common to all three patterns of arm elevation is combined deltoid and supraspinatus action.* The relative responsibility of these two muscles, however, still is in doubt.

It has been commonly assumed that abduction of the arm is initiated by the supraspinatus and continued by the deltoid.[21] Codman[10] believed that the deltoid could not abduct the arm without the supraspinatus. This interpretation is based on clinical experience with large rotator cuff ruptures. Such a lesion deprives the person of the ability to lift the arm, yet once the arm has been passively raised to the horizontal the patient can maintain that arm position, though strength is reduced.

Three findings contradict the probability

*References 22, 23, 26, 38, 52.

that abduction is initiated by the supraspinatus: muscle size, EMG patterns, and cuff mechanics.

The muscle is anatomically too small to lift the arm independently. While it could accomplish the first 30 degrees, a 200% effort would be required to reach the horizontal position. In contrast, the size and leverage of the deltoid would allow the arm to be raised with an effort of 55% of maximum.

Dynamic EMG shows that the middle and anterior deltoids and supraspinatus function synchronously.[23,32,38] Through such a combined action, the calculated intensity of each muscle is 35% of maximal strength. This level of muscular effort would be compatible with long endurance demands.

Infraspinatus and subscapularis. Participation by the other rotator cuff muscle also has been identified. Presumably they contribute to the force couple that facilitates arm elevation.[22,38,52] Studies of normal[22,38,46,52] and athletic[3,26] arm function, as well as assessment by axillary and suprascapular nerve blocks,[11,12] leave the role of the infraspinatus and subscapularis during arm elevation in question. Electromyographically, the infraspinatus is the next most active rotator cuff muscle after the supraspinatus muscle, while the subscapularis is more selective.[23,24,26] Because of their potential contribution to glenohumeral joint stability, enhancing these muscles' participation in arm elevation is very desirous. Anatomically, both muscles have fan-shaped distribution of their fibers. This enables the upper fiber to roughly parallel the alignment of the supraspinatus and thus contribute a similar function. In addition, the lower fibers angle downward to introduce a depressive action. The basic function of these two muscles and the teres minor is humeral rotation on the glenoid.[52]

Infraspinatus activity is stimulated by elevating the arm with some degree of elbow flexion. This introduces an internal rotation torque that must be restrained if hand position is to be preserved. The teres minor would also participate in this action. EMG studies indicate that the infraspinatus is the more active muscle in this pair.[23,26]

Subscapularis activity relates to its ability to provide internal rotation. Deceleration of external rotation is a common stimulus.[23] It often functions in company with the other internal rotators of the shoulder, such as the pectoralis major, teres major, and latissimus dorsi.

Horizontal Extension and External Rotation

This motion synergy is commonly used to create a propulsive force in sports. It provided the cocking[2,21] phase of pitching,[23,26] throwing,[2] and tennis serve and is also a significant

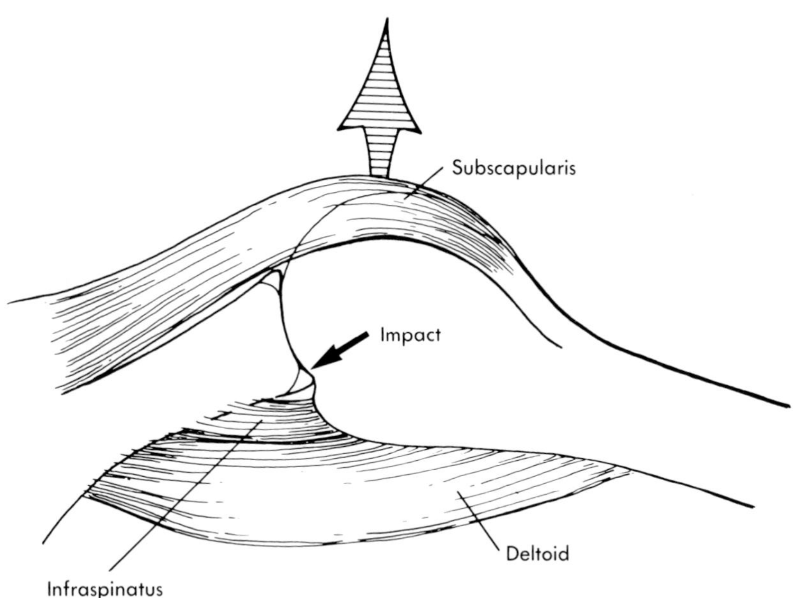

FIG. 32-9. Horizontal extension and external rotation. Posterior deltoid induced impact *(small arrow)* and anterior shear *(large arrow)* countered by infraspinatus and subscapularis muscle action. (From Rowe CR: The shoulder, New York, 1988, Churchill Livingstone, Inc.)

part of most strokes in swimming.[6,45,51] Both posterior impingement and anterior subluxation are likely complications.

As the middle and anterior deltoids support arm weight, the posterior deltoids increases its activity to draw the humerus backwards (horizontal extension) (Fig. 32-9). Two force patterns result: compression and anterior shear.

At the beginning of posterior deltoid action, the muscle's line of pull is primarily longitudinal, making compression the major force. Alignment of the muscle tends to concentrate the force at the posterior margins of the humeral head and glenoid fossa. During rapid motion this can be an abrupt and destructive impact of considerable intensity.

The muscle's origination along the length of the scapular spine and insertion at the midhumeral shaft places the posterior deltoid's line of pull a considerable distance behind the glenohumeral joint center. This distance increases as horizontal extension becomes greater. An anterior shear force is induced that increases in intensity as hyperextension proceeds. External rotation accentuates the anterior subluxation tendency by directing the angulated humeral head against the anterior capsule.

Protective forces are available from three rotator cuff muscles: infraspinatus, teres minor, and subscapularis. The infraspinatus is a primary motor for both external rotation and hyperextension. Hence it can reduce the intensity of posterior deltoid action. Also, because it lies adjacent to the joint margin, its actions prevent humeral subluxation. The teres minor, as an external rotator, also reduces the deltoid response.

Subscapularis activity at the end of the hyperextension and external rotation effort provides an anterior restraint against humeral displacement. This synergistic sequence is displayed in the EMG analysis of a baseball pitch (Fig. 32-10). The sternal pectoralis major also provides a protective force as its tendon crosses the anterior joint surface when the arm is both hyperextended and externally rotated. Hence, initiation of the motion combined with decelerating forces involves a complex synergy and sequence of muscle action.

Internal Rotation and Horizontal Flexion

Acceleration to complete the throwing or propulsive act and then follow-through are performed by the following sequence of cocking, acceleration, and follow-through. Muscle activity is stimulated by tension at the end of the cocking phase. EMG recordings show that the major muscle contributing to acceleration is the subscapularis.[23,26] Participation of the sternal pectoralis major and latissimus dorsi was less consistent. The latter muscle was strongly used by professional pitchers, while amateurs called on the pectoralis major.[19] Athletic use of the teres major has not been assessed, but EMG studies of basic arm function identified its action in internal rotation and adduction.[52] This implies that the teres major would be a logical participant in the acceleration to follow-through motion sequence.

During follow-through the weight of the

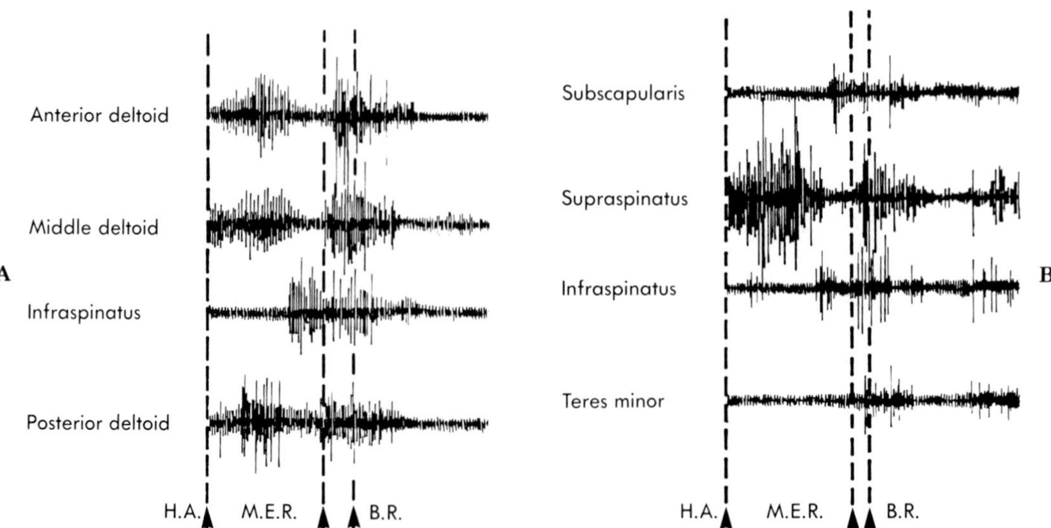

FIG. 32-10. Muscle action during a typical baseball pitch. **A,** Deltoid. **B,** Rotator cuff. Phases of pitching: *H.A.*, hands apart; *M.E.R.*, maximum external rotation; *B.R.*, ball release. (From Rowe CR: The shoulder, New York, 1988, Churchill Livingstone, Inc.)

arm creates a distractive force at the shoulder from the pendulous momentum present. The antagonistic action identified in the infraspinatus, teres minor, supraspinatus, and latissimus dorsi[19] acts to decelerate the force and serve to maintain shoulder joint integrity.

Scapulothoracic Articulation

Five muscles directly control the scapula. Functional division of the trapezius into upper, middle, and lower units expands the number to seven. The major and minor rhomboids will be considered as one. Hence, functional concern revolves around six muscle units: levator scapulae; upper, middle, and lower trapezius; rhomboids; and serratus anterior. Synergistic action of the muscles varies with the scapular motion desired.

Motor controls of the scapula

- Levator scapula
- Trapezius (upper, middle, and lower)
- Rhomboids
- Serratus anterior

Among the scapula's potential functions, upward rotation in conjunction with arm elevation is the primary clinical concern. The other actions complete the arm's versatility with their significance varying according to the person's occupation or sport.

Although each scapular motion can be performed independently for testing, they normally are an integral component of arm function.

Upward Rotation

Rotation of the scapula is defined by the direction the glenoid moves. Upward rotation is an essential component of arm elevation. Two muscles are recognized as the upward rotators of the scapula: trapezius and serratus anterior. Normally, the trapezius and serratus act together, but either also can accomplish scapular rotation independently, though the strength of arm elevation will be less. Independent action by the trapezius is well documented by clinical experience. Isolated loss of the trapezius is a less frequent occurrence. Recent experience with two patients indicated incomplete arm elevation resulting from limited scapular rotation by the serratus. Lack of posterior stabilization allowed the serratus muscle length to be dominated by scapular abduction.

Within the trapezius, Inman et al[22] found that only the upper segment displayed consistent action in both abduction and flexion. Reduced participation by the lower trapezius in all but the last segment of flexion leaves the scapula free to move anteriorly. These limitations in the contribution of the trapezius to flexion places an added burden on the serratus anterior. This is particularly true in swimming, where maximal upward reach is used to increase one's stroke.

To attain maximal scapular rotation, both the trapezius and serratus anterior must be effective. EMG analysis of swimming demonstrated that the serratus worked at 75% of its maximal muscle test capability.[39] This is too strenuous for a lengthy effort. A similar high level of activity was identified during voluntary arm elevation in all three basic planes, whether the elbow was flexed or extended.[38] Raising the arm to 90 degrees averaged 41% of maximum, while reaching full elevation increased the effort to 66% of maximum. During pitching, there also is a short period of serratus activity that exceeds 100% of the manual muscle test (MMT). The relative intensity of the serratus consistently was greater than that of the trapezius, which progressed from 34% to 42% maximum. According to Weber's data the two muscles are of equivalent size (12.8 and 12.6 cm^2) and thus should have similar force potentials.[58] The greater effort by the serratus suggests that it is less well developed to meet the functional demands imposed on it. Adequate training is thus particularly significant if one is to lessen the threats of impingement. Maximal overhead reach puts all the muscles in a relatively inefficient situation because of fiber shortening. Activities in flexion reduce the ability of the lower trapezius to contribute, resulting in a higher demand on the serratus. A 75% effort by the serratus cannot be maintained during prolonged swimming sessions, hence better training is indicated.

Retraction (Adduction)

Drawing the scapula back toward the vertebral midline accentuates horizontal extension of the arm. A synonym for this action is scapular adduction. The cocking phase of pitching and pulling relies on such assistance. Several swimming strokes also use this action.

Direct muscle control is provided by the middle trapezius and rhomboids. The latissimus dorsi also retracts the scapula incidental to complete arm extension.

Protraction (Abduction)

Advancement of the scapula anteriorly on the thorax has been called both"protraction" and "scapular abduction" (moving away from the vertebral column). The latter term, however, leads to confusion when scapular and humeral motions are considered together. Hence the older term "protraction" is being adopted again. Protraction is the function of the serratus anterior. There also may be some assistance by the sternal pectoralis major as it horizontally flexes the arm. Follow-through in throwing,[2] pitching,[3] tennis serve, and crawl strokes[10,51] include scapular protraction.

Depression

Descent of the scapula is used to elevate the trunk while the arms are stabilized. The site of arm fixation varies. During gymnastics an overhead bar, ring, or underlying platform is used. Immediate muscular control is provided by the inferior digitations of the serratus anterior and the lower trapezius. Additional force of considerable magnitude is gained from the two large thoracohumeral muscles: sternal pectoralis major and latissimus dorsi.

Scapula motion

- **Upward rotation**
  Trapezius
  Serratus anterior
- **Retraction**
  Middle trapezius
  Rhomboids
- **Protraction**
  Serratus anterior
- **Depression**
  Lower trapezius
  Inferior portion of serratus anterior

Arm Torque

To understand the relationships between arm function and muscle action, some simple rules of mechanics must be appreciated.

Raising the arm from the side of the body moves its center of gravity (c/g) away from this neutral line. A moment arm (or lever) has been created. This is seen as a demand torque to which the muscles must respond. As arm elevation increases, the functional lever is lengthened, leading to a correspondingly greater torque (Fig. 32-11).

These changes follow the cosine law of trigonometry. The maximal arm lever occurs at 90 degrees elevation. This decreases 71% at the 45-degree position and 50% of maximum with the arm elevated 30 degrees. The significance of these numbers relates to the changing demands arm weight places on the shoulder's abducting musculature.

Flexing the elbow 90 degrees reduces the arm torque 22% because the forearm and hand are opposite the elbow joint. This postural change, however, introduces an internal rotation torque. Hence, while the deltoid demand was lessened, a need for infraspinatus activity was added. Such postural variations can be used in the design of therapeutic exercises, for performance of a sport, or for basic daily use.

Muscle Forces

Muscles provide the body's active force to create or restrain motion. They function through bony levers. As a result, muscle strength is a torque ($F \times L = T$), as was arm demand. Both muscle force (F) and lever lengths (L) are modified by joint position.

The maximal force a muscle can produce is proportional to the number of motor cells it contains. These slender fibers (50 μm diameter) are counted indirectly by measuring the muscle's physiologic cross-section. If all the fibers have a longitudinal arrangement, a simple transverse (anatomic) section is sufficient. Pennate muscles have oblique fibers. This means one must count several bundles to attain the perpendicular area of all its fibers, a task that can only be done by detailed anatomic dissection.

The type of muscle action is a second strength variable. Isometric contractions provide the basic force. Eccentric action (contraction versus passive lengthening) has been found to produce the same amount of use.[48] In these two forms of muscle action (isometric and eccentric) the resulting force is a combination of both active and passive tension (Fig. 32-12). The latter arises from the collagenous sheaths enveloping each muscle fiber.[17] Concentric (shortening) contractions lack the advantage of passive tension and thus produce proportionally less force (13% to 20%).[48]

Speed further reduces concentric force. Motion at 214 degrees per second decreases maximal strength by 50%.[41]

Lever length is the final determinant of muscle effectiveness. It varies with joint position. The greater the perpendicular distance between the muscle's line of pull and the ful-

Factors in muscle force analysis

- Number of motor cells in muscle
- Type of contraction
- Speed of contraction
- Lever length

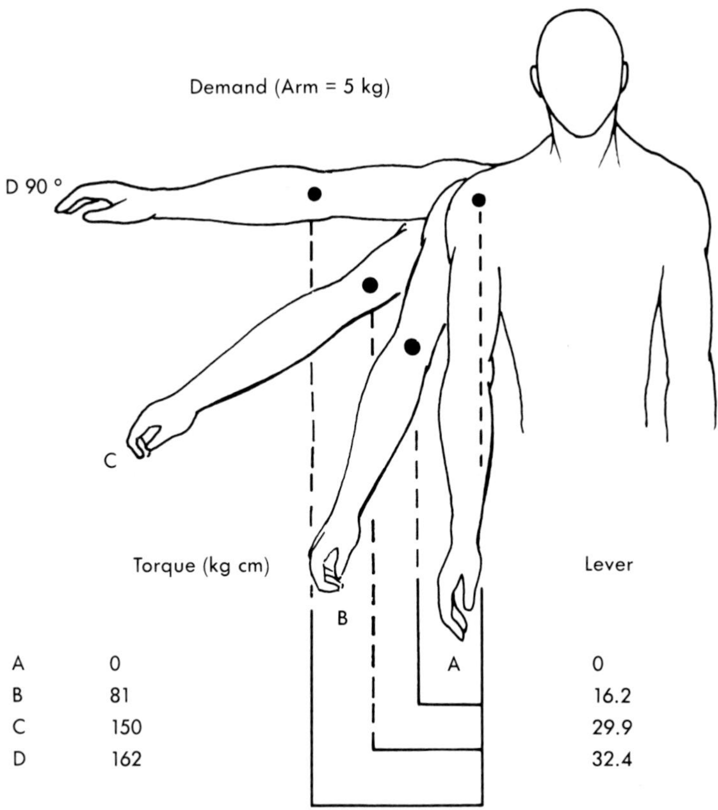

FIG. 32-11. Shoulder torque introduced by arm position. Weight is consistent but leverage increases with greater elevation. *A* = 0 degrees, *B* = 30 degrees, *C* = 45QoW, *D* = 90 degrees. (From Rowe CR: The shoulder, New York, 1988, Churchill Livingstone, Inc.)

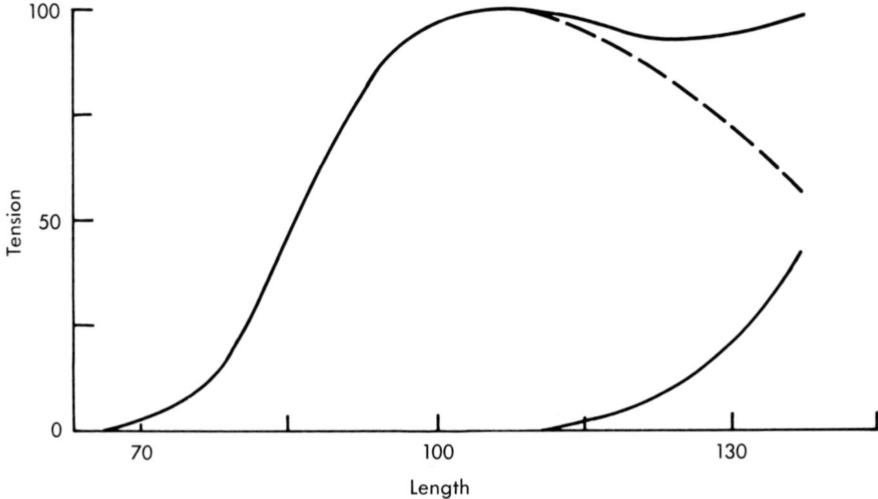

FIG. 32-12. Length tension relationships of muscle. *Top curve*, total tension; *dotted line*, active tension; *lower curve*, passive tension as muscle is pulled beyond resting length (100%). (From Rowe CR: The shoulder, New York, 1988, Churchill Livingstone, Inc.)

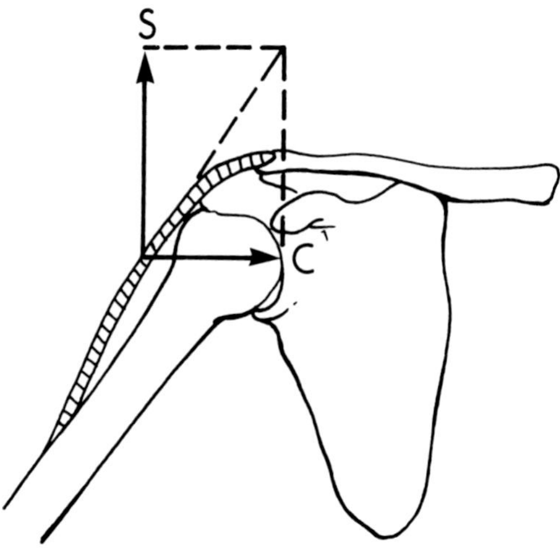

FIG. 32-13. Joint forces induced by muscle action (middle deltoid is the model). *C*, compression (perpendicular to plane of joint); *S*, shear (parallel to joint). (From Rowe CR: The shoulder, New York, 1988, Churchill Livingstone, Inc.)

crum of motion, the more effective is the muscle's force.

At the onset of arm elevation in the scapular plane, only the middle deltoid has an effective lever. Abduction to 60 degrees increases the muscle's leverage by 60%. It then remains relatively stable. The anterior deltoid with much of its origin on the clavicle, starts with an insignificant abduction lever, but rapid and continual arm elevation moves a greater proportion of the muscle lateral to the joint center. By 90 degrees it has surpassed that of the middle deltoid. In the resting position the origin of the posterior deltoid on the scapular spine places most of the muscle mass medial to the shoulder joint center. This alignment does not significantly improve until the arm has abducted 120 degrees. These improvements in mechanical leverage counter the effects of shortened muscle fiber (sarcomere) length. They also accommodate the increase in arm demand so that elevation strength is maintained. In contrast, lever length for the supraspinatus remains fairly constant throughout the range of arm elevation. This means there is no leverage advantage available to compensate for the reduction in muscle fiber length. Consequently, the supraspinatus becomes progressively less effective.

Shoulder Joint Forces

As muscles act to control the arm they create forces within the joint. These forces are classified by their alignment to the joint surface as either compression or shear (Fig. 32-13). Those directed toward the center of the joint (i.e., perpendicular to the plane of the glenoid fossa) are called "compression." Shear forces are parallel to the joint surface.[43]

The line of pull of most shoulder muscles is oblique to the plane of the glenoid fossa. As a result, both compression and shear forces accompany muscle action. The compressive forces contribute to joint stability as they drive the humeral head into the glenoid socket. In contrast, shear forces threaten the stabilizing tissues by the sliding strains created. The magnitude of the forces is determined by the intensity of muscle action. The amounts of shear and compression vary as the muscle's alignment changes.

During arm function the forces within the shoulder joint are related to two major muscle groups: deltoid and rotator cuff. They differ markedly in their patterns of compression and shear.

Deltoid

The deltoid changes from a vertical to horizontal muscle as the arm is elevated. This alters the relative dominance of shear and compression force produced. During scapular plane abduction, the force patterns of the anterior and posterior components are similar to that of the middle head. With the arm at rest, the middle deltoid's line of pull is 27 degrees to the glenoid face. As a result, at the initiation of abduction, the dominant direction of deltoid pull is vertical, creating significant upward shear (89% of the muscle's total force versus a compression value of 45%) (Fig. 32-14). Further elevation progressively makes the muscle's line of pull more horizontal. Shear is reduced and compression increased. Above 60 degrees abduction, compression exceeds shear.

Rotator Cuff

Force patterns of the rotator cuff muscle contrast sharply with the deltoid. Their dominant directions are horizontal and downward. The supraspinatus is basically horizontal (Fig. 32-15). As a result, compression is the dominant joint force generated. There is a much smaller vertical shear, equaling 34% of the muscle force.

All three of the other rotator cuff muscles have a mean downward alignment (Fig. 32-16). While their precise direction has not been measured, it approximates 45 degrees for the infraspinatus and subscapularis and 55 degrees for the teres minor.[41] Their inferior shear force (71% to 82%) would counteract that of the deltoid. Inman noted that during

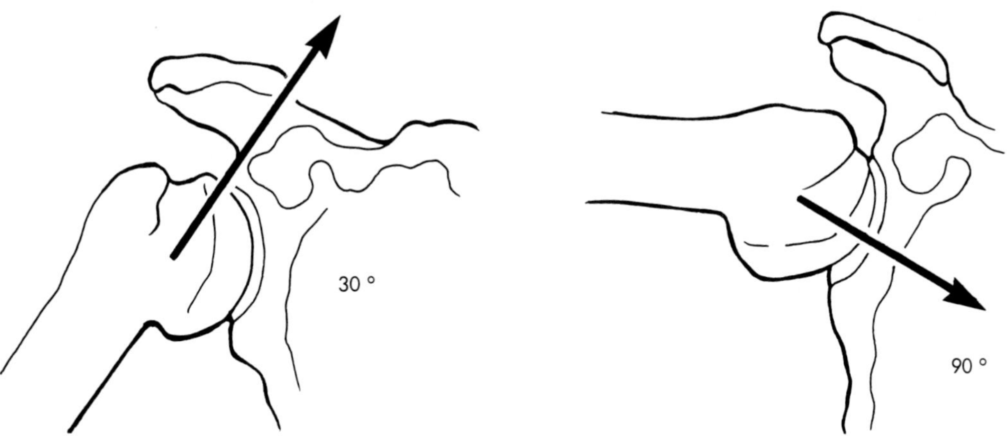

FIG. 32-14. Direction of the joint forces with shoulder in **A,** 30-degree. **B,** 90-degree scapular abduction. (From Rowe CR: The shoulder, New York, 1988, Churchill Livingstone, Inc.)

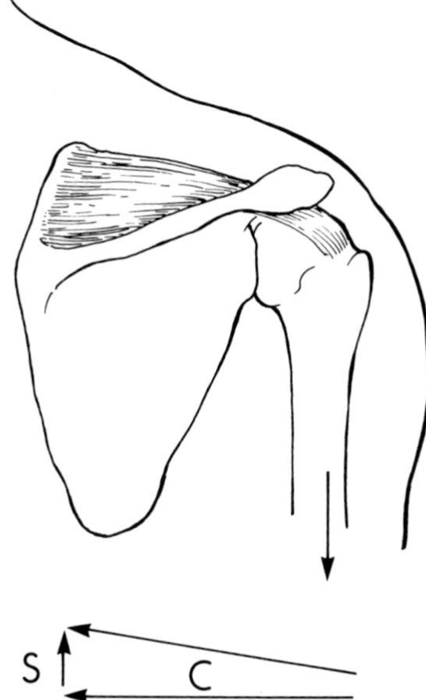

FIG. 32-15. Supraspinatus joint forces, compression dominant. (From Rowe CR: The shoulder, New York, 1988, Churchill Livingstone, Inc.)

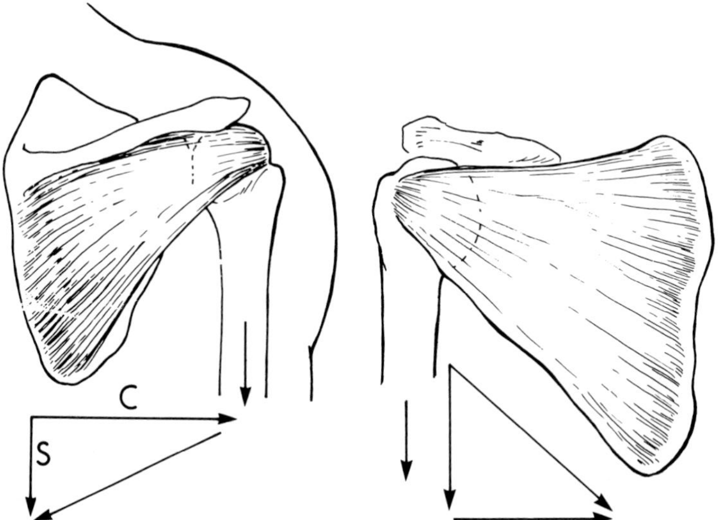

FIG. 32-16. Depressor muscles of the rotator cuff: shear force is strong and downward. **A,** infraspinatus. **B,** subscapularis. (From Rowe CR: The shoulder, New York, 1988, Churchill Livingstone, Inc.)

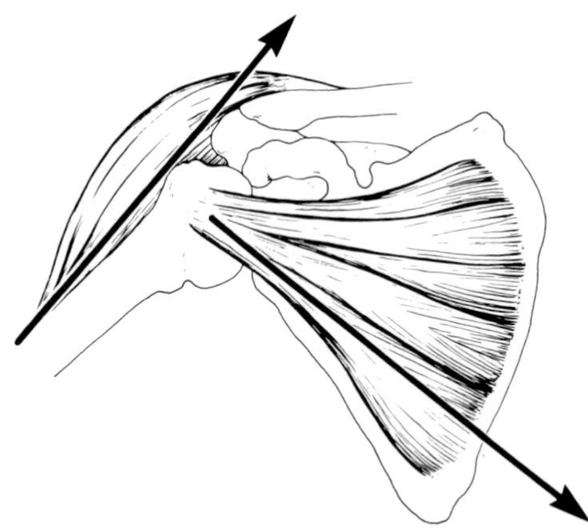

FIG. 32-17. Inman force couple between deltoid and depressor muscles in the rotator cuff. (From Rowe CR: The shoulder, New York, 1988, Churchill Livingstone, Inc.)

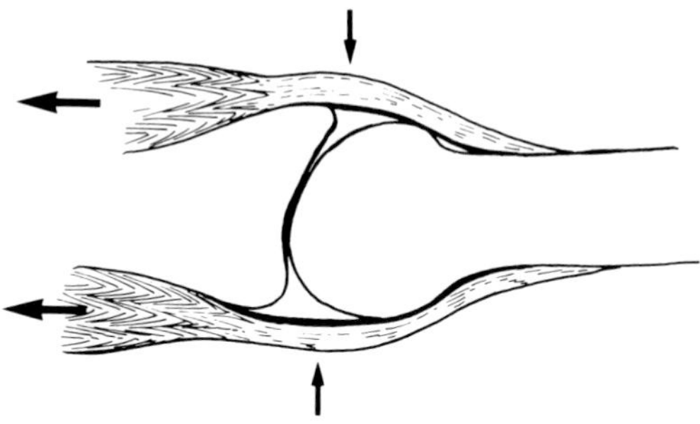

FIG. 32-18. Rotator cuff muscle action creates compressive and encircling shear forces to stabilize the humeral head of the glenoid fossa. (From Rowe CR: The shoulder, New York, 1988, Churchill Livingstone, Inc.)

routine arm elevation the deltoid and rotator cuff contracted synchronously. He called this action "the shoulder-force" couple with the upward and downward forces in balance (Fig. 32-17). Inman also postulated that arm abduction could not occur without rotator cuff coordination.[22]

The combined effect of such muscle action was calculated by Inman et al[22] as creating a shoulder joint compression force equaling body weight. These authors also found that peak joint force occurred at 90 degrees, while maximal shear was at the 60-degree position.

Biceps Role in Rotator Cuff Tears

The role of the biceps at the shoulder has been controversial.[5,16] EMG analysis during pitching demonstrated that the biceps functions predominatly at the elbow rather than at the shoulder during throwing.[53] The similarity of the biceps and brachialis firing patterns supported this finding. Biceps activity correlated with motion, occurring as the elbow flexed during late cocking and as the elbow decelerated during follow-through. The heads of the triceps worked together, also correlating with elbow motion.

The biceps does make a small functional contribution to the shoulder during abduction and flexion when the arm is externally rotated and supinated.[5,16] Evaluation of the lateral biceps (long head) action in shoulders with rotator cuff tears revealed that the muscle may be a significant contributor to both flexion and abduction in the compromised shoulder.[53] This was supported by the significantly increased activity of the lateral biceps during shoulder flexion and abduction with a torn rotator cuff. Before this study, a consistent intraoperative finding had been an enlarged biceps tendon in association with a major rotator cuff tear. The increase in EMG activity along with the observed enlargement of biceps tendon width would implicate a use-induced hypertrophy of the tendon. Therefore it is suggested that the practice of sacrificing interscapular portion of the biceps tendon for grafting material or tenodesis during rotator cuff repair should be examined more discriminately.

Dynamic Shoulder Stability

As identified by the muscle force pattern at the shoulder, the function of the rotator cuff is to reduce the shearing strain introduced by deltoid action. Contouring of the tendons around the humeral head adds a direct restraining force.

Muscle action transforms the tissue into straighter, tense bands (Fig. 32-18). Both compression and shear forces are created to stabilize the humeral head on the glenoid. The favorable balance between compression and shear force makes shoulder elevation to 90 degrees the optimal position of joint stability.

THE ELBOW

Elbow Mobility

The elbow is limited by bony constraints, joint geometry, capsule, ligaments, and muscles. Normal elbow hinge motion includes 5 degrees of hyperextension and 150 degrees of flexion. Axial rotation of the radius about the ulna averages 130 degrees (75 degrees of pronation and supination to 55 degrees). Elbow extension is limited by four factors. Two are skeletal impingement between the forearm and the humerus (i.e., the radial head against the anterior capitellum) and impact of the coronoid process against the trochlea. Two other limitations relate to the soft tissue. These include tension of the anterior capsule and the musculature. The range of forearm rotation occuring at the elbow also is modified by the soft tissues.[1] Total rotation from supination to pronation in the intact arm is around 130 degrees. When the muscles are removed from a cadaver, the range increases to 190 degrees, and when the ligaments are cut, the range increases to 210 degrees.[1]

Instant Centers of Elbow Motion

The axis of elbow flexion and extension passes through the trochlea. The instant center of rotation occurs within a 2 to 3 mm zone at the center of the trochlea.[36] The axis of rotation is internally rotated 3 to 8 degrees relative to the plane of the epicondyles, and its perpendicular axis has a lateral opening angle of 4 to 8 degrees relative to the long axis of the humerus.[1]

The carrying angle that is formed by the long axes of the humerus and ulna in the frontal plane averages 10 to 15 degrees in men and 15 to 20 degrees in females. Because the trochlea is not orthogonal to the humerus, the carrying angle changes, being greatest at full extension and diminishing during flexion.

The longitudinal axis of forearm rotation or supination-pronation runs proximally from the distal end of the ulnar center to the center of the radial head. The ulna remains fixed with the radius rotating over the ulnar shaft during pronation and supination.

Movement of the elbow joint occurs about two basic planes, the transverse and longitudinal axis. Isometric muscle contraction often occurs to maintain or check the position of the elbow in space as the limb is moved at the shoulder.

Elbow Muscle Control

Flexion

There are three primary elbow flexor muscles: brachialis, biceps, and brachioradialis. Being superficial, mobile, and large, the biceps brachii is most conspicuous. The biceps, by inserting on the radius, acts first as a supinator and then flexes the elbow. With the forearm pronated, the biceps is less active because its functional leverage is less. The biceps also acts to decelerate elbow extension.

The brachialis, which lies deep to the biceps, is of similar size. Its more pennate form leads to a greater physiologic cross section (45%), which compensates for the shorter lever length. The insertion of the brachialis on the ulna makes the actions of this elbow flexor independent of forearm position.

Brachioradialis action also is sensitive to forearm rotation but in a reverse relationship. Supination laterally displaces the muscle so that its flexion capability is much reduced. Conversely, middle position and pronation put the brachioradialis in a very favorable flexor position on the anterior surface of the joint. While its leverage is good, the muscle is small (36% of the biceps).

Elbow flexors

- Brachialis
- Biceps brachii
- Brachioradialis

The pronator teres as well as the finger and wrist flexors and extensors have limited elbow flexion capability.

Extension

The medial head of the triceps and anconeus are most active during elbow extension with the lateral and long head of the triceps supplementing the extension force.[54] There is increased activity of the triceps with increasing elbow flexion resulting from its secondary action as a decelerator and from an increasing stretch reflex.

Elbow extensors

- Triceps
- Anconeus

Forces

Muscles create the force needed to lift the arm and move it from one position to another. Incidental to that action, forces are created within the joint. Some contribute to stability while others threaten joint integrity. The balance of joint forces depends on arm position and the pattern of responding muscles.

The forces created within the elbow joint are dependent on the joint position. This is because the line of action of the arm muscles change during flexion and extension. The maximal elbow flexion strength occurs at 90 degrees with decreasing force during extension. Because the flexor muscles have such a poor mechanical advantage with the elbow in relative extension, the isometric forces have to be greatest in this position. Flexor muscle

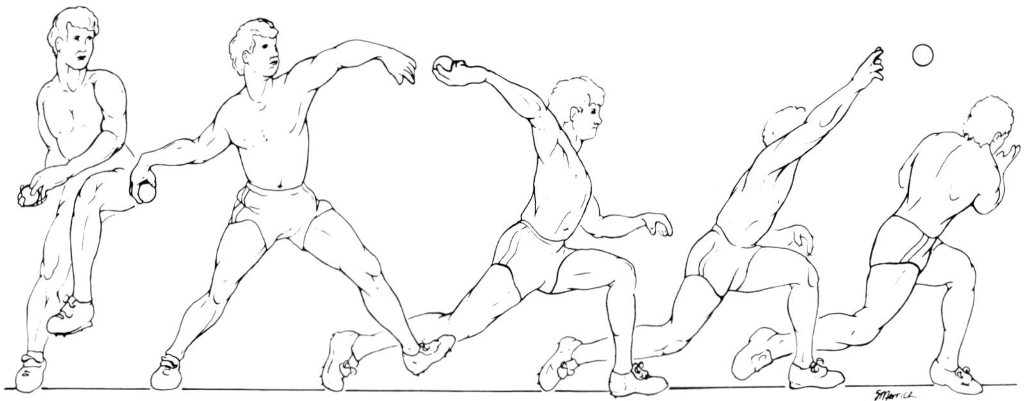

FIG. 32-19. Phases of the pitch, from left to right: wind-up, early cocking, late cocking, acceleration, follow-through.

action introduces a posterosuperior compressive force across the distal humerus.

Elbow Stability

Unlike the unconstrained glenohumeral joint, the elbow is one of the most stable joints secondary to its bony interlocking anatomy. Stability is enhanced and supported by the static soft tissue stabilizers.

The radial collateral ligament lies on the axis of rotation and therefore is taut throughout elbow motion. In contrast, the ulnar collateral ligament components will be taut during different positions of elbow motion.[1]

During extension, varus stress is shared between the bony anatomy and lateral collateral ligament complex. Valgus stress is shared between the bony anatomy and medial collateral ligament (anterior component). During flexion, the bony anatomy provides the majority of varus stability, whereas the medial collateral ligament provides the majority of stability to valgus stress.

ATHLETIC SHOULDER FUNCTION

Athletic injuries to the shoulder are common. It was observed that athletes often had selective weakness of specific rotator cuff muscles rather than generalized muscle impairment. This led investigators to question whether Inman's conclusions regarding single plane motion and analysis could be applied to sport-specific activities.[18,24,26]

The basis of the difference found during athletic endeavors was one of functional demand. Casual elevation of the arm in any of the basic planes presents a prolonged three-dimensional challenge to stabilize the arm in space. Consequently, the humeral rotator muscles act in synchrony with the deltoid, which is raising the arm. The EMG data have demonstrated that the rapid and precise motion patterns characterizing the individual sports stimulate more selective muscle action as well as specific periods of great intensity.

The concept of the separate and independent action of the deltoid and rotator cuff helped to explain selective muscle weakness seen in the throwing athlete. Therefore a specific rehabilitation program to individually strengthen the rotator cuff muscles in the throwing athlete was devised.[37] This program has remained in effect in both prevention and rehabilitation, and it is used by both amateur and professional athletes.

While each sport has its own phasic pattern, there is also a commonality among them.[41] With the exception of swimming, each arm cycle begins with a gentle approach to the appropriate starting position. Subsequently, the shoulder structures are "cocked" to provide a tense, highly forceful unit ready for an accelerated release.[54] Once the critical effect has been accomplished, the muscles respond to decelerate the limb so that residual force will not cause injury. In this sequence, baseball pitching provides the clearest model, but the same pattern is evident in the other sports under different phasic terms.

Throwing

Phases of Throwing Motion

During a baseball pitch the deltoid is responsible for arm elevation with active forward flexion and abduction of the humerus.[2,22] In most sports only a moderate level of muscle effort is required. The exceptions are high activity in swimming and the tennis backhand stroke. The baseball pitch has been divided into five stages described as follows (Fig. 32-19).

STAGE I
Windup or preparation stage, ending when the ball leaves the gloved hand.
STAGE II
Early cocking stage, a period of shoulder abduction and external rotation, that begins as the ball is released from the nondominant hand and terminates with foot-ground contact.
STAGE III
Late cocking stage, arm function continuing until maximal external rotation at the shoulder is attained.
STAGE IV
Acceleration stage, starts with internal rotation of the humerus and ends with ball release.
STAGE V
Follow-through stage, starts with ball release and ends when all the motion is complete.

All heads of the deltoid (anterior, middle, and posterior) experienced peak activity in early cocking when the arm was elevated to 90 degrees. Subsequently, in late cocking, the activity of the deltoid diminished as the rotator cuff muscles increased their action. This sequential pattern of muscle activity, beginning with the deltoid and ending with the rotator cuff, contradicts the obligatory synergy proposed by Inman. It also emphasizes and demonstrates the importance of the rotator cuff in throwing, and it demonstrates that in late cocking the primary force is generated by the rotator cuff.

The supraspinatus has been thought to play an important role in humeral abduction. Its action in pitching demonstrated peak activity in late cocking when the arm already is abducted and most prone to subluxation.[55] The supraspinatus contributes to the stability of the joint by drawing the humeral head toward the glenoid.[4,31,43] This correlated with the compressive force pattern Poppen noted at the glenohumeral joint in abduction.[43] The markedly greater use of the supraspinatus muscle by the amateur pitchers compared to the professionals is a strong endorsement for preliminary conditioning.[19] Fatigue from overuse could readily subject the amateurs to shoulder injury. As the athlete becomes proficient, efficient and economical use of the muscles takes place, preventing overuse and injury.

The infraspinatus and teres minor are responsible for external rotation of the shoulder.[4,31] Their action contributes to stability by drawing the head toward the glenoid fossa. The activity patterns were similar for both muscles, with peak activity in late cocking and follow-through, though both lagged behind the supraspinatus in timing.

The subscapularis has its peak activity in late cocking when eccentrically contracting to protect the anterior joint, which is under extreme tension. It then continues to function as an internal rotator to help carry the arm across the chest during acceleration and follow-through.[25]

Professional throwing athletes demonstrated selective use of the individual rotator cuff muscles.[19] The professional pitchers were able to use the subscapularis muscle exclusively among the rotator cuff muscles during the acceleration phase of pitching. This was in contrast to the amateurs who tended to use all the rotator cuff and biceps muscles. The proper, coordinated motion of the trunk, shoulder, and elbow by the professional renders the supraspinatus, infraspinatus, teres minor, and biceps unnecessary for acceleration. Repetitive activities such as pitching can lead to muscle strains and tendonitis.[44] Overuse syndromes may occur earlier and more often in the athlete who uses his muscle unnecessarily. Efficient muscle use learned through training may improve endurance and avoid an injury that is secondary to overuse.

The pectoralis major and latissimus dorsi function together to act as internal rotators and eccentrically contract to protect the joint along with the subscapularis during late cocking.[24] Further increase of their activity during acceleration indicates that intense internal rotation and forceful arm depression provide the principle propulsive force.

The serratus anterior controls the scapula to provide a stable glenoid to serve as a secure platform for the humeral head.[4,22] This provides a stable platform with which the humeral head articulates. Serratus anterior activity is important for both upward and scapular protraction during late cocking. This allows the scapula to keep pace with the humerus, which is horizontally flexing and externally rotating. The relatively low level of trapezius activity during the cocking and acceleration phases implies that this muscle primarily provides supplementary scapular stabilization to enhance the rotational action of the serratus anterior during pitching. During follow-through the adductive action of the trapezius serves to decelerate scapular protraction.

Throwing Shoulder with Impingement

Analysis of the shoulder in throwers with subacromial impingement demonstrated discrepancies in the pattern of muscle use between the impingers and normals.[35] During late cocking, deltoid activity continued in the impingers while decreasing in the normals. A lower level of supraspinatus action renders it less able to assist the deltoid during cocking. Presumably this dynamic imbalance results from supraspinatus inhibition to reduce tension on an injured tendon.

The internal rotators (subscapularis, pectoralis major, and latissimus dorsi) and serratus anterior also had dramatic differences during both early and late cocking in the impinged shoulders. Their reduced activity may contribute to increased external rotation, superior humeral migration, and impaired scapular rotation, which would predispose or aggravate the impingement syndrome.

The data provide evidence that the neuromuscular differences seen may account for the initial or persistent impingement problems in the throwing athlete. Complete reconditioning and retraining of these muscles must be accomplished as part of a preventive or rehabilitative program.

Throwing Shoulder with Instability

Evaluation of the patients with an isolated diagnosis of glenohumeral instability revealed differences from the normals.[18] The increased activity of the biceps during acceleration with instability was mild, but it could represent a compensatory mechanism to help stabilize the humeral head against the glenoid. This is consistent with the difference occurring in late cocking and acceleration when the arm is most prone to subluxation.

The mild enhancement of supraspinatus activity throughout cocking and acceleration may help to stabilize the joint in the instability patient by drawing the humeral head toward the glenoid.

The pectoralis major, subscapularis, and latissimus dorsi all demonstrated marked decreased activity during the pitch in patients with instability. Inhibition of the synergistic activity of these muscles allow for persistent or accentuated external rotation. This neuromuscular difference is postulated to be a factor in producing or maintaining chronic anterior instability.

Decreased serratus anterior activity in the instability patient diminishes horizontal protraction of the scapula, which normally begins during late cocking. Early fatigue of the serratus anterior will then add to the stress on the anterior restraints.

As part of a conservative or postsurgical rehabilitative program, the thrower with subluxation should strengthen and retrain the muscles about the shoulder. Data have been provided to support the internal rotators and scapular protractors as key points of focus in patients with instability.

Upon careful clinical evaluation of throwing athletes with impingement findings, many were found to have underlying anterior instability. Clinically, we found that when both entities were present, the instability problem had to be addressed primarily or the symptoms persisted (see Chapter 33).

Swimming

The swimming strokes are broken down into the pull-through and recovery phases as described by Richardson et al[45] (Fig. 32-20, 32-21, and 32-22). EMG studies of shoulder activity during swimming also emphasized the importance of the rotator cuff. The supraspinatus, infraspinatus, and middle deltoid were predominantly recovery phase muscles. They function to abduct and externally rotate the extremity in preparation for a new pull-through phase similar to the cocking phase of throwing. This position places the arm at risk for subacromial impingement.[20] The serratus anterior also has an important function during recovery. It allows the acromion to rotate clear of the abducting humerus and pro-

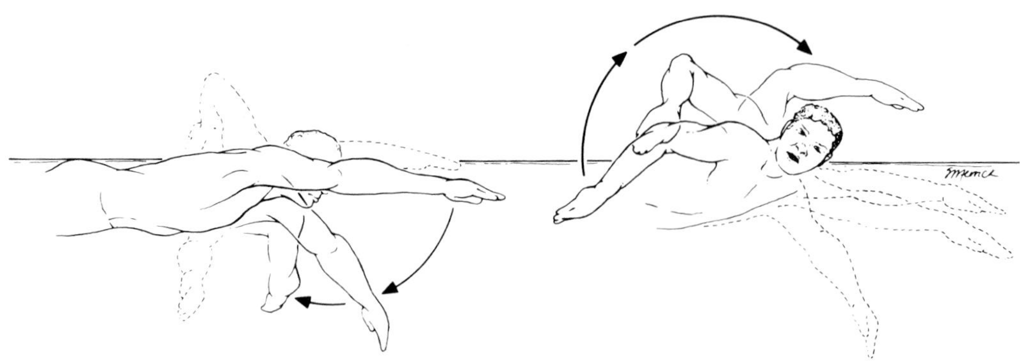

FIG. 32-20. Phases of the freestyle stroke, from left to right: pull-through, recovery.

vides a stable glenoid on which the arm may rotate as in throwing. The dry land data indicate that the serratus anterior works at nearly maximal levels to accomplish this. If over the course of a number of cycles this muscle fatigues, scapular rotation may not coincide with humeral abduction and impingement may precipitate. The biceps exhibited erratic action during all the strokes and functioned primarily at the elbow as occurred in pitching. The latissimus dorsi and pectoralis major were found to be propulsive muscles with action similar to the acceleration phase of throwing. The swimming study indicated that particular attention must be paid to the rotator cuff and serratus anterior in an effort to decrease the common problem of swimmer's shoulder impingement syndrome.[9]

Tennis

The tennis serve is divided into five categories corresponding to the baseball pitch[34] (Fig. 32-23).

Both the forehand and backhand ground strokes are divided into three stages (Figs. 32-24 and 32-25):

STAGE I
Racquet preparation stage begins with shoulder turn, ending with the initiation of weight transfer to the front foot.

STAGE II
Acceleration stage initiates with weight transfer to the front foot accompanied by forward racquet movement, culminating at ball impact.

STAGE III
Follow-through stage begins at ball impact and ends with completion of the stroke.

The tennis serve requires a complex sequence of muscle activity with phases similar to those observed in baseball pitching. Compared to pitching, deltoid muscle function is low during cocking because abduction is contributed to by trunk rotation. The tennis serve acceleration and follow-through phases demonstrated muscle patterns and activity that were similar to those observed in throwing.

The tennis serve was very similar to the overhead throw, and thus a conditioning program as outlined for pitchers may be used for tennis players. Emphasis should be placed on the rotator cuff and serratus anterior.

Analysis of the forehand ground stroke revealed a similar passive windup sequence. Again, trunk rotation provided a force for shoulder motion. In follow-through there was a marked decrease in activity among the accelerating muscles and a concomitant increase in the external rotators responsible for deceleration. The backhand ground stroke was similar in concept but opposite in muscle activity to the forehand. Follow-through demonstrated deceleration with increased activity of the internal rotators.

Golf

Shoulder activity during a right-handed golf swing was evaluated.[25]

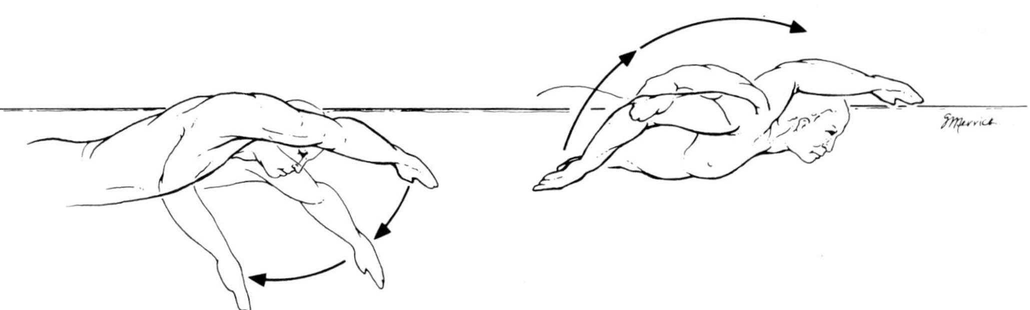

FIG. 32-21. Phases of the butterfly stroke, from left to right: pull-through, recovery.

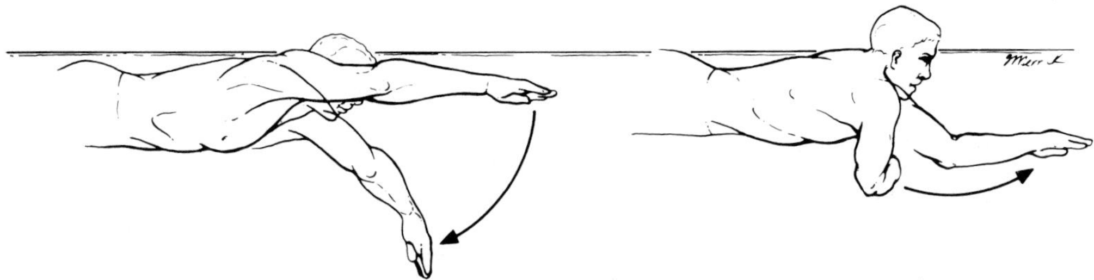

FIG. 32-22. Phases of the breaststroke, from left to right: pull-through, recovery.

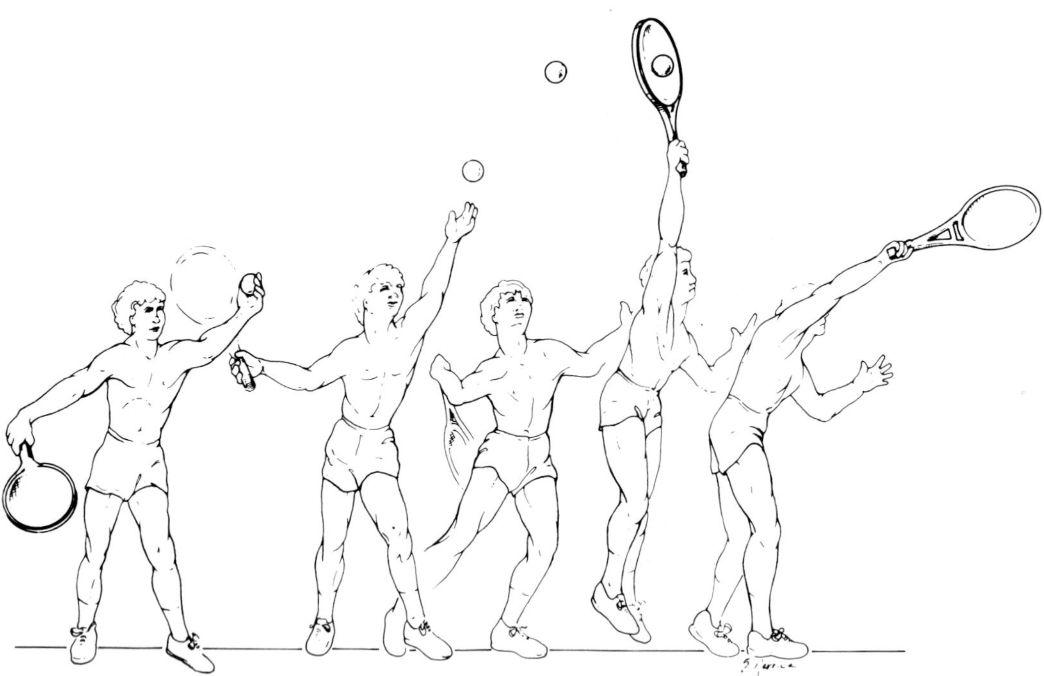

FIG. 32-23. Phases of the tennis serve, from left to right: wind-up, early cocking, late cocking, acceleration, follow-through. (From Morris M, et al.: Am J Sports Med 17(2), 1989.)

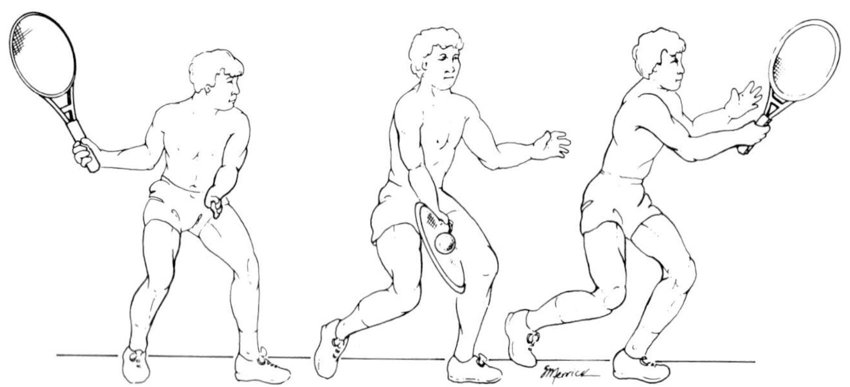

FIG. 32-24. Phases of the tennis forehand, from left to right: preparation, acceleration, follow-through. (From Morris M, et al.: Am J Sports Med 17(2), 1989.)

The phases of the golf swing are divided as follows (Fig. 32-26):

TAKEAWAY
This phase begins with the initiation of motion in the address position to the end of the backswing.

FORWARD SWING
Phase lasting from the end of the backswing until the club becomes horizontal.

ACCELERATION
Phase lasting from the point at which the club is horizontal until ball contact.

FOLLOW-THROUGH
Phase lasting from ball contact until the end of motion.

Analysis of the golf swing revealed a different pattern of action in its four phases.[25] Relative quiescence of the deltoid and dominance of rotator cuff muscle activity was observed. This may be explained by the limited elevation of the arm in the golf swings compared to pitching, swimming, or tennis. Again, rotator cuff activity was seen to be dictated by motion demands and not in obligatory synergy with the deltiod. The subscapularis was more active than any other muscle throughout the swing. In addition, the rotator cuff muscles showed as much activity on the

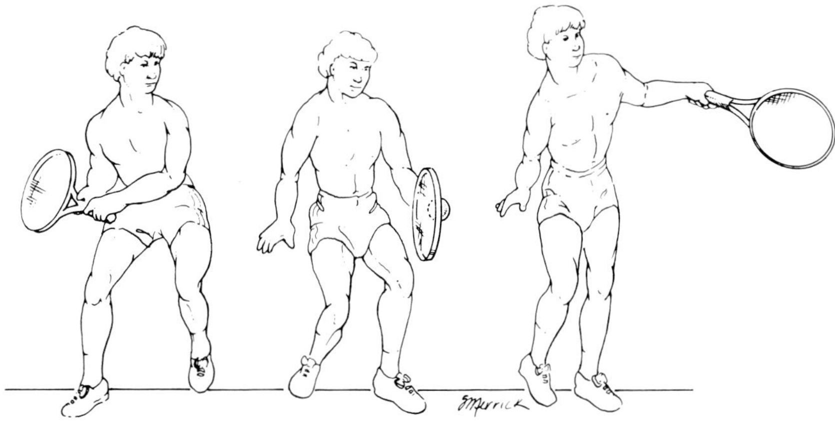

FIG. 32-25. Phases of the tennis backhand, from left to right: preparation, acceleration, follow-through. (From Morris M, et al.: Am J Sports Med 17(2), 1989.)

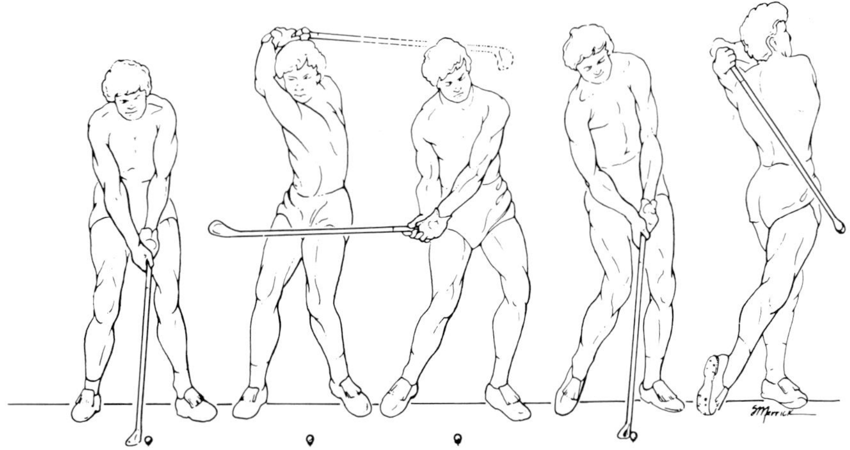

FIG. 32-26. Phases of the golf swing, from left to right: take-away, forward swing, early acceleration, late acceleration, follow-through. (Modified from Jobe FW: Am J Sports Med 17(6), 1989.)

right shoulder as the left shoulder. The latissimus dorsi and pectoralis major provided power bilaterally and showed marked activity during acceleration. As part of a training program, the golf player should emphasize the rotator cuff, pectoralis major, and latissimus dorsi in both arms.

ATHLETIC ELBOW FUNCTION

Throwing

Analysis of the muscles about the elbow during a pitch included the extensor digitorum communis (EDC), brachioradialis, flexor carpi radialis (FCR), flexor digitorum superficialis (FDS), extensor carpi radialis longus (ECRL), extensor carpi radialis brevis (ECRB), pronator teres, and supinator.[50]

The windup or preparation phase had relatively low activity in all groups as the forearm was slightly pronated and flexed and the wrist extended. Muscle activity was highest in the EDC, ECRB, and pronator teres. There was little difference between the fast ball and the curve.

Early cocking is terminated as the front foot touches the ground and the hand and ball are positioned back as far as possible. The elbow is flexed, the wrist and metacarpophalangeal joints extended, and the forearm slightly pronated. Muscle activity is of moderate intensity in the wrist extensors (ECRB and ECRL), metacarpophalangeal extensors (EDC), brachioradialis, and pronator teres when a fast ball is thrown. Activity is markedly lower in the brachioradialis when a curve ball is thrown, suggesting that less elbow flexion is required for its delivery.

Late cocking is terminated by maximal humeral external rotation and 90 degrees of abduction. The wrist is extended, the elbow flexed, and the forearm pronated to 90 degrees with increased forearm pronation when the fast ball is thrown. There is an increased activity in the wrist extensors and supinator when the curve ball is thrown. This suggests that with the curve ball, the ball is positioned differently in the hand, and the forearm slightly more supinated.

Acceleration is an explosive, short stage. The elbow is extended and the wrist and metacarpophalangeal joints are flexed to propel the ball forward. The difference between the fast ball and curve is most apparent at acceleration because the ECRL and ECRB activity is higher with the curve ball. This probably is a reflection of the different posture necessary at the release point of the curve.

Follow-through is terminated by maximal pronation of the forearm as the humerus is internally rotated and adducted accross the chest. The wrist extensors again demonstrate more activity when the curve ball is thrown.

The results showed low to moderate activity in all muscles during all phases of the pitch. The function is more likely positioning to accept the transfer of energy from the larger trunk and girdle structures. The most notable difference between the fast ball and the curve ball is an increase in the ECRL and ECRB activity during late cocking, acceleration, and follow-through of the curve as compared to the fast ball. This probably is a reflection of the different posture necessary at the release point of a curve.

Tennis

Analysis of elbow function in tennis players revealed predominant activity of the wrist extensors in all strokes.

The muscles evaluated include the biceps, triceps, brachialis, extensor digitorum communis (EDC), extensor carpi radialis longus (ECRL), extensor carpi radialis brevis (ECRB), pronator teres, and flexor carpi radialis (FCR).

The ground strokes were divided into the following four phases:

PHASE I
This phase is racquet preparation, which begins with the first motion of the backswing and ends with the first forward motion of the racquet.

PHASE II
This phase is acceleration, which begins with forward racquet movement and ends with ball contact.

PHASES III AND IV
These phases are follow-through, which begins with the ball contact and ends with completion of the stroke. Phase III is early follow-through, which is the first 25% of the time in the phase, and phase IV is late follow-through, which is the last 75% of the time.

The serve was divided into the following six phases:

PHASE I
This phase is wind-up, which begins with the first motion of the racquet and until ball release from the nonracquet hand.

PHASES II AND III
These phases are cocking that initiates with ball release and continues to the point of maximal external rotation in the serving shoulder. Phase II is early cocking, which is the first 75% of the time, and phase three is late cocking, which is the last 25% of the time.

PHASE IV
This phase is acceleration, and it starts with forward motion of the arm and continues until ball contact.

PHASES V AND VI
These phases are follow-through, beginning with ball contact and continuing until completion of the stroke. Early follow-through (phase five) is the first 25% of the time in the phase, and late follow-through (phase six) is the last 75% of the time.

During the ground strokes, the muscles appear to stabilize the arm as a rigid extension of the racquet. The racquet-arm unit then accepts the transfer of energy from the shoulder and trunk as they rotate and as body weight shift occurs.

The muscles at the elbow act to control elbow flexion and extension, forearm rotation, and the four motions of the wrist (fexion, extension, radial, and ulnar deviation).

The triceps and brachialis function only to control the elbow hinge. They showed low to moderate activity throughout the ground strokes. This implies that the muscles have a positioning function and that the inherent stability of the elbow joint provides the resistance against the forces of the stroke.

The biceps has two functions: to perform flexion at the elbow and to control forearm rotation. The biceps showed low to moderate activity during the ground strokes except for an increase in activity during forehand acceleration and early follow-through. Brachialis activity remained low during these phases. This implies that in addition to its role in positioning the elbow in flexion, the biceps was serving to stabilize forearm rotation.

The pronator teres showed increased activity during forehand acceleration. This synergistic activity with the biceps appears to stabilize the forearm against rotation.

Wrist and grip stability are found in a position of extension and radial deviation. The highest elbow activity during the ground strokes was in the muscles that control the wrist. The radial wrist extensors, ECRB and ECRL, were active in both strokes.

The EDC also showed high activity during the backhand where resistance of the flexor moment, brought on by acceleration and ball contact, was required.

The role of the muscles about the elbow is different during the serve than during the ground strokes. Instead of acting as an extension of the racquet, their role is to act much like the springs of a catapult, cocking the racquet and then contributing to its acceleration forward.

During the cocking of the racquet, the primary muscle action relates to wrist control. The ECRB, EDC, and ECRL all showed high activity. The elbow and forearm positions were achieved passively at the elbow by shoulder position and gravity.

During acceleration the primary site of muscle action was found to be at the elbow and forearm. The triceps showed its only phase of high activity in any stroke as it provides power by extending the elbow. The increased activity of the pronator teres provided position and power at the forearm.

The biceps showed a significant increase in activity in late follow-through. Its action appeared to be deceleration of the supination/extension movement brought on in the acceleration phase.

The major function during ground strokes is stabilization of the elbow, forearm, and wrist with major activity at the wrist. During the serve the muscles' function is to produce movement at three sites: the elbow, forearm, and wrist. From this motion, cocking and acceleration of the racquet is obtained.

Power in the serve comes from increased activity in the triceps and pronator teres. The predominant activity of the wrist extensors in all the strokes may be one cause for their frequent injury.

SUMMARY

The muscles of the shoulder and elbow act according to their mechanical qualities and are function or sport specific. Separating the professional from the amateur athlete further refined this principle and demonstrated that individual muscles of the rotator cuff act independently.

Evaluation of the different sports revealed that while the rotator cuff function is important in all, the emphasis and role of the individual muscles varied. The importance of serratus anterior muscle activity to stabilize and protract the scapula was a consistent finding. At the elbow, the major demand is placed on the muscles controlling the wrist. Thus it is critical to understand the demands placed upon the upper extremity in a particular sport or activity to treat pathologic conditions.

REFERENCES

1. An K, and Moorey B: Biomechanics of the elbow. In Morrey B, editor: The elbow and its disorders, Philadelphia, 1985, WB Saunders Co.
2. Atwater AE: Biomechanics of overarm throwing movements and of throwing injuries, Exerc Sport Sci Rev 7:43, 1979.
3. Basmajian JV, and Bazant FJ: Factors preventing downward dislocation of the adducted shoulder joint, J Bone Joint Surg 41A: 1182, 1959.
4. Basmajian JV, and Deluca CJ: Muscles alive: their functions revealed by electromyography, Baltimore, 1985, Williams & Wilkins, p. 265.
5. Basmajian JV, and Latif A: Integrated actions and functions of the chief flexors of the elbow: a detailed electromyographic analysis, J Bone Joint Surg 39A:1106, 1957.
6. Batterman C: Mechanics of the crawl arm stroke, Swimming World 7:4, 1966.
7. Bechtol CO: Biomechanics of the shoulder, Clin Orthop 146:37, 1980.
8. Boone DC, and Azen SP: Normal range of motion in joints in male subjects, J Bone Joint Surg 61A:756, 1979.
9. Clancy WG: Shoulder problems in overhand overuse sports, Am J Sports Med 7:138, 1979.
10. Codman EA: The shoulder. Brooklyn, N.Y., 1934, G Miller & Co.
11. Colachis SC, Jr, Strohm BR, and Brecher VL: Effects of axillary nerve block on muscle force in the upper extremity, Arch Phys Med Rehabil 50:647, 1969.
12. Colachis SC, Jr, and Strohm BR: Effects of suprascapular and axillary nerve blocks on muscle force in upper extremity, Arch Phys Med Rehabil 52:22, 1971.
13. Doody SG, Freedman L, and Waterland JC: Shoulder movements during abduction in the scapular plane, Arch Phys Med Rehabil 51:595, 1970.
14. Dvir Z, and Berne N: The shoulder complex in elevation of the arm: a mechanism approach, J Biomech 11:219, 1978.
15. Freedman L, and Munro RR: Abduction of the arm in the scapular plane: scapular and glenohumeral movements, J Bone Joint Surg 48A:1503, 1966.
16. Furlani J: Electromyographic study of the biceps brachii in movements of the glenohumeral joint, Acta Anat 96:270, 1976.
17. Garfin SR et al: Role of fascia in maintenance of muscle tension and pressure, J Appl Physiol 51(2):317, 1981.
18. Glousman RE et al: Dynamic EMG analysis of the throwing shoulder with glenohumeral instability, J Bone Joint Surg 70A:220, 1988.
19. Gowan ID et al: A comparative EMG analysis of the shoulder during pitching: professional vs. amateur pitchers, Am J Sports Med 15:586, 1987.
20. Hawkins RJ, and Hobeika PE: Impingement syndrome in the athletic shoulder. Symposium on injuries to the shoulder in the athlete, Clin Sports Med 2:391, 1983.
21. Hollingshead WH: Anatomy for surgeons, vol 3, The back and limbs, New York, 1958, Hoeber-Harper.

22. Inman VT, Saunders JB de CM, and Abbott LC: Observations on the function of the shoulder joint, J Bone Joint Surg 26:1, 1944.
23. Inman VT, and Saunders JBDeCM: Observations on the function of the clavicle, Calif Med 65:158, 1946.
24. Jobe FW et al: An EMG analysis of the shoulder in pitching: a second report, Am J Sports Med 12:218, 1984.
25. Jobe FW, Moynes DR, and Antonelli DJ: Rotator cuff function during a golf swing, Am J Sports Med 14:388, 1986.
26. Jobe FW et al: An EMG analysis of the shoulder in throwing and pitching: a preliminary report, Am J Sports Med 11:3, 1983.
27. Johnston TB: The movements of the shoulder joint, Br J Surg 25:252, 1937.
28. Jones DW, Jr: The role of shoulder muscles in the control of humeral position (an electromyography study), master's thesis, Cleveland, 1970, Case Western Reserve University.
29. Kent BE: Functional anatomy of the shoulder complex, Phys Ther 51:867, 1971.
30. Lucas DB: Biomechanics of the shoulder joint, Arch Surg 107:425, 1973.
31. MacCowaill MA, and Basmajian JV: Muscles and movements: a basis for human kinesiology, New York, 1977, Robert Krieger Publishing.
32. Maki S, and Gruen T: Anthropometric study of the glenohumeral joint, vol 1, Transactions, 22nd Annual Meeting of the American Orthopaedic Research Society, 1976, p. 173.
33. Matsen FA III: Biomechanics of the shoulder. In Frankel VH, and Nordin M, editors: Basic biomechanics of the skeletal system, Philadelphia, 1980, Lea & Febiger, p. 221.
34. McCormick J et al: An EMG analysis of shoulder function in tennis players, Unpublished study, Biomechanics Laboratory, Centinela Hospital, Inglewood, Calif., 1985.
35. Miller L et al: EMG analysis of shoulders in throwers with subacromial impingement, Unpublished study, Biomechanics Laboratory, Centinela Hospital, Inglewood, Calif., 1985.
36. Morrey B, and Chao E: Passive motion of the elbow joint, J Bone Joint Surg 58A:501, 1976.
37. Moynes DR: Prevention of injury to the shoulder through exercises and therapy: symposium on injuries to the shoulder in the athlete, Clin Sports Med 2:413, 1983.
38. Nuber GW et al: EMG analysis of classical shoulder motion, Trans Orthop Res Soc 11:1986.
39. Nuber GW et al: Fine wire electromyography analysis of muscles of the shoulder during swimming, Am J Sports Med 14:7, 1986.
40. Perry J: Normal upper extremity kinesiology, Phys Ther 58:265, 1978.
41. Perry J: Anatomy and biomechanics of the shoulder in throwing, swimming, gymnastics and tennis: symposium on injuries to the shoulder in the athlete, Clin Sports Med 2:247, 1983.
42. Poppen NK, and Walker PS: Normal and abnormal motion of the shoulder, J Bone Joint Surg 58A:195, 1976.
43. Poppen NK, and Walker PS: Forces at the glenohumeral joint in abduction, Clin Orthop 136:165, 1978.
44. Richardson AB: Overuse syndromes in baseball, tennis, gymnastics and swimming: symposium on injuries of the shoulder in the athlete, Clin Sports Med 2:379, 1983.
45. Richardson AB, Jobe FW, and Collins HR: The shoulder in competitive swimming, Am J Sports Med 81:159, 1980.
46. Saha AK: Theory of shoulder mechanism: descriptive and applied. Springfield, Ill, 1961, Charles C Thomas, Publisher.
47. Saha AK: Mechanics of elevation of glenohumeral joint: its application in rehabilitation of flail shoulder in upper brachial plexus injuries and poliomyelitis and in replacement of the upper humerus by prosthesis, Acta Orthop Scand 44:668, 1973.
48. Schmidt GL: Biomechanical analysis of knee flexion and extension, J Biomech 6:79, 1973.
49. Shevlin MG, Lehmann JF, and Lucci JA: Electromyographic study of the function of some muscles crossing the glenohumeral joint, Arch Phys Med Rehabil 50:264, 1969.
50. Sisto D et al: An electromyographic analysis of the elbow in pitching, Am J Sports Med 15:260, 1987.
51. Slater-Hammel AT: An action current study of contraction-movement relationships in the tennis stroke, Res Q 20:424, 1949.
52. Sugahara R: Electromyographic study of shoulder movements, Jpn J Rehabil Med 11:41, 1974.
53. Ting A et al: EMG analysis of lateral biceps muscle action in shoulders with rotator cuff tears, Unpublished study, Biomechanics Laboratory, Centinela Hospital, Inglewood, Calif., 1986.
54. Travill AA: Electromyographic study of the extensor apparatus of the forearm, Anat Rec 144:373, 1962.
55. Turkel SJ et al: Stabilizing mechanisms preventing anterior dislocation of the glenohumeral joint, J Bone Joint Surg 63A:1208, 1981.
56. Wadsworth TG: The elbow, New York, 1982, Churchill Livingston, Inc.
57. Walker PS: Human joints and their artificial replacements. Springfield, Ill., 1977, Charles C Thomas, Publisher.
58. Weber EF: Ueber die Langenverhaltnisse der Fleischfasen der Muskeln im allgemeinen, Ber Verh K Sach Ges Wissensch, Math-Phys, 1851, p. 63.

ADDITIONAL READINGS

Adelsberg S: The tennis stroke: an EMG analysis of selected muscles with rackets of increasing grip size, Am J Sports Med, 14:139, 1986.

Anderson M: Comparison of muscle patterning in the overarm throw and tennis serve, Res Q 50:541, 1979.

Ballesteros MLF, Buchtal F, and Rosenfalck P: The pattern of muscular activity during the arm swing of natural walking, Acta Physiol Scand 63:296, 1965.

Basmajian JV: Primary anatomy, Baltimore, 1964, Williams & Wilkins.

Bateman JE: Cuff tears in athletes, Orthop Clin North Am 4:721, 1973.

Bost FC: The pathological changes in recurrent dislocation of the shoulder, J Bone Joint Surg, 1942.

Carlson BR: Relationship between isometric and isotonic strength, Arch Phys Med Rehabil 51:176, 1970.

Clarys JP: A review of EMG in swimming: explanation of facts and/or feedback information. In Hollander AP, Huijing P, de Goat G, editors: Biomechanics and medicine in swimming. Champaign, Ill, Human Kinetics, p. 123, 1983.

Clarys JP, Jiscott J, and Lewillie L: A cinematographical, electromyographic and resistive study of water polo and competition front crawl. In Cerguighlini S, Verano A, Wastenmueller J, editors: Biomechanics III. Basel, 1972, Springer-Verlag, p. 446.

Cotton RE, and Rideout DF: Tears of the rotator cuff: a radiological and pathological necropsy survey, J Bone Joint Surg 46B:314, 1964.

Counsilman JE: Forces in swimming two types of crawl stroke, Res Q 26:127, 1955.

deAndrade MS, Grant C, Dixon A StJ: Joint distention and reflex muscle inhibition in the knee, J Bone Joint Surg 47A:313, 1965.

De Freitas V, Vitti M, and Furlani J: Electromyographic study of levator scapulae and rhombodius major muscles in movements of the shoulder and arm, Electromyogr Clin Neurophysiol 20:205, 1980.

deLuca CJ, and Forrest WJ: Force analysis of individual muscles acting simultaneously in the shoulder joint during isometric abduction, J Biomech 6:385, 1973.

Demster W: Space requirements of the seated operator, WADC Tech Rep 55-159, Washington DC, 1955, US Dept Commerce, Office of Technical Services.

DePalma AF: Surgery of the shoulder, Philadelphia, 1973, JB Lippincott Co.

DiStefano V: Functional anatomy and biomechanics of the shoulder joints, Athl Training 12:141, 1977.

Dupuis R et al: Forces acting on the hand during swimming and their relationships to muscular, spatial and temporal factors. In Teraud J, Bodingfield EW, Nelson RC, et al, editors: International series on sports sciences 8: Swimming III, Baltimore, 1979, University Park Press, p. 110.

Ekholm J et al: Shoulder muscle EMG and resisting moment during diagonal exercise movements resisted by weight-and-pulley-circuit, Scand J Rehabil Med 10:179, 1978.

Gainor BJ et al: The throw: biomechanics and acute injury, Am J Sports Med 8:114, 1980.

Hagberg M: Electromyographic signs of shoulder muscular fatigue in two elevated arm positions, Am J Phys Med 60:111, 1981.

Haggmark T, Jansson E, and Svane B: Cross-sectional area of the thigh muscle in man measured by computed tomography, Scand J Clin Lab Invest 38:355, 1978.

Hawkins RJ, and Kennedy JC: Impingement syndrome in athletes, Am J Sports Med 8:151, 1980.

Haxton HA: Absolute muscle force in the ankle flexors of man, J Physiol (Lond) 103:267, 1944.

Hitchcock HH, and Bechtol CO: Painful shoulder, J Bone Joint Surg 30A:263, 1978.

Jensen RK, and Blanksby B: A model for upper extremity forces during the underwater phase of the front crawl. In Lewillie L, and Clarys JP, editors: Proceedings of the second international symposium on biomechanics in swimming, Baltimore, 1974, University Park Press, p. 145.

Jobe, FW: Serious rotator cuff injuries. Symposium on injuries to the shoulder in the athlete, Clin Sports Med 2:407, 1983.

Jobe FW, and Moynes DR: Delineation of diagnostic criteria and a rehabilitation program for rotator cuff injuries, Am J Sports Med 10:336, 1982.

Kadandji I: The physiology of the joints, ed 2, vol 1, The elbow: flexion and extension, Baltimore, 1970, Williams & Wilkins.

Katz DR: EMG comparison of two serratus anterior manual muscle tests: a pilot study, University of Southern California, Physical Therapy Department, 1983.

Kulund DN et al: Tennis injuries: prevention and treatment, Am J Sports Med 7:249, 1979.

London J: Kinematics of the elbow, J Bone Joint Surg 63A:529, 1981.

Matasen FA: Biomechanics of the shoulder. In Bateman JE, editor: The shoulder and neck, ed 2, Philadelphia, 1978, WB Sanders Co.

McLaughlin HL: Rupture of the rotator cuff, J Bone Joint Surg 44A:979, 1982.

Miyashita M: Arm action in the crawl stroke. In Lewillie L, and Clarys JP, editors: Proceedings of the second international symposium on biomechanics in swimming, Baltimore, 1974, University Park Press, p. 167.

Morrey BF: The elbow and its disorders, Philadelphia, 1985, WB Saunders Co, p. 56.

Morrey BF, Chao EY: Recurrent anterior dislocation of the shoulder. In Black J, and Dumbleton JH, editors: Clinical biomechanics: a case history approach. New York, 1981, Churchill-Livingston, p. 24.

Moseley HF, and Overgaard B: The anterior capsular mechanism in recurrent anterior dislocation of the shoulder, J Bone Joint Surg 44B:913, 1962.

Nelson RC, and Pike NL: Analysis and comparison of swimming starts and strokes. In Morehouse C, and Nelson RC, editors: Swimming medicine IV, Baltimore, 1977, University Park Press, p. 347.

Penny JN, and Welsh RP: Shoulder impingement syndrome in athletes and their surgical management, Am J Sports Med 9:11, 1981.

Priest JD, and Nagel DA: Tennis shoulder, Am J Sports Med 4:28, 1976.

Rathburn JB, and Macnab I: The microvascular pattern of the rotator cuff, J Bone Joint Surg 52B:540, 1970.

Reeves B: Experiments on the tensile strength of the anterior capsule structures of the shoulder in man, J Bone Joint Surg 50B:858, 1968.

Saha AK: Anterior recurrent dislocation of the shoulder, Acta Orthop Scand 68:479, 1967.

Saha AK: Dynamic stability of the glenohumeral joint, Acta Orthop Scand 42:491, 1971.

Schleihauf RE: A hydrodynamic analysis of swimming propulsion. In Terauds J, and Bedingfield EW, editors: Swimming III, Proceedings of the third international symposium on biomechanics in swimming, Baltimore, 1978, University Park Press, p. 70.

Seirig A, and Baz A: A mathematical model for swimming mechanics. In Lewillie L, and Clarys JP, editors: Swimming, water polo and diving, Brussels, 1970, University Libre.

Shoo MJ, and Perry J: The shoulder girdle muscles in transfer: an electromyographic study, Resident Seminars, Rancho Los Amigos Hospital, Downey, Calif, 1978.

Slocum DB: The mechanics of some common injuries to the shoulder in sports, Am J Surg 98:394, 1959.

Staples OS, and Watkins AL: Full active abduction in traumatic paralysis of the deltoid, J Bone Joint Surg 25:85, 1943.

Steindler A: Kinesiology of the human body under normal and pathological conditions, Springfield, Ill., 1970, Charles C Thomas.

Sullivan WE et al: Electromyographic studies of biceps brachii during normal voluntary movement at the elbow, Anat Rec 107:243, 1950.

Sullivan PE, and Portney LG: Electromyographic activity of shoulder muscles during unilateral upper extremity proprioceptive neuromuscular facilitation patterns, Phys Ther 60:283, 1980.

Tarbell T: Some biomechanical aspects of the overhead throw. In Cooper JM, editor: CIC symposium on biomechanics, Indiana University, 1970, Chicago, 1971, Athletic Institute.

Tullos HS, and King JW: Throwing mechanism in sports, Orthop Clin North Am 4:709, 1973.

Van Linge B, and Mulder JD: Function of the supraspinatus muscle and its relationship to the supraspinatus syndrome, J Bone Joint Surg 45B:750, 1963.

Weiner DS, and Macnab I: Superior migration of the humeral head, J Bone Joint Surg 52B:524, 1970.

Williams PL, and Warwick R: Gray's Anatomy, ed 36, Philadelphia, 1980, WB Saunders Co.

Yoshizawa M, et al: Electromyographic study of two styles in the breaststroke as performed by top swimmers. In Smussen E, and Jorgensen K, editors: International series on biomechanics 2B, biomechanics VI-B. Baltimore, 1978, University Park Press.

CHAPTER 33 Diagnosis and Treatment of Shoulder Injuries in Throwers

Ralph A. Gambardella
Frank A. Jobe

A wide variety of injuries can afflict the shoulder girdle in baseball.[24,54] The throwing athlete places unusually high demands on the shoulder joint. This joint is the link in transferring force generated from the trunk to the arm and thereby imparting speed to the baseball. The shoulder is greatly adapted to this function by the multiple planes of motion (i.e., scapular, sagittal, and coronal) available to it. However, these large degrees of freedom also make this joint more susceptible to injury.

Many injuries in the shoulder girdle are caused by the repetitious act of throwing and are therefore considered overuse problems rather than acute injuries.[40] Because overuse problems are more associated with the repetition of the throwing act, it is understandable that the majority of problems are going to afflict the pitcher rather than a player in a different position. Although this chapter focuses on many of these overuse problems created by the act of throwing, it is important to remember that shoulder injuries also occur as a result of direct contact and acute injury associated with that type of contact. Acute anterior shoulder dislocations as well as recurrent shoulder subluxation problems have been known to occur as a result of head-first sliding, with the arm caught in an abducted and externally rotated position. In addition, acromioclavicular joint separation can easily occur with blows to the superior aspect of the shoulder girdle as outfielders crash into walls and barriers attempting to catch fly balls.

There are five basic classifications of shoulder injuries involving the throwing athlete.

The first is the subacromial space complex of injuries and involves impingement syndromes, rotator cuff tendonitis, bicipital tendonitis, and subdeltoid bursitis. The second classification is glenohumeral instability and includes both anterior and posterior subluxation or dislocation problems as well as labrum injuries[33]; by far the most common problem is that of anterior subluxation. Acromioclavicular joint problems, neurovascular entrapment syndromes, and injuries to the physis in adolescents round out the more common overuse syndromes that occur in the throwing athlete. It is important to remember that instability often causes problems with the subacromial space and therefore the first two classifications often co-exist.

Classification of shoulder throwing injuries

- Subacromial space problems
- Glenohumeral instability
- Acromioclavicular problems
- Neurovascular entrapment syndromes
- Physeal injuries

The most critical problem confronting the clinician is the realization that the various types of shoulder injuries can be present in combination. The clinician must identify and address each particular problem to successfully treat the injured athlete. In many throwers it is not unusual to have rotator cuff tendonitis, anterior subluxation, and a labral injury. Therefore it is of paramount importance to obtain a detailed history and perform a comprehensive physical examination. The advent of new techniques, including arthroscopic evaluation, has enhanced our understanding of these complex problems, allowing the physician to make a more accurate diagnosis.[2,29] It is only with an accurate diagnosis that a successful treatment and rehabilitation program can be outlined for the athlete.

FUNCTIONAL ANATOMY

The shoulder girdle is made up of four functional joints. They are the glenohumeral joint, the acromioclavicular joint, the sternoclavicular joint, and the scapulothoracic complex. Whereas normal motion in most humans would allow for 160 degrees of forward flexion and abduction, the throwing athlete often exhibits increased shoulder motion and in particular *increased external rotation* in the abducted plane. Shoulder abduction occurs as a combination of both glenohumeral and scapulothoracic motion in a 2:1 ratio. While this ratio may differ in throwers, large deviations from this ratio caused by fatigue or injury place additional demands on the ligamentous structures as well as the muscle tendon units.

The glenohumeral joint is a very unstable joint, and the stability in the joint is enhanced anteriorly by the glenoid and humeral head retroversion. In addition, stability both anteriorly and posteriorly is enhanced by the glenoid labrum and fibrous structures that increase the coverage of the humeral head, thereby enhancing the stability in all planes. Of particular importance are the capsular reinforcements, which have been described as the glenohumeral ligaments of the shoulder. In the throwing athlete the importance of the anterior inferior glenohumeral ligament in the prevention of anterior and anteroinferior instability has now been well documented. The rotator cuff adds support and restraint to the glenohumeral joint and is of particular importance with the follow-through phase of the throwing mechanism. Finally, the biceps tendon also has a role as a humeral head depressor and, in addition, in throwing, has been shown to be an important decelerator of the forearm.

The subacromial space is a fixed space containing the subdeltoid bursa and loose fibroconnective tissue. This space is bounded superiorly by the undersurface of the acromion, inferiorly by the superior border of the rotator cuff, laterally by the deltoid, and medially by the coracoacromial ligament. Alterations in the subacromial space caused by osteophyte formation along the undersurface of the acromion, thickening of the rotator cuff or subdeltoid bursa, or alterations of the coracoacromial ligament can all cause problems to the shoulder in the throwing athlete.

THROWING MECHANICS

The throwing mechanism has been divided into five phases: (1) windup, (2) early cocking, (3) late cocking, (4) acceleration, and (5) follow-through[28,34] (Fig. 33-1). Highest stresses on the anterior and inferior capsular structures occur during phase 3, when maximal abduction and external rotation are attained.[37] In addition, very high stresses are imparted to posterior capsular structures during phase 5. These large stresses are counterbalanced by intense periods of muscle activity by the shoulder girdle muscles.[11]

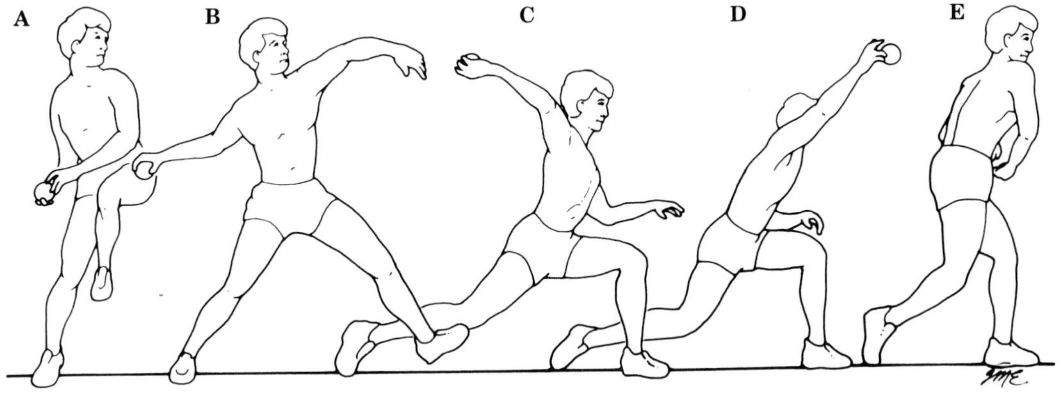

FIG. 33-1. Mechanics of throwing. **A,** Windup. **B,** Early cocking. **C,** Late cocking. **D,** Acceleration. **E,** Follow through.

Peak muscle activity is measured in percentages of manual muscle strength tests (MMT) with 100% MMT being the peak 1 second electromyographic signal during a manual muscle strength test. During the baseball pitch the deltoid exhibits peak activity in early cocking (42% MMT) with a second peak occurring at follow-through (43% MMT).[26,27] Supraspinatus peak activity (45% MMT) occurs at late cocking, with a less intense peak at follow-through. The supraspinatus contributes to joint stability by compressing the humeral head toward the glenoid.

The subscapularis is most active (115% MMT) in late cocking, when the shoulder is in maximal external rotation and again in deceleration as the arm is internally rotated (151% MMT).[30]

MECHANISM OF INJURY: IMPINGEMENT VERSUS INSTABILITY

Although there appear to be patients who are seen clinically as either "pure impingers" or "pure subluxators," most appear with symptoms and physical findings indicative of both problems. In the throwing athlete, the primary event is probably anterior subluxation or instability. This occurs associated with the terminal stage of windup when the shoulder is abducted and maximally rotated. With the repetition of the throwing act, the high stresses generated on the anterior capsule during phase 3 lead to stretching of the anterior capsule and, in particular, the anterior inferior glenohumeral ligament (Fig. 33-2). As this complex stretches and flattens, the shoulder will start to subluxate. Whether or not this primary instability is caused solely by mechanical breakdown or is a result of rotator cuff muscle fatigue and imbalance is unknown. However, this early istability initiates a cascade of events leading to both impingement and labral problems.

As instability progresses, abnormal demands are placed on the rotator cuff. Alterations in force are generated at the joint level, and an abnormal firing sequence of the shoulder girdle muscles occurs. This occurs particularly because of an imbalance in the scapular rotators (i.e., serratus, rhomboids, etc.), which are overworking and firing out of sequence in an effort to keep the humeral head in the glenoid. The inability of the muscles to act in synchrony leads to chronic irritation of the rotator cuff and in particular the supraspinatus as it passes under the acromion and coracoacromial arch during phases 3 and 4 of the throwing act. In addition, the supraspinatus is overworking in an attempt to stabilize the subluxating humeral head.[14] It does this by acting as a humeral head depressor. This may explain the greater electromyographic maximal activity seen in the supraspinatus with amateur pitchers than that seen in the professional thrower.[15]

Subacromial mechanical impingement can result in subdeltoid bursitis, rotator cuff tendonitis, and bicipital tendonitis. Within the joint, as this impingement and instability continue, one can see the development of partial rotator cuff tears and posterior labrum tears. The labrum injury often consists of a fraying along the posterior superior edge of the labrum but can also include a bucket handle type of lesion. Another finding in the joint often seen arthroscopically is a roughened area of articular cartilage on the humeral head that is smaller and posterior to the normal

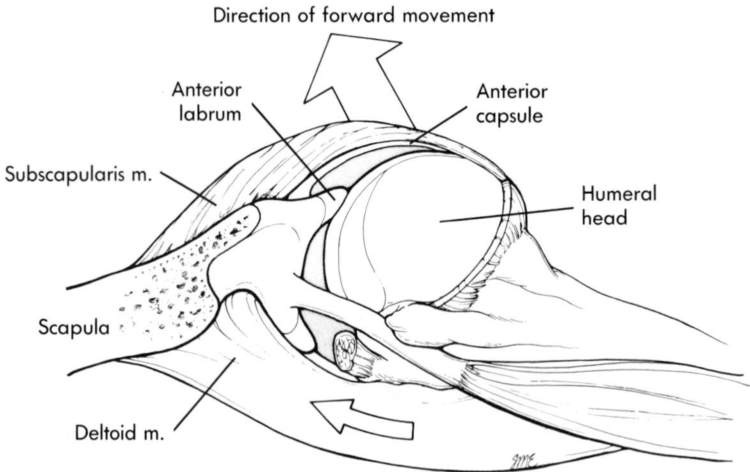

FIG. 33-2. Phase three of the throwing motion. Highest stresses are placed on the anterior and inferior capsule and labrum.

location of the classic Hill-Sachs lesion. Whereas the Hill-Sach's humeral defect is thought to be secondary to an anterior dislocation,[19] chondromalacic changes seen just inferior to the bare area are most likely caused by levering posteriorly against the posterior glenoid as the humeral head subluxates anteriorly.

Instability may be associated with anterior labral thinning and attenuation of the anterior inferior glenohumeral ligament. However, as instability progresses to recurring dislocation, frank tearing of the anterior labrium and the classic Bankhart lesion can occur.[5]

Consequences of subacromial impingement

- Subdeltoid bursitis
- Rotator cuff tendonitis
- Bicipital tendonitis

DIAGNOSIS

History

The clinical history becomes extremely important in the diagnosis of shoulder injury in the athlete because it will give the astute clinician important clues necessary to make the appropriate diagnosis.[53] A detailed history becomes extremely important when physical examination shows signs of both impingement and instability.

First, it is important to determine whether the onset of the problem occurred acutely with one particular throw or whether there was an accumulation and gradual onset of symptoms associated with the repetitive act of throwing. Although many athletes may try to attribute their problem to one particular game or event, it is important to quiz the patient in an effort to determine if there were other subtle symptoms or problems that may have led to the onset of what the patient may often feel is an acute injury. For example, on questioning many throwers may state that before noticing the onset of pain with each throw, they may have experienced shoulder soreness or stiffness after activity for several weeks.

The location of the pain both anatomically and by particular phase of throwing is also important.[23,32] Many anterior subluxators will experience pain posteriorly in phase 3 of throwing with the arm at 90 degrees of external rotation. Pain with full forward flexion is common in impingement. Pain with forward flexion across the chest seen in phase 5 of throwing can indicate an acromioclavicular joint problem. Many throwers who are experiencing anterior subluxation will describe a feeling of weakness, giving way, or a "dead arm," especially in phase 3. Attempts should also be made to elicit symptoms of clicking, which may be mechanical in nature, as seen in a bucket handle labrum tear.

Pain radiation from the neck to the shoulder or pain associated with neck range of motion may indicate a cervical problem. In addition, pain radiation below the elbow, especially with unrelated elbow pathologic findings, is often seen in cervical radiculopathy. Associated sensory or motor deficits should also be noted.

The history of how the athlete's problem has been treated is very important in trying to determine an appropriate course of action. This is especially true because many of these patients have been seen and treated for several weeks by primary care physicians before evaluation. Response to rest, oral antiinflammatory medication, and physical therapy should be recorded. Of paramount importance is to determine exactly what has been done in terms of physical therapy. Often therapy may have consisted only of the use of modalities such as ice, ultrasound, and heat rather than a comprehensive rotator cuff exercising program. This information is important in determining whether and when surgical intervention is indicated.

Finally, remember that shoulder pain that is not activity related may also be secondary to malignancy (Pancoast's tumor) or neurovascular syndromes or referred from cardiac or diaphragmatic problems.

Physical Examination

A complete physical examination consists of inspection, palpation, recording range of motion and muscle strength, and an assessment of joint stability. The examination should begin with a visual inspection of the upper torso, which can only be accomplished if all the patient's clothing above the waist is removed.

Inspection

Whereas most physicians have been taught to look for symmetry, this may be misleading when inspecting an athlete's shoulder. This is because throwing athletes typically exhibit hypertrophy of the shoulder girdle musculature. This hypertrophy can also make palpation of underlying structures more difficult. However, generalized hypertrophy also enhances recognition of specific muscle wasting, as seen with more chronic problems involving specific neurologic deficits. An example would be the wasting of the supraspinatus and infraspinatus muscles seen as a result of suprascapular nerve entrapment. Visualization of the acromioclavicular joint may detect prominences consistent with previous acromioclavicular joint separation or injury.

Palpation

After inspection, palpation of anatomic landmarks should be performed to elicit areas of tenderness. Anterior structures that can be palpated include the acromioclavicular joint, coracoid process, biceps tendon, and anterior capsule. The biceps is often best palpated with the patient supine and the arm held by the examiner to relax the deltoid. In this position the tendon becomes a subcutaneous structure and even in normal patients palpation may be mildly uncomfortable. In these instances comparison with the contralateral shoulder can be helpful. In the supine position the anterior capsule can also be palpated. The insertion of the supraspinatus into the greater tuberosity can be palpated just inferior to the anterolateral tip of the acromion. With the patient standing with the hand in an anatomic position (palm forward) the supraspinatus insertion into the greater tuberosity sits just inferior to the lateral tip of the acromion. Posterior structures that can be palpated for tenderness include the vertebral border of the scapula with its associated rhomboid muscles, posterior capsule, and teres minor. The latter two structures are best palpated with the patient prone. Tenderness along the trapezius and paracervical musculature may be seen in athletes with associated cervical problems.

Range of Motion

Evaluation of shoulder range of motion should consist of recording forward flexion,

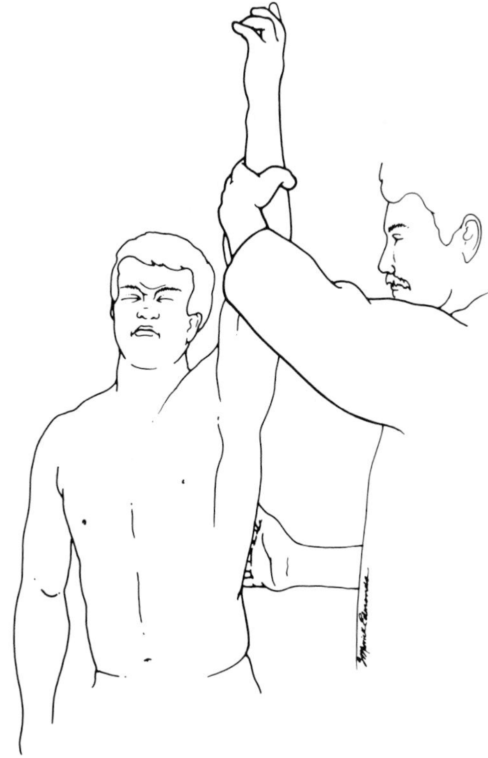

FIG. 33-3. Impingement sign. Pain with full forward flexion.

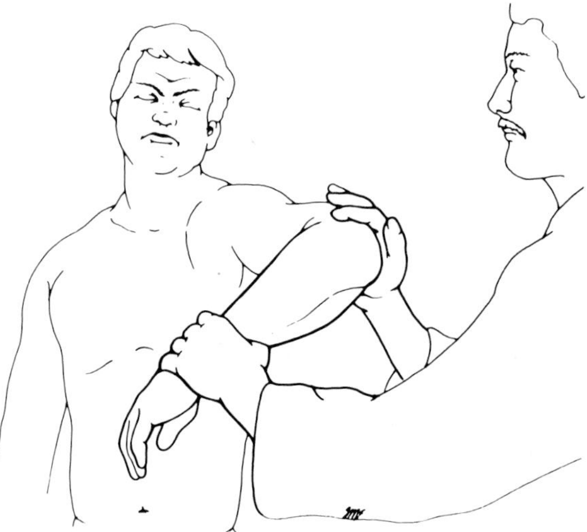

FIG. 33-4. Hawkins sign. Pain with forward flexion and internal rotation.

abduction, abduction/external rotation, internal rotation, forward flexion across the chest, and extension. Throwing athletes normally will exhibit an increase in external rotation with a concomitant decrease in internal rotation when compared to the contralateral shoulder. When one examines abduction, visualization of the scapula from the posterior aspect is important. Incongruent and uneven scapulothoracic motion may be the earliest sign in athletes with glenohumeral instability. Pain elicited in the fully forward flexed position has been described as a positive impingement test (Fig. 33-3). This finding can also be demonstrated by first stabilizing the scapula and then allowing forward flexion and internal rotation of the humerus to bring the supraspinatus under the coracoacromial ligament complex as described by Hawkins and Hobeika (Fig. 33-4).[18] Horizontal adduction across the chest should be evaluated for tightness of posterior capsular structures and may also elicit discomfort in the acromioclavicular joint indicative of acromioclavicular joint arthrosis.

Strength Evaluation

Muscle strength can be evaluated usually by manual motor testing, although more specific evaluation with the assistance of isokinetic testing may also be indicated. The supraspinatus test is performed by applying manual resistance while the shoulder is abducted 90 degrees and forward flexed 30 degrees and with the athlete's thumbs pointing toward the floor (i.e., forearm internally rotated) (Fig. 33-5). This test may be recorded as positive for eliciting pain only or for pain and weakness and as such may be helpful in the detection of rotator cuff tears. Weakness of the serratus anterior muscle can be elicited by having the patient do a push-up against the wall and observing for winging of the scapula.

Stability Evaluation

Glenohumeral instability is best examined with the patient supine. Patient cooperation is extremely important in terms of allowing the muscles about the shoulder girdle to relax in order to allow examination of the underlying capsular structures. The apprehension test is performed with the patient supine and

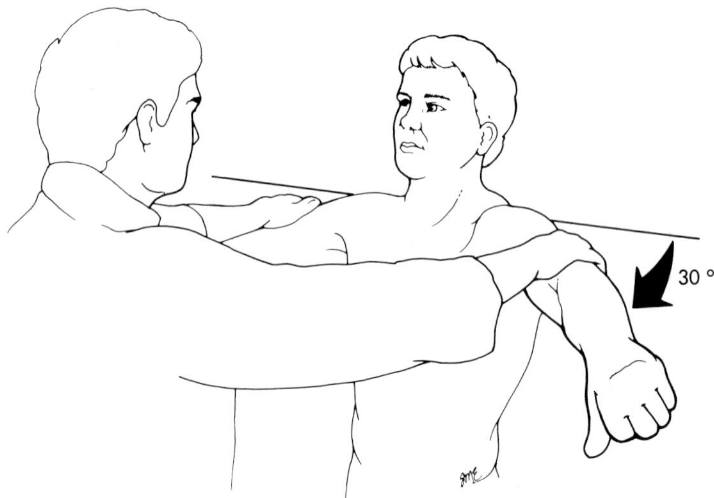

FIG. 33-5. Supraspinatus test. Arms abducted 90 degrees, forward flexed 30 degrees, and internally rotated 180 degrees (thumbs pointing to floor). Manual resistance causes pain and/or weakness.

the arm abducted 90 degrees and maximally externally rotated. In this position, patients with recurrent anterior dislocation problems will exhibit immediate apprehension and try to prevent the examiner from bringing the arm into this position. These patients will also complain of pain along the anterior capsule with the shoulder in this position. However, patients who are having a problem with anterior subluxation and, in particular, the throwing athlete will exhibit a different response to the apprehension test. In the thrower whose shoulder is mildly anteriorly subluxating, the maximally abducted and externally rotated position will often produce discomfort but not apprehension. Pain may be experienced both anteriorly and posteriorly. A "relocation test" can then be performed to confirm this diagnosis. The relocation test is done by first performing the apprehension maneuver and then repeating the same maneuver with a posteriorly directed force generated along the shaft of the humerus using the examiner's hand in an effort to eliminate the anterior subluxation (Fig. 33-6). With the humeral head now being held in place, with the force being generated posteriorly as the arm is brought into an abducted and externally rotated position, the patient has no pain. Subtle degrees of anterior and posterior instability can also be evaluated with the patient's shoulder in a supine position. With the humeral head held between the thumb anteriorly and fingers posteriorly, the examiner can apply forces anteriorly or posteriorly to elicit capsular laxity. In addition, posterior labral injuries may be detected by adding an axial load along the shaft of the humerus. As the head is then directed posteriorly with the addition of this compressive force, a palpable and sometimes audible click can be elicited supportive of a posterior labral tear.

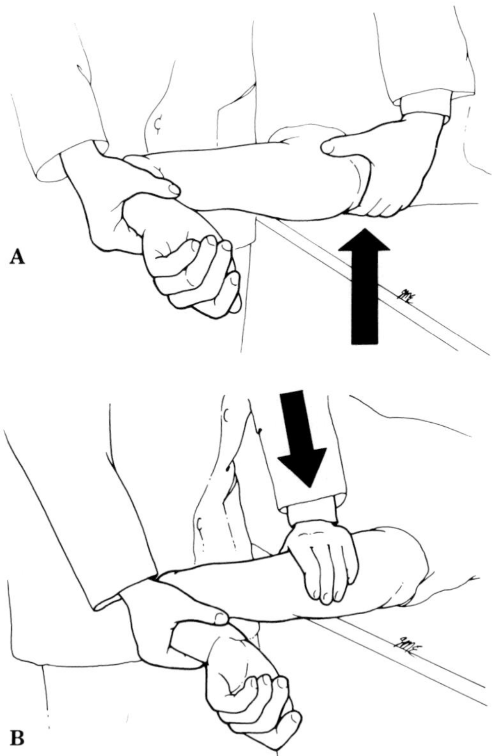

FIG. 33-6. Relocation test. **A,** Arm maximally abducted and externally rotated; patient complains of pain. **B,** Arm maximally abducted and externally rotated with force directed posteriorly; patient's pain eliminated.

Roentgenographic Examination

Routine roentgenographic views of the shoulder should include a true anteroposterior view as well as views in internal and external rotation, a transaxillary lateral view, and a scapular notch view. The scapular notch view has been found to be particularly helpful in evaluating possible impingement, because the various anatomic variants in the acromion can be identified.

CONDITIONING AND REHABILITATION

A comprehensive conditioning program is required by the athlete who desires optimal performance. This program must include flexibility, strengthening, and endurance activities. The athlete who is involved in throwing activities must in addition to general conditioning perform sports-specific upper extremity and endurance exercises.[35]

The **warm-up period** is important because it allows increased efficiency of body functions by raising body temperatures. This can be done by jogging or cycling type of activities. In addition, the shoulder can benefit from local application of heat in the form of hot packs, whirlpool, and so on before stretching during the warm-up period, since this may enhance blood flow to the shoulder. In the thrower, shoulder **stretching exercises** should be limited to those involving the posterior capsule. This is because the throwing shoulder normally has an increased range of external rotation in the abducted plane. Anterior stretching, particularly in the abducted position may further damage an already attenuated capsule and should be avoided. It is not unusual for a thrower to have limited internal rotation, and posterior capsular stretching is important in preventing injury.

Strengthening of the shoulder girdle musculature is important both for maintenance and as part of a rehabilitation program after injury. Strengthening of the deltoid and rotator cuff muscles is mandatory, but it has become increasingly important to also exercise the scapular stabilizers (i.e., serratus, rhomboids, teres major, latissimus, and trapezius). Progressive isotonic and isokinetic exercises are done to achieve maximal performance levels.

All conditioning programs should include a **cool-down period** after activity (i.e., throwing). This often takes the form of cryotherapy with application of ice to the shoulder for 10 to 15 minutes and may be accompanied by elevation or massage or both. The application of cold results in decreased blood flow to deeper structures and reduction of metabolic activity. This is believed to reduce swelling and further degradation of inflamed tissues.

A successful rehabilitation program for the athlete's shoulder must be individualized to the player's problem.[25] Many factors, such as severity and chronicity of the problem, as well as expected performance levels, must be assessed to determine length of rehabilitation. All successful therapy programs must also be integrated with a progressive throwing program to return the athlete to preinjury status. Our rehabilitation program consists of three phases. Phase 1 involves the use of modalities to reduce pain, inflammation, and edema. This is followed by a range of motion program placing only minimal stress on the involved structures. Phase 2 involves specific stretching of tightened capsular structures and isotonic strengthening activities, and phase 3 leads to further isokinetic exercises. At this time the athlete can begin a progressive shoulder throwing program, advancing back to preinjury status with the addition of maintenance stretching and strengthening exercises. The time frame involved must be individualized and needs to be continually reviewed and revised jointly by the athlete, trainer, therapist, and physician.

IMPINGEMENT SYNDROMES

Shoulder impingement is very common in the throwing athlete.[9,18,22] Anatomically, this syndrome involves the subacromial complex, consisting of the undersurface of the acromion, subdeltoid bursa, coracoacromial ligament, rotator cuff, and biceps tendon. The rotator cuff and long head of the biceps act as humeral head depressors, preventing humeral head migration with subsequent mechanical impingement occurring against the bony roof and coracoacromial ligament. The subdeltoid bursa normally allows smooth gliding with glenohumeral motion. As the arm is abducted from 80 to 125 degrees, the greater tuberosity comes in close proximity to the anterior acromion.

Pathophysiology

A simple imbalance of the rotator cuff with relative weakness of the supraspinatus allows the vertical force of the deltoid to produce more of a compressive force as the arm is abducted. This can establish subdeltoid bursal thickening and further supraspinatus irritation. The area of the supraspinatus involved has been described by Rathburn and Macnab[38] as an area of relative hypovascularity, and further irritation, thickening, and fibrosis can occur. In addition, inflammation of the long head of the biceps tendon can occur as it passes through the groove as this critical area again passes beneath the coracoacromial arch. Therefore supraspinatus tendonitis and bicipital tenosynovitis can occur independently of one another or in combination.

Impingement leading to rotator cuff disease can occur along two separate pathways. The three stage impingement classification described by Neer[3] delineates the pathway of the general population where aging may produce rotator cuff pathology irrespective of throwing athletes. In stage 1 edema and hemorrhage of the rotator cuff (particularly the supraspinatus) occur. This progresses with repeated trauma to stage 2 changes of thickening and fibrosis. Both stages 1 and 2 are reversible. However, further deterioration results in stage 3 changes with osseous degeneration and eventual tear formation. The second classification delineates the pathway of rotator cuff disease seen in the younger athletic throwing population. Remember that this is specific to the thrower and is initiated by underlying primary arterior glenohumeral instability.

History

The athlete with impingement syndrome will often have a history of a painful arc of motion. In particular, abduction from 80 to 125 degrees with the arm internally rotated will reproduce symptoms. Most patients will describe pain as sharp and activity related. As in most inflammatory processes, pain will usually increase after activity. Some patients may in addition complain of night pain, especially when sleeping with the arms overhead. Depending on which structures are inflamed, slight differences in history can be noted. Patients with bicipital tenosynovitis will complain of pain in the anterior quadrant of the shoulder, especially along the bicipital groove. This pain occurs often just before ball release (end of phase 4). Athletes with supraspinatus tendonitis tend to localize pain deeper in the shoulder or laterally at the deltoid.

Physical Examination

Visual inspection of shoulder abduction usually reveals asynchrony when viewed posteriorly. The scapulothoracic incongruent motion is the athlete's subtle attempt to reposition the humeral head beneath the acromion in an effort to clear the inflamed tissues. This can also lead to scapulothoracic bursitis.[44] Visible atrophy of the supraspinatus or infraspinatus may or may not be seen. A painful arc of motion can be elicited with abduction from 60 to 125 degrees. Tenderness can be palpated over the supraspinatus at the greater tuberosity (just lateral to the acromion) or biceps tendon if the groove is involved. A positive impingement test either in the forward flexed position (Neer) or in 90 degrees of forward flexion with the humerus internally rotated (Hawkins) is usually present. The isolated supraspinatus test may be positive for either reproducing pain or for eliciting both pain and weakness. In pure impingement syndromes there will be no physical findings suggestive of glenohumeral instability, but in the thrower subtle instability should always be suspected.

Treatment

Nonoperative Treatment

Over 90% of all impingement syndromes respond to conservative management.[25,31] This takes the form of a physical therapy program of rotator cuff strengthening exercises in combination with the use of nonsteroidal oral antiinflammatory agents. Injection of corticosteroids should be used sparingly and only in combination with an ongoing exercise program, because they have been shown to reduce tensile strength and may lead to further osseous deposition. The physical therapy program should be individualized. Strengthening of the supraspinatus, infraspinatus, and teres minor are performed based on the primary structures involved as determined by physical examination. We recommend that all rotator cuff exercises be performed with the arm at the side to prevent further irritation of these inflamed structures. Exercises for the scapular rotators (i.e., serratus, rhomboids, teres major) should also be performed to help regain scapulothoracic congruent motion. The use of ultrasound, in particular phonophoresis, can complement a therapy program. Phonophoresis can be especially effective in bicipital tenosynovitis.

Operative Treatment

When conservative management has failed, surgical options have traditionally included isolated coracoacromial ligament resection or anterior acromioplasty.[16,36] Although these procedures have produced good results overall, Tibone reported poor results after acromioplasty in the throwing athlete.[46] Although both procedures can now be done arthroscopically, there is no reason to believe results will improve. The reason for this is that in the thrower, glenohumeral instability may be present in addition to impingement. In the presence of instability, impingement procedures do not help, because the humeral head can continue to migrate and thereby compress the rotator cuff because of capsular laxity. It is therefore of primary importance when contemplating a surgical decompression of the subacromial space that glenohumeral instability is ruled out as a diagnosis. This often necessitates a diagnostic shoulder arthroscopy before performing acromioplasty. Stage 3 changes require open surgical repair.[47]

GLENOHUMERAL INSTABILITY

Recurrent anterior subluxation of the shoulder is the single most important problem in the throwing athlete, and the diagnosis can be the most difficult to make.[41] In the 1950s and 1960s, Rowe and Zarins,[42] like Blazina and Saltzman,[6] started to report on throwers with a "dead arm syndrome" and associated this with transient subluxation. Others have subsequently shown that severe stresses are placed on the anterior capsular structures during phase 3 of throwing, which can result not only in injury to the capsule leading to instability, but also in injury to the labrum. The key restraint in phase 3, in which the arm is maximally abducted and externally rotated, is the anterior inferior glenohumeral ligament, as shown by Turkel and associates[49] and more recently by Warren.[50,51] The insertion of this ligament into the labrum is often the site of tearing.

History

The common complaint of the athlete with anterior subluxation is that the shoulder feels as if it were "dead" in the cocking position.

Few throwers may actually be aware that the shoulder is slipping or popping, but many can describe only vague complaints of feeling "something is not right" in the shoulder. Much more commonly, sharp pain or weakness or both may be the only symptoms with which the athlete presents.[13] Clicking or popping may be present and may indicate the presence of associated labrum tears.

Location of the athlete's pain can also be misleading. Athletes with moderately severe anterior instability will complain of pain anteriorly along the glenohumeral joint in the late cocking phase of pitching. In these patients the apprehension test is almost uniformly positive. Also, in these patients up to 40% according to Rowe and Zarins[42] had roentgenographic evidence of Hill-Sachs lesions and, in addition, changes noted along the glenoid rim. However, in the athlete who has only mild anterior glenohumeral instability, the presenting symptom may be only pain, and, in fact, the pain felt in the cocking phase can be either posterior rather or anterior. Patients do not complain of giving way or slippage but may complain of symptoms consistent with an impingement. This posterior pain is secondary to inflammation within both the rotator cuff and capsule and may be related also to traction of the posterior structures as the arm moves from the late cocking position and begins to accelerate. Howell et al[21] have shown that in the maximally abducted and externally rotated position the center of the humeral head is approximately 4 mm posterior to the center of the glenoid and as the arm then forward flexes and rotates in acceleration, the humeral head glides anteriorly, producing sheer stress on the glenoid and the labrum. One should remember also that increased laxity results in diminished clearance for structures under the coracoacromial arc and the athlete will then have impingement symptoms.

Physical Examination

Shoulder motion should be carefully assessed, because often patients with evidence of anterior subluxation will have a loss of external rotation in the maximally abducted position. A positive apprehension sign in this position will be present in the moderate to severe subluxator; however, it is usually absent in more mild cases of instability. In the presence of mild instability, the patient may exhibit a positive relocation sign as described earlier. Tenderness may be palpated posteriorly along the glenohumeral capsule, and tenderness may also be elicited along the insertion of the supraspinatus. A positive impingement test and other physical findings consistent with impingement may often be present.

Physical findings in instability

- Loss of external rotation in abducted positions
- Apprehension sign
- Relocation sign of Jobe
- Anterior or posterior glenohumeral capsular tenderness
- Supraspinatus tenderness

Roentgenographic Evaluation

Roentgenographic evaluation may be helpful in patients wth anterior instability. Again, in the more severe cases of instability, plain roentgenograms, including a true anteroposterior view of the shoulder, a West Point axillary view, and Stryker notch views, have been helpful in detecting the presence of Hill-Sachs lesions. However, in athletes with mild or moderate anterior instability, routine roentgenograms, sophisticated CT scans with and without contrast, and Magnetic Resonance Imaging (MRI) techniques have been helpful.

Operating Room Evaluation

Examination with the patient under anesthesia and diagnostic shoulder arthroscopy are often necessary to confirm the diagnosis. At the time of arthroscopic evaluation, the anterior subluxation of the humeral head can be seen and demonstrated in the abducted and externally rotated position. Abnormalities of the anterior labrum are often present. These labral changes may consist of flattening and thinning anteriorly with an absence of the normal anterior inferior glenohumeral ligament or may consist of actual tears in the labrum as described in the classic Bankhart lesion. Bucket handle tears or flap tears may occur. In a few of these patients simple arthroscopic resection of the labrum tear may improve symptoms,[1] but this does not alter the instability, and many of these athletes will go on to develop recurrent problems with throwing. Therefore athletes must be cautioned that arthroscopic labral resection alone usually will not allow the thrower to return to throwing. As a result of the impingement syndrome that may be present secondarily, associated arthroscopic findings may include fraying of the posterior labrum and of the supraspinatus portion of the rotator cuff.[3] Andrews and associates[4] have further identified a series of glenoid labrum tears related to the long head of the biceps. In their series the majority of tears were located over the anterosuperior portion of the glenoid labrum near the origin of the tendon of the long head of the biceps into the glenoid. In general, one should be cautioned that despite the presence of arthroscopic findings consistent with impingement, the initiating event is usually that of anterior glenohumeral instability.

Arthroscopic findings in instability

- Anterior subluxation of humeral head
- Flattening and thinning of anterior labrum
- Labral tears
- Attenuation of anterior inferior glenohumeral ligament

Treatment

The treatment of the majority of patients with mild anterior subluxation revolves around a well-supervised shoulder rehabilitation program done in conjunction with a physical therapist. This program will only be successful if the athlete stops throwing completely during this period of rehabilitation. Selection of the proper exercise program will vary with each patient, but the importance of exercising scapular rotators, the serratus anterior, as well as the rotator cuff musculature is now being realized. Rehabilitation also is not complete without a supervised gradual return to throwing with attention to proper throwing mechanics.

Nonoperative Treatment

The rehabilitation program consists of three phases. In phase 1 range of motion exercises are performed, but care is taken to avoid undue stress to the anterior capsule. This is accomplished by performing exercises with the shoulder in the scapular plane. External rotation exercises are done with the arm by the side and limited to 45 degrees. Both external rotation, internal rotation, abduction, flexion, and extension exercises are performed using rubber tubing and progressing to free weights. Mobilization of the posterior capsule is also important.

In phase 2 emphasis on eccentric strengthening is begun and isokinetic strengthening and endurance training are started. Again, these exercises are done with the arm at the side.

In phase 3 stress is gradually applied to the anterior capsule by allowing isokinetic internal rotation and external rotation exercises to be performed with advancing degrees of shoulder abduction. When strength and endurance testing demonstrates 80% of function compared to the uninvolved side, then sports-specific activities such as a progressive throwing program can be initiated.

Operative Treatment

The surgical treatment of moderate and severe anterior glenohumeral instability has centered around repair of the Bankhart lesion when present and various anterior capsular reconstructive procedures.[7,20,43,48] Although these procedures have generally met with uniform success, the ability of the professional thrower to return to his or her previous level of activity has been dismal. Because of these inconsistent results in the professional thrower the anterior capsulolabral reconstruction was devised. The goal of this surgical procedure is to reconstruct the anterior inferior glenohumeral ligament complex with minimal disruption of anatomic structures, thereby allowing both reinforcement of the anterior capsule and early return of full motion so necessary for the pitcher's successful return.

Anterior capsulolabral reconstruction (Fig. 33-7)

Surgical technique. An 8 to 10 cm axillary incision is made beginning 1 cm inferior to the tip of the coracoid. The deltopectoral groove is identified and split, retracting the cephalic vein laterally. The conjoined tendon is retracted medially. The subscapularis is then split in line with its fibers along the lower one fifth of its width. This is done to preserve as much neurovascularity of the muscle as possible. With the anterior capsule now exposed, a T-type of incision is made, reflecting capsule off the glenoid side both superiorly and inferiorly. If the capsule is redundant inferiorly, then the inferior flap should be carefully reflected from the glenoid down to the most inferior portion. This must be done with the utmost caution to prevent damage to the axillary neurovascular structures. Three drill holes are then placed along the anterior glenoid from the 3 o'clock to 5 o'clock position. Next, the inferior flap is pulled superiorly and sutured along the anterior glenoid, re-creating the anterior inferior glenohumeral ligament and labrum. This is done using nonabsorbable no. 1 Ethibond sutures. The superior flap is then sutured in position, reinforcing the anterior capsule.

There are several important technical points to remember in performing this procedure. First, it is mandatory to re-create the

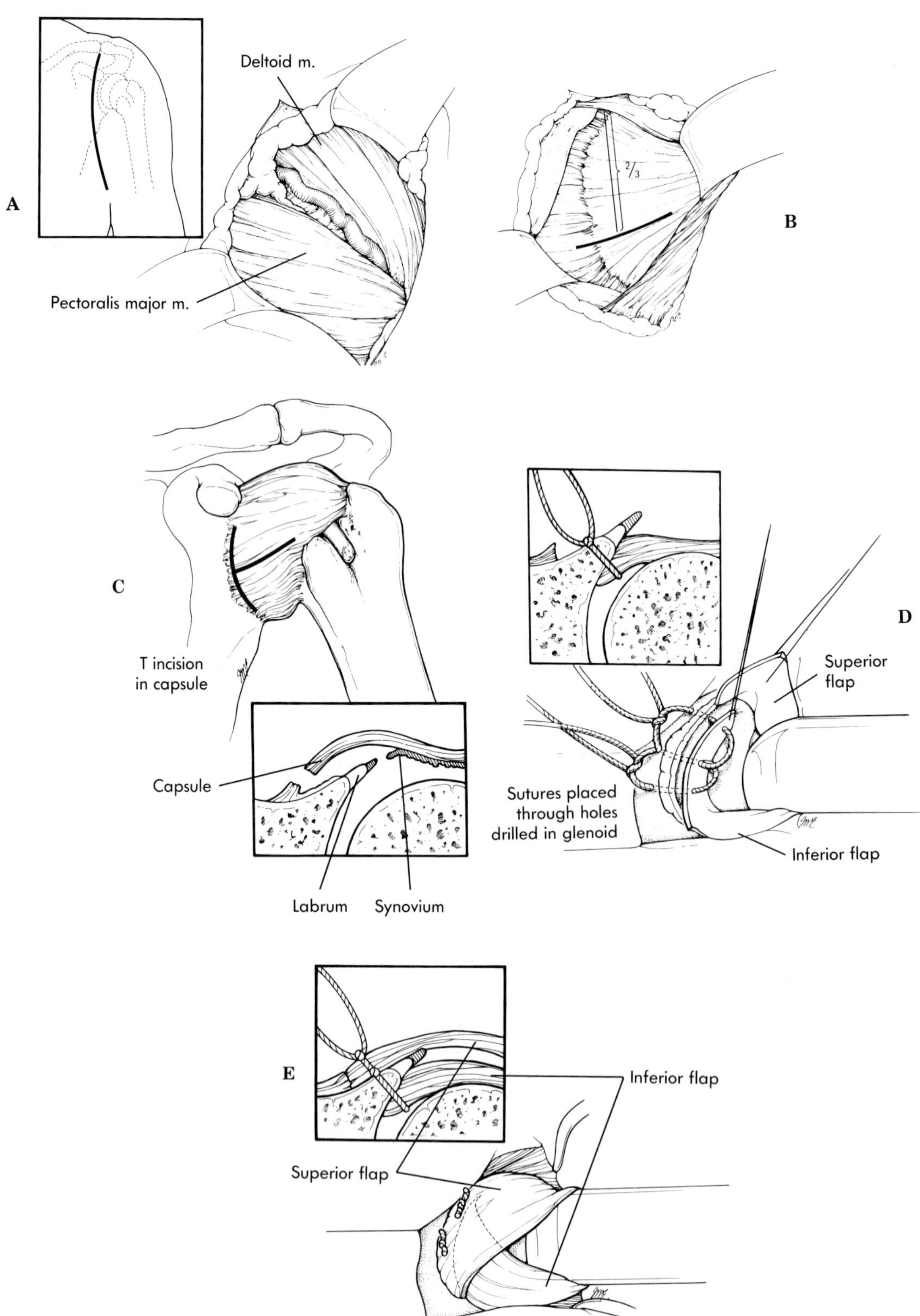

FIG. 33-7. Anterior capsulolabral reconstruction. **A,** Skin incision, delto-pectoral groove. **B,** Subscapularis split. **C,** Capsular T-type incision. **D,** Holes placed in glenoid from the 3 o'clock to the 5 o'clock position. **E,** Flaps tied into place.

anterior inferior glenohumeral ligament and thereby provide a new labral soft tissue bumper. Second, it is important to cause minimal disruption of normal anatomy. This means that the subscapularis must be split rather than completely resected as in the classic Bankhart repair. Exposure may be limited medially by the intact coracobrachialis.

Postoperative rehabilitation. Postoperatively, the patient is immobilized in an abduction splint at approximately 90 degrees of abduction and 45 degrees of external rotation for 2 weeks. During this time the splint may be removed to allow the shoulder to adduct and to allow passive abduction. In addition, active elbow range of motion is encouraged as well as forearm strengthening activities such as squeezing a softball. Isometric exercises may also be performed during this period.

At 2 weeks the patient is no longer required to use the abduction splint and the patient is started on a progressive active and passive range of motion program with emphasis placed on protecting the anterior repair. Active external rotation with the arm by the side and the elbow flexed 90 degrees can also be performed with the use of rubber tubing. Shoulder shrugs and supraspinatus strengthening activities can be begun at this time. At 6 weeks, shoulder flexion strengthening exercises may be added, as well as the use of the upper body ergometer for endurance training. By 8 weeks, the patient should have regained a full range of motion. Resistive exercises are continued and isokinetic strengthening activities can begin the third and fourth months but should be done with faster speed and in a position of flexion to protect the anterior joint capsule.

At 4 months, isokinetic strengthening may begin for flexion and abduction, and, in addition, training at slower speeds may be initiated. Progressive strengthening activities should be performed with emphasis on eccentric modes. At 4 to 5 months after surgery isokinetic testing may be performed. If the isokinetic testing shows 80% or above compared to the other involved shoulder, then a progressive shoulder throwing program can be initiated. As the shoulder throwing program is initiated, it is important to continue strength, flexibility, and endurance training.

The throwing program usually will require approximately 3 months to perform. This program involves progressive tossing of a ball with increasing distance and duration, initially on an alternate-day program and then progressing to a throwing-2-days, resting-1-day sequence. When the athlete returns to the mound the throw should be at half speed, emphasizing accuracy and technique. The athlete then progresses from half speed to three-fourths speed, with eventual return to a normal pitching regimen. It is this smooth progression from one phase to another under close supervision that will determine when an athlete will actually return to full competition. The time frame involved is variable and must be individualized to the athlete's need and condition of the shoulder. Rapid progression from one phase to the next without adequate rest and reassessment by the athlete, therapist, and physician will only result in delays, complications, and ultimate failure. Usually one year or more of rest is necessary before the athlete can compete.

Throwing program

- Alternate day, light tossing
- Throw 2 days and rest 1 day
- Half speed from mound
- Three fourths speed from mound
- Full return

ACROMIOCLAVICULAR JOINT PROBLEMS

The acromioclavicular joint provides support for the upper portion of the shoulder. The articulation is not a direct one, because a disc of fibrocartilage is present between the two bones. The joint is stabilized primarily by the coracoclavicular ligament. However, the forward and backward motion of the distal clavicle is further controlled by the coracoacromial ligament, whose importance in throwing has previously been discussed.

Abduction and external rotation of the shoulder cannot occur without axial rotation of the clavicle, which produces sheer forces at the acromioclavicular joint. In addition, the follow-through phase of throwing is associated with positioning the arm in a degree of forward flexion across the chest. This produces high compression forces at the acromioclavicular joint as well. Accumulation of these stresses in the throwing athlete results in degenerative changes in the fibrocartilaginous disc, as well as on the articular surfaces of the joint.

History and Physical Examination

The athlete typically experiences pain at the acromioclavicular joint associated with phase 3 (late cocking) or phase 5 (follow-through of the throwing motion). Pain is usually sharp and very specific. Associated bicipital symptoms are common.

Physical examination reveals tenderness to palpation at the acromioclavicular joint, usually anteriorly. Forward flexion at shoulder level across the chest will reproduce symptoms. Remember that the acromioclavicular joint symptoms may exist with impingement as well. Roentgenographically, degenerative changes may be present, with sclerosis and lytic irregularities often noted in the distal clavicle. Degenerative bone spurs may also be present on either side of the joint inferiorly. Interestingly, no correlation has been found between the degree of degenerative changes and symptoms.

Treatment

Mild symptoms may respond to rest, oral antiinflammatory agents and a mobilization program. Bathing the acromioclavicular joint with a corticosteroid solution may also reverse acute symptoms and provide long-lasting relief. In athletes whose condition does not respond to nonoperative management, surgical resection of the distal clavicle has provided good relief.[8]

The amount of bone resected is critical, because the clavicle provides attachment for both shoulder girdle musculature (deltoid and pectoralis) and ligamentous structures (coracoclavicular ligament). The proper amount of bone resection should still retain maximal length with these attachments and yet provide complete clearance in the remaining joint to prevent impingement throughout a complete range of motion of the shoulder. Laboratory studies undertaken have shown weakness of muscles in the surgically treated patient. Functionally, throwers have been able to return to their previous level of activities without problems.

NEUROVASCULAR ENTRAPMENT SYNDROMES

Neurovascular entrapment syndromes are relatively rare in the thrower, but when they occur they may cause significant loss of function and may end the athlete's career. These syndromes can be further divided into those involving the thoracic outlet, those involving the suprascapular nerve, and those involving the quadrilateral space.

Thoracic Outlet Syndrome

Thoracic outlet problems in the thrower can be manifested by various nonspecific complaints and often confusing and vague physical signs.[45] Athletes may complain of diffuse muscle aching or easy fatigability. Pain and paresthesias involving the neck or entire upper extremity may be present. Complaints of weakness, numbness, tingling, and temperature changes, as well as nocturnal complaints, are all possible.

Physical examination should include Adson's test and the hyperabduction maneuver of Wright and Lipscomb,[52] as well as the costoclavicular maneuver described by Baker and Thorberry. Roentgenograms may indicate the presence of cervical ribs. Electromyographic studies, including nerve conduction velocity studies, and vascular studies may be necessary to make a definitive diagnosis.

Many thoracic outlet problems can be relieved with nonoperative management emphasizing proper posture, as well as shoulder girdle muscle strengthening. Axillary artery occlusion and venous thrombosis may require anticoagulants or surgery.[52] Surgical release of the anterior scalene muscles and cervical rib excision have also been described as treatment for thoracic outlet problems not improved by more conservative management.

Suprascapular Nerve Entrapment

The suprascapular nerve is a motor nerve originating from roots C5 and C6 and passing to the upper border of the scapula, where it then passes through the scapular notch covered by the transverse scapular ligament. It is at this level that the supraspinatus muscle is innervated. The nerve then passes around the neck of the scapular spine before providing innervation to the infraspinatus muscle. It is at this point where entrapment usually occurs in the thrower and appears as an isolated infraspiratus atrophy.

Athletes may be seen with vague posterior or posterolateral shoulder pain. Because the supraspinatus and infraspinatus are not functioning properly, other problems, such as rotator cuff tendonitis, bicipital tenosynovitis, and bursitis, may also be present. On physical examination one should observe wasting of either the infraspinatus alone or in combination with the supraspinatus, depending on the level of entrapment.

Treatment must include a period of rest from throwing in an effort to relieve further irritation to the nerve. Often, rest in combination with a flexibility and strengthening program for the atrophied rotator cuff muscles as well as the scapular rotators will be all that is necessary. In cases of long-term entrapment with significant atrophy, surgical release at either level may be performed, but these procedures have not enjoyed much success in our experience. Interestingly, there are pitchers who have been able to continue throwing even at a professional level despite chronic wasting of the infraspinatus musculature from long-standing entrapment problems. This is because during normal throwing the infraspiratus only functions at 30% MMT. If the athlete can restrengthen the remaining infraspiratus muscle despite entrapment, he will be able to throw at preinjury levels.

Quadrilateral Space Syndrome

The quadrilateral space is formed superiorly by the teres minor, inferiorly the teres major, medially by the long head of the triceps, and laterally by the neck of the humerus. Through this space pass the posterior circumflex vessels and the axillary nerve. Compression of these structures can occur in the abducted externally rotated position of the arm, which is seen in the terminal cocking phase of throwing. Fibrous bands can also be present in this space, which can further entrap these structures. The thrower is seen with nonspecific shoulder pain and only occasionally with paresthesias. The symptoms appear to coincide with phase 3 of the throwing motion when the arm is maximally abducted and externally rotated.[39] As such, patients may note symptoms only associated with a particularly hard throw. Physical examination of the shoulder is quite normal, although again this problem may coexist with other more common shoulder disorders. Tenderness directly over the quadrilateral space often is present but may be confused with the tenderness seen in this area with the more common teres minor tendonitis. Electromyography is usually negative, although rarely a mild denervation pattern may be seen in the deltoid. The diagnosis is confirmed by subclavian arteriography at which time the posterior circumflex artery can be seen to occlude with humeral abduction and external rotation.

In patients who remain symptomatic, surgical decompression through a posterior shoulder approach has been effective. This is a rare entity and only a few cases in throwers exist, but surgical decompression has been successful in the throwers treated.

ADOLESCENT INJURIES

Adolescent shoulder injuries occur via the same basic mechanisms as in the adult, but the physeal growth plate changes the types of injuries seen. Capsular structures about the shoulder joint have greater strength than the epiphyseal plate, therefore the plate becomes the most vulnerable spot for injury. There are several growth plates about the shoulder including those of the acromion, coracoid, proximal humerus, and glenoid, with many of the growth plates staying open beyond the age of 18 years.

Little League Shoulder

Little league shoulder is a term coined by Dotter[12]; it is manifested by shoulder pain in the throwing athlete associated with throwing activities. Pain is usually about the shoulder and deltoid in a nonspecific pattern and is worse after activity and especially after hard throwing. Physical examination is usually normal with the exception of palpable tenderness over the proximal humerus physis. Patients may also exhibit signs of impingement.

The diagnosis can usually be made with the aid of roentgenograms that reveal widening of the proximal epiphyseal plate of the humerus.[10] Often, comparison roentgenograms of the opposite limb are necessary. Callus bone formation may subsequently occur secondary to periosteal reaction. It is felt that this physeal fracture occurs because of the relative weakness of the zone of hypertrophy in the physis, which is subject to both sheer and torque as the shoulder moves from abduction and external rotation to internal rotation as one goes from phase 2 to phase 5 of pitching.[17] The athlete will respond to a period of rest, allowing this stress fracture to heal, and the athlete can return to playing without problems as long as attention is paid to conditioning and the prevention of overuse.

Other injuries in the adolescent include those seen in the adult, such as impingement and instability problems.

REFERENCES

1. Andrews JR and Carson W: The arthroscopic treatment of glenoid labrum tears in the throwing athlete, Orthop Trans 8:44, 1984.
2. Andrews JR et al: Arthroscopy of the shoulder: technique and normal anatomy, Am J Sports Med 12:1, 1984.
3. Andrews JR et al: Arthroscopy of the shoulder in the management of partial tears of the rotator cuff: a preliminary report, Arthroscopy 1:117, 1985.
4. Andrews JR et al: Glenoid labrum tears related to long head of the biceps, Am J Sports Med 13:337, 1985.
5. Bankart ASB: The pathology and treatment of recurrent dislocation of the shoulder joint, Br J Surg 26:23, 1939.
6. Blazina ME and Saltzman JS: Recurrent anterior subluxation of the shoulder in athletes—a distinct entity, J Bone Joint Surg 51A:1037, 1969.
7. Bost F and Inman V: The pathologic changes in recurrent dislocation of shoulder: a report of Bankhart's operative procedure, J Bone Joint Surg 24:595, 1942.

8. Cahill BR: Osteolysis of the distal part of the clavicle in male athletes, J Bone Joint Surg 64:1053, 1982.
9. Cahill BR: Understanding shoulder pain, Instr Course Lect 34:332, St Louis, 1985, The CV Mosby Co.
10. Cahill BR et al: Little league shoulder, J Sports Med 2:150, 1974.
11. Cain PR et al: Anterior stability of the glenohumeral joint: a dynamic model, Am J Sports Med 15:144, 1987.
12. Dotter WE: Little leaguer's shoulder: a fracture of the proximal epiphyseal cartilage of the humerus due to baseball pitching, Guth Clin Bull 23:68, 1953.
13. Garth WP et al: Occult anterior subluxations of the shoulder in noncontact sports, Am J Sports Med 15:579, 1987.
14. Glousman et al: Diagnostic electromyographic analysis of the throwing shoulder with glenohumeral instability, J Bone Joint Surg 70A:220, 1988.
15. Gowan ID et al: A comparative electromyographic analysis of the shoulder during pitching: professional versus amateur pitchers, Am J Sports Med 15:586, 1987.
16. Ha'eri G and Wiley AM: Shoulder impingement syndrome: results of operative release, Clin Orthop 168:128, 1982.
17. Hansen NM: Epiphyseal changes in the proximal humerus of an adolescent baseball pitcher, Am J Sports Med 10:380, 1982.
18. Hawkins RJ and Hobeika PE: Impingement syndrome in the athletic shoulder, Clin Sports Med 2:391, 1983.
19. Hill HA and Sachs MD: The grooved defect of the humeral head: a frequently unrecognized complication of dislocation of the shoulder joint, Radiology 35:690, 1940.
20. Hill JA et al: The modified Bristow-Helfet procedure for recurrent anterior shoulder subluxations and dislocations, Am J Sports Med 9:283, 1981.
21. Howell SM et al: Normal and abnormal mechanics of the glenohumeral joint in the horizontal plane, J Bone Joint Surg 70A:227, 1988.
22. Jackson DW: Chronic rotator cuff impingement in the throwing athlete, Am J Sports Med 4:231, 1976.
23. Jobe CM and Jobe FW: Painful athletic injuries of the shoulder, Clin Orthop 173:117, 1983.
24. Jobe FW: Thrower problems, Sports Med 7:139, 1979.
25. Jobe FW and Moynes DR: Delineation of diagnostic criteria and a rehabilitation program for rotator cuff injuries, Am J Sports Med 10:336, 1982.
26. Jobe FW et al: An EMG analysis of the shoulder in throwing and pitching, Am J Sports Med 11:3, 1983.
27. Jobe FW et al: An EMG analysis of the shoulder in pitching: a second report, Am J Sports Med 12:218, 1984.
28. King JW et al: Analysis of the pitching arm of the professional baseball pitcher, Clin Orthop Rel Res 67:116, 1979.
29. Lombardo SJ: Arthroscopy of the shoulder, Clin Sports Med 2:309, 1983.
30. Moynes DR et al: Electromyography and motion analysis of the upper extremity in sports, Phys Ther 6:1905, 1986.
31. Neer CS: Anterior acromioplasty for the chronic impingement syndrome in the shoulder: a preliminary report, J Bone Joint Surg 54A:41, 1972.
32. Norwood LA et al: Anterior shoulder pain in baseball pitchers, Am J Sports Med 6:103, 1978.
33. Pappas AM et al: Symptomatic shoulder instability due to lesions of the glenoid labrum, Am J Sports Med 11:279, 1983.
34. Pappas AM et al: Biomechanics of baseball pitching: a preliminary report, Am J Sports Med 13:216, 1985.
35. Pappas AM et al: Rehabilitation of the pitching shoulder, Am J Sports Med 13:223, 1985.
36. Penny JN and Welsh RP: Shoulder impingement syndromes in athletes and their surgical management, Am J Sports Med 9:11 1981.
37. Perry J: Anatomy and biomechanics of the shoulder in throwing, swimming, gymnastics and tennis, Clin Sports Med 2:247, 1983.
38. Rathburn JB and Macnab I: The microvascular pattern of the rotator cuff, J Bone Joint Surg 52B:540, 1970.
39. Redler MR et al: Quadrilateral space syndrome in a throwing athlete, Am J Sports Med 14:511, 1986.
40. Richardson AB: Overuse syndromes in baseball, tennis, gymnastics and swimming, Clin Sports Med 2:379, 1983.
41. Rockwood CA: Subluxation of the shoulder: the classification, diagnosis and treatment, Orthop Trans 4:306, 1980.
42. Rowe CR and Zarins B: Recurrent transient subluxation of the shoulder, J Bone Joint Surg 63A:863, 1981.
43. Rowe CR et al: The Bankart procedure: a long-term end-result study, J Bone Joint Surg 60A:1, 1978.
44. Sisto DJ and Jobe FW: The operative treatment of scapulothoracic bursitis in professional pitchers, Am J Sports Med 14:192, 1986.
45. Strukel RJ et al: Thoracic outlet compression in athletes, Am J Sports Med 6:35, 1978.
46. Tibone JE: Shoulder impingement syndrome in athletes treated with an anterior acromioplasty, Clin Orthop 188:134, 1985.
47. Tibone JE et al: Surgical treatment of tears of the rotator cuff in athletes, J Bone Joint Surg 68A:887, 1986.
48. Torg JS et al: A modified Bristow-Helfet-May procedure for recurrent dislocation and subluxation of the shoulder: report of two hundred and twelve cases, J Bone Joint Surg 69A:904, 1987.
49. Turkel SJ et al: Stabilizing mechanisms preventing anterior dislocation of the glenohumeral joint, J Bone Joint Surg 63A:1208, 1981.
50. Warren RF: Subluxation of the shoulder in athletes, Clin Sports Med 2:339, 1983.
51. Warren RF: Instability of shoulder in throwing sports, Instr Course Lect 34:337, St Louis, 1985 The CV Mosby Co.
52. Wright RS and Lipscomb AB: Acute occlusion of the subclavian vein in an athlete: diagnosis, etiology and surgical management, J Sports Med 2:343, 1975.
53. Yocum LA: Assessing the shoulder: history, physical examination, differential diagnosis, and special tests, Clin Sports Med 2:281, 1983.
54. Zarins B et al: Injuries to the throwing arm, Philadelphia, 1985, WB Saunders Co.

CHAPTER 34 Prevention and Rehabilitation of Shoulder Injuries in Throwing Athletes

Karen Middleton

The upper extremity is the primary site of acute and chronic injuries from throwing. The volatile action of the throwing mechanism places high stresses and demands on the shoulder and elbow. As a result, shoulder and elbow problems are common among throwers. Baseball pitchers usually experience shoulder or elbow pain from the physiologic overload of the repetitive high-frequency, high-velocity demand on the upper extremity. According to King et al,[14] 50% of all baseball players experience sufficient elbow or shoulder joint symptoms to keep them from throwing for various periods during their careers.

The coordinated sequence of throwing is influenced by such variables as glenohumeral and scapulothoracic motion,[16] flexibility of the joint capsule, and proper muscle balance and symmetry. To prevent recurrent injury and subsequent compensation in performance, maintenance of normal surrounding joint musculature and flexibility is paramount. To understand throwing injuries and to consider rehabilitation of such injuries and prevention of recurrence of injury, one must first consider the anatomic shoulder mechanics and the proper mechanics of throwing.

BIOMECHANICAL CONSIDERATION OF INJURY

Anatomic Shoulder Aspects

The shoulder region is a complex of 20 muscles, three bony articulations, and three soft tissue moving surfaces that permit the greatest mobility of any joint area of the body.[14] Stability and mobility of the glenohumeral and scapulothoracic joints work together with associated movements of the acromioclavicular and sternoclavicular joints to provide both power and coordination required of shoulder movement in the throwing act. Support and stabilization of the shoulder depend on muscles and ligaments.[22] The dynamic support of the shoulder is derived from the anterior, superior, and posterior musculature. The rotator cuff musculature, along with the glenohumeral joint ligaments, supports the humeral head in the glenoid cavity. The importance of the rotator cuff in glenohumeral support and assistance in abduction and rotation of the joint is often overshadowed by one's consideration of the larger, more powerful muscles of the shoulder girdle. The key role of the rotator cuff as the essential stabilizer of the glenohumeral joint and as the major decelerator of the arm during the throwing act cannot be overemphasized.

Mechanics of Throwing

The mechanics of throwing have been described by Tullos and King,[25] Jobe et al,[11] Pappas,[19] McLeod,[17] King et al,[14] and Prentice and Cooma.[20] McLeod[17] describes the pitching mechanism as an act divided into five phases: windup, cocking, acceleration, release and deceleration, and follow through. Important in the consideration of the mechanical analysis of the movement of the arm is the involvement of the entire body. The windup is a balance phase that prepares the pitcher for the proper body alignment and weight shift to lead into the cocking phase. In this phase, kinetic energy is stored and the pitchers have the opportunity to "hide" the ball from the batters. During the windup, the opposite knee is lifted upward and the body placed in a position so that all segments of the body (legs, hips, trunk, and arms) contribute to the throw. Cocking is the next phase that applies tension on the accelerator muscles. The opposite leg is extended forward and planted just left of midline of the path to the plate. The hips follow, internally rotating, to provide maximal thrust. At this point, the arm is abducted and in extreme external rotation, and the shoulder and trunk progress forward to provide extrinsic loading to the pitching arm. Forward movement of the ball occurs in the acceleration phase. The body continues its forward motion and the pectoralis major and latissimus dorsi fire to horizontally adduct and internally rotate the arm. The arm "drags" behind as tremendous force is applied. During this acceleration, a considerable extension force is placed on the elbow joint. The deceleration phase is stated to be two times greater than acceleration forces.[11] The humerus has a high rate of internal rotation during the deceleration phase. The rotator cuff musculature is instrumental in decelerating the motion of the arm and stabilizing the humerus in the glenoid cavity. In the follow-through phase, there is a stretch of the rotator cuff and a reduction of tension on the posterior shoulder structure. A smooth transition is provided from the violent phase of deceleration to recovery.

Other throwing sports require special consideration because of the differences in technique and the weight of the projectile to be thrown over a given distance. The body is exposed to unique forces in various sports. For example, comparisons of throwing a football and throwing a baseball reveal that the football is heavier, the windup in throwing a football is less than a baseball, the forward fling is shorter, and the follow through is in a different arc and not as powerful.[4] Discussions of rotator cuff problems are addressed by Gambardella and Jobe in Chapter 33.[13] Comparisons are made of throwing a baseball, hitting a tennis serve, and hitting a golf ball in discussions of rotator cuff problems.

Sports medicine researchers through the U.S. Olympic Committee have analyzed the mechanism of throwing in members of the U.S. water polo team.[21] Patterns of throwing in water polo are similar to those of baseball with a positioning phase, a windup, a throw, and follow through. Rollins et al[21] describe specific modifications in water polo:

> The initial stance includes holding the ball out of the water, positioning the opposite arm in front for balance, and an eggbeater motion of the legs to maintain position. The windup includes cocking of the throwing arm, vertical upward push with the kick leg, ball push-off, and a pull with the opposite or steadying arm. During the moment before throwing, the ipsilateral hip is abducted, and the contralateral hip is flexed. Greater elbow flexion and external humeral rotation are related to increased ball velocity.

Research and Clinical Findings

Injuries to the upper extremity caused by the throwing motion in sports have stimulated progressive research and analysis. High-speed cinematography and dynamic electromyography (EMG) with computer-assisted analysis have allowed study of the complex throwing act. The muscle activation pattern of the shoulder during each phase of throwing was outlined in studies by Jobe et al.[11,12] The supraspinatus, infraspinatus, teres minor, subscapularis, and anterior, middle, and posterior portions of the deltoid muscle were observed in five pitchers. An acceleration phase of 0.1 seconds was noted; next came a follow-through phase in which there were significant muscular contractions of all the muscle groups to decelerate the arm. In the later electromyographic study, the activities of the pectoralis major, biceps, triceps, latissimus dorsi, seratus anterior, and brachialis muscles were examined. Large rotational torques are produced in the humerus with each phase of the throw.[17] The rapid acceleration and deceleration forces that occur often predispose the throwing arm to injury. The forces involved in each phase may lead to injuries that may be musculotendinous, articular, capsular, or neural. Inflexibility of the shoulder can cause a limitation of extension and external rotation. When the shoulder is externally rotated with a lack of motion, stress can occur to the anterior capsule to cause a microinjury or macroinjury with resultant inflammatory response. Injury occurs when the stress tolerance of the tissues is exceeded. With the shoulder in horizontal extension, abduction, and external rotation in the cocking phase, irritation of the biceps tendon or "impingement syndrome" may result.

During acceleration, the strong anterior musculature distracts the humeral head anteriorly on the glenoid rim. If the posterior muscles are weak or the capsule lax, the overload of the anterior force can cause compressive stress and injury to the anterior superior glenoid labrum. The deceleration phase is the most active phase, with intense firing of all the muscles, particularly those of the rotator cuff.[9] With extrinsic overload, the rotator cuff frequently has resultant tears at the superior cuff area, which are manifested as an impingement type of pain in evaluation of the shoulder.

The clinical diagnosis of a pathologic condition is arrived at through a correlation of the functional anatomy and physical examination. The procedure of (1) history taking; (2) physical examination consisting of inspection, palpation, and assessment of range of motion and flexibility, stability, strength, and nerve involvement; and (3) special tests and roentgenographic evaluation helps in formulation of a diagnosis.

Diagnostic Arthroscopy

Shoulder arthroscopy allows examination with the patient anesthetized and has provided an excellent method of evaluating and diagnosing shoulder pathologic conditions in throwing athletes.[24] Diagnostic and surgical arthroscopic techniques are described by Andrews and Carson,[1] who stress the attention to be given to patient position and technical detail. The physician is able to examine the glenohumeral joint intraarticularly and identify shoulder pathologic conditions, such as tears of the glenoid labrum, partial tears of the rotator cuff, partial tears of the biceps tendon, and joint osteophytes. Arthroscopic examination has been invaluable for confirming clinical findings in correlation with mechanisms of the injury. Andrews and Carson[2] have noted glenoid labrum tears related to the long head of the biceps through arthroscopic examination of throwing athletes. Also reported was the high frequency of tearing of the anterosuperior aspect of the glenoid labrum. This was hypothesized to be a result of the force of the biceps tendon eccentrically contracting during the follow-through phase to decelerate the elbow and provide compressive force to the glenohumeral joint. Arthroscopy has provided an increased knowledge of the pathologic processes of the shoulder joint.

PREVENTION

Proper Throwing Mechanics

"Bad habits" of throwing are often developed at a young age during early participation in any given sport. Little League players who are anxious and enthusiastic about their sport are often encouraged by parents and coaches to increase the frequency of throwing with less emphasis on the quality of throwing and with no knowledgeable instruction available. Thus, set patterns of faulty throwing mechanics become set kinematics for the individual. Proper body mechanics are of primary importance in avoiding injury from repetitive, high-velocity throwing. Coaches must concentrate on proper pitching technique for an individual thrower who experiences chronic arm problems. Biomechanical analysis with the use of high-speed cinematography is invaluable for detecting problem points during the throwing act. This is also a valuable tool in the rehabilitative phase so that once a player overcomes an injury, faulty mechanics can be corrected to prevent reinjury. In a work with JR Andrews, Johnny Sain,[23] professional baseball pitching coach, stresses the following points in the mechanics of pitching: (1) avoidance of overextending the arm and shoulder, (2) avoidance of overextending the planted leg, and (3) pointing the planted leg in the proper direction. This avoids "opening up" or "staying closed" too long, causing a compensation of the body in the delivery of the throw. The shoulder is abducted 90 degrees with proper pitching motion. With the overhead, three-quarter, or sidearm delivery, the body lean or trunk side flexion, as well as elbow flexion, differs; however, the shoulder remains at 90 degrees of abduction. If the throwing arm is abducted to a much greater degree than this, impingement problems are likely. The throwing act that is mechanically sound lessens the chance of injury and promotes an increased longevity of the thrower in his or her sport.

Year-Round Conditioning and Postinjury Maintenance

Essential to ball players is an off-season program and year-round conditioning. Players who are injured during spring training as a result of poor conditioning come to the real-

A

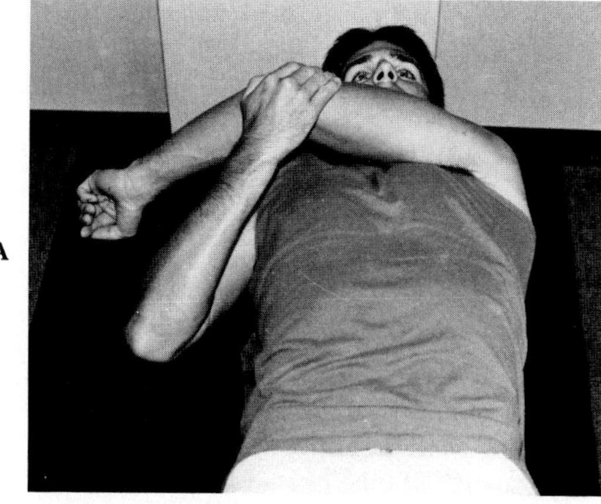

B

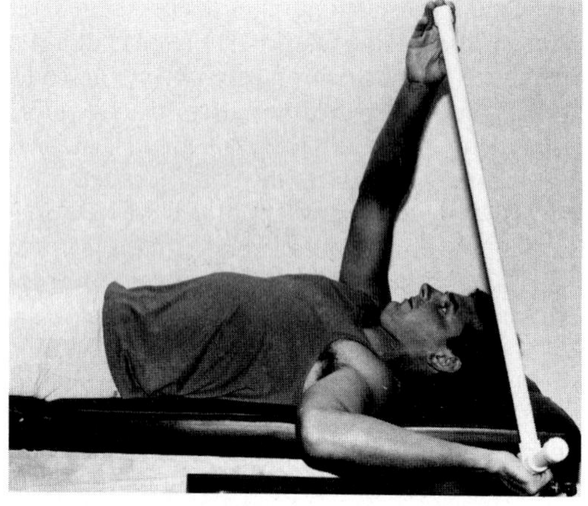

FIG. 34-1. Shoulder flexibility. **A,** Assessment with arms stretched in a horizontal adducted position. **B,** Supine external rotation performed at 90 degrees of abduction.

ization that they cannot expect to get in shape right before spring training and throw well without a high risk of injury. Players should progress back gradually so that they are not throwing "too hard, too fast, too far, too quickly," predisposing themselves to injury. Off-season conditioning programs address conditioning, strength training, and flexibility. It is of utmost importance that a structured flexibility and strength program and a good throwing program be followed. A year-round program helps to prevent injury, and a maintenance program helps to prevent recurrence.

Flexibility and stability of the shoulder are paramount in the dynamic throwing act. The joint capsule must allow range of motion and flexibility to provide a fluid delivery. Optimal abduction and external rotation are needed in the cocking phase, as well as freedom of movement in all positions. Flexibility is assessed and performed in horizontal adduction and combined abduction and external rotation (Fig. 34-1).

External rotation flexibility exercises are performed at three different angles for abduction: 90 degrees, approximately 135 degrees, and full abduction. This is performed with the athlete lying supine with the arm in one of the various positions for external rotation. A T-bar or any similar apparatus is utilized to actively assist stretching in external rotation. Each repetition is held for a count of five, with at least 25 repetitions performed. Flexibility exercises should be performed before and after throwing and should also be performed in conjunction with any weight-training program. A good balance between the anterior and posterior musculature must exist so that the shoulder will not be predisposed to injury. In addition to any anterior strengthening that a player may perform, special emphasis must be given to the posterior musculature (e.g., the rotator cuff).

REHABILITATION

Rehabilitative Goals

The goal of any rehabilitation program is return to an optimal preinjury status. A good rehabilitation program is directed toward achieving full range of motion, improving flexibility, increasing strength, and regaining power, coordination, endurance, accuracy, and timing for the activity. An eclectic approach of rehabilitative techniques allows one to formulate the best program according to the unique deficiencies of each individual. For full rehabilitation, one must not only achieve all components; but also reaccomplish the specificities of the sport. The specific adaptation to imposed demand (SAID) principle allows one to rehabilitate functionally by performing the activity. In addition to the activity itself being performed, the specific amount of concentric versus eccentric work is functionally addressed. Coleman et al[7] propose a performance profile–directed simulated game as an objective, functional evaluation of a baseball pitcher's return to throwing. The simulated game includes a 15-minute warm-up period and then 50 to 80 pitches thrown with progressive velocity. The breakdown of these 50 to 80 pitches corresponds to how the pitcher performs in a game. There are an average of 12 to 18 pitches thrown per inning, including 6 to 10 fastballs, thrown in an average of five to eight innings with a rest period of 9 minutes between innings.

The excessive demand and stress of throwing may lead to a spectrum of injuries ranging from minimal to maximal severity of pathologic conditions. Mild injuries with resultant inflammatory response and symptomatic pain

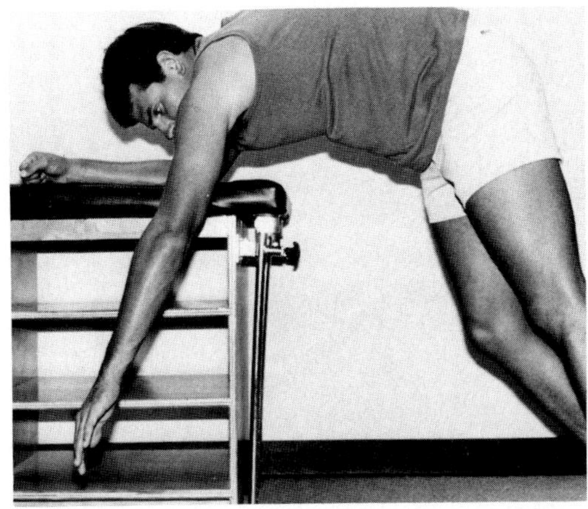

A

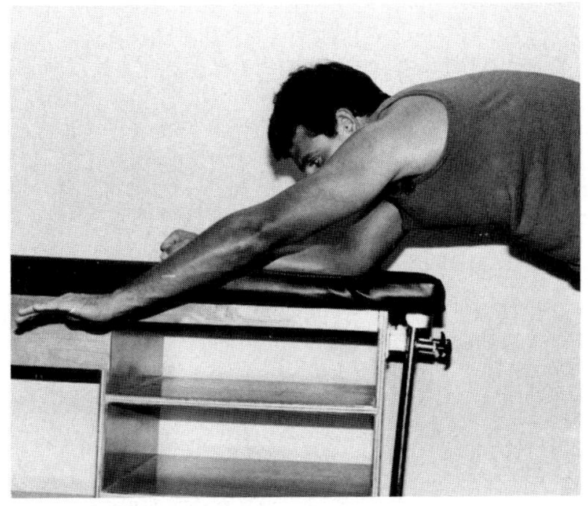

B

FIG. 34-2. Codman's excercises. **A,** Circumduction excercises (clockwise and counterclockwise circles) also stimulate mechanoreceptors of the joint, which helps to decrease shoulder discomfort. **B,** Pendulum swings encourage increased movement of the humeral head in the glenoid cavity.

may lead to a moderate or severe chronic problem if continued overdemand is placed on the shoulder without appropriate treatment in the early phase of injury. Mild overuse injuries, such as muscular strains, tendonitis, or bursitis, respond well to a period of rest from activity and conservative measures and treatments, such as ice, electrical muscle stimulation, moist heat, ultrasound, transcutaneous electrical nerve stimulation, antiinflammatories, exercise, and a gradual return to activity. If a continued overuse problem becomes chronic and severe, a cycle may result of increased pain and inflammation leading to shoulder tightness, muscular weakness, and imbalance with additional problems of compensation in activity that increases abnormal biomechanics.

Flexibility

Loss of shoulder flexibility results from muscular tenderness, muscular tightness, or capsular tightness. Inflexibility of the glenohumeral joint of the injured throwing shoulder can be assessed in positions of horizontal adduction and combined abduction and external rotation with the scapula stabilized. With loss of flexibility, movement is tight at the end range with a deficit of motion as compared to the uninvolved extremity. Codman[6] defines the synchronous movement of the shoulder girdle as "scapulohumeral rhythm," which is a 3:2 ratio of glenohumeral motion and scapular rotation. With glenohumeral joint tightness and loss of motion, compensation of the scapulothoracic joint occurs in an effort to perform a specific movement. Codman's exercises of circumduction and pendulum swings encourage increased movement of the humeral head in the glenoid cavity (Fig. 34-2).

A thrower needs full range of motion with good flexibility and movement positions. Active-assisted flexion can be performed in a supine position, as well as with rope and pulley exercises, which can assist in obtaining full flexion and a combination of abduction and external rotation motion (Fig. 34-3).

Abduction and external rotation are needed to perform the cocking position. Deficiency of these motions causes loss of throwing efficiency and velocity with resultant compensatory mechanics. Flexibility must be stressed when there is a loss of motion of the throwing shoulder. External rotation stretching is one of the most important exercises to perform. In the supine position, the athlete performs this active-assisted external rotation stretch in three abducted positions: 90 degrees, approximately 135 degrees, and full abduction (Figs. 34-2 to 34-4).

Inflexibility of the posterior musculature seen with horizontal adduction as well as internal rotation creates increased stress to the posterior shoulder structures on follow through. Internal rotation exercises, performed to stretch the rotator cuff, and good posterior flexibility are achieved with the horizontal adduction stretch (Fig. 34-5). The athlete should perform 25 repetitions of these motions three times daily. Proprioceptive neuromuscular facilitation (PNF) techniques are also effective in increasing flexibility. Techniques may be used to provide relaxation of antagonist muscles and increase agonist muscle action to gain range of motion.[15] Various mobilization techniques also help to stretch the joint capsule and loosen up the throwing

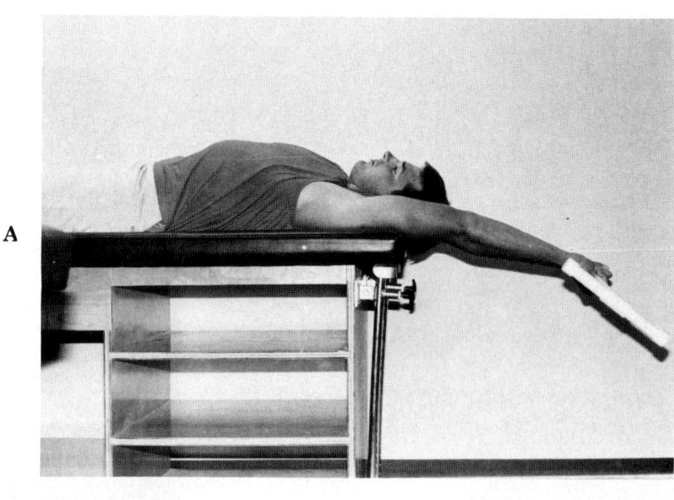

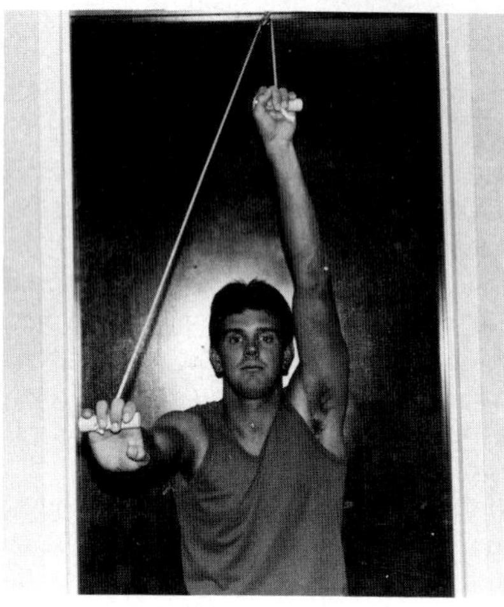

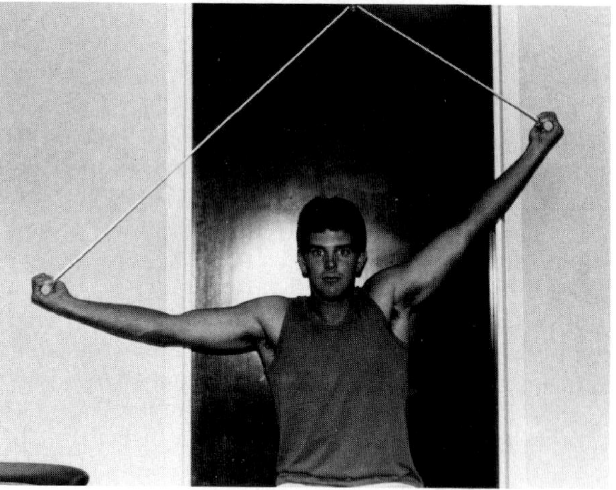

FIG. 34-3. Active-assisted flexion. **A,** Supine position performed. **B,** Over-the-door rope and pulley used in flexion position. **C,** Active-assisted exercise to obtain combination of full abduction with external rotation motion.

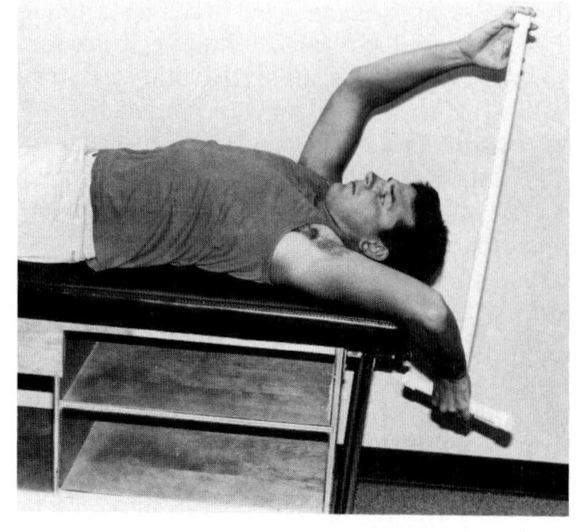

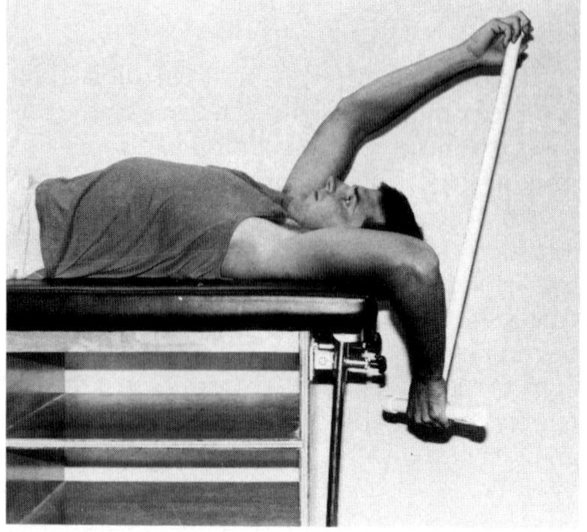

FIG. 34-4. Supine external rotation stretch. **A,** 135 degrees of abduction. **B,** 180 degrees of abduction.

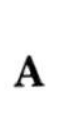
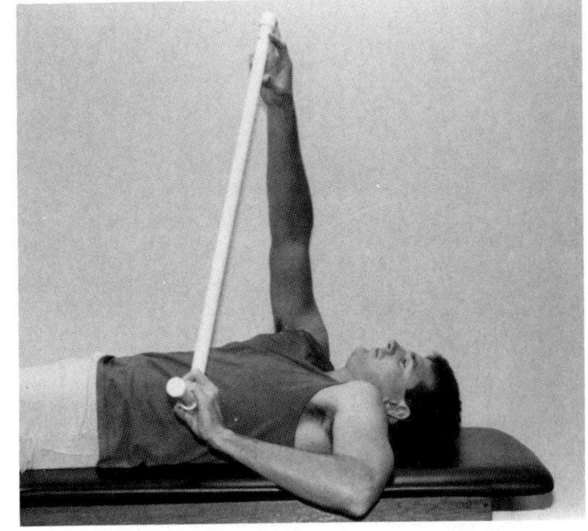
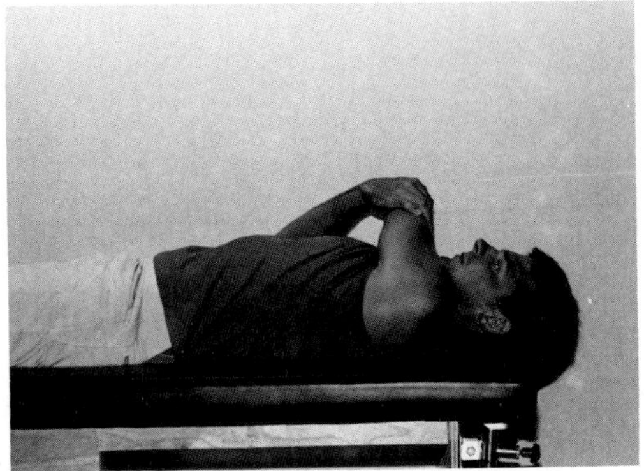

B

FIG. 34-5. A, Internal rotation is performed to stretch the rotator cuff. **B,** Horizontal adduction stretch.

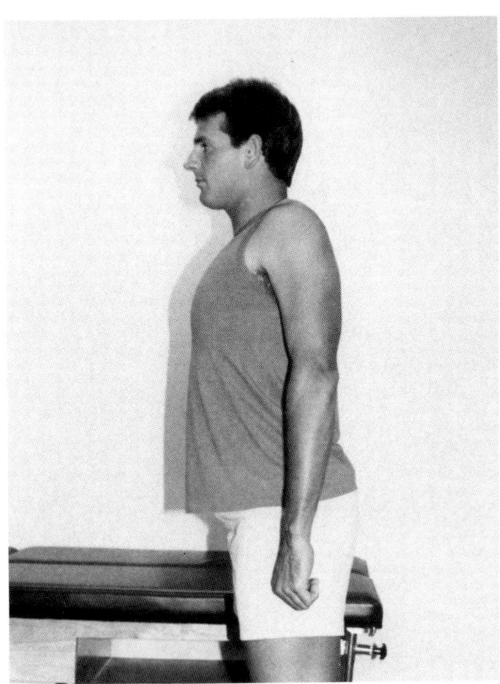

FIG. 34-6. Shoulder shrugs performed.

shoulder.[8] Numerous variations of stretches that are performed by each individual ball player, according to specific needs, are all part of the total routine of stretching. Impromptu "dugout stretches" are additionally important and effective. Flexibility exercises are essential for the throwing arm because the arm is propelled through an arc of motion limited to the range of passive mobility. To minimize the level of stress to the shoulder, flexibility and dynamic muscle balance are needed to provide proper synchronous motion.

Strength

Once a normal return of passive and active range of motion has been achieved, a strengthening program that focuses on muscular deficits of the shoulder is given priority. Goals of increasing strength and endurance in integrated muscle action of the athlete are accomplished by a *high repetition–low weight program.* Five sets of 10 repetitions are performed of each specific exercise outlined for the individual. Weight progression and rehabilitation of the injured throwing arm are initially increased gradually, beginning without weight on active movements and increasing from 1 to 5 pounds (0.45 to 2.45 kg) in weight. The exercises are performed in a concentric/eccentric manner with a slow lifting and a slow lowering technique. The strength/endurance exercises are performed three times daily. Heavier weights and weight-training machines, which may be used in strength programs for the uninjured shoulder, should not be used in the case of the injured shoulder until full range of motion, flexibility, strength, and throwing capabilities have been achieved.

Exercises for stabilization of the scapula are very important for the throwing shoulder. The shoulder shrug with scapular abduction is one exercise good for strengthening the scapula stabilizers. The shoulders are "brought up into a shrug," held for a count of two, pinched backward, held for a count of two, and then relaxed slowly to the starting position (Fig. 34-6).

Isometrics performed in different positions through full range of motion can also help strengthen the shoulder. Exercises can be

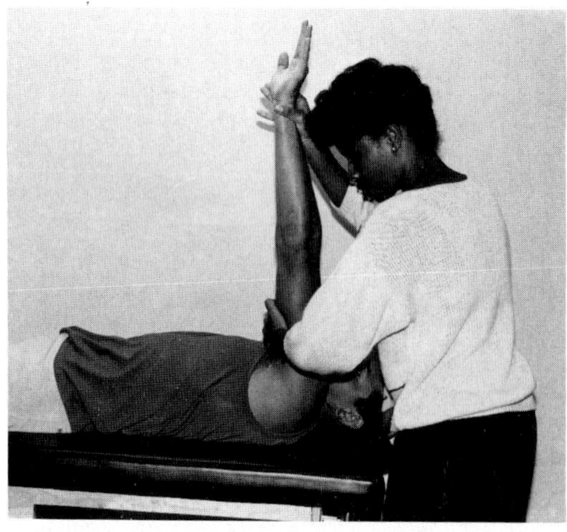

FIG. 34-7. Exercise of isometric co-contraction for joint stabilization.

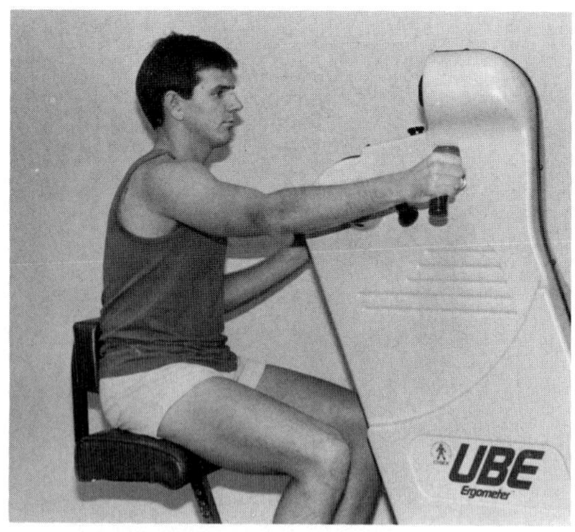

FIG. 34-8. Cybex upper body ergometer (UBE) for shoulder girdle endurance and strengthening.

A

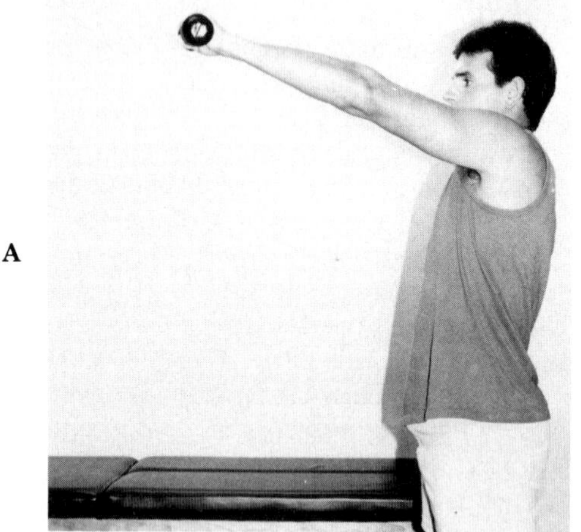

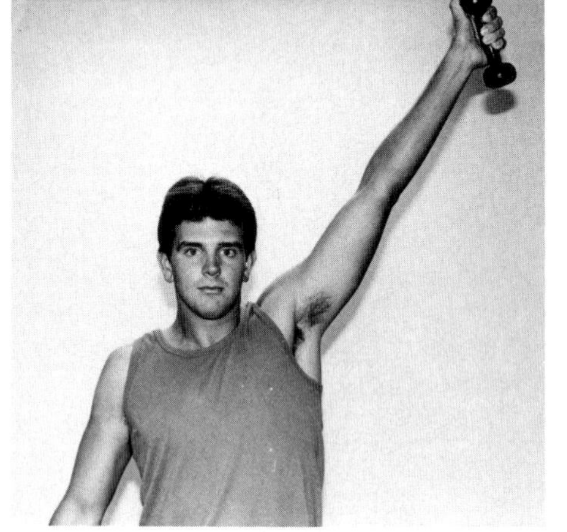

B

FIG. 34-9. Primary strengthening of the deltoid. **A,** With active forward flexion. **B,** With active abduction.

A

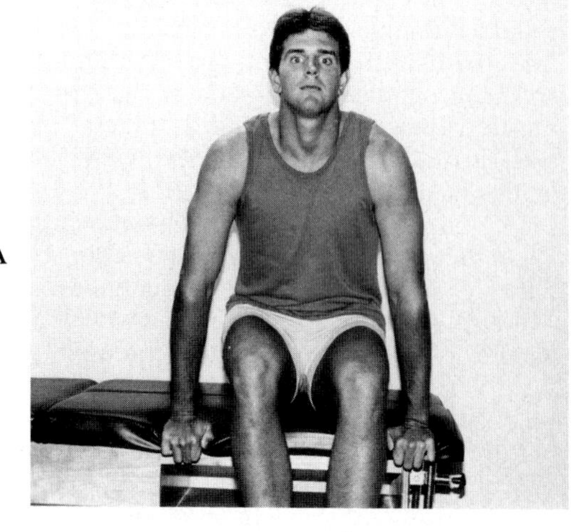

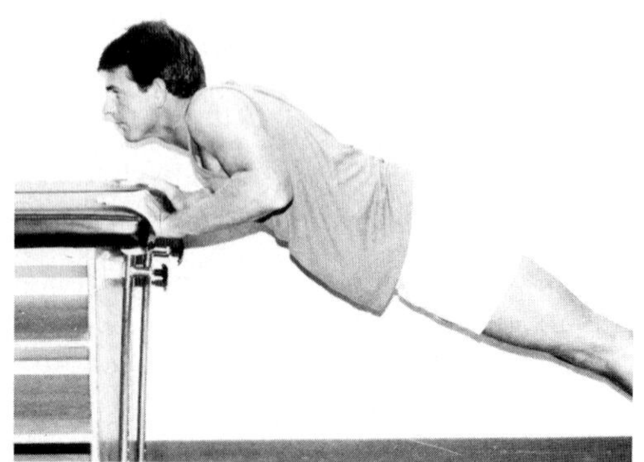

B

FIG. 34-10. Exercises to develop endurance and strength of the shoulder depressors, horizontal adductors, and internal rotators. **A,** Sitting dips. **B,** Modified push-ups.

performed individually, holding isometric contractions for at least six counts. Isometric co-contractions can be performed against controlled manual resistance for increased joint stabilization (Fig. 34-7).

Another variation for achieving shoulder girdle endurance and strength is exercising with the upper body ergometer (UBE) (Fig. 34-8).

Primary strengthening of the deltoid is performed in forward flexion and abduction from the standing position (Fig. 34-9).

Jobe et al[11] studied the peak activity of the deltoid, elevating and holding the arm at 90 degrees during the cocking phase. While in the acceleration phase, the pectoralis major, latissimus dorsi, and serratus anterior are all active. Exercises of sitting dips and push-ups develop endurance and strength of the shoulder depressors, horizontal adductors, and internal rotators (Fig. 34-10, *A*).

The modified push-up reduces stress on the anterior aspect of the shoulder (Fig. 34-10, *B*).

Biceps curls and triceps extensions are additional exercises for upper extremity strengthening (Fig. 34-11).

Rotator Cuff Program

Soft tissue injuries, such as tendonitis or partial tearing of the rotator cuff, often respond well to the conservative treatment of a rehabilitative patient program. Patients who have not benefited solely with exercise have been cited to return successfully to sports participation following arthroscopic treatment and a structured rehabilitation program.[2,3] The rotator cuff is composed of the supraspinatus, infraspinatus, teres minor, and subscapularis. Return to throwing depends on the effectiveness of a program of strengthening of the posterior cuff muscles. The subscapularis muscle, which provides dynamic support for medial (internal) rotation, has not been reported to be involved in the rotator cuff tears that have been seen during surgery of throwing injuries.[3] Electromyographic analysis of muscle action reveals pertinent information that is incorporated into rehabilitation philosophies.[10,12,13] Specific rotator cuff exercises noted in this chapter are derived from a study by Blackburn et al[5] that analyzed the supraspinatus, infraspinatus, and teres minor muscles in a functional position. The level of muscle stimulation was measured in a series of rotator cuff exercises in various positions, including standing and prone positions. The results of the study indicated that the supraspinatus muscle is involved when the arm is elevated in any position. The stimulus produced in the muscles was maximal when the individual exercised in the prone position. While the athlete is utilizing gravity in the prone position, the mechanism of throwing

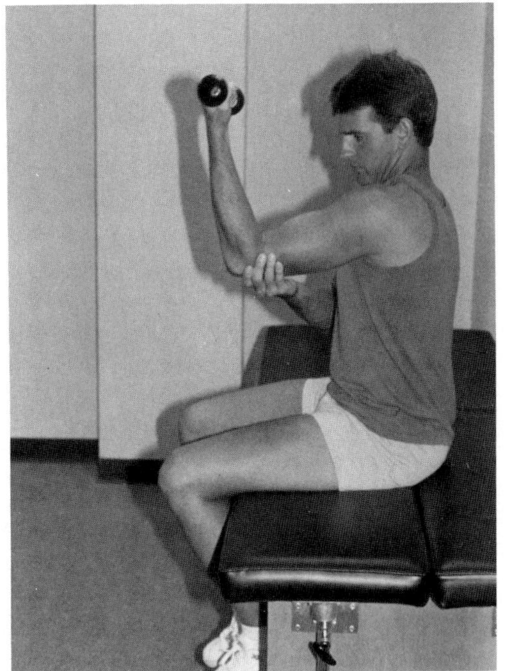

A

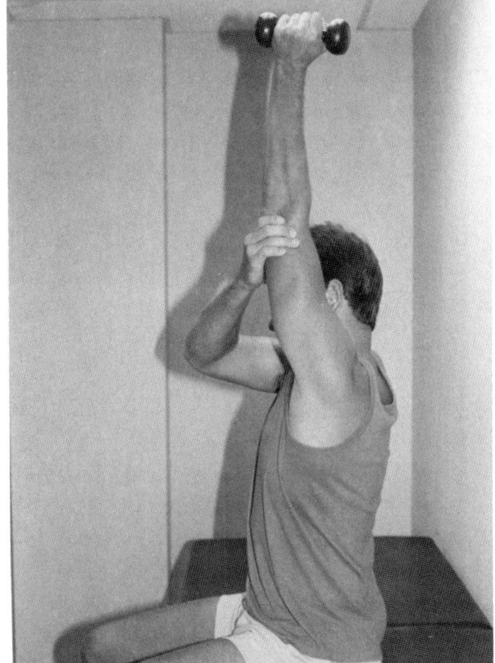

B

FIG. 34-11. Upper extremity strengthening. **A,** For biceps, performed with biceps curl exercise. **B,** For triceps, performed with triceps curl exercise.

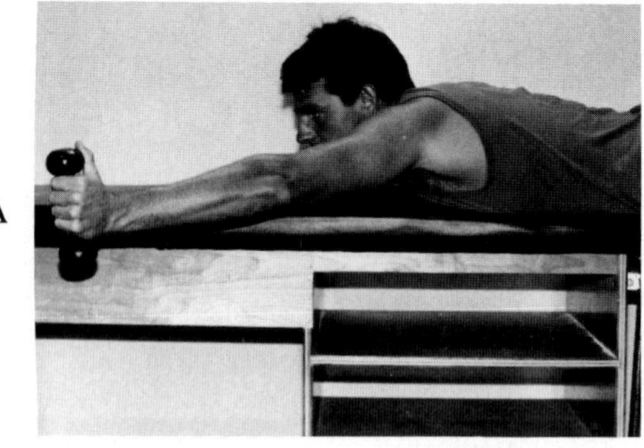

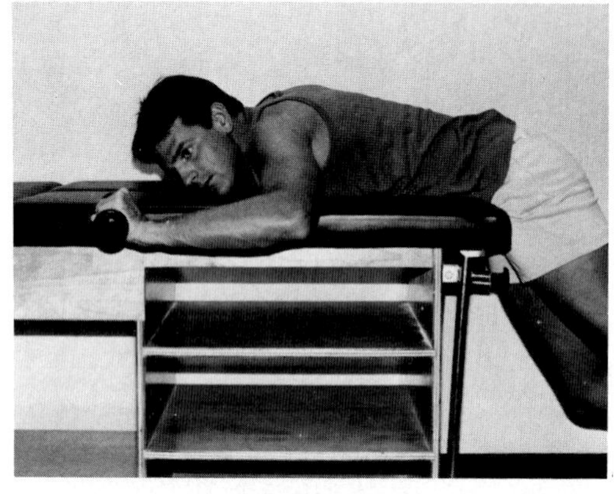

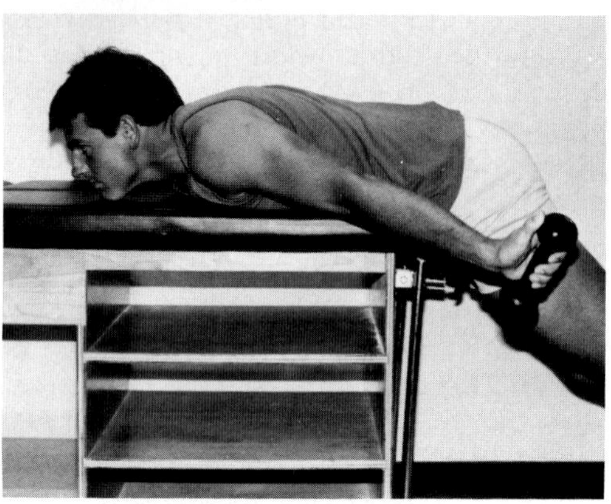

FIG. 34-12. Optimal positions for exercising rotator cuff. **A,** Prone horizontal abduction at 100 degrees with arm in externally rotated position. **B,** Prone external rotation strengthening position. **C,** Prone extension with arm in externally rotated position.

can be mimicked and the specificity of the exercise will be correlated to the act of throwing.[5]

Specific optimal positions for exercising the rotator cuff that provide maximal recruitment of the supraspinatus, infraspinatus, and teres minor follow:

1. With the patient prone and the arm externally rotated (thumb pointed up), lift the arm into horizontal abduction at 100 degrees to eye level, pause for two counts, and lower the arm slowly (Fig. 34-12, *A*).
2. With the patient prone and the arm externally rotated, lift the arm into pure abduction, pause for two counts, and lower the arm slowly.
3. With the patient prone (90/90 degrees), the arm supported in 90 degrees of abduction with elbow flexed to 90 degrees and the forearm hanging off the table, lift the arm into external rotation as high as possible, pause for two counts, and lower the arm slowly (Fig. 34-12, *B*).
4. With the patient prone (for increased work of the infraspinatus and teres minor), lift the arm into complete extension, then pause for two counts, and lower the arm slowly (Fig. 34-12, *C*).

Eccentric Work

Eccentric work is important because deceleration of the arm in motion requires eccentric contractions. The inertia unit is an excellent exercise modality for eccentric work. By utilizing various functional positions, the extremities are strengthened in an eccentric mode. Coordination and timing are additional factors that may be improved with this interval workout (Fig. 34-13).

Exercising with rubber tubing may provide similar benefits. Functional positions in diagonal patterns may be used for increasing strength in a functional mode (Fig. 34-14). In addition, various isokinetic units provide the capacity to exercise in an eccentric mode in a velocity spectrum workout.

Proprioceptive Neuromuscular Facilitation

Proprioceptive neuromuscular facilitation (PNF) can be an effective exercise modality. The clinician may use a variety of techniques

A 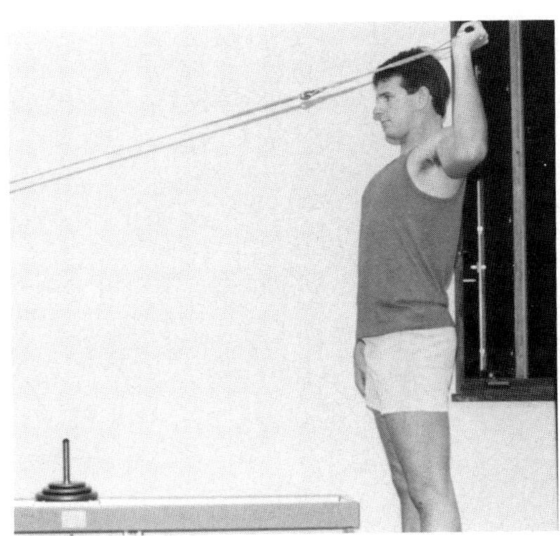

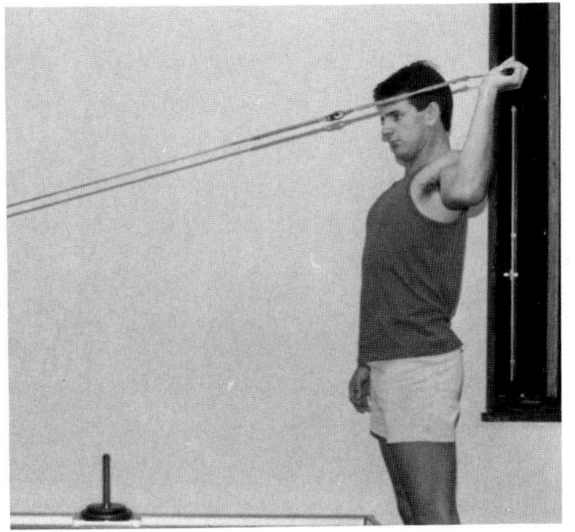 B

FIG. 34-13. Eccentric contraction exercises for deceleration of the arm. **A,** Impulse inertia unit used for strengthening. **B,** Interval eccentric exercise in functional position.

A 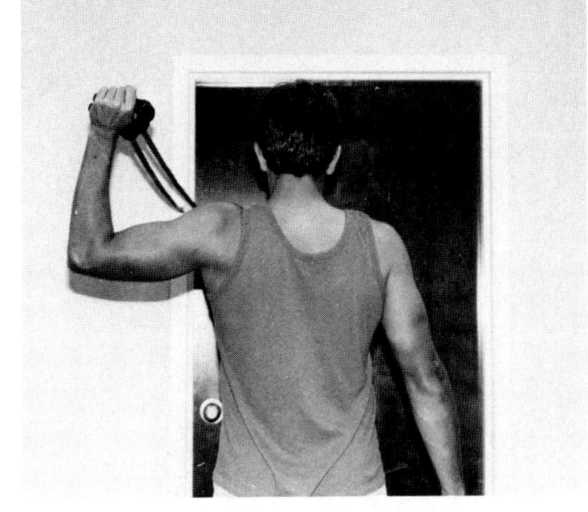

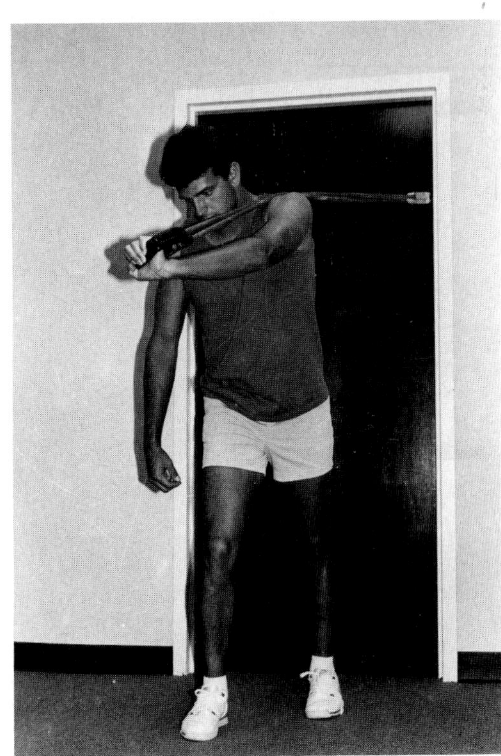 B

FIG. 34-14. Rubber tubing exercises. **A,** For strengthening. **B,** For function.

to achieve optimal strength, endurance, and coordination of the shoulder. These techniques are composed of rotational and diagonal patterns, similar to motions of most sports activities.[20] Strengthening techniques include repeated contraction, where the weak components are facilitated in the range to provide a more coordinated motion; slow reversal and slow reversal hold, which involve an isotonic contraction of the antagonist followed by an isotonic or isometric contraction of the agonist to develop strengthening within the range with normal reciprocal timing of muscle response (Fig. 34-15); and rhythmic stabilization to produce isometric co-contractions and stability of the agonist and antagonist muscle groups.[15]

Return to Throwing

After a thrower has regained full flexibility and adequate muscle strength, an aggressive return to throwing minimizes the chances of reinjury. Pitching involves the entire body; therefore it is essential that attention be given to strength and flexibility of the trunk and lower extremity as well. The interval throwing program (ITP) is an after-injury or after-surgery program modified in design by Dr. George Medich, former major league pitcher.

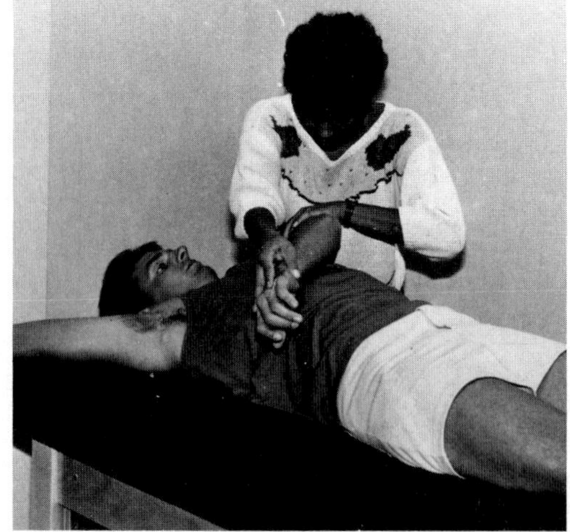

A

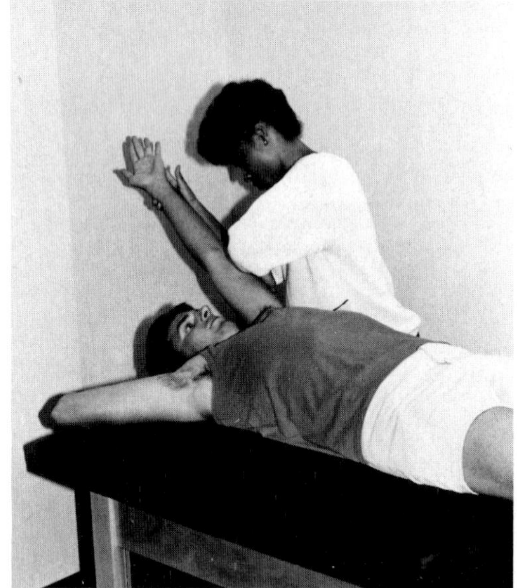

B

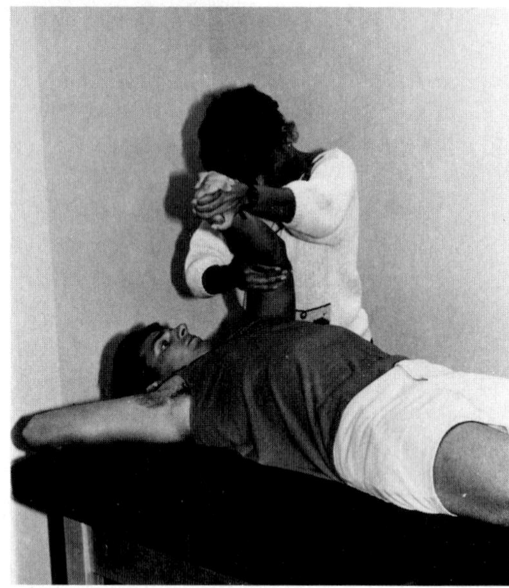

C

FIG. 34-15. Proprioceptive neuromuscular facilitation (PNF) techniques performed with the throwing arm. **B,** PNF allows work in rotational and diagonal positions to be performed. **C,** Isometric co-contractions performed in supine position against manual resistance.

Focus is given to proper total body warm-up and stretching, proper throwing mechanics, and progression through graduated throwing distances.[18] The throwing program varies with each individual according to his or her needs without a set timetable in terms of progression at each level or time of completion. The "crow-hop" (hop, skip, and throw) method is recommended for proper throwing mechanics to discourage flat-footed tossing from the beginning. Along with the proper body mechanics to decrease stress on the throwing arm, each level of throwing should be achieved without pain or complication before the next level is initiated. This decreases the incidence of reinjury and facilitates the rehabilitative process. The objective of each phase is for the athlete to throw 50 balls pain-free at the specific distance, with a goal of throwing at a distance of 180 feet 50 times without pain and then progressing to unrestricted throwing (Fig. 34-16).

Any one of several isokinetic units available (i.e. Biodex, Cybex, Kin Com, Lido) may be used to assess strength and endurance at high speeds, once the patient is back to a desirable level of throwing (Fig. 34-17). The units may also be used as a high-speed conditioning tool in utilizing diagonal patterns three times weekly to augment the lightweight exercise

45' Phase

Step 1: A) Warm-up throwing
B) 45' (25 throws)
C) Rest 15 minutes
D) Warm-up throwing
E) 45' (25 throws)

Step 2: A) Warm-up throwing
B) 45' (25 throws)
C) Rest 10 minutes
D) Warm-up throwing
E) 45' (25 throws)
F) Rest 10 minutes
G) Warm-up throwing
H) 45' (25 throws)

60' Phase

Step 3: A) Warm-up throwing
B) 60' (25 throws)
C) Rest 15 minutes
D) Warm-up throwing
E) 60' (25 throws)

Step 4: A) Warm-up throwing
B) 60' (25 throws)
C) Rest 10 minutes
D) Warm-up throwing
E) 60' (25 throws)
F) Rest 10 minutes
G) Warm-up throwing
H) 60' (25 throws)

90' Phase

Step 5: A) Warm-up throwing
B) 90' (25 throws)
C) Rest 15 minutes
D) Warm-up throwing
E) 90' (25 throws)

Step 6: A) Warm-up throwing
B) 90' (25 throws)
C) Rest 10 minutes
D) Warm-up throwing
E) 90' (25 throws)
F) Rest 10 minutes
G) Warm-up throwing
H) 90' (25 throws)

120' Phase

Step 7: A) Warm-up throwing
B) 120' (25 throws)
C) Rest 15 minutes
D) Warm-up throwing
E) 120' (25 throws)

Step 8: A) Warm-up throwing
B) 120' (25 throws)
C) Rest 10 minutes
D) Warm-up throwing
E) 120' (25 throws)
F) Rest 10 minutes
G) Warm-up throwing
H) 120' (25 throws)

150' Phase

Step 9: A) Warm-up throwing
B) 150' (25 throws)
C) Rest 15 minutes
D) Warm-up throwing
E) 150' (25 throws)

Step 10: A) Warm-up throwing
B) 150' (25 throws)
C) Rest 10 minutes
D) Warm-up throwing
E) 150' (25 throws)
F) Rest 10 minutes
G) Warm-up throwing
H) 150' (25 throws)

180' Phase

Step 11: A) Warm-up throwing
B) 180' (25 throws)
C) Rest 15 minutes
D) Warm-up throwing
E) 180' (25 throws)

Step 12: A) Warm-up throwing
B) 180' (25 throws)
C) Rest 10 minutes
D) Warm-up throwing
E) 180' (25 throws)
F) Rest 10 minutes
G) Warm-up throwing
H) 180' (25 throws)

Step 13: A) Warm-up throwing
B) 180' (25 throws)
C) Rest 10 minutes
D) Warm-up throwing
E) 180' (25 throws)
F) Rest 10 minutes
G) Warm-up throwing
H) 180' (50 throws)

Step 14: unrestricted throwing activities/throwing velocity now can be increased to game competition levels.

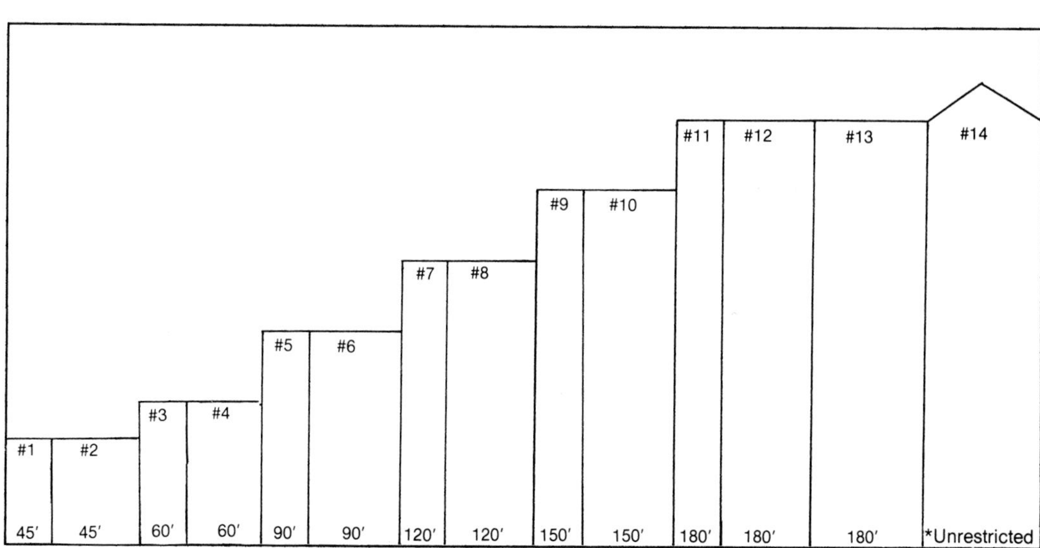

FIG. 34-16. Interval throwing program.

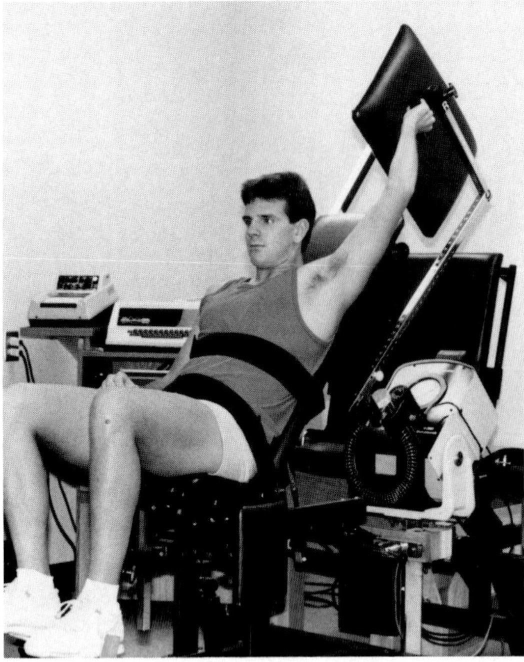

FIG. 34-17. Isokinetics may be utilized at spectrum speeds for increased neuromuscular training.

program. Remembering that this isokinetic mode of the Cybex concentric, the eccentric work done by the posterior rotator cuff should be supplemented with proper teaching with weights, rubber tubing, or an eccentric exercise device.

Maintenance of dynamic muscle balance and flexibility is paramount to meet the unique demands of the throwing shoulder. Specific individual deficits must be addressed to achieve optimal rehabilitation. Understanding the mechanism of throwing and what muscles perform during this complex act allows the sports medicine practitioner not only to treat throwing injuries, but also to prevent them.

REFERENCES

1. Andrews JR and Carson WG: Arthroscopy of the shoulder: technique and normal anatomy, Am J Sports Med 12:1, 1984.
2. Andrews JR and Carson WG: Glenoid labrum tears related to the long head of the biceps, Am J Sports Med 13:337, 1985.
3. Andrews JR and McLeod WD: Mechanisms of shoulder injuries, Phys Ther 66:1906, 1966.
4. Axe MJ: Comparison of baseball and football throwing. Injuries to the Throwing Arm Conference, Phoenix, 1985.
5. Blackburn TA, McLeod WD, and White B: EMG study of rehabilitation of the rotator cuff. AAOS meeting, Nashville, 1987.
6. Codman EA: The shoulder, Boston, 1934, Thomas Todd Co, p 42.
7. Coleman AE, Axe MJ, and Andrews JR: Performance profile–directed simulated game: an objective functional evaluation for baseball pitchers, J Orthop Sports Phys Ther 9:101, 1987.
8. Fauls D: Warm-up and cool-down stretching techniques. In Zarins B, Andrews JR, and Carson WG, editors: Injuries to the throwing arm, Philadelphia, 1985, WB Saunders Co, p 266.
9. Gaines BJ et al: The throw: biomechanics in acute injury, Am J Sports Med 8:2, 1980.
10. Jobe FW and Moynes DR: Delineation of diagnostic criteria in a rehabilitation program for rotator cuff injuries, Am J Sports Med 10:336, 1982.
11. Jobe FW et al: EMG analysis of the shoulder in throwing and pitching: a preliminary report, Am J Sports Med 11:3, 1983.
12. Jobe FW et al: EMG analysis of the shoulder in pitching: a second report, Am J Sports Med 12:218, 1984.
13. Jobe FW et al: Electromyography and motion analysis of the upper extremity in sports, Phys Ther 66:1905, 1986.
14. King JW, Bielsford HJ, and Tullos HS: Analysis of the pitching arm of the professional baseball pitcher, Clin Orthop 67:116, 1969.
15. Knott M and Voss DE: Proprioceptive neuromuscular facilitation: patterns and techniques, New York, 1956, Harper & Row Publishers, Inc.
16. Lehmkuhl LD and Smith LK: Brunnstrom's clinical kinesiology, Philadelphia, 1988, FA Davis Co, p 219.
17. McLeod WD: The pitching mechanism. In Zarins B, Andrews JR, and Carson WG, editors: Injuries to the throwing arm, Philadelphia, 1985, WB Saunders Co, p 266.
18. Medich G: The interval throwing program, Sports Med Update 2:1, 1987.
19. Pappas AM: Biomechanics of baseball pitching, Am J Sports Med 13:216, 1985.
20. Prentice WE and Cooma E: The use of proprioceptive neuromuscular facilitation techniques in the rehabilitation of sports-related injury, Phys Ther 21:26, 1986.
21. Rollins J et al: Water polo injuries to the upper extremity. In Zarins B, Andrews JR, and Carson WG, editors: Injuries to the throwing arm, Philadelphia, 1985, WB Saunders Co, p 30.
22. Rothman RH, Marvel JP, and Heppenstall RB: Anatomic considerations in the glenohumeral joint, Orthop Clin North Am 6:341, 1975.
23. Sain J and Andrews JR: Proper pitching techniques. In Zarins B, Andrews JR, and Carson WG, editors: Injuries to the throwing arm, Philadelphia, 1985, WB Saunders Co, p 30.
24. Taylor K: Shoulder arthroscopy, Sports Med Update, winter 1988.
25. Tullos HS and King JW: Throwing mechanism in sports, Orthop Clin North Am 4:709, 1973.

CHAPTER 35 Evaluation, Treatment, and Prevention of Elbow Injuries in Throwing Athletes

James R. Andrews
Scott P. Schemmel
James A. Whiteside

The elbow in the throwing athlete when uninjured works as a finely tuned articulation to deliver the final momentum to the forearm, hand, and eventually to the object being thrown with great acceleration. In contradistinction, when injured, the elbow in the throwing athlete presents with symptoms of pain, tenderness, swelling, and limitation of motion, all in response to repetitive valgus vector forces and stresses. When impaired, the elbow responds very much like the shoulder in that momentary prolapse and pain during acceleration and at release point prevent the thrower from achieving both normal velocity and control. The biomechanics, however, that produce comparable findings of the shoulder and of the elbow are related but have dissimilarities.

The elbow joint is unique in that it allows for flexion and extension because of the ulnar hinge relationship with the humerus and rotation because of the radiocapitellar and radioulnar articulations. To understand the pathophysiologic etiology of elbow problems in pitchers, quarterbacks, and javelin throwers, one must visualize the mechanics of throwing, something that has been documented in baseball pitchers. Thus the baseball pitcher serves as an excellent clinical model for the study of other throwers.

BIOMECHANICS

A thorough understanding of elbow joint biomechanics is essential for any physician involved in the treatment of the throwing athlete. This knowledge, combined with a comprehensive grasp of elbow anatomy, serves as the cornerstone for the diagnosis and treatment of elbow injuries.

Slocum[45] was one of the first to classify throwing injuries into medial tension and lateral compression phenomena. Numerous articles that followed confirmed and expanded on this concept. Essentially, all pathologic conditions of the elbow resulting from the repetitive act of throwing can be related to the excessive tensile and compressive forces that are generated about this joint. Throughout this chapter, as evaluation, treatment, and prevention of elbow injuries are discussed, the biomechanical concepts presented here should be referred to.

Throwing athletes, regardless of their specific sport, suffer similar injuries to the elbow. The pathophysiology of these injuries has been best described in baseball players generally and pitchers specifically. Analysis of the pitching mechanism allows for the most comprehensive understanding of throwing mechanics. This mechanism consists of several phases: wind-up, cocking, acceleration, deceleration, and follow-through.[27,31,50]

Five phases of pitching

- Wind-up
- Cocking
- Acceleration
- Deceleration
- Follow-through

Wind-Up

The first phase of the pitching mechanism is the wind-up. In this phase the pitcher prepares for delivery of the ball by assuming correct body posture and balance. Initially, both feet are planted. The weight is then shifted back on to the ipsilateral leg with the contralateral leg brought up into a "tucked" position with the hip and knee flexed to about 90 degrees. The hips and shoulders are externally rotated 90 degrees or greater to the intended line of the throw. The elbow is flexed, the forearm pronated, and the wrist extended. During this preparatory phase there is little activity in any of the muscle groups about the elbow or in the forearm[44] (Fig. 35-1, *A*).

Cocking

The wind-up phase is followed by the cocking phase, which as the name implies involves positioning or "cocking" the body, arm, and ball in such a manner to provide the optimum acceleration for ball delivery. The contralateral leg is extended out of its "tucked up" position and planted out in front of the body. This initiates internal rotation of the previ-

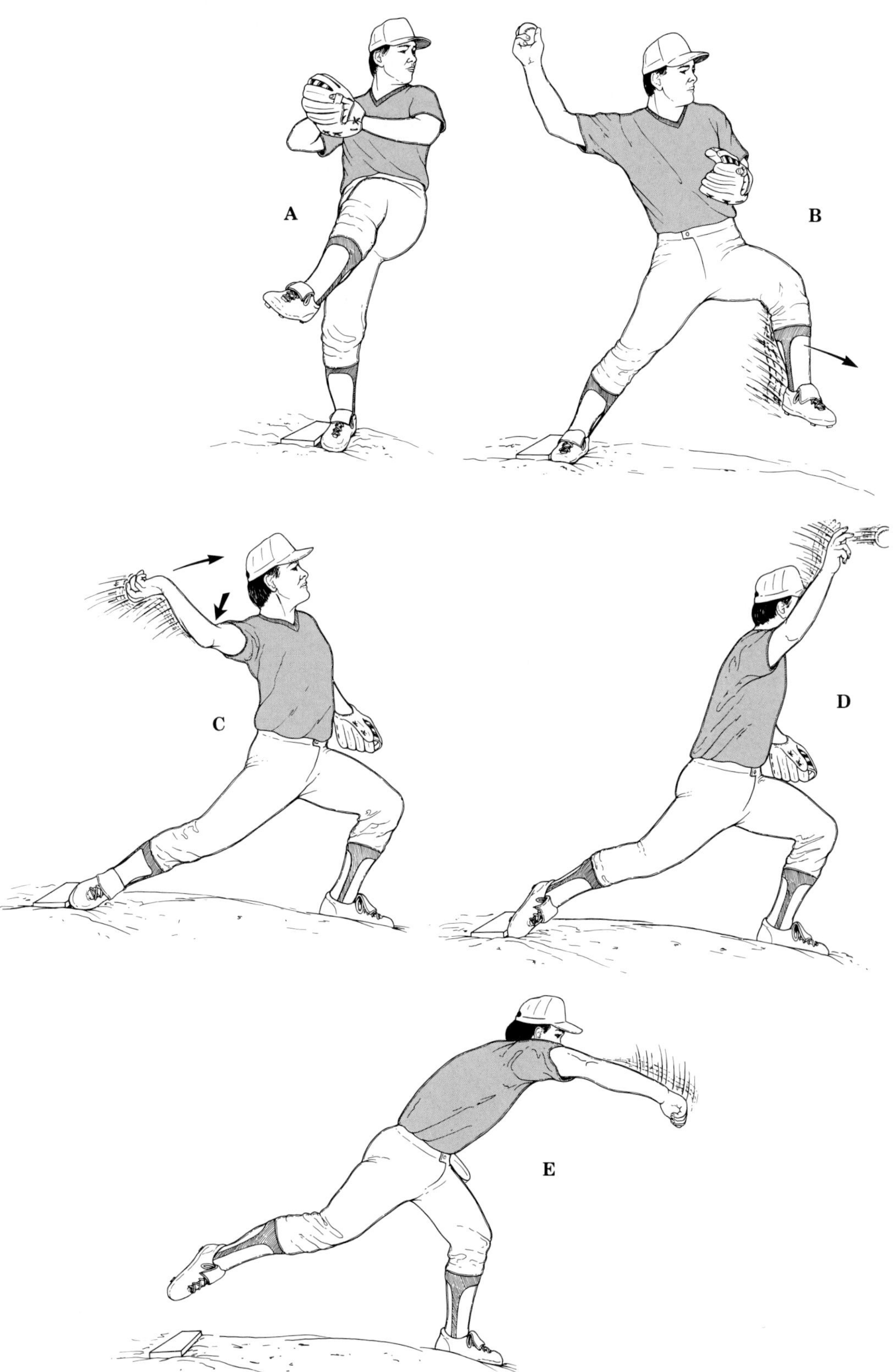

FIG. 35-1. Five phases of pitching. **A,** Wind-up. **B,** Cocking phase. **C,** Acceleration phase. **D,** Deceleration and ball release. **E,** Follow-through.

ously externally rotated pelvis and is followed by internal rotation of the shoulder and a forward thrusting of the chest. The humerus is brought up into a 90-degree abducted position and is maximally externally rotated. The elbow is flexed approximately 90 degrees, and the wrist and metacarpophalangeal joints are extended.[44] The forearm is slightly pronated initially and is fully pronated by the end of this phase for a fast ball, though less so for a curve ball. Electromyographic (EMG) studies and high-speed motion analysis indicate that minor changes in forearm rotation as well as in wrist and finger position are the primary determinants of the spin placed on the ball during the delivery of the pitch.[44] This concept was recognized by astute pitching coaches long before technical analysis was possible.[39] These minor changes are in contrast to the highly improbable proposed active pronation or supination of the forearm during the high-speed event of ball acceleration and release.[1,38] By assuming the cocking posture, the hand and ball are positioned far behind the arm and body. This allows for extrinsic tension to be applied to those muscle groups that will be used subsequently to accelerate the ball in the next phase. In the terminal stage of cocking, the shoulder and chest smoothly move forward, with the hand and ball left behind, thus maximally increasing the extrinsic muscle tension already developed.

The muscle activity about the elbow during the cocking phase is moderately intense.[44] Principal muscles involved in assuming the position include the wrist extensors, the metacarpophalangeal joint extensors, and the brachioradialis and pronator teres. A curve ball requires less activity in the brachioradialis and pronator teres than does a fast ball; however, a curve ball requires more supinator and wrist extensor activity than does a fast ball.[44] Interpretation of these variances for the different pitches is being evaluated on an ongoing basis.[6] Decreased EMG activity in the brachioradialis does not necessarily indicate less elbow flexion for a curve ball. It simply reflects less flexion force with no dependence on elbow angle. The fine technical differences in muscle use and joint positioning with the delivery of various pitches and throwing techniques will be fully delineated only after further integration of EMG studies and high-speed motion analysis (Fig. 35-1, *B*).

Muscle activity and pitch selection

- Curve ball: more supinator/wrist extensor activity
- Fast ball: more brachioradialis/pronator teres activity

Acceleration

The acceleration phase is that component of the pitching mechanism that occurs between the cocking phase and ball release. Acceleration refers specifically to the forces that are imparted to the ball and not the various arm segments during the phase. The trunk and, at times, the humerus go through deceleration phases during acceleration of the ball. Over the course of approximately 50 to 80 msec, the ball is accelerated from a stationary position to a speed in excess of 80 miles per hour.[31] This first involves the transfer of momentum generated within the body of the pitcher as he moves forward through this phase. This momentum is transferred in a "whip-like" fashion sequentially from the trunk to the shoulder, the humerus, the elbow, and the forearm. Finally, the momentum is imparted to the hand and ball as the release point is approached.

The forward motion at the chest and shoulder that was present at the termination of the cocking phase is stopped, and the pitcher moves his trunk forward as he transfers his weight onto the forward-planted contralateral foot and leg. This allows for an orderly transfer of the anterior momentum from the legs to the trunk and into the shoulder. At the same time, during the first half of this acceleration phase, the anterior muscles, primarily the pectoralis and subscapularis, contract to accelerate the humerus anteriorly along a horizontal plane. Also the shoulder internal rotators, subscapularis, latissimus dorsi, and teres major contract to start the internal rotation of the humerus. Thus at this point in the acceleration phase tremendous forward forces are generated in the humerus. The forearm, hand, and ball, however, are essentially "left behind." This results in the elbow being placed in a position of extreme valgus, generating significant tensile forces across the medial side of the elbow joint and compressive loads at the lateral side of the joint.

At the halfway point of this phase, the rate of adduction of the humerus is decreased by imposition of a deceleration from the teres minor, infraspinatus, and supraspinatus muscles. As the humerus decelerates, it allows for a transfer of momentum to the forearm, thus adding to the rate of internal rotation and further accelerating the ball. As the forearm and wrist accelerate, the centrifugal force generated begins to impose an extension force across the elbow joint. If left unprotected at this point, the elbow would rapidly and forcibly hyperextend. However, the rate of extension is regulated by the active participation of the elbow flexors, particularly the biceps and the brachialis muscles. At this point in the acceleration phase, a large degree of torque is present at the elbow joint and is coupled with a high rate of extension, both of which combine to cause relatively high shear forces to be imposed on the articular cartilage. It is these shear stresses that can initiate articular surface degeneration in the joint.

As the release point is approached, the forearm, hand, and ball are accelerated to their maximum velocity, which occurs at the end of the acceleration phase. The grip on the ball is loosened, and over the next 6 to 10 msec the ball leaves the hand.[31] Because of the high rate of forearm internal rotation and elbow extension, the hand will rotate down off the ball, and, through proper positioning of the fingers, the pitcher can impart the desired spin. This is called the "release point," and from this moment on the relative arm motion must be decelerated (Fig. 35-1, *C*).

Deceleration

The momentum developed throughout the acceleration phase results in an outward force on the arm of approximately 300 pounds as the deceleration phase is entered.[31] This 300-pound force must be opposed through active muscle contraction to maintain some appositional stability of the glenohumeral joint and to oppose the forward motion of the shoulder. In addition to the distracting force on the glenohumeral joint, the internal rotation forces in the humerus generated through the acceleration phase must be opposed. The external rotators of the shoulder, as well as the posterior deltoid, contract to stop the arm. The deceleration forces are significantly large and act over a very short duration of time, making them very difficult to measure, but in general, the deceleration torques generated about the shoulder are greater than those of the acceleration phase.[31]

In summary, the forces that must be counteracted through deceleration include humeral internal rotation, glenohumeral distraction, and elbow extension. Essentially all the shoulder muscles contract violently at this point; in addition, large muscle groups, particularly the biceps, brachialis, and brachioradialis, contract in an attempt to slow elbow extension velocity. If the elbow extension velocity is not decelerated entirely, hyperextension injuries common to the elbow can occur. Additionally, if the elbow extension is decelerated too rapidly, the extremely high flexion forces required can overstress the long head of the biceps muscle and its tendon (Fig. 35-1, *D*).

Follow-Through

Finally, in the follow-through phase of throwing, the body moves forward with the arm, reducing the distraction forces applied to the shoulder and relieving the tension generated in the rotator cuff muscles. As the shoulder, trunk, and ipsilateral leg move forward in the follow-through, the pitcher is able to maintain his balance and position himself for his next action or reaction.

Although the pitching mechanism has been observed and analyzed by many authors over the last 25 years, only recently has the specific muscle activity occurring about the elbow during the various phases of pitching been identified.[44] Recent EMG analysis, combined with high-speed photography carried out by Jobe et al,[44] has increased our understanding of the muscle forces generated about the elbow during the throwing act. Measurable muscle activities about the elbow have been shown to be only mild to moderate throughout all phases of pitching.[44] It appears that the muscles act to position the elbow and forearm into a posture that will allow maximum transfer of the energy and momentum developed by the large muscles of the shoulder girdle and trunk. Rapid, forceful contraction of the muscles about the joint as a means of enhancing ball delivery does not seem to occur. In addition, forceful contractions of muscles about the joint as a means of altering ball delivery (i.e., as with a curve ball) does not seem to occur. Rather, ball grip, combined with minor changes in muscle activity levels that allow for an alteration in elbow and wrist positioning before ball release, appears to be all that is necessary to generate the desired changes in ball delivery that are seen with different types of pitches.

Pitch selection mechanics

- Ball grip affects pitch type
- Forceful muscle contraction to alter joint movement *does not* occur

It has been often theorized that forceful firing of the flexor-pronator mass to promote rapid forearm pronation and wrist flexion contributes to medial elbow morbidity.[1] This has been associated particularly with little league elbow as well as pathologic changes in pitchers who compete at higher levels. However, recent EMG studies (discussed previously), combined with our knowledge of forces generated across the throwing elbow biomechanically, leads us to believe that medial elbow morbidity is less likely to be caused by forceful, active contraction of the flexor-pronator muscle group mass and more likely to be secondary to significant passive distraction generated across the elbow during the acceleration phase of throwing.

Although there are minimal differences in muscle activity about the elbow in the delivery of a curve ball versus a fast ball, they result in differences in angular forces at the elbow. It does appear that torque generation in the elbow varies with different types of pitches. In terms of valgus forces placed on the elbow, the fast ball develops greater torque in the elbow than either the slider or the curve ball.[31] The fast ball results in a rate of elbow exension that is relatively smooth and well controlled throughout its full range of motion. However, in delivery of the curve ball or slider, the rate of elbow extension exceeds that of the fast ball, generating greater shear forces on the elbow joint surfaces. These shear forces are most pronounced with the curve ball, less pronounced with the slider, and even less pronounced with the fast ball.[31] With this in mind, it may be that the curve ball places greater stresses across the elbow without active contribution of those shear forces from the arm and forearm musculature (Fig. 35-1, *E*).

Elbow shear forces

Curveball >Slider > Fastball

FUNCTIONAL ANATOMY

The anatomy of the elbow should be studied in respect to the stability it offers in resistance to large valgus and extension forces generated by the act of throwing. The ulnar collateral ligament has been shown to be the primary stabilizer of the elbow.[32,41,48] Secondary stabilizers are both bony and soft tissue structures.[32] Bony contributions include the articulations of the olecranon, olecranon fossa complex, and the radial head and capitellum. The secondary soft tissue stabilizer is primarily the forearm flexor-pronator muscle mass arising from the medial epicondyle of the humerus. Rather than simply noting where these structures exist relative to one another, it is important to understand how they function to stabilize the joint against the previously noted forces.

Elbow stability

Primary

- Ulnar collateral ligament

Secondary

- Bony articulations: olecranon, olecranon fossa complex, radial head, and capitellum
- Soft tissue: flexor-pronator muscle group

Osseous Structures

Humeroulnar Articulation

The humeroulnar joint provides for elbow flexion and extension. The humeral contribution consists of the trochlea, the coronoid fossa anteriorly, and the olecranon fossa posteriorly. The trochlea is covered by hyaline cartilage over a 330-degree arch, and it projects anteriorly from the shaft of the humerus at an angle of approximately 30 degrees. In the AP plane, the trochlea has a 6-degree valgus slope, which, along with the proximal ulna, determines the carrying angle at the elbow. A 3- to 5-degree internal rotation of the trochlea in respect to the epicondylar line has been described.[33] It appears to result in a 5-degree external rotation of the ulna in terminal extension and a 5-degree internal rotation in initiating flexion from full extension. The ulna's contribution to this joint consists of the following: (1) the trochlear notch for articulation with the trochlea, (2) the olecranon process for articulation with the olecranon fossa, and (3) the coronoid process for articulation with its corresponding fossa in the humerus. The trochlear notch has a 30-degree posterior inclination that corresponds with the 30-degree anterior rotation of the distal humerus. This configuration allows for up to 150 degrees of flexion through the humeroulnar articulation.

In the throwing athlete, it is not the hyaline cartilage–covered trochlea or the trochlear notch that serves as the primary site of bony pathologic change. Unlike the articular surfaces of the radius and the capitellum, the articular surfaces of the trochlea and trochlear notch rarely serve as the source of condylar defects, chondromalacia, or articular loose bodies. Rather, it is the olecranon process, the corresponding olecranon fossa, and, to a lesser extent, the coronoid fossa that are affected.[2,52] These frequently mentioned valgus stresses are stabilized in a secondary manner by the olecranon within the olecranon fossa over the last 30 degrees of extension. These valgus stresses result in the abutment of the medial aspect of the olecranon process against the medial olecranon fossa. Hyperextension forces cause straight posterior and posterolateral abutment of the olecranon in the olecranon fossa, leading to subsequent osteophyte formation in these areas. These changes are discussed further under posterior injuries. Anteriorly, abutment of the coronoid process within the coronoid fossa can result in osteophyte formation on the coronoid process or within the fossa itself (Fig. 35-2).

Radiocapitellar Articulation

Unlike the trochlear ulnar articulation, the radiocapitellar joint is essentially unconstrained. The capitellum is hemispheric and covered by hyaline cartilage. The radial head, with its hyaline cartilage surface, is concave and articulates with the capitellum. It is free to rotate about the capitellum in pronation and supination. Rotation can be completed through an arch of 160 to 170 degrees. As with the trochlear ulnar joint, radiocapitellar joint pathologic change is determined by the force patterns developed in the throwing elbow. The radiocapitellar joint is a site of compression loads and serves as a secondary stabilizer to these valgus forces.[32,41] Articular cartilage changes, including dramatic chondral defects, can be found in both the radial head articular cartilage and in that of the capitellum.

Proximal Radioulnar Articulation

The proximal radioulnar articulation consists of the radial head, the annular ligament, and the radial notch of the ulna. Contact of this articulation covers only one fifth of the radial head at any one time, with the annular ligament providing the remainder of coverage and support to this joint. The radioulnar joint is a very infrequent source of bony pathologic change in the throwing elbow.

Ligamentous Structures

The ligamentous anatomy about the elbow reflects the dominant forces that occur at this joint, not only in the act of throwing but also in its everyday use at work and at home. For most activities, primary stresses placed across the elbow are in a valgus direction with varus stresses to the elbow being infrequent.[33]

Radial (Lateral) Collateral Ligament

These types of stresses are reflected in the phylogenetic development of the radial collateral ligament, which varies in size and course from individual to individual (Fig. 35-3).

The radial collateral ligament originates from the lateral epicondyle and inserts pri-

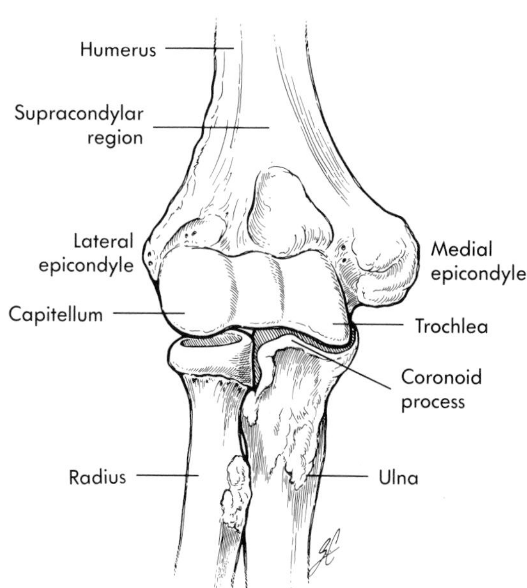

FIG. 35-2. Frontal view of elbow, showing the large coronoid fossa, smaller radial fossa, and trochlea medial to the capitellum.

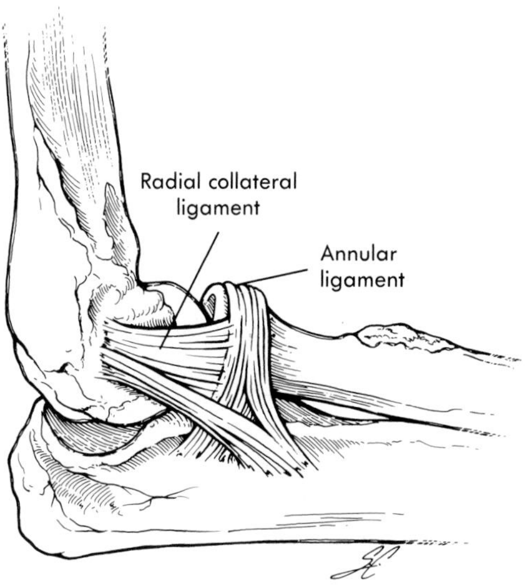

FIG. 35-3. Radial collateral ligament is often less well defined surgically than anatomically.

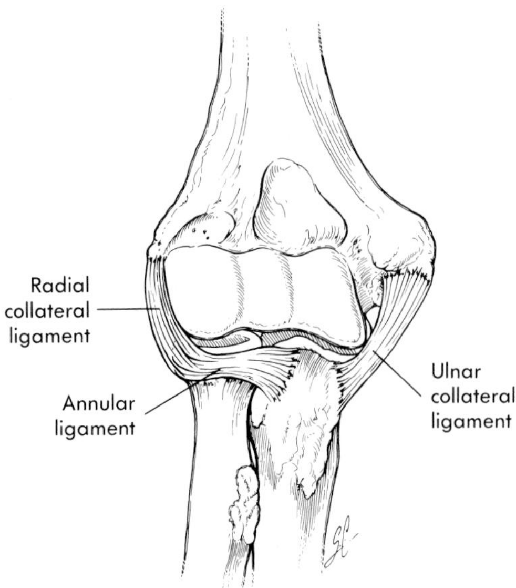

FIG. 35-4. Frontal view reveals distal attachment of the ulnar collateral ligament to the medial margin of the coronoid process and a portion of the radial collateral ligament/annular ligament complex attachment to the lateral margin of the ulna.

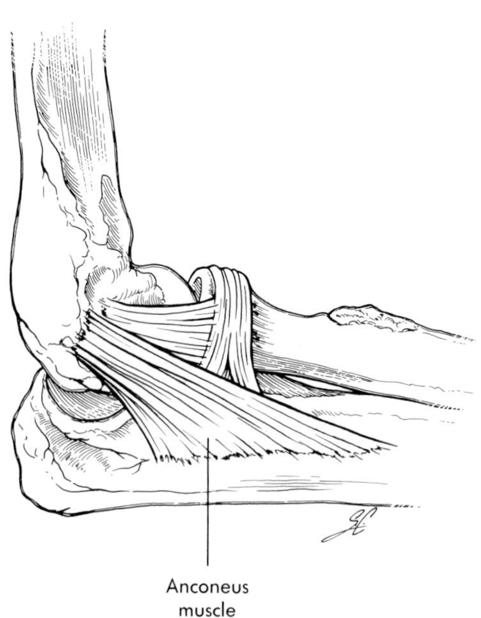

FIG. 35-5. Anconeus muscle acts as a secondary support structure to the radial collateral ligament.

marily into the annular ligament around the radius, where a few nonfunctional fibers also attach to the radial notch of the ulna (Fig. 35-4). This ligament does not perform the function of a true ligament with bone-to-bone attachments. However, the anconeus muscle, with its origin just posterior to that of the radial collateral ligament on the lateral epicondyle of the humerus, inserts onto the radial border of the ulna and assumes the function of a dynamic collateral ligament attaching bone-to-bone. Thus the anconeus appears to aid in elbow stabilization against a varus stress[48] (Fig. 35-5).

Radial collateral ligament

- Origin: lateral epicondyle
- Insertion: annular ligament; radial notch of ulna
- Supplements: anconeus muscle
- Function: weak stabilizer against varus stress

Ulnar (Medial) Collateral Ligament

In contrast, the ulnar (medial) collateral ligament is a well defined and consistent structure that would be more aptly considered as a ligamentous complex. The ulnar collateral ligament consists of an anterior oblique component that originates from the undersurface of the medial epicondyle of the humerus and inserts into the ulna just posterior to the coronoid process. The posterior oblique component arises from the same point and passes posterior and distal and inserts into the ulnar surface of the mid-olecranon. A less well developed transverse ligament courses from the insertion of the posterior oblique to the insertion of the anterior oblique bundle and deepens the trochlear notch of the ulna.

Ulnar collateral ligament components

- Anterior oblique
- Posterior oblique
- Transverse

The anterior oblique ligament is taut in both flexion and extension. It does not lie on the axis of elbow flexion, but, because of its rectangular shape, its anterior fibers are taut in extension while its posterior fibers become taut in flexion.[41] Thus, as a whole, the anterior oblique component is taut throughout the full range of motion. Conversely, the posterior oblique segment of this ligament is taut only in flexion and is slack in extension. Sectioning of the posterior oblique ligament does not alter the stability of the elbow to valgus stress if

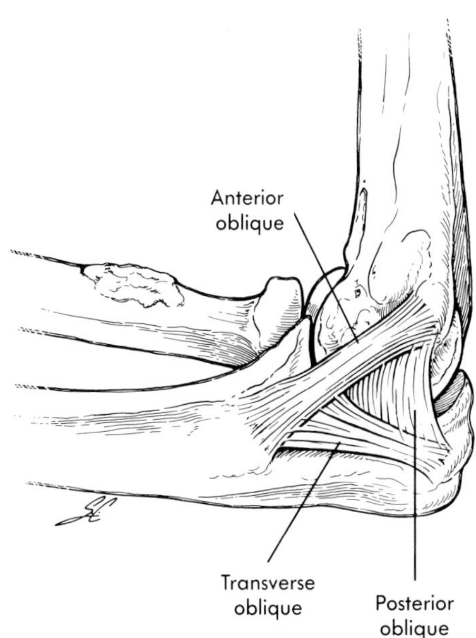

FIG. 35-6. Normal anatomic alignment of the three components of the ulnar collateral ligament.

the anterior oblique ligament is intact. Furthermore, sectioning of the anterior oblique ligament results in elbow instability even when the posterior oblique component is intact.[41] The transverse oblique ligament represents essentially a thickening of the joint capsule and plays no real role in joint stability (Fig. 35-6).

The ulnar collateral ligament is the cornerstone of the throwing elbow, and its importance and that of the anterior oblique fibers in the stabilization of this joint against the forces incurred in throwing cannot be overemphasized. The incompetence of this structure, acute or chronic, is the initiator for much of the morbidity associated with the throwing elbow.

Musculotendinous Structures

The remaining structures about the elbow—the musculotendinous insertions and origins and the major nerves and vessels—will not be exhaustively covered here because they are well known to the surgeon. Some of this anatomy is reviewed elsewhere in this chapter during presentation of nerve entrapment syndromes about the elbow. There are, however, some pertinent anatomic entities that deserve discussion.

Flexors

The flexors of the elbow joint—the brachialis, biceps, brachioradialis—are not commonly involved in the generation of symptoms at the elbow. Their role in elbow deceleration is essential in the throwing act, and it is through this mechanism that they are subject to repetitive forces that may result in symptoms. The most common musculotendinous unit about the elbow involved in throwing pathologic change is that of the superficial flexor-pronator group. This muscle group, which takes its tendinous origin from the medial epicondyle, consists of the flexor carpi radialis, flexor digititorum sublimis, pronator teres, palmaris longus, and flexor carpi ulnaris muscles. This common flexor-pronator muscle mass serves as a dynamic secondary stabilizer of the elbow against valgus forces. As such, the forces that produce pathologic changes within this structure are primarily tensile ones.[13,24]

Extensors

On the lateral side of the elbow the brachioradialis, extensor carpi radialis longus and brevis, and a portion of the common extensor tendons originate from the distal humerus. As noted earlier, the brachioradialis serves as a flexor of the elbow, and, in the throwing athlete, its importance lies in its deceleration of elbow extension that occurs during the throwing act. The extensor carpi radialis longus and brevis are important because they relate to the lateral epicondylitis phenomenon that occurs in many athletes.[13,24,34]

Growth and Ossification Centers

In Little League and adolescent elbows, the yet unfused secondary center of ossification of the medial epicondyle is subject to the same valgus forces as in the mature athlete; as a result, separation or fragmentation of this growth center can occur.[1,12] It is not within the scope of this chapter to fully review the development of the secondary centers of ossification about the elbow.[21] Briefly, however, it is important to note that the capitellum, trochlear, and lateral epicondylar growth centers unite into one common growth center before their union with the distal humerus. The capitellar growth center first appears at approximately 1 year of age; the trochlear and lateral epicondylar growth centers appear around age 10. These three centers fuse together at approximately 13 years in the female and 15 years in the male and subsequently unite to the distal humerus at approximately 16 years of age in both sexes. The trochlear growth cartilage rises from two separate secondary ossification centers, which should not be mistaken for fragmentation of this growth cartilage during this time. The medial epicondylar growth center's appearance and time of ultimate union with the humerus is the most variable. It usually appears between the ages of 7 and 8 in the female and 8 and 9 in the male. It is the last of the growth centers to fuse to the distal humerus, doing so at approximately age 14 in the female and 18 in the male. In comparison with the other growth centers about the distal humerus, it is more strongly subjected to repetitive tensile loads accompanying the throwing act than are the other growth centers. As such, it is the growth center that is most predisposed to injury in throwing sports.[1,38] Finally, the radial head growth center appears in the female and male at approximately ages 6 and 7 and fusion occurs at ages 14 and 16, respectively.

Neuroanatomy

Although tardy ulnar nerve palsy and ulnar neuritis as related to the throwing elbow are discussed under nerve lesions, a detailed understanding of the course of the nerve and its anatomic relationships at the elbow is imperative.[21] In the arm, the ulnar nerve pierces the medial intermuscular septum, passes from the anterior to the posterior compartment of the arm, and lies on the front of the medial head of the triceps muscle. The superior ulnar collateral artery passes with the ulnar nerve behind the medial epicondyle. The nerve enters the forearm after passing posterior to the epicondyle and dives between the two heads of origin of the flexor carpi ulnaris muscle that arise from the ulna and humerus. The lateral bed of the ulnar nerve as it passes behind the medial epicondyle directly overlies the medial aspect of the olecranon and the olecranon tip. It is important to realize this close approximation in differentiating the various causes of ulnar neuritis in the throwing elbow. In addition to these classic causes of ulnar nerve pathologic change in the elbow (which are well described in many textbooks), it is important to understand that pathologic changes that take place on the medial border of the olecranon, as well as its tip, can have a direct effect on the ulnar nerve.

PHYSICAL EXAMINATION

The ancient medical dictum that obtaining a factual chronicle of events surrounding an injury is essential to a successful diagnosis holds great truth in the care of the throwing athlete with elbow problems. It is not sufficient just to know the general area of involvement and that pitching aggravates the problem. Rather, the history must produce specifically *what* the problem is—pain and its characteristics and/or restriction of motion and disability. Then, as clearly as can be noted, the history must produce *where* the primary location of this symptom complex is, *when* it was first observed, and *when* it became a limiting factor. The mechanisms that precipitated the problem need to be determined. *How* did it happen? Was the onset acute or insidious, in only one phase of throwing, or after changing playing position, training, or technique? In addition to basic information of age, length of time in sport, and level of sports participation, the projected timetable of the athlete should be documented (e.g., red-shirted this season, need to report for winter league, and so on) in order to fashion a treatment regimen that is suitable for all concerned within the bounds of judicious, expert care.

Inspection

This initial phase of examination requires exposure of the trunk and arms in a comfortable, unobstructed setting to evaluate the neck, shoulder, and upper arm as subtle sites of pathologic change that can affect the elbow. A measurable exercise-induced muscular hypertrophy is often noted in the triceps, biceps, and extensor and flexor forearm muscles bilaterally as a result of weight training. However, unilateral hypertrophy is usually noted in the sport-dominant arm. In the anatomic, extended position, the pitching arm may appear longer and bigger and may have a carrying angle of 10 to 15 degrees greater than the nondominant arm. Confirmation of variances, if needed, can be made roentgenographically.

Common throwing arm changes

- Unilateral muscle hypertrophy (triceps, biceps, forearm flexors, forearm extensors)
- Increased carrying angle
- Flexion contracture

Visualization

Visualization of the exposed skin about the elbow may contribute to the diagnosis by allowing for the detection of the following: (1) areas of contusion or ecchymoses, (2) redness caused by cellulitis, (3) scarring secondary to healed burns or surgery, (4) blanching from vascular insufficiency, (5) petechiae from platelet deficiencies, (6) eczematoid or psoriatic rashes, and (7) rheumatoid nodules. Further information can be obtained by noting uneven surface contours resulting from bulging as in olecranon bursitis, posterior dislocation, or a depression in the antecubital space as a result of rupture of the bicipital tendon from its insertion on the radius.

Range of Motion

Range of motion about the elbow is measured in flexion/extension and pronation/supination. Ordinarily, except in congenital laxity and Marfan's syndrome, the elbow extends only to 0 degrees and flexes to about 150 degrees, or less if impeded by increased muscle mass. Hyperextension of the elbow, though common in gymnasts, is rare in throwers. Instead, incomplete extension (flexion contracture) tends to occur and often is asymptomatic. This flexion contracture can result from either capsular sprain, flexor muscle mass strain anteriorly, or intraarticular loose bodies; whereas, the inability to completely flex indicates triceps strain, capsular tightness, and loose bodies.

Possible causes of elbow flexion contracture

- Repetitive capsular sprain
- Flexor muscle strain
- Intraarticular loose bodies

Pronation and supination should allow for about 150 degrees of forearm rotation. Failure to do so may reflect radiocapitellar osteochondritis, loose bodies, or motor nerve entrapment with resulting biceps, pronator teres, pronator quadratus, and supinator muscle paresis. As causes of decreased range of motion, consideration should also be given to edema and other swelling as a result of muscle fatigue and increased forearm fascial compartment pressure resulting from overuse.

Palpation

Superficial palpation of the region about the elbow revealing skin temperature and sensation comparable to that of the uninvolved extremity indicates intact neurovascular systems. When contracted, forearm muscles should produce a firm, even tone without localized herniation of a fascial defect or a ganglion. The medial supracondylar area should be palpated for epitrochlear lymphadenopathy, which is indicative of systemic or malignant disease. Brachial artery pulsation should be palpated, and deep tendon reflexes of the biceps, triceps, and brachioradialis muscles should be obtained by percussion.

Deep palpation about the elbow may reveal sites of unreported tenderness resulting from traction osteophyte formation on the medial side of the humeral ulnar joint, or swelling adjacent to the head of the radius caused by increased intracapsular pressure, or in the distal, medial area of the humerus from an anomalous supracondylar process. For completeness, palpation is systematically carried out over the medial, anterior, lateral, and posterior aspects of the elbow in order to determine the specific areas of pain and/or limited motion.

Stability

Integrity of elbow function depends on the ligamentous structures medially, laterally, and anteroposteriorly. Medially, there is a well-developed ulnar collateral ligament (medial collateral ligament) that is divided into three portions: (1) the all-important anterior oblique, (2) the less important posterior oblique, and (3) the functionally unimportant transverse oblique ligament. Because of its unique positioning, the anterior oblique ligament is taut throughout the full range of motion and is the prime stabilizer on the medial side against valgus stress during acceleration and deceleration phases of pitching. The posterior oblique ligament is taut only in flexion and plays a secondary role in medial stability, as does the radiocapitellar joint laterally, which acts as a buttress to guard against extreme valgus deformation.

To test for **medial stability,** the elbow is stressed by placing a valgus pressure on the distal forearm held at 20 to 30 degrees of flexion, a position that allows for disengagement of the olecranon from its fossa. The medial opening is determined and compared to that of the uninvolved side. With the elbow position maintained, the examiner's hands are reversed, and varus stress is applied to the forearm to test for **lateral stability.** After hyperextension and posterior dislocation, medial instability is to be expected, even if it is not apparent, because of disruption of the anterior oblique ligament.

On the lateral aspect of the elbow, some stability is maintained by the radial collateral ligament that arises from the lateral epicondyle and is inserted into the annular ligament about the proximal radius. Significant additional support comes from the extensor muscle mass and the anconeus muscle that inserts on the ulna.

Anterior stability depends very little on the integrity of the trochlear-olecranon complex. Instead, control of anterior displacement relies especially on the ulnar collateral ligament, the anterior capsule, and, to a lesser extent, the radial collateral ligament. There are no ligaments to control posterior displacement. Proper alignment, then, depends on the anterior capsule and the abutment of the radial head and the coronoid process of the ulna against the adjacent humerus.

Further stability is obtained by muscular competency and interaction of the three primary flexors of the elbow (the biceps, the brachialis, and the brachioradialis muscles); the primary extensor (the triceps muscle); the pronators (the pronator teres and pronator quadratus muscles); and the supinator and the biceps muscles. Together with the medial flexor and lateral extensor forearm muscle groups, muscular stability is added to the principal ligamentous support.

Localization of Pain

The elbow is most vulnerable to soft tissue injury by the production of a considerable valgus stress in the phases of cocking, acceleration, and deceleration of the pitching motion. The elbow, when subjected to repeated episodes of traction stress, can cause soft tissue microscopic tearing, fluid and inflammatory cell accumulation, and acute pain. Chronic pain and limitation of motion result from repeated bleeding insults to the stressed area, which attempts to heal by inflammation, followed by fibrous scarring, and later by calcification. Localization of the most painful site requires identification of the underlying anatomy.

Medial

Using the medial epicondyle as a landmark, palpation for tenderness is begun locally and then distally over the flexor-pronator muscle tendinous mass. This area most commonly is subject to fatigue, with microtears caused by excessive valgus tensile forces that scar and result in flexion contractures.

Deep to the flexor muscle mass, the anterior oblique portion of the ulnar collateral ligament is a frequent source of ligamentous sprains caused by chronic stress. Its integrity is determined by performing the valgus stress test of the forearm with the elbow slightly flexed. The posterior oblique ligament lies posterior and inferior to the medial epicondyle and is less commonly involved in medial traction injuries. Medial discomfort can also be elicited by percussion over the ulnar nerve above, in, and below the ulnar groove. The combination of flexor muscle mass strain, ulnar collateral ligament sprain, and ulnar neuritis is frequently encountered, since all three can be produced by the same valgus stress forces.

Other sources of medial pain are as follows: (1) medial epicondylitis caused by injury of the tendinous origin of the flexor-pronator muscle mass; (2) avulsion fractures of the medial epicondylar ossification center, often occurring in young pitchers; (3) ulnar traction spurs arising from the coronoid process of the ulna and the medial epicondyle of the humerus; and (4) osteochondral loose bodies.

Sources of medial elbow pain

- Flexor-pronator tendon origin inflammation
- Anterior oblique portion of ulnar collateral ligament sprain
- Ulnar neuritis
- Avulsion fractures
- Osteochondral loose bodies
- Traction spurs (coronoid process or medial epicondyle)
- Flexor-pronator muscle strain

Lateral

Laterally, the site of pain may be located at the lateral epicondyle, denoting overload tendonitis of the common extensors, but it is predominantly located at the extensor carpi radialis brevis. Although more commonly noted in racquet sports (tennis elbow), lateral epicondylitis does occur after prolonged pitching with fatigue, a condition that allows for excessive forearm pronation and wrist flexion after release in the deceleration motion phase. True extensor musculature strains are infrequent and tend to occur in the poorly conditioned or older batting and throwing athlete.

When valgus stress occurs medially, compression of the radiocapitellar articulation occurs laterally, resulting in osteochondrosis (Panner's disease) in the young athlete and articular fragmentation and bony overgrowth in the capitellum and radial head in the mature athlete. Progression to loose body formation does occur. Therefore careful palpation of the area proximal to the radial head needs to be performed.

Tenderness about the supinator muscle suggests compression entrapment of the posterior interosseous branch of the radial nerve. Increased proximal tenderness can indicate injury to the radial nerve (radial tunnel syndrome). If fullness deep to the anconeus muscle and posterior to the lateral epicondyle is

Sources of lateral elbow pain

- Lateral epicondylitis
- Radiocapitellar impingement/degeneration
- Posterior interosseous nerve entrapment

noted, hemarthrosis of an acute injury or effusion of a chronic irritation is a probability.

Posterior

Valgus stress in throwing produces a shearing force posteriorly in the olecranon fossa that initiates formation of spurs, osteophytes, and loose bodies and later leads to degenerative changes, all of which may be tender to palpation (Figs. 35-7 and 35-8). Extension overload (extensor valgus overload syndrome) in the deceleration and follow-through phases can produce localized pain and tenderness by impingement of the olecranon on the posteromedial aspect of the olecranon fossa. To test for valgus overload–produced pain, the partially flexed forearm is brought into a valgus position and then forcefully extended to abut the olecranon and its medial fossa in order to reproduce symptoms that may be difficult to localize otherwise. Acute, forceful hyperextension of the elbow can result in avulsion fractures of the tip of the olecranon, whereas chronic overuse tends to produce triceps tendonitis, which may lead to contracture. Direct posterior trauma can produce characteristic swelling of olecranon bursitis, which may become very painful when infected. Loose bodies need to be sought in the posterior compartment medially and laterally.

Sources of posterior elbow pain

- Loose bodies
- Degenerative changes of the olecranon and olecranon fossa
- Triceps tendonitis
- Olecranon avulsion
- Olecranon bursitis

Anterior

The location of anterior elbow pain is not limited to the antecubital fossa where bicipital tendon strains and avulsions are encountered. Hypertrophied muscles of the medial forearm wrist flexors, the lateral elbow flexors, and the brachioradialis can become swollen and tender from fatigue after exercising. Muscle hypertrophy and exercise-induced edema can create a syndrome of anteromedial pain secondary to increased pressure within the fascial planes of the forearm. Diffuse anterior elbow tenderness can be attributed to anterior capsulitis, which is seen after an incidental

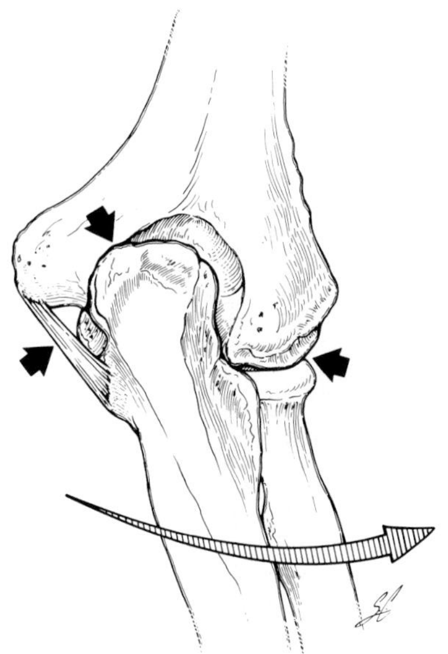

FIG. 35-7. Posterior view of elbow, illustrating the three major sites of trauma in valgus extension overload stress.

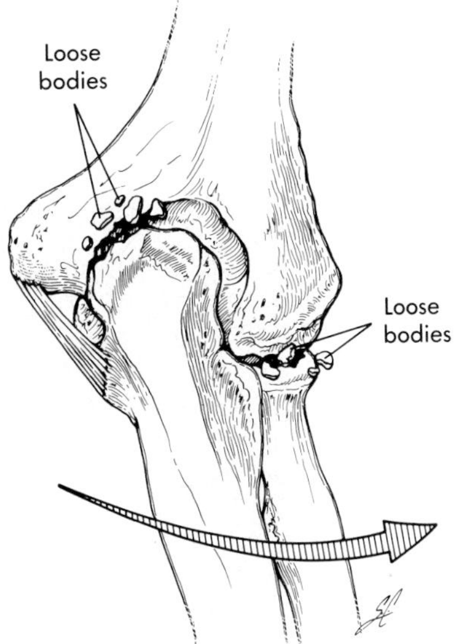

FIG. 35-8. Posterior view of the elbow reveals stretching of the ulnar collateral ligament and osteophyte formation as a result of chronic valgus extension overload stress.

hyperextension injury but usually not with repetitive throwing. Although mostly anteromedial in location, vague postexertional discomfort can be a finding in the pronator teres syndrome as a result of entrapment of the median nerve at the level of the pronator teres. When this occurs, typically, parethesias of the thumb and index finger are also noted.

Sources of anterior elbow pain

- Biceps strain/avulsion
- Flexor-pronator exertional compartment syndrome
- Pronator syndrome
- Anterior capsulitis

ROENTGENOGRAPHIC EVALUATION

Accurate interpretation of roentgenographic studies performed on the throwing elbow requires both a comprehensive knowledge of the broad spectrum of afflictions that are possible at this joint and a thorough physical examination. As a result of extensive overlap in the various clinical entities occurring within the region of the elbow, roentgenographs, stress studies, arthrograms, and CT arthrography often play an important role in determining the working diagnosis and subsequent treatment (see Chapter 14). Roentgenographs alone, without careful correlation with physical findings, can be a source of misinformation rather than an aid to diagnosis.[40]

Standard Views

The initial roentgenographic evaluation of the injured elbow in the throwing athlete should consist of an AP radiograph comprising a 90-degree flexed lateral view and two oblique views. An axial radiograph, which is taken with the elbow flexed to 110 degrees, the arm lying on the cassette, and the beam

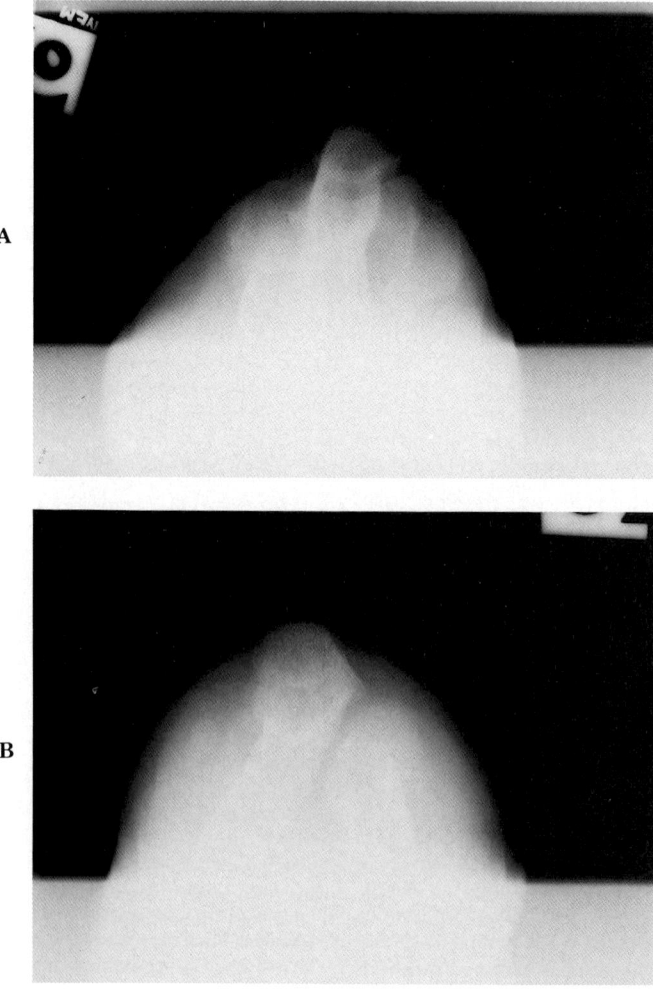

FIG. 35-9. Normal axial views of **(A)** immature and **(B)** mature elbow.

angled 45 degrees to the ulna, should also be obtained (Fig. 35-9). This roentgenogram allows for the best view of the olecranon as it articulates with the trochlea and puts the medial aspect of the olecranon in profile. Of note in most skeletally mature elbows in high-caliber pitchers is the generalized humeral hypertrophy that is present (Fig. 35-10). This was initially described in tennis players by Jones[26] and noted also in baseball players by Jobe.[24] Because this finding represents an adaptive change of exercise, it is not felt to be pathologic or directly responsible for any other pathologic conditions occurring about the elbow.

Medial

Because the medial elbow is subjected to tensile loads during throwing, the bony pathologic changes identified on roentgenograms are directly related to this phenomenon. In the youngster whose growth centers are fully present but not yet fused, the medial epicondyle can show various effects of the applied forces. These changes include fragmentation and accelerated growth of the epicondyle and, on occasion, the frank separation and subsequent displacement of the epicondyle through the growth apophysis.[1,12,30,38] Comparison roentgenograms may be helpful in fully delineating the magnitude of these changes. As the elbow matures, the separation can be more peripheral and not involve the entire epicondyle.[38,54] In the fully mature skeleton, smaller avulsion fragments can also occur directly off the epicondyle.

On routine views, radiopaque densities may be identified in the ulnar collateral ligament. These densities represent calcifications and later ossifications within the tendon substance that occur in advanced stages of the overuse pathology spectrum. Traction spurring may also be seen on the proximal medial ulna at the site of the medial collateral ligament insertion[8,10,16,22,45] (Fig. 35-11). This may be accompanied by a "kissing lesion" from the inferior medial surface of the trochlea (Fig. 35-12).

Anterior

Anteriorly in the elbow, any spurring of the coronoid process should be noted on lateral roentgenograph as should any calcification occurring in the anterior capsule or tendinous insertions of the elbow flexors (Fig. 35-13). These calcifications can occur as the result of tension injuries developing in those structures during elbow deceleration.[22,45]

Lateral

Laterally the compressive and shear forces to which the radius and capitellum are exposed lead to characteristic radiographic findings.[43] These findings primarily consist of os-

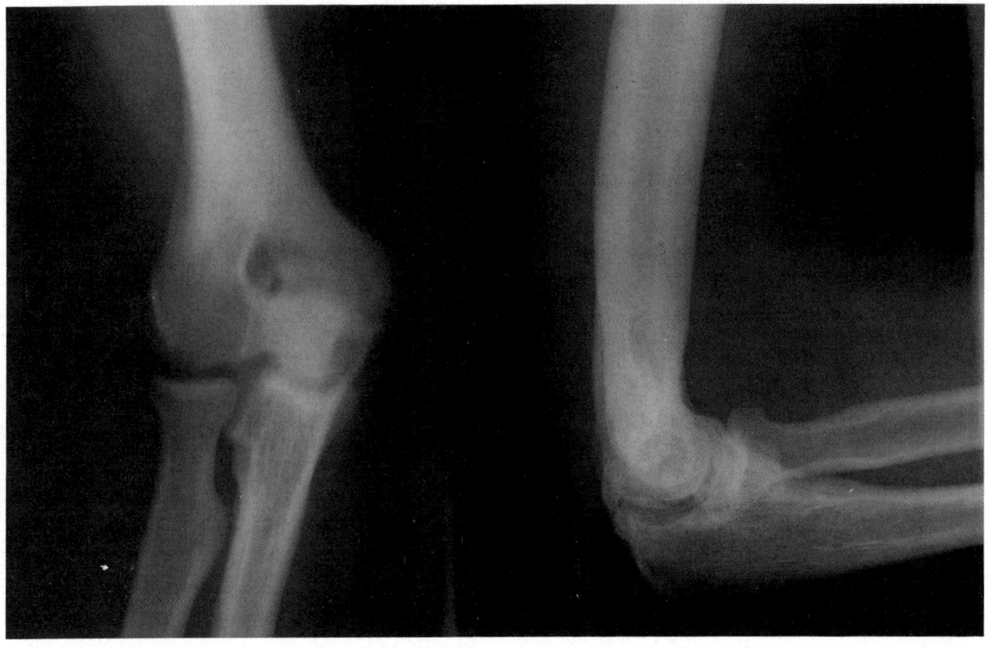

FIG. 35-10. Humeral hypertrophy of the dominant arm is a common finding in throwing athletes. Note also posterior compartment pathologic change.

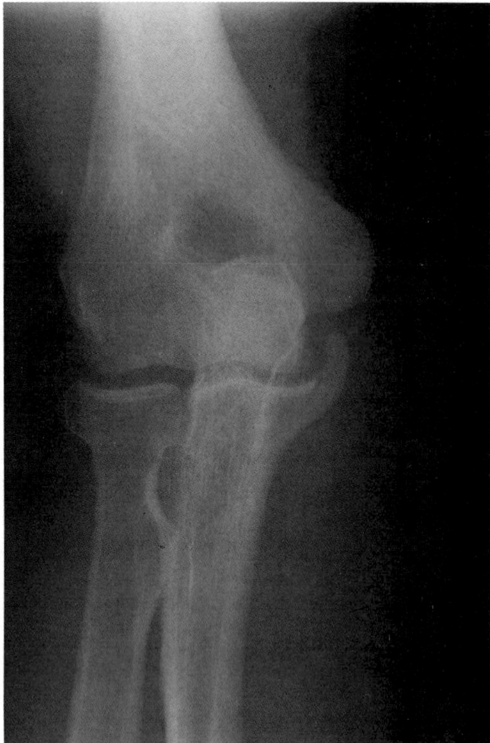

FIG. 35-11. Traction spurring in a professional pitcher of the medial coronoid with calcification of the ligament.

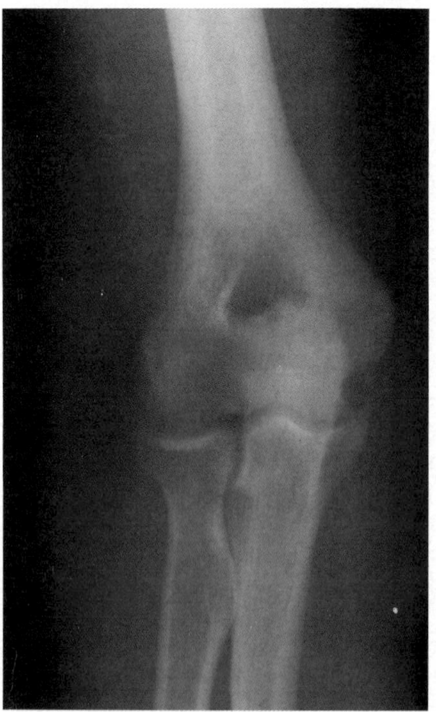

FIG. 35-12. Traction spurring of proximal ulna at site of ulnar collateral ligament insertion with "kissing lesion" of trochlea. Note calcification in the substance of the ligament.

teochondritis dissecans of the capitellum, radial head hypertrophy, and occasionally an osteochondral defect or fracture from the capitellum or radial head[1,2,24,27,38] (Fig. 35-14). Further elaboration on the cause of these changes will be covered later in this chapter. Osteochondral fragmentation of the capitellum and radial head hypertrophy are ominous signs for competitive athletes.[2,8,22,47] In the osteochondritic lesion, a portion of the capitellum will show irregular ossification and rarefaction within a crater. This crater may have a sclerotic rim, and a loose body may be noted. The lateral roentgenograph shows flattening of the capitellum.[53] The lucencies in the capitellum may be seen better on oblique views and arthrotomograms (Fig. 35-15). More recently, CT arthrography has been helpful in identifying these lesions in the capitellum as well as in locating any intraarticular loose bodies.[2]

Posterior

Posteriorly the olecranon and the olecranon fossa are the sites of bony pathologic changes. The compressive loads generated between the medial wall of the fossa and the corresponding medial tip of the olecranon result in degenerative changes and osteophytes.[2,22,27] This so-called valgus extension overload syndrome is a manifestation of combined valgus and compressive forces developing in the throwing elbow.[52] The posterior osteophyte, thus formed,

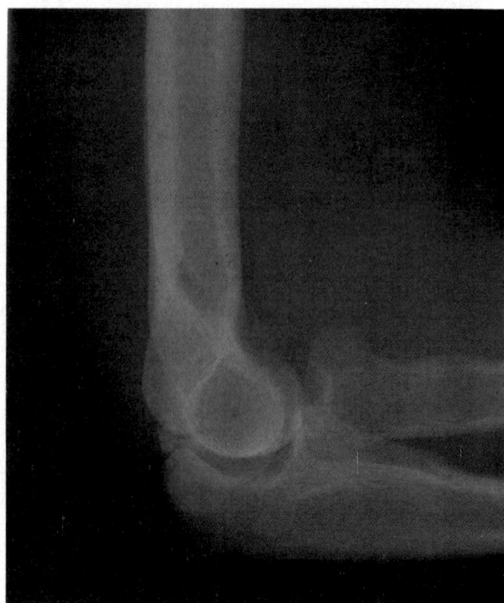

FIG. 35-13. Calcification in the anterior capsule of a baseball pitcher. Note the posterior compartment loose body.

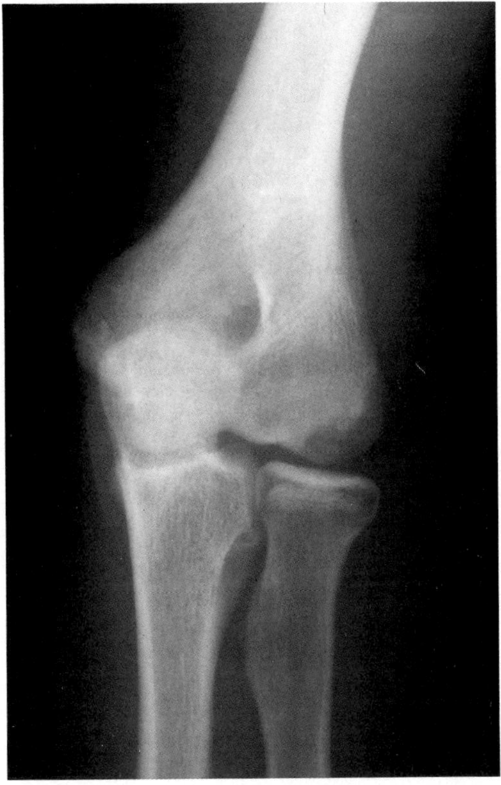

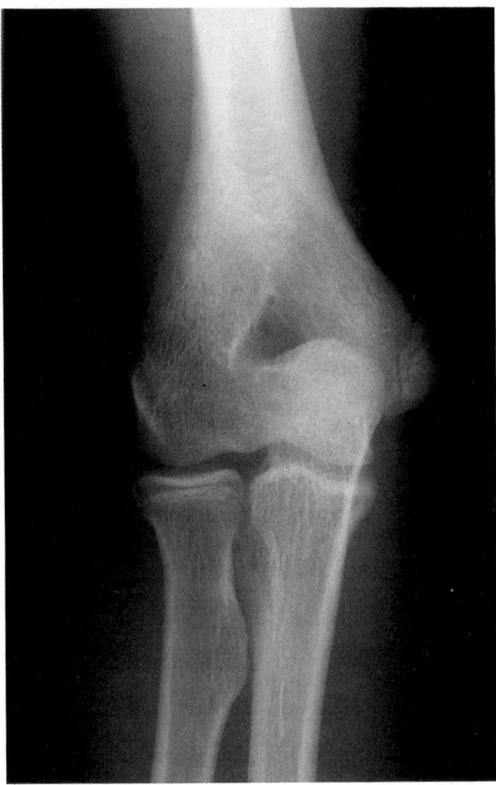

FIG. 35-14. Osteochondritis dissecans of capitellum and radial head hypertrophy in 15-year-old right-handed pitcher. Normal left side for comparison.

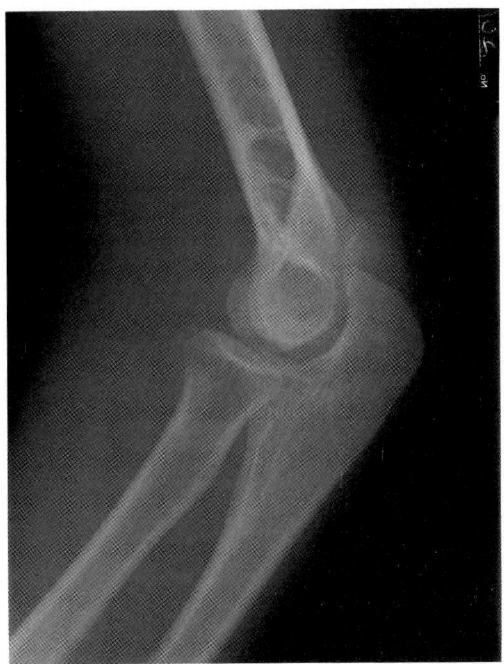

FIG. 35-15. Osteochondritis of capitellum in 13-year-old female basketball player seen only on oblique view with forearm supination.

can be fractured off and serve as a source of loose bodies.[2,22,24,27] These osteophytes are best identified on the axial view as described earlier.[52] Straight posterior osteophytes are more readily apparent and often can be identified on a routine flexed lateral view.[43]

Magnetic Resonance Imaging (MRI)

MRI studies of the elbow in the thrower have not yet been reported; the nature of the predominantly bony lesions about the elbow may limit the role of MRI in this effort. In acute soft tissue injuries, such as ulnar collateral ligament rupture, current adjuvants to plain films, including stress views and arthrograms, are quite helpful in confirming the diagnosis (to be described in the section covering this injury). However, as the resolution of MRI scanning continues to improve, the ability of this diagnostic modality to significantly contribute to our evaluation of the injured elbow will be substantial.

INJURIES

A distinction can be made between injuries of the elbow in the throwing athlete and the throwing injuries of the elbow. Throwing injuries of the elbow refer to the "overuse syndromes" that occur as a result of repetitive stresses that the structures about the elbow incur as a result of throwing over many months or years. Although the clinical manifestations of a throwing athlete's symptoms may be acute at onset, essentially all of these injuries are the result of pathologic changes occurring at the subclinical level over various periods of time. The cumulative pathologic changes occurring in the anatomic structures about the joint eventually exceed the body's ability to repair or compensate for them, thus resulting in presentation of the athlete to the trainer or the physician with his or her symptoms. These "overuse injuries" differ from acute, traumatic injuries to the elbow that occur as a result of a single injury or episode. These traumatic injuries refer specifically to accidents or injuries not caused by the act of throwing itself that the throwing athlete may incur to his dominant elbow in the course of his athletic event or during daily living. An example of this injury might include an acute rupture of the ulnar collateral ligament caused by a valgus force resulting from an attempt to tag out a runner on a base path. Another example might be an asymptomatic subluxing ulnar nerve that suffers a direct blow when it is in its subluxed position on the medial epicondyle, or a posterior dislocation of the elbow in an athlete that may or may not be related to his athletic participation. Although these types of injuries can occur in the general population, their presentation in the dominant elbow of a throwing athlete requires special consideration if these individuals are to continue to participate at a high level of competition.

Naturally, success in the treatment of the throwing athlete's elbow is closely correlated with the accuracy of the diagnosis. Diagnostic acumen, in turn, depends on a thorough knowledge of those factors already discussed in this chapter—biomechanics, anatomy, and radiography, combined with a thorough examination.

In discussing the various clinical entities about the elbow, it is convenient to group the lesions into medial, lateral, posterior, and anterior injuries. These areas can be further subdivided into bony versus soft tissue injuries or combinations thereof; even further subdivision into the skeletally mature or immature athlete is also helpful. However, because of unique considerations, the immature elbow will be discussed separately in this chapter.

Medial Elbow Injuries

Ulnar Collateral Ligament Injury (noncontact)

Ulnar collateral ligament (UCL) rupture in the throwing athlete, most commonly the baseball pitcher, will often present as an acute event of moderate-to-severe medial elbow pain that occurs specifically during the act of throwing. It is often accompanied by a "pop" heard by the athlete. It is not uncommon for the injury to occur on a cold day following inadequate warm-up. The athlete will complain of acute medial elbow pain and may have concomitant signs of ulnar nerve irritation. Medial elbow ecchymosis may be found on examination. When a history similar to this is obtained, until proved otherwise, the diagnosis must be torn ulnar collateral ligament. A high index of suspicion of a tear is paramount for the prompt diagnosis and initiation of treatment for this injury.

Findings in acute ulnar collateral ligament injury

- Moderate-to-severe medial elbow pain
- Onset during throwing
- "Pop" felt or heard by athlete
- Medial elbow ecchymosis
- Ulnar nerve symptoms
- Positive elbow arthrogram (complete tears)
- Positive gravity stress test (under anesthesia)

In the acutely injured thrower, the physical examination for instability can be inhibited by muscular spasm and pain. The close proximity of the various anatomic structures (namely, the flexor-pronator flexor mass, the ulnar collateral ligament, the ulnar nerve, and the medial olecranon fossa and process) makes differentiation by palpation very difficult. The **gravity stress test** has been described as a means of determining medial elbow instability.[41,54] This test is carried out by having the patient lie in a supine position on a table in the radiology suite. The patient's involved arm is abducted 90 degrees at the shoulder and is maximally externally rotated. The elbow is flexed approximately 20 degrees to clear the olecranon from its fossa. The force of gravity will open the medial elbow in the face of instability. An AP radiograph is obtained, and any opening of the medial elbow is determined (Fig. 35-16). Unfortunately, regional or general anesthesia is often required to complete the gravity stress test without too much patient discomfort. Therefore this test

A 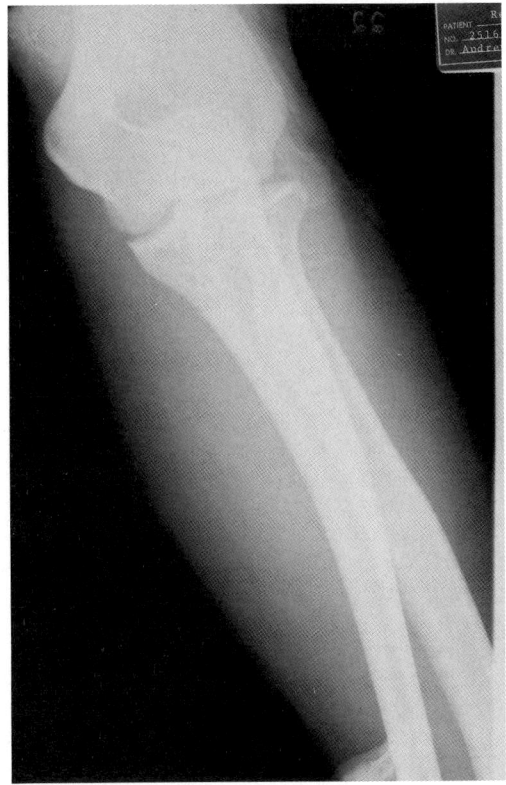

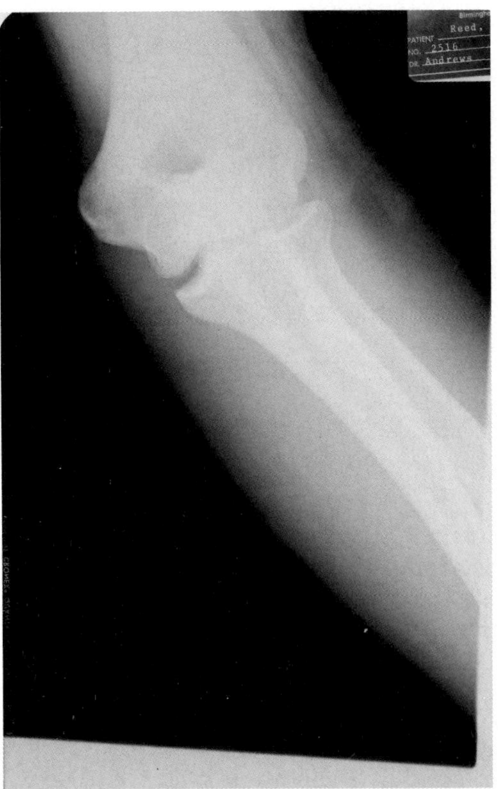 B

FIG. 35-16. A, AP radiography of the elbow before stressing. **B,** The elbow after a valgus stress is applied. Note the widened medial joint space.

cannot always be used to determine the integrity of the ulnar collateral ligament before an anesthetic is administered. We have found use of an **elbow arthrogram** to be very helpful in determining the status of the ulnar collateral ligament. It has been our experience that an elbow arthrogram showing leakage of dye through the medial joint capsule indicates not only a tear of the capsule itself but also a tear in the anterior oblique fibers of the ulnar collateral ligament and is thus consistent with medial elbow instability (Fig. 35-17). This arthrographic finding has been confirmed by the gravity stress test and under direct observation in those individuals who have undergone subsequent examination under anesthesia and surgical repair.

Although the athlete may perceive of this injury as a singular episode, in reality the pathologic processes occurring within the ligament structure have been chronically at work. These progressive destructive changes can occur in overuse syndromes when activity is not abated. These changes include edema and inflammation initially, followed by fibrotic scar formation within the ligamentous structure, and finally calcification and in some cases ossification of this scar tissue. Because these pathologically altered tissues cannot serve the function of the ulnar collateral ligament in its resistance to the repetitively applied valgus forces, the ligament will ultimately fail. In some cases, only minimal stress, rather than throwing the "high hard one," leads to final rupture. Almost all patients with acute ulnar collateral ligament injuries have a history of pain and tenderness over the medial aspect of the elbow—pain that was associated with throwing for months or years before the acute episode. Many have had corticosteroid injections into the medial aspect of the elbow in an attempt to alleviate these symptoms, and this may play some role in the ultimate weakening and failure of the ulnar collateral ligament.[23,36,46]

Acute ulnar collateral ligament insufficiency in the throwing athlete, if left untreated, will almost universally result in chronic ulnar collateral ligament insufficiency. In Jobe's report[25] on the reconstruction of the ulnar collateral ligament in athletes, his first 16 patients included eight who

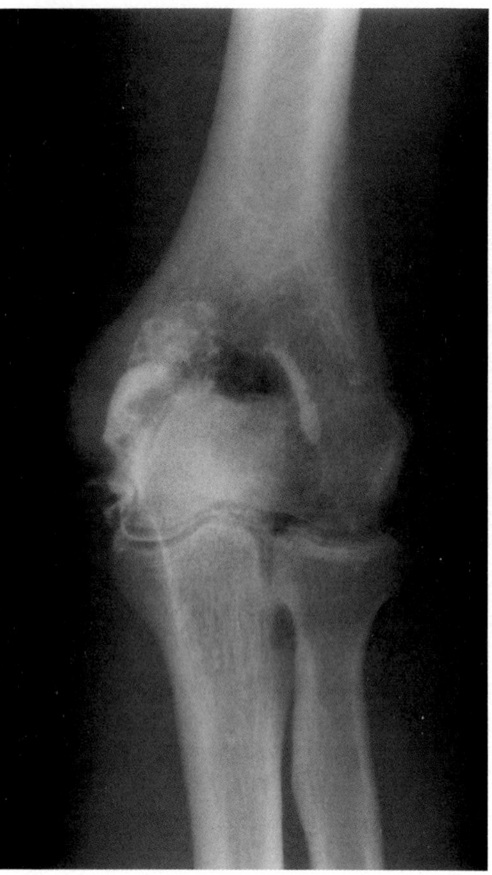

FIG. 35-17. Positive arthrogram demonstrates dye leakage from the medial joint. Close anatomic relationship of the ulnar collateral ligament and medial joint capsule result in their concomitant injury.

had a history of rupture occurring as a sudden catastrophic event. On clinical examination, these patients had valgus instability as determined by a positive gravity medial stress test. All elected to undergo a period of rehabilitation in an attempt to avoid surgery, but, as all conservative measures were ineffective, after an average of 7 months postinjury, all of the patients chose to have effective ulnar collateral ligament reconstruction.

As noted previously, a ruptured ulnar collateral ligament in the throwing athlete does not commonly occur in normal healthy tissue, even if it presents as an acute injury. However, this injury pattern can and does occur in teenage throwers who experience a singular acute and complete tear of their anterior oblique fibers. Typically, at the time of surgery, the ligament is found to have torn through normal tissue or to have avulsed off its origin or insertion (Fig. 35-18). In these cases, direct repair is an appropriate option. In the adult athlete most of the ligaments are found at the time of surgery to be attenuated and scarified, making primary repair difficult, if not contraindicated. In these instances, the surgeon must be prepared to reconstruct the ligament in the same manner in which such reconstruction is performed in repairing chronic ligamentous insufficiency.

Primary repair. The medial aspect of the elbow is approached through a curvilinear incision centered just anterior to the medial epicondyle. As the incision is deepened through the subcutaneous tissue, the medial antebrachial cutaneous nerve should be identified and protected throughout the remainder of the procedure. The ulnar nerve should be identified proximal to the cubital tunnel, and its courses should be traced to the two heads of the flexor carpi ulnaris. Care should be taken in the initial identification of the nerve to assure that it has not undergone an anterior dislocation directly into the operative field. The ulnar nerve should be decompressed and routinely transposed. The forearm flexor muscle mass is dissected off the medial epicondyle sharply upward. With reflection of this muscle mass, the underlying ulnar collateral ligament will be exposed and identified. Usually, the anterior oblique band of the ulnar collateral ligament, as well as capsular tissue both anterior and posterior to this band, will be completely disrupted. In many cases midsubstance tears of the ligament do not occur; instead avulsion injuries off of either the medial epicondylar origin or at the insertion point into the medial aspect of the coronoid process of the ulna are present. If the tendon appears healthy, a midsubstance tear of the anterior oblique band is repaired with a 2-0 Ticron suture or a similar nonabsorbable suture, and the capsule is then repaired with an absorbable suture. If the anterior oblique ligament is disrupted through an avulsion injury from either the humerus or the ulna, it can be repaired back to this bony structure through drill holes. Postoperatively the patient is splinted for 10 days in 90 degrees of elbow flexion. At this point a functional brace, which allows elbow flexion from 30 to 60 degrees, is applied. Over the next 5 weeks the brace is removed three times a day for range of motion exercises, with the goal being full range of motion by 6 weeks. At 6 weeks postoperatively, progressive resistance exercises are initiated and continued through the twelfth week. At this point, functional activities, including a well-supervised and controlled interval throwing program, are started. This pro-

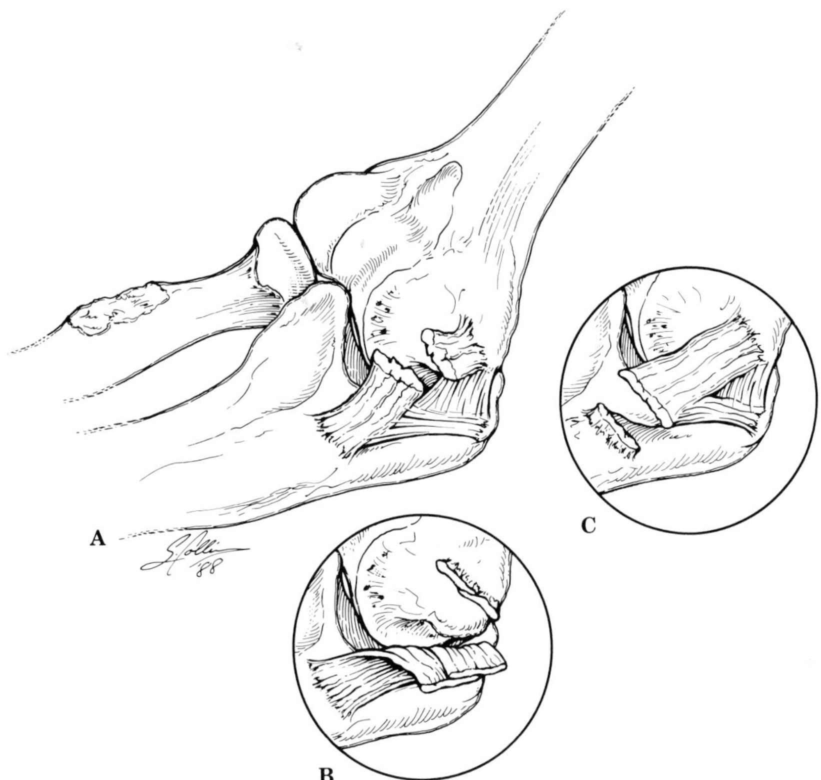

FIG. 35-18. Three views of tearing of the anterior oblique portion of the ulnar collateral ligament. **A,** Midsubstance, **B,** at the medial epicondyle, and **C,** at its insertion into the ulna.

gram will be completed on an individual basis over a 1- to 3-month period. A return to competitive throwing is thus accomplished at 4 to 6 months postoperatively. It is our opinion that prompt repair of this injury and proper postoperative rehabilitation allow the throwing athlete the best chance for return to his or her previous level of activity.

Chronic Ulnar Collateral Ligament Insufficiency

The pathologic processes of the overuse syndrome can result in progressive attenuation of the ulnar collateral ligament. This "stretching out" of the structure leads to ligamentous insufficiency even in the absence of a singular catastrophic episode of ligament failure. However, in most cases there is a history of medial elbow problems. Some athletes report a previous severe injury, suggestive of acute ligament rupture, which was not diagnosed or where definitive treatment was not carried out. Typically, these athletes present later with the same clinical findings as throwers with progressively attenuated ligaments: tenderness over the medial aspect of the elbow, posteromedial pain, and roentgenographic changes consistent with valgus extension overload.[25,52]

Jobe[25] has described reconstruction of the ulnar collateral ligament, using autogenous tendon grafts in an attempt to allow for a return of the throwing athlete to his previous level of competition. Using this technique, 10 of 16 throwing athletes successfully returned to their previous level of throwing capability, while one athlete was able to return only to a lower level of throwing capability. Schwab et al[41] have also described good results with a procedure for osteotomy of the medial epicondyle with transfer to a proximal and anterior position on the humerus in the reconstruction of a chronically lax ulnar collateral ligament.

Ligament reconstruction. The surgical technique for ulnar collateral ligament reconstruction uses the same approach as that previously described for primary repair. The flexor-pronator muscle mass is reflected off the medial epicondyle, beginning posteriorly and medially and reflecting this structure anteriorly and distally. This dissection is completed when there is adequate exposure of the entire ulnar collateral ligament from origin to insertion. The ulnar nerve is mobilized proximally from the medial intermuscular septum in the arm and is freed distally to where it enters the interval between the two heads of the flexor carpi ulnaris. The anterior oblique and the posterior oblique bundles should be identified and inspected. A 3.2 mm drill bit is used to develop osseous tunnels in both the distal humerus and proximal ulna. Entrance to these tunnels should correspond to the point of origin of the ligament from the medial epicondyle and point of insertion of the anterior oblique fibers to the proximal ulna. The palmaris longus is the preferred tendon for reconstruction; however, in its absence, either the plantaris or a toe extensor tendon is suitable. If placed correctly, some part of the reconstructed tendon should be taut throughout the full range of motion without acting as a tether either to full flexion or to extension. The flexor-pronator muscle mass is sutured back to the medial epicondyle through drill holes, and the ulnar nerve is transposed anteriorly in the subcutaneous fashion. The nerve is stabilized in this position by two nonconstricting fascial slings formed from the flexor muscle fascia (Fig. 35-19).

Postoperatively the patient's elbow is immobilized at 90 degrees of flexion for 2 weeks, after which light active progressive resistance exercises are initiated for the shoulder and elbow. At 4 weeks, resistance is increased, with gradual progression to maximum resistance being reached at 4 months. At this point, functional activities, including a well supervised and controlled interval throwing program, may be initiated. Patients return to throwing activities at 6 to 12 months based on individual progress.

The surgical technique and postoperative regimen is further described in the works of Jobe,[25] Schwab,[41] and Woods.[54]

Medial Epicondylar Fracture

Like most injuries on the medial aspect of the elbow in the throwing athlete, medial epicondylar fractures, although occurring acutely, are a result of chronic tensile overload. The forces applied to the medial epicondyle through both the ulnar collateral ligament and the origin of the flexor-pronator muscle mass result in adaptive changes within the epicondyle. These changes include the overgrowth of the medial epicondylar apophysis in the adolescent, as well as its occasional fragmentation, which is noted in the section on Little League elbow.[6,12,30,38] These same forces no doubt exist throughout the baseball pitcher's career, and, when they ex-

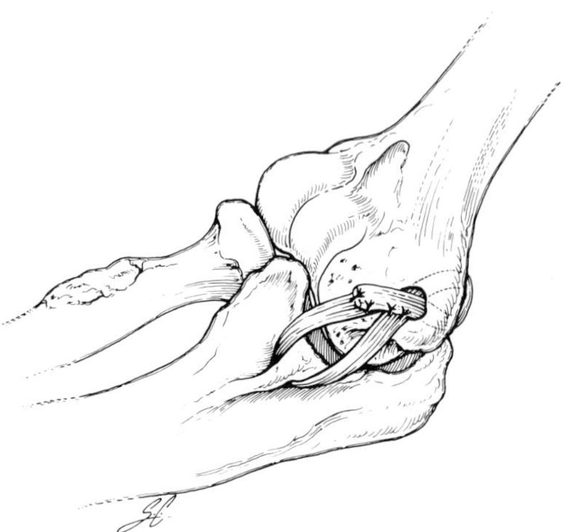

FIG. 35-19. An example of figure-eight reconstruction of chronic ulnar collateral ligament insufficiency using an autogenous tendon graft.

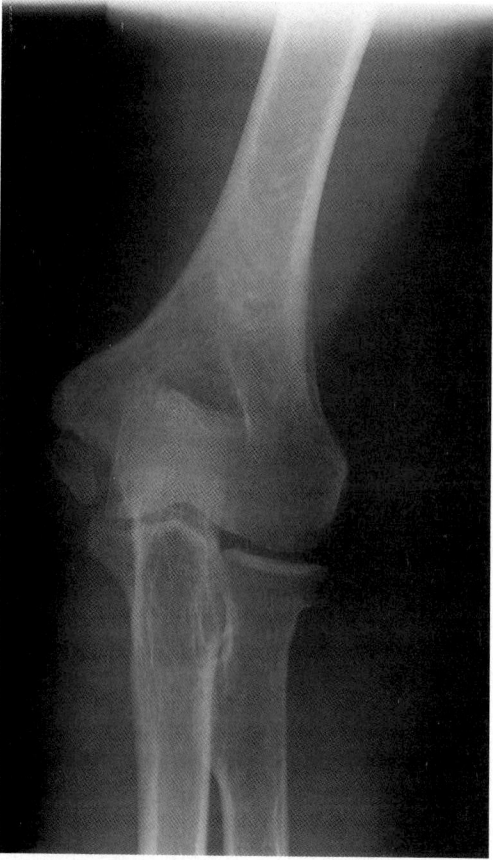

FIG. 35-20. Fracture in a youth through the growth plate of the medial epicondyle with minimal medial instability.

ceed the body's ability to adapt or repair itself, these fractures occur.[2,8,24,27]

The medial epicondylar apophysis is the last of the growth centers about the distal humerus to fuse with the metaphysis; it occurs at around age 14 in females and as late as age 17 in males.[21] Most medial epicondylar fractures in individuals in this age group will penetrate the apophyseal growth plate, with the entire fragment being displaced. The fragment will include the origin of the flexor-pronator muscle and may or may not include the attachment of the ulnar collateral ligament. We have seen complete avulsions of the medial epicondyle where the fracture does not include the ulnar collateral ligament (Fig. 35-20). The ulnar collateral ligament attaches to the base of the medial epicondyle, and, in some cases, is spared in regard to this specific type of injury. Regardless of its degree of displacement, in the throwing athlete it should be anatomically reduced and secured internally with K-wires or an interfragmentary screw (Fig. 35-21). Although minimal and even moderate displacement of the medial epicondylar apophysis would be clinically acceptable for some individuals, the resulting laxity of the ulnar collateral ligament in the throwing athlete could be disabling in the individual's sport. In addition, epicondylar apophyseal displacement can alter the relationship of the ulnar collateral ligament to the elbow joint axis of rotation. Subsequent tethering of the joint by the ligament can result in loss of flexion and/or extension.

Medial epicondylar avulsion fracture

- Anatomic reduction in the throwing athlete
- No displacement acceptable

In the skeletally mature elbow, the medial epicondylar fracture is less frequently a large fragment but more often a smaller bony lesion, which in some cases can even be comminuted or fragmented[2,38] (Fig. 35-22). This, however, does not assure that the ulnar collateral ligament's origin on the medial epicondyle remains intact or that the ulnar collateral ligament has not failed in its midsubstance.[11,54] It is extremely important in the face of a medial epicondylar fracture, regardless of its size or its relative displacement, to determine the integrity of the ulnar collateral ligament. This can be quite difficult in the

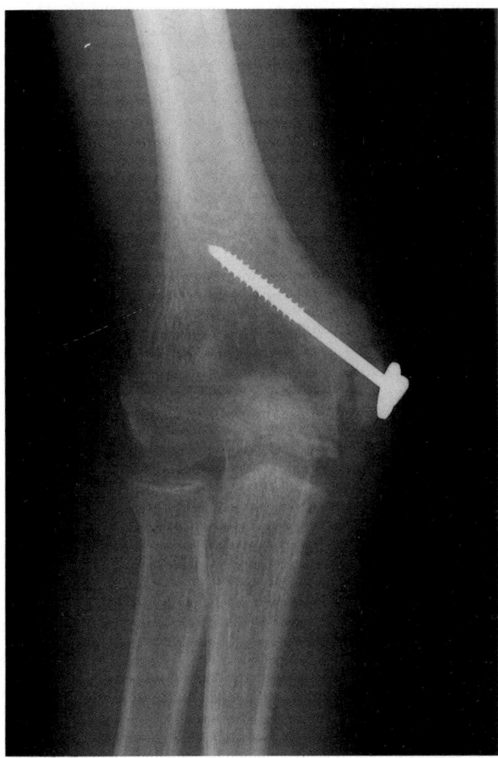

FIG. 35-21. Postoperative roentgenogram demonstrating reduction and fixation of medial epicondylar Salter I fracture by interfragmentary screw.

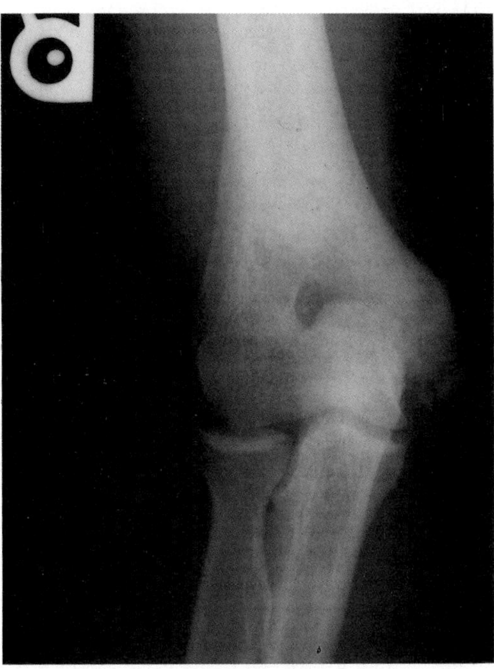

FIG. 35-22. Chronic avulsion fragmentation of the medial epicondyle in a professional baseball pitcher. Although currently asymptomatic, this player had a history of intermittent medial elbow pain.

case of an acute injury in which muscular pain and spasm cause the patient to guard the elbow. An elbow arthrogram, as described in the section on ulnar collateral ligament injury, is also indicated in this circumstance in order to establish the competence of this ligament.

Any throwing athlete who shows ulnar collateral ligament incompetence of the throwing elbow will require open repair or reconstruction of this structure.[25,54] The surgical technique and postoperative treatment of these patients are described under the section on isolated ulnar collateral ligament repairs. Treatment of the accompanying medial epicondyle fracture will depend on its size and comminution. The fracture fragment can be reduced and fixed to the distal humerus; if it is small or fragmented, it can be excised at the time of ulnar collateral ligament reconstruction. Berkley[11] has observed that medial epicondylar fracture fragments that involve the ulnar collateral ligament must be anatomically reduced, since even small degrees of rotational displacement can result in a functional lengthening of the ulnar collateral ligament and subsequent instability in the throwing elbow.

Substantial medial epicondyle fractures will occur in some instances without ulnar collateral ligament involvement. There seems to be a paucity of attention in the current literature to the treatment of these fractures. Berkley[11] has suggested that stable, nondisplaced fractures should be immobilized at 90 degrees of flexion for 3 to 4 weeks, with subsequent actively protected range of motion. Fractures that are displaced more than 1 cm in elbows that are stable to valgus stress should be treated with open reduction and internal fixation. Jobe[24] has stated that any such fracture displaced more than 2 mm should be reduced, and our clinical experience leads us to agree.

Muscle and Tendon Injuries

Flexor-pronator strain. Slocum[45] noted that the fibers of the flexor-pronator muscle group were particularly susceptible to overloading because of valgus strain of the arm during the act of throwing. He felt that this muscle group underwent a state of temporary myostatic contracture secondary to fatigue and that this prevented its return to normal resting length. If the individual athlete continued to throw despite these myostatic contractures, microscopic tears would take place within the muscle substance and would result in secondary fibrosis and a permanent loss of elbow extension. King,[27] in his description of physical findings in the professional baseball pitcher, noted not only hypertrophy of the dominant upper extremity musculature from the shoulder through the forearm but also the now commonly recognized flexion contractures at the elbow present in these high-calibre pitchers. Over 50% of the pitchers examined showed fixed deformities in flexion at the elbow. He also noted valgus deformities of the elbow as a second common finding occurring in approximately 30% of the pitchers. Elbow flexion contractures have been identified in pitchers as young as those participating in Little League. Two major studies evaluating Little Leaguer's elbow show a 12% and 5% prevalence of elbow flexion contractures in these young athletes.[20,30] These percentages undoubtedly increase as the pitchers continue their careers and expose their medial muscle groups to this chronic repetitive tensile loading. Despite the prevalence of flexion contractures in high-level pitching, an elbow flexion contracture in a young pitcher with a sore medial elbow should *not* be disregarded. As noted by Slocum,[45] early elbow flexion contractures are a result of myostatic muscle activity and spasm. With appropriate rest and abstinence from throwing, this can be a reversible physical finding. The goal should be to limit the extent of pathologic change and its subsequent cumulative effect on the medial flexor-pronator muscle group.

Flexion contracture in growing athletes must not be ignored!

Flexor-pronator complete tear. Acute, complete, or extensive tearing of the belly of the flexor-pronator muscle is believed to be a rare lesion (Fig. 35-23). In an analysis of 100 symptomatic baseball players conducted by Barnes and Tullos,[8] only two cases of flexor forearm muscle rupture were identified. Primary operative muscle repairs were unsuccessful. The postoperative rehabilitation period was lengthy, and the players were never able to return to an effective asymptomatic level of throwing. Fortunately, lesser degrees of pronator muscle mass strain are symptomatic for a short period of time and will respond to a protocol of physical therapy combined with icing. Occasionally, ossification will occur within the muscle belly near its origin. This is seldom symptomatic, but if it does prove to be painful it can be excised without injury to the underlying joint capsule or ulnar collateral ligament.

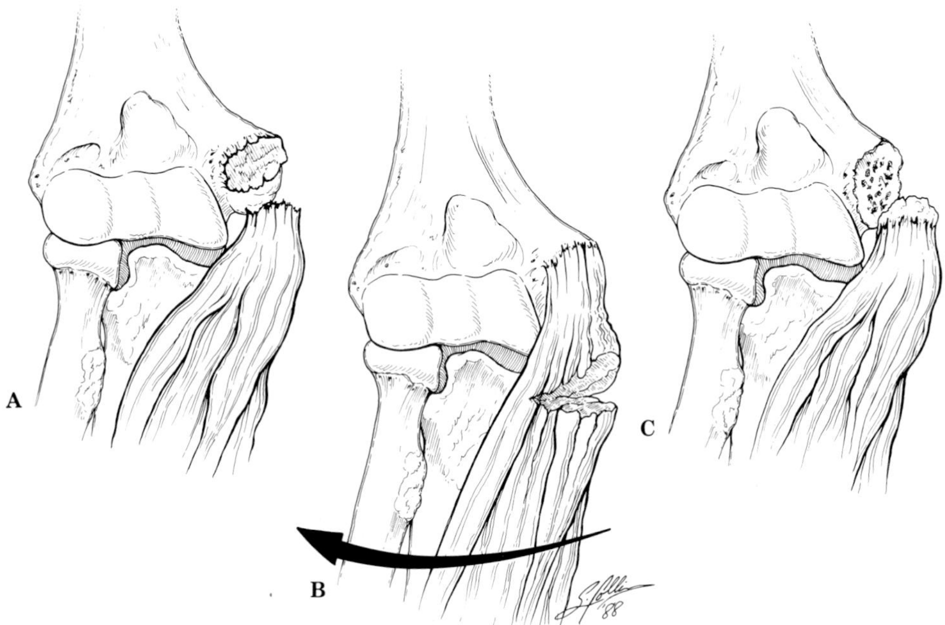

FIG. 35-23. Flexor-pronator muscle mass under valgus stress may **(A)** tear away from its origin on the medial epicondyle, **(B)** tear in midsubstance, or **(C)** avulse adjacent bone from its origin.

Medial epicondylitis. Because of repetitive tensile forces applied to the flexor-pronator muscle mass, medial epicondylitis is a frequent finding in the throwing athlete. The tensile forces generated in the throwing act primarily exert their pull directly at the flexor-pronator origin from the medial epicondyle; thus tenderness will develop at this insertional point. Similar to that for minor muscle belly injuries, these symptoms should respond to a physical therapy program combined with an eccentric stretching and strengthening protocol, as outlined in the rehabilitation section of this chapter (see p. 809).

Traction spurs. One additional lesion that is amenable to surgical intervention is a traction spur, which can develop on the ulna just medial to the ulnar coronoid process, immediately adjacent to or associated with the ulnar collateral ligament.[10,16,22,38] This traction spurring or calcific mass can develop either independently of the ulnar collateral ligament or within the substance of the ligament itself. Should the traction spur or calcific mass prove to be painful, it can be excised through an incision in the flexor-pronator muscle; great care should be taken to identify and protect the ulnar collateral ligament insertion into the ulna.[10,16,22] One must be sure that the integrity of this ligament remains intact and that removal of the spur does not subsequently result in medial elbow instability.

Nerve Injury

Considerable attention is paid to medial traction and lateral compression forces as primary causes of pathologic states of the elbow in the throwing athlete. Often, however, repetitive throwing motion and the consequences of medially and laterally applied forces concurrently produce subtle neuropathies that mimic other injuries. About the elbow, the ulnar, medial, radial, and musculocutaneous nerves are exposed to direct trauma and are indirectly susceptible to inflammation as the result of the following: (1) local tight fibrous tissue and muscular hypertrophy; (2) anomalous muscles; (3) anatomic vascular, and neural variations; (4) bony irregularities; and (5) abnormally lax or tight connective tissue.

Factors in nerve injury

- Muscular hypertrophy
- Fibrous bands
- Anomalous muscle
- Anatomic, vascular, or neural variations
- Bone irregularity
- Lax or tight connective tissue

Ulnar Nerve

The ulnar nerve, the continuation of the medial cord of the brachial plexus in the middle of the arm, pierces the medial intramuscular septum, passes alongside or deep to fibers of the medial head of the triceps muscle and is located in a superficial groove (ulnar sulcus) between the olecranon and the medial epicondyle. Without giving off branches proximal to the elbow, the ulnar nerve enters the forearm between the humeral and ulnar heads of the flexor carpi ulnaris muscle. A thickening of this fibrous connection (arcuate ligament of the cubital tunnel) between the two heads causes a compression entrapment and, along with the arcade of Struthers in the distal arm and the ulnar groove of the medial epicondyle, are common sites for ulnar neuritis (Fig. 35-24). Near the elbow, motor innervation is given off to the flexor carpi ulnaris and the ulnar half of the flexor digitorum profundus muscles. Repetitive, overhand throwing tends to accentuate normal stretching of the ulnar nerve, especially during the cocking phase of flexion and external rotation and in the acceleration phase with valgus stress on the ulnar collateral ligament. During these motions, which result in increased traction, any mechanically tethering of the ulnar nerve along its course can cause a friction type of neural dysfunction, i.e., medial epicondylar separations, ulnar traction spurs, and irregularities in the ulnar groove. More commonly, with flexion friction, ulnar neuritis is the result of recurrent subluxation or infrequent dislocation of the ulnar nerve out of the ulnar sulcus or groove. Although occurring normally in 16% of the general population, subluxation of the ulnar nerve is noted especially in congenitally lax throwing athletes.[14] Individually, either hypertrophy of forearm flexor musculature or increased forearm fascial compartment pressure can compress the ulnar nerve, especially in the region of the arcuate ligament. The medial head of the triceps and anomalous anconeus epitrochlearis muscles can also hypertrophy and locally entrap the ulnar nerve.

The indecorous-sounding **tardy ulnar nerve neuritis syndrome** is a late developing traumatic ulnar neuropathy that can occur in pitchers and is usually reported years after compression injuries caused by epicondylar fractures and constriction of fibrous bands between the heads of the extensor carpi ulnaris muscle.

Initially, the athlete complains of posteromedial elbow pain and intermittent parethesias in the fourth and fifth fingers, aggravated by throwing but improved by rest. Sensory deficits may be noted in the ulnar half of the ring finger, little finger, palmar hypothenar area, and specifically in the dorsoulnar aspect of the hand. Clinical signs of muscular weakness are late findings. Variation of neural anastomoses with the median nerve (Martin-Gruber) makes hand and finger configuration deficits difficult to interpret. The laboratory finding of decreased ulnar nerve EMG activity and velocity may lag behind symptoms and a positive Tinel's sign.

Median Nerve

Medial and lateral roots from the brachial plexus unite to form the median nerve. The nerve accompanies the brachial artery down

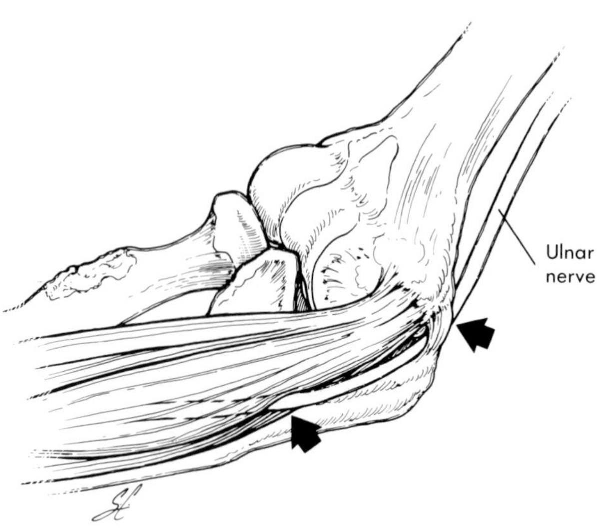

FIG. 35-24. Two common sites of ulnar nerve compression: proximally at the cubital tunnel and distally between the two heads of the flexor carpi ulnaris.

the arm and courses under the supracondylar process (if present) and the infrequently present ligament of Struthers—without giving off branches—to lie medially at the elbow, deep to the bicipital fascia and superficial to the brachialis muscle. The median nerve enters the forearm between the two heads of the pronator teres and gives motor branches to the pronator teres, flexor carpi radialis, palmaris longus, and flexor digitorum superficialis muscles. Arising from the median nerve distal to the level of the epicondyles is the pure motor branch, the anterior interosseous nerve. The anterior interosseous nerve then passes through the forearm and innervates the flexor pollicis longus, the medial half of the flexor digitorum profundus, and the pronator quadratus. The main branch of the median nerve continues deep to the tendinous origin of the flexor digitorum superficialis and eventually enters the carpal tunnel at the wrist. Entrapment, which produces compression, friction, or increased traction, can occur from muscle hypertrophy and anatomic variations when there is repetitive throwing. In the shoulder, infrequently the median nerve can be divided by anomalous suprascapular and posterior humeral circumflex arteries, a condition which results in neurologic deficits in the hand. More importantly, there are several sites of median nerve involvement about the elbow. Infrequently, fractures about the supracondylar area and the aberrant ligament of Struthers from the anterior medial supracondylar process can occur, causing inflammation. In the proximal forearm, the median nerve can be constricted by the terminal fibers of the biceps tendon (lacertus fibrosis) by, in or under the hypertrophied pronator teres, and by the thickened flexor digitorum superficialis arch (flexor superficialis bridge).

Potential sites of median nerve compression

- Anomalous suprascapular and postior humeral circumflex arteries
- Ligament of Struthers
- Lacertus fibrosis
- Pronator teres
- Flexor digitorum superficialis arch

Pronator teres syndrome is caused by repetitive athletic pronation movements, forced gripping, or direct trauma, which cause compression of the median nerve at the pronator teres level and to a lesser extent by entrapment in the lacterus fibrosis or at the flexor superficialis bridge. Symptoms may vary, but characteristically, there are vague postexertional pains in the proximal volar aspect of the forearm, together with paresthesia of the thumb, index, and long fingers. Also found are a negative Phalen test (wrist flexion that does not produce median nerve hand involvement), late occurring weakness in the medial-innervated intrinsic muscles and sensory changes in the hand, and normal function of extrinsic muscles innervated by the anterior interosseous nerve. Because EMG nerve studies may not be diagnostic, clinical maneuvers can enhance symptoms. Resisted pronation of the flexed elbow at 90 degrees with progression to full extension intensifies pain in the proximal forearm because of compression of the median nerve at the level of the pronator teres. Resisted supination with the elbow flexed heightens forearm discomfort because of compression at the lacertus fibrosis, and resisted flexion of the long finger magnifies volar symptoms because of compression at the flexor digitorum superficialis arch.

The **anterior interosseous nerve syndrome** is less commonly known than, but can occur with, the pronator teres syndrome in athletic overuse situations and in crush injuries. In the throwing athlete who complains of poor mechanical function of the thumb, index, and long fingers, a presumptive diagnosis of anterior interosseous nerve syndrome can be made from the position of the thumb and index finger in a pinch maneuver. The distal phalanx of the index finger is hyperextended with hyperflexion of the proximal interphalangeal joint. The thumb assumes a position of hyperextension of the interphalangeal joint and hyperflexion of the metacarpophalangeal joint. In addition, the area of pulp contact of the thumb with the finger is more proximal. These attitudes are the result of lack of function of the long flexors of the thumb and index fingers. The weakness of the pronator quadratus can be determined by comparing the amount of resisted forceful supination of the forearm in the flexed position with that in the extended position. There are no cutaneous sensory fibers to evaluate in the anterior interosseous nerve. Congenital soft tissue variations and Martin-Gruber anastomoses with the ulnar nerve tend to complicate the determination of the site of primary pathologic change.

Radial Nerve

As the largest branch of the brachial plexus, the radial nerve is the continuation of the posterior cord. The radial nerve winds posterior to the humerus and comes to lie anteriorly. In the arm, it supplies the three heads of the triceps, the anconeus muscles, and the sensory nerves to the arm and forearm. Having reached the lateral side of the arm, the radial nerve pierces the lateral intramuscular septum and runs between the brachialis and brachioradialis muscles. In the distal third of the arm, it innervates the brachioradialis and the extensor carpi radialis longus muscles. Usually at the level of the radiocapitellar joint of the elbow, the radial nerve bifurcates into a superficial and a deep branch. After giving off a motor branch to the extensor carpi radialis brevis muscle, the superficial branch of the radial nerve continues distally in the forearm to supply sensation over the radiodorsal area of the hand, thumb, index finger, long finger, and one half of the ring finger.

The deep branch of the radial nerve at the elbow is the posterior interosseous nerve. It passes between the two heads of the supinator, deep to the arcade of Frohse, into the supinator muscle, which it innervates. Distally, the posterior interosseous nerve supplies a superficial group of muscles: the extensor digitorum communis, extensor digiti quinti, extensor carpi ulnaris, and a deep group of muscles: the abductor pollicis longus, extensor pollicis longus and brevis, and the extensor indicis proprius.

Areas of compression of the radial nerve about the elbow can occur around the lateral epicondyle and in the radial tunnel, which extends from the radial head to the supinator muscle. Such areas of entrapment at times may be the result of Monteggia-type dislocations or fractures of the radius and a congenital fibrous band located anterior to the radial head, anomalous radial recurrent vessels, and the hypertrophied external carpi radialis brevis muscle. However, the most common site of compression is either the posterior interosseous branch or the radial nerve as it enters the arcade of Frohse, which is a fibrous thickening of the supinator muscle, or the hypertrophied muscle itself. Compression at this level produces motor dysfunction but no cutaneous sensory deficits comparable to the purely motor anterior interosseous nerve counterpart. Forearm muscle hypertrophy; repetitive, forceful elbow motion; wrist flexion and extension; and congenital variations in the throwing athlete cause entrapment, increased traction, and friction.

The athlete may present with deep aching of the extensor muscle mass after throwing or batting or after direct trauma to the lateral elbow. If injury occurs to the radial nerve before deep branching, sensory parethesia along the superficial radial nerve distribution may be noted. If the insult to the radial nerve at this level is severe, there may be inability to extend the wrist and fingers; sensory deficits in the thumb, index, and long fingers; and loss of brachioradialis muscle function. High involvement of the posterior interosseous nerve may yield only loss of extension at the metacarpophalangeal joints of the thumb and fingers.

Analogous to tardy ulnar nerve syndrome, tardy posterior interosseous nerve syndrome with symptoms occurring years after the initial injury is now a recognized entity.

Anterior lateral elbow pain can be enhanced clinically by resisted supination of the forearm with the elbow in full extension. This provocative maneuver compresses the supinator muscle. Lidocaine injection into the radial tunnel is diagnostic of radial nerve injury if the extensor pain is relieved and posterior interosseous nerve palsy results.

In the differential diagnosis of lateral elbow pain, systemic disease such as diabetes, periarteritis nodosa, and heavy metal poisoning need to be considered along with lateral epicondylitis or tennis elbow.

Musculocutaneous Nerve

Often overlooked on the lateral aspect of the elbow and forearm is the contribution of the musculocutaneous nerve that is formed from the splitting of the lateral cord of the brachial plexus. It pierces and innervates the coracobrachialis and courses between the brachialis and the biceps muscles to the lateral side of the arm. The musculocutaneous nerve exits the deep fascia lateral to the biceps at the elbow and continues into the forearm as a lateral antebrachial cutaneous nerve distally to the thenar eminence. The biceps and the greater part of the brachialis muscles are supplied by the motor branches of the musculocutaneous nerve.

Entrapment of the musculocutaneous nerve can occur at the level of the bicipital aponeurosis, resulting from repetitive forceful pronation of the forearm and extension of the elbow in the deceleration phase of throwing after ball release. Also the nerve is susceptible to direct trauma and the pressure of muscle hypertrophy as are the other nerves about the elbow.

A vague description of discomfort over the lateral antebrachial cutaneous nerve distribution in the forearm is often the initial complaint of the athlete. There may be palpable tenderness anteriorly, the local pressure over the bicipital aponeurosis may magnify symptoms. Not to be disregarded is the role of the biceps and brachialis muscles in controlling elbow extension in the deceleration phase of throwing. It is imperative to test the strength of flexion of the forearm in a pitcher with control problems in order to rule out musculocutaneous nerve entrapment.

Medical Treatment of Soft Tissue Injuries

Rest is the medical treatment most often prescribed for soft tissue injuries about the elbow caused by repetitive throwing. Actually, rest for the throwing athlete means refraining from the offending throwing action and, after diagnosis, institution of supervised, therapeutic exercise (passive, active, and resisted). Except when casting for fractures and splinting for postsurgical cases, immobilization is considered an enemy of the elbow. Medical treatment is directed toward safely and effectively restoring full range of motion, developing muscular strength and endurance, and attaining previous levels of flexibility and proficiency while maintaining cardiovascular fitness and total body well-being. Methods and modalities of treatment have changed over the years, but basic principles of therapy have persisted. After supportive measures, formal medical treatment for inflammation resulting from sprains, strains, contusions, and surgery about the elbow essentially is implementation of a formal rehabilitation program. The inflammatory reactive process can develop from direct trauma, but more often it results from repetitive, excessive stress placed on ligamentous, muscular, articular, or nervous tissue; this produces microtrauma, edema, weakness, tightness, limited motion, and pain. Should throwing continue, ligamentous injury, nerve irritation, and muscular imbalance become apparent, and abnormal biomechanics ensue, often initiating new symptoms. This disuse cycle is obviated by judiciously adhering to the guideline of not "working through" undiagnosed pain.

The primary treatment for elbow pain is **cryotherapy.** Ice in a ziplock bag or a commercial ice pack is applied directly to the involved area and held in place with an elastic wrap for 20 to 30 minutes. A sling may be needed for comfort. Heat is to be avoided early because, although comforting, it produces local swelling, whereas ice produces local anesthesia that permits motion and reduces swelling and edema.

As part of the clinical assessment, the degree of elbow (1) flexion/extension, (2) forearm pronation/supination, and (3) the valgus carrying angle are measured. Flexion contracture, increased carrying angle, and incomplete supination are frequently encountered in athletes who have been throwing for several years. An estimate of medial and lateral stability as compared to the uninvolved arm is noted in response to stress with the elbow flexed at 20 to 30 degrees to free the olecranon from its fossa.

Motion

Once the pathologic condition is ascertained, a patient-specific agressive therapeutic exercise program is devised with the goal of expediently returning the athlete to action within the propriety of sound medical judgment. The principle idea in the rehabilitation or treatment scheme (the terms are essentially interchangeable) is to restore range of motion. The foundation of this protocol is simple: slow **passive stretching,** followed by **active stretching** through the available range of motion, using pain as a guide. These motions should be held for 6 to 10 seconds and done in sets of 10 to 12, repeating them at least three times a day. **Proprioceptive neuromuscular facilitation (PNF)** is also used to regain range of motion. PNF depends on proprioceptor stimulation of the muscle when it is maximally stretched and then completely shortened in the functional position. The technique requires substantial knowledge and should be employed initially by professional therapists and trainers.

Flexibility about a joint literally refers to ease of movement through the range of motion. Ordinarily after injury, as the range of motion returns to normal, the ability to bend or extend with facility follows. Although range of motion and flexibility are not synonymous, they must be congruous. For the athlete, flexibility implies the propitious use of full range of motion.

Strength

The second principle in therapeutic exercise is to restore strength, which is known to be measurably decreased within 48 hours after injury and the beginning of inactivity. Strength, the power to resist a force, is defined as static (isometric) when there is no joint movement or dynamic (isotonic) when motion ensues. To produce strength, muscles contract and shorten concentrically and lengthen against resistance eccentrically. The prime example is the biceps/brachialis group that flexes the elbow in the wind-up phase (concentric contraction) and acts to resist elongation in elbow extension (eccentric contraction) during the decleration phase of throwing.

Concentric and eccentric muscular contractions play equally significant roles in athletic endeavors, a fact not to be overlooked in rehabilitation protocols. In various training modes, overflow from concentric strength training gains to eccentric strength training gains, and vice versa, does occur.[19] Uniquely, eccentric contractions require lower muscular energy per unit of tension than concentric contractions. Also, because of both noncontractile and contractile tissue working in elongation, eccentric muscles contract at approximately 36% greater mean tension than can be achieved concentrically. In general, using eccentric (negative) rehabilitation techniques offers an alternative to conventional concentric (positive) methods; however, each has a precise functional significance. As mentioned, the eccentric action of the biceps/brachialis musculature in controlling deceleration must be intricately meshed with concentric muscular action in acceleration to provide the trajectory and velocity components of performance. Therefore, once adequate range of motion and flexibility is achieved, therapeutic exercise must be directed toward enhancing sports-specific functional activities.

There are three main types of muscle-strengthening exercises. **Isometric exercise** is performed by contracting muscle groups without associated joint movement. This technique requires two thirds maximum effort held for 6 seconds in multiple sets of ten. Isometric exercise is most efficacious in early rehabilitation before full range of motion is restored and when insufficient strength may prevent use of other equipment.

Isotonic exercise typically is performed with free weights and is characterized by variable speed and fixed weight. Based on the DeLorme principle, weight is lifted six to ten times until fatigue occurs. Over time, muscle strength increases, and more weight is added to overload the muscles. This is referred to as progressive resistance exercise (PRE) and is the gold standard of muscle-strengthening programs. In contrast to maintenance programs, isotonic exercises are performed daily by the injured athlete.

Isokinetic exercise is characterized by fixed speed and accommodative resistance as exhibited in the Orthotron and Cybex equipment. These machines provide equivalent resistance to that which the athlete exerts through the entire range of motion. The advantage over isotonic exercise is that slow speed isokinetic exercise (60 degrees per second) stimulates muscle strength at more functional levels.

Variable resistance equipment, like Nautilus, now is in vogue in fitness centers, health spas, and high school, college, and professional team training rooms. To use these machines, the athlete must produce near maximum force through the available range of motion. For colleges, the weight room with free weights, power racks, and Nautilus-like machines serves as a recruiting tool. However, unless properly instructed in the use of these machines, athletes may sustain musculoskeletal injuries from improper use. Also, the progression from specific therapeutic exercises to freelance weight training after injury should be done only with the knowledge and direction of the physician/therapist/trainer team.

Manual resistance can be used to produce isometric or isokinetic exercise. Although not truly consistent in the amount of resistance, manual resistance, whether self-imposed or one-on-one, can be easily adapted to the use of specific muscle groups.

Modalities

Physical therapy modalities are useful adjuncts to exercise therapy. Electrical stimulation of muscles can be advantageous early as a counter measure to pain and later in rehabilitation for re-education of muscular contraction. The use of heat, in the form of hydrocollator packs (150 to 160 degrees), warm whirlpools (105 to 110 degrees), paraffin baths, and ultrasound should be considered after the acute phase of injury when muscle spasm occurs and increased flexibility and range of motion are needed in order to return to functional activity.

Modalities used in elbow rehabilitation

- Electrical stimulation
- Cryotherapy
- Heat
- Ultrasound

Caution, however, is suggested when using the many modalities now available. Just as the physician must carefully individualize aggressive therapeutic exercise, the proper and successful use of rehabilitative modalities rests on the expertise of skilled professional therapists and trainers.

Exertional Compartment Syndrome

Exertional compartment syndromes rarely occur in the throwing athlete. Despite numerous professional athletes involved in throwing who have very well developed flexor-pronator muscle groups, there are no extensive studies in the literature on this problem. Bennett[10] reported a syndrome in which a pitcher was unable to continue throwing for more than two or three innings because of marked pain and swelling over the flexor-pronator muscle group. On examination, he found this athlete to have distinct fullness over the pronator teres. He described a compartment release that consisted of a cruciate division of the fascia of the flexor-pronator muscle group, which provided relief of these symptoms. On close evaluation of his report, however, it appears that he may have been referring to a pronator teres syndrome with proximal forearm pain secondary to compression of the median nerve; this seems likely, as he specifically implicates the lacertus fibrosis and the proximal fascial arcade of the flexor digitorum sublimis. If in doubt, these lesions could be differentiated and confirmed on the basis of nerve conduction studies or compartment pressures, with appropriate treatment being directed to the lesion once the diagnosis has been established.

Acute Traumatic Injuries to the Medial Elbow

Ulnar Collateral Ligament Rupture

Contact injuries. Ulnar collateral ligament rupture differs from the rupture of the isolated ulnar collateral ligament resulting from overuse (noncontact) in the throwing athlete. The contact injury occurs when the forearm and elbow are forced into marked valgus deviation by a single applied force or blow (contact), as in the football quarterback whose forearm is hit during cocking, acceleration, or at release of the ball while attempting a pass. It has also been described in baseball infielders who extend the arm to tag a passing runner whose body force exerts a marked valgus overload on the infielder's medial elbow[35] (Fig. 35-25).

Mechanisms of ulnar collateral ligament injury

- Noncontact: acute injury (pitching)
- Noncontact: chronic injury (pitching)
- Contact: acute injury (football)
- Associated with posterior elbow dislocation

Regardless of the causing mechanism, this is a serious injury for any throwing athlete, as there is evidence that absence of a functional ulnar collateral ligament adversely affects throwing performance.[25] This diagnosis must be specifically ruled out by appropriate tests, including the elbow arthrogram and a gravity stress test, if possible. If the diagnosis is confirmed, surgical intervention is indicated.

The surgical approach for this lesion is similar to that described for ulnar collateral ligament repair (see p. 800). The associated pathologic state at surgery may differ from patient to patient when this ligament has been ruptured by a singular traumatic event. Whether there is additional anatomic disruption depends on the degree of force applied to the medial aspect of the elbow. This includes flexor-pronator origin avulsions, intramuscular disruption, and disruption of the soft tissues, all of which stabilize the ulnar nerve within the cubital tunnel.[35] Care must be taken to immediately identify the ulnar nerve above the level of the elbow and to trace it into the area of ecchymosis and tissue disruption to assure that it has not been displaced directly into the surgical field. In any event, the ulnar nerve should be decompressed and transposed because leaving it in its anatomic location will result in excessive fibrosis developing about the nerve. The flexor-pronator muscle mass is reapproximated to the medial epicondyle through drill holes. The results of repairing the ulnar collateral ligament acutely warrant using this approach rather than reconstructing the ligament using a free autogenous graft.[35]

Elbow dislocation. Elbow dislocations have been treated successfully by reduction, limited immobilization, and early range of motion therapy. In most cases, only minor sequelae usually result from this standard form of treatment. There is, however, a reported 9% to 14% incidence of recurrent elbow dislocation following a posterior fracture dislocation.[51] This recurrent dislocation appears to be caused by the instability that results from disruption of the ulnar collateral ligament at the time of the initial dislocation (Fig. 35-26).

Tullos et al[48] have shown that the anterior oblique ligament band of the ulnar collateral ligament was torn in 34 of 37 patients in whom a posterior elbow dislocation had occurred earlier. Disruption of this ligament was diagnosed by a positive stress test and confirmed at the time of acute surgical repair following initial dislocation. With this high rate of ulnar collateral ligament injury associated with posterior elbow dislocations, it is imperative to test for the integrity of the ulnar collateral ligament in any patient, particularly the throwing athlete. Should the throwing athlete suffer this injury in the dominant arm, acute repair of the ligament following reduction of the dislocation is indicated if the athlete

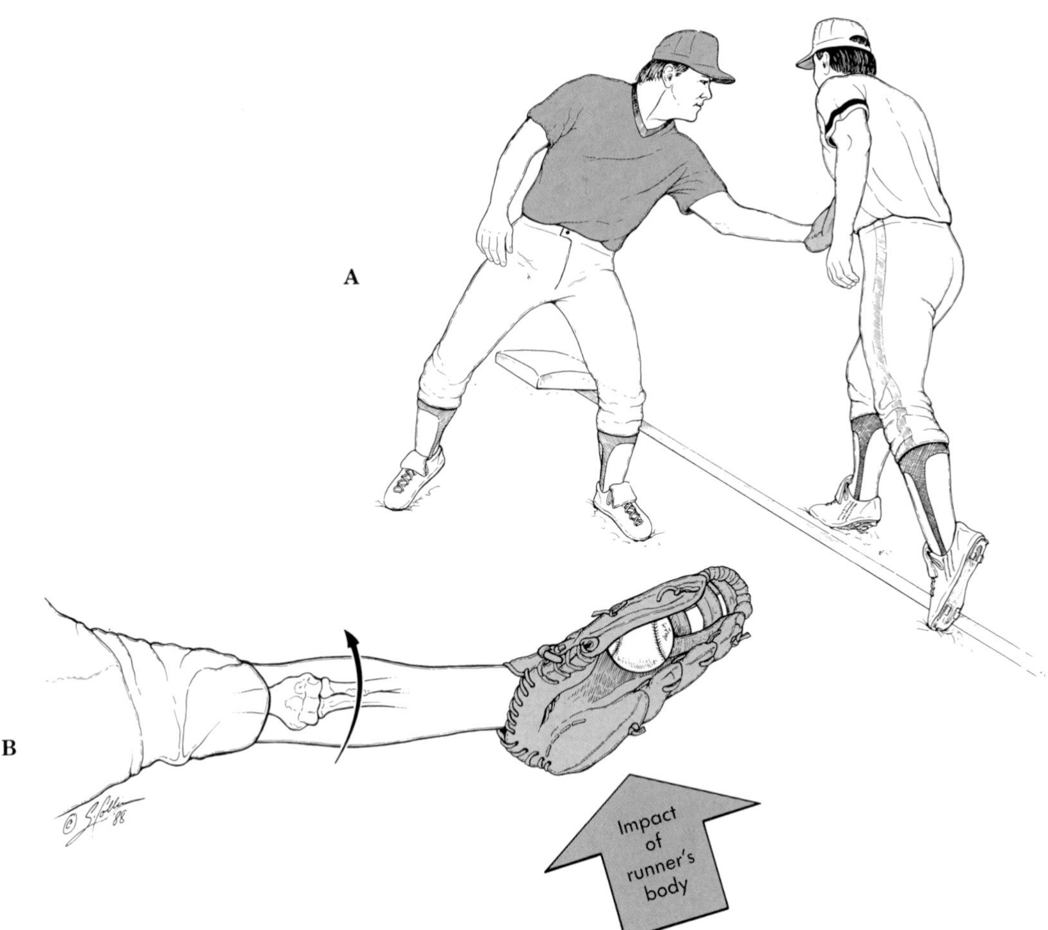

FIG. 35-25. A, Example of a forceful valgus stress applied to the ulnar collateral ligament of the extended elbow. **B,** Close-up, composite drawing of first baseman's glove and bony anatomy of the elbow and the production of valgus traction medially and compression laterally.

desires the best chance for return to his or her previous level of throwing activity.

Ulnar Nerve Contusion

The section of this chapter that deals with nerve entrapment syndromes about the elbow describes the clinical presentation and subsequent management of irritation of the ulnar nerve caused by compressive and tensile forces occurring about the nerve and associated with the act of throwing. However, the athlete can incur an injury to the ulnar nerve independently of these irritating forces. This refers specifically to a direct blow being applied to the ulnar nerve while it is subluxed from its posterior position in the cubital tunnel anterior to the medial epicondyle. In this position, the nerve is "unprotected" and can be injured directly rather than indirectly, as occurs in the repetitive act of throwing.

Recurrent dislocation of the ulnar nerve as the elbow is moved through a range of motion has been identified in up to 16% of the general population. The nerve may either sublux onto the medial epicondyle or completely dislocate anterior to the medial epicondyle. Childress[15] found that those nerves that subluxed on the medial epicondyle but did not translocate anterior to it were at greater risk of direct injury; whereas the completely dislocating ulnar nerve was at increased risk for friction neuritis.

A direct blow to the ulnar nerve in its subluxed position is acutely painful and may be the initiating factor in a chronic ulnar nerve irritation. The initial injury should be treated with rest, ice, and a gradually increasing mobilization as the acute episode subsides. As far as possible or as appropriate in the athlete's sport, protective padding should be used; if

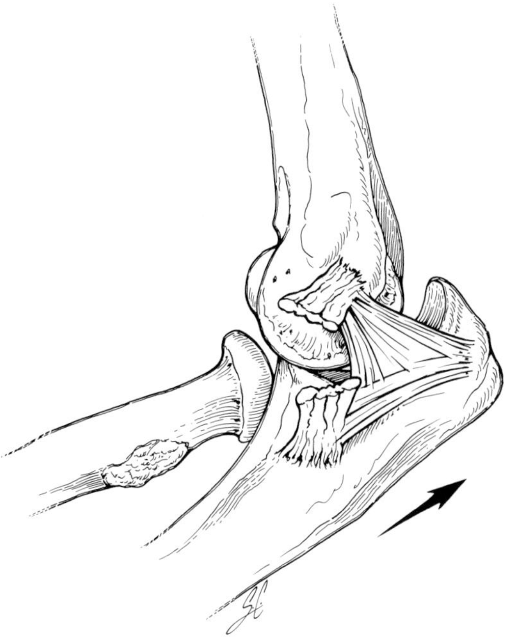

FIG. 35-26. Posterior dislocation of the elbow after midsubstance tear of the anterior oblique portion of the ulnar collateral ligament.

recurrent ulnar neuritis develops as a result of this initial injury, formal anterior transposition of the nerve is indicated.

Lateral Elbow Injuries

Bony Injuries

Slocum's[45] list of lateral compression injuries of the elbow resulting from baseball pitching are as follows: traumatic osteochondritis dissecans, fracture of the capitellum, and traumatic arthritis. The first of these, osteochondritis dissecans, is discussed in depth in that part of this chapter concerned with the skeletally immature elbow in the throwing athlete. As described by Slocum, the forces at work on the outer side of the elbow include compression caused by valgus overload, rotational forces resulting from pronation and supination of the forearm, and extension forces that are applied during the deceleration phase of the throwing act. Much of the literature that concerns lateral elbow problems in the throwing athlete refers specifically to the skeletally immature elbow. It is noteworthy that there is an absence of reports identifying bony lateral lesions as a significant source of pathologic change in mature throwing athletes.

Lateral compression injuries

- Traumatic osteochondritis dissecans
- Fracture of the capitellum
- Traumatic arthritis

An analysis of 100 symptomatic baseball players by Barnes and Tullos[48] included 50 elbow injuries, of which 11 were symptomatic secondary to loose bodies, only one of which originated from the radiocapitellar articulation. Indelicato[22] reported on 25 professional baseball players who underwent a reconstructive surgical procedure on their dominant elbow. None of the players in the study had any roentgenographic evidence of lateral compartment disease. In 20 of the 25, good results were obtained; however, in two of the five with unsatisfactory results, loose bodies were removed from the posterior compartment, and the radiohumeral joint was visualized at that time. Significant articular degeneration in the radiohumeral joint was noted in these two cases.

This is not to say that radiocapitellar lesions do not occur or have not been reported. However, we have recently evaluated the radiographs of 65 professional baseball pitchers participating at various levels of competition ranging from class A baseball to the major leagues.[40] These pitchers were randomly selected and roentgenographically evaluated, using a routine throwers' series of roentgenograms (previously described) as part of their preseason physical evaluation. Interestingly, in none of these radiographic evaluations were any capitellar or radial head injuries identified. We cannot conclude that radiocapitellar lesions occur only in the adolescent or skeletally immature throwing athlete, but we think the infrequency of capitellar and radial head injuries in skeletally mature athletes may be because athletes who incur such injuries during their career are unable to continue to compete. These individuals, therefore, are victims of the natural selection process in high-calibre throwing. Slocum[45] felt that the predominance of the lateral elbow injury in the skeletally immature thrower may be because of increased ligamentous laxity about the elbow in this age group and the smaller surface area of articulation between the capitellum and radius, resulting in greater stress concentration on these joint surfaces.

When chondral defects are noted in the skeletally mature pitching elbow, they can arise from either the radial head articular cartilage or the capitellum. In some cases, these chondral defects can be quite large, with both osseous and cartilagenous components affected, while in other cases they will be small osseous lesions or strictly cartilagenous loose bodies not identified on conventional roentgenograms.[2]

Chondromalacia of the capitellum and accompanying classically described softening, fibrillations, and fractures have been identified arthroscopically. Use of CT-arthrography (Fig. 35-27), which is now routinely employed in the evaluation of a high-caliber throwing athlete with elbow pain, helps delineate any lateral compartment changes. A definitive diagnosis is best accomplished through arthroscopic visualization of the radiocapitellar articulation.[4] As will be discussed in a later section on that topic, elbow arthroscopy has become a safe and effective technique in both the evaluation and treatment of elbow injuries of the throwing athlete. It allows for complete inspection of the joint, including the radiocapitellar articulation. Previously, when open techniques were used to treat other lesions in the throwing athlete, this articulation was not well visualized. Thus the integrity of the radiocapitellar joint was not confirmed, and the pathologic change within this articulation contributing to unsatisfactory results was only speculative.

In the skeletally mature elbow, chondral lesions and loose bodies can be safely removed, in most cases, through an arthroscopic approach.[4] Despite their origin from the radiocapitellar articular surfaces, these loose bodies can often be found lying in the posteriolateral compartment of the elbow. Thus it is necessary to carry out a complete evaluation of an elbow during arthroscopy regardless of the presenting or obvious complaints and roentgenographic findings. In the skeletally mature elbow, debridement of the articular defects is carried out in order to promote a fibrocartilagenous healing response. It does not seem to be advantageous to pin back osteocartilaginous loose fragments from these joint surfaces. The surgical technique for the arthroscopic treatment of these injuries is further delineated under the section on elbow arthroscopy.

Soft Tissue Injuries

Tendonitis on the lateral aspect of the elbow in the throwing athlete is uncommon. In the general population, lateral epicondylitis oc-

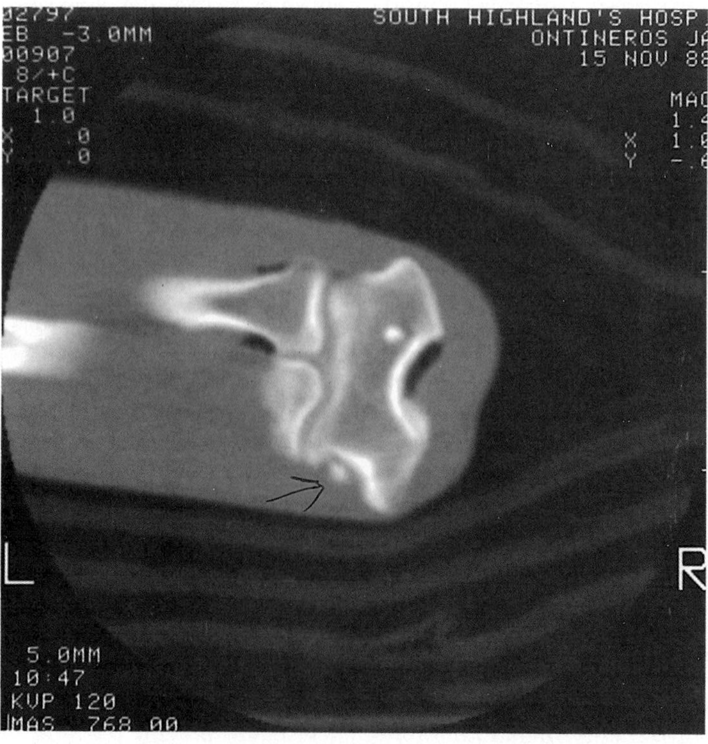

FIG. 35-27. CT scan following air-contrast arthrography reveals a tear in the capsule on the ulnar aspect of a right elbow.

curs seven times more frequently than medial epicondylitis and is a common presenting complaint in racquet sports.[34] Lateral epicondylitis occurring in the throwing athlete is an overuse-type syndrome, more likely related to forearm and wrist biomechanics than to valgus-related stresses applied directly across the elbow. The lateral elbow pain of tendonitis must be differentiated from that of the radial tunnel syndrome, which also is a rare finding in throwing athletes.

The treatment for this condition remains essentially a nonsurgical one. Physical therapy plays a major role and should include ice massage with wrist extensor and flexor stretching; in addition, an eccentric reconditioning program should be used as described in the rehabilitation section of this chapter.

Posterior Elbow Lesions

Lesions in the posterior elbow, specifically at the olecranon and olecranon fossa, are probably the most common type of injury in the throwing athlete. Fortunately, most reports in the literature, combined with our personal experience, indicate that these lesions are not only amenable to surgical treatment but also are ones in which the athlete has a good chance of returning to his or her previous levels of throwing.[2,8,10,22] In Barnes[8] study of 100 symptomatic baseball players, 50 of whom had elbow injuries, 10 of the 50 had posterior compartment bodies that were removed surgically, resulting in all 10 of them returning to their previous level of throwing. In a review of 25 cases of correctable elbow lesions in professional baseball players, Indelicato[22] reported that 14 of 25 underwent surgical removal of loose bodies from the posterior compartment, yielding complete satisfaction in 12 of 14 cases.

Bony Injuries

Valgus extension overload conditions. Except for triceps tendonitis (discussed later), posterior elbow pathologic change is primarily bony in nature. With the exception of a rare traction-induced stress fracture of the olecranon tip, these bony injuries are believed to result from the rapid and forceful extension and valgus forces applied to the elbow in the late acceleration and complete deceleration phases of throwing.[27] It should be recalled that as the forearm and wrist accelerate through the later stages of the acceleration phase of throwing, the centrifical force that is generated begins to impose an extension force across the elbow joint. At this point in the acceleration phase, a large degree of torque and a high rate of extension are present at the elbow joint. These two forces combine to cause a relatively high shear force to be imposed on the articular cartilage of the posteromedial olecranon and, more particularly, on the corresponding medial wall of the olecranon fossa. This is known as valgus extension overload.[52] Any valgus instability, even if minor, will lead to further abutment of the posteromedial olecranon against the olecranon fossa. In addition, the tip of the olecranon process impinges into the olecranon fossa in the posterior aspect of the humerus, and repetitive impingements can cause osteophytic bone formation directly at the tip of the olecranon and in the fossa itself. Thus both the tip and the posteromedial aspect of the olecranon can serve as sites of bony osteophytes that may subsequently fracture and become the source of loose bodies. Osteophyte and loose body formation can also arise in the olecranon fossa itself. If not specifically sought out, posteromedial corner osteophytes are sometimes overlooked. These osteophytes are the result of valgus extension overload (as noted previously). They can be delineated by the axial view taken as part of the routine radiographic study (Fig. 35-28). The osteophytes not only serve as a source of loose bodies but also, because of the nature of their position, they can result in friction irritation on the undersurface of the ulnar nerve as it passes directly over the posteromedial portion of the joint while it rests in the cubital tunnel. Forced extension of the elbow during physical examination can produce complaints of posterior elbow pain caused by straight posterior osteophytes. However, the posteromedial osteophytes of the valgus extension overload syndrome may not be symptomatic unless a valgus component to the extension is added. With the valgus force applied to the forearm as the elbow is brought into extension, the patient's symptoms relative to these osteophytes can be reproduced.

The treatment of posterior elbow pain in the presence of posterior and posteromedial osteophytes is initially conservative (Fig. 35-29). Attempts are made through rest, ice, and various physical therapy modalities to alleviate the thrower's symptoms to a point where he or she can return to the pre-injury activity. However, if symptoms persist despite these measures, surgical intervention is indicated. We have found arthroscopic excision of osteophytes and removal of loose bodies to be a successful and reproducible technique for the treatment of these lesions.[7] Occasionally with the valgus extension overload syndrome,

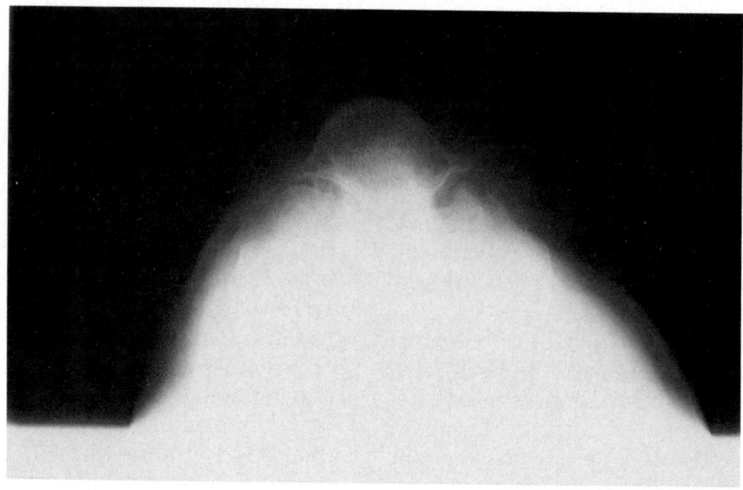

FIG. 35-28. Axial view demonstrates significant posterior osteophytes both medially and laterally.

purely cartilagenous hypertrophy is noted in the posteromedial aspect of the olecranon fossa complex. Although these lesions are not seen radiographically, at the time of arthroscopy they can be readily identified and removed. Using the arthroscopic techniques, thorough debridement of the posterior compartment is achieved. More exacting removal of the offending pathologic tissue is possible through arthroscopic techniques than with open surgery. This allows for maximum retention of bone to act as a secondary stabilizer against the valgus forces of the throwing act. Although the operative procedure does not alter the repetitive forces that initiated the development of the pathologic condition, it does offer the competitive athlete a chance to return to his or her previous level of throwing, symptomatically improved, but with the knowledge that the changes as well as the symptoms may recur. Postoperative care for arthroscopic debridement of the posterior compartment includes a posterior splint for 2 to 3 days, followed by range of motion activities and a stretching and strengthening program once range of motion has been achieved. In general, throwing athletes are able to resume their previous activity approximately 6 to 8 weeks postoperatively.

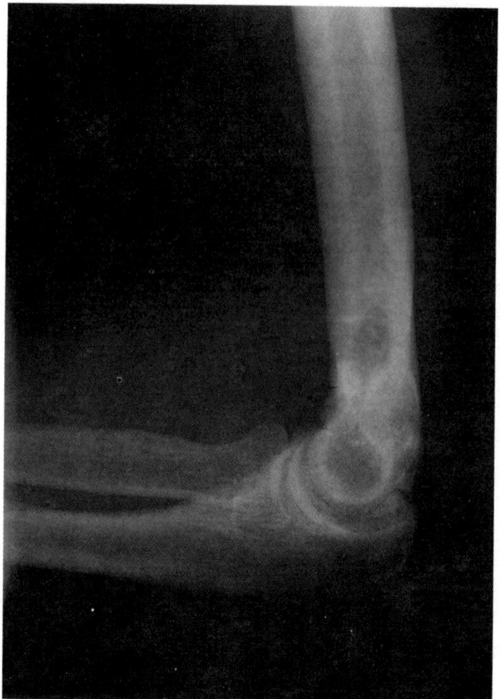

FIG. 35-29. Posterior osteophytes are well visualized on a 90-degree flexion lateral view. This osteophyte has fractured away from the olecranon tip.

Fractures. Fractures of the olecranon include avulsions of the tip of the olecranon caused by acute traction through the insertion of the triceps tendon and stress fractures caused by repetitive extensor action.[10,16,45] The avulsion injuries can be treated symptomatically with immobilization; however if they prove to be persistently painful despite conservative treatment, they may require surgical excision. The rare olecranon stress fracture may also require surgical intervention when painful. Often asymptomatic, actively throwing athletes have been identified with the lesion on routine evaluation.

Soft Tissue Conditions

Triceps tendonitis. Triceps tendonitis, although occurring less frequently than medial epicondylitis or lateral epicondylitis, is seen on occasion.[13,24,45] It, like the other tendonitis problems of the elbow, should respond to rest and proper physical therapy modalities (outlined in the rehabilitation section of this chapter). However, like other forms of tendonitis, it may be slow to respond and may prove to be frustrating for both the treating physician and the athlete who wishes to return promptly to his or her previous asymptomatic level of activity.

Anterior Elbow Lesions

Most anterior elbow problems in the throwing athlete are soft tissue in nature. Those lesions, affecting the anterior aspect of the elbow, include biceps tendonitis and anterior capsular strain accompanied by periosteal reaction and bony hypertrophy or spur formation. Hypertrophy of the coronoid process is also seen (Fig. 35-30). The biceps tendon is exposed to large eccentric loads during the deceleration phase of the throwing act.[31] With the brachioradialis and brachialis, the biceps tendon serves to decelerate the elbow to prevent marked, forced hyperextension secondary to the tremendous centrifical forces generated at ball release. Preseason conditioning should include an eccentric biceps strengthening program to train this musculotendinous unit to perform in the manner expected of it during the throwing act. Rest, physical therapy modalities, and stretching and strengthening programs are prescribed for bicipital tendonitis. Both the anterior joint capsule and the brachialis insertion on the anterior aspect of the elbow are exposed to these same tensile forces during elbow extension and may also become symptomatic. With repetitive elbow flexion, bony anterior elbow lesions arise from the abutment of the coronoid process into the coronoid fossa. Osteophyte formation and loose body generation can occur from either surface. If symptomatic, these lesions are amenable to arthroscopic excision.

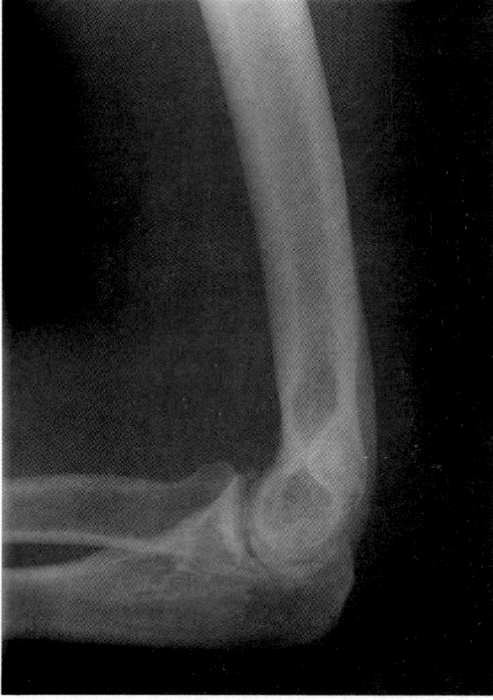

FIG. 35-30. Note the spurring of the coronoid process and subtle reactive changes at the coronoid fossa as a result of abutment by the spur.

THE SKELETALLY IMMATURE THROWING ATHLETE

The degree of skeletal maturity of the athlete's elbow is determined roentgenographically by correlating chronologic age with the appearance and fusion of the secondary centers of ossification of the distal humerus, olecranon, and radial head. Although there may be variability in development because of genetic, nutritional, and hormonal factors, maturation usually proceeds in an orderly, predictable fashion. Comparable application of acute or repetitive trauma sufficient to produce pathologic changes at one age may yield different clinical and radiologic findings at another age. For the immature athlete, intrinsically, it is bone age that determines the characteristic changes that the trauma of throwing produces. Extrinsically, the causes of change are force, caliber, frequency, and the biomechanics of throwing. In the young athlete, as in the more mature one, the five different phases of throwing produce equivalent shearing and compressive forces laterally and traction forces medially. Also, full or hyperforced extension produces increased pressure posteriorly and stretching anteriorly.

Repetitive microtrauma produces progressive physiologic changes in soft and bony tissue that can become painful, ultimately compromising strength and motion. Potentially the most injurious component of throwing in the immature elbow occurs during the early acceleration phase when the forward-moving shoulder imparts a valgus stress on the trailing elbow. This valgus stress imparts a medial pull or stretch on the soft tissue structures and their bony attachments and a compression with shearing of the capitellum laterally on the radial head. In the follow-through phase, as the valgus elbow extends, increased pressure is exerted on the posteromedial olecranon as it impinges the olecranon fossa. These forces inflict different sequelae at arbitrarily selected but convenient subdivisons of immaturity. This multiplicity of information has led to confusion of the nomenclature and classification of pathologic states in the elbow in the immature athlete. In contradistinction to the shoulder, where little league shoulder is described by Dottier[17] as one entity (epiphyseal fracture of the proximal humerus), several pathologic conditions are loosely combined under the umbrella of little league elbow.

Medial Problems

First brought to medical attention by Brogdon,[12] little league elbow is seen roentgenographically as cortical thickening, medial epicondylar enlargement, fragmentation, beaking, and separation in response to overuse. Clinically called medial epicondylitis, little league elbow occurs predominately between ages 9 and 12 and, when recognized and treated early, seldom becomes debilitating. Technically, the entity is classified as a **medial traction apophysitis,** since throwing produces tension stress force across the epiphyseal plate in an area of bone that does not contribute to humeral length and that, at this age, is extracapsular.

Roentgenographic findings in little league elbow

- Cortical thickening
- Medial epicondylar enlargement, fragmentation or beaking
- Separation of the medial epicondyle

In addition to the flexor-pronator muscle group, the medial apophysis gives origin to the two major stabilizing portions of the ulnar collateral ligament: (1) the anterior oblique band, which is taut both in flexion and extension, and (2) the posterior band, which is taut in flexion only. Medial stability is often overlooked if the elbow is not tested clinically by active stressing or passively by the roentgenographic gravity medial stress technique. Traction medial apophysitis during throwing clinically produces medial tenderness and swelling, decreased extension, and localized pain on valgus stressing. Aggravation of symptoms is noted on resisted flexion/exten-

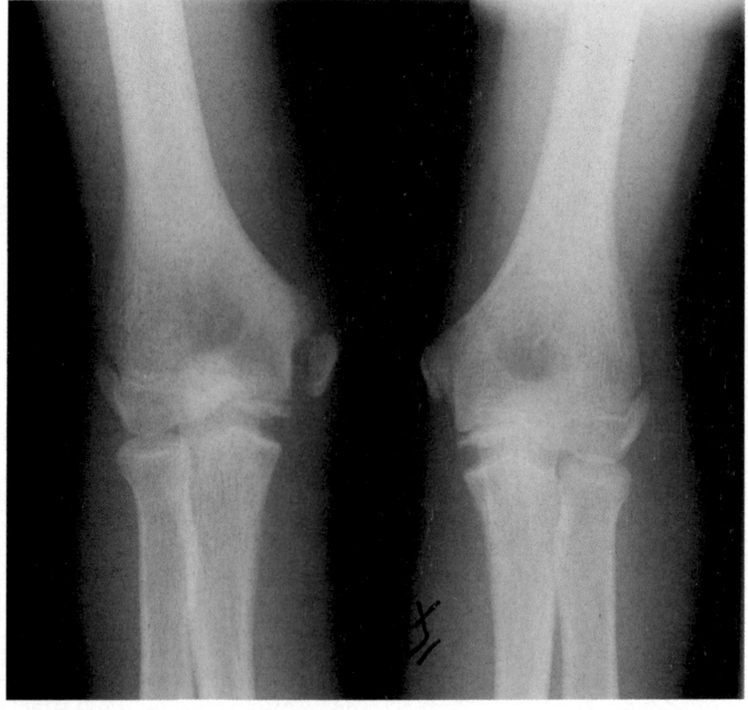

FIG. 35-31. Salter I medial epicondylar fracture through the apophysis in a 12-year-old right-handed shortstop. Injury occurred with a hard throw to first base. Left arm for comparison.

sion and pronation of the wrist. Roentgenographically, with continued throwing despite medial symptoms, greater irregularity of the epiphyseal plate develops, along with increased displacement of the apophysis. Subsequently, or with a forceful throw, significant avulsion occurs, which usually displaces the apophysis distally (Fig. 35-31). However, the fragment, often accompanied by a small piece of metaphyseal bone, may migrate into the joint or become attached to the coronoid process. True avulsion is indicated when the injured elbow has 5 ml or more of displacement compared to the uninvolved elbow. Reapproximation is needed, yet some controversy still exists as to whether surgical replacement yields better results than conservative methods. Nevertheless, an incarcerated joint fragment requires manipulation or extraction.

Fusion of secondary centers of ossification of the medial epicondyle occurs last in the distal humerus. As maturation continues, confusion may develop on discerning an avulsion fracture if irregularity and fragmentation of the ossification center normally occurs. Once fused, avulsion of a fragment or of the entire epicondyle can occur as a result of a single throw in a player with a heavy throwing history. Fibrous nonunion does result and may be painful. Ectopic bone, traction osteophytes, and spurring are evidence of sustained trauma and are seen concurrently with increased valgus deformity.

Repetitive traction stress forces in the skeletally more mature young adult may produce inflammation at the origin of the flexor-pronator muscle—epicondylar interface—resulting in microscopic or macroscopic avulsion of the musculotendinous insertion. Less frequently, tearing of the proximal muscle fibers is found. Such strains and muscular avulsions are clinically indiscernible, with differentiation being merely didactic.

As in the mature athlete, ulnar neuropathy in the young athlete can result from traction produced in the throwing motion, irritation from subluxation out of the ulnar groove, or compression from fascial adhesions secondary to lateral avulsion fractures. The incidence of ulnar nerve involvement increases with maturity of the thrower and the number and velocity of the throws.

Lateral Problems

The major throwing-related trauma that can occur to an immature athlete's elbow laterally centers around the capitellum. In a 1929 study, Panner[37] reported on three children (ages 7, 10 and 10) with a capitellar pathologic condition similar to osteochondritis dissecans but without loose body formation. Believing that such a pathologic condition was accident-related, he concluded that, while trauma might be the incidental cause, another essential factor must exist in order for the disease to develop, yet he had no assurance as to what that factor was. He believed that the entity now commonly known as osteochondrosis of the capitellum or Panner's disease was comparable to the pathologic change associated with Osgood-Schlatter's, Koehler's, and Calvé-Perthes' diseases. In osteochondrosis, typically there is rarefaction and blurring of the structures, initially leading to diminished size and fuzziness of the edges of the ossification center. The clinical symptoms are mild, and there is no corpora libera formation. Recovery is slow but complete.

The lateral epicondyle is subject to far less pathologic change in the immature elbow than the medial epicondyle, primarily because of the nature of the throwing motion. However, in the follow-through phase, sufficient forceful extension traction is produced to occasionally cause avulsion of the lateral apophysis along with a fragment of the condyle, the origin of the extensor muscles of the forearm and wrist, and the radial collateral ligament. Clinically, the findings may mimic an extension-type supracondylar fracture. Caution is indicated in making a radiologic diagnosis of avulsion of the lateral apophysis in the young athlete because there is normally a separation of the ossification center and the metaphysis of the humerus in youth.

Woodward[53] reports Mayo Clinic experience of capitellar lesions, two thirds of which were baseball pitching–initiated symptoms occurring between the ages of 9 and 15 years. In that report, irregular ossification and rarefaction with a crater formation was noted along with flattening of the capitellum and loose body formation. His radiographic diagnosis was osteochondritis dissecans with some familiar and constitutional tendencies. Woodward distinguished osteochondritis dissecans from the osteochondrosis of Panner. The latter is noted at an earlier age, involves the whole ossification center of the capitellum, forms no loose bodies, and requires only conservative treatment. Woodward reported that after surgical removal of loose bodies (when needed) in osteochondritis dissecans, the prognosis for the return to normal function was good.

Adam's[1] study clearly demonstrated that in addition to the recognized entity of medial apophysitis, Little League elbow occasionally involved osteochondritis of the capitellum and the head of the radius. Gugenheim,[20] however, failed to recognize roentgenographic evidence of aseptic necrosis of the capitellum or the radial head in his study of 595 Little League pitchers. Ellman,[18] Tullos and King,[49] and Larson,[30] concluded that conditions described as osteochondrosis or osteochondritis dissecans both result from compression forces that develop during throwing as a secondary component of medial valgus stress. In 1930, Kirby[28] reported on two pitchers (ages 19 and 24) in whom he found lateral foreign bodies that were pieces of cartilage chipped from the head of the radius as the head was "brought backward suddenly with great force against the condyle of the humerus."

Since Koonig[29] in 1889 coined the term "osteochondritis dissecans" to mean a dissected piece of articular cartilage (in the knee), its etiology has been depicted as either hereditary, vascular, or traumatic.

A possible clarification of this picture was presented by Singer and Roy[42] who concluded that osteochondrosis and osteochondritis dissecans are stages of the same entity with different bone ages at onset and that the level of activity is responsible for the variable roentgenographic findings. They postulated that early trauma resulted in vascular supply disruption and further damage which, by the age of 13 or 14, progressed to loose body formation and secondary changes in the radial head, followed ultimately by arthritic degeneration.

It is not the intent here to ignore polarization of opinions regarding the cause and subsequent pathologic state of the medial and lateral compartment of the elbow as a result of throwing. Instead, it seems prudent to agree that the classic definition of Brogdon[12] of medial epicondylitis (apophysitis) be reserved for the term "Little League elbow" and, to avoid confusion, lesions (lateral, posterior, and anterior), whether osteochondrosis or osteochondritis dissecans, be considered as secondary entities. Also there should be agreement that, compared to medial lesions, lateral lesions present at an older age, occur less frequently, and may have debilitating long-lasting consequences.

Posterior Problems

The posterior oblique portion of the ulnar collateral ligament, which distally is attached to the medial olecranon, is taut in flexion and lax in extension. The radial collateral ligament laterally attaches to the annular ligament and not to the radius. Combined, these two ligaments provide only minimal stability for the immature elbow joint. This leaves the posterior elbow particularly vulnerable to exertional trauma. In 1941, Bennett[9,10] was the first to recognize that the mechanics of throwing could produce stress sufficient to result in cartilaginous changes of the olecranon and the adjacent humerus. Wilson and Andrews et al[52] showed that in the early acceleration phase of pitching excessive valgus stress is applied to the elbow, causing wedging of the olecranon into the olecranon fossa and the formation of posteromedial osteophytes and loose bodies.

During the follow-through phase of throwing, impingement more posteriorly on the olecranon tip can occur. More importantly, however, in this phase the forceful contraction of the triceps occurs with stress being applied to its insertion into the olecranon.

Roentgenographic findings depend on bone development at the time of repetitive stress. Early, there is noted irregular ossification of the secondary centers and traction apophysitis. Later, avulsion fractures occur with loose body formation. There may be nonunion of the secondary ossification centers and lack of fusion between the ossified center and the olecranon. In the young adult, major or minor avulsions of the triceps tendon at the olecranon insertion may develop, especially in athletes with hypertrophied musculature. Heterotropic bone formation may occur at that level and may limit extension.

Anterior Problems

The anterior capsule of the immature elbow is susceptible to hyperextension stress as seen in young pitchers with generalized laxity, poor strength, and improper mechanics. Symptoms of capsulitis may be masked by concurrent tenderness of the distal biceps, brachialis, and flexor group muscles.

Anteriorly, early roentgenographic changes are trochlear hypertrophy accompanied by subtle changes in the ossification centers. Subsequently, osteochondritis of the trochlea is noted and is followed by loose body formation. Trochlear osteophytes may develop later. Coronoid osteophyte formation, after ossification is complete in males at about age 13, is caused by the repetitive anterior hyperextension stress of throwing.

Treatment

The treatment of elbow injuries in the immature athlete begins with an understanding

TABLE 35-1 Summary of findings in the medial, lateral, posterior, and anterior elbow in the immature athlete

Children 7-10	Little League 9-12	Pony League 13-14	High School 15-18	College/Professional 19+
Medial				
Increased cortical thickening of humerus Hypertrophy of arm muscles	Fragmentation, beaking, separation, hypertrophy, asymmetry, and increased density of medial epicondylar epiphysis (Brogdon[12]) (classic little leaguer's elbow) Ulnar neuropathy	Avulsion and *fatigue* Fracture of medial epicondylar epiphysis	Avulsion fracture of entire medial epicondyle Fracture fragment of medial epicondyle Valgus deformity	Nonunion of medial epicondyle to humerus Ectopic bone formation Traction osteophytes and spurs Avulsion of flexor-pronator muscles at origin
Lateral				
Osteochondrosis of capitellum (Panner)	Early osteochondritis of capitellum Apophyseal separation and fragmentation of lateral epicondyle	Erosion, deformity, and osteochondritis dissecans of capitellum Deformity, hypertrophy, and osteochondritis of head of radius Premature closure of radial head epiephysis	Overgrowth of radial head Radiocapitellar joint incongruity	Osteochondritis dissecans and avulsion fracture of radial head (Kirby[28]) (baseball pitcher's elbow) Loose bodies Degenerative arthritic changes Flexion contractures
Posterior				
Triceps hypertrophy	Osteochondritis and hypertrophy of olecranon Irregular ossification of secondary centers of ossification olecranon	Traction apophysitis Avulsion fracture of olecranon	Nonunion of secondary centers of ossification and olecranon Nonunion of olecranon physis Posteromedial osteophytes, spurs, and loose body formation	Avulsion of triceps at insertion Hypertrophic bone formation at triceps insertion Degenerative arthritic changes
Anterior				
	Trochlear hypertrophy Subtle changes in ossification centers of trochlea	Osteochondritis of trochlea	Osteochondritis dissecans; osteophytes of trochlea Loose bodies Coronoid osteophyte formation	Degenerative arthritis changes

of the developmental bony anatomy. Pappas[38] has observed that during childhood most throwing problems are related to the development of secondary epiphyses in the medial epicondyle, trochlea, capitellum, and olecranon. Characteristically, these lesions can be self-limiting once throwing is eliminated. Once pain-free, gradual return to baseball is permitted after the athlete completes rehabilitation techniques to improve strength and flexibility.

As secondary ossification centers fuse, fragmentation, avulsions, and physeal separations occur. Partial immobilization is necessary and each situation must be individualized for possible surgical intervention. Pappas[38] notes that the capitellum is particularly susceptible to avascular necrosis and compression deformation leading to loose body formation. Surgical removal of osteocartilaginous fragments is recommended only as a means of restoring range of motion. Often, lesions of the capitellum are found to be refractory to treatment, leading to disability.

Avulsion of secondary centers may require surgical repair since some result in painful nonunion. Nevertheless, for the immature athlete, stress reactions medially, compression forces laterally, inpingement posteriorly, and stretching anteriorly are rehabilitated in a generic fashion just as in the mature athlete. Patience is paramount (Table 35-1).

ARTHROSCOPY OF THE ELBOW

Arthroscopy has proved to be a very useful adjuvant in the diagnosis and treatment of elbow injuries in the throwing athlete. It has helped us gain a more thorough understanding of the diverse pathologic changes that can occur within the symptomatic throwing elbow. Accurate diagnoses are often difficult because of the close anatomic relationship in the elbow area of structures involved in throwing injuries and the amount of overlap in their clinical presentation when injured. Although most of the problems occurring about the elbow result from overuse and involve soft tissue, the ability to identify or rule out specific intraarticular cartilagenous and osteocartilagenous entities is very valuable. Previous reports in the literature have noted the difficulty in determining the reasons for unsatisfactory results when open operative intervention has been carried out for a seemingly symptomatic lesion.[22] When possible and appropriate, combining an arthroscopic examination of the elbow joint with any elbow procedure in the throwing athlete allows us to fully document the status of all compartments and joint surfaces. This enables us to develop a more accurate diagnosis and prognosis for the individual patient and serves as a means by which we can more accurately assess the results of our surgery.

Indications

Current indications for elbow arthroscopy include the treatment of most intraarticular elbow pathologic states previously treated through arthrotomy.[3,5,7] For the throwing athlete, this would consist of debridement of any acute, traumatic, chondral, or osteochondral lesions, including treatment of osteochondritis dissecans when indicated by the patient's symptoms and age. Anterior osteophytes in the region of the coronoid process impinging in the coronoid fossa or any hypertrophy of the coronoid process can be debrided. In addition, posterior osteophytes, either those found directly posterior on the tip of the olecranon or those found classically with valgus extension overload can also be addressed. Loose bodies, from whatever source, are optimally treated by arthroscopic extraction (Fig. 35-32). Loose body extraction is the procedure for which arthroscopy is most commonly and successfully used in the treatment of the throwing athlete. In addition to these

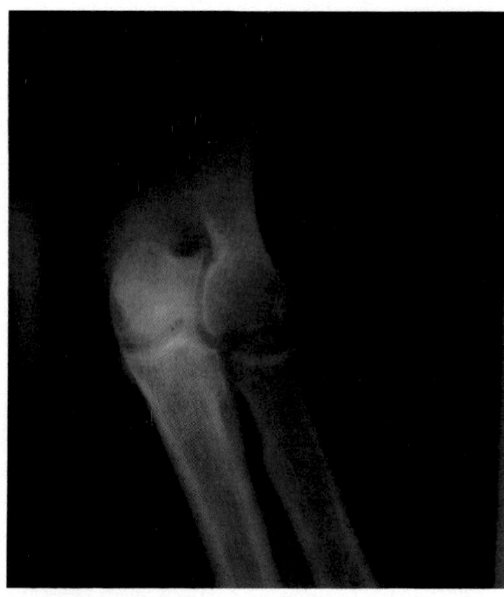

FIG. 35-32. Loose bodies can be found in any area of the elbow joint and are one of the primary indications for elbow arthroscopy.

indications, arthroscopic evaluation of the elbow should be completed in any throwing athlete in whom a definitive diagnosis for persistently disabling pain has not been made, and it should also be completed as part of the workup and treatment in any athlete undergoing elbow surgery for a soft tissue problem (such as anterior transposition for ulnar neuritis or removal of extraarticular painful bony deposits) in whom the diagnosis is unclear.

Indications for arthroscopy in throwers

- Debridement of chondral, osteochondral injuries
- Loose body removal
- Osteophyte debridement (coronoid fossa/process, olecranon fossa/process)
- Diagnostic dilemma

Surgical Technique

The patient is placed on a standard surgical table with the forearm and wrist supported in a wrist gauntlet that is connected to an overhead pulley system suspended from the end of the table. The shoulder is abducted to 90 degrees, allowing the entire arm to extend over the side of the table. With the elbow at 90 degrees of flexion, excellent access to both medial and lateral aspects of the elbow can be achieved. The elbow can be extended as necessary for the posterior portal placement, which is commonly done with the elbow at 30 degrees short of full extension. Full pronation and supination of the forearm is possible.

Positioning of the arm in this manner not only allows for excellent access but also, because of the 90 degrees of elbow flexion, enhances protection of the neurovascular structures in the antecubital fossa. The important neurovascular structures running across the front of the elbow (median nerve, brachial artery, and radial nerve) are relaxed in this position and are more easily displaced away from the direct operating field as the various portals are made and instruments are introduced. For excellent control of bleeding without obstruction to the operating field, a tourniquet is placed as far proximally as possible on the arm during elbow arthroscopies.

After routine sterile prep and drape, the procedure is initiated by first identifying the bony landmarks about the elbow. These include the medial and lateral epicondyle, radial head, and the tip of the olecranon. Using these palpable bony structures as landmarks and keeping in mind the underlying soft tissue anatomy, standard arthroscopic portals can be established in a reproducible and safe method. These portals include the antrolateral, antromedial, straight lateral, posterolateral, and posterior sites, which are usually established in this sequence.[3,5,7]

More than any other joint, the elbow requires predistention to allow for safe and effective penetration of the capsule. With joint distention, the vital structures are further "pushed away" from the joint, and the tough anterior capsule is tensed to allow for penetration with the trocar. Predistention is accomplished by directing an 18-gauge spinal needle into the joint through the lateral "soft spot" directly over the anconeus muscle. Saline is introduced from a 40 cc syringe, and back flow is confirmed.

Portals

Anterolateral Portal

The anterolateral portal is located approximately 3 cm distal and 1 cm anterior to the lateral epicondyle. This portal will be just anterior to the radial head at the joint line. Following predistention, a #11 surgical scalpel is used to make a small incision through the skin only. The blunt trocar is then directed towards the center of the joint and will penetrate the deep fascia overlying the extensor carpi radialis brevis. The lateral antebrachial cutaneous nerve will pass approximately 1 cm lateral and posterior to this portal.

The deep branch of the radial nerve before penetrating the supinator muscle will be approximately 1 cm anterior and medial to this portal. The superficial branch of the radial nerve is slightly more medial.

Via this portal, the arthroscopic anatomy best visualized is on the medial aspect of the elbow anteriorly. This includes the coronoid process and coronoid fossa. The medial joint capsule is well seen and through it hemorrhage in the ulnar collateral ligament is sometimes noted. Visualization of the radiocapitellar interface via this portal is limited.

Anteromedial Portal

The anteromedial portal is established approximately 2 cm distal and 2 cm anterior to the medial epicondyle. As with the anterolateral portal, when the trocar is introduced into the elbow, it should be directed towards the middle of the joint. The trocar will penetrate the deep fascia overlying the tendinous portion of the pronator teres muscle. The median nerve will be located approximately 1 cm lateral to this portal. Before arthroscopic evaluation of any elbow, a complete history and examination for previous elbow surgery, in general, and ulnar nerve transposition, in particular, should be completed. It is not uncommon for baseball pitchers to have had a previous ulnar nerve transposition. If a nerve transfer has been done, an anteromedial portal should not be established. The brachial artery will be just lateral to the median nerve and farther away from the instruments. The medial antebrachial cutaneous nerve will be 1 cm medial to this site. This portal allows excellent visualization of the radiocapitellar joint.

Straight Lateral Portal

The straight lateral portal is placed through the lateral "soft spot" of the elbow. This soft spot is bordered by the capitellum, trochlea notch of the ulna, and head of the radius. It is the area in which elbow aspiration is commonly done. Introduction of a trocar into the elbow from this portal penetrates the deep fascia over the anconeus muscle. As previously described, an 18-gauge needle is initially placed into this portal site for predistention of the elbow joint. Later, a formal portal is made at this site for the introduction of the arthroscope and visualization of the underlying bony anatomy, including the trochlea and trochlear notch. It is important to visualize this articulation at the time of elbow arthroscopy in order to determine the presence of any loose bodies or fragments between these joint surfaces. The arthroscope can be directed from this portal into the posterior elbow.

Posterolateral Portal

The posterolateral portal is located in line with the lateral epicondylar ridge, approximately 3 cm proximal to the olecranon tip. This point is located on the lateral edge of the triceps tendon. With the arthroscope in the straight lateral portal and the lens directed posteriorly, an 18-gauge spinal needle is placed into the posterior elbow compartment under direct arthroscopic visualization. The skin portal is made, and the trocar and sheath are then directed towards the olecranon fossa. This portal can be used in conjunction with the straight posterior portal and the straight lateral portal for visualization and instrumentation of the posterior aspect of the elbow.

Straight Posterior Portal

The posterior portal is placed proximal to the tip of the olecranon in the midline of the triceps. Correct proximal-to-distal placement is determined once the offending pathologic condition has been arthroscopically identified. An 18-gauge spinal needle penetrates the triceps fascia and is directed towards the pathologic area. Once the needle is arthroscopically identified, a small skin incision is made at the point of needle entry and the trocar and sleeve are inserted, following the same path as the needle. This path usually is approximately 3 cm proximal to the tip of the olecranon. The arm should be placed at 30 degrees short of full extension at the elbow before marking this portal and introducing a trocar. This arm position will be maintained while working in the posterior elbow. The posterior portal sheath perforates the deep fascia of the triceps as it is directed towards the olecranon fossa. The ulnar nerve will lie at least 2 cm medial to the portal site. Directly through this portal, the olecranon tip, the posterior aspect of the trochlea, and the olecranon fossa can be visualized. This portal serves as access for instrumentation into the posterior joint, while visualization is accomplished with the arthroscope in the posterolateral portal. Arthroscopic evaluation is not complete until all intraarticular structures have been visualized. A minimum of three portals (the anterolateral, straight lateral, and posterolateral) are necessary to complete this task. The establishment of additional portals will be determined by the individual pathologic condition present. In reviewing the appropriate portal selection for various procedures within the elbow joint, certain points should be remembered. Radiocapitellar chondromalacia or loose fragments are best visualized through the anteromedial portal with instrumentation through the anterolateral portal. Coronoid fossa and coronoid process osteophytes are visualized with the arthroscope through the anterolateral portal and are instrumented through the anteromedial portal. The straight lateral portal is employed for inspection of the trochlea of the humerus and its articulation with the trochlear notch for identification of any loose bodies within this area. The arthroscope is introduced through this portal into the posterior compartment to aid in the establishment of the posterolateral portal. However, the posterior and posterolateral portals into the olecranon fossa are best used for posterior compartment visualization, with instrumentation occurring through the corresponding unoccupied portal. With this technique, the osteophytes at the tip of the olecranon, the posterior medial olecranon, and olecranon fossa changes can be visualized and excised.

By following the previously discussed guidelines and by maintaining a conscious appreciation of the course of the underlying anatomic structures, reproducible, safe evaluation and treatment of intraarticular elbow pathologic states in the throwing athlete can be accomplished.

REFERENCES

1. Adams JE: Injury to the throwing arm, Cal Med 102(2):127, 1965.
2. Andrews JR: Bony injuries about the elbow. In The throwing athlete, instructional course lectures, 34, St Louis, 1985, The CV Mosby Co.
3. Andrews JR and Angelo RL: Elbow arthroscopy. In The elbow, ed 2, Wadsworth Inc, (in progress).
4. Andrews JR and Carson WG: Arthroscopy of the elbow. In Zarins, Andrews, and Carson editors: Injuries to the throwing arm, Philadelphia, 1985, WB Saunders Co.
5. Andrews JR and Carson WG: Arthroscopy of the elbow, Arthroscopy I, Injuries to the Throwing Arm, 1985, Philadelphia, WB Saunders Co.
6. Andrews JR and McLeod WD: Work in progress.
7. Andrews JR, St Pierre RK, and Carson WG: Arthroscopy of the elbow, Clin Sports Med 5(4):653, October 1986.
8. Barnes DA and Tullos HS: An analysis of 100 symptomatic baseball players, Am J Sports Med 6(2):62, 1978.
9. Bennett GE: Shoulder and elbow lesions of the professional baseball pitcher, JAMA 510, August 16, 1941.
10. Bennett GE: Elbow and shoulder lesions of baseball players, Am J Surg 98:484, 1959.
11. Berkeley ME, Bennett GE, and Woods GW: Surgical management of acute and chronic elbow problems. In Zarins, Andrews and Carson editors: Injuries to the throwing arm, Philadelphia, 1985, WB Saunders Co.
12. Brogdon BG and Crowe NE: Little leaguer's elbow, USAF Hospital, Lackland Air Force Base, Texas Department of Radiology 83:(4), 671, 1960.
13. Cabrera JM and McCue FC III: Nonosseous athletic injuries of the elbow, forearm and hand, Clin Sports Med 5(4):681, October 1986.
14. Childress HM: Recurrent ulnar nerve dislocation at the elbow, J Bone Joint Surg (Am) 38:978, 1956.
15. Childress HM: Recurrent ulnar nerve dislocation at the elbow, Clin Orthop 108:168, 1975.
16. DeHaven KE and Evarts CM: Throwing injuries of the elbow in athletes, Orthop Clin North Am 4(3):801, July 1973.
17. Dottier WE: Little leaguer's shoulder: Fracture of proximal epiphyseal cartilage of humerus due to baseball pitching, Guthrie Clin Bull 23:68, 1953.
18. Ellman H: Osteochondrosis of the radial head, J Bone Joint Surg (Am) 54:1960, 1975.
19. Ellenbecker TS, Davies GJ, and Rowenski MJ: Concentric versus eccentric isokinetic strengthening of the rotator cuff, Am J Sports Med 16(1):64, 1988.
20. Guggenheim JJ et al: Little league survey: the Hughston study, Am J Sports Med 4(5):189, 1976.
21. Hollinshead WH: Anatomy for surgeons: the back and limbs, vol 3, Philadelphia, 1982, Harper & Row, Publishers Inc.
22. Indelicato PA et al: Correctable elbow lesions in professional baseball players: a review of 25 cases, Am J Sports Med 7(1):72, 1979.
23. Ismail Am, Balakrishnan R, and Rajakumar MD: Rupture of patella ligament after steroid infiltration, J Bone Joint Surg (Br) 51:503, 1969.
24. Jobe FW and Newber G: Throwing injuries of the elbow, Clin Sports Med 5(4):621, October 1986.
25. Jobe FW, Stark H, Lombardo SJ: Reconstruction of the ulnar collateral ligament in athletes, J Bone Joint Surg (Am) 68(8):1158, October 1986.
26. Jones HH et al: Humeral hypertrophy in response to exercise, J Bone Joint Surg (Am) 59(2):204, March 1977.
27. King JW, Brelsford HJ, and Tullos HS: Analysis of the pitching arm of the professional baseball pitcher, Clin Orthop 67:116, November/December 1969.
28. Kirby FJ: Foreign bodies in the elbow joint, JAMA 404, August 9, 1930.
29. Koonig F: Lehrbuchder Allgemeine Chirugic fur Aerzten and Studirende, Berlin, 1889 A Hirschwald, p 751.
30. Larson RL et al: Little league survey: the Eugene study, Am J Sports Med (4)5:201.
31. McLeod WD: The pitching mechanism. In Zarins, Andrews, and Carson editors: In injuries to the throwing arm, Philadelphia, 1985, WB Saunders Co.
32. Morrey BF and An KN: Articular and ligamentous contributions to the stability of the elbow joint, Am J Sports Med, 1983.
33. Morrey BF, editor: The elbow and its disorders, Philadelphia, 1985, WB Saunders Co.
34. Nirshl RP: Tennis elbow, Orthop Clin North Am 3(4):787, 1973.
35. Norwood LA, Shook JA, and Andrews JR: Acute medial elbow ruptures, Am J Sports Med 9(1):16, 1981.
36. Noyes FR and Grood ES: Effect of intra-articular portico steroids on ligament properties: a biomechanical and histological study in rhesus knees, Clin Orthop Corr, 123:197, 1977.
37. Panner HJ: A peculiar affectation of the capitellum humeri resembling Calve-Perthes' disease of the hip, Acta Radiol 10(3):234, 1929.
38. Pappas WM: Elbow problems associated with baseball during childhood and adolescence, Clin Orthop 164:30, April 1982.
39. Sain J: Proper pitching techniques. In Zarins, Andrews, and Carson editors: Injuries to the throwing arm, Philadelphia, 1985, WB Saunders Co.
40. Schemmel SP et al: Radiographic changes in the asymptomatic professional baseball player (manuscript in preparation).
41. Schwab GH et al: Biomechanics of elbow instability: the role of the medial collateral ligament, Clin Orthop Corr, 146:42, January/February 1980.
42. Singer KM: Radiographic evaluation of the throwing elbow. In Zarins, Andrews and Carson editors: Injuries to the throwing arm, Philadelphia, 1985, WB Saunders Co.
43. Singer KM and Roy SP: Osteochondrosis of the humeral capitellum, Am J Sports Med 12:351, 1984.
44. Sisto DJ et al: An electromyographic analysis of the elbow in pitching, Am J Sports Med 15(3):211, 1987.
45. Slocum DB: Classification of elbow injuries from baseball pitching, Texas Med 64:48, March 1968.
46. Sweetnam R: Editorial: corticosteroid arthropathy and tendon rupture, J Bone Joint Surg (Br) 51:397, 1969.
47. Tivnon MC, Anzel SH, and Waugh TR: Surgical management of osteochondritis dissecans of the capitellum, Am J Sports Med 4:121, 1976.

48. Tullos HS et al: Adult elbow dislocations: mechanism of instability. In Anderson LD editor: Instructional course lectures, St Louis, 1986, The CV Mosby Co.
49. Tullos HS and King JW: Lesions of the pitching arm in adolescents, JAMA 220:264, 1972.
50. Tullos HS and King JW: Throwing mechanism in sports, Orthop Clin North Am 4(3):709, July, 1973.
51. Wheeler DK and Linscheid RL: Fracture: dislocation of the elbow, Clin Orthop 50, 1967.
52. Wilson FD et al: Valgus extension overload in the pitching elbow, Am J Sports Med 11(2):83, 1983.
53. Woodward AH and Bianco AJ: Osteochondritis dissecans of the elbow, Clin Orthop 110:35, 1975.
54. Woods EW and Tullos HS: Elbow instability and medial epicondyle fractures, Am J Sports Med 5(1):23, 1977.

CHAPTER 36 Tennis Injuries

Robert R. Nirschl

Racquet and throwing sports are common producers of overuse injuries. Tennis, a complex neurophysiologic sport, involves the actions of running, catching, hitting, and throwing in many body segments. Although tennis injuries commonly occur in the upper extremity, the experience at the Virginia Sportsmedicine Institute reveals many tennis-related injuries involving the lower extremities and trunk. In addition, recreational athletes often have preexisting deficiencies or abnormalities, such as arthritic changes and muscular weakness, which are vulnerable to sport abuse.

Overall, our experience reveals a 50% split between upper and lower extremity problems. Lateral tennis elbow; shoulder tendonitis (supraspinatus); medial tennis elbow; ulnar nerve dysfunction (zone 3 medial epicondylar groove compression); and ulnar side wrist problems (triangular fibrocartilage complex [TFCC] and distal radioulnar joint) are the most common in the upper extremity. More common lower extremity problems include ankle sprain; knee maladies (patellofemoral joint, meniscal, and tendonitis problems are most common); lower leg overuse in association with pronated feet (shin splints, plantar fasciitis, Achilles tendonitis, fatigue strain); and muscle tendon strains or pulls (gastrocnemius, Achilles, quadriceps, hamstrings, and thigh adductors). Trunk problems, including abdominal muscle strain, lumbar

Common upper extremity tennis injuries

- Lateral tennis elbow
- Shoulder tendonitis
- Medial tennis elbow
- Ulnar nerve dysfunction
- TFCC injury
- Distal radioulnar joint dysfunction

strain, rhomboid and levator scapular strain, lumbar disk syndrome, and aggravation of cervical and lumbar osteoarthritis, are also not unusual. This chapter is directed to upper extremity problems. In general, lower extremity injury solutions are similar to the treatment protocols used in other running sports, although some variations are needed concerning show wear, conditioning, tennis sport techniques, and equipment.

ETIOLOGY OF SHOULDER AND ELBOW TENDONITIS

Many variables have been suggested or identified concerning tendonitis injury. My observations, and those of others,[10,17,21,22] include the following:

1. Overuse (play exceeding three times per week; poor technique and equipment)
2. Age 35 to 55 most common for tennis elbow and shoulder tendonitis
3. Constitutional factors (mesenchymal syndrome, gout, estrogen deficiency, and hereditary mechanical issues)
4. Inadequate conditioning (lower and upper extremities)
5. Postural deficiencies (thoracic kyphosis with tight shoulder adductors and internal rotators)

Variables contributing to tendonitis

- Overuse
- Age
- Constitutional factors
- Inadequate conditioning
- Postural deficiencies

A survey of teaching tennis professionals reveals that their major frustrations in teaching include students who use tennis as a conditioning tool, poor racquet preparation, and the perception that tennis is primarily an upper body sport.[2,4] These conceptual errors are common injury producers.

PATHOLOGIC CONSIDERATIONS OF SHOULDER TENDONITIS AND LATERAL AND MEDIAL TENNIS ELBOW

Common Misconceptions

The concepts of pathologic change concerning these common tendonitis problems are often misunderstood. In my opinion, traditional surgical approaches have perpetrated continuing confusion.

Lateral Tennis Elbow

The traditional surgical concepts (muscle slide[11] and Bosworth's[5]) concentrate the surgical effort on the extensor aponeurosis, orbicular ligament, and lateral joint soft tissues. Transverse incisions of these tissues have obscured the origin of the extensor brevis, thereby negating accurate identification of pathologic tissue.

Medial Tennis Elbow

Muscle slide by transverse incision obscures pathologic changes in the medial epicondylar origin of the pronator teres and flexor carpi radialis. Excess release also harms normal tissue and increases the potential for valgus instability.

Rotator Cuff Tendonitis

The concept of primary impingement[14] has focused on the size of the coracoacromial arch. Surgical techniques (acromioplasty and release of coracoacromial ligament) have tended to distract from the identification and treatment of the primary pathologic problem in the rotator cuff (usually supraspinatus).

Spectrum of Tendonitis

A diagnosis of tendonitis is not in itself sufficient to organize an adequate treatment plan. The spectrum of pathologic change in tendonitis is substantially varied. The basic pathologic categories for repetitive microtrauma include the following:

1. Inflammation only (changes are reversible to normal tissue)
2. Pathologic alteration: angiofibroblastic degeneration (modifiable but not reversible to normal tissue)
3. Angiofibroblastic degeneration plus rupture
4. Associated changes: (a) fibrosis; (b) soft (hydroxyapatite) calcification; (c) hard (bony exostosis) calcification; (d) iatrogenic cortisone alteration

Tendonitis stages

- Inflammation only
- Pathologic alteration—angiofibroblastic degeneration
- Angiofibroblastic degeneration plus rupture

The basic categories for tendon macrotrauma include (1) partial mechanical dissociation with continuity and (2) complete mechanical dissociation without continuity.

NOTE: Angiofibroblastic degeneration is not noted in sudden violent macrotrauma to an otherwise normal tendon.

It is commonly accepted that the pathologic pattern of chronic tendonitis is etiologically based upon repetitive mechanical microtrauma (tendon dissociation), with the resultant tissue being the product of the healing reaction. Because angiofibroblastic changes are not commonly noted after major macrotrauma (for example, Achilles rupture), other explanations must be sought. In my opinion, angiofibroblastic change is a degenerative process rather than a reparative process. Goldie[8] has previously reported similar changes but did comment upon the process. A likely cause of this degeneration is anoxia and infarct secondary to vascular compromise.[14,23] Rupture through angiofibroblastic tissue with secondary fibrosis is also common. Combinations of mechanical dissociation from macrotrauma and tissue degeneration of microtrauma are also possible; one concept is not mutually exclusive of the other. Overall, however, the common problems referenced (shoulder tendonitis and tennis elbow) are characteristically chronic tendonitis from repetitive microtrauma.

With such a wide variability in the pathologic spectrum, it is quite clear that the treatment plan must be individualized to the specifics of pathologic change for consistent success.

CONCEPTS OF TENDON OVERUSE

The basic mechanical processes of tendon overuse include (1) intrinsic—tendon stress from intrinsically produced tensile forces (primarily repetitive muscle contractile tension); (2) extrinsic—(a) compression (abrasion or impingement) or (b) stretch (secondary to forces outside the musculotendonous unit); and (3) combinations.

Tendonitis common to racquet and throwing sports characteristically occurs by intrinsic overload. In analysis of tennis elbow with reference to tennis mechanics, extrinsic overload is rarely noted.

SECONDARY ROLE OF IMPINGEMENT IN SHOULDER TENDONITIS

In the analysis of the etiology of shoulder tendonitis, the supraspinatus is subject to major repetitive intrinsic overload in the cocking, acceleration, and follow-through phases of the tennis serve and overhead stroke. Young athletes in a variety of other sports, such as swimming and throwing, have similar intrinsic overload. Objective evidence of coracoacromial arch stenosis is commonly lacking, further supporting the observation that intrinsic overload is likely the key factor in the etiology of rotator cuff tendonitis from athletic activities. As reported by Neer,[15] in older age groups subacromial changes may ultimately occur, but in my opinion, this phenomenon is more likely secondary to upward humeral migration with reactionary changes occurring via secondary impingement.

In my observation, tennis-induced shoulder tendonitis most commonly occurs in the supraspinatus tendon by intrinsic overload during the serve and overhead strokes. The primary factors in progressive sequencing appear to be the following:

1. Eccentric loading of the supraspinatus tendon during acceleration and follow-through phases of tennis serve and overhead or throwing motions
2. Fatigue progressing to physiologic weakness
3. Inflammation, vascular compromise, permanent tendon change (angiofibroblastic degeneration), with occasional progression to rupture (partial or complete). (Pathologic change will result in both physiologic and structural weakness.)
4. Loss of humeral head control and upward humeral migration. (NOTE: the rotator cuff is a key stabilizer in humeral head control.)
5. Secondary impingement
6. Subdeltoid bursitis
7. Fibrosis with progression to rupture
8. Humeral greater tuberosity exostosis and/or erosion; subacromial exostosis
9. Acromioclavicular osteoarthritis commonly noted after the fifth decade. (NOTE: Acromioclavicular osteoarthritis may occur independently of rotator tendonitis but is commonly associated.)

In young athletes (in racquet sports, swimming, throwing, etc.) major fibrosis and bony exostosis are the exceptions. In the sixth and seventh decades in recreational athletes, associated subacromial changes occur, but these are still the minority (10%, in my experience). This finding is supported by the classic 1972 report of Neer,[15] in which only 25% of patients were noted to have subacromial changes. Older recreational athletes are more likely to sustain full thickness rotator cull tears; major upward humeral migration is common in this situation.

On the basis of present clinical observations, the concept of primary impingement as advanced by Neer is unlikely in the majority of cases. At most, Bigliani's report[3] on cadaver dissections would support coracoacromial arch compromising acromial variation of 40%. My surgical observation, as indicated, notes a subacromial compromise of approximately 10% (almost always noted after the fifth decade and rarely noted before the fifth decade). Although an occasional patient may have an acromial variant sufficient enough to cause primary impingement, I conclude that the majority of cases of rotator cuff tendonitis (certainly in the younger racquet-sport group) are caused primarily by intrinsic musculotendinous overload, just as in tendonitis of other body areas. This conclusion is also supported by the successful clinical response of the majority of rotator cuff cases to rehabilitative exercise (e.g., a change in the acromial bony anatomy is not achieved by exercise).

DIAGNOSTIC KEYS

The keys to the diagnosis of tendonitis are well recognized by most physicians. Signs of local palpable tenderness and pain upon specific stress to the musculotendinous unit in question are major diagnostic aids. Classic historical onset of pain in anatomic patterns following multiple repetitions solidifies the diagnosis.

Laboratory aids include sonography, magnetic resonance imaging (MRI), computerized axial tomography (CAT) scan, arthrogram, and routine roentgenogram in individualized circumstances.

With reference to the shoulder, the following points seem appropriate.

1. A positive impingement sign does not imply that impingement is the cause of symptoms (e.g., pinching a tender Achilles tendon does not imply that pinching is the causative factor). The clinician should confirm the diagnosis by seeking a positive supraspinatus stress test.

2. The large majority of shoulder tendonitis problems does not reflect full thickness tear. A normal arthrogram therefore does not imply the absence of major pathologic change.

3. Major weakness of surrounding scapular muscles and thoracic muscles is common. Tendonitis and muscle strain of these groups are often present and should be identified.

TREATMENT CONCEPTS

The healing response after injury follows a basic sequence: (1) inflammatory exudation and/or hemorrhage; (2) cellular invasion; (3) collagen and ground substance production; and (4) maturation and strengthening.

The basic concepts for the treatment of tendonitis are designed to control or enhance these aspects of the biologic healing response. Implementation of these concepts takes the following form[6,16,17,19]: (1) relief of pain and inflammation; (2) promotion of healing; (3) promotion of general fitness; (4) control of force loads; and (5) surgery as needed.

Treatment stages

- Relief of pain and inflammation
- Promotion of healing
- Promotion of general fitness
- Control of force loads
- Surgery as needed

These concepts are germane to all sports injuries. Each sport, however, is unique, and the individualized variations in specific implementations are numerous.

Relief of Pain and Inflammation

Our treatment of protocol incorporates the principles of "PRICEMM," which stands for Protection, Rest, Ice, Compression, Elevation, Medication, and Modalities. It is designed to minimize any harmful excesses of inflammatory exudation, hemorrhage, and diminished oxygen perfusion.

It should be noted that rest is defined as absence from abuse, not absence from activity. Antiinflammatory medication is helpful regarding inflammation and exudation, but it does not provide a stimulus for cellular response and maturation and must therefore be used only in the perspective of a larger treatment plan. With reference to the modalities of physical therapy, the most helpful modality in our experience, other than ice and heat, is high voltage electrical stimulation.[18]

Promotion of healing techniques

- Rehabilitative exercise
- High-voltage electrical stimulation
- Central aerobics and general conditioning
- Absence of abuse

Promotion of Healing

The goal in this category is to enhance the proliferative invasion of vascular elements and fibroblasts, followed by collagen deposition and ultimate maturation. This is accomplished by (1) central aerobics and general conditioning exercise and (2) absence from abuse.

The initiation of these programs occurs after inflammation and pain control are secure (usually 1 to 3 weeks for tennis elbow and shoulder tendonitis).

Rehabilitative exercise often involves the use of multiple resistance systems in proper sequence. The concepts of endurance training are used (namely, many repetitions and low resistance). The resistance systems include water, calisthenics, isometrics, isotonics (weight resistance), isoflex (elastic tension cord resistance), and isokinetics (hydraulic resistance).[24]

Each resistance system has its own characteristic and must be properly sequenced for maximal effect (Fig. 36-1).

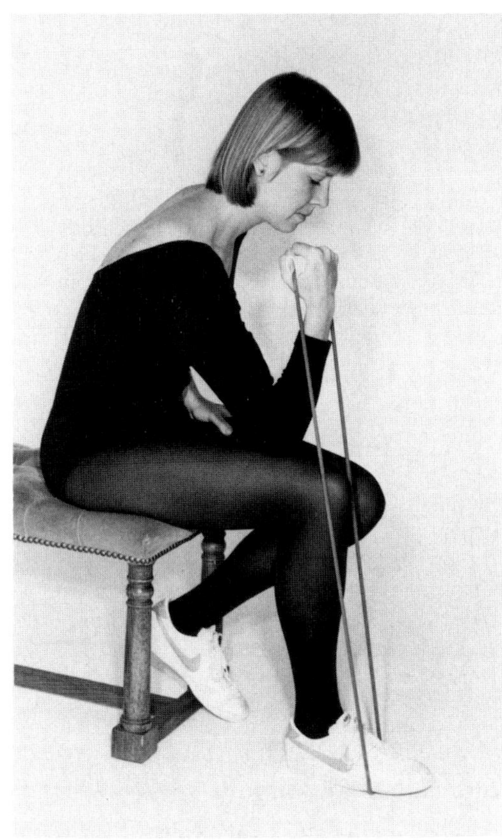

FIG. 36-1 Isoflex muscle resistance exercises. Elastic tension cord exercises. Elastic tension cord exercises of varying resistances in proper sequence with isometric, isotonic, and isokinetic techniques are important to the rehabilitative effort. (From Nirschl R: Muscle and tendon trauma: tennis elbow. In Morrey BF; The elbow and its disorders, Philadelphia, 1985, WB Saunders Co.).

High-voltage electrical stimulation is theorized to reduplicate some aspects of the piezoelectric effect.

Central aerobics exercise increases general blood supply and therefore likely enhances peripheral oxygen perfusion.

General Body Conditioning

General body conditioning offers many advantages in enhancing rehabilitation for specific body-part injury:

1. Central and peripheral aerobics, providing the opportunity for increased regional perfusion
2. Neurophysiologic synergy and overflow, providing neurologic stimulus to injured tissue
3. Minimization of weakness of adjacent uninjured tissue (domino effect)
4. Fat and weight control

It is the goal therefore to offer a maintenance or enhancement program for body fitness and also provide an additional stimulus for the healing of injured tissue.

Control of Force Loads

In addition to tissue improvement, it is highly appropriate to minimize or eliminate potential injury-producing abusive force loads either during rehabilitation, at the time of sports return, or during activities of daily living. The basic concepts for implementation are the following: (1) counter-force bracing; (2) improved sports technique; (3) control of activity duration and frequency; and (4) proper equipment.

Bracing

Counterforce control of intrinsic overload of the elbow and shoulder tendons is appropriate (Fig. 36-2). The counterforce concept of constraining key muscle groups while maintaining muscle balance has proved quite helpful. Elbow counterforce bracing has been noted by Groppel[9] to decrease elbow angular acceleration and decrease EMG muscle activity. Blatz[4] has reported on counterforce bracing of the biceps for shoulder tendonitis. We have also noted some anecdotal success in relief of activity-related rotator cuff pain in some patients.

Improved Sports Technique

Certain activities allow a variety of techniques to accomplish certain goals. In tennis, inadequate techniques serve to concentrate abusive force loads to the upper extremity (especially medial and lateral elbow). Those techniques that place priority on lower body par-

A

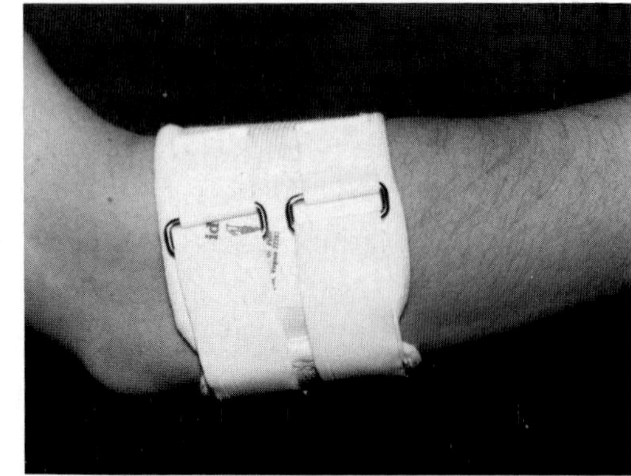

B

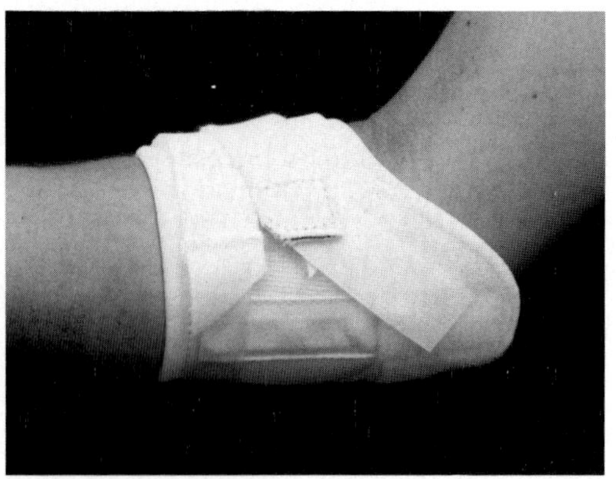

C

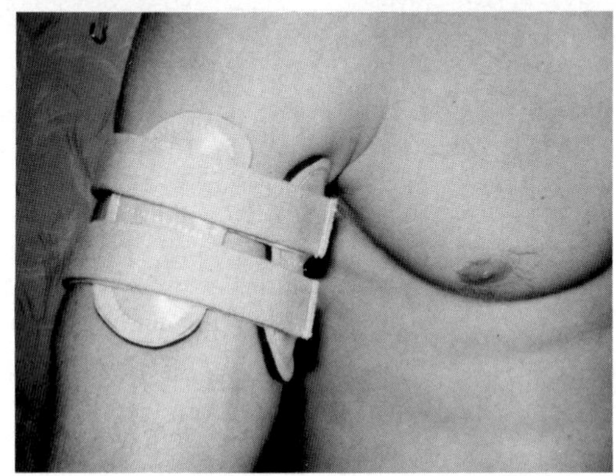

FIG. 36-2 A, Lateral counterforce elbow brace. Counterforce bracing it used to decrease pain and control abusive force overloads. Adequate design includes multiple tension straps and wide bracing for full patient control. Curved contours allow accurate fit to key areas in the conically shaped extremities. **B,** Medial counterforce elbow brace. Medial protection adds extra support for the common flexor origin. **C,** Biceps counterforce brace. Counterforce support of the biceps has subjective relief of activity-related rotator cuff pain in some patients. (Courtesy of Medical Sports Inc., Arlington, VA.)

ticipation have proved to be effective in decreasing the potential for injury (Fig. 36-3 and 36-4).

Control of Intensity and Duration of Activity

Abusive training techniques commonly result in injury.

Equipment

In tennis, the racquet plays a large role in force loads. Much research needs to be done in this area. Present clinical observation suggests that a midsized (90 to 100 square inches of hitting zone) graphite composite lightweight medium flex racquet offers best protection.

Good quality synthetic string with string tension at the racquet manufacturer's recommended low range for the specific racquet in question seems best to control abusive force loads.

Appropriate grip size has been correlated with the hand size. Use of the anthropometric hand measurement of the ring finger described initially by this author in 1973 has worked well[17] (Fig. 36-5).

SURGICAL CONSIDERATIONS

Indications for Surgery

If rehabilitation is unsuccessful or if the damage on clinical evaluation of the acute injury eliminates rehabilitation as a viable approach, surgical intervention is considered. For this topic, shoulder tendonitis and tennis elbow are discussed.

The criteria for surgery for any chronic tendonitis is basically an inability to heal and/or to mature pathologic tissue (for example, an-

A 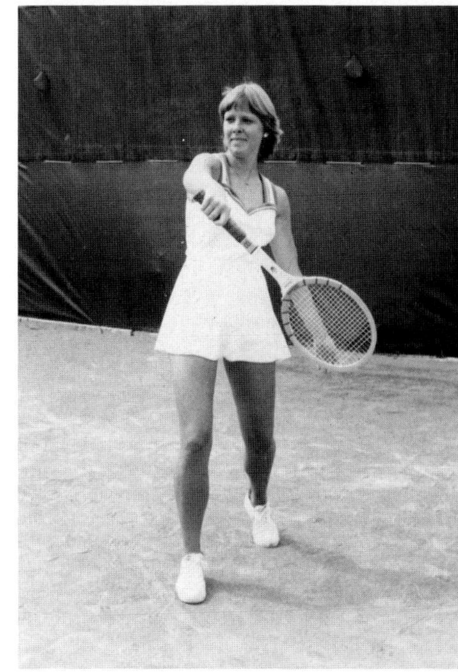  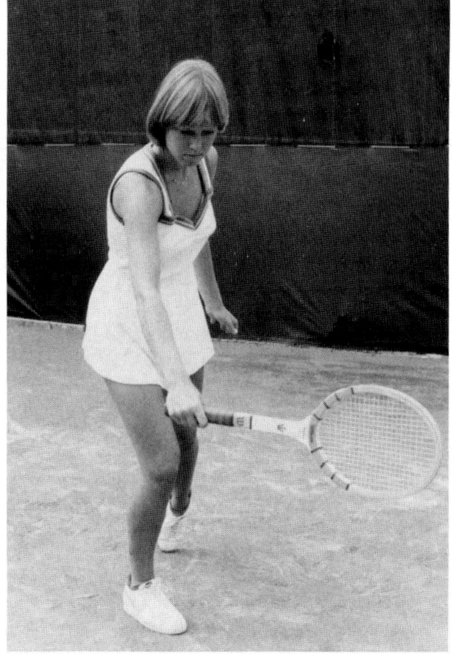 B

FIG. 36-3 Faulty backhand tennis stroke. Poor body weight transfer increases abusive force loads to the vulnerable forearm muscle groups. **B,** Quality backhand tennis stroke. Proper lower body and shoulder action is protective to the forearm muscle groups.

A 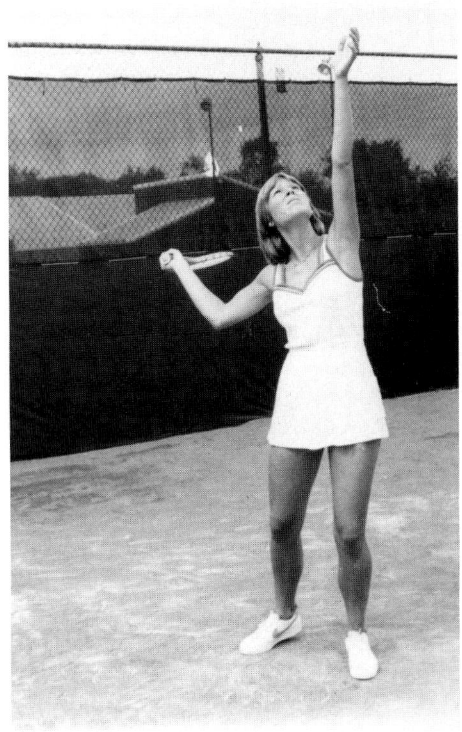 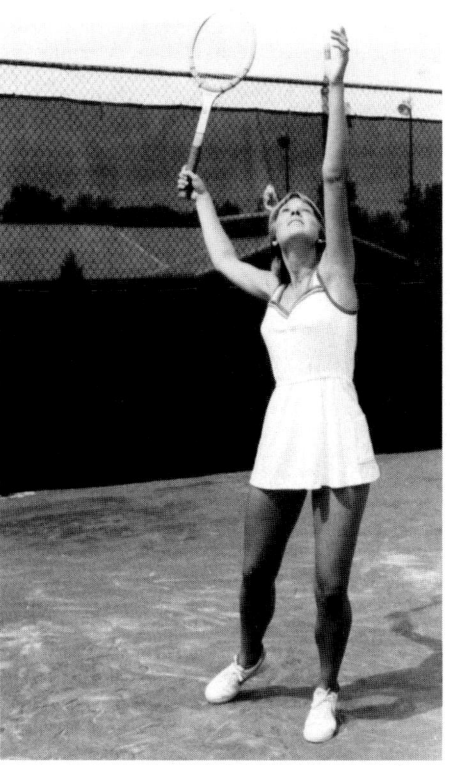 B

FIG. 36-4 Elevated technique to protect shoulder and medial elbow. **A,** The 90-degree-angle position is most derogatory because the shoulder shear forces are greatest in this case. In addition, forces on the medial elbow are greater. Therefore, this position increases the chances of injury to both the shoulder and medial elbow. **B,** High arm elevations are more protective to the shoulder tendon cuff (shoulder scapular elevation releases the tight coracoacromial canal and diminishes rotator cuff shear forces). Higher elevations also diminish medial elbow force load. (From Nirschl R and Sobel J: Tennis elbow prevention and treatment, Arlington, Va., 1989, Medical Sports Publishing.

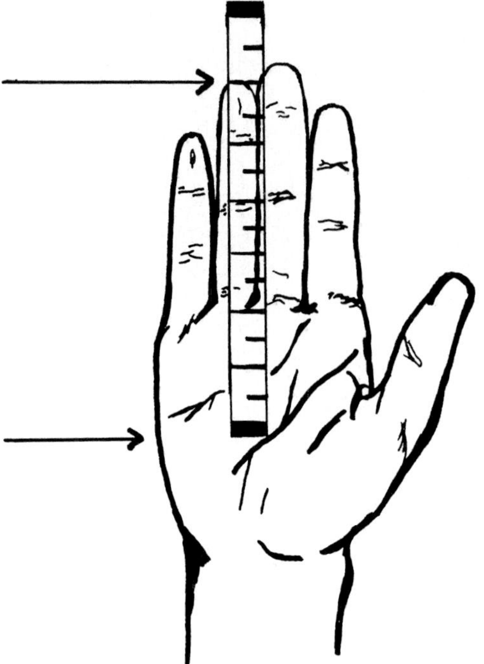

FIG. 36-5 Hand size measurement to determine proper grip handle size. Measurement of the ring finger along the radial border from the proximal palmar crease to the ring finger tip is a good technique for determining proper grip handle size. (From Nirschl RP, and Sobol J: Tennis elbow: prevention and treatment, Arlington, Va, 1989 Medical Sports Publishing.

giofibroblastic degeneration, fibrosis, calcification, iatrogenic cortisone changes, or combinations) by nonsurgical methods. The following are clinical guidelines for surgical selection:

1. Failed quality rehabilitative program. (NOTE: In my observation, most rehabilitative programs are currently of poor quality.)
2. Altered quality of life
3. Constant pain or rest pain
4. Objective laboratory changes (roentgenogram, arthrogram, MRI, sonogram)
5. Persistent weakness, atrophy, and dysfunction

A quality rehabilitation program, of course, includes the concepts of inflammation control, promotion of healing, general conditioning, and control of abusive forces. In most instances, patients referred to the author for surgery have not had a quality rehabilitation program. In these circumstances, a trial of the full rehabilitation program is prescribed before a final consideration for surgery.

In the event surgery is undertaken, the hallmarks of good surgical concept and technique include the following:

1. Identification of the symptoms causing the pathologic change
2. Resection of the pathologic tissue
3. Tendon closure by repair of circumambient adjacent normal tissue
4. Protection of normal tissue (for example, avoidance of excessive tissue dissection)
5. Appropriate postoperative rehabilitation

To implement these principles, specified techniques have been developed.

Concepts of Shoulder Surgery

As noted in the section on secondary role on impingement, my present conclusions are that restoring health to the rotator cuff is the highest priority. Enlarging the coracoacromial arch is appropriate with proper indication but does not ensure healing of the rotator cuff. In my view, the traditional acromioplasty had been unnecessarily punishing to normal structures (e.g., acromion, deltoid, and coracoacromial ligament) without benefit to the stated goal of restoring health to the injured rotator cuff.

Author's Preferred Technique

The concept of individualization of surgery cannot be overemphasized. No one technique will ever suffice for each situation but must be adapted to the findings. The usual basic pathologic findings that I have noted at surgery are the following:

1. Supraspinatus full-thickness angiofibroblastic degeneration occurs just lateral to the bicipital groove, extending from the humeral head greater tuberosity proximally 2 inches. Erosions, calcification, and/or partial-to-complete tendon ruptures are common associated findings.
2. The coracoacromial ligament is invariably normal in appearance.
3. Acromioclavicular (AC) osteoarthritis is present in approximately 75% of patients 50 years and older.
4. Greater tuberosity exostosis and/or erosion is present in approximately 25% of patients 50 years and older.
5. Biceps tendon alteration occurs in approximately 10% of patients after age 50. Biceps rupture is unusual but does occur on occasion.
6. Identifiable subacromial exostosis or an anterior acromial hook variant is present in approximately 10% of patients.
7. Occasional superoanterior labrum tears occur in throwing-sport athletes, but they are uncommon in racquet-sport athletes.

The surgical treatment as noted varies dependent upon the findings. If surgical selection has been correct (via clinical examination, roentgenogram, sonogram, arthrogram, CAT scan, or MRI), the patient will have supraspinatus angiofibroblastic degeneration with or without varying degrees of erosion, fibrosis, and/or rupture. Full-thickness elliptic resection of the pathologic tissue is performed with tendon closure for primary intrinsic overload tendonitis.[18]

In my opinion, the coracoacromial ligament is an important structure, functioning as a passive constraint to upward humeral migration. The ligament is therefore not resected unless major tightness is present or exposure is needed. In the usual situation, the front 30% edge of the coracoacromial ligament is released. Even in those cases of major rotator cuff rupture requiring AC joint resection for exposure or osteoarthritis, some segment of the ligament is often retained.

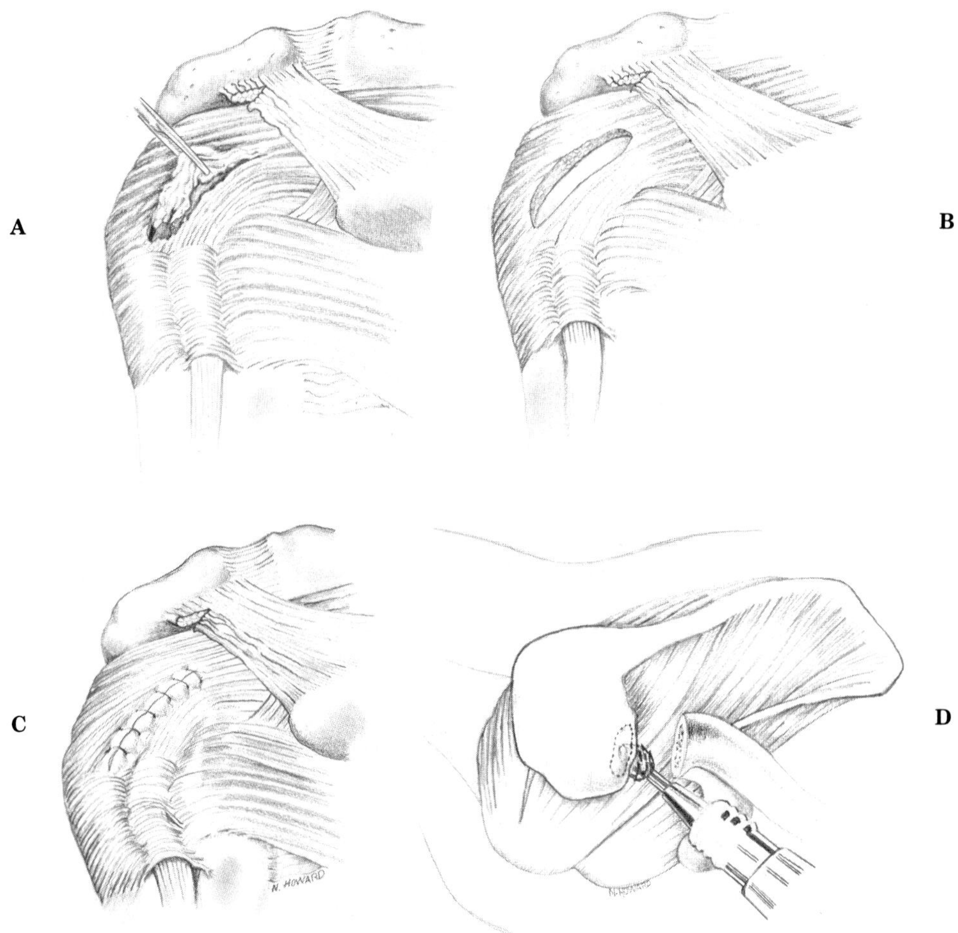

FIG. 36-6. A, Resection and repair of rotator cuff pathology. Shoulder surgery—identification of tendon showing pathologic change. The supraspinatus tendon is typically involved in angiofibroblastic degeneration and fibrosis. Resection of full-thickness degenerative changes (with or without rupture) is important to successful pain relief. **B,** Resection of tendon—partial release of coracoacromial ligament. The angiofibroblastic degeneration is removed by full-thickness elliptic excision. Unless otherwise needed, only the anterior 30% edge of the coracoacromial ligament is released. **C,** The resection defect is repaired with absorbable sutures. **D,** Partial acromioplasty. In those cases in which an objectively demonstrated subacromial spur is present (10% in the author's experience), a horizontal abrasion removal is undertaken. The deltoid origin is preserved. Not all cases require resection of the distal clavicle. (From Nirschl R: Rotator cuff surgery, vol 38, chapter 42. In: Instructional course lectures, American Academy of Orthopedic Surgery, 1989).

To protect normal tissues, such as the deltoid, the incision is placed at the level of the AC joint and directly parallel to the fibers of the deltoid. Under no routine circumstances is the deltoid incised from its origin on the acromion (Fig. 36-6).

If additional pathologic changes are present, these are treated as indicated:

1. Resection of AC joint for osteoarthritis.

2. Resection of greater humeral tuberosity bony exostosis.

3. Resection of pathologic bursal tissue but retention of normal bursal tissue.

4. Removal or smoothing of the underside of acromion by abrasion technique. NOTE: It is unnecessary and, in my opinion, undesirable (via harm to deltoid origin) to use the traditional acromioplasty technique. The traditional technique increases postoperative morbidity and delays rehabilitation. Overall, supplemental surgery for the AC joint greater tuberosity and subdeltoid bursa is relatively common, but the necessity of any type of acromial surgery is 10% or less.

5. Resection of any pathologic segment of the long head of biceps. It is unnecessary to expand the surgery by tethering the biceps in the groove. This concept offers no advantage, increases postoperative morbidity, and delays rehabilitation. If full biceps rupture has previously occurred, only debridement is undertaken unless the circumstance is unusual. Biceps surgery is indicated in approximately 10% of patients.

6. If major rotator cuff rupture is of such magnitude as to compromise repair, an autogenous patch graft (iliotibial band) is indicated. Currently, for rotator cuff tears greater than 3 cm, a patch graft offers increased security of repair and is undertaken.

7. Unrepairable tears. Massive unrepairable tears are debrided only. This offers pain relief, and function (strength, endurance, and active motion arcs) will be compromised to varying degrees. NOTE: Function in these circumstances can, however, be surprisingly good for activities of daily living.

Postoperative Protocol

A typical postoperative protocol is the following:

1. The patient spends 1 day in the hospital.

2. The patient wears a sling for 7 to 10 days.

3. High-voltage electrical stimulation and motion exercise are started 2 to 3 days postoperatively.

4. External rotation beyond neutral is restricted for 4 weeks. All other motions, active and passive, are initiated promptly with respect to patient comfort. Continuous passive motion is commonly used starting 5 to 7 days postoperatively.

5. At 4 weeks, 75% of normal active range is often present.

6. Full functional power return varies, dependent upon findings. Controlled return to tennis is usually initiated at 2 months. If the quality of the remaining tissue is good and the repair is firm, return to racquet sports is usual. Tears that do not allow repair of normal tendon to normal tendon have a diminishing prognosis for return. NOTE: Early results with the autogenous tendon patch graft are encouraging for improved prognosis in those patients who have compromised quality of tendon tissue.

Role of Arthroscopy

Arthroscopy currently offers the greatest opportunity in the diagnostic dilemma of subluxation versus pure tendonitis. This problem is more prevalent in the throwing sports than in the racquet sports.

An arthrogram with a CAT scan appears helpful, but diagnostic confirmation of a superior labrum tear and semidefinitive treatment by arthroscopic debridement offer an additional advantage.[2] Final conclusions at this time, however, would be premature.

The premise of arthroscopic debridement of the coracoacromial arch has been advanced by Ellman.[7] This approach, in my opinion, is flawed by total acceptance of the concept that primary impingement is the key etiologic factor in all cases of rotator cuff tendonitis. There are currently no objective criteria to clinically substantiate the presence of acromial variation or coracoacromial ligament impingement. Appropriate specific indications for this procedure are therefore undeveloped.

In addition, Andrews[1] has pointed out that arthroscopic debridement of the rotator cuff itself is least successful when the identified pathologic change was minimal. This finding is likely related to the technical inability of arthroscopic technique to accurately identify the extent of supraspinatus pathologic change. In my experience, angiofibroblastic degeneration is full thickness, and complete resection should be undertaken for best results. Arthroscopy, however, offers no opportunity for full-thickness resection, repair of defects that occur after resection, or repair of ruptured tendons. The ability to assess the coracoacromial space for true evidence of stenosis is basically nonexistent as well, and all of these recognition factors are further visually compromised by the technical problem of rapid fluid accumulations.

Overall, therefore, arthroscopic technique is limited in its approach to the rotator cuff. Reported success to date with limited debridement may more likely be dependent upon enforced postoperative rest and a high-quality postoperative rehabilitation program. In addition, arthroscopy offers no major rehabilitative advantage over the author's preferred technique of resection and repair.

Further review and refinement of the arthroscopic technique may bring consistent future success if the disadvantages can be eliminated.

Tennis Elbow

The etiologic factors and pathologic changes discussed for shoulder tendonitis are likewise germane to lateral and medial tennis elbow. Intrinsic musculotendinous overload results in the same sequences of pathologic change. The activities of tennis most likely to initiate difficulty are the backhand stroke for the lateral elbow and the serve and/or late forehand stroke for the medial elbow.

The usual pathologic sequences for tendon change are (1) inflammation, (2) progression to angiofibroblastic degeneration, and (3) progression to partial and/or complete rupture.

Tendon degeneration sequence

- Inflammation
- Angiofibroblastic degeneration
- Partial or complete rupture

The tissues most commonly involved in the author's experience are described as follows.

Lateral Tennis Elbow

In patients who had demonstrated pathologic change (98%), the extensor carpi radialis brevis was involved in 100% of cases; the anterior edge extensor aponeurosis (finger extensors) in 35%; the bony exostosis of the lateral epicondyle in 20%; and the radial nerve in less than 1%. Partial rupture of the extensor brevis tendon was noted in approximately 15% of our surgical series. NOTE: Combinations of the above are not unusual.

Medial Tennis Elbow

In patients who had demonstrated pathologic change (93%), the pronator teres and flexor carpi radialis were involved in 100% of our series; and the flexor carpi ulnaris in 10%. Partial rupture of tendons was noted in 3%.

Associated medial elbow abnormalities (surgical cases—racquet sports). Ulnar nerve dysfunction occurred in 60% of our series; medial collateral ligament sprain in 2%; osteocartilaginous loose bodies in 1%; and triceps tendonitis in 1%. NOTE: In baseball pitchers, the associated abnormalities of ulnar nerve dysfunction, medial collateral ligament sprain, osteocartilaginous loose bodies, and triceps tendonitis are statistically higher.*

Author's Surgical Indications

Surgical indications for tennis elbow are similar to those discussed for shoulder tendonitis. Again, the technique must be individualized to the circumstance. The basic concept is to identify pathologic change, resect abnormal tissue, and repair adjacent healthy tissue. Harm to normal structures is avoided (e.g., muscle slides, or orbicular ligament and synovial fringe incision).

Lateral tennis elbow. The incision extends from an inch proximal and just anterior to the lateral epicondyle to the level of the radial head. The interface between the extensor longus and extensor aponeurosis is identified, and a splitting incision is made between. The extensor longus is retracted anteriorly, bringing the extensor brevis origin into view. The brevis origin normally attaches to the underside anterior edge of the aponeurosis distal to the epicondyle, at the anterior ridge of the epicondyle, and to the distal humeral ridge. In the properly selected case, a dull, grayish edematous tissue will be noticed instead of the normal glistening tendon.[20]

This pathologic tissue often encompasses the entire origin of the extensor brevis to the level of the lateral joint line. In approximately 35% of cases, pathologic change will be noticed in the anterior underside of the extensor aponeurosis; this is also removed. If pathologic changes do occur in the extensor aponeurosis, it is unusual to have an area greater than 15% involved. Calcific exostosis of the lateral epicondyle is present in 20% of the cases. If these changes are observed, the anterior aspect of the extensor aponeurosis is partially peeled off the lateral epicondyle, and the bony exostosis is removed.

A small longitudinal opening is routinely made in the synovium anterior to the radial collateral ligament for inspection of the lateral compartment. In the classic case, it is rare

*References 12, 13, 19, 25, 26.

to find any changes in the lateral joint compartment, synovial fringe, or orbicular ligament.

Two or three drill holes are placed through cortical bone to the cancellous level to enhance vascular supply. The extensor brevis maintains some soft tissue attachments at the level of the radial head; thus, minimal brevis retraction takes place. It is therefore unnecessary to suture the remaining brevis to retain proper mechanical length. This finding is pertinent to the retaining of normal strength after healing has occurred (Fig. 36-7).

Medial tennis elbow (author's technique). The surgical concepts of medial tennis elbow are the same as those for the lateral (such as excision of angiofibroblastic pathologic tissue without harm to normal structures). In addition, ulnar nerve dysfunction may be an associated problem, and surgical treatment may be required to resolve this difficulty as well.

The majority of pathologic changes are present in the origin of the pronator teres and flexor carpi radialis close to their attachment to the medial epicondyle.[19] Pathologic change into the flexor carpi ulnaris also occurs occasionally. On rare occasion, rupture into the medial joint with secondary pseudobursal formation has been observed.

The incision is longitudinal, approximately 3 inches in length, and parallels the medial epicondylar groove starting approximately 1 inch proximal and just posterior to the medial epicondyle. Care is taken to avoid a sensory nerve branch just distal and anterior to the epicondyle. A thin muscle layer may mask the pathologic changes underneath. It is important to have a clear understanding of the pa-

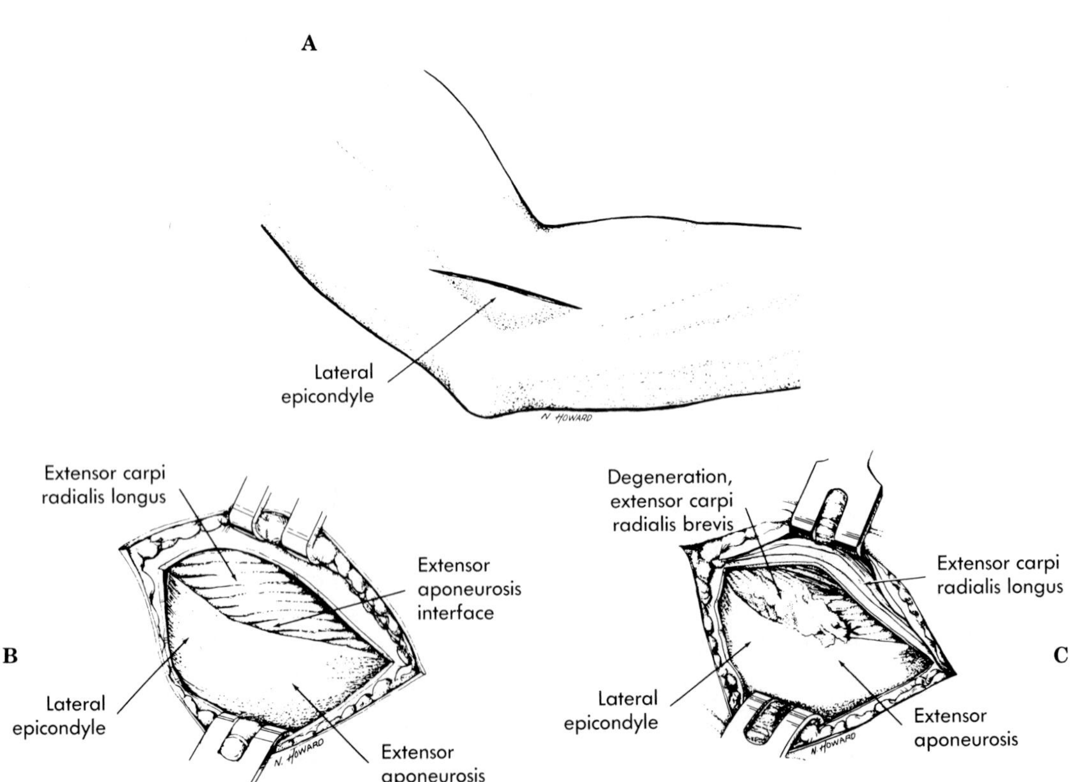

FIG. 36-7. The author's surgical technique for lateral tennis elbow tendonitis. **A,** Incision is slightly anterior to lateral epicondyle and extends from the level of the radial head to 1 inch proximal to the lateral epicondyle. **B,** Interface between extensor carpi radialis longus and extensor aponeurosis is identified. **C,** Extensor carpi radialis longus is retracted anteriorly and origin of extensor carpi radialis brevis comes into view. The normal origin includes some attachment of the brevis to the anterior edge of the extensor aponeurosis as well as the anterior lateral epicondyle and distal anterior lateral condylar ridge. If surgical indications are correct, changes of grayish edematous tendon alteration should be visible without the use of optical assistance.

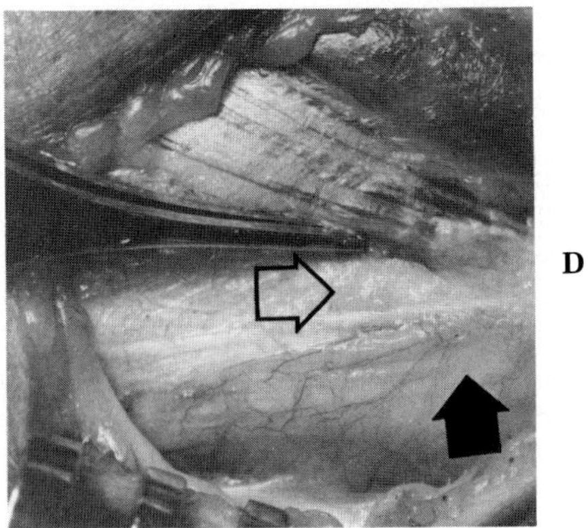

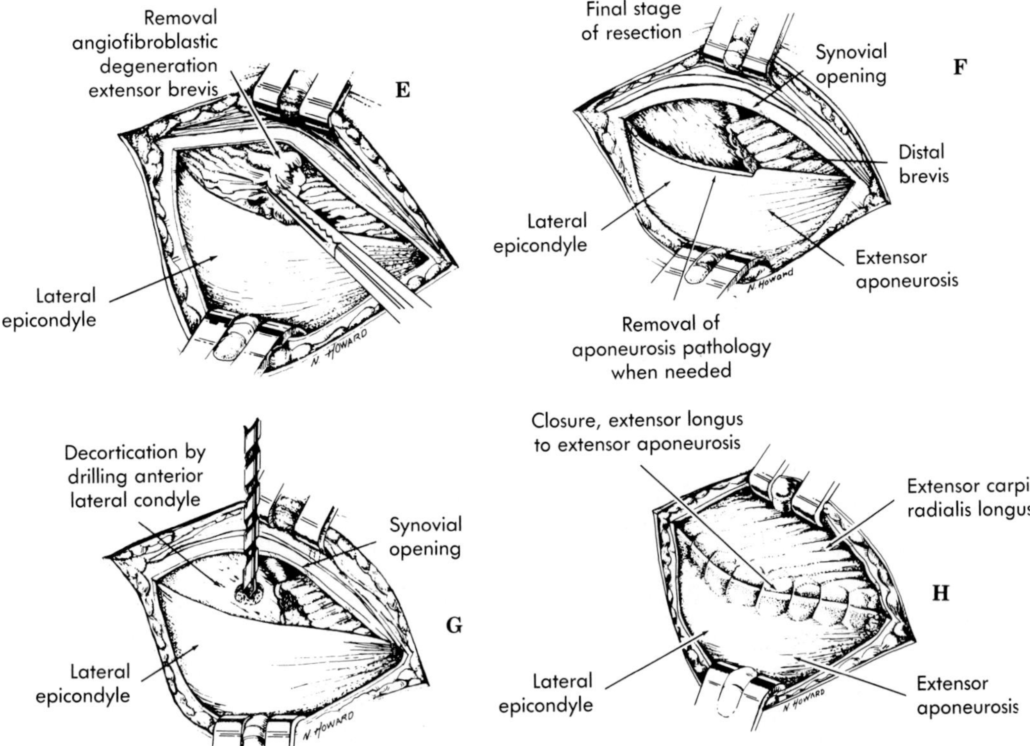

FIG. 36-7, cont'd. D, Gross visual appearance of angiofibroblastic change. Dark arrows identify normal tendon appearance of inferior edge of extensor carpi radialis longus. Open arrow identifies grayish homogeneous changes in extensor brevis characteristic of angiofibroblastic hyperplasia. **E,** Removal of angiofibroblastic degeneration of extensor brevis. In the typical case, the extensor aponeurosis and lateral epicondyle are not disturbed. **F,** Final stage of angiofibroblastic resection. All pathologic tissue is removed. In approximately 35% of cases some alteration is noted in the anterior edge of the extensor aponeurosis. The pathologic change is removed if present. A small opening in the synovium is made to inspect the lateral compartment, but it is rare to identify any pathologic changes. **G,** Vascular enhancement. To enhance vascular supply, three holes are drilled through the cortical bone of the anterior lateral condyle to cancellous bone level. **H,** Repair. The extensor longus is now firmly repaired to the anterior margin of the extensor aponeurosis. Because the extensor brevis is still attached to the underside of the extensor longus, it is unnecessary to suture the distal brevis. Note that a firm attachment of the extensor aponeurosis to the lateral epicondyle is maintained at all times. (From Nirschl R: Prevention and treatment of elbow and shoulder injuries in the tennis player, Clin sports med, 7(2), April 1988.

tient's primary area of tenderness before the anesthetic is given, since this area of tenderness precisely locates the area of pathologic change.

A longitudinal incision is made in the tendon origins at the prime area of tenderness, extending from the medial epicondyle distally for about 2 inches. The tendons are spread, and the lesion will come clearly into view if the surgical indications are correct. All excision of pathologic tissue is performed longitudinally and elliptically, including resection to the joint in the occasional indicated case. All normal tissue attachments of the medial epicondyle are left intact. (CAUTION: The common flexor origin is a key medial stabilizer, and indiscriminate release of normal tendon attachment can lead to medial instability). The resulting elliptic dead space is then closed with absorbable suture (usually 0 to 1 size) (Fig. 36-8).

Ulnar Nerve

So that a logical treatment sequence is established, the medial epicondylar groove is divided into three zones: zone 1, proximal to the

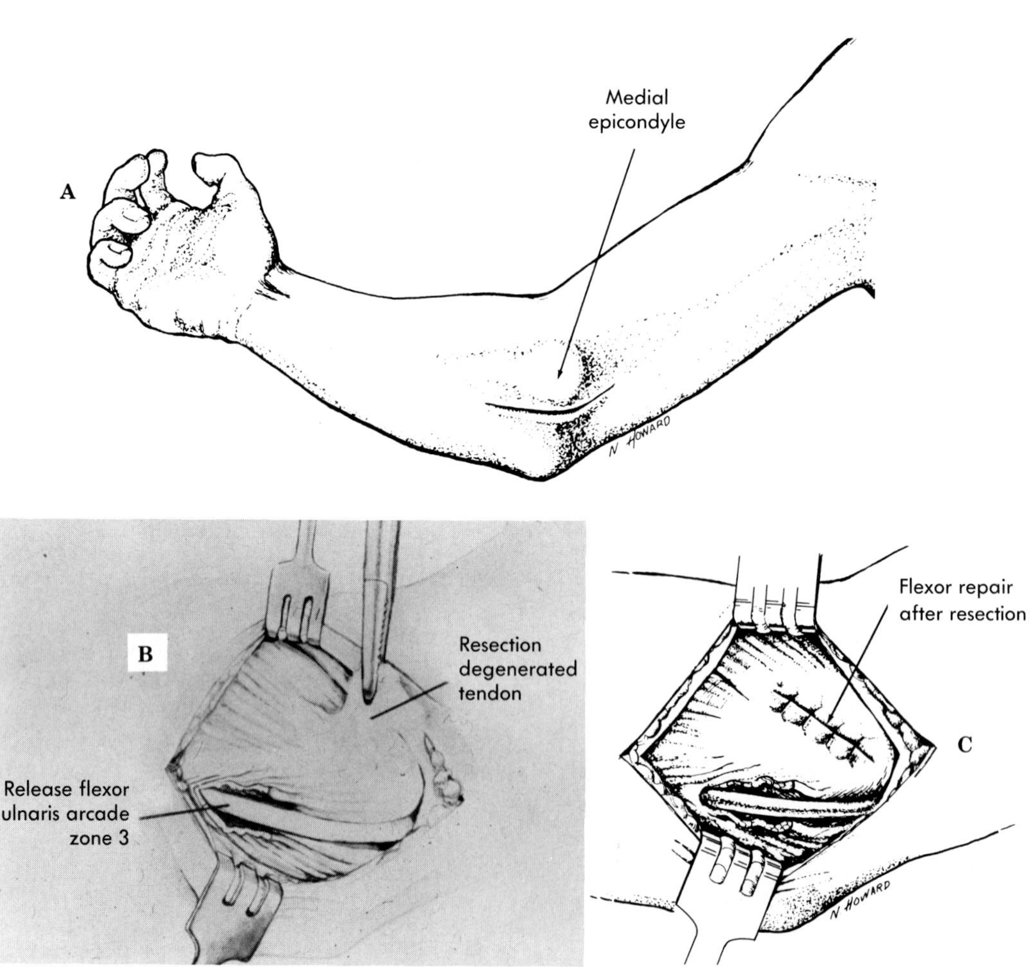

FIG. 36-8. Surgery for medial tennis elbow. **A,** Incision is made as depicted. Care is taken to avoid harm to the sensory cutaneous nerve just anterior to the medial epicondyle. **B,** Resection of angiofibroblastic degeneration. The angiofibroblastic changes are usually in the origin of the pronator teres and flexor carpi radialis. The pathologic tissue is removed in longitudinal and elliptic fashion, leaving attachments of normal tissue intact. If dysfunction of the ulnar nerve has been noted clinically, decompression of the ulnar nerve in zone 3 of the medial epicondylar groove is done. If specific indications for ulnar nerve transfer are present, anterior subcutaneous transfer is undertaken. **C,** Medial epicondylar attachments of normal tissue are not disturbed. (From Nirschl R: Muscle and tendon trauma: tennis elbow. In Morrey BF: The elbow and its disorders, Philadelphia, 1985, WB Saunders Co.)

medial epicondyle; zone 2, at the medial epicondyle; and zone 3, distal to the medial epicondyle.[20] Overall, nerve dysfunction usually occurs by either compression or tension forces. The majority of ulnar nerve symptoms in the racquet sports occurs by compression in zone 3. Compression from osteophytic spurs, loose bodies, or rheumatoid synovitis can occur in zone 2, and zone 1 compression may be caused by a tight medial intermuscular septum.

Tension forces can occur with a subluxating or dislocating ulnar nerve (either congenital, traumatic, or iatrogenic); skeletal valgus (usually from fracture malunion); or medial ligament rupture with secondary dynamic valgus instability (common in throwers). A hostile scar environment from prior disease, trauma, or surgery may result in combinations of compression and tension.

My present indications for anterior ulnar nerve transfer are for dysfunctions, primarily secondary to tension problems, and include the following: (1) nerve subluxation or dislocation from the epicondylar groove; (2) skeletal valgus; (3) dynamic valgus ligamentous instability; (4) unresolvable hostile environment; and (5) necessity of surgical exposure to the medial elbow compartment.

In my experience, 60% of those patients operated upon for medial tennis elbow, in the racquet sports, will have symptoms reflective of ulnar nerve dysfunction. In most instances, the offending problem is compression dysfunction at zone 3 of the medial epicondylar groove. Decompression of this zone by release of the flexor ulnaris arcade will generally resolve the symptoms. If the indications for ulnar nerve transfer are present, transfer is undertaken. The author's preference is anterior subcutaneous transfer with easy relaxed angles. Release of the proximal motor branch with a small amount of flexor ulnaris muscle aids in the attainment of a relaxed angle distally (Fig. 36-9).

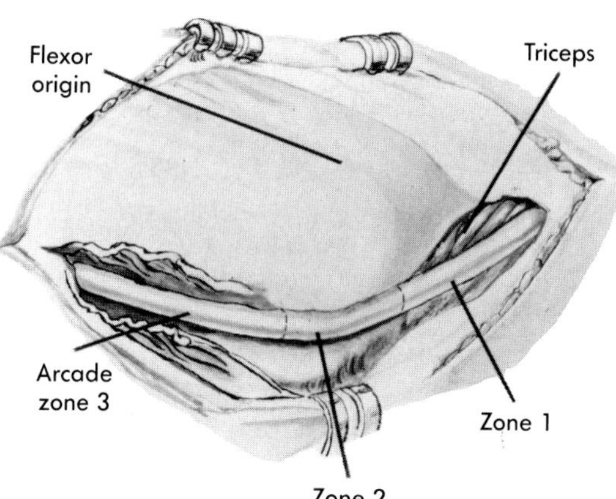

FIG. 36-9. Medial epicondylar ulnar nerve zones. The most common ulnar nerve clinical problem in the racquet-sport athlete is compression in zone 3. Surgical decompression is the treatment of choice in those patients who have specific criteria for ulnar nerve transfer. (From Nirschl R: Muscle and tendon trauma: tennis elbow. In Morrey BF: The elbow and its disorders, Philadelphia, 1985, WB Saunders Co.)

Posterior Tennis Elbow

Triceps tendonitis as an isolated entity is relatively uncommon. It is more often associated with posterior compartment osteoarthritis, osteocartilaginous loose bodies, or lateral tennis elbow. Surgical intervention is quite straightforward, with a longitudinal incision in the triceps tendon usually at or close to its olecranon attachment. Elliptic excision of the angiofibroblastic changes, as in the medial tennis elbow approach, is undertaken.

Postoperative Care

For lateral, medial, and posterior tennis elbow, the postoperative course is similar. The elbow is protected at 90 degrees for 1 week in a counterforce elbow immobilizer. The immobilizer is light and allows active use of the wrist, hand, and shoulder as the patient's tolerance permits (Fig. 36-10).

Postoperative regimen

- Immobilize at 90 degrees for 1 week
- Week 2—begin range of motion work
- Week 3—begin strength work
- Week 6—begin sport technique work

Implementation of limbering exercises for 2 weeks is then followed by strength and endurance resistance exercises, usually starting at 3 weeks after surgery. Strength resistance exercises include isometrics, isotonics, isoflex, and isokinetics in proper sequence and intensity. Resistance exercise is continued until full strength returns. Full strength in the dominant arm is approximately 10% greater than in the nondominant arm in the average person and 20% greater in the competitive racquet and throwing-sport athletes. Usually full strength return on average requires 4½ months for lateral and 5½ months for medial tennis elbow. Although full racquet and throwing-sport competitive activity is not recommended until full strength returns,

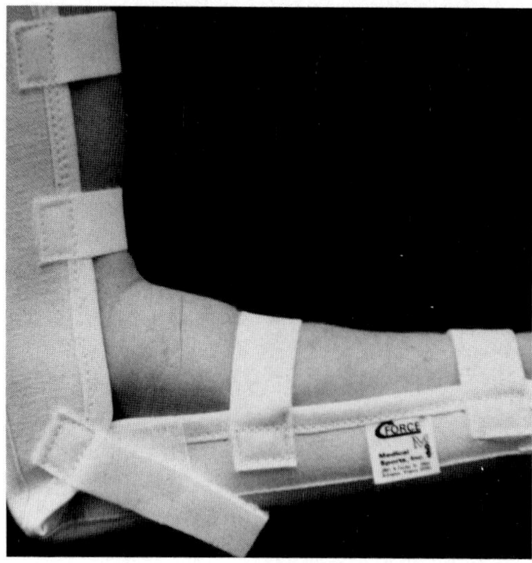

FIG. 36-10. Elbow immobilizer. The Velcro Fastening Elbow Immobilizer increases patient comfort and enhances the rehabilitative effort. (Courtesy of Medical Sports, Inc., Arlington, VA).

modified sport technique patterns are often initiated starting at 6 weeks after surgery.

Results

Our present experience with the described elbow surgical techniques encompasses approximately 500 cases. Of these, 85% experienced complete pain relief, and 12% experience partial pain relief with or without mild strength deficits but improved over the preoperative condition, and 3% of patients experienced no pain relief or strength improvements. None of the failure group were noted to have increased pain or strength deficits secondary to surgery.

Complications have been unusual, with the exception that 0.6% had temporary superficial infection, and 1% of patients have noticed a loss of extension of up to 5 degrees.

SUMMARY

Tennis is both a lower and an upper body sport. This chapter has focused on the upper extremity injuries of shoulder tendonitis and tennis elbow. Trunk and back problems and leg injuries occur in 50% of tennis injuries.

Quality rehabilitation for shoulder tendonitis and tennis elbow tendonitis include relief of pain, promotion of healing, a general fitness program, and control of abusive overloads. If rehabilitation fails and proper indications are present, surgical correction is highly effective for resolution of symptoms and return to tennis.

REFERENCES

1. Andrews JR: Personal communication, February, 1987.
2. Andrews JR, Carson WG, and Ortega K: Arthroscopy of the shoulder: technique and normal anatomy, Am J Sports Med 12:1, 1984.
3. Bigliani L: Analysis of acromial variations, Orthop Trans 10:216, 1986.
4. Blatz D: Personal communication, March, 1986.
5. Bosworth DH: The role of the orbicular ligament in tennis elbow, J Bone Joint Surg 37A:427, 1955.
6. Curwin S, and Stanish WD: Tendonitis: its etiology and treatment, Lexington, Mass. 1984, The Collamore Press.
7. Ellman H: Arthroscopic decompression of the subacromial space. Presented to the annual meeting of the AAOS, San Francisco, January 1987.
8. Goldie I: Epicondylitis lateralis humeri: a pathological study, ACTA Chir Scand (suppl 339) 1964.
9. Groppel J, and Nirschl RP: A biomedical and EMG analysis of the effects of counter-force braces on the tennis player, Am J Sports Med 14:195, 1986.
10. Gruchow HW, and Pelltier D: An epidemiologic study of tennis elbow, Am J Sports Med 7:234, 1979.
11. Hohmann G: Das Wesen und die Behandlung des Sogenannten Tennisellen Bogens, Munch Med Wochenschr 80:250, 1933.
12. Indelicato PA, et al: Correctable elbow lesions in professional baseball players: a review of 25 cases, Am J Sports Med 7:72, 1979.
13. Jobe FW: Thrower problems, Sports Med 78:139, 1979.
14. Mosley HF, and Goldie I: The arterial patterns of the rotator cuff, J Bone Joint Surg 45B:780, 1963.
15. Neer CS: Anterior acromioplasty for the chronic impingement syndrome in the shoulder: a preliminary report, J Bone Joint Surg 54A:41, 1972.
16. Nirschl RP: Tennis elbow, Orthop Clin North Am 4:787, 1973.
17. Nirschl RP: Arm care, Arlington, Va., 1983, Medical Sports Publishing.
18. Nirschl RP: Shoulder tendonitis. In Pettrone FA, editor: AAOS Symposium on Upper Extremity Injuries in Athletes, St. Louis, 1986, The CV Mosby Co.
19. Nirschl RP: Soft-tissue injuries about the elbow, Clin Sports Med 5:637, 1986.
20. Nirschl RP, and Pettrone FA: Tennis elbow: the surgical treatment of lateral epicondylitis, J Bone Joint Surg 61A:832, 1979.
21. Priest JD, Braden J, and Gerbierich JG: The elbow and tennis (Part I), Phys Sport 9(4):80, 1980.
22. Priest JD, Braden J, and Gerbierich JG: The elbow and tennis (Part II), Phys Sport Med 8(1):77, 1980.
23. Rathbun JB, and MacNab T: The microvascular patterns of the rotator cuff, J Bone Joint Surg 52B:540, 1970.
24. Sobel J, and Nirschl RP: Conservative treatment of tennis elbow, Phys Sports Med 9:42, 1981.
25. Wilson FD, et al: Valgus overload in the pitching arm, Am J Sports Med 11(2):83, 1983.
26. Woods GW, Tullos HS, and King JW: The throwing arm: elbow joint injuries, Am J Sports Med 1:43, 1973.

CHAPTER 37 Prevention and Rehabilitation of Racquet Sports Injuries

Janet Sobel
Frank Pettrone
Robert Nirschl

FACTORS IN INJURY

A survey[20] conducted among teaching tennis professionals about their major frustrations with their students revealed a number of factors that these professionals consider as frequent causes of injuries among tennis players. The most commonly observed problems include:

- Students using tennis as a means of achieving cardiovascular and/or musculoskeletal fitness
- "Getting the racquet back too late" as a result of poor timing, poor conditioning, or poor appreciation of the sport's mechanics
- The common misperception of tennis as an upper body sport

Interestingly, it is the same three errors that are among the leading factors contributing to injury in tennis players.

Using Tennis to "Get in Shape"

Tennis, indeed to a greater extent than many other sports, requires full body involvement and is based on a **link system** of force transfer: from the legs, through the trunk, into the arms, to the racquet. Failure or error in timing, strength, or form at any link along the way is likely to set one up for injury to a more distal link in the progression.[9]

So often today people are deciding to start getting into shape, and tennis looks like an attractive avenue. Unfortunately, novices often bring onto the court some combination of old injuries that were never adequately rehabilitated, day-to-day posturally induced muscle weakness and flexibility deficits, poor cardiovascular condition, and a generally slow-moving body. The injuries that result are often products of these inadequacies. Treating upper extremity injuries incurred in raquet sports must therefore involve a close and thorough evaluation of the individual's overall fitness level. An injury prevention program must also address these issues.

Predisposing factors to injury in recreational tennis players

- Previous injury with inadequate rehabilitation
- Day-to-day posturally induced muscle weakness
- Flexibility deficits
- Poor cardiovascular condition

Injury History

All too often, when a patient presents with an arm injury, the focus of attention is the arm and the remainder of the body is neglected. As a result, the real cause is overlooked and goes uncorrected. Then, despite complete rehabilitation of the arm injury, the player is plagued with one injury after another every time he or she returns to playing. For example, an old high school knee injury that was not adequately restored may well throw off the player's timing, agility, and power. The body will compensate to make up for this deficiency during a match, setting up the shoulder, elbow, or wrist for potential injury. Whenever a player has an arm injury, particularly when there is no other apparent etiology the player's injury history needs to be extensively reviewed.

Perception of Tennis as an Upper Body Sport

As previously mentioned, proper tennis mechanics involve using the body as a link system. Quality stroke mechanics in any shot obtain power from quick footwork, knee action from flexion to extension, pelvic rotation, forward weight transfer, and full shoulder motion. Control is derived from hitting with a firm elbow and wrist (Fig. 37-1). Faulty strokes move the lower body minimally and use the arm as the primary power source. When the upper body is repeatedly used for power, it becomes vulnerable to overuse injury. This is the most common form of injury in the arms with tennis.

Components of quality stroke mechanics

- Power from quick footwork
- Knee action from flexion to extension
- Pelvic rotation
- Forward weight transfer
- Full shoulder motion
- Firm elbow and wrist position

Racquet Back Too Late

Getting the racquet back too late is often a result of poor understanding of the mechanics of the sport or slowness in getting to the ball on time. It inevitably results in improper swing techniques: late strokes, using the forearm muscles as the primary power source, and impacting the ball with excessive wrist action.

Heredity and Physical Variables

Some individuals are more likely to sustain overuse injuries, regardless of the quality of

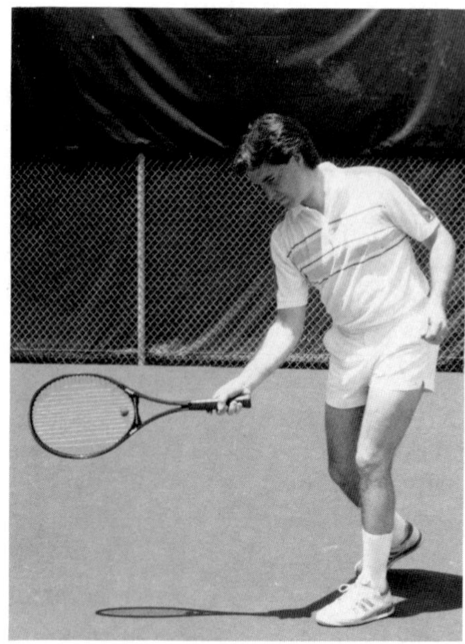

FIG. 37-1. Quality stroke mechanics.

their strokes, based on certain aspects of their physical makeup. These factors, with respect to the upper extremity in the racquet sports, include:

- *Individual variations in anatomic design:* Increased carrying angle at the medial aspect of the elbow is a factor to consider in susceptibility to medial tennis elbow. Acromial slope may be a factor in vulnerability to shoulder rotator cuff tendonitis and wear-and-tear changes.
- *Chemical makeup:* Hormonal variation in women as a result of gynecologic factors (hysterectomy, menopause) may make them more susceptible to tendonitis.[13] Certain individuals' tissue quality is less capable of withstanding higher force loads and less efficient at healing.
- *Age:* Upper extremity injuries are seen with much higher frequency in 35- to 55-year-old players.[16,24]

Postural Considerations

An individual's posture throughout daily activities plays an enormous role in the vulnerability to upper back and shoulder injuries in the racquet sports. The typical desk worker's posture has exaggerated anteroposterior spinal curves, with the head forward. The muscle imbalances that commonly result include weak abdominal and upper back muscles and tight pelvic, lower back, and anterior shoulder muscles.

It becomes virtually impossible for the muscles to overcome their imposed inadequacies when called on to do so during tennis. Tight pelvic muscles will not allow the needed excursion of pelvic rotation and trunk extension. Tightness across the anterior area of the shoulder prevents the needed range for good form in overheads and serves. Weak upper back muscles are inadequate scapula retractors and rotators and often necessitate overload of the arm and forearm to generate power.

If we do not address and correct the poor posture of everyday living when it is seen in a player, we are perpetuating inefficient energy use, unnecessary strain on all body parts, and injury susceptibility.

Equipment and Environment

Certain racquet characteristics play a significant role in the upper extremity injury in tennis. The market has opened up a multitude of options in size, shape, materials, and stringing of tennis racquets. Prevention or rehabilitation of a player's injury should include a discussion of the racquet currently being used by the athlete.

Racquet evaluation should include the following questions:

What racquet are you now using, and how long have you been playing with that racquet?

So often, a player's injury (especially at the elbow) dates to within 1 month after starting to play with a new racquet. Either the racquet itself may not be a good one for the player's arm or the arm cannot adjust to the differences.

Racquet evaluation

- Length of time using racquet
- Racquet material
- Racquet head size
- String tension
- Grip size

What is the racquet material?

Racquet material is not likely to significantly affect the shoulder or wrist. However, the introduction of metal racquets created an epidemic of tennis elbow injuries because of their poor vibration-absorbing nature. In fact, a study of 534 players in China found an incidence of tennis elbow highest with aluminum racquets (62%) or twice as high as with any other material. This same study found one and one-half times the injury rate with medium-weight racquets than with lightweight ones.[24] Graphite and ceramic composites are currently considered to be the best in terms of vibration absorption and thus the most protective against tennis elbow.

What racquet head size are you using?

The oversized racquets have enormous appeal for many older people, beginners, and those who have problems getting to the ball quickly. Unfortunately, this larger head size makes the arm susceptible to injury because of the torque effect on shots hit off-center. The midsize racquet is preferable when considering injury avoidance in the upper extremity.

What is the string tension?

Higher stringing tension generally offers more control but increases the torque and vibration in the arm. Our recommendation for injury prevention is to stay at the lower end of the manufacturer's recommendation.

What is the size of the grip?

It is remarkable how few recreational players know what the measurement of their racquet's grip is or whether it is appropriate for them. They are generally advised by the salesperson to use what is comfortable. Sometimes they will use whatever grip size is available in the racquet they want! The result is

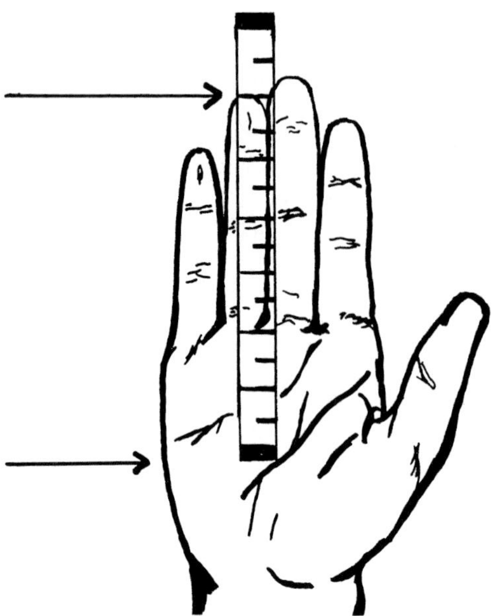

FIG. 37-2. Nirschl technique for proper handle size: measure from proximal palmar crease to the top of the ring finger.

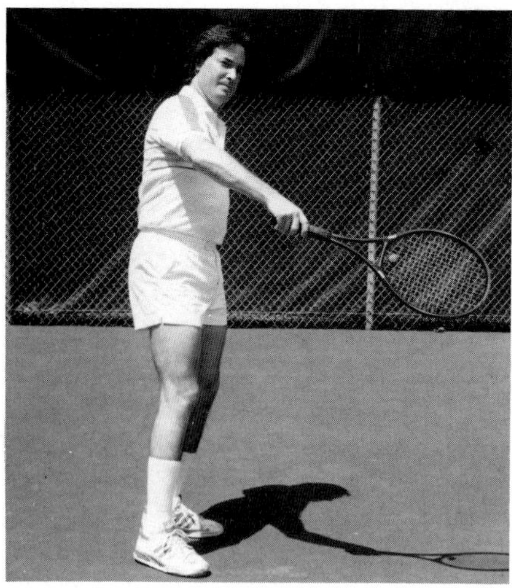

FIG. 37-3. Faulty backhand with the front shoulder up, using forearm muscles for power and excessive wrist action.

unnecessary injuries. A grip too small lessens control and sets the stage for excessive wrist motion. A grip too large puts the wrist muscles at a mechanical disadvantage. A good measure of grip size[15] is given in Fig. 37-2.

At this time, the guidelines for racquet selection for nontournament players in terms of arm protection against abusive force overloads are given in the box below.

Guidelines for racquet selection by nontournament players

- Head size: midsize
- Material: graphite composite (fiberglass, ceramic)
- Handle: leather grip, size as measured
- Weight: well-balanced, light
- Stringing material: synthetic nylon (restring every 6 months)
- String tension: lowest range of manufacturer's recommendation

All the above factors need to be addressed as part of a patient's treatment for an upper extremity injury. Further, to fully evaluate and offer meaningful help to avoid reinjury, we must investigate the possible causative factors in the patient's game. Regardless of the quality or extensiveness of the rehabilitation, reinjury is inevitable if the player repeats the same faulty patterns that created the forces causing the initial injury. Because it is unrealistic for us to get out with every patient and analyze his or her game, we have found it helpful to become familiar with some of the teaching pros in our area who can work with the patient.

■ ■ ■

A brief discussion of the most common tennis injuries and their most likely causes follows.

MECHANISMS OF INJURY

Elbow

Lateral Tennis Elbow

By far the most common upper extremity tennis injury is lateral tennis elbow, an overuse tendonitis of the extensor tendons, primarily the extensor carpi radialis brevis. In the inexperienced player, this is often a result of a faulty backhand, where the ball is hit with the front of the shoulder up and the power source is the forearm muscles (Fig. 37-3). A two-handed backhand is far more protective and should be considered in these players (Fig. 37-4). A late forehand with resulting wrist snap to bring the racquet head to hit the ball is another factor in these players. Highly skilled players are vulnerable to lateral tennis elbow in their serve: the ball is often impacted with full power and speed with the forearm

Biomechanical factors in lateral tennis elbow

- Faulty backhand using wrist extensors for power
- Late forehand with wrist snap
- Serve with forceful forearm pronation and wrist snap

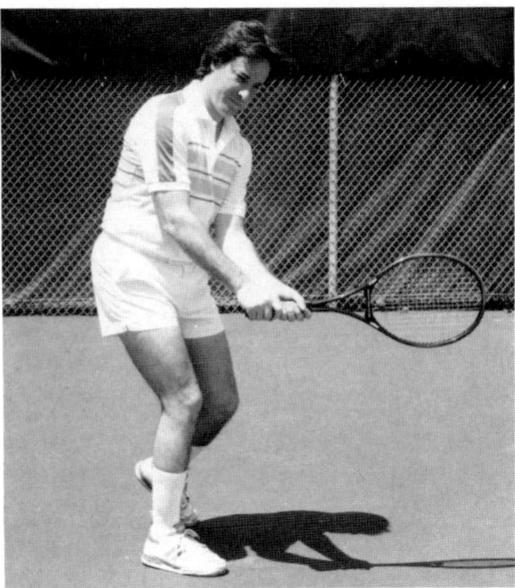

FIG. 37-4. The two-handed backhand is protective of the extensor tendons.

in full pronation and wrist snap, thus increasing the load on the already taut extensor tendons. The frequency and intensity of the tournament level player's schedule enhance the overload effect, because there is often no chance between matches for recovery or rest.

Medial Tennis Elbow

Medial tennis elbow occurs with significantly less frequency in the racquet sports than does lateral tennis elbow. In the experienced player, medial tennis elbow is often a result again of the late forehand with its resultant wrist snap to bring the racquet head forward quickly. These players also may improperly try to impart topspin on the ball by pronating over it, again overloading the medial tissues.

Medial tennis elbow can also result from the quality serve and overhead motions. In the back-scratch position, there is tremendous valgus stress on the medial tissues. These structures are susceptible to injury as the racquet head accelerates upward to impact with pronation and, finally, wrist snap. This combination of valgus stretch, pronation, and wrist snap with the high repetition and intensity of the competitive player may lead to medial overload. Medial tennis elbow may, in some cases, lead to ulnar nerve compression and dysfunction.

Posterior Tennis Elbow

Triceps tendonitis is rare in the racquet sports but may result from sharply extending the elbow excessively, primarily in the serve but sometimes with improper forehand or backhand ground strokes.

Shoulder

Rotator Cuff Tendonitis

The rotator cuff is subject to injury in the well-executed tennis serve and overhead smash and sometimes in the high backhand volley. The rotator cuff is responsible for creating external rotation in the serve and for maintaining the position of the humeral head. In the follow-through, the posterior components of the rotator cuff are eccentrically loaded to decelerate the arm. If the rotator cuff strength is inadequate to handle the load, it may be susceptible to injury. The rotator cuff is vulnerable also in the highly skilled player by virtue of the sport-induced muscle imbalance in and of itself: the strength ratio of external rotators to internal rotators tends to be quite low (65%), and these muscles have difficulty overcoming the powerful upward pull of the deltoid on the humeral head when the arm is raised, or the enormous forces pulling the arm forward in the follow through.

In a serve with inadequate shoulder elevation, the shoulder structures may be subject to excessive friction. The faulty serve is often characterized by inadequate knee and lower back action, the pelvis parallel to the net, a twisting arm, and inadequate arm elevation at impact. The key then to protect the shoulder tissues is high elevation above the horizontal. In the older population, arthritic changes may develop in the shoulder complex. Grinding the soft tissues against these changes by rotation in the range of 90 degrees of abduction can only lead to further problems. It is especially important to check the rotator cuff function in these players, because an inadequate cuff may allow excessive displacement of the humeral head with resultant added wear and tear. A vicious cycle may result:

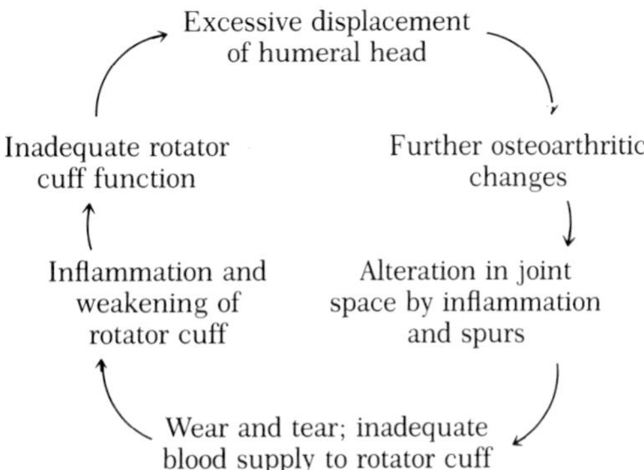

Improving the blood supply and nutrition to the cuff, as well as its strengthening and improved performance, can then help break the cycle and lessen the rate or extent of the changes.

Stretch Injuries

The shoulder and scapular muscles are subject to tension or stretch injuries in the serve or overhead motions. At impact with the ball, the deltoid is pulled to its extreme and overstretch may result in tendonitis as the deltoid is heavily loaded eccentrically and pulls on its insertion at the proximal humerus. The potential cephalad subluxation of the humerus in this position may result in traumatic synovitis after excessive repetition.

Scapula

Bursitis may occur at the inferior angle of the scapula with poor lower body and trunk mechanics in the serve: inadequate pelvic rotation and back movement may lead to excessive shoulder movement in the cocking position, with resultant friction at the bursa.

Forearm

Forearm injuries are rarely seen in the racquet sports and will therefore be considered only briefly. **Pronator teres syndrome,** in which the player complains of volar forearm pain after playing can result from forceful repetitious pronation with tight gripping. Symptoms may involve the median nerve and are reproduced by gripping tightly with resisted pronation from the elbow at 90 degrees to full extension. **Compression of the dorsal branch of the radial nerve** along its path may result in an aching pain over the extensor mass in the proximal aspect of the forearm with possible distal radiation or paresthesias along the radial nerve. The player is likely to experience tenderness approximately four fingerbreadths distal to the lateral epicondyle over the supinator.

Wrist

Wrist **ulnar collateral ligament sprain** may result from exaggerating "laying the wrist back." This is an error beginners often make in taking their instructors too literally. Cocking the wrist back rigidly at ball impact is a weak position for the wrist and allows no pliability for shock absorption, leaving the ulnar collateral ligament vulnerable at ball impact. The quality position puts the wrist at its greatest mechanical advantage. This is the position the wrist is in for a handshake.

Lack of wrist firmness during play can be injurious to the distal aspect of the radioulnar joint, where pronation and supination occur. This may be seen on late forehand ground strokes with a floppy wrist, ending with supination in the follow-through, or with excessive wrist roll, resulting in a synovitis at this joint. Grip size, stroke technique, and forearm muscle strength need to be addressed in players with these problems.

REHABILITATION PRINCIPLES

After upper extremity injury, a comprehensive rehabilitation program includes the following components:

1. Relief of pain and inflammation
2. Protection against abuse in sports and activities of daily living
3. Promotion of healing
4. Rehabilitation exercise to the injured part and conditioning to the adjacent part
5. Maintenance or enhancement of overall fitness level
6. Sport-specific exercise and restoration of functional performance
7. Return to sports

Pain and Inflammation Relief

The hallmark of the phase of pain and inflammation relief is **PRICEM:**

***P*rotect** the injured part against further damage. This implies avoiding motions that stress or compromise the injured tissue.

***R*est** in this context means avoiding further abusive overload, not absence of activity. In fact, we encourage the player to maintain as high an activity level as possible while staying away from those activities that may further aggravate the injured part. Absolute rest (e.g., immobilization) should be avoided if medically reasonable. Although it undoubtedly helps to eliminate abuse, absolute rest also encourages atrophy, deconditions tissue, lessens vascular supply to the area because of reduced demand, and is detrimental to the healing process. To determine the appropriate type and level of activity, pain offers the best guide. Reproducing the pain that prompted seeking medical attention should be interpreted as interfering with the needed "rest" of the injured part.

***I*ce** is indicated as long as the signs of inflammation persist, which may mean throughout all rehabilitation and sports return. It encourages local vasoconstriction, lessens the inflammatory response, slows local metabolism, and helps to relieve pain and muscle spasm through counterirritation and slowed nerve conduction velocity.

***C*ompress and *E*levate** if appropriate to assist venous return and minimize swelling.

***M*edications and *M*odalities:** It has been our experience that a brief early course of antiinflammatory medications in conjunction with therapeutic modalities helps to speed the rehabilitation process.

NOTE: It has also been our experience that an arm that has had several cortisone injections is significantly more difficult to rehabilitate. If at all possible, cortisone injections should be used only with the following guidelines:

Avoid cortisone injection directly into tendon

No more than 3 injections in the same location

The primary indication for injection is when pain is so intense that it compromises compliance with the rehabilitation exercise program and/or significantly compromises activities of daily living, when nonsteriodal, antiinflammatory drugs are ineffective

A 7 day rest period is recommended after injection before resumption of the exercise program.

Modalities

We have found the physical therapy modalities given in the box to be most effective.

Useful modalities for upper extremity injuries

- Electrical stimulation
- Ultrasound
- Ice
- Heat

Electrical stimulation (ES) is effective in pain reduction, enhancing circulation, quieting muscle spasm, and decreasing swelling and inflammation. Continuous stimulation with a high pulse rate (at least 100 pps) for 20 to 40 minutes is recommended for these goals. Electrical stimulation also can be very effective in muscle reeducation and lessening muscle disuse atrophy postoperatively. For these goals, the stimulation parameters would differ. Further, ES may play a role in stimulating the body's biologic healing process by virtue of the electrical current itself. In recent years, several new stimulators have been introduced such as interferential and neuroprobe. As the supportive data on each are sparse, it is up to the users and patients to determine which is most effective for the specific need.

Ultrasound is a deep-heating agent in which sound waves are absorbed by the tissue, producing heat as well as nonthermal effects resulting from a vibration of molecules. It is thought to increase cell membrane permeability, resulting in better transport of metabolic products. It may help enhance connective tissue extensibility by enhancing collagen fiber separation. Ultrasound is thus very good before exercise, because it makes the tissue more susceptible to remodeling by tensile forces. It is also quite effective in managing muscle spasm. It is of questionable value over bony areas because bone picks up sound waves, causing an intense deep pain. Therefore using ultrasound over a bony area is rarely effective, because it is too painful for the athlete to get a therapeutic dosage. Ultrasound should not be used over the growth lines of children and adolescents.

Phonophoresis uses the ultrasound to drive whole molecules of an antiinflammatory medication (usually steroids) through the skin into the inflamed tissues. Great caution must be used if the medium is a steroid, however, because of its potentially dangerous effects. Steroids have been found to lessen collagen and ground substance production and decrease the tensile strength of tendons, and they may lead to failure of weight-bearing tissue under stress. In our opinion, the potential benefits of phonophoresis cannot justify its use in view of these dangers, especially where cortisone injections have already been tried.

Transverse friction massage is considered by many to be an effective way of increasing circulation to tissue and lessening excessive or abnormal scar tissue formation. Here the area is massaged deeply across the direction of its fibers. It can unfortunately be very painful and should probably be saved for situations of chronic tissue damage where the goal is to bring the tissue to an acute, more manageable state.[45] There is no experimental or clinical research available at this time that substantiates the value of transverse friction massage.

Heat applications promote vascular supply to an area and may help with muscle relaxation. In inflamed tissue, however, they are indicated only when heating the part for exercise, because they will otherwise tend to cause further swelling.

The duration of the "rest" period varies, based on the severity and nature of the problem and the individual's needs. All too often, the athlete misinterprets the pain and inflammation relief gained from the rest period as a sign that he or she can return to play and then immediately on return rediscovers the pain. The reason is clear: absence from abusive activity will generally relieve pain. However, steps must be taken to rehabilitate the injured part to restore the quality of the tissue and condition it for the demands of the sport.

Promotion of Healing and Rehabilitative Exercises

We continue to protect against abusive overload and minimize inflammation, often by continuing ice, electrical stimulation, and protective activity, with superimposed rehabilitative exercise. The ice, electrical stimulation, and sometimes antiinflammatory medicines are helpful as needed to minimize pain and inflammation through the exercise period and allow for more effective work on rehabilitative exercises. The goals of these early exercises are to enhance oxygenation and tissue nutrition; to prevent or minimize neurophysiologic reflex inhibition, (thus minimizing unnecessary atrophy), to align collagen fibers along the lines of stress and inhibit excessive scar formation, and to stimulate the joint mechanoreceptors, all while protecting the healing fibers against excess stress or reinjury.[7] These exercises involve very low-intensity, submaximal effort and progress gradually and methodically, primarily based on our knowledge of biologic healing time factors and the patient's pain. As the exercises progress, the goals become reconditioning and restoration of strength, endurance, and flexibility for functional performance.

Several studies in the past 10 years point to the necessity of rehabilitation exercises after injury. A study by Cruchow and Pelletier[5] in 1979 found that tennis players who had not had resistance training had an increased incidence of tennis elbow complaints. Further, tennis players who exercised after tennis elbow had a 31% recurrence versus those who did not exercise, who had a 41% recurrence.

Throughout this effort, we need to address the individual's overall fitness level, including aerobic and anaerobic capacity, coordination and agility, correction of lingering deficits from old injuries, and overall strength, endurance, and flexibility of other body parts. Particular attention should be paid to:

- Strength throughout a flexible range of motion of the gluteals, abdominals, and upper back
- Endurance of the shoulder rotator cuff, forearm, and grip (if not an injured part)
- Correcting quadriceps—hamstrings, ankle dorsiflexion and plantar flexion, hip internal-external rotation, abdominal, lower back, and shoulder internal-external rotator muscle imbalances

It has been our experience that no one form of strengthening exercise can possibly answer all the needs of a quality rehabilitation effort. Thus the exercise program invariably involves overlapping of isometrics, isotonics, rubber tubing exercises (Isoflex), and isokinetics for strengthening and endurance work. Flexibility is generally done manually. Its sequencing and intensity are highly specific to the part of the body and the nature of the tissue. Thus flexibility will be discussed individually with each body part.

Isometrics are helpful early in rehabilitation because they can effectively decrease swelling (through the pumping action of the muscle), they do not irritate the joint because there is no motion, and they prevent neural disassociation (the muscle contractions stimulate the mechanoreceptor system).[8] We begin with multiangle isometrics in limited motion arcs at submaximal intensity, progressing to maximal intensity isometrics in the shortened, middle, and lengthened positions. These can be done throughout the day; a good general guideline is the "rule of 10s": 10 repetitions, 10 seconds hold per repetition, 10 times per day. If a particular angle is painful, it can be worked around, with the patient taking advantage of the overflow of benefits to 15 degrees on either side of the exercise angle.[11]

Midrange isotonics begin on a daily basis with very high repetitions and no weight, progressing to full range and then gradually increasing the weight and decreasing the repetitions, with the eventual goal of a strength training regimen performed two or three times per week. To start, then, the goal is to mold the fiber alignment along the lines of stress and to prepare the damaged tissue to effectively handle the greater loads to come. Such an isotonic program stimulates the body's own biologic healing and allows for early controlled eccentric loading. The advantages of eccentric loading in rehabilitating overuse injuries are (1) it creates less compressive forces across the joint; (2) it may offer greater tendon loading[21]; and (3) it makes the muscles work as they will need to in the sport. Many of the loads to the upper extremity musculotendinous units in the racquet sports are eccentric ones (e.g., the wrist extensors and posterior rotator cuff in the serve). Their inadequacy against the multiple repetitions of eccentric loads throughout their range of motion is a major factor in their high injury rate.

Once the exercises can be done with 1.4 kg (3 pounds), **Isoflex,** or rubber tubing, exercises are initiated and done on alternate days with the isotonics. The progression variables here are the repetitions, range of motion, rate of exercise, and placement of the anchor end of the tubing for resistance intensity. Once slow motion repetitions are mastered, timed high-speed endurance bouts follow. The Isoflex and isotonic programs complement each other well in that we can alternate endurance and strength training. Whereas isotonics generally work best in the muscle's midrange, Isoflex works the end range.

Once good control of the injured part through a reasonable range of motion is demonstrated, **isokinetics** are initiated. The available variables in isokinetic exercises are range, speed, intensity of effort, and duration. We start with short bouts, limited range, and submaximal effort in the middle speeds, working toward full motion arc endurance bouts throughout a velocity spectrum, with emphasis on the higher speeds. These take the best advantage of what isokinetics have to offer: most racquet sport movements occur at higher speeds. In following the SAID (specific adaptation to imposed demands) principle[23] of neurophysiologic patterning, we need to exercise appropriately to prepare for the sport's demands. Higher speed exercise is likely to impose less compression forces on the joint, since fewer fibers can be recruited and thus less torque can be generated.

The principles and techniques of **proprioceptive neuromuscular facilitation (PNF)**[12] are applicable with all of the above forms as well as with the manual resistance of a partner, therapist, or coach. These exercises place specific demands on the neuromuscular mechanism through stimulation of the proprioceptors in order to elicit a specific desired response. Three motion components (flexion-extension, abduction-adduction, and internal-external rotation) combine to form a diagonal pattern: antagonistic movement patterns comprise the two movements of each diagonal. The components are selected to create movement patterns of facilitation that will work muscles from their fully lengthened to their shortened state.[12]

An excellent overall upper body exercise form is cycling with the arms. This can be performed using either a specifically designed upper body exerciser (UBE, Lumex Corp.) or sitting on the floor behind a stationary bicycle, pedaling with the arms. Low-resistance, high-speed endurance bouts or sprint workouts can be developed based on the individual's needs.

Sport-Specific Exercise and Progressive Return

The need for exercises per se is completed once the following criteria are met:

- Full pain-free range of motion
- Strength and endurance tests demonstrate adequate balance of muscles around the joint and normal strength of the injured tissue

Full restoration of strength and mobility is critical before sport-specific exercises and return to play. If strength and mobility are not restored, we can safely assume that the deficits will persist and may predispose the player to future problems. Once rehabilitation is completed, we can address the specific demands of the sport with emphasis on coordinated interaction of antagonists and supporting muscles; agility, skill, and speed drills; and performance training (see the section on an Injury Prevention Program). At this time it is hoped that the preinjured status of the rest of the body has been maintained or enhanced and that deficits elsewhere that may have set the stage for the injury have been effectively addressed. On sports return, the player should be offered some specific guidelines to deal with future problems. A sense of how to interpret the body's warning signals and when and how to respond gives the player some control over minimizing the likelihood of furthering an injury. Using a pain scale such as the following can be helpful[3,14*]:

- Phase I: Soreness after activity, usually gone in 24 hours
- Phase II: Mild soreness and stiffness before activity, which disappears once warmed up; mild soreness after activity
- Phase III: Stiffness before and mild pain during activity but not enough to alter activity
- Phase IV: Pain during play that alters ability to perform
- Phase V: Constant pain, even at rest

Whenever possible, return to sport is controlled by manipulating the variables of duration, frequency, types of strokes, and intensity of competition. By interplaying and progressing these components methodically, any injury-promoting factors can be identified and addressed. The player begins with short bouts on the court, using nonabusive strokes.

---

*Phases I and II are usually self-limiting and will respond to antiinflammatory measures. Phase III requires activity modification and antiinflammatory measures. If ignored, it is likely to worsen. Phases IV and V require medical attention, major activity modifications, and full rehabilitation.

Increasing time on the court is then alternated with introducing more challenging strokes until full-duration play with all strokes is tolerated. Finally, he or she can return to competitive play. The rehabilitation exercises should be continued three times per week through sport return until well after the player is fully back and asymptomatic.

INJURY-SPECIFIC REHABILITATION

Application of the above principles to the most common tennis injuries needs to be highly individualized to what is appropriate for the particular patient's situation. The following discussion presents guidelines based on what has been most successful in our experience and is in no way intended to be a formula. In fact, we are most successful using this only as a basic framework for modifications based on the patient's input and feedback. It is constantly reevaluated and altered to achieve our goals as efficiently and thoroughly as possible; and with each patient the process is different.

Lateral Tennis Elbow

Lateral tennis elbow generally is manifested by extreme tenderness just anterior and distal to the lateral epicondyle (extensor carpi radialis brevis) and weakness and/or pain with stress testing, wrist extension, third finger extension, and grip. Occasionally supination is involved. Symptoms are intensified when testing is done with the elbow straight, because the tissues are further stressed in this position.

Rehabilitation should follow these guidelines:

- Avoid actions or activities of daily living that reproduce the lateral elbow pain. This often includes shaking hands, picking up a coffee cup, and turning a key. In tennis, some players may be able to continue easy hitting but the backhand must be avoided.
- Wear a counterforce brace for any activities that are potentially abusive (e.g., extensive writing or typing, hand shaking, occupational stresses, needlework). The brace is worn during exercises and return to play.
- Heat, electrical stimulation, and ice are the modalities we have found most effective. Usually four to six sessions over 2 or 3 weeks are sufficient.
- Exercises begin with daily repetitions (no weight) of wrist extension, pronation, and supination and elbow flexion within pain-free motion arcs. Full range exercises and weight are added on to tolerance until 1.4 kg (3 pounds) is comfortable, at which time alternate-day Isoflex exercises begin (five repetitions to start). The Isoflex exercises are wrist extension, pronation, supination, and radial and ulnar deviation.
- Instruct the patient to squeeze a tennis ball and open the fingers against the resistance of a rubber band several times throughout the day. These exercises are done first with the elbow bent at the side and progress over time until they can be done with the arm out straight.
- Isokinetics throughout a velocity spectrum rehabilitation program[17] from 60 degrees/second up to 210 degrees/second and then back down to 48 degrees/second. Early 5-second bouts should progress to 30-second bouts.
- Arm cycling and leg work are done for strength and agility.
- Flexibility exercises to the wrist are added last, once the arm is relatively pain free. We have found that early stretching of damaged tendons delays healing and slows the rehabilitative effort. The strength exercises are done through the fullest possible pain-free motion arcs, but flexibility exercises per se are done last.
- Grip testing: the dominant arm should test out approximately 20% to 25% stronger than the nondominant arm. Tests should be done with the elbow bent and straight.
- Isokinetic testing at 60 degrees/second should demonstrate certain relationships:
  - Dominant arm 15% to 25% higher than nondominant (recreational players will show less difference, tournament players more difference)
  - Flexors strongest group, then pronators, then supinators, with extensors weakest; extensors should be 60% to 70% of flexors
  - Supinators should be 80% to 90% of pronators
- Progressive sports return: Following the concepts of a gradual methodical progressive return, a program such as the following is recommended[15]:
  - 15 minutes, forehand only
  - 30 minutes, forehand only
  - 30 minutes, forehand and backhand (two-handed)
  - 45 minutes, forehand and backhand
  - 45 minutes, all strokes
  - Serve
  - Full play
  - Competitive play

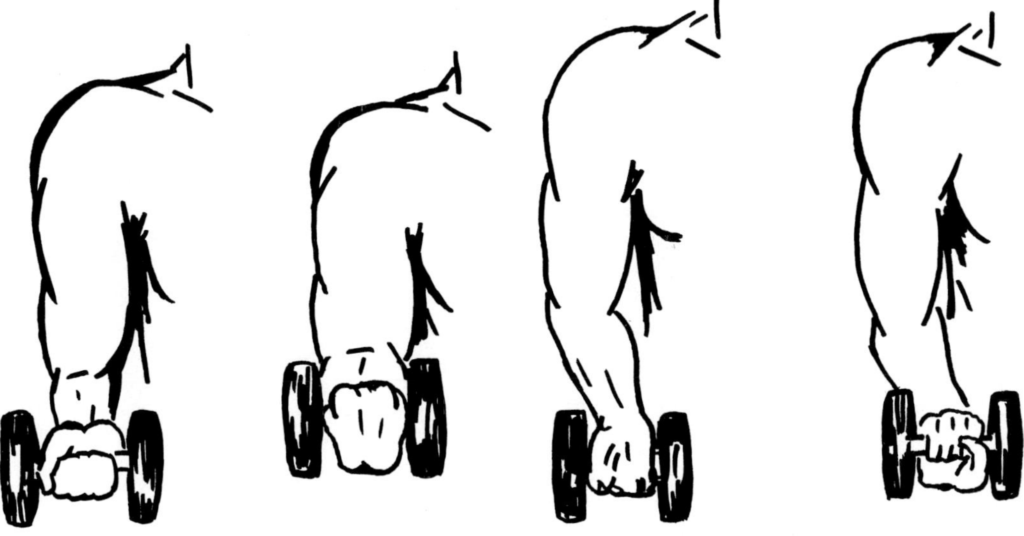

FIG. 37-5. Wrist flexion.

FIG. 37-6. Wrist extension.

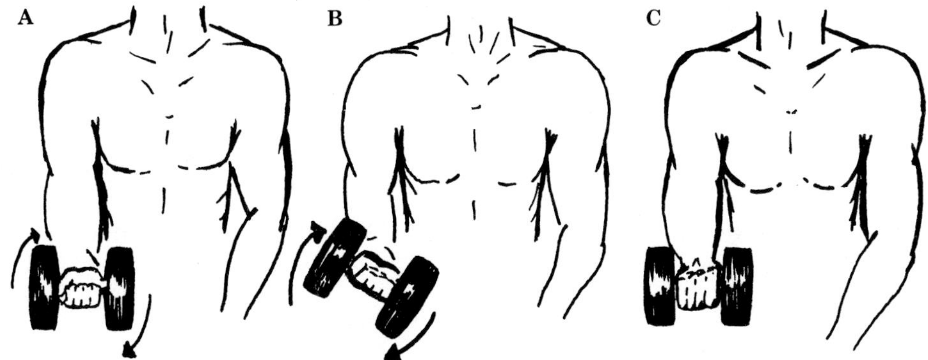

FIG. 37-7. Pronation-supination. **A,** Full supination. **B,** Supinated pronation. **C,** Full pronation.

Medial Tennis Elbow

Medial tennis elbow is manifested by tenderness over the medial epicondyle and may or may not involve ulnar nerve symptoms; as well as pain and/or weakness on wrist flexion, finger flexion, grip, and pronation.

Activities involving tight gripping, strengthening exercises with the wrist fully extended (e.g., Nautilus biceps curls, push-ups), and fly machines should be avoided.

Exercises are as with lateral tennis elbow but include wrist flexion (Figs. 37-5 to 37-9). Sports return should follow a progression such as the following[15]:

15 minutes, backhand and lobs
30 minutes, backhand and lobs
30 minutes, backhand, lobs, and forehand (no topspin)
45 minutes, backhand, lobs, and forehand
45 minutes, all strokes
Serve
Full play
Competition*

Rotator Cuff Tendonitis

Shoulder rotator cuff tendonitis often is manifested by:

Shoulder pain that is aggravated in activities of daily living by lying on that side (thus compromising vascular supply to the supraspinatus)[18]; holding the arm in the 90- to 110-degree range (e.g., driving with arm on back of seat); and hyperextension with internal rotation (e.g., putting on a coat or pulling wallet away).

Visible wasting of the cuff muscles around the scapula as compared with the uninvolved side. Since the injury most commonly occurs in the dominant shoulder, the atrophy is particularly dramatic.

*Late strokes must be avoided throughout.

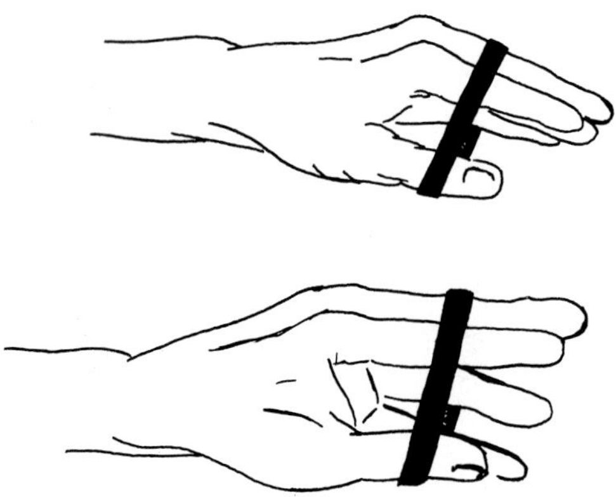

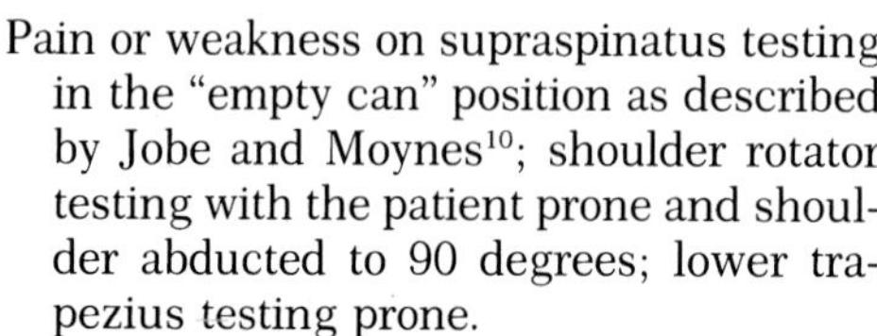

FIG. 37-8. Rubber band for finger extensors.

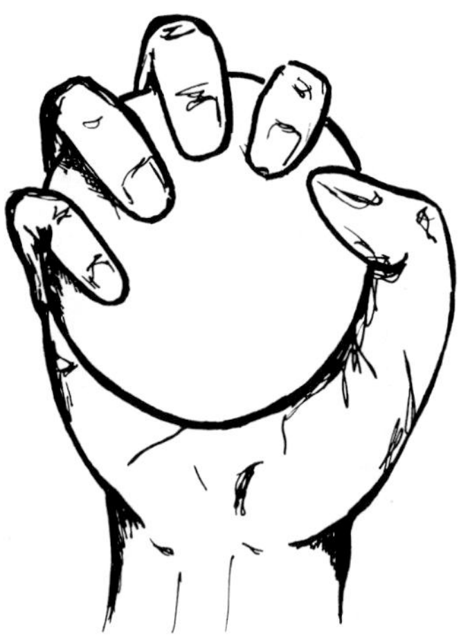

FIG. 37-9. Tennis ball squeeze.

Pain or weakness on supraspinatus testing in the "empty can" position as described by Jobe and Moynes[10]; shoulder rotator testing with the patient prone and shoulder abducted to 90 degrees; lower trapezius testing prone.

The rehabilitation program should include:

Avoiding activities with the arm fully overhead or hyperextended with internal rotation or adducted across the chest at 90 degrees; avoiding sleeping on the involved side.

Electrical stimulation, ultrasound, heat, and ice.

Postural correction: the slumped posture itself tends to collapse the shoulder joint so that there is less freedom of movement. With inflammation present, the effects become even worse, sometimes carrying over to the other tissues. Further, the slumped posture creates a detrimental muscle imbalance as discussed on p. 845. Thus emphasis on good posture throughout the player's day is critical to rotator cuff tendonitis resolution and avoidance of recurrence.

Early flexibility exercises. Unlike with other areas of tendonitis, we begin these immediately to the shoulder, because shoulder flexibility exercises do not stretch (and therefore irritate) the injured tissue. The purpose of these exercises is to maintain full motion arcs for strengthening exercises, to prevent capsular adhesions, and to correct the muscle imbalances of poor posture. These include Codman's pendulum exercises with a cuff weight, PNF diagonals and techniques, gentle mobilization if needed, and passive static and dynamic stretching.

Rehabilitation exercises of the rotator cuff muscles in a protected position. The cuff weaknesses must be corrected first to avoid further abnormal joint mechanics and further damage. Rehabilitation exercises are given in the box on p. 855.

Rehabilitation exercises are done with high repetitions and low weight. Cybex standing internal-external rotations in a modified neutral position of the shoulder (again to avoid wringing out the vascularity to the cuff) are started early in the treatment at submaximal midspeed bouts, progressing to high-speed duration bouts. External rotators' strength must be emphasized because their weakness as a rule is the greatest muscle imbalance at the shoulder and at the same time the demands on them (concentric and eccentric) in swinging are enormous.

Once manual muscle testing of each of the rotator cuff muscles in their independent action is demonstrated, we begin shoulder conditioning exercises that presuppose the integrity of the cuff (e.g., military press, PNF diagonals through increasing motion arcs, triceps press, prone internal-external rotations, prone overhead lifts, and horizontal lifts).

Exercises to strengthen the biceps for their potential role as humeral head depressors.[1]

Exercises to strengthen the upper and lower trapezius and serratus anterior. These upwardly rotate the scapula, thus altering the angle of the glenoid fossa and maintaining optimal deltoid length.

Upper body cycling.

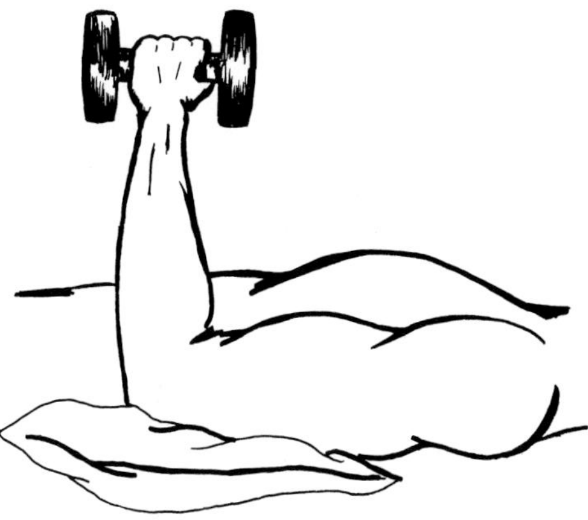

FIG. 37-10. Supine rotation.

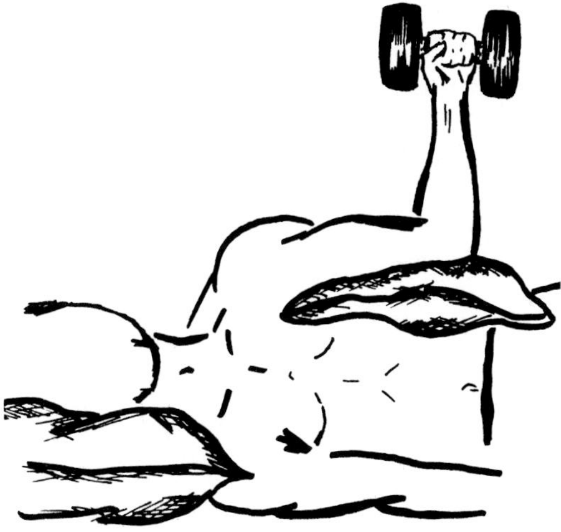

FIG. 37-11. Sidelying external rotation.

Criteria for return to play include:

Full pain-free motion arcs that meet the demands of the sport

An isokinetic test that demonstrates normal strength, normal torque curve shapes, and adequate balance of agonist-antagonist muscle relationships

Graduated return to play with a progression such as[15]:

- 15 minutes, forehands
- 30 minutes, forehand and backhand
- 45 minutes, forehand and backhand
- 45 minutes, all strokes
- Serve
- Full play
- Competition

Technique modifications as needed

Continued ice after play and continuing the exercises on a maintenance program

Basic rehabilitation exercises for rotator cuff muscles

Supine internal rotation (Fig. 37-10)

Exercise benefits:	Subscapularis, infraspinatus, teres minor
Starting position:	Lie on back, involved arm close at side, elbow bent 90 degrees. Support arm on a small pillow or towel roll.
Exercise action:	Slowly rotate arm inward toward abdomen, then slowly rotate back out again.

Sidelying external rotation (Fig. 37-11)

Exercise benefits:	Infraspinatus, teres minor, subscapularis
Starting position:	Lie on good side; hold involved elbow bent to 90 degrees with pillow between arm and side.* Involved hand holds weight on stomach.
Exercise action:	Holding elbow close to side, externally rotate arm so that hand points to ceiling. Hold 2 seconds, and then slowly lower.

Empty can (Fig. 37-12)

Exercise benefits:	Supraspinatus
Starting position:	Sitting or standing, raise arm out to side and forward 30 degrees in front of body (arm parallel to floor). Internally rotate shoulders so that thumb points down as in emptying a can.
Exercise action:	Keeping elbow straight, slowly lower arm to thumb at waist level. Hold 2 seconds, and then raise to starting height.

Prone horizontal abduction (Fig. 37-13)

Exercise benefits:	Rhomboids, middle trapezius, external rotators
Starting position:	Lie on bench on stomach with involved arm hanging to floor, thumb pointing toward ceiling, hand at eye level.†
Exercise action:	Raise arm out to side as high as you can.

*The pillow is necessary to avoid wringing out the vascular supply when the arm is fully internally rotates.[22]
†An electromyographic study done by TA Blackburn Jr et al found this position to elicit the greatest overall activity in the posterior rotator cuff.[2]

INJURY PREVENTION PROGRAM

A supplemental program for any sport is designed to contribute to the prevention of injuries and enhance performance. Many factors need to be addressed in designing a preventive program.

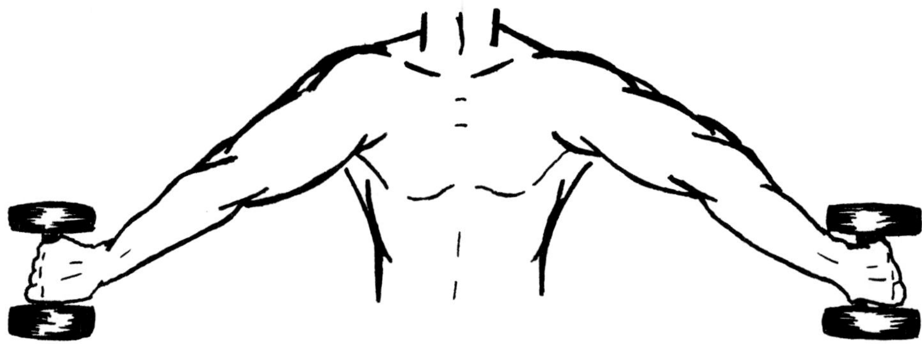

FIG. 37-12. Empty can.

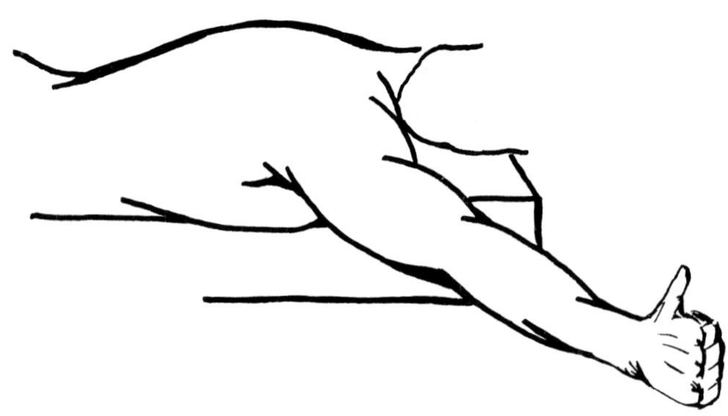

FIG. 37-13. Prone horizontal abduction.

Specificity of Training

Address the specific needs of the individual as determined by injury history, current fitness level, level of sports participation, and specific tests of his or her strength, flexibility, and endurance. Thus sports preparation may well involve any or all of these categories of exercise:

- *Rehabilitative exercise:* to stimulate healing of injured or vulnerable tissue and return it to its normal state
- *Conditioning exercise:* to get in shape, improving the performance ability of a normal body part
- *Sports exercise:* to enhance skill level, with progressive competition

The goal here is to get the player in shape for the sport, that is, to prepare him or her for maximal performance participation and to minimize injury risk.

General Fitness Level

Overcome the imbalances created by the individual's daily activities and fill in the fitness gaps. Never has the significance of well-rounded physical fitness been appreciated as it is now. True physical fitness includes a well-balanced integration of musculoskeletal strength, flexibility, and endurance; neuromuscular and cardiovascular efficiency; good nutrition; and weight control. Unfortunately, no one sport does all this, and supplemental work is needed to create a fully conditioned, healthy athlete. Tennis as a sport encompasses substantial body involvement and therefore promotes reasonably, but not totally, balanced development of muscular strength, flexibility, and endurance. Further, tennis stimulates coordinated eye-hand skills, agility, and reaction times. The effects in the area of cardiovascular and respiratory (aerobic) training are limited, however, because of brief activity bursts separated by long, minimal-activity intervals. Recommended aerobic supplements to choose from are walking, jogging, or running; bicycling; swimming; Nordic track or cross-country skiing; aerobics classes; and rowing. For the athlete to enhance the current level, the chosen activity would have to be done maintaining the target heart rate, four or fives times per week, 30 minutes at a time.

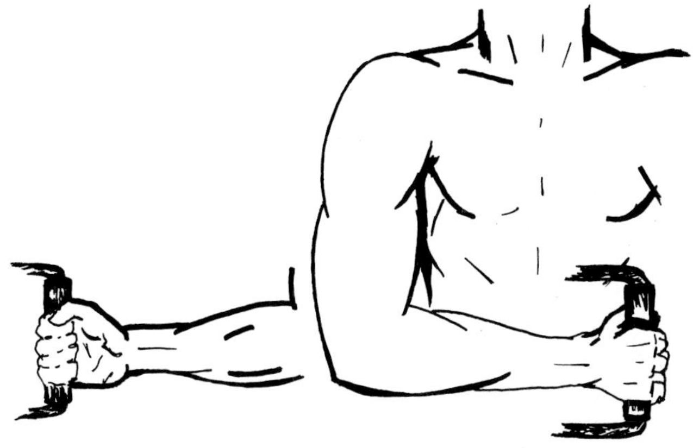

FIG. 37-14. Isoflex, or rubber tubing.

Strength Program

The most common strength deficits in most people are:

- Legs: hip flexors, hamstrings, and groin, especially in their extreme motion limits; ankle dorsiflexors and evertors
- Trunk: Lower and upper abdominals
- Arms: shoulder external rotators and flexors, triceps, wrist extensors, grip

Thus a supplemental strength program for a tennis player should first test the individual for weaknesses in these areas and then include exercises for the following as dictated by their tests:

Gluteals, hamstrings (e.g., curls, crunches, hyperextensions, squats)
Abductors and adductors
Gastrocnemius muscles, dorsiflexors and evertors of the ankle
Abdominals (e.g., bicycle, reverse curls, crunches, crunch-twisting)
Scapular retractors (e.g., rowing, push-ups, horizontal abduction)
Rotator cuff (e.g., internal-external rotations, supraspinatus)
Triceps (e.g., French curl, overhead press)
Wrist extensors
Finger extensors (e.g., work against a rubber band)
Grip (e.g., squeeze a tennis ball)

Guidelines for an isotonic free-weight program would be:

12 to 15 repetitions; increase by 1 kg (2 pounds) once this is comfortable for three consecutive exercise sessions
2 seconds to raise, 2 seconds to hold, 3 seconds to lower
Full motion arcs

For players who travel a lot, we recommend an isoflex, or rubber tubing, program, such as that given in the box (Fig. 37-14).

Flexibility Program

Goals

The goals of flexibility exercises for tennis are[19]:

Injury prevention during sports participation. All the motion demands that may be encountered on the court must be met comfortably beforehand to avoid getting into unmanageable positions while playing. Equally as important is strength throughout the motion extremes.

Overcoming the imbalances imposed by the sport. Tennis is actually one of the better sports in terms of challenging all the body parts in their motion extremes.

Good form. The player with good form avoids compensating for an area of inflexibility with excessive motion in another body part.

Lessening the work effort by the antagonist.

Common flexibility deficits in most people include:

Legs: Gastrocnemius, hamstrings, iliotibial band, soleus, adductors
Trunk: Lower back, pectorals
Arms: Anterior area of shoulder, shoulder flexors, wrist extensors

A recommended flexibility program for anyone should be based on findings on the following tests:

1. Shoulder internal rotators, pectorals
2. Shoulder inferior joint capsule
3. Wrist flexors (should be 90 degrees) and extensors (should be 80 degrees)
4. Hamstrings (These are best tested lying on the back with the hip of the test leg bent 90 degrees so that the thigh is perpendicular to floor. Normal hamstring flexibility allows the knee to be straightened fully so that the whole leg is

Isoflex exercise program

Shoulder external rotation
Exercise benefits: External shoulder rotators (infraspinatus and teres minor)
Starting position: Stand with feet comfortably spread. Hold Isoflex handle in exercise hand, waist high, with loop in other hand on hip.
Exercise action: Keeping exercise elbow at side, place firm tension on Isoflex by pulling handle away from exercise hip with exercise hand. Slowly externally rotate handle outward as far as possible.

Shoulder internal rotation
Exercise benefits: Anterior deltoid, pectoralis, teres major, latissimus dorsi, subscapularis
Starting position: Loop Isoflex around doorknob. Stand to the left of the door. Hold Isoflex handle in right hand just to side of right hip.
Exercise action: Place firm tension on Isoflex by moving further from the doorknob if necessary. Pull handle away from right hip with right hand. Now, slowly internally rotate handle inward as far as possible.

Extensor wrist curl
Exercise benefits: Forearm extensors
Starting position: Sit in chair and place Isoflex under right foot. Hold handle in right hand, palm down. Support forearm on thigh with wrist and hand extended beyond knee.
Exercise action: From wrist-down position, slowly raise hand and bend wrist backward as far as possible.

Flexor wrist curl
Exercise benefits: Forearm flexors
Starting position: Sit in chair and place Isoflex under right foot. Hold handle in right hand, palm up. Support forearm on thigh with wrist and hand extended just beyond knee.
Exercise action: From wrist-back position, slowly curl wrist up.

Trunk twist
Exercise benefits: Quadratus (back flank muscles); oblique abdominals
Starting position: Stand on Isoflex loop with right foot. Hold Isoflex handle in right hand with right arm extended down right side.
Exercise action: Lift Isoflex handle up and out to right side approximately 15 cm (6 inches) while bending from the waist as far to the left as possible. Slowly twist the trunk to the left and backward as far as possible. Hold for 3 seconds. Relax and return to starting position. Repeat to the opposite side.

Back extension
Exercise benefits: Midline, paralumbar muscles; quadratus lumborum
Starting position: Hold Isoflex in front of body so handle is between both feet. Bend forward approximately 90 degrees (less if you are unable to bend to 90 degrees). Grasp either side of loop with hands. NOTE: The lower the loop is grasped, the greater the exercise efficiency.
Exercise action: Holding firmly to Isoflex loop, slowly uncurl back to full starting position. Hold for 3 seconds. Relax and return to starting position.

Hip flexion
Exercise benefits: Iliopsoas, rectus femoris, sartorius; quadriceps
Starting position: Secure Isoflex anchor strap to right ankle with attach zone facing forward. Stand with left foot on Isoflex with handle to outside of foot. Pull right leg forward until mild tension occurs.
Exercise action: Holding knee straight and ankle up, pull right leg forward and up as far as possible.

Ankle plantar flexion
Exercise benefits: Calf muscles
Starting position: Secure Isoflex anchor on right foot with attach zone on the bottom of the foot. Sit on floor with knee straight. Hold Isoflex handle in both hands at waist level.
Exercise action: Pull foot and ankle up as far as possible. Firmly holding Isoflex handle, point toe and ankle down as far as possible.

Ankle dorsiflexion
Exercise benefits: Ankle dorsiflexor
Starting position: Secure Isoflex anchor strap on right foot with the attach zone on top of foot. Place Isoflex loop under chair leg; sit on floor away from chair until mild tension on Isoflex occurs.
Exercise action: Slowly pull toes and ankle up as far as possible.

Flexibility exercise program

- Supine hamstring stretch for hamstring and calf muscles
- Supine hip twist for hip rotators, abductors, lower back
- Alternate knee-to-chest for lower back, gluteals, hip rotators
- Sitting groin stretch for groin, inner thigh
- Sitting figure-4 stretch for hamstrings, lower back, Achilles tendon
- Spinal twist for spinal muscles, hips
- Quadriceps stork stretch for iliopsoas, quadriceps
- Standing adductor stretch for groin
- Trunk side bend for iliotibial band
- Wall stretch for gastrocnemius, soleus
- Pendulum stretch for shoulder
- Triceps overhead stretch
- Horizontal adduction stretch for posterior area of shoulder
- Forearm stretch for wrist flexors and extensors

Dynamic stretches for tennis

- Swing the racquet in controlled but full motion arcs.
- Reach arms up alternately (as if climbing a ladder at the highest rungs).
- Holding a racquet with hands overhead, bend side to side.
- Hold a racquet behind your back with arm fully overhead, elbow fully bent ("back scratch" position as in serve). Racquet handle is held by dominant arm, and nondominant arm grabs the head. Pull the head down, thus stretching the inferior capsule of the dominant arm.
- "Punch" across body with arms at shoulder height.
- In forward-bent position, knees bent and legs wide apart, lunge from side to side.
- Holding a racquet, rotate trunk, twisting side-to-side with arms at shoulder level and then overhead.

Supplemental exercise program

Area for improvement	Exercise
Serve and overheads	Pullover, triceps, French curl, shoulder flexion-extension, rotator cuff
Grip strength and racquet control	Forearm muscles, wrist extensors, tennis ball squeeze
Court movement and acceleration	Quadriceps, gluteals, hamstrings, abductors, adductors, gastrocnemius, soleus, squats

straight and perpendicular to floor.)

5. Hip flexors (Thomas test)
6. Long sitting toe touch for lower back, hamstrings, gastrocnemius, and soleus

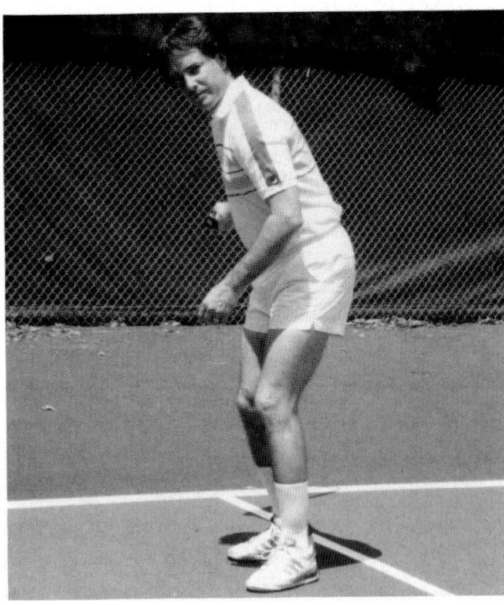

FIG. 37-15. Agility drills.

Exercises

The exercise program given in the box is designed to meet the goals discussed above for tennis. These should be done only after a proper warm-up. It is not necessary to do all the exercises; select those that are appropriate as determined from testing.* In each exercise, the following procedure should be advised:

Stretch as far as you can, going just short of pain.

Then inhale deeply and as you exhale, stretch a bit farther, still without pain.

Hold this fully stretched position for 20 seconds, breathing easily.

Relax.

Repeat this procedure three times for each stretch.

In addition to the static stretching, dynamic stretching (see box) is very effective, after warming up, before playing. In a controlled manner, with exaggerated but flowing motions, the part is actively moved through the

*NOTE: A highly individualized evaluation is essential to determine where functional deficits exist. A number of misconceptions and much time have been wasted from the lack of specificity and vagueness of many exercise programs.

To enhance specific tennis skills, a supplemental exercise program (see box) should include exercises specific to the demands of the sport.[22]

Agility and tennis drills

Agility drills

Run the lines sideways (first within singles, then between doubles lines), touching down at each side.
Jump rope.
Do side-to-side jumps over 20 to 30 cm (8- to 12-inch)
Use balance board.

Tennis drills

Hit the ball, with player and ball staying in the alley (Fig. 37-15).
Practice ball toss alongside a pole, tossing the ball parallel to the pole.
Instructor hits while the player is running forward. Player must split step and go in either direction.

motion extremes. The motions of the sport are mimicked but without the stresses of impact or weight bearing.

Finally, agility and tennis drills (see box) should be included. In general, a teaching tennis professional is the best resource on such drills.

REFERENCES

1. Andrews J: Shoulder arthroscopy, AAOS instructional course lectures, Las Vegas, 1985.
2. Blackburn T et al: Presentation at AAOS sports medicine national meeting, Nashville, 1985.
3. Blazina HE et al: Jumper's knee, Orthop Clin North Am 412:665, 1973.
4. Chamberlain G: Cyriax's friction massage: a review, J Orthop Sports Phys Ther 4(1):16, 1982.
5. Cruchow HW and Pelletier D: An epidemiologic study of tennis elbow, Am J Sports Med 7:234, 1979.
6. Cyriax J: Textbook of orthopaedic medicine, vol 1, Baltimore, 1969, The Williams & Wilkins Co.
7. Davies G: A compendium of isokinetics in clinical usage, LaCrosse, WI, 1984, S & S Publishers.
8. deAndrade JR et al: Joint distension and reflex muscle inhibition in the knee, J Bone Joint Surg 47A:313, 1965.
9. Groppel J: Tennis for advanced players, Champaign, IL, 1984, Human Kinetics Publishers.
10. Jobe F and Moynes D: Delineation of diagnostic criteria and rehabilitation program for rotator cuff injuries, Am J Sports Med 10:336, 1982.
11. Knapik JJ et al: Angular specificity and test mode specificity of isometric and isokinetic strength training, J Orthop Sports Phys Ther, 4:2, 1983.
12. Knott M and Voss D: Proprioceptive neuromuscular facilitation, New York, 1968, Harper & Row, Publishers.
13. Nirschl R: Mesenchymal syndrome, Va Med Monthly 96:659, 1969.
14. Nirschl R: Tennis elbow, Orthop Clin North Am 4(3):787, 1973.
15. Nirschl R: Arm care, Arlington, VA, 1983, Medical Sports Publishing.
16. Nirschl R and Pettrone F: Tennis elbow, J Bone Joint Surg 61A:832, 1979.
17. Quillen WS: Application of isokinetic exercises in rehabilitation, In Davies G: A compendium of isokinetics in clinical usage, LaCrosse, WI, 1984, S & S Publishers.
18. Rathburn J and McNab J: The microvascular pattern of the rotator cuff, J Bone Joint Surg 52B:540, 1970.
19. Sobel J: Supplemental exercises for throwing, swimming, gymnastics: Paper presented at AAOS symposium on upper extremity injuries in athletes, Washington, DC, 1984.
20. Sobel J: Unpublished data, 1987.
21. Stanish W: Tendinitis: its etiology and treatment, Lexington, MA, 1984, Collamore Press.
22. Stone W and Kroll W: Sports conditioning and weight training, ed 2, Boston, 1986, Allyn & Bacon, Inc.
23. Wallis EL and Logan GA: Body conditioning through exercise, Englewood Cliffs, NJ, 1964, Prentice-Hall.
24. Yang and Peng: J Formosan Med Assoc, 1984.

CHAPTER 38 Upper Extremity Gymnastic Injuries

Garron G. Weiker

Since Charles Froland introduced gymnastics to the Harvard College program in 1825, the United States has seen a continued and steady growth of participation in the sport. In recent years, probably because of extensive television coverage of Olympic competition, the number of gymnastic participants has grown in exponential proportions. There are no readily available accurate figures of the number of participants, but conservative estimates[27,32] place the number at well over 500,000 in more than 2,000 private clubs across the nation. In addition, there are many gymnasts participating in high school, intercollegiate, and privately owned membership gyms.

The actual number and distribution of injuries within the sport is not well defined despite the efforts of several authors in recent years.[11,29,33] In club gymnastics, an injury incidence of 11.9/100 participants over the course of a 9-month period was noted. Of these, 12.5% of the overuse problems and 20% of acute injuries involved the upper extremity. More than 50% of the injuries involved the upper extremity in the small number of males seen in this study (Fig. 38-1). A review of women's intercollegiate gymnastics noted an injury rate of 94% (66 of 70 gymnastics-competing seasons) where 20 of the 66 reported injuries involved the upper extremity. Of these 26, 10 involved the supraspinatus tendon, 4 involved the wrist, and 4 involved the elbow.[29] In a study of club-level gymnasts, high school gymnastics programs, and two collegiate programs, there were 39.8 injuries per 100 participants in a gymnastics-competing season. Of these, 31% occurred in the upper extremity. Although these numbers are not sufficient to comfortably define the upper extremity injury problems related to gymnastics, they do indicate a definite problem worthy of consideration by any physician dealing with gymnasts.

Evaluation of gymnastics problems is complicated by the extreme variability of experience and exposure. Male and female competitors participate in different events as well as different numbers of events. The age of participation ranges from 2 to 22, and the level of activity varies from "bouncing babies" programs to elite international competition. Coaching varies from physical education majors assigned to coach school gymnastics to highly qualified full-time professionals. Facilities vary from temporarily assembled mats and equipment to permanent built-in practice and competition areas within the major private clubs.[10] Care of athletes also varies extensively, from programs with affiliated physicians who have a dedicated interest in the

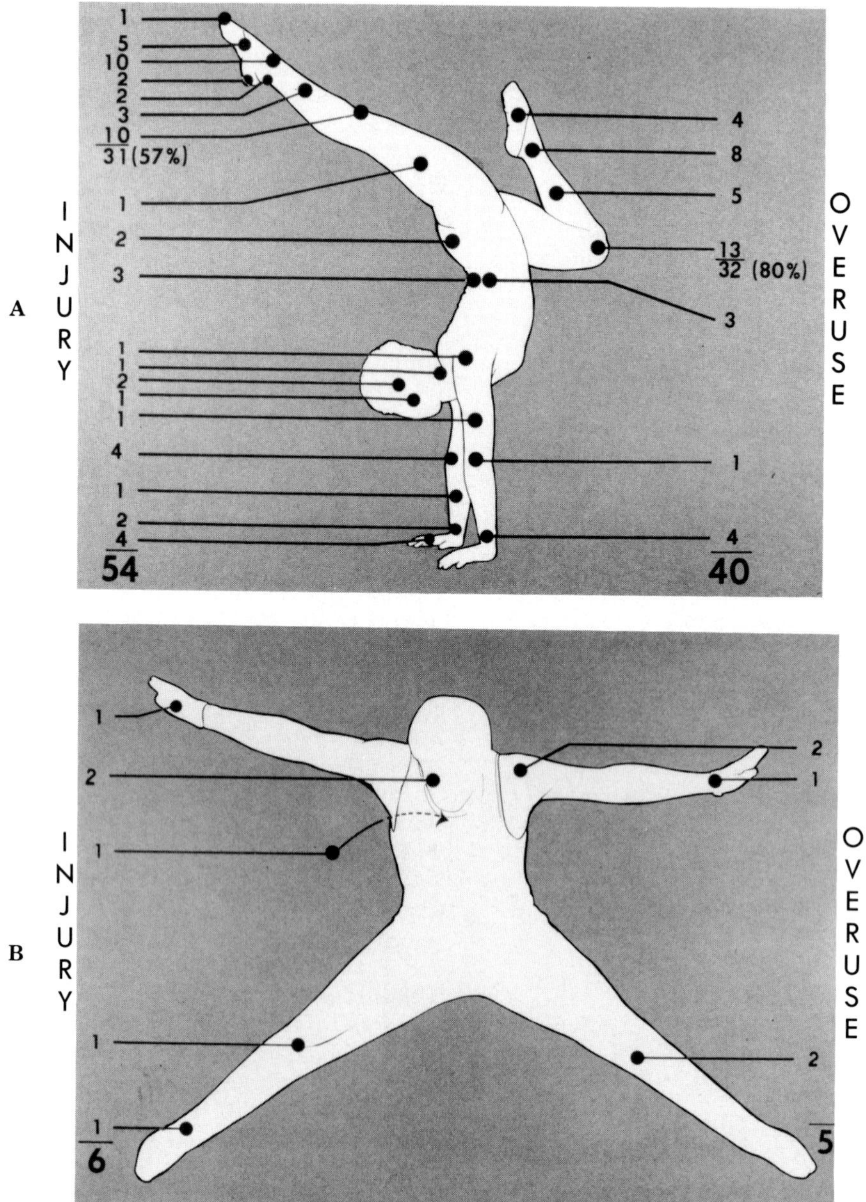

FIG. 38-1. Overuse injuries (on right) and acute injuries (on left) in 9 months of club gymnastics. **A,** Female. **B,** Male. (Reprinted with permission. Weiker GG: Club Gymnastics. Symposium on Gymnastics. Clinics in Sports Med 4(1):39, January 1985.)

sport to programs that have no specific method of dealing with medical problems incurred during gymnastics. Because of these differences, programs have an equally variable injury rate and injury pattern.

The basic mechanical activity of gymnastics is common to all programs despite this wide variation in exposure, risk, and care. Gymnastics requires extensive use of and places high stress on the upper extremity. The combination of strength, flexibility, and speed used in the sport subjects the upper extremity to high tension, impact shock, rotational stress, and compression loads. Weight-bearing compression, with or without associated impact, sets gymnastics apart from all other sports. The unavoidable stresses are accentuated by the effort to maintain graceful poise. Hyperextension of the elbow in various pose positions is considered an integral part of gymnastics (Fig. 38-2).

Acute injuries to the upper extremity are well documented in many sports but, as noted by Matheson,[18] stress fractures and other overuse injuries are rare with the exception of specific entities such as little league elbow and shoulder. Contrary to that general pattern in sporting activities, gymnasts do develop overuse injuries of the upper extremity.*

Although gymnastics does inherently place the upper extremity at risk, it is apparent that training techniques and facilities also play a part in the incidence of injury. Any physician dealing with gymnasts would be wise to review the Gymnastics Safety Manual[36] and the articles by Ganim[10] and Aronen[2]. Proper attention to flexibility, strength, training, and coaching techniques, as well as selection, placement, and maintenance of equipment, plays a role in determining the incidence of problems.

---

*References 2, 5, 8, 11, 17, 21, 22, 24, 25, 26, 27, 31, 33, 37.

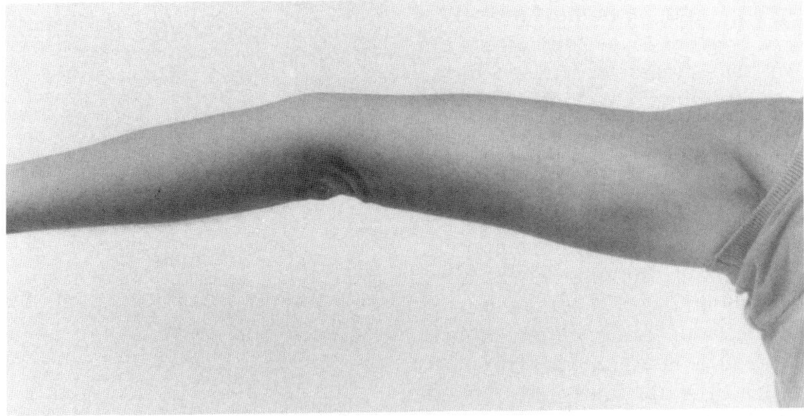

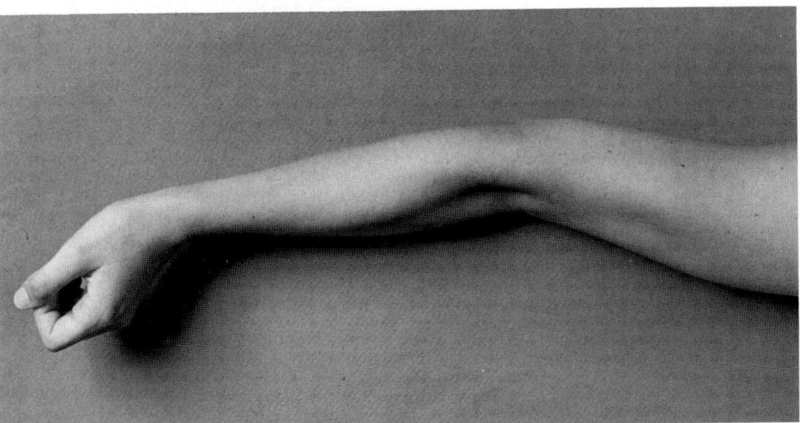

FIG. 38-2. Examples of physiologic hyperextension of the elbows in two gymnasts.

Factors in gymnastics injuries

- Flexibility
- Strength training
- Coaching technique
- Equipment
  - Selection
  - Placement
  - Maintenance

SHOULDER

Problems in the gymnast's shoulder are more frequently related to overuse than to acute injury and are more often encountered in male competitors. This disparity is probably related to the difference in females' flexibility, gymnastics apparatus, and techniques. Women's events are primarily developed to demonstrate grace, rhythm, flexibility, and balance, but the majority of men's events are designed to emphasize power and strength. Maneuvers such as the iron cross, repetitive dislocates on rings, giant swings on the high bar, and programs on the pummel horse, parallel bars, and floor all place high stress on the male gymnast's shoulders. The accentuation of flexibility training in young females who are inherently loose jointed does increase the risk of chronic instability problems in the female gymnast.

As with most overuse syndromes, chronic problems in the gymnast's shoulder may be traced to overtraining, improper technique, inadequate conditioning, inadequate warm-up, inherent anatomic abnormalities, or lack of rehabilitation after acute injury. The most common causes of acute injury are missed moves, falls from the apparatus, and inadvertent contact with apparatus, people, or stationary objects.

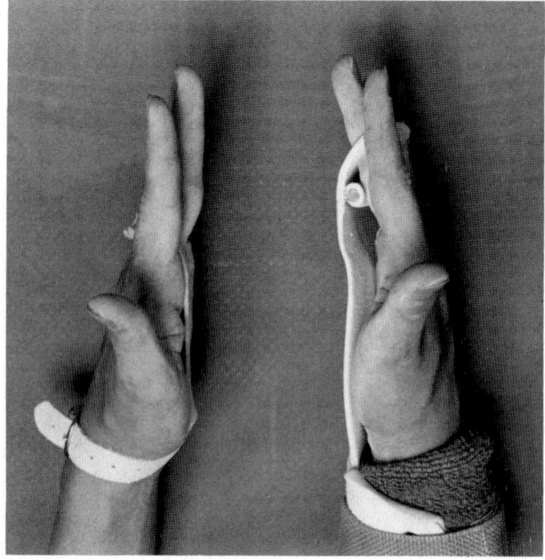

FIG. 38-3. Profile view of traditional grip on left and the doweled grip on the right.

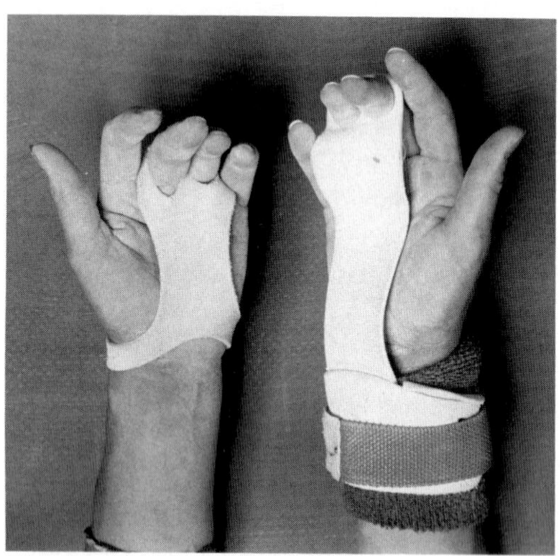

FIG. 38-4. Palmar view of traditional grip on left and the doweled grip on the right.

Overuse injury etiologies

- Over-training
- Improper technique
- Inadequate conditioning
- Inadequate warm-up
- Anatomic abnormalities
- Rehabilitation deficiencies following acute injury

An aspect of the sport that is in a state of flux at this time is repetitive giant swings, which place stress on the shoulder. Use of this maneuver was relatively limited until the advent of the doweled grip, which allows a much better grip. The increased grip enables the gymnast to perform higher-velocity and more frequent giant swings as well as other swinging maneuvers. This problem has primarily been related to male gymnasts, since the doweled grip was used only by them until recently. Presently female gymnasts are making the transition to the doweled grip on uneven parallel bars, and we can anticipate an increase of shoulder stress phenomena among female gymnasts (Fig. 38-3, 38-4, 38-5).

Overuse Problems

Impingement Syndrome

Impingement syndrome is an area fraught with great confusion in the orthopaedic lit-

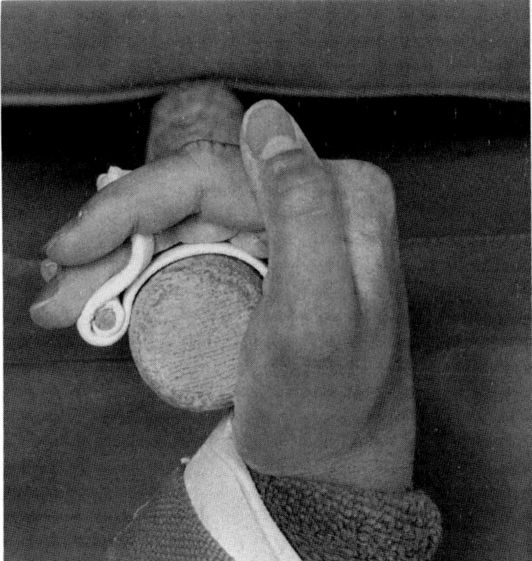

FIG. 38-5. Staged view showing the additional gripping power that the dowel offers.

erature today. There are multiple tests that diagnose the syndrome, multiple explanations of its causes and pathophysiology, and therefore, multiple suggestions for treatment. The confusion is caused by attempting to find an acceptable definition and explanation that crosses all barriers. The impingement syndrome seen in the 50-year-old nonathletic individual (with a pathologic condition of the rotator cuff and pain on shoulder abduction) is not necessarily the same entity seen in the 14-year-old athlete (with pain on flexion of the internally rotated shoulder). It is possible that a thrower's shoulder (with supraspinatus tendon pain in 30 degrees flexion and resisted external rotation)[13] is an entirely separate entity.

Despite this controversy, we do see a specific entity in gymnasts that is commonly referred to as impingement syndrome. The general complaint is pain on forward flexion with neutral or internal rotation. The athlete classically has pain when swinging on the bars or rings and in certain positions of handstands. The classic presentation is discomfort initially noted after activities and eventually noted throughout and after activity. To date I have seen no associated rotator cuff tears or irreversible lesions. It appears that athletes with impingement syndrome are incapacitated early enough with typical stage I edema, inflammation, and pain that they seek medical help. The use of nonsteroidal antiinflammatory medication in conjunction with activity modification and rehabilitation has proved effective.

Stage I impingement treatment

- Nonsteroidal antiinflammatory medication
- Activity modification
- Rehabilitation

The gymnast is initially withheld only from practicing the events that are causing primary difficulty. During that first 2-week period he or she performs a range of motion exercise program in all parameters and a strengthening program designed primarily to balance the shoulder musculature. Each program is individually tailored after examination and is designed to accentuate any areas of detectable weakness. When the gymnast returns to the gym the only modification that has proved necessary is to slightly widen the hand placement on the bars, vaulting horse, floor, and beam.

Biceps Tendonitis and Subluxation

Although biceps tendonitis may overlap with impingement syndrome, it is occasionally seen as a specific entity in the male gymnast. The athlete complains of pain in the anterior aspect of the shoulder and on examination has tenderness over the biceps groove, a positive Speed test, and negative impingement tests. A subluxing biceps tendon presents as the sensation of something moving within the shoulder during dislocates and power moves on the rings, pommel horse, and/or parallel bars. The localizing signs are over the biceps tendon, and arthrography occasionally shows a shallow bicipital groove with redundancy of the overlying sheath.

In both biceps tendonitis and subluxation, it appears that faulty technique and inadequate musculature are the primary cause. To date these patients have uniformly responded to conservative rehabilitation efforts; therefore surgical intervention has not been necessary. A program of rest, ice, nonsteroidal antiinflammatory medication, and range of motion/strengthening exercises has proved effective.[2,13,14]

Chronic Instability

Performing the desired gymnastic maneuvers accentuates hypermobility of the shoulders, allowing the full spectrum of instabilities to be seen. As with other athletes, in gymnasts the most frequent instability is anterior subluxation and the most frustrating is the multidirectional instability seen in loose-jointed females. The natural selection of physiologi-

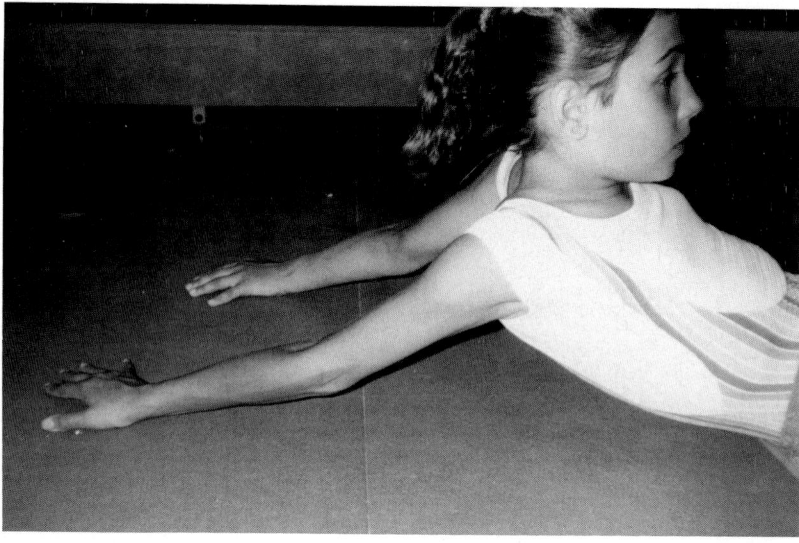

FIG. 38-6. Typical exercise to increase shoulder flexibility. This position may cause symptoms in the gymnast with unstable shoulder.

cally hypermobile individuals and the maximum range of motion used in gymnastics increase the risk of developing symptomatic instability. One particular exercise that is routinely performed by gymnasts to increase shoulder mobility causes instability complaints (Fig. 38-6). Those patients with complaints of instability usually have physiologic hypermobility associated with poor technique and/or muscle strength about the shoulder girdle. Rarely is there a history of acute traumatic dislocation or subluxation.

Rehabilitation and minor modification of technique have uniformly proved to successfully alleviate these complaints. The program involves general muscle strengthening of the entire shoulder girdle with accentuation of the internal rotators and modification of warm-ups to avoid extremes of shoulder motion. The inherent conflict of restricted motion caused by surgical stabilization and the need for extremes of motion in competition mitigate the need for operative intervention. Surgical stabilization of the shoulder is likely to end the athlete's career.

Miscellaneous

There is an entity that treating physicians should be aware of in the male gymnast's shoulder. Fulton[9] originally described "**Ringman's** shoulder," which was reported as a roentgenographic finding on routine shoulder studies. This entity is represented by an area of benign hypertrophy at the humeral insertion of the pectoralis major and latissimus dorsa. It has been described as a corticodesmoid-like lesion on roentgenographic appearance and is a common finding that has no clinical significance in the male gymnast. One case of a gymnast who had osteochondrosis of the proximal humeral physis or little league shoulder came to my attention.[1] On close questioning the gymnast admitted that he had also been throwing extensively at home with his father in hopes of becoming a pitcher in baseball the next year. I am not aware of any reported cases of gymnastics-related overuse injuries to the proximal humeral physis.

Acute Injuries

Contusions and Strains

The most commonly seen acute problems of the shoulder in gymnastics are related to contusion and muscular strain. Contusions are generally the result of a fall from the apparatus or inadvertent contact with an obstacle in the gym. Attention to general safety precautions can prove highly effective in preventing these injuries. Careful arrangement of the apparatus, padding of fixed obstacles, avoidance of horseplay and other distractions in the gym, and generous use of spotting are

Safety precautions to prevent injury

- Careful placement of apparatus
- Padding of fixed obstacles
- Avoidance of horseplay
- Generous spotting

all beneficial. Strains are, as in most sports, primarily related to inadequate warm-up, excessive training past the point of fatigue, and inadequate rehabilitation of previous injuries. They are not critical injuries and respond well to the usual conservative measures.

Subluxation or Dislocation

Acute subluxation or dislocation of the shoulder generally is a result of a missed move and/or a fall from the apparatus. Again, the most effective way to prevent this type of injury is aggressive strength training, avoidance of distractions in the gym, good coaching, and judicious use of spotting during practice.

Treatment

Treatment of the acute problems about the shoulder is relatively standard. Phase I consists of 7 to 14 days of rest, ice massage, and if necessary for comfort, a sling. Afterward, a formal active and passive range of motion program is started in conjunction with progressive resistance exercises. The gymnast should not be allowed to go back to full-scale activities in the gym until the shoulder has full and equal range of motion as well as normal strength. Before full recovery the gymnast can work out in the gym, go through calisthenics and warm-ups as tolerated, and perform tailored activities that do not put the shoulder into the position of risk. The only exception to this treatment protocol is an acute dislocation or subluxation. Because of the nature of this sport, a minimum of 4 to 6 weeks in a sling and swath should be required before initiating range of motion and strengthening exercises. Conditioning can be maintained during that period of time either by deep water running with a flotation vest or the use of an exercise bike.

Summary

Although shoulder complaints are not rare in gymnastics, the shoulder joint has not been the site of major problems. I have not seen the need to operate on the shoulder of any gymnast and have not been aware of any gymnast who has felt it necessary to discontinue the sport because of shoulder problems. Persistent impingement syndrome or recurrent dislocations could necessitate surgical intervention, but the latter would probably be the end of a gymnastic career.

ELBOW

Chronic problems in the gymnast's elbow appear to be related to the use of the extremity for weight-bearing support. Acute elbow injuries are the consequences of falls and high-velocity tumbling. The average female gymnast has extension ranging from 3 to 12 degrees of recurvatum and accentuated valgus inclination of the elbow. It is apparent in motion studies that the female gymnast tends to lock the elbow in a mechanically stable position taking advantage of that hyperextension to tolerate the load. The male gymnast tends to rely more on the strength of his triceps but still works primarily in full extension. Acute injuries are usually the result of a fall on the outstretched arm and occur more frequently in less experienced gymnasts. Coaches routinely teach gymnasts how to "bail out" when they miss or lose control of a maneuver. The natural reflex is to reach out and break a fall with the outstretched arm. Bailing out replaces that natural reflex with the learned response of tucking the arms in and rolling on impact. Thick pads around the apparatus and generous use of spotting also decrease the frequency of elbow injuries.[23]

Overuse Problems

Benign Problems

Several benign problems occur around the elbow as a result of inadequate conditioning, excessive workouts, or inappropriate training techniques. These include tendonitis at the triceps insertion comparable to a "jumper's knee" of the elbow, olecranon bursitis caused by repetitive contact, and chronic synovitis.[12,23] Both medial and lateral epicondylitis is seen, but medial is much more common. This is probably related to the increased valgus causing high-traction forces precipitated by weight-bearing maneuvers. The power moves such as the iron cross and other fixed-support moves used by the male gymnasts also exert high valgus load. All of these overuse problems are treated effectively with ice, strengthening of the elbow and wrist, modification of training techniques, and relative rest during the acute phase.

Elbow overuse injuries

- Triceps tendonitis
- Olecranon bursitis
- Chronic synovitis
- Medial epicondylitis
- Lateral epicondylitis

Osteochondritis Dissecans

The most dramatic of the overuse syndromes in the gymnast's elbow is osteochon-

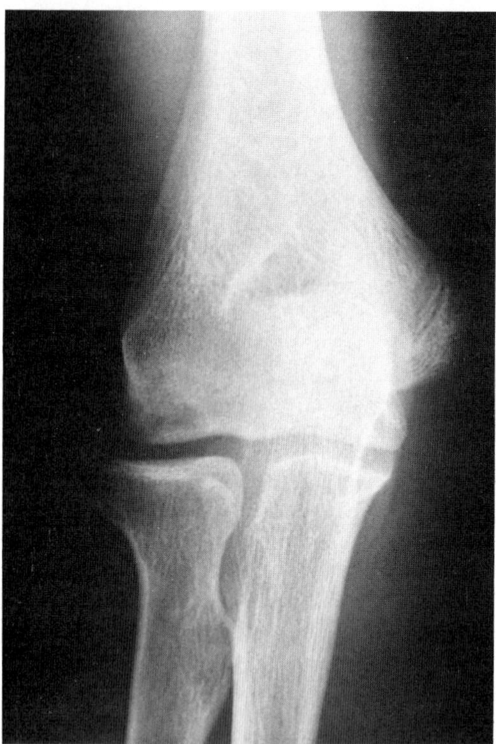

FIG. 38-7. Sixteen-year-old female gymnast with osteochrondritis dissecans lesion visible in the capitellum.

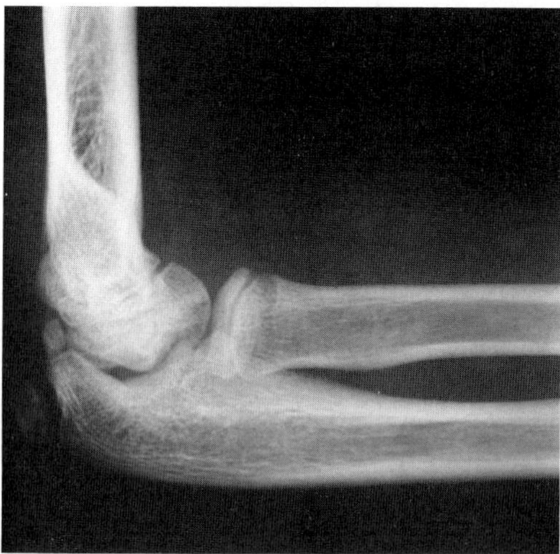

FIG. 38-8. Twelve-year-old female gymnast with osteochrondritis dissecans of the capitellum seen on lateral plain film.

dritis dissecans of the capitellum (Panner's disease). On occasion associated enlargement of the radial head is found, much as is seen in little league elbow. Goldberg,[12] Singer,[28] and Priest[23,25] have all reported cases of osteochondritis dissecans of the capitellum. Their experience and mine indicates that this entity tends to occur most frequently in very successful, aggressive, young gymnasts who are rapidly progressing through the various levels of competitive skills. Although seen in both male and female gymnasts, it is seen predominantly within the female population. (Fig. 38-7).

The presentation of osteochrondritis dissecans is usually pain that is variable in severity and initially noted following activities, then gradually progresses to the point that it bothers the gymnast throughout activities. The first complaints are usually related to vault and floor exercise. Fifty percent of my patients with osteochrondritis dissecans have described mechanical sensations of catching within the joint by the time of their first visit. Standard roentgenograms may or may not show a lesion that is typically centered on the capitellum in the position of contact with the radial head in full extension. The lesion is typical of osteochondritis dissecans of the lateral condyle. An area of lucency, a sclerotic margin, and often a sclerotic central fragment can be seen (Fig. 38-8). Occasionally a loose body is actually detected on plain films.

The most effective means of evaluating this entity has been double-contrast arthrotomography to define the lesion and demonstrate whether there is a defect in the overlying articular surface (Fig. 38-9). If the study shows no evidence of surface defect, a trial of physical therapy is instituted. Vaulting and tumbling are avoided for 3 to 6 months while the gymnast works on range of motion and strength. Progress is monitored by observation, symptomatology, and roentgenograms to see if the lesion heals spontaneously. Recent evaluation with both CT scan and MRI have shown excellent demonstration of the lesion but have offered no significant additional information over that of the arthrotomogram.

Arthroscopy is recommended for those patients who are having definite mechanical symptoms and/or demonstrate definite loosening of the fragment. The lesion is readily visualized with standard elbow arthroscopic technique. The fragment is excised and the bed curetted down to bleeding bone. Postoperatively the patients are placed in a sling for 7 to 10 days for comfort's sake only, and then started on an active-only range of motion program. As soon as full motion has been obtained progressive resistance exercises are initiated. Because of the nature of gymnastics, I do not recommend resection of the radial

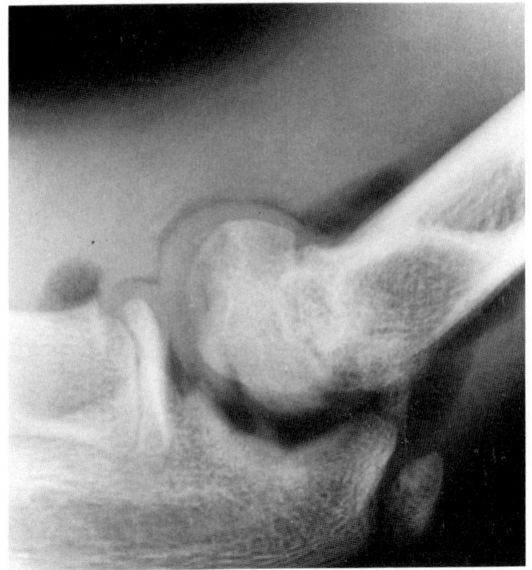

FIG. 38-9. Arthrotomogram of patient in Fig. 38-8 demonstrating a defect in the articular cartilage.

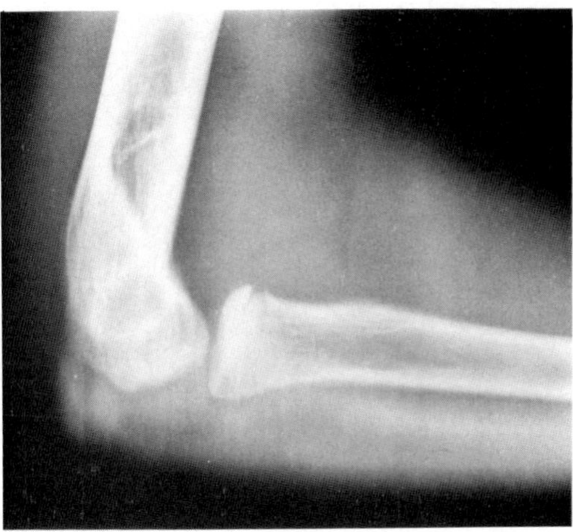

FIG. 38-10. Lateral tomogram of patient who demonstrated a chondral defect on the surface of the radial head.

head. In the one case that demonstrated involvement of the radial head, the surface was debrided with a chondral abrader and then the standard postoperative course was followed (Fig. 38-10).

Singer[27] reported on 7 cases of osteochondritis dissecans of the capitellum in 5 patients ranging from ages 11 to 13. He noted the change in capitellar vascular supply from poorly collateralized end vessels in ages 5 to 19, to excellent collateral supply in the adult. It was also his belief that cases of this nature are limited to children in that high-risk group of ages 11 to 13. Of the 5 patients he treated, 4 returned to full competition and 1 chose to quit gymnastics rather than undergo treatment.

I have treated 10 female patients who had osteochrondritis dissecans. Five of these patients were initially treated conservatively with the program previously noted. Three of the 5 patients healed satisfactorily and returned to full competition without difficulty. Two of the 5 patients developed mechanical symptoms and underwent surgical intervention along with the other 5 cases who presented initially with mechanical symptoms. Of the 7 elbows (in 6 females), the first 3 were treated with diagnostic arthroscopy, arthrotomy, debridement, and curettement. All 3 of these patients subsequently returned to full competitive symptom-free activity within 6 months. The slowest recovery (6 months) was a patient whose elbow had a large lesion of approximately 1 cm in diameter. After debridement, the radial head could be seen to dip into the defect on extension and then go through a major shift as it rode up and out of the defect. This shift gradually cleared over 6 months, and at the 2-year follow-up, there was normal motion of the elbow and no functional difference between the operated elbow and the nonoperated elbow. The remaining four procedures were performed arthroscopically and gained full range of motion, full function, and full return to activity within 4 months.

Case example

A male patient with osteochrondritis dissecans sought treatment 18 months after the onset of symptoms. At that point he had an extensive lesion involving nearly 50% of the capitellar surface and associated enlargement and deformity of the radial head. He subsequently saw several other orthopaedic surgeons, all of whom recommended intervention and/or cessation of gymnastics. He and his family elected to stay in the sport without treatment, but after another year he quit because of inability to perform and was lost to follow-up.

Vaulting. My associates and I in the Musculoskeletal Research Department of the Cleveland Clinic Foundation have been evaluating pressure across the upper extremity in vaulting for the past 2 years. Early data gained by coordinating high-speed video and upper extremity forces recorded on an instrumented vaulting horse have demonstrated several interesting facts[34] (Fig. 38-11). The gymnasts exert a force through the upper extremities that averages 2½ to 3½ times their body weight with each vault. The actual force

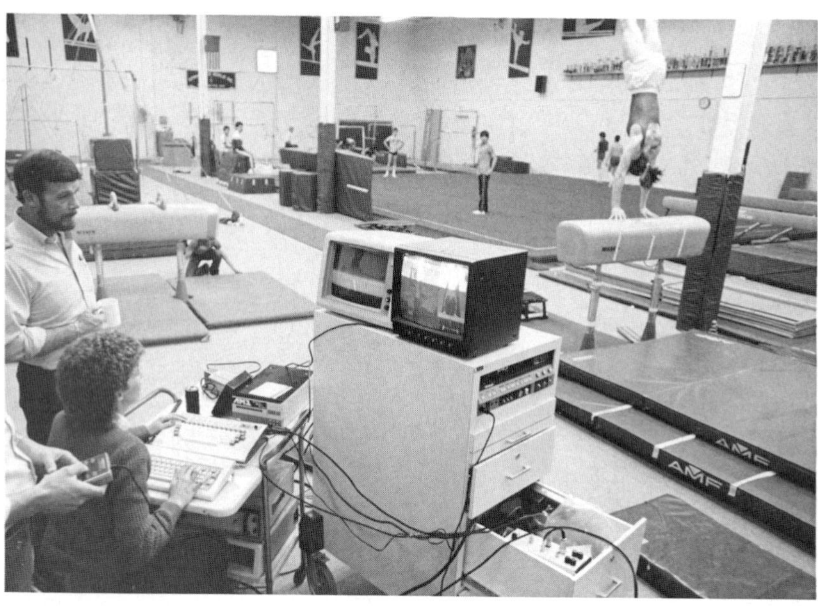

FIG. 38-11. Monitoring system wired to an instrumented vaulting horse to determine forces generated.

A

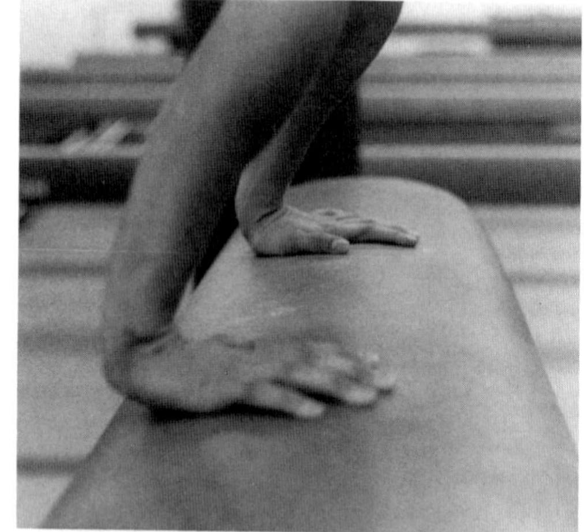

B

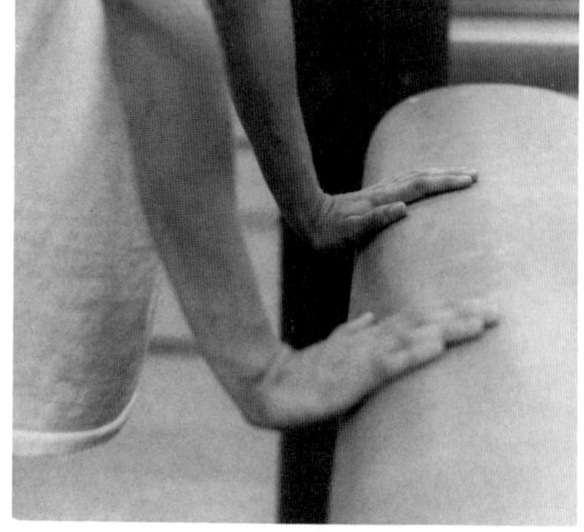

FIG. 38-12. Comparison of contact position on horse. **A,** Hands at leading edge. **B,** Correct hand location.

transmitted is largely dependent on technique. A low angle of attack at the time of contact with the horse markedly accentuates the forces, as does contact close to the leading edge of the vaulting horse (Fig. 38-12). Vaulting with the elbow fixed in full extension tends to cause higher peak readings than does the technique of slight flexion (5 to 15 degrees) and reextension on impact. Vaulting with the hands supinated so that the fingers point toward the ends of the horse causes increased load when compared to vaulting with the fingers straight ahead in the line of the body motion (Fig. 38-13). These are all early findings based on a preliminary system of measurement and are not yet in a form satisfactory for formal presentation and publication.

▪ ▪ ▪

All of the anecdotal information relating to osteochondritis dissecans of the elbow is presented to demonstrate several points. First of all, this is a unique entity that is seen almost exclusively in baseball pitchers and gymnasts. Second, body weight and vaulting techniques are critical in relation to impact loading of the elbow. We anticipate that technique on floor exercise and beam is equally important in determining the degree of load through the elbow. Third, complaints of chronic elbow pain in the gymnast warrant careful consideration and evaluation. Any gymnast who complains of elbow pain that persists for more than a week should have full and adequate evalua-

A

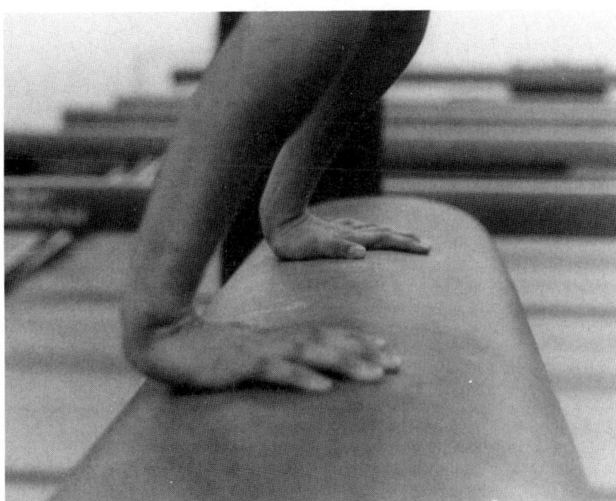

B

FIG. 38-13. A, Hands in incorrect supinated position. **B,** Hands in correct alignment.

tion, including standard roentgenograms. Fourth, the treatment of this lesion is much easier if the diagnosis is made early. However in those cases in which it is made late, the surgeon should feel comfortable in going ahead with debridement of the lesion and adequate rehabilitation. A high percentage of these athletes should return to full competitive status with appropriate treatment.

Medial Epicondylitis

Use of the upper extremity as a weight-bearing member in athletes with a high degree of valgus elbow alignment causes compression loads across the radiocapitellar joint. It also places chronic traction stress on the medial collateral ligament complex and the medial epicondyle. Chronic medial epicondylitis and medial collateral ligament sprains are a common problem in young gymnasts and are frequently ignored unless a knowledgeable person works closely with the gymnastics program.

Icing, strengthening, stretching, and technique adjustments on floor exercises and vaulting will generally allow rapid recovery. It is usually unnecessary to take time out from gymnastics. Treatment should be initiated only after adequate evaluation to rule out osteochondritis dissecans. Goldberg[12] also notes a problem with synovitis in the elbow of these athletes. This again should respond to ice, nonsteroidal antiinflammatory medication, a mild modification of activities to decrease the maximum stresses across the elbow, and a strengthening program.

Acute Injuries

Medial Epicondyle Fracture

Fracture of the medial epicondyle is not a surprising injury in this group of aggressive young athletes with open physeal plates and valgus inclination of the elbow. The best approach to prevention includes proper falling technique to avoid landing on the outstretched arm, thick mats, and liberal use of spotters. Regrettably, when this injury does occur in the gymnast the medial epicondyle is frequently displaced and trapped. Surgical reduction and fixation are often required.[23] In patients who do not have significant displacement, conservative treatment is appropriate with a brief period of immobilization (10 to 20 days) followed by early range of motion exercises. The rehabilitation program should initially be limited to active range of motion only and progress should be followed closely. Strengthening can begin when the patient has regained motion of no less than 5 degrees to 130 degrees. Resumption of gymnastics is

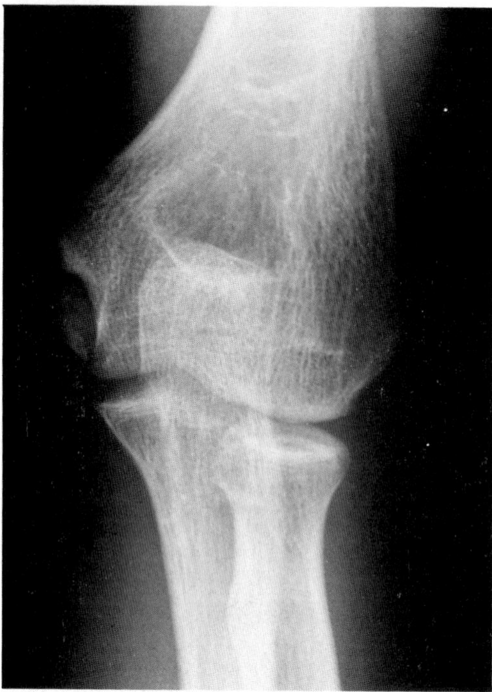

FIG. 38-14. Anteroposterior view of elbow showing nonunion of medial epicondylar fracture after approximately 6 months of conservative care.

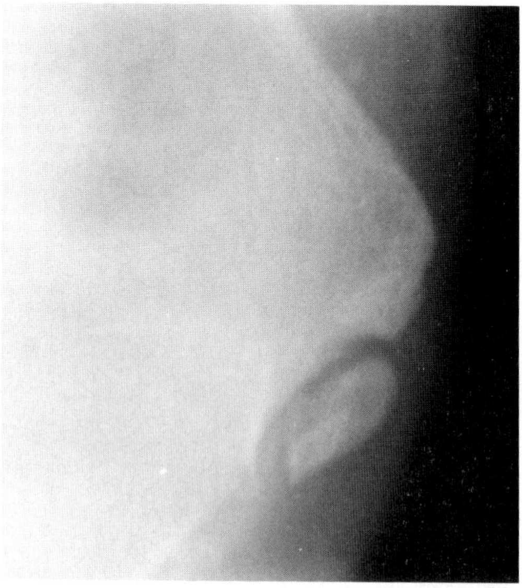

FIG. 38-15. Magnification view of same lesion in Fig. 38-14.

allowed when the patient has achieved full range of motion and full strength comparable to the contralateral side. In Priest's series,[24] over 80% of gymnasts were able to return to competitive activity after major injuries to the elbow.

Case example

A gymnast of national caliber was treated conservatively for medial epicondylar fracture and subsequently was unable to regain adequate motion despite intensive physical therapy. At 6 months the roentgenograms showed a nonunion of part of the medial epicondyle but did not show major displacement or any evidence of entrapment (Fig. 38-14, and 38-15). The elbow was stable on examination but lacked 30 degrees of extension and 20 degrees of flexion. Surgical exploration of the elbow revealed a heavy fibrous band tethering from the nonunion site to the olecranon. When the nonunion was taken down and the band transected, the patient immediately had full range of motion without restriction. Internal fixation of this fracture and subsequent standard postoperative rehabilitation have resulted in essentially full range of motion and return to full competitive level (Fig. 38-16). The standard methods of treatment for the medial epicondylar fracture may be followed in gymnasts, but residual loss of motion warrants surgical exploration.

Supracondylar Fracture

The mechanism of injury, resultant deformity, and associated problems are no different in the gymnast than in any other child sustaining a supracondylar fracture of the humerus. The treating physician should use whatever method of closed reduction and immobilization, closed reduction and internal fixation, or open reduction internal fixation that he or she feels most comfortable with. The only modification from the standard treatment is emphasis on more aggressive early active range of motion. Passive range of motion machines and continuous range of motion machines for the elbow have not proved satisfactory in my experience.

Radial Head Fracture

Fractures of the radial head are very rare in gymnasts, but when they do occur they should be treated conservatively but aggressively. The elbow should be rested during the period of initial discomfort and then aggressive active range of motion initiated as soon as it can be tolerated. Operative intervention should be restricted to open reduction and internal fixation with the miniature fragment set if necessary to regain satisfactory anatomic configuration. At all costs, resection of the radial head *should be avoided* in the gymnast. In no case in my personal experience, in my conversations with other orthopaedists who treat gymnasts, or in any literature concern-

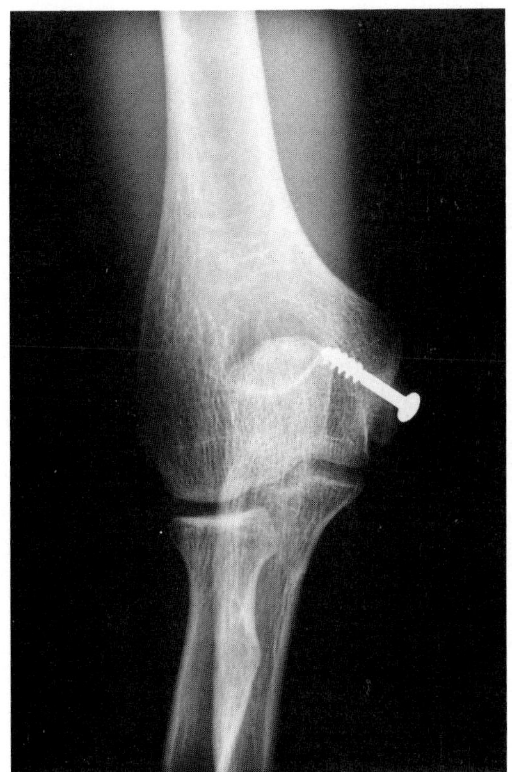

FIG. 38-16. Postoperative anteroposterior view of the same elbow seen in Figs. 38-14 and 38-15.

ing radial head fracture[23] did a gymnast return to acceptable competitive level after resection of the radial head. This operation should be resorted to only as a salvage procedure if the decision has already been made to withdraw the athlete from gymnastics.

Dislocation

Dislocation of the elbow is usually caused by a fall on the extended arm and is generally lateral or posterolateral. Rarely a straight posterior dislocation is encountered. Patients should be splinted as they lie and transported to an emergency room. Roentgenograms should be taken and the neurovascular status carefully documented. The elbow can then be carefully reduced by closed technique. Repeat roentgenograms should be taken to confirm both the reduction and to rule out possible associated fractures. The limb is immobilized in a posterior plaster slab or sling and swath for 7 to 21 days. Josefsson[15] reviewed 30 simple dislocations and confirmed the general clinical impression that surgical repair of the ligaments offered no additional stability over the nonoperative treatment. Range of motion was definitely superior in the nonsurgical treatment group. Grossly unstable elbows should be placed in a cast for 2 to 3 weeks and minimally unstable elbows for 1 week. When immobilization is discontinued the patient should be placed on a active-only range of motion program along with ice treatment 3 to 5 times a day for 20 to 30 minutes. Frequent monitoring of progress and constant reinforcement is needed to encourage the athlete not to attempt various means of passive motion. Despite the most careful and aggressive treatment some athletes with this injury will fail to regain full extension. Mehlhoff[20] noted 28% of elbow injuries were dislocations and that the average adult lost 12.3 degrees extension after dislocation. Aronen,[2] Josefsson et al,[15] Mehlhoff,[20] Taylor and Shively,[30] and Priest[23] all confirmed the need for a shortened period of immobilization and aggressive active range of motion work following the immobilization.

Gymnasts who fail to regain full extension are forced to either drop out of the sport or accept a decreased level of performance. Despite the general teaching to the contrary, it has been my experience that it is possible to regain full extension with surgical intervention (Fig. 38-17). In 4 elbows explored 9 months or more after dislocation, contracture of the anterior capsule proved to be the limiting factor in all cases. Transverse capsulotomy performed through a lateral incision allows full extension on the operating table. Postoperatively, the elbows are casted in full extension. After 3 weeks in full extension the cast is bivalved and the patient allowed to remove it 3 times a day for active flexion exercises. After 6 weeks the cast is removed and the patient is placed on an active flexion/extension range of motion program. Six months after surgery all 4 of these patients returned successfully to competitive gymnastics or gymnastics coaching. Two of them have recurvatum of 5 degrees and 3 degrees, which is within 1 degree of the contralateral elbow. One of the patients has full extension of 0 degrees compared with a contralateral elbow that has 5 degrees of hyperextension. The fourth patient lacks 2 degrees of extension compared with a contralateral elbow that has 2 degrees of hyperextension.

Elbow dislocation in the gymnast should be treated as follows: (1) Fully evaluate and perform closed reduction, (2) Immobilize for 1 to 3 weeks, (3) Initiate aggressive active-only range of motion exercises, and (4) perform an anterior capsulotomy if adequate extension has not been obtained by 6 months. In no case has residual instability been a problem.

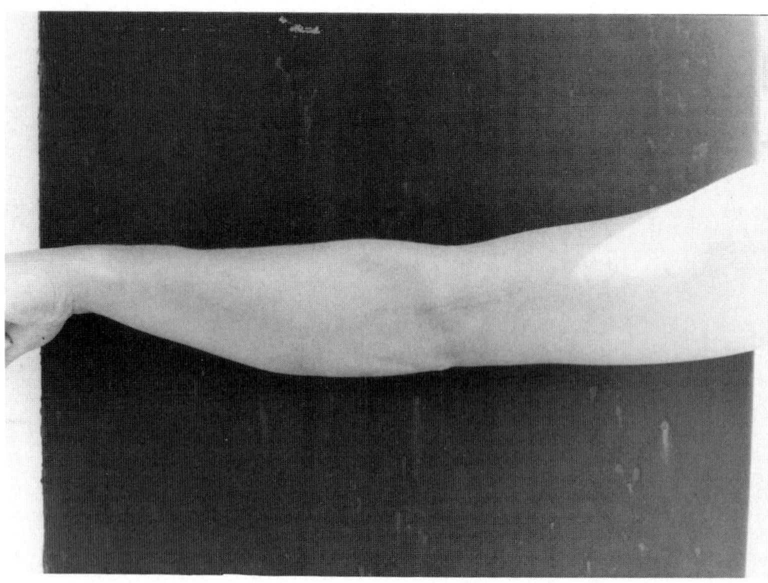

FIG. 38-17. Postoperative extension of elbow in 30-year-old female coach who lacked 30 degrees of extension after conservative treatment of posterolateral elbow dislocation.

Treatment of elbow dislocation

1. Evaluate carefully and perform closed reduction
2. Immobilize 1 to 3 weeks
3. Aggressive active-only ROM program
4. Anterior capsulotomy if adequate extension has not been obtained at 6 months

Contusions

As with other joints, contusions about the elbow are a frequent occurrence and may involve any aspect of the joint, including the ulnar nerve in its groove. These injuries generally occur secondary to contact with apparatus, floor, stationary obstructions, or other people. They are best avoided by proper layout of the gym, proper attention to technique, avoidance of distractions, and the use of spotters. Treatment is initiated with 1 to 3 days of rest, ice, and nonsteroidal antiinflammatory medication. Then active range of motion exercises are instituted until full range of motion is obtained. Progressive resistance exercises are done until the athlete has full range of motion and full strength as compared with treatment of the contralateral elbow. Only then is he or she allowed to return to gymnastics.

WRIST

Problems of the wrist are so endemic in gymnastics that dorsal wrist pain has been described as a normal and direct result of the sport.[2] The complexity of the wrist with its multiple bones, joints, bursae, and tendons has resulted in confusion in the literature (see Chapter 21). Injuries are commonly discussed according to subjective criteria with little objective proof of the underlying pathologic condition. Terms such as "dorsal wrist pain," "dorsiflexion wrist jam syndrome," "wrist splints," "adventitial bursitis," "dorsal wrist capsulitis," and "multiple tendonitis" have appeared in the literature.* The exact pathologic conditions underlying many of the wrist problems have not been well defined.

Although complaints of wrist pain are common in gymnasts, they should not be ignored. A thorough history focusing on the types of maneuvers and the wrist positions that cause the greatest pain should be followed by a thorough physical examination to localize tenderness, identify pain parameters, and demonstrate any of the multiple provocative tests for tendonitis. Routine roentgenograms and diagnostic local anesthetic injections will occasionally offer the answer, but refractory cases require fluoroscopy, arthrography, bone scanning, MRI, CT, cineroentgenography

*References 2, 5, 7, 16, 18, 20, 25, 26, 37.

and/or arthroscopy. The choice of specific techniques for evaluation needs to be individualized according to clinical suspicion.

Overuse Problems

Dorsal Wrist Pain

An entity frequently seen in gymnasts is pain in the dorsum of the wrist with maximum dorsiflexion. The patient usually complains of pain on vaulting, floor exercises, or the pommel horse. He or she had no history of specific acute trauma and frequently no history of a recent technique change. This entity is often described as "dorsiflexion jam syndrome," "dorsal impaction syndrome," or "dorsal capsulitis." The particular problem appears to be primarily endemic in gymnasts; however, it has recently been reported in divers who enter the water with the wrists in dorsiflexion and the hands cupped to decrease their entry splash. It has also been reported in several instances in skaters who have had repetitive falls onto the dorsiflexed hand while practicing maneuvers.

Physical examination reveals diffuse pain over the dorsum of the wrist that is accentuated by active or passive dorsiflexion. Examination, including neurovascular evaluation, yields findings within normal limits. Routine roentgenograms have consistently proved to be normal, and there have been no reviews in the literature that use MRI or bone scanning in this group of patients. Teitz[31] has noted the presence of dorsal spurs on the lunate and the distal end of the radius that appear to oppose on wrist dorsiflexion. This has not been confirmed in other articles nor in my experience. There is some speculation[27] that this problem is accentuated by the use of overly soft mats, twisting maneuvers such as the Sukahara vault, twisting maneuvers on the beam, and the high repetitions of today's training.

Dorsal wrist pain

- Diffuse dorsal pain
- Pain increased with active or passive dorsiflexion
- Normal results on routine physical examination
- Normal results on routine roentgenograms

The paucity of experience with more advanced diagnostic imaging and evaluation is related to the frequent occurrence of the problem and relative ease with which it is treated. It is difficult to validate the expense incurred

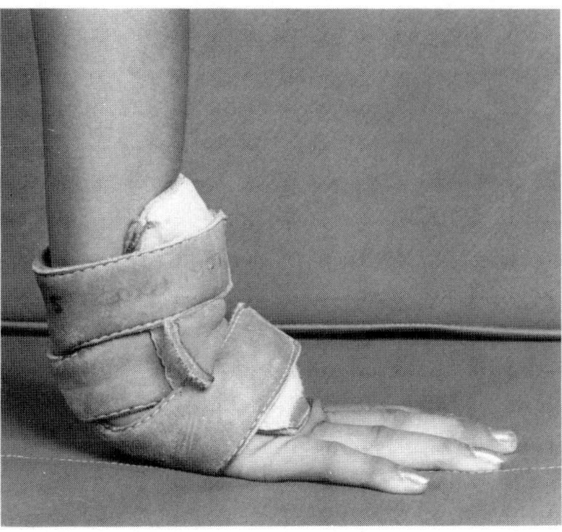

FIG. 38-18. A commercially available dorsiflexion block. (Courtesy of R.B.J. Athletic Specialties, Spanish Fork, Utah.)

by state of the art testing for a problem that can be adequately managed despite the lack of scientific understanding. Treatment involves a combination of the standard modalities used for overuse syndromes and avoidance of the maximum dorsiflexed position. This is accomplished by decreasing the intensity of training, icing before and after activities, nonsteroidal antiinflammatory medication, physical therapy, and dorsiflexion blocks. Increased range of motion and strength for wrist extensors and flexors are the primary goal of physical therapy. Limitation of dorsiflexion may be accomplished simply by taping a rectangular piece of ethafoam to the dorsum of the wrist or by a commercial device that straps into place and limits dorsiflexion (Fig. 38-18). In addition, coaches are encouraged to review the gymnast's technique and modify floor, vault, pommel horse, and beam techniques to decrease maximal dorsiflexion positioning.

Distal Radius Stress Fracture

Stress fractures of the distal radius including the epiphysis and metaphysis have been reported.[26,27] This entity is much like dorsiflexion jam syndrome with the gymnast reporting an insidious onset of wrist pain related to weight-bearing and impact-loading activities. Examination reveals volar or dorsal tenderness over the distal radius either at the physis or the epiphysis. Roentgenograms in 50% of the cases reported by Roy, Cains, and Singer[27] demonstrated widening of the physeal plate, an epiphyseal fracture line, or sclerosis about the physeal plate. The other

50% of the cases were diagnosed on the similarity of symptoms without roentgenographic change. Read[26] noted one difference in clinical presentation when he reported tenderness over the distal radius on the volar aspect. In neither of these studies was the use of bone scans described, so the actual diagnosis of those cases with no specific roentgenographic changes is open to speculation.

I have found that it is extremely difficult to separate the dorsiflexion jam syndrome from distal radial stress fracture or a continuum phase possibly occurring between the two entities. Again, additional scientific study has been slow in development, since these entities respond well to simple conservative treatment.

The standard treatment is ice, range of motion and strengthening exercises, and partial rest with avoidance of high-impact and twisting loads. All of the reported cases have healed spontaneously without surgical intervention or aggressive treatment. In chronic cases the long-term result and the rate of healing seem to be the same whether or not the wrist is placed at rest. Those cases seen and diagnosed early do seem to heal faster if placed at rest.

Chronic Wrist Sprain

Bartolozzi et al[3] recently reported a review of chronic wrist problems in intercollegiate gymnasts. The initial symptoms were very similar to those discussed under dorsiflexion jam syndrome and distal radial stress fractures. Roentgenographic evaluation revealed a tendency toward ulnar drift of the wrist with some degree of aberrant wrist development. The authors speculated that these changes were related to high-impact and weight-bearing loads over a long course of gymnastics during the childhood. Arthrography and arthroscopy demonstrated disruption of the radioulnar triangular fibrocartilage. Arthroscopic debridement of the triangular fibrocartilage should alleviate the symptoms. Chronic sprain of the ulnar collateral ligaments presents with localized tenderness over the ulnar styloid and the ulnar side of the wrist. The treatment is the same as that suggested for dorsiflexion jam syndrome.

Tendonitis

Tendonitis about the gymnast's wrist has been found in the abductor pollicis longus, extensor pollicis longus, extensor carpi ulnaris, and the more proximal portion of the abductor pollicis longus. Dorsal radial tendonitis is initially seen as classic de Quervin's tenosynovitis with pain on ulnar deviation and rotational activities of the wrist. On examination there is generally a sense of fullness overlying the tendons and a positive result to Finkelstein's test. The tendonitis variant of the more proximal abductor pollicis longus tendon and associated adventitial bursa[37] has been initially described as localized crepitation proximal to the wrist in addition to the classic findings of de Quervain's tenosynovitis (Fig. 38-19).

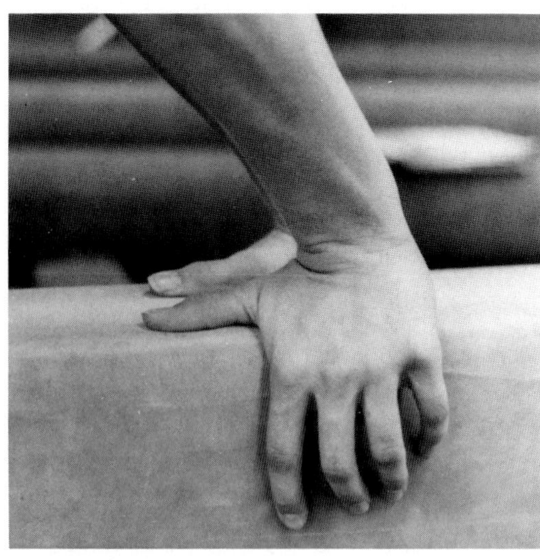

FIG. 38-19. Position of hand on beam that causes symptoms of both ulnar sprains and radial tendonitis.

All of these entities have been effectively treated with an initial period of complete rest, ice, and nonsteroidal antiinflammatory medication. The gymnast gradually returns to activity while he or she goes through intensive physical therapy to increase the range of motion and strength of the wrist. In the rare refractory case it has been necessary to perform a surgical release of the tendon sheath. In all cases operated on at this institution, recovery has been complete and the gymnasts have resumed full competition.

Carpal Stress Fractures

Tenderness and pain localized over the carpals that is not responsive to the usual conservative measures should be fully evaluated with routine roentgenograms as well as either bone scan, CT scan, or MRI. Stress fracture and aseptic necrosis of the capitate, carpal scaphoid, and lunate have been described[17,21,31] A bone scan that shows positive findings for carpal stress fracture should be followed by a period of rest with splinting or casting. After 4 to 6 weeks of protected rest the gymnast is placed on a strengthening, stretching, and graduated return to activity program. Follow-up roentgenograms should always be obtained to evaluate the healing progress, particularly if avascular necrosis is present.

Ganglia

Gymnasts appear to be neither more prone nor more resistant than the general population to the development of ganglia about the wrist. The treatment of a symptomatic ganglion in a gymnast is also the same as generally accepted with the exception that the associated disability may require earlier aggressive intervention. Volar wrist ganglia are initially seen with the classic symptoms of localized pain and tenderness but seldom causes a major problem for the gymnast. Dorsal wrist ganglia are frequently associated with other wrist complaints and present a major problem. The dorsiflexion block braces used for the jam syndrome and distal radial stress fracture put pressure directly on the ganglia, which limits the use of the block braces.

Forearm "Splints"

Gymnasts occasionally have complaints of aching pain in the forearm that is exacerbated by activities (particularly weight bearing) in the gym. Deep palpation reveals tenderness between the radius and ulna and the patient experiences discomfort with maximal dorsiflexion of the fingers and wrist. The pathophysiology of this entity has not been well defined, but it appears to be similar to the shin splint syndrome of the lower extremities. Whether this is traction-related irritation of the radioulnar syndesmosis, periostitis, or myositis is still unknown, but the treatment is definitely conservative. Activity modification to decrease impact loading and weight-bearing, ice, and nonsteroidal antiinflammatory medication, will initially clear the symptoms. After resolution of the symptoms, strengthening, stretching, short-term circumferential taping, and graduated return to activities are initiated. Forearm splints usually present early in the season and resolve as conditioning is completed. Gymnasts who have experienced this problem in previous years are strongly encouraged to avoid loss of forearm conditioning. They can either work the weight program during the off season or, as is typical in club gymnastics, continue in the sport year-round. To date there have been no serious sequelae reported as a result of wrist pain.

Forearm splints

- Aching forearm pain
- Pain exacerbated by activity
- Seen early in season
- Tenderness found on deep palpation between radius and ulna
- Pain with active wrist and finger dorsiflexion

Acute Injuries

Acute trauma to the gymnast's wrist is not uncommon but is generally not significantly different from that seen in other sports and activities.

Fracture of the Scaphoid

As with other activities, carpal scaphoid fractures generally result from a fall on the dorsiflexed hand with the arm extended and supinated behind the back. Gymnasts should not sustain this injury if they have learned to tuck and roll rather than putting their arm back to protect themselves. They present with the classic pain on ulnar and radial deviation as well as pinpoint tenderness over the anatomical snuff box. Roentgenograms usually reveal normal findings in the early stages and show delayed visualization of the fracture line in 2 to 3 weeks. Suspicion of carpal scaphoid fracture warrants bone scan or tomography. Treatment, as in other sports, is initiated with a long-arm thumb spica cast. This is reduced to a short-arm thumb spica cast after 3 weeks and subsequently to a short-arm splint or cast at approximately 6 to 8 weeks. Adjustments in timing of cast transitions are dependent on the roentgenographic appearance. Return to gymnastics is anticipated at 10 to 12 weeks after the injury.

Distal Radial Fracture

Colles' fractures, reverse Colles' fractures, and Salter's fractures I through IV have been seen in gymnasts. The treatment is identical to that used for those injuries in any other group of young patients.

Fracture Related to the Doweled Grip

One injury that is unique to gymnastics is the high speed–flexion rotation fracture dislocation of the wrist or distal forearm. This particular entity was unheard of until recent years when the doweled grip became popular. This style of grip has a dowel built into it at approximately the level of the middle phalanx. (See Figs. 38-3, 38-4, and 38-5). The dowel

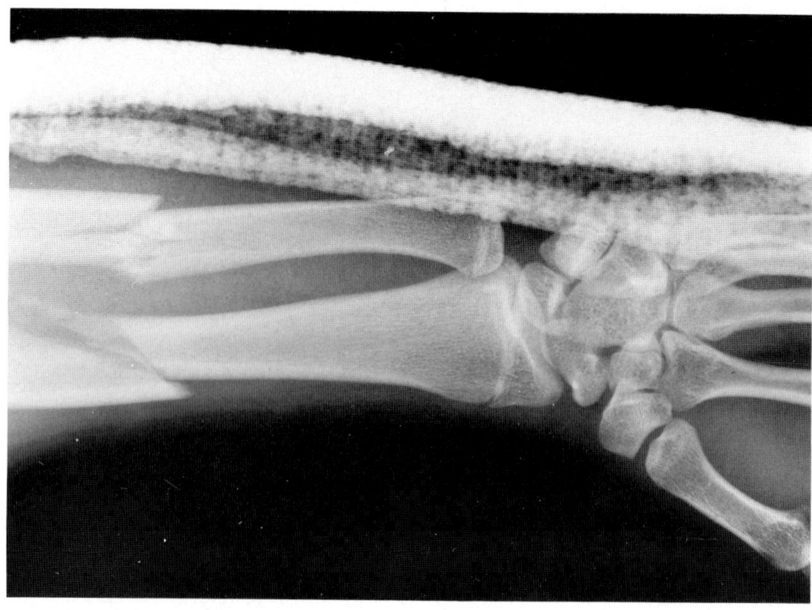

FIG. 38-20. Anteroposterior roentgenogram of a 16-year-old female gymnast who sustained a comminuted radius and ulna fracture when her doweled grip caught on the high bar.

allows excellent purchase on the bar and allows giant swings of greater intensity and frequency than had previously been done. I am aware of several cases reported anecdotally and one in the literature[2] in which the dowel apparently caught on the bar while the gymnast's momentum continued in a giant swing fashion. This resulted in the hand's being trapped to the bar as the body continued to revolve around it, causing a dorsal fracture dislocation of the wrist.

This entity has previously been a unique problem of male gymnasts, since only they were using the dowel. It is now becoming common for gyms to convert the uneven parallel bars to the smallest-diameter bar allowed by competition rules and to have their female gymnasts use dowel-grips also. In one recent case an accomplished 16-year-old female gymnast sustained a comminuted both-bone forearm fracture while performing giant swings on a high bar (Fig 38-20). Her description of the injury was very clear because she was aware that the grip caught, but was unable to stop her momentum. Treatment of these injuries is beyond the scope of this chapter in that it needs to be individualized to the specific trauma encountered and is best managed by the hand specialist. Precautions against fractures involve being certain that the grips fit the gymnasts correctly, are well cared for, in good repair, and are adequately chalked. The grips need to be carefully fitted according to the manufacturer's directions and frequently checked for any stretching. If they fit too loosely the leather can fold over and lock to the bar (Fig. 38-21). Female gymnasts should *not* be allowed to work out on the men's high bar because of the smaller diameter. Regular cleaning of the bars to avoid chalk buildup will decrease the likelihood of grip stick.

Proper use of chalk

- Chalk hands and grip before each swinging-activity session
- Clean bars of caked chalk to avoid buildup

HAND

With the exception of skin problems, injuries to the hands of gymnasts are not unique nor particularly frequent.[19] The author has seen Bennett's fractures, proximal interphalangeal joint (PIP), fractures and dislocations, mallet finger deformities, metacarpal fractures, gamekeeper's thumb, and jammed fingers in gymnasts. All of these have occurred as unique specific trauma normally related to contact with apparati or the floor. No specific treatment recommendations are required beyond those used for other athletes with comparable injury.

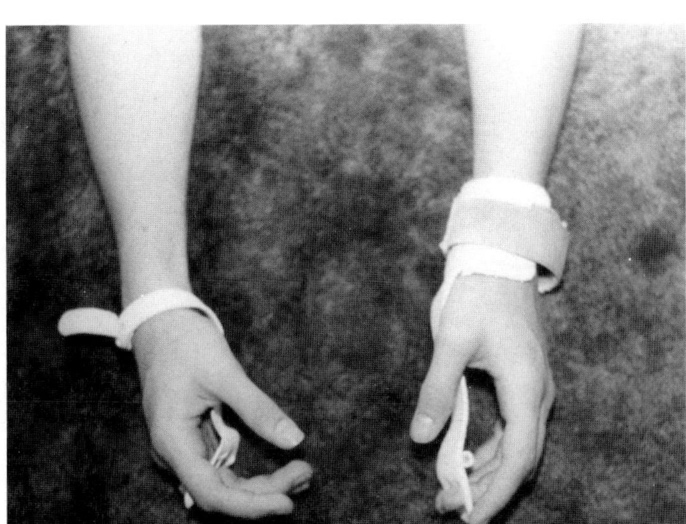

FIG. 38-21. Fit of doweled grip should be fitted tight enough that the fingers cannot reach full extension. There should be no laxity of the grip.

Skin Problems

Skin problems on the hand that are unique to gymnasts warrant consideration. Calluses on the palm and the palmar aspect of the fingers are the natural consequence of the work on bars, rings, and pommel horse (Fig. 38-22). When the calluses become tender they should be pared with an emory board or sandpaper and massaged with a moisturizing cream after workouts. Grips that are properly fitted, well maintained, and well chalked decrease the friction and therefore the severity of callus formation. Return to the gymnasium after any prolonged period of inactivity predisposes the gymnast to blisters. They are best prevented by gradual return to apparatus and wise use of grips and chalk. When blisters do occur the normal physiologic skin cover should be left in place as long as possible. Once the skin does break, the gymnast should be instructed to keep the hands clean and dry.

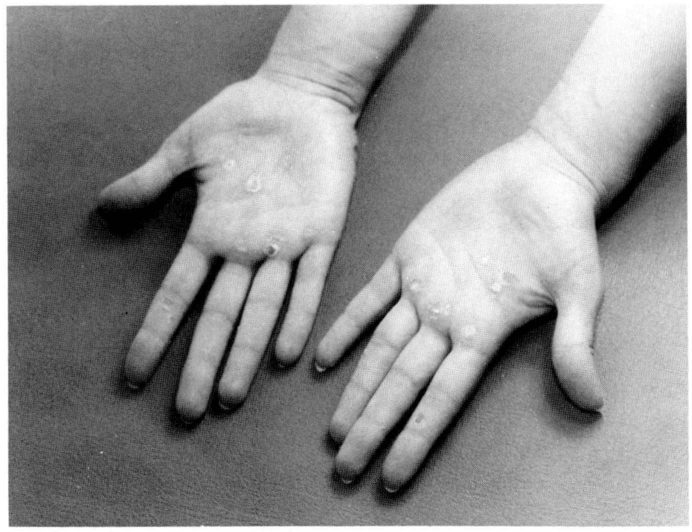

FIG. 38-22. Calluses on palmar aspect of a gymnast's hands. These are typical.

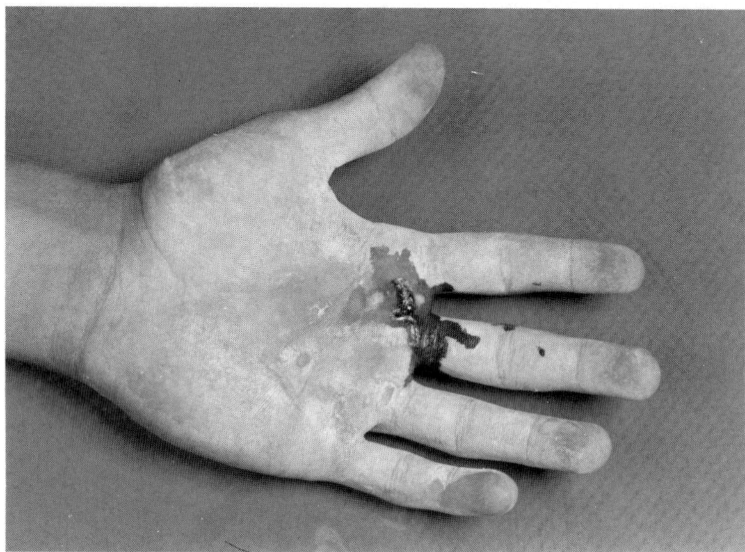

FIG. 38-23. Acute tear on a male gymnast's hands. This occurred while working the pommel horse with no grips and inadequate chalk.

Skin Tears

The primary skin problem of the gymnast's hand is referred to as "tears." This problem occurs when friction overload causes callused skin to shear loose from its underlying attachments (Fig. 38-23). Prevention of tears is presently based on a combination of experience and folklore handed down within the gymnastic community. Routine care of the palms includes keeping the calluses trimmed, limiting workouts when so-called hot spots develop, wearing properly fitted and well-maintained grips, and using moisturizing cream after workouts. The proper use of chalk has long been a standard part of gymnastics and has two primary components. First, the hands and grip should be freshly chalked before each use of swinging-type apparatus. Second, the bars should be routinely cleaned to avoid a buildup of caked chalk, which becomes sticky and increases friction.

When a gymnast sustains a tear it is usually a result of continuing to participate despite warning signs. Visible fissuring of the skin or the presence of hot spots, which indicate blistering beneath the callus, require rest. Tears should be kept clean, aggressively moistured, and monitored for the possibility of infection. Once the tear has sealed and is no longer painful the gymnast then returns to the apparatus with gradual progression to "retoughen the hands."

UPPER EXTREMITY PROBLEMS IN THE GYMNASTICS COACH

In most sports the coach is involved primarily on a mental level with instruction and strategy. The gymnastics coach is extensively involved in practice verbally, mentally, and physically. The physical act of spotting to aid maneuver development and protect from injury is a large part of the job. In addition to the well-recognized low back pain, nasal fractures, and multiple contusions incurred by spotters, we see multiple problems in the upper extremities. Philosophically, it is important to remember that not only does the coach sustain injuries similar to those of the gymnasts but also the treatment must be equally aggressive. The coach's ability to perform his or her job requires athletic ability and a sound body.

Shoulder

The coach's shoulder takes a great deal of stress while spotting, especially when working with young, inexperienced gymnasts. Coaches have been treated for biceps tendonitis, supraspinatus tendonitis, chronic AC joint arthritis, rotator cuff tears, and acute rupture of the pectoralis major.

Elbow

The crossed-arm position used to spot tumbling tricks puts high stress on the medial side of the elbow.[4] Those stresses are often superimposed on long-standing elbow problems from the coach's days of competition. The coach initially complains of medial epicondylitis types of symptoms or intraarticular symptoms related to long-standing osteochondritis dissecans lesions. Inflammation of the ulnar collateral ligament, de Quervain's tendonitis, and finger injuries are also all common problems among coaches.

The important thing to remember in dealing with this group of individuals is that although the coaches are not performing the tricks, they are sustaining much the same stresses and loads as the participating gymnasts. Problems need to be taken seriously and treated as aggressively as is the competitive athlete.

SUMMARY

In this chapter we have reviewed multiple problems that occur in the upper extremities of gymnasts. If nothing else is clear, you should be aware that these problems do exist, and many of them have a career-ending potential. The physician involved in sports medicine needs to be aware of the problems and unique characteristics of this group and be readily accessible to the gymnast. The participants are generally young, very enthusiastic, extremely dedicated, subjected to significant peer pressure, and conditioned to accept pain as a normal part of the sport.

Equipment is critical to the prevention of these injuries, and the involved physician should be aware of the following general principles.

1. The gym must be laid out with adequate space between apparatus and adequate padding on all fixed obstacles.
2. Every inch of the floor should be padded with adequate matting and the bases of all apparatus protected with pads.
3. The floor exercise area should have adequate spring to decrease impact loading, but not so soft that it allows abnormal dorsiflexion of the wrists or catching of the hands in rotational maneuvers.
4. The beams must be adequately spaced and their surfaces in excellent repair.
5. Bars and vault must be cleaned frequently to avoid the accumulation of chalk or any other substance that would cause stickiness.
6. Chalk boxes must be readily available and placed throughout the gym.
7. Gymnasts on the swinging apparatus should be wearing well-fitted grips in good repair.
8. Ice should be readily accessible to the gymnasts.

The physician who treats gymnasts should also be aware of the general principles of training and monitor the patients under their treatment. The physician should take the following steps to avoid injuries:

1. Encourage logical, graduated progression of training regimens.
2. Encourage strength training throughout the year.
3. Encourage meticulous attention to technique.
4. Encourage the avoidance of distractions within the gym.
5. Recommend modification of intensity in programs as needed for specific problems.
6. Modify individual gymnasts' programs for specific problems.

In the injury incidence studies done thus far the most important factor in prevention of injuries has been the use of spotters.[22,23,24,33] Coaches adequately trained in spotting techniques should be encouraged to routinely spot their athletes during all stages of trick development and the majority of time for established tricks.

REFERENCES

1. Adams JE: Little league shoulder: osteochondrosis of the proximal humeral epiphysis in boy baseball pitchers, Cal Med 105:22, 1966.
2. Aronen JG: Problems of the upper extremity in gymnasts. Symposium on Gymnastics. Clin Sports Med 4(1):61, 1985.
3. Bartolozzi AR et al: Wrist pain syndrome in the gymnast: pathogenetic, diagnostic, and therapeutic considerations. (Research award paper presentation). American Orthopaedics Society for Sports Medicine, thirteenth annual meeting, Orlando, Fla, June 29 to July 2, 1987.
4. Boone T: Helping hand can equal sore elbow, Phys Sportsmed p 41, January, 1976.
5. Chambers RB: Orthopaedic injuries in athletes (ages 6 to 17): comparison to injuries occurring in 6 sports. Am J Sports Med 7(3):195, 1979.
6. Cooney WP: Bursitis and tendonitis in the hand, wrist, and elbow: an approach to treatment, Minn Med 491, August 1983.
7. Cooney III WP: Sports injuries to the upper extremity: how to recognize and deal with some common problems, Sports Injuries 76(4):45, 1984.
8. Dobyns JH, Sim FH, and Linscheid RL: Sports stress syndromes of the hand and wrist, Am J Sports Med 6(5):236, 1978.
9. Fulton MN, Albright JP, and El-Khoury GY: Cortical desmoid-like lesion of the proximal humerus and its occurrence in gymnasts (Ringman's shoulder lesion), Am J Sports Med 7(1):57, 1979.
10. Ganim RJ: Gymnastics safety for the physician.

Symposium on Gymnastics. Clin Sports Med 4(1):123, January 1985.
11. Garrick JG: Epidemiology of women's gymnastics injuries, Am J Sports Med 8(4):261, 1980.
12. Goldberg MJ: Gymnastics injuries. Symposium on Sports Injuries. Orthop Clin North Am 11(4):717, October, 1980.
13. Jobe FW: Differential diagnosis of shoulder. The shoulder in the athlete. Paper presented at AAOS forxyninth annual meeting, Los Angeles, August 28, 1983.
14. Jobe FW and Moynes DR: Delineation of diagnostic criteria and rehabilitation program for rotator cuff injuries, Am J Sports Med 10(6):336, 1982.
15. Josefsson PO et al: Surgical versus non-surgical treatment of ligamentous injuries following dislocation of elbow joint, J Bone Joint Surg 69A(4):605, 1987.
16. Kirby RL: Flexibility and musculoskeletal symptomatology in female gymnasts and age-matched controls, Am J Sports Med 9:3, 160, 1981.
17. Manzione M, and Pizzutillo PD: Stress fracture of the scaphoid waist. a case report, Am J Sports Med 9(4):268, 1981.
18. Matheson GO et al: Stress fractures in athletes: a study of 320 cases, Am J Sports Med 15(1):46, 1987.
19. McCue FC III et al: Hand and wrist injuries in the athlete, Am J Sports Med 7(5):275, 1979.
20. Mehlhoff TL: Early mobilization recommended for simple elbow dislocation, News bulletin, Am Acad Orthop Surg 6(1):22, 1987.
21. Murakami S, and Nakajima H: Aseptic necrosis of the capitate bone in two gymnasts. Am J Sports Med 12(2):170, 1984.
22. Pettrone FA, and Ricciardelli E: Gymnastic injuries: the Virginia experience 1982-1983, Am J Sports Med 15(1):59, 1987.
23. Priest JD, and Weise DJ: Elbow injury in women's gymnastics, Am J Sports Med 9(5):288, 1981.
24. Priest JD: Elbow injuries in sports, sports medicine fitness and nutritioin corner, Minn Med, p 543, 1982.
25. Priest JD: Elbow injuries in gymnastics. Symposium on gymnastics. Clin Sports Med 4(1):73, January, 1985.
26. Read MTF: Stress fractures of the distal radius in adolescent gymnasts, Brit J Sports Med 15(4):272, 1981.
27. Roy S, Caine D, and Singer KM: Stress changes of the distal radial epiphysis in young gymnasts, Am J Sports Med 13(5):301, 1985.
28. Singer KM and Roy SP: Osteochondrosis of the humeral capitellum, Am J Sports Med 12(5):351, 1984.
29. Snook GA: Injuries in women's gymnastics: a 5 year study, Am J Sports Med 7(4):242, 1979.
30. Taylor AA and Shively RA: Bilateral elbow dislocations with intra-articular displacement of the medial epicondyles, J Trauma 20(4):332, 1980.
31. Teitz CC: Sports medicine concerns in dance and gymnastics, Clin Sports Med 2(3):571, 1983.
32. Weiker GG: Introduction and history of gymnastics, Clin Sports Med 4(1):39, 1985.
33. Weiker GG: Club gymnastics. Symposium on gymnastics. Clin Sports Med 4(1):39, 1985.
34. Weiker GG, Grabner M, and Campbell K: Pressure across the elbow during gymnastic vaulting. Unpublished.
35. Whiteside JA et al: Fractures and refractures in intercollegiate athletes: an eleven-year experience, Am J Sports Med 9(6):369, 1981.
36. Wettstone E, editor: Gymnastics safety manual, University Park, 1977, Pennsylvania State University Press.
37. Wood MB et al: Abductor pollicis longus bursitis, Clin Orthop 93:293, June 1973.

CHAPTER 39 Evaluation, Treatment, and Prevention of Upper Extremity Injuries in Golfers

John R. McCarroll

The golf swing is physically demanding and has contributed to various injuries. The person who does not play golf may imagine it is less taxing than other sports.* However, it is not. Injuries are frequent and result in sprained wrists, aching shoulders, and sore elbows; most injuries are related to the golf swing.[3–5]

The frequency of golf injuries to the upper extremity has received little attention in the literature. There have been reports of fractures of carpal bones, especially the hook of the hamate secondary to impact with the end of the club.[10] There are many incidences of ulnar and median neuropathies along with tendonitis as a result of various injuries during different parts of the golf swing.[7,9] One study of professional golfers reported that in the upper extremity, in right-handed golfers, the left wrist was most frequently injured, followed by the left hand, the left shoulder, and the left elbow[3–5] (Table 39-1).

BIOMECHANICS

To evaluate, treat, and prevent golf injuries, one must understand the golf swing. I like to break the golf swing into three parts: take-away, impact, and follow-through.

Take-Away

Take-away (Fig. 39-1) consists of the setup and movement to the top of the back swing. During this time, golfers take their grip, stand properly, and align themselves over the ball. They then rotate the shoulders, trunk, hips, and knees while the head remains stationary. This action is accomplished by hyperabduction of the left thumb in the right-handed

*EDITORS' NOTE: Walking and swinging golf clubs at an 18-hole, 3-hour pace generate a heart rate increase of approximately 20% on a flat course, and a hilly course can effect a 40% rise in pulse rate (unpublished data, Nicholas Institute of Sports Medicine and Athletic Trauma).

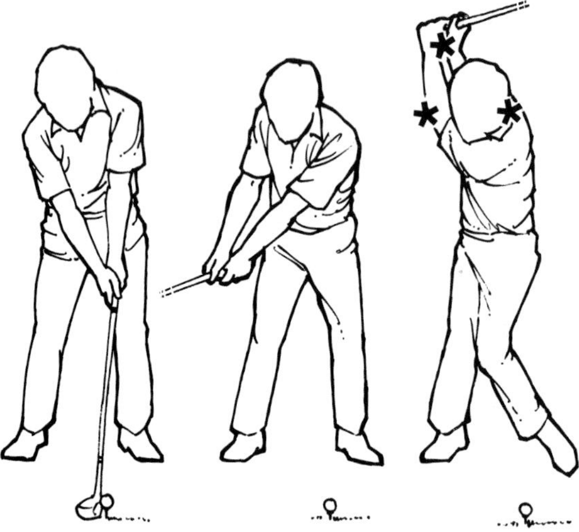

FIG. 39-1. Take-away.

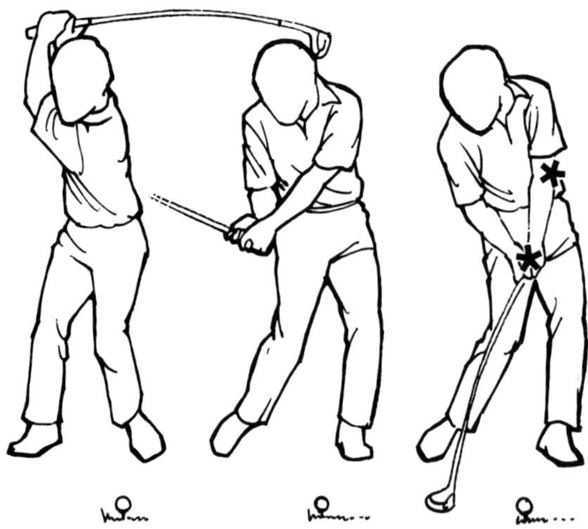

FIG. 39-2. Impact.

golfer, radial deviation of the left wrist at the top of the back swing, and dorsiflexion of the right wrist. The marks in Fig. 39-1 represent areas of stress to the wrist, elbow, and shoulder during this phase of the golf swing.

Impact

Impact (Fig. 39-2) consists of preimpact and impact phases (downswing and acceleration). As the player starts to hit the ball, the right wrist is in maximal dorsiflexion; the left thumb is hyperabducted; the left ulnar nerve, right elbow, and forearm flexors are stretched; and the left hip is rotated. At impact, the left wrist and hand are thrust into the ball, compression occurs at the right wrist, and the left elbow extensor mass contracts.

TABLE 39-1 Injuries to the upper extremity in professional golfers

	Men (%)	Women (%)	Total (%)
Left wrist	16.1	31.3	23.9
Left hand	6.8	7.5	7.1
Left shoulder	10.9	3.0	6.9
Left elbow	3.1	4.5	3.8
Left thumb	5.2	1.5	3.3
Right wrist	1.5	4.5	3.1
Right elbow	4.2	1.5	2.8
Right shoulder	0.5	4.5	2.5

Data from McCarroll JR and Gioe TJ: Phys Sportsmed 10:64, 1982.

TABLE 39-2 Injuries to the upper extremity in recreational golfers

	Men (%)	Women (%)	Total (%)
Left elbow	22.2	28.6	23.2
Left wrist	9.4	5.2	8.7
Left shoulder	7.5	13.0	8.3
Left hand	5.2	6.5	5.4
Right elbow	1.0	3.0	2.2

Follow-Through

The **follow-through** phase (Fig. 39-3) consists of the time after impact and follow-through. After the player hits the ball while pivoting, the left forearm supinates, the right forearm pronates, the lumbar and cervical areas of the spine rotate and hyperextend, hip rotation is completed, and there is a complete weight shift to the left side of the body with rotation of the knees to the left and inversion of the left ankle.

EPIDEMIOLOGY

Injuries to the upper extremity may arise in any phase of the golf swing. In a study of professional golfers[5] the wrist and shoulder were the most affected parts of the upper extremity during take-away. The wrist was most affected in the impact phase, followed by the elbow and hand, and the shoulder and elbow were the most affected in the follow-through phase.

The incidence of golf injuries to the upper extremity was reported in two articles. One article[5] on professional right-handed golfers shows that the left wrist was injured in 23.9% of the golfers, followed in incidence by the left

TABLE 39-3 Mechanisms of injury[5]

	Percent
Too much play or practice	21.4
Poor swing mechanics	14.4
Hit ground or large divot	12.8
Pain just starts with no cause	9.2
Hit by ball	8.6
Overswing (swing too hard)	7.9
Poor warm-up	4.9
Hit object other than ball	4.7
Grip or swing change	3.4
Fall	3.1
Twist during swing	2.9
Fell out of golf cart	2.4
Miscellaneous (hit by club, bitten by snake)	4.1

Data from McCarroll JR and Gioe TJ: Phys Sportsmed 10:64, 1982.

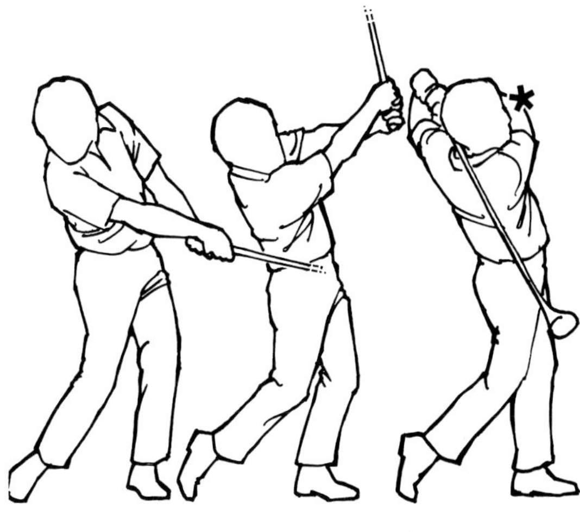

FIG. 39-3. Follow-through.

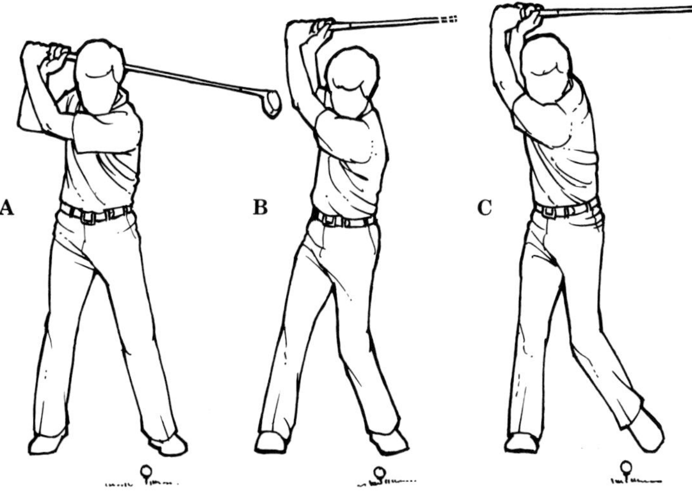

FIG. 39-4. Three golfers. **A,** Golfer showing bent elbow and poor swinging mechanics. **B,** Golfer showing poor weight shift and poor swinging mechanics. **C,** Golfer showing correct swing position at top of take-away.

hand, left shoulder, left elbow, and left thumb (Table 39-1). In a recently completed but as yet unpublished study I did of recreational golfers the incidence of injuries to the upper extremity differs, with the elbow being the most commonly injured. This is related to poor swing mechanics (Table 39-2).

The mechanism of injury (Table 39-3) is most commonly related to the golf swing. The most common mechanism of injury is too much play or practice, causing overuse syndrome to the upper extremity. In the professional golfer[5] these injuries are most commonly caused by the repeated stress of practice, but in the recreational golfer these can be the result of poor swing mechanics (Fig. 39-4). Bending of the left elbow on take-away causes the elbow to be extended sharply into the ball at impact, causing increased stress to the forearm and resulting in tennis elbow (Fig. 39-4, *A*). In the middle golfer (Fig. 39-4, *B*), the poor weight shift, or so-called reverse pivot, causes unnecessary stress on the joints, tendons, and muscles of the upper extremity. The golfer on the right in Fig. 39-4, *C* shows the proper swing that reduces the stress on the upper extremity. Other mechanisms of injury, such as hitting trees, roots, or hard ground, can also cause injuries. These are summarized in Table 39-3.[5]

Just as the incidence, type, and mechanisms of injuries varied, so did the treatment of these injuries. Although specific injuries and their treatment are discussed later in this

TABLE 39-4 Treatment of golf injuries

Type	Professional (%)	Recreational (%)	Total (%)
Rest	16.0	30.8	24.7
Physical therapy	16.9	12.0	14.1
Medication	10.7	9.5	9.9
Injection	10.2	9.2	9.6
Ice	6.3	10.8	9.0
Heat	8.5	7.6	8.0
Chiropractor	6.5	0.7	3.1
Braces (tennis elbow)	5.8	8.5	7.4
Surgery	5.8	3.4	4.4
Traction	1.7	0.7	1.2
Acupuncture	1.6	0.4	0.9

Data from McCarroll JR and Gioe TJ: Phys Sportsmed 10:64, 1982.

chapter, we would like to summarize the various types of treatment that these golfers received. In the professional golfer[5] physical therapy was the most commonly prescribed treatment, followed by rest. In the recreational golfer more time was given for rest and physical therapy was second. These findings are summarized in Table 39-4. However, in the professional golfer, 54.3% of the men and 53.7% of the women are still bothered by their injuries.[5] Of the recreational golfers, 44.6% are still bothered by their injury.

SPECIFIC GOLF INJURIES

It would be redundant to repeat the physical findings, treatment, and other tests of such common disorders seen in other parts of this text as carpal tunnel syndrome, rotator cuff impingement, lateral epicondylitis (tennis elbow), and ulnar nerve subluxation or entrapment, because these are very common injuries in golf and are covered well in other chapters. This discussion will emphasize a few injuries that may be unique to golf.

Fracture of the Hook of the Hamate

The hook of the hamate is a long, thin bone that is subject to injury as it projects toward the palmar surface of the hand. Fractures occur in golf when the grip of the club strikes the hook of the hamate and fractures it. The athlete complains of wrist pain and weak grip. Clinical examination shows tenderness to pressure over the hook of the hamate. Roentgenograms should include anteroposterior, lateral, and oblique views of the wrist. These routine roentgenograms often do not show a fracture, and many times a carpal tunnel view of the wrist is needed. If these films do not show a fracture but the injury is still suspected, then a bone scan or CT scan may be helpful. Since the ulnar nerve and flexor digitorum profundus to the small finger are all so close to the fracture site, the patient may experience symptoms of ulnar nerve impingement or tendonitis. Fracture of the hook of the hamate may also lead to rupture of the ring finger flexor tendon from chronic inflammatory changes.[10]

In the acute nondisplaced fracture, the treatment is a short arm cast and rest for 6 weeks. The incidence of nonunion of this fracture is high, and in a badly displaced fracture or in a nonunion, the excision of the hook itself is indicated.[10]

de Quervain's Disease

de Quervain's disease is a common condition I have seen in at least five professional golfers as a result of repetitive practice. de Quervain's disease is a tenosynovitis of the first dorsal compartment of the wrist. The diagnostic sign of it is Finkelstein's test. This is performed with the thumb and hand forcibly deviated toward the ulnar side of the wrist. There is exquisite pain over the radial styloid process and the common sheath of the abductor pollicis longus and extensor pollicis brevis tendon. This test is also similar to the mechanisms that are involved in hitting the golf ball. At preimpact and impact this causes repeated stress and synovitis in golfers. Conservative treatment of de Quervain's disease involves splints, ice, and antiinflammatory medication. Only in resistant cases is injection or operative treatment considered.

Traumatic Arthritis

Traumatic arthritis is very common in the small joints of the hand, especially in professional and avid golfers because of the con-

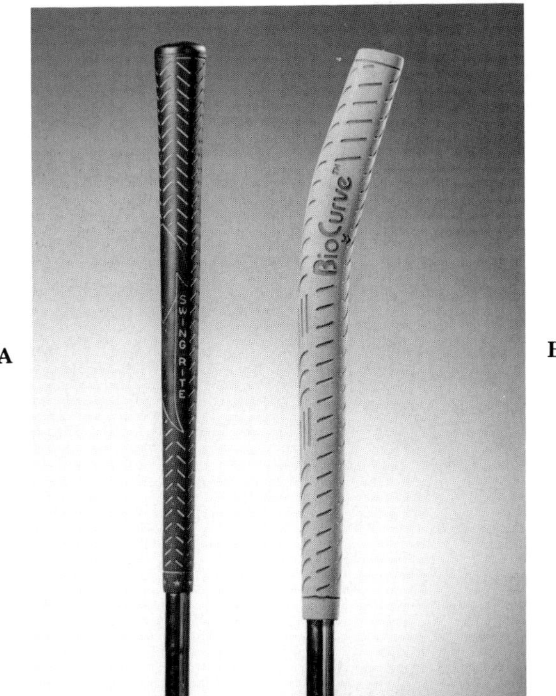

FIG. 39-5. Two golf clubs and their grips. **A,** The swing right grip is the standard accepted golf grip. **B,** The Bio-Curve grip is the new curved grip that prevents certain hand, arm, and elbow injuries.

stant stress of striking the ball. This can be treated with antiinflammatory drugs and grip changes. However, there are special grips that reduce the torque and stress on the hands and forearms (Fig. 39-5) for those players with these conditions, but these grips are not yet legal under the United States Golf Association's rules.

Miscellaneous Conditions

Other conditions such as tendonitis, ligamentous sprains, and carpal tunnel syndrome may occur in the wrist and hands of golfers. These are discussed in Chapters 26, 27, and 31.

Epicondylitis

The golfer may suffer two very common elbow injuries, medial and lateral epicondylitis. The diagnosis and treatment of these injuries in racquet and throwing sports are well covered (Chapter 17). We will not repeat the signs, symptoms, and treatment but will try to describe how these occur in golf and how by correcting the poor swing mechanics these problems may be prevented or resolved. Fig. 39-4 shows a golfer with the left elbow bent on the backswing, or take-away. When he tries to hit the ball he snaps or throws the hand and forearm at the ball, causing excessive and incorrect stress on the extensor muscles of the forearm and their origins at the lateral epicondyle. Also at impact the golfer may "roll" the wrist or supinate the left forearm, causing increased torque on these muscles and lateral epicondylitis in the left arm of the right-handed golfer. This can be prevented by proper address, take-away, and swing mechanics, as well as the proper medical treatment.

Medial epicondylitis, sometimes referred to as "golfers' elbow," usually occurs over the medial epicondyle of the right elbow in the right-handed golfer. This is caused by "hitting from the top." In this situation, instead of pulling the club through with the left side using the legs, back, shoulder, and other muscles, the golfer throws the club from the top of the backswing, or take-away, down into the ball at impact. This is very similar to hitting a forehand in tennis or a "kill" shot in racquetball. It causes extreme stress on the flexor muscles, especially at the attachment on the medial epicondyle. Injury to the ulnar nerve must be evaluated during the physical examination. Treatment is symptomatic, using ice, counterforce bracing, physical therapy, or antiinflammatory medication and injections. Occasionally, surgery is necessary (surgical techniques are discussed in Chapter 17). The need for surgery can often be prevented by correcting the athlete's swing mechanics.

Shoulder Impingement Syndrome

The most common injury to the shoulder in golf is that of rotator cuff impingement syndrome. This problem is discussed in detail in Chapter 8.

PREVENTION OF GOLF INJURIES

Biomechanics

In preventing golf injuries, one should start with the golf swing. As in any sport, proper mechanics are extremely important. The teaching golf professional, using years of experience and such devices as video recording, can correct the mechanisms of the golf swing to prevent injuries and to change abnormal stress applied to various body parts.

Equipment Considerations

The next step in preventing golf injuries is the use of proper equipment. Proper size and shape of the grip are necessary to ensure proper swing mechanics and to relieve torsional stress at impact. The stiffness of the shafts and the length and weight of the club may also play an important role. Many manufacturers are trying to make equipment to relieve specific problems, such as special grips for arthritic or injured golfers. The most recent is the Bio-Curve grip (Fig. 39-5), which decreases torsional stress to the arm and hand. Unfortunately, these clubs have not yet been approved by the United States Golf Association and therefore are not in common use. The club professional is again the expert in these areas and should assist the golfer in these aspects.

Golf equipment considerations

- **Grip**
  - Size
  - Shape
- **Club**
  - Stiffness
  - Length
  - Weight

Conditioning and Golf

Golf is an activity demanding a very high degree of refined motor skills. There are many frustrated golfers trying to play when they are not in shape. The weekend golfer and even the professional golfer must condition the body before going to the course or must assume the risk of injury. Golf is a strenuous game, and weakness in the upper extremity that will not withstand the stress of hitting or swinging at a golf ball will contribute to the occurence of an injury. Too many golfers ruin the entire golf season with injuries to the shoulder, elbow, or wrist, as well as other injuries. Injuries, sore muscles, and frustrating days on the golf course can be eliminated by a preseason, regular season, and off-season conditioning program.

Recent studies add scientific data to the need for a conditioning program. Jobe et al,[1] in a study of bilateral shoulder muscle activity during the golf swing using electromyography and high-speed photography, showed that an understanding of muscle firing patterns might help the golfer to prevent injuries and develop appropriate training and conditioning programs. They studied the swings of seven adult male right-handed professional golfers and found that all portions of the deltoid muscles were inactive on the right side during the golf swing. The deltoid was likewise inactive on the left except for a brief spurt from the anterior portion during the milliseconds immediately preceding ball contact.

The rotator cuff muscles on the left, the supraspinatus, fired at a low level throughout the swing as did the infraspinatus. The latter had a slightly larger burst of activity immediately after ball contact. The subscapularis was more active than any other muscle throughout the golf swing. The cuff muscles on the right side showed as much activity overall as those on the left. In addition, the latissimus dorsi and pectoralis major seemed to provide power bilaterally, with marked activity during the preimpact, or acceleration, phase. Jobe et al also showed that the left shoulder of the right-handed golfer does not provide more drive than the right. To achieve greater distance it would seem that a golfer should concentrate on exercising the rotator cuff bilaterally as well as the latissimus dorsi and pectoralis major.

To perform at one's optimal level, to hit the ball farther, to make more consistent contact with the ball, to lessen one's chance of injury, and to improve overall endurance, one must follow certain types of conditioning programs.

Stretching

Stretching exercises are used to maintain complete range of motion of various body parts, not just the upper extremity. Without maximal attainable range of motion and flexibility, the golfer may be injured when swing-

TABLE 39-5 Nautilus workout program for golf

Exercise	Muscles developed	Skills involved
Hip and back	Buttocks, lower	Driving power Walking endurance
Leg extension	Quadriceps	Driving power Walking endurance
Leg curl	Hamstrings	Hip turn Driving power
Double shoulder (lateral press)	Deltoids	Club control Impact velocity
Double shoulder (seated press)	Deltoids, triceps	Shoulder turn Club extension
Pullover	Latissimus dorsi	Shoulder turn Club extension
Wrist curl	Forearm flexors	Club head control Impact power Acceleration
Reverse wrist curls	Forearm flexors	Club head control Impact power Acceleration

Data from Peterson J: Conditioning for a purpose, the West Point way, West Point, NY, 1977, Leisure Press.

ing or taking a divot. It is extremely important to have a good warm-up program involving flexibility stretching for the body. These exercises are well illustrated and explained in Jobe's works[1,2] and that of Spackman.[8]

Strength

Golf is not only a strength game like many sports; strength in itself will not enable the individual to hit the ball better or longer. However, it will allow the skilled player to strike shots with more consistently explosive power over extended periods. Any golfer with a weak area, for example, the shoulder, is at risk for injury. There are various muscles that need to be strengthened to improve basic skills. Driving power involves the buttocks, quadriceps, hamstrings, and lower back muscles. The hip turn involves the lower back muscles and hip flexors. Impact velocity, or swinging the club through the ball, requires well-formed latissimus dorsi and triceps muscles. Control of the club through take-away, impact, and follow-through requires strength in the deltoids, triceps, biceps, forearms, and hand flexors.

A typical Nautilus or Universal gym workout is summarized in Table 39-5.[7] The golfer who does not have specialized exercise equipment can use weighted clubs, chairs, or other household items. These programs are well described by Jobe et al[1] and Spackman[8] in their monographs.

Cardiovascular Training

Cardiovascular exercise for endurance is another essential part of conditioning. Climbing hills and walking 18 holes are impossible without having the heart and lungs to respond to strenuous exercise, especially in very hot, humid weather. Following a preseason conditioning program of jogging and bicycling, walking and staying out of the golf cart will help build endurance and help with overall fitness.

SUMMARY

The golf swing is physically demanding and has contributed to various types of injuries. The wrist, shoulder, and elbow are frequently injured. These injuries may be prevented or reduced by a combination of proper conditioning, treatment, and proper swing mechanics.

REFERENCES

1. Jobe FW, Moynes DR, and Antonelli DJ: Rotator cuff function during a golf swing, Am J Sports Med 14:388, 1986.
2. Jobe FW and Moynes DR: 30 Exercises to better golf, Inglewood, CA, 1986, Crampton Press.
3. McCarroll JR: Golf. In Schneider RC, Kennedy JC, and Plant ML, editors: Sports injuries: mechanisms, prevention and treatment, Baltimore, 1985, The Williams & Wilkins Co.
4. McCarroll JR: Golf: common injuries from a supposedly benign activity, J Musculoskel Med 3(5):9, 1986.
5. McCarroll JR and Gioe TJ: Professional golfers and the price they pay, Phys Sportsmed 10:64, 1982.

6. Peterson J: Conditioning for a purpose, the West Point way, West Point, NY, 1977, Leisure Press, p 280.
7. Roberts J: Injuries, handicaps, mashies, and cleeks, Phys Sportsmed 6:121, 1978.
8. Spackman RB: Conditioning for golf, Murfreesburo, IL, 1974, Schwebel Printing.
9. Stover CN, Wiren G, and Topaz SR: The modern golf swing and stress syndrome, Phys Sportsmed 4:42, 1976.
10. Torisu T: Fracture of the hook of the hamate by a golf swing, Clin Orthop 83:91, 1972.

CHAPTER 40 Upper Extremity Swimming Injuries

Peter J. Fowler

Injury to the shoulder is the most common problem facing competitive swimmers of all ages. The repeated strong demands made on the upper body stress the shoulder muscles and their tendons far in excess of normal usage and design. Anatomic features and biomechanical forces may combine in the swimmer to produce "swimmer's shoulder." This term refers to tendonitis of the rotator cuff, usually the supraspinatus and/or the biceps tendon, and was first used in the clinical literature by Kennedy and Hawkins in 1974.[6] They reported that 3% of the competitive swimmers surveyed had experienced shoulder pain. Recent papers have quoted a history of shoulder pain in 50% of swimmers.[11] Intensity of training schedules has increased significantly and, coupled with biomechanical factors, may be a causal factor in the increased incidence of swimmer's shoulder. Understanding these factors can assist swimmers and their coaches to plan training programs that reduce its incidence. An informed coach is the best ally a sports physician can have; it is much easier to prevent an injury than to work with an injured athlete.

SWIMMING STROKES

There are four competitive swimming strokes: the front crawl, backstroke, breaststroke, and butterfly. Seventy-five percent of propulsion comes from the arms in the front crawl, backstroke, and butterfly. In the breaststroke the arms and legs contribute equally. The freestyle event in competitive swimming is open to any stroke, usually the front crawl is chosen. In this chapter we use the term "freestyle" and "front crawl" synonymously.

ANATOMIC FEATURES

The shoulder joint is the most mobile joint in the human body and has little bony support or protection. It relies on its capsule, the surrounding ligaments, and the rotator cuff muscles, as well as larger muscles, such as the pectoralis major and the serratus anterior for the stability that allows the arm to function with power and precision throughout its range of motion.

The four rotator cuff muscles work in a force couple combination with the deltoid and long head of the biceps to contain the head of the humerus in the glenoid fossa.

The supraspinatus muscle inserts on the uppermost facet of the greater tuberosity. It acts as a fulcrum for the deltoid during abduction and is active throughout that movement. It also assists the other rotator cuff muscles to resist any upward displacement of the humeral head in other arm actions. The infraspinatus and the teres minor are external rotators. In the horizontal plane, the infraspinatus extends the humerus. The infraspinatus muscle also works in combination with the supraspinatus and the subscapularis to depress the humeral head.

The primary internal rotator of the shoulder is the subscapularis. It stabilizes the head of the humerus by resisting anterior or inferior displacement in the glencid fossa and, as previously mentioned, exerts a depressive force on the humeral head in combination with the supraspinatus and the infraspinatus.

Active in forward flexion of the shoulder, the long head of the biceps also has an important role in stabilizing the head of the humerus. This function should not be overlooked in shoulder mechanics.

The scapular muscles, the serratus anterior, the rhomboids, and the trapezius work constantly in the swimming arm action. If they fatigue, especially the serratus anterior, the scapula may have relative downward tilt, altering the mechanics of the glenohumeral joint. This in turn can contribute to the onset of impingement tendonitis.

Scapular muscles active in swimming arm action

- Serratus anterior
- Rhomboids
- Trapezius

TENDONITIS

Overwork

The shoulder joint is least stable, and therefore most vulnerable to injury, in the overhead position. Swimming puts continuous repeated demands on the shoulder in this position. The muscles of the rotator cuff may work excessively hard to contain and stabilize the humeral head, and the workload may fatigue them. Superior migration of the humeral head may occur with cuff fatigue, increasing subacromial loading. This, in turn, may be a precipitating factor in the onset of tendonitis.

Impingement

Soft Tissue Factors

The supraspinatus and the biceps tendons are particularly susceptible to impingement. Their tendons insert on or cross the humerus directly below the coracoacromial arch, formed by the coracoid process, the rigid coracoacromial ligament, and the anterior acromion. When the arm is in abduction, forward flexion, and internal rotation, the head of the humerus moves under the arch and the tendons may be impinged. This position is assumed in the catch phase of all competitive strokes. Repeatedly the tendons are impinged against the arch, which may result in a mechanical irritation and an inflammatory response or tendonitis.

The inflammation may further compromise the available space under the coracroacromial arch. If untreated, the inflammatory process can go on to include the subacromial bursa and the acromioclavicular ligament.

Osseous Contributing Factors

In 1986, Bigliani and his associates[1] reported a study attempting to discover a correlation between acromial shape and full-thickness tears. They examined the acromions of 140 cadavers and classified them according to shape, angle of anterior slope, and the presence of anterior spurs.

Three acromial shapes were identified: type I, flat; type II, curved; and type III, hooked. There were variations in the angle of the slope from 13.1 to 28.7 degrees, and there were rotator cuff tears in 70% of the acromions with bony spurs.

Bigliani's findings suggested an anatomic factor in refractory tendonitis that does not respond to conservative management. A type III acromion in a competitive swimmer may precipitate impingement because the dimensions of the coracoacromial arch are already decreased. A tendonitis would be more easily

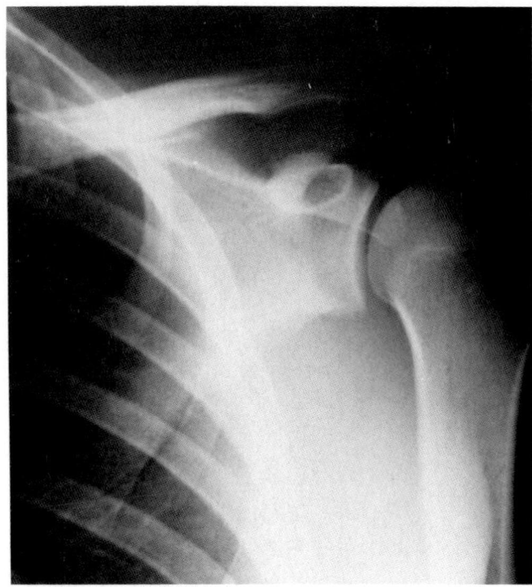

FIG. 40-1. A lateral scapular view taken with the tube directed 10 degrees caudal.

developed and more resistant to treatment. The type III slope described by Bigliani can be seen on roentgenogram using a lateral scapular view taken 10 degrees caudally (Fig. 40-1). However, further studies are required to confirm its association with refractory tendonitis.

Staging

Neer and Welsh[9] have provided clinicians with a chronologic framework for the progression of tendonitis. Stage I, edema and hemorrhage, is most often seen in athletes under 25 years. Stage II, fibrosis and tendonitis, occurs in athletes between 25 and 40, while Stage III most often develops in those over 40. Osteophytes form under the acromion,[8] and tendon ruptures, either partial or complete, can occur. However, in the competitive athlete these stages can occur at any age.

Hypovascularity

Rathbun and Macnab's[10] study of the functional relationship between arm position and blood supply to the supraspinatus and the biceps tendon is well known. In adduction and neutral rotation, the tendons are stretched tightly over the head of the humerus and their blood supply is compromised. In abduction the vessels fill, restoring full circulation. This "wringing out" mechanism, or repeated hypovascularity, may contribute to early degenerative changes in the tendon. It occurs in the area of the tendon most vulnerable to impingement, compounding the potential for damage by repetitive stress.

Increased Shoulder Joint Laxity

Overwork as a factor in tendonitis in competitive swimmers has already been described. However, if the athlete has loose or lax shoulers, the muscles of the rotator cuff may already be working hard just to contain the humeral head. The added rigor of training makes additional demands on already fatigued or fatiguing muscles. Increased laxity should not be overlooked as a contributing factor in an athlete with resistant tendonitis.

In 1982, Fowler and Webster[3] evaluated 188 competitive swimmers between 13 and 26 years of age. There was a control group of 50 recreational athletes not bothered by shoulder pain. Each subject had a formal history taken, recording any episodes of shoulder pain. They were assessed for positive signs of tendonitis and for posterior, inferior, and anterior instability or increased laxity.

Anterior instability was tested using the "apprehension test." A positive response was recorded if the athlete displayed any sign of pain or anxiety. The sulcus sign was used to recognize inferior instability.

Posterior laxity was evaluated using the "load and shift" test conducted in two positions, sitting and supine. While supine, the athlete lies on the examining table with the shoulder to be inspected free. The arm is supported in the 90-degree abducted position and force is then applied to the humerus posteriorly (Fig. 40-2). In the second test, with the athlete sitting, the shoulder girdle is stablized with one hand and forearm while the other hand translates the humerus posteriorly (Fig. 40-3).

The index for posterior laxity was based on the excursion of the humeral head with respect to the posterior glenoid fossa. In many normal asymptomatic individuals the proximal humerus can be translated posteriorly 50% of the glenoid width. Any movement greater than that, in this study, was classified as excessive posterior laxity.

Fifty percent of the 188 swimmers had a history of shoulder pain. Almost 55% of the swimmers and 52% of the control participants had some degree of posterior laxity in one or both shoulders. These results suggest that *swimming does not predispose an athlete to increased posterior laxity*. Twenty-five percent of the swimmers had a history of tendonitis and increased posterior laxity; the ten-

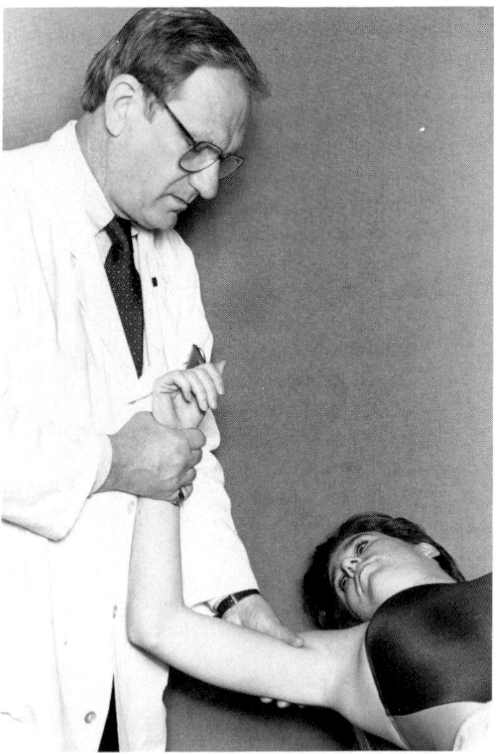

FIG. 40-2. A clinical test for posterior laxity. The abducted position mimics the position of the arm in many sporting activities.

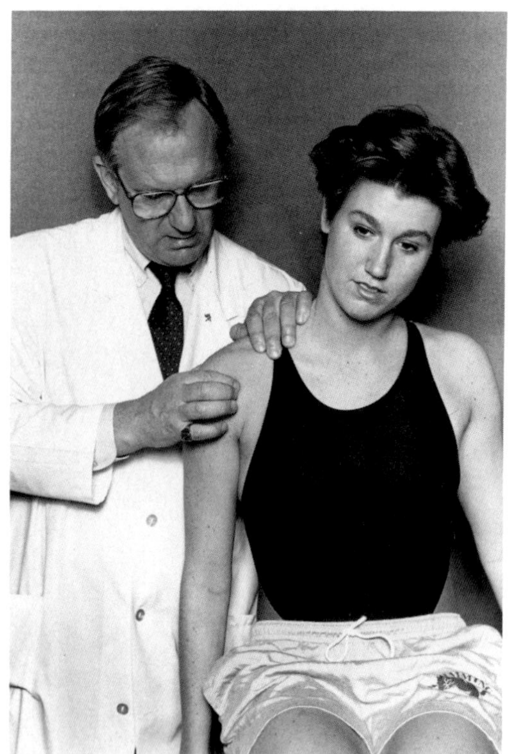

FIG. 40-3. A test for posterior laxity. Ensure that the patient maintains proper posture. Care should be taken when grasping the humeral head; this area may be tender.

donitis was always in the lax shoulder. There does seem to be a relationship between tendonitis and posterior laxity.

Shoulder Strength Imbalance

Many of these same swimmers demonstrated weakness of the external rotators when gross manual testing was performed. Forty athletes had weakness on one or both shoulders. Thirty-three had both weakness and a history of tendonitis in that shoulder.

This prompted a second study[4] to determine rotation strength about the shoulder. One hundred and nineteen swimmers and 51 controls all between 13 and 26 years of age were tested on the Cybex II Dynamometer. The controls were competitive athletes participating in sports that did not primarily require arm rotation strength.

Internal and external rotation strength were measured in neutral, 90 degrees abduction, and 90 degrees flexion. There was a significant difference in the torque ratio between the two groups in abduction and neutral (Table 40-1). The difference in the ratio was attributable to the swimmers' greater strength in internal rotation. There was no significant difference in external rotation strength between the two groups.

TABLE 40-1 Internal external rotation ratio

Position	Swimmers	Control
90 degrees abduction	62.1	78.2
Neutral	53.7	65.8

Shoulder strength imbalances noted in swimmers

- Very strong internal rotators
- Normal strength external rotators
- Abnormal ratio of internal to external rotators

This study indicates that swimmers have an imbalance in rotation strength ratios when compared to other athletes. This is probably

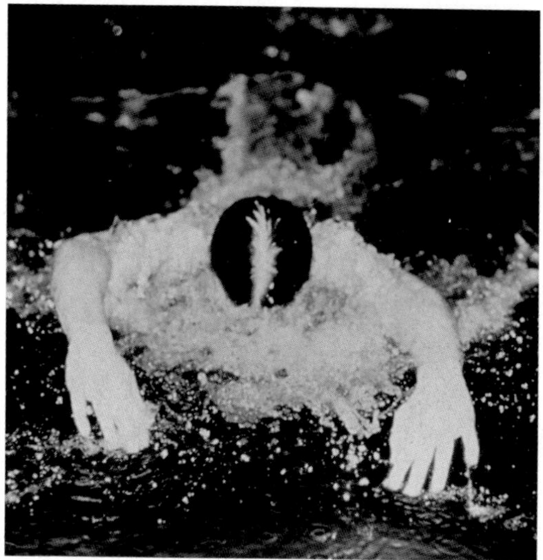

FIG. 40-4. The reach or arm entry position for the butterfly stroke. This arm position is similar for all 4 competitive strokes.

because of the emphasis in their training programs, both swimming and on land, in strengthening the internal rotators and extensors to improve swimming speed and endurance.

Modifying training programs to include external rotation strengthening to restore the normal strength ratio should be a preventive measure against tendonitis. Evaluation of external rotation strength in swimmers with a resistant tendonitis can give the clinician added information of value concerning the effectiveness of conservative management.

Impingement Positions in Swimming Strokes

In 1981 Webster[11] circulated a questionnaire to age-group swimmers in the Province of Ontario. Its aim was to formulate a profile of the athlete with tendonitis.

Of the 155 responses, 48.4% reported present or past episodes of shoulder pain. Ninety-nine percent used the front crawl as their main practice stroke. Analysis of the front crawl arm position at the time they experienced pain seemed to correlate with the biomechanical factors in tendonitis (Table 40-2).

At entry and the first half of the pull phase, the shoulder is in forward flexion, abduction, and internal rotation. This forces the head of the humerus toward the anterior acromion and coracoacromial ligament and may impinge the supraspinatus and the biceps tendons (Fig. 40-4).

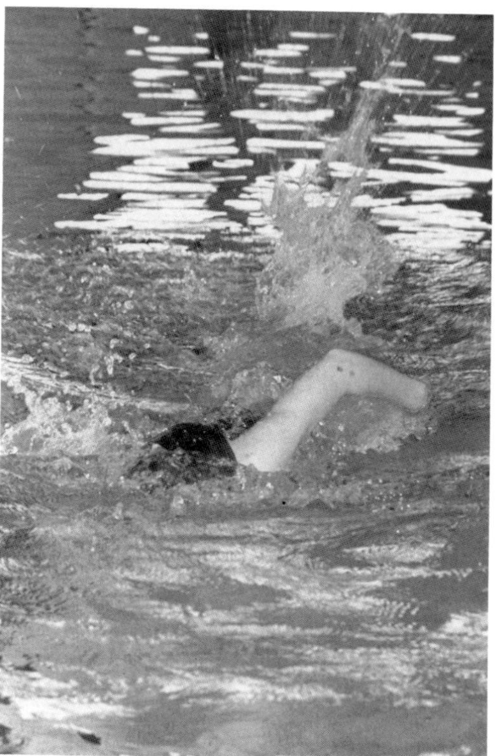

FIG. 40-5. The recovery phase of the freestyle stroke. The amount of subacromial loading in this position is in part determined by the amount of internal rotation of the humerus and the degree of abduction of the arm. The swimmer should turn the torso to recover the arm from the water.

Lateral impingement may be associated with the recovery phase. The shoulder is in abduction and internal rotation, and the head of the humerus comes up against the lateral border of the acromion (Fig. 40-5). This is particularly true when the shoulder leads the rest of the arm. When the head leads the arm through recovery, there is less potential for lateral impingement.

During the end of the pull phase, the shoulder is in adduction and internal rotation, corresponding to the "wringing out" mechanism (Fig. 40-6).

TABLE 40-2 Pain during front crawl arm cycle

Position	Percentage
Entry/first half pull phase	44.7
End of pull	14.3
Recovery	23.2
Throughout cycle	17.8

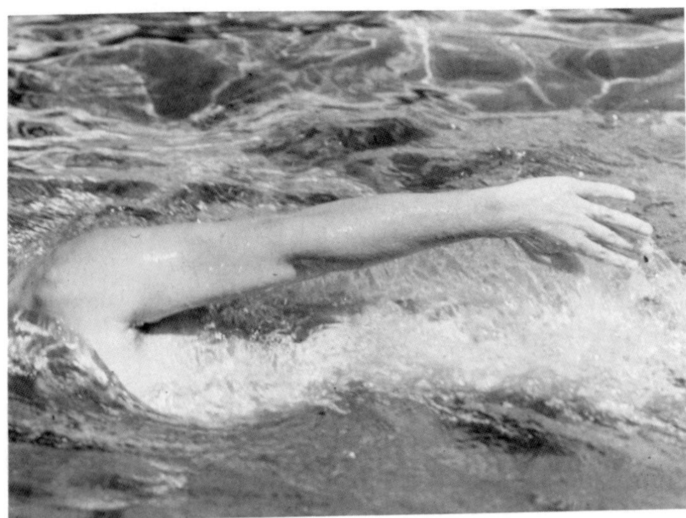

FIG. 40-6. The end of the pull phase is similar for all strokes with the exception of the breaststroke. The area of wringing out of the supraspinatus tendon is the same vulnerable area.

SUMMARY

Overwork, impingement, and hypovascularity are three main factors that contribute to impingement tendonitis in the competitive swimmer. Although the anatomic factors predispose some swimmers to tendonitis, changing training programs and modifying stroke technique can be used effectively both as preventive measures to reduce its incidence and as part of treatment to control its progress.

SHOULDER INSTABILITY

Anterior Instability

Pain from shoulder instability alone is seen in competitive swimmers but not as often. *Anterior instability* is usually secondary to a traumatic incident in another sport. The arm is seldom in the provocative position in any swimming stroke as compared to the throwing mechanism. An exception is the usual backstroke turn where the arm can be levered anteriorly (Fig. 40-7). An alternative type of backstroke turn can biomechanically alleviate this problem. Anterior instability and its evaluation and treatment are discussed in a separate section of this volume (see Chapter 7).

Multidirectional Instability

In contrast to anterior instability, swimmers with frank posterior instability may have pain from dislocating their shoulders in the swimming stroke cycle. The at-risk position of forward flexion and internal rotation occurs in all strokes. Those with multidirectional instability, congenital or acquired, are susceptible to this. This pain must be differentiated from those suffering from painful tendonitis who have concomitant increased laxity.

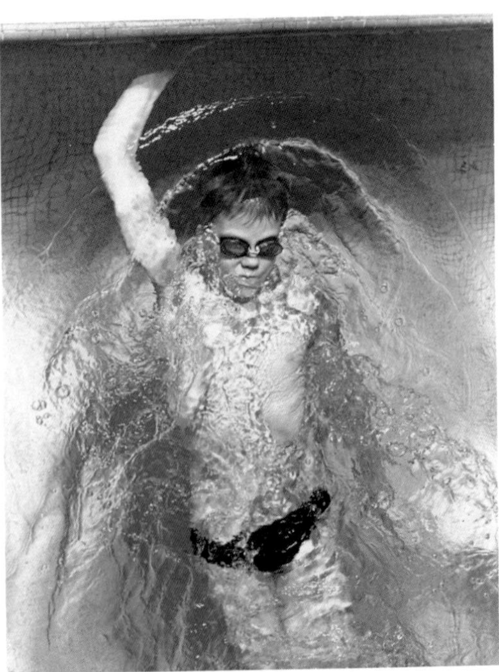

FIG. 40-7. In the standard backstroke turn when the arm touches the wall, the humerus is abducted and externally rotated. The hand remains on the wall around which the body pivots. The head of the humerus may be pried anteriorly if there is anterior laxity.

EVALUATION OF SWIMMERS FOR TENDONITIS

Palpation of the supraspinatus tendon medial to its insertion on the greater tuberosity will elicit tenderness if the tendon is inflamed. If the long head of the biceps is involved, there will be tenderness over the bicipital groove.

Those with supraspinatus tendonitis often demonstrate the classic "painful arc" syndrome. There is pain with active abduction between 60 and 100 degrees. Symptoms of a biceps tendonitis can be reproduced by resisting forward flexion of the straight arm while the forearm is supinated. The presence of a biceps tendonitis can be indicative of a refractory supraspinatus tendonitis.

Clinical pain is often reproduced by placing the shoulder in the impingement aggravated position. In the test described by Neer, the examiner further stresses the already forward flexed arm. This test drives the head of the humerus against the anteroinferior border of the acromion (Fig. 40-8).

A second test, often more appropriate in swimmers, has the examiner internally rotate the arm that is already 90 degrees forward flexed (Fig. 40-9). This pushes the head of the humerus against the coracoacromial ligament, aggravating an inflamed tendon and reproducing pain.

Clinicans should look for muscle weakness about the shoulder, particularly in the external rotators. With the patient's arm in external rotation and adduction and the elbow flexed 90 degrees, the examiner applies an internal rotation force, which the patient resists (Fig. 40-10). Gross weakness will be readily apparent. This test is often accompanied by pain.

The generalized laxity of the swimmer is assessed particularly as it relates to the shoulder. Increased laxity or frank instability needs to be documented as it contributes to a tendonitis progression or may in fact be the total cause of the pain. In anterior instability, the "apprehension" test is very helpful. The patient lies supine on the examining table. The examiner abducts the arm 90 degrees, then externally rotates the humerus. A positive sign is when the patient exhibits a feeling of anxiety, often with pain, or will not allow further external rotation. This feeling may be alleviated by applying posterior pressure on the upper arm, keeping the humeral head contained.

Posterior translation can be assessed with the patient supine, while the examiner holds the arm 90 degrees abducted and applies posterior pressure to the upper humerus (see Fig. 40-2). Movement of the humeral head 50% of the glenoid width is considered normal, and motion greater than that, while not necessarily abnormal, would influence the mechanics of the shoulder by creating an increased work load to the rotator cuff. If the shoudler is unstable, applying an axial load may reproduce the symptoms the patient is having while swimming. This would be pain from the instability itself.

A second test has the patient sitting while the examiner stabilizes the shoulder girdle with one hand and applies posterior pressure

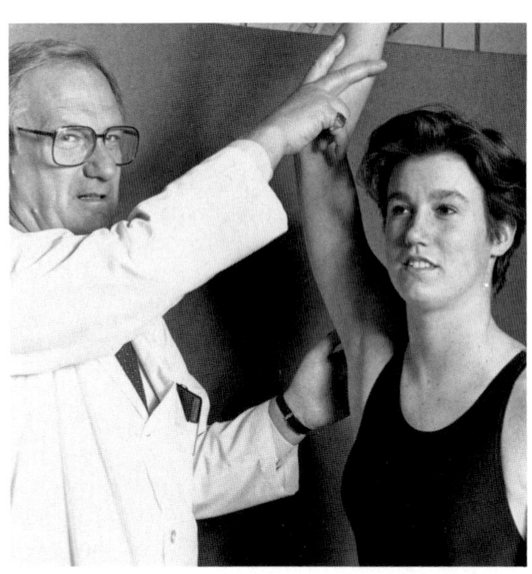

FIG. 40-8. Pressure is applied to the fully forward flexed humerus. Pain may be reproduced if already inflamed tendons are impinged against the anterior acromion.[8]

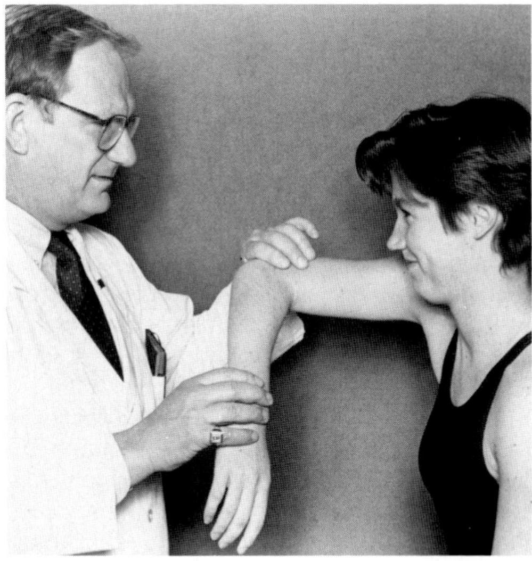

FIG. 40-9. In this test the tendons are impinged under the coracoacromial arch. Care must be taken when using this test as very little pressure will elicit the painful response.

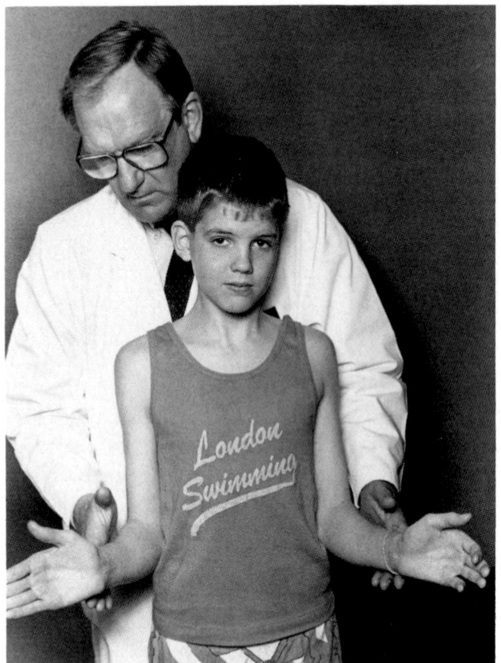

FIG. 40-10. This manual test is appropriate for a gross determination of external rotation muscle strength. A similar resistance test may be performed with the arm abducted to 90 degrees.

to the humeral head with the other hand. The amount of movement is assessed (see Fig. 40-3).

The presence of a sulcus with inferior traction indicates instability in this direction.

The progression of tendonitis is insidious. Pain becomes generalized about the shoulder and is often present at night or at rest. The athlete tends to avoid painful positions and subtle changes in stroke mechanics develop to minimize pain. In other activities as well, athletes will modify all positions that aggravate the symptoms.

Over time there may be a gradual loss of range of motion at the shoulder followed by muscle weakness. Wasting of the supraspinatus and the infraspinatus may become evident. In a mature athlete this may signal either degeneration of the rotator cuff tendon or a partial cuff tear. Cuff tears are seldom seen in age-group swimmers and are rare in all athletes under 25 years of age.

Clinical classification of tendonitis is based on Blazina's[2] categories for Jumper's Knee. In grade I tendonitis the athlete has pain after the activity; in grade II, pain occurs during and after the sport but is not disabling. A grade III tendonitis describes disabling pain during and after activity, while in a fourth and most serious category the condition is so severe that the athlete has pain with daily activities.

PREVENTION

Stress syndromes about the shoulder are easier to prevent than treat, and the principles for prevention should be incorporated into the athlete's training program early.

Work Load

Overwork is one of the primary causes of tendonitis and is often the result of increased intensity of the training sets. Putting athletes through rigorous training sessions before they are ready or through on "extra hard" practice at the beginning of training may do more than show swimmers how much work they need to do. Either of these can trigger the onset of tendonitis.

Training should gradually increase the demand on the swimmers as the schedule progresses. Each training session can be designed so the difficult portion of the practice is earlier in the workout, before the swimmer begins to over-tire. Practice can continue with emphasis on stroke drills, alternating strokes with leg work, and start-and-turn technique to provide the swimmers with relative rest to the structures at risk. With proper instruction, swimmers can learn to guard against the damaging effects of fatigue using increased awareness and good stroke mechanics to minimize the potential for injury.

Strengthening

Imbalance in muscle strength about the shoulder results from emphasis on specific muscle groups during pool and dry-land training, and it contributes to overwork for the cuff muscles. A balanced exercise program that includes external rotation strengthening may reduce the incidence of tendonitis, particularly that associated with increased posterior laxity. The training program should not overlook exercises for the biceps and the scapular muscle. As in the swimming stroke, one should avoid painful subacromial loading positions when doing weight training. Using paddles while swimming is a method of increasing resistance. Paddles must be used with caution because the increased leverage can overload the rotator cuff muscles.

Stretching

Stretching should be done regularly and well as part of the daily training warm-up. Three times weekly is insufficient. In 1981 Griep[5] studied the relationship between shoulder flexibility and the incidence of tendonitis in swimmers. He measured shoulder flexibility in a group of 168 swimmers and recorded the information by gender and by stroke most frequently used. At the end of 6

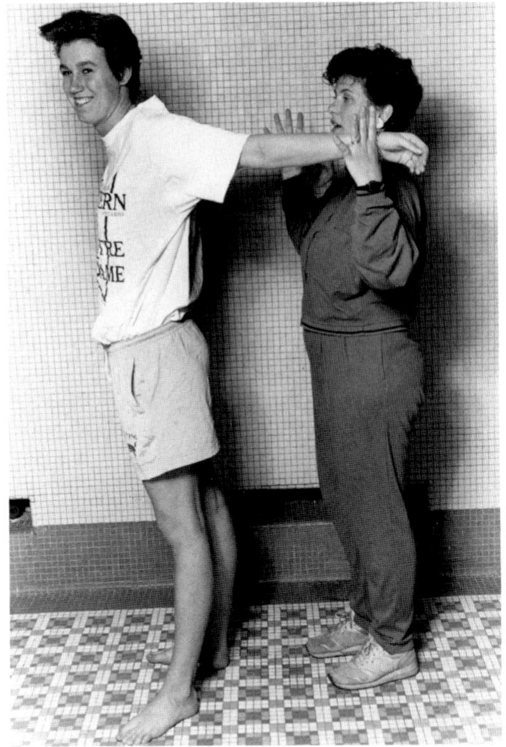

FIG. 40-11. Neuromuscular fascilitated stretching with a partner requires a knowledge of proper technique.[5a]

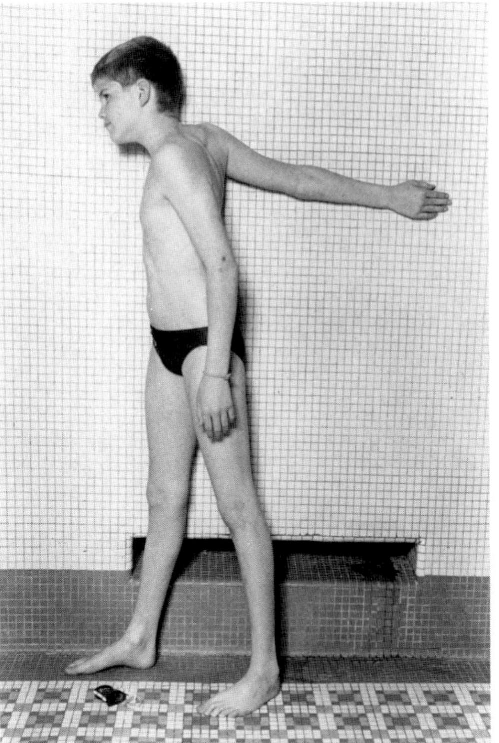

FIG. 40-12. When stretching alone, one can accomodate all of the same muscle groups as stretching when with a partner.

months Griep was able to predict with 93% accuracy which swimmers would develop tendonitis. Regardless of category, the swimmers with restricted flexibility were more likely to develop a tendonitis than those who maintained flexibility with a stretching program.

Swimmers over age 15 should be sufficiently mature to stretch in pairs (Fig. 40-11). The stretching techniques can be either passive or proprioceptive neuromuscular facilitated (PNF).[5a] In the passive type of stretch the partner stretches very slowly to the limit of the pain-free range, then holds the position. In PNF stretching the swimmer to be stretched moves to the limits of range. The partner then maintains that position while the swimmer contracts against the partner's resistance. This is then repeated a variable number of times. Partner stretching has to be done very carefully because overstretching of the soft tissues can increase the irritation to the tendons of the rotator cuff.

Swimmers under the age of 15 are less likely to understand the pitfalls of pairs stretching. For safety reasons they should be taught to stretch on an individual basis (Fig. 40-12).

Stroke Mechanics

Poor stroke mechanics can be a large factor in tendonitis. The coach should analyze the performance of the strokes that cause pain and modify them. Swimmers must be made aware that poor technique not only slows them down but puts them at risk for injury. Analysis of changing stroke technique during fatigue situations is essential. Insufficient body roll in freestyle or backstroke can contribute to lateral shoulder impingement. In the freestyle the swimmer may be told to attain a high elbow position during the recovery. The high elbow position must be achieved with body roll rather than muscle activity. Forcing the elbow into a higher position without body roll may induce subacromial humeral head impingement.

In the "catch" phase of all strokes one is preparing for maximal propulsion. Over-reach with excessive internal rotation may cause undue subacromial loading and excessive activity for the cuff muscles to contain the humeral head. Also, excessive internal rotation at the end of the stroke may intensify the "wringing out" phenomenon.

There is contradictory evidence that breathing patterns affect the incidence of tendonitis[11]. Breathing to alternate sides keeps the swimmer from leaning constantly on to the same shoulder.

Finally, the importance of the coach can not be overemphasized. The coach can conduct an ongoing stroke analysis and guide the swimmer away from stroke errors that contribute to impingement tendonitis. Altering body roll, reach, and degree of shoulder internal rotation can reduce both the frequency and the length of time the shoulder is in the precarious position. The coach plans the training program and monitors the athlete's performance, preventing overwork and fatigue of the rotator cuff.

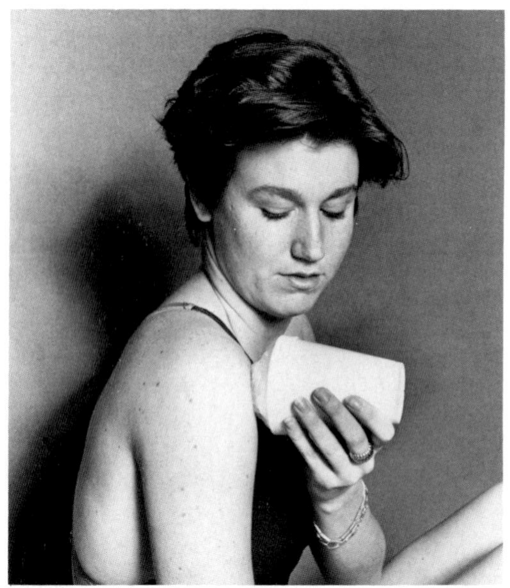

FIG. 40-13. Cold applied to the shoulder is a most effective therapy. Ice cups, crushed ice in plastic bags, or cold packs may be used.

TREATMENT

Tendonitis

Grade I

A grade I tendonitis responds well to management.[2]

Swimmers are told to increase the time spent in both the prepractice stretch and in the pool warm-up. Stretches should pay attention to all structures, including the anterior ones. Appropriate stretching can restore lost range of motion, increase the blood flow, and reduce the potential for further impingement injury. In the pool, warm-up should be prolonged, at a very slow pace and in pain-free strokes. Additional arm warm-ups should be done after kicking sets. A swimming warm-down is recommended after the training session.

Treatment of grade I tendonitis

- Increase prepractice strength and warm-up times
- Emphasize pain-free strokes
- Encourage swimming warm-down period after training session
- Use cryotherapy to reduce pain and inflammation
- Correct external rotation weakness

After the practice the athlete should ice the sore shoulder for no more than 15 minutes to reduce pain and inflammation. Ice cups are the simplest and most effective way to do this (Fig. 40-13). If the swimmer has weakness of the external rotators this should be corrected. The exercises should work the external rotators beginning in adduction and progressing to varying degrees of abduction. This improves the control of the glenohumeral joint, which in turn results in more efficient muscle work and a better performance potential. The swim practice should be as pain-free as possible. If the swimmer has pain only when the work load is too heavy, the load must be reduced for a time and then gradually increased. If only one stroke causes symptoms, the athlete should discontinue it temporarily. Once the symptoms have subsided, the stroke, with any faults corrected, can be gradually introduced back into the training program.

Grade II

A grade II tendonitis requires rest, physiotherapy, and perhaps medication, in addition to the previous management. Rest does not mean total absence from the sport. One can work on strokes that do not elicit pain or concentrate on leg work. In the latter case, kick boards should not be used because they place the shoulder in the pain-provoking position. For aerobic training, running and cycling can supplement the shorter swim workout.

Treatment of grade II tendonitis

- Relative rest (emphasize leg work and pain-free stroke)
- Antiinflammatory medicine
- Physiotherapy modalities (ultrasound, TENS)
- Strengthening program
- Mobilization techniques

A short course of antiinflammatory medication in conjunction with these measures will help improve symptomatic relief.

At this stage or in the grade III tendonitis, the athlete may be referred for physiotherapy. The therapist will assess the athlete's shoulder to determine intensity and duration of pain, range limitations, and any loss of strength in the muscles of the arm and the shoulder girdle.

Treatment is determined by the assessment findings and may include the use of modalities such as ultrasound, interferential therapy, or transcutaneous electrical nerve stimulation (TENS). Loss of range is treated with passive mobilization techniques and range of motion exercises. If there is an imbalance in muscle strength or significant weakness in any muscle group, the therapist will plan an appropriate strengthening program. Depending on the nature and presentation of the pair, joint range, and weakness, the exercises will be isometric, isotonic, or where possible, isokinetic. However, an effective treatment program can be developed using only free weights and/or rubber surgical tubing.

The exercises should not reproduce pain. Often the pain is felt only in certain positions and the exercises can be done around such positions. If, however, the exercise is painful throughout range it should be discontinued or decreased in repetition or resistance to the level at which it is pain-free.

If the treatment program is successful, the athlete gradually returns to the full program but is advised to continue with therapy until the preinjury level of activity is attained.

If the tendonitis is not responding to treatment and there is still painful response to the impingement aggravating test, a steroid injection into the subacromial space may be considered. Such injections should never be used routinely. If the situation merits its use, the athlete's swimming load should be decreased following the injection and gradually return to former levels over 4 to 6 weeks.

Grade III

In some cases none of these measures is successful and the athlete progresses to a grade III stage or beyond, with the tendonitis becoming refractory. At this time, options available to the athlete include a change of sports or surgery. Unless a high-caliber career is possible at the national or international level, most young swimmers correctly select the former option and in most instances should be encouraged to. Surgical options include resection of the diseased segment of tendon, along with adjacent subacromial bursal tissue if involved and/or decompression of the same area.

Before selecting surgery as an option, the clinician should make clear to the athlete that the postoperative recovery period involves a serious personal commitment. During that time, rehabilitation will include a progressive exercise program to restore range of motion and balance muscle strength. The athlete's cooperation and compliance to the program will directly effect its outcome. The return to the pool should begin with slow swimming progressive to interval training and guided stroke modification, as well as an overlap period from formal rehabilitation. The importance of the coach to the athlete's successful return to sport cannot be overemphasized.

Grade IV

A grade IV clinical presentation, pain with all activity, is most often seen in the mature athlete. It may indicate a tear of the rotator cuff. Conservative treatment may not satisfactorily relieve these symptoms. Although the diagnosis may be made clinically, imaging techniques such as arthrography, ultrasonography, and magnetic resonance imaging may give confirmation. Arthroscopy of the shoulder joint and the subacromial space can help identify such lesions as partial thickness tears and thickened subacromial bursae. Although not a frequent cause of pain, particularly in younger swimmers, superior quandrant labral tears, anterior or posterior, can cause pain in the swimmer and be successfully treated with arthroscopic excision[7].

In younger athletes, bursectomy alone can provide relief, followed by appropriate rehabilitation. A more radical decompression to include resection of the anteroinferior acromion and a portion of the coracoacromial ligament is usually recommended. Repair of a torn rotator cuff is done to provide symptomatic relief and prevent progressive tearing. This may be noted in the older swimmer competing at the master level. It is unlikely that the athlete will return to the preinjury level of participation, and this should be made clear preoperatively.

Formal physiotherapy plays a significant role postoperatively, because range of motion is often lost and muscle strength, endurance, and power deteriorate. Classically the abductors and the external rotators are the weakest groups, but all muscle groups about the shoudler girdle must be included in the program.

Anterior Instability

Stroke modification and balance-strengthening exercises are the primary conservative

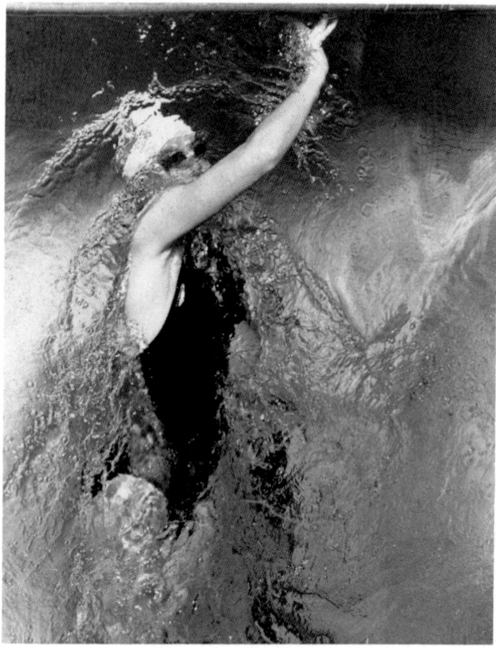

FIG. 40-14. The modified backstroke turn avoids the provocative position. Care must be taken not to turn more than 90 degrees before touching the wall to avoid disqualification.

treatments available to the swimmer with anterior instability.

The turn in the backstroke in particular brings on the symptoms, reproducing the sensation that the joint is dislocating. The traditional turn can be modified by having the swimmer reach across the body to touch the pool wall. This is followed by a somersault to come out of the turn (Fig. 40-14). If symptoms do not subside, examination under anesthesia and/or arthroscopy can assist in diagnosing intraarticular lesions such as the Bankhart or Hill-Sachs. An anterior stabilization procedure can provide relief and return athletes to preinjury levels if they regain their motion and strength.

Multidirectional Instability

Persistence with a nonoperative program is suggested for prolonged periods of multidirectional instability. Stroke modification, correction of strengthening deficits, and alteration of training programs, all designed to minimize the magnitude and incidence of abnormal motion, can be used successfully in most cases. Surgical treatment possibilities include an inferior capsular shift, a "reefing procedure" to the posterior cuff and capsule, and a glenoid osteotomy. Such procedures should be considered only when nonoperative treatment has been completely exhausted. Restriction of motion by these procedures will undoubtedly terminate a competitive swimming career at a high competitive level. Such treatment can realistically be undertaken to provide symptomatic relief for daily activities and to allow the athlete to participate in recreational swimming and other sports.

SUMMARY

Swimmer's shoulder is most commonly pain experienced from tendonitis. The etiology of this tendonitis in a competitive swimmer may be complex. It requires the combined effort and cooperation of the athlete, coach, therapist, and physician for successful prevention and management.

REFERENCES

1. Bigliani NU, Morrison DS, and April EW: The morphology of the acromion and its relationship to rotator cuff tears, Orthop Tran 10(2):216, 1986.
2. Blazina ME: Jumper's knee, Orthop Clinic N Am 4(3):65, 1980.
3. Fowler PJ and Webster MS: Shoulder pain in highly competitive swimmers, Orthop Trans 7(1):170, 1983.
4. Fowler PJ and Webster MS: Rotation strength about the shoulder: establishment of internal to external strength ratios. Presented at the American Orthopaedic Society for Sports Medicine annual meeting, Nashville, July 1985.
5. Griep JF: Swimmer's shoulder: the influence of flexibility and weight training, Phys Sport med 13(8):92, 1985.

5a. Holt LE: Scientific stretching for sport, pamphlet, LE Holt.

6. Kennedy JC, and Hawkins RJ: Swimmer's shoulder, Phys Sports med 2(4):35, 1974.
7. McMaster WC: Anterior glenoid labrum damage: a painful lesion in swimmers, Am J Sports Med 14(5):383, 1986.
8. Neer CS: Anterior acromioplasty for the chronic impingement syndrome in the shoulder, J Bone Joint Surg 54A:41, 1972.
9. Neer CS and Welsh RP: The shoulder in sports, Orthop Clin N Am 8:585, 1977.
10. Rathburn JB and Macnab I: The microvascular pattern of the rotator cuff, J Bone Joint Surg 52B(3):544, 1970.
11. Webster MS, Bishop P, and Fowler PJ: Swimmer's shoulder, undergraduate thesis, Waterloo, Ont. 1981, University of Waterloo.

PART VIII Disabled Athletes

CHAPTER 41 Sports Medicine and the Physically Disabled

John G. Yost
Lana K. Minnigerode
Howard J. Ellfeldt

As we near the twenty-first century, the physically disabled are making a larger and larger impact on society as a viable and productive force. Before World War II, 80% of paraplegics died within 3 years from complications of paraplegia.[4,6] Today, 80% of paraplegics have a normal life expectancy. This turnaround is largely the responsibility of Sir Ludwig Guttman. He showed that if the paraplegic is well nursed in early states, with avoidance of pressure sores and kidney infections, the individual can eventually learn to take care of himself or herself.[4]

HISTORY

Dr. R. W. Jackson, an orthopedist with deep interest in disabled athletes, has described the historical advances initiated by Sir Ludwig.[6] Guttman introduced archery as a therapeutic measure for paraplegic war veterans at the Spinal Injuries Center, at Stoke Mandeville Hospital, in England. In 1950, international competition among disabled sportsmen first occurred when Dutch paraplegic archers competed against an English team. The competition was such a success that it was repeated the next year, with more countries invited and more activities added. The Games had reached such proportion in 1960 that the site was moved from Stoke Mandeville to Rome, Italy. Thus, the first wheelchair olympics were held immediately after the regular Olympics.

The Games were moved to Tokyo, Japan, the site of the Olympics in 1964. In 1968, the Mexican government would not support the wheelchair games and they were held in Tel Aviv, Israel. In 1972, 1000 competitors from 38 countries participated in the Games held in Heidelberg, West Germany. Toronto, Canada was the host city in 1976, with 1500 athletes from 44 countries competing. In 1980, the International Coordinating Council was formed. This became the governing body for sports for athletes disabled from any cause. That year, the Olympic Games for the Physically Disabled were held in Arnheim, Holland. It was the second largest athletic event that year, with 2500 competitors.

A surge of interest from other groups of disabled persons paralleled the development of sports for individuals with spinal paralysis. Amputee athletes were included in participation in the wheelchair games and developed their own rules and regulations. Blind athletes became organized on a worldwide basis, with local, regional, national, and international competitions. The Cerebral Palsy Association for Sport has become active and organized on an international basis.[6] In 1984, demonstration events by disabled athletes were included in both the Summer Olympic Games in Los Angeles and in the Winter Olympic Games in Sarajevo.

Today, a wide variety of sports can be enjoyed by the disabled athelete[4] (Table 41-1).

Illness and injury were feared in the early days of sports for the disabled, but they have not materialized. The disabled athlete who trains for an event is no more liable to injury than his or her able-bodied counterpart.[4,12] In fact, serious injury is *less* common in the handicapped skier than in the average nonhandicapped skier.

In order to prevent any one individual or team from gaining unfair advantage, an equitable medical classification was developed for the physically disabled. All competitors in the same class should have an equal degree of disability.[7] Classification is done by an international team of doctors who are certified by the medical panel to ensure proper athlete classification before the records are allowed to stand.[4]

For blind athletes, there are two classes. Those with more than 10% visual acuity are in a class separate from those with less than 10% visual acuity. If individuals can appreciate differences between light and dark or distinguish shadows, they are at a significant advantage.[6]

Classification of blind athletes

- >10% Visual acuity
- <10% Visual acuity

Amputee athletes are subdivided into 12 categories of limb disablement, to take into account various combinations of upper and lower extremity limb loss. Neurologic disorders may be classified on either anatomic (location and nature of spinal cord lesions) or functional (the quantity and quality of active muscle mass) basis.[6]

The wheelchair games include all neurologic and paralyzing disorders, and six categories have been established. Basically, the category or class of participation depends on the level of spinal cord involvement. Quadriplegic athletes are divided into three categories: those without triceps, those with triceps, and those with some function in the hands (resulting from a lesion at the level of the first thoracic vertebra and sparing of intrinsics or from a central cord lesion). Paraplegic athletes with no trunk muscles are in a category above those with abdominal musculature, and both are above those with some hip extension or flexion. Two systems are used in the United States. The National Wheelchair Athletic Association (NWAA) system, used for its organized competitions, has five classes (Fig. 41-1). The National Wheelchair Basketball Association (NWBA) uses a three-class system[10] (Fig. 41-2).

Skiing for the physically disabled began in Germany during World War II (1942).[3] Skiing, as a form of rehabilitation for returning American amputees, started in 1944. This movement was pioneered by Gretchen Fraser.[9] Equipment was very crude and ill-fitted initially. However, crutches with attached skis developed into outriggers with skis in the 1950s, and other equipment for handicapped skiers was introduced thanks to the interest of Mr. Paul Leimkuehler, a prosthetist who lost his leg in World War II. Many individuals with various disabilities have been taught skiing and have benefitted in rehabilitation of their spinal cord injury, cerebral palsy, multiple sclerosis, muscular dystrophies, deafness, blindness, and mental retardation.[9] In 1968, Dr. Paul Brown and Dr. William Stonek began a ski school that now exists as the Winter Park Handicap Ski Program. A well-fitted prosthesis can allow some below-knee amputees to use normal equipment, but for others and above-knee amputees, three-track skiing is used.

Special adaptive equipment exists for athletes with cerebral palsy and myelodysplasia, such as the ski bra. A ski bra attaches to the tips of the skis preventing the tips from crossing. This allows a snow plow position of the skis, aiding control and maneuverability. Canting wedges can be installed between the sole of the ski boot and the ski, aiding skiers with residual deformities, such as club feet, muscle imbalance, or bony abnormalities in the foot or lower leg.[9]

Blind skiers, usually working one-on-one with an instructor, are required to wear a ski vest indicating their disability. Ski sledding is popular with paraplegics and bilateral short above-knee amputees. The Arroya ski sled was perceived in the handicap ski program at Winter Park. Careful attention to seat, backrest, cushioning, leg, and lapcover with a roll bar results in a safe, efficient ski sled. While learning, sit-skiers are attached by tether to an able-bodied instructor. Organizations in-

TABLE 41-1 List of competitions

Wheelchair Games	Blind Games	Amputee Games
Track	Track	Track
Field	Field	Field
Swimming	Swimming	Swimming
Archery	Bowling	Table tennis
Weight lifting	Pentathlon	Rifle shooting
Fencing	Goal ball	Bowling
Table tennis	Wrestling	Football kicking
Rifle shooting	Skiing	Slalom
Snooker		Pentathlon
Slalom		Volleyball
Pentathlon		Skiing
Basketball		

volved in skiing for the disabled are listed in the box.[9]

Organizations and equipment manufacturers involved in skiing for the handicapped

American Athletic Association for the Deaf (AAAD)
3916 Lantern Drive
Silver Springs, MD 20902

Blind Outdoor Leisure Development (BOLD)
533 E. Main Street
Aspen, CO 81611

Children's Hospital
NHSRA Chapter
1056 E. 19th Avenue
Denver, CO 80218

Horizons for the Handicapped
P.O. Box 2143
Steamboat Springs, CO 80477

International Committee of Sports for the Deaf (CISSO)
Secretariat CMSH82
CH-1861
Les Mosses, Switzerland

International Stoke-Mandeville Games Federation (ISMGF)
Stoke-Mandeville Sports Stadium
Harvey Road
Aylesbury, Buckinghamshire
England

National Association for Sports for Cerebral Palsied (NASCP)
66 E. 34th Street
New York, New York 10016

Special Olympics
1701 K. Street NW, Suite 303
Washington, DC 20006

Winter Park Recreational Association
P.O. Box 36
Winter Park, CO 80482

BENEFITS OF EXERCISE

Psychologic and physiologic benefits from exercise have been studied in disabled athletes.[1,6,11,12,17]

Disabled athletes are more oriented toward achieving cognitive goals than their able-bodied peers, a finding attributed to the years of hard work spent proving themselves. Improved body image is another anticipated benefit, with improved psychosocial adjustment.

Physical benefits include increased endurance and more efficient work. In wheelchair propulsion, trained subjects used fewer arm strikes to achieve faster speed against greater resistance. Thus, increased power of arm strike leads to greater work efficiency, with reduction in metabolic cost. In a study of strength scores in retarded children, they showed an initial score 1.5 SD below their nonretarded peers. After a 10-month period of exercises, the children showed a virtually complete correction of low strength scores and improvement in balance and posture.[12]

Wheelchair users vary widely in levels of cardiopulmonary fitness and muscular strength. Elite wheelchair athletes rated 9% below able-bodied athletes, expressed as VO_2 max per unit body mass, and were 50% above sedentary wheelchair users, in one study.[6] Wheelchair athletes have been shown to possess muscles with larger fiber areas than Olympic athletes.[17] The relative populations of different fiber types is genetically determined. Wheelchair athletes who have muscles with a high percentage of type I fibers perform better in marathon racing; and those with a higher percentage of type II fibers, especially type IIb are more likely to succeed in wheelchair sprinting.[1,17] The level of spinal cord lesion is a less important determinant of maximum oxygen intake than is habitual physical activity. With habitual physical activity, forearm physical work capacity increased by 50%. Dynamic strength and endurance (lifting weights) increased by 19% and 80%, respectively.[6]

RECENT ACCOMPLISHMENTS

Through the work of Will Cloney, Director of the Boston Marathon Committee, and Paul DePace, Chairman of the National Wheelchair Marathon, organized wheelchair marathon competition was started.[1]

Rich Hansen, a Canadian wheelchair athlete, wheeled around the world, 24,901 miles over a 2-year period. This was done to raise awareness of the abilities of disabled athletes and to raise funds for spinal cord research.[8]

In 1977, Bob Hall won the first official wheelchair marathon in 2 hours, 40 minutes, and 10 seconds. Sharon Rohn, the only female competitor, finished the 26-mile, 285-yard course in 3 hours and 40 minutes. In 1980, Curt Brinkman won in 1 hour and 55 minutes, and Sharon Limpert was the first woman to finish in 2 hours, 49 minutes, and 4 seconds. In 1986, Andre Viger won the Boston Marathon for wheelchair athletes in a time of 1 hour, 43 minutes, and 25 seconds. The top 13 men finished under 2 hours. Candace Cable-Brooks had the best time for women—2 hours, 9 minutes, and 28 seconds.

Water skiing for wheelchair users is an uncommon activity, but not because of lack of desire. Lack of equipment had been a prob-

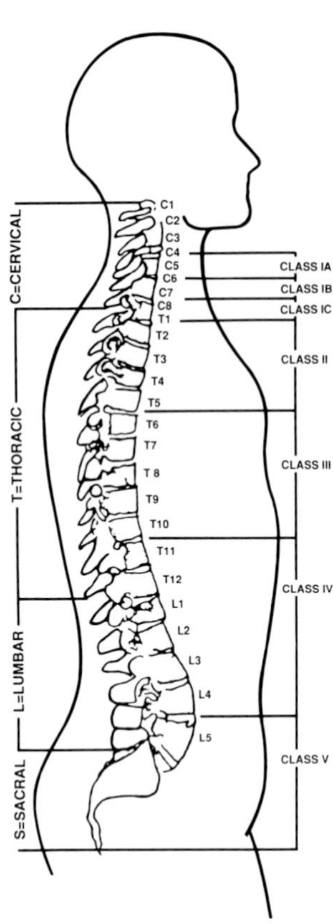

CLASS IA

All cervical lesions with complete or incomplete quadripelgia who have involvement of both hands, weakness of triceps (up to and including grade 3 on testing scale) and with severe weakness of the trunk and lower extremities interfering significantly with trunk balance and the ability to walk.

CLASS IB

All cervical lesions with complete or incomplete quadriplegia who have involvement of upper extremities but less than IA with preservation of normal or good triceps (4 or 5 on testing scale) and with a generalized weakness of the trunk and lower extremities interfering significantly with trunk balance and the ability to walk.

CLASS IC

All cervical lesions with complete or incomplete quadriplegia who have involvment of upper extremities but less than IB with preservation of normal or good triceps (4 or 5 on testing scale) and normal or good finger flexion and extension (grasp and release) but without intrinsic hand function and with a generalized weakness of the trunk and lower extremities interfering significantly with trunk balance and the ability to walk.

CLASS II

Complete or incomplete paraplegia below T1 down to and including T5 or comparable disability with total abdominal paralysis or poor abdominal muscle strength (0-2 on testing scale) and no useful trunk sitting balance.

CLASS III

Complete or incomplete paraplegia or comparable disability below T5 down to and including T10 with upper abdominal and spinal extensor musculature sufficient to provide some element of trunk sitting balance but not normal.

CLASS IV

Complete or incomplete paraplegia or comparable disability below T10 down to and including L5 without quadriceps or very weak quadriceps with a value up to and including 2 on the testing scale and gluteal paralysis.

CLASS V

Complete or incomplete paraplegia or comparable disability below L2 with quadriceps in grades 3-5.

FIG. 41-1. National Wheelchair Athletic Association classification system.

lem, but with the development of Kan-Ski, by Royce Andes in California, and marketing of E-ski, by Phil Carpenter in Louisiana, more disabled athletes are turning into water skiers. Competitions now exist including slalom, wake cross, and trick-ski events.

Weight lifting championships for men and women are held throughout the country and internationally. A lifter in the 65-kilo class lifted 170 kilos (374.7 pounds). An 85-kilo class lifter successfully set a national record with a lift of 202.5 kilos (446.2 pounds). Jon Brown, an American paraplegic, has successfully bench-pressed 585 pounds.

Ice picking is a sport for disabled persons in which long-blade ice sledges and shortened cross-country poles called "picks" are used. A recent 5-mile race was won in a time of 38 minutes and 20 seconds.[16] Sledge hockey is Canada's newest winter sport for the disabled. The sledge has an oval-shaped metal frame with two blades under the seat and a runner in the middle, under the front. The player is anchored to the sledge with a seat belt and ankle strap.[18] Players are propelled using shortened hockey sticks with sharpened metal picks affixed to one end. The rules are very similar to those of ice hockey.

A national bass tournament for the physically disabled is held in Texas and sponsored by POINT (Paraplegics on Independent Nature Trips). Grand prize in 1986 was a $6000 boat and motor. Seventy-six entrants from 10 different states competed.[13] The tournament was won by a quadriplegic without finger function. He casted with the rod strapped to his hand while reeling with the other hand.

PREVENTATIVE MEASURES

With the rapid development of sports for disabled athletes has come an equally rapid

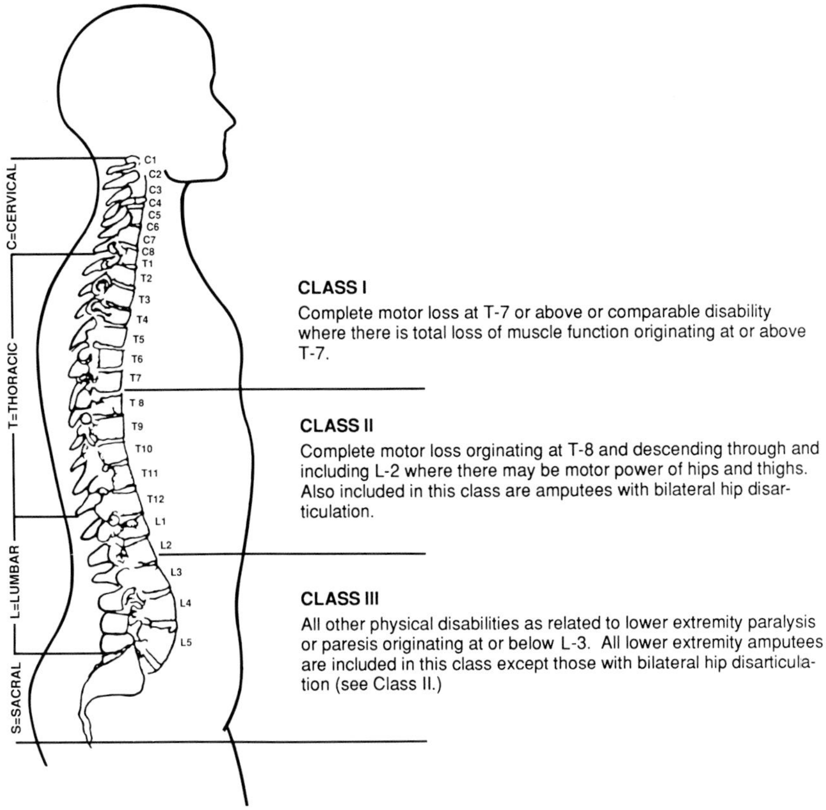

FIG. 41-2. National Wheelchair Basketball Association classification system.

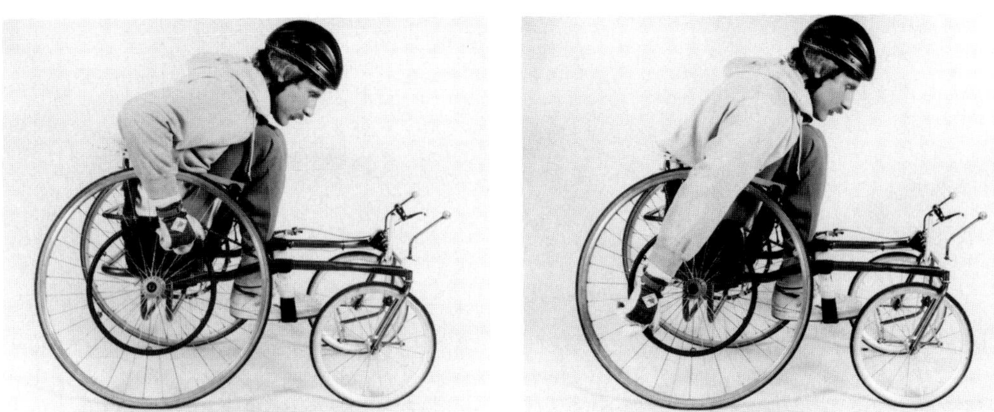

FIG. 41-3. Racing wheelchair with athlete strapped in. Proper propulsion technique for a paraplegic with wrist extension power is demonstrated.

evolution in wheelchair design. Today's racing wheelchair is built like a racing bicycle, with lightweight aluminum frames, pneumatic tubular tires, and large rear wheels, with a maximum diameter of 70 centimeters. There can be only one handrim attached to each of the driving wheels. Small handrims (25 centimeters in diameter) are used to attain a high-gear ratio. With a small handrim, the chair becomes harder to push, but the potential for speed is maximized[11] (Fig. 41-3). No chains, levers, gears, or other mechanical devices are permitted for propulsion. The maximum length for a racing wheelchair is 120

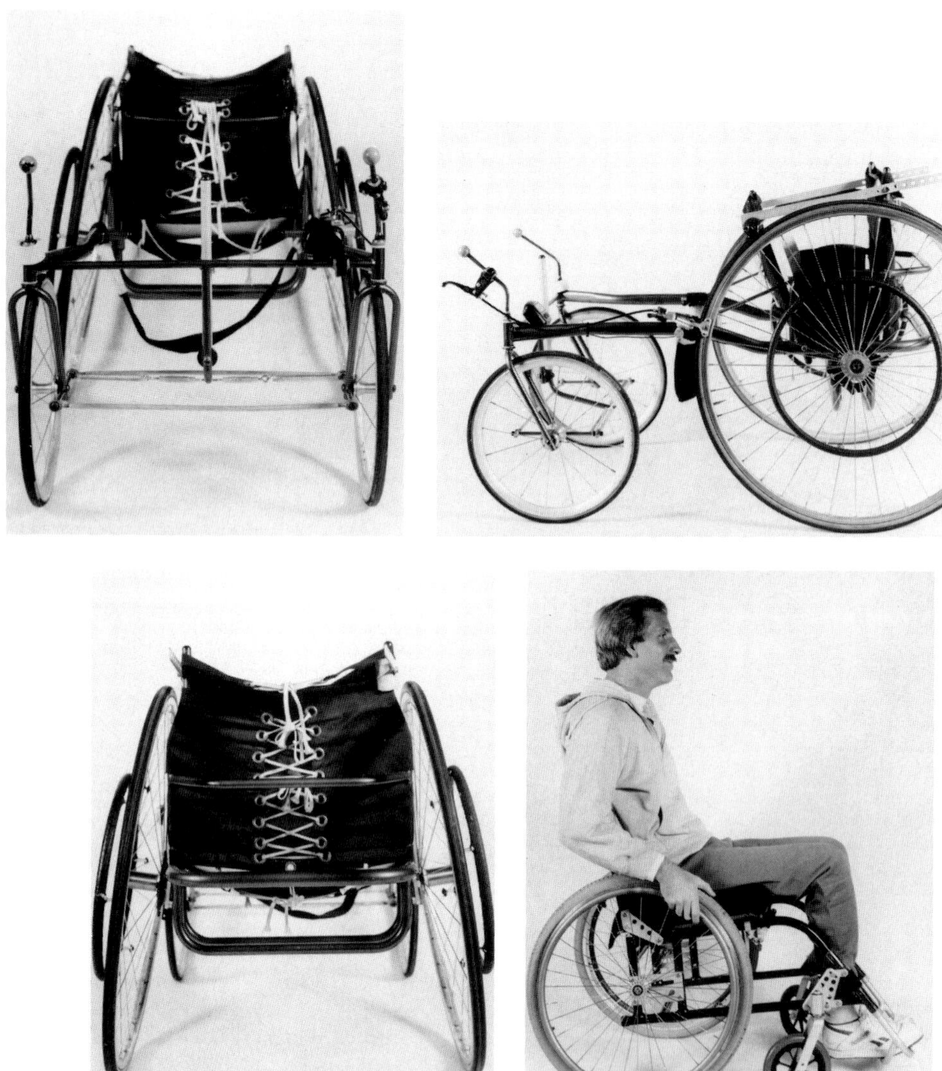

FIG. 41-4. A to **C,** Front, side and back views of a racing wheelchair. **D,** Basketball wheelchair, side view.

centimeters, and no part of the wheelchair can protrude beyond the width of the distance between the outer edges of the handrims or tires, whichever is widest. No part of the wheelchair can serve the sole purpose of reducing wind resistance.[14] Today, a racing wheelchair is capable of attaining speeds of 30 to 35 mph. Changing the position of the rear axle in relation to the athlete's center of gravity affects wheelchair maneuverability, stability, pushing difficulty, and turning ability. Rear wheel camber, angling the top portion of the wheels inward, adds side stability. Most sport wheelchairs are equipped with anti-tip devices on the back of the chair, which help prevent the chair from tipping backward if the athlete shifts back in the chair during use. Examples of chairs are included (Fig. 41-4).

Racing wheelchair design

- Lightweight aluminum frame
- Pneumatic tubular tires
- Large rear wheels (maximum diameter 70 cm)
- Small handrim
- Rear wheel camber
- Anti-tip devices

Certain precautions and equipment are necessary for safe, effective training and competition. Guidelines for equipment, racing protocol, and safety are set by the National Wheelchair Athletic Association.[14,15]

The forces applied to the hands during racing are great. Heavily taped gloves are necessary to allow sustained pushing with a minimum of soft tissue injury. Generally, racers wear snug-fitting handball gloves, heavily wrapped with athletic tape, Elastoplast, and cloth friction tape (for padding and adhesion), at those points on the hand at which the greatest forces are applied (Fig. 41-5).

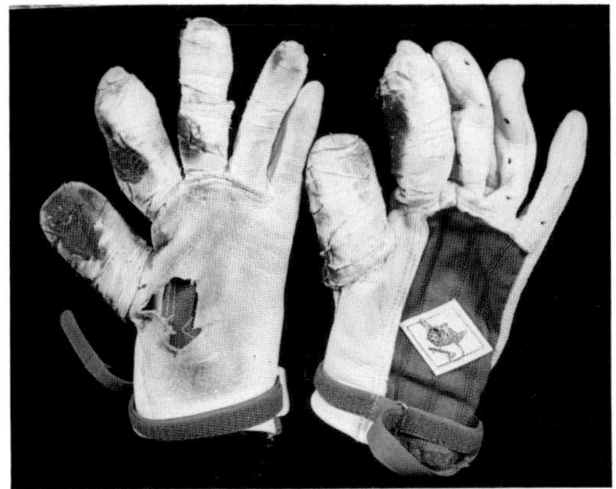

FIG. 41-5. Snug fitting handball gloves are used to protect the hand. Areas of increased pressure are reinforced with tape, Elastoplast, or cloth friction tape.

Contact on the inner aspect of the arm with the top of the tire causes friction burns. This is especially common in the novice competitor. As an athlete becomes more experienced, the best configuration of body position, handrim diameter, and camber are found and friction burns become less of a problem. To prevent injury, athletes wear tube socks or wrist bands to protect the inner aspect of the arm.

Strapping is used to add sitting stability for the individual with a relatively high level of paralysis. This consists of a binder or belt around the athlete and the back of the wheelchair. Strapping is used to control the unwanted motion of spastic lower extremities. In roadracing, straps are used to secure the lower extremities to the wheelchair, so that they cannot fall to the ground. If strapping is incorrect, the feet and legs can be injured and the athlete could also be thrown from the wheelchair (Fig. 41-6). At high speeds, this could result in serious injury. A race official is responsible to rule on the safety of the wheelchair and the athlete before the race.

Athletes wth impaired sensation should inspect their bodies after each work-out for pres-

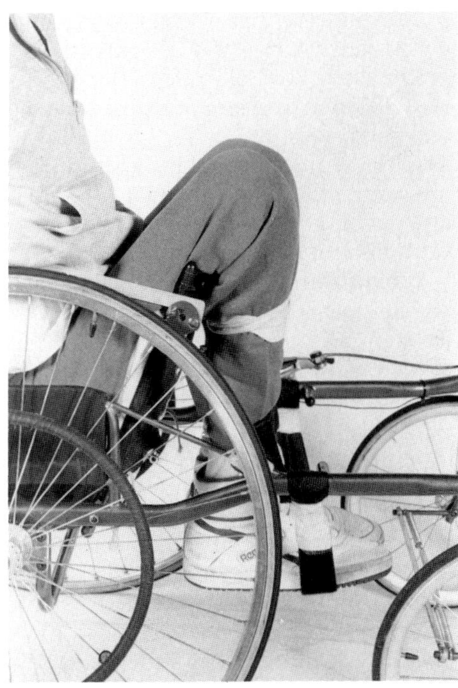

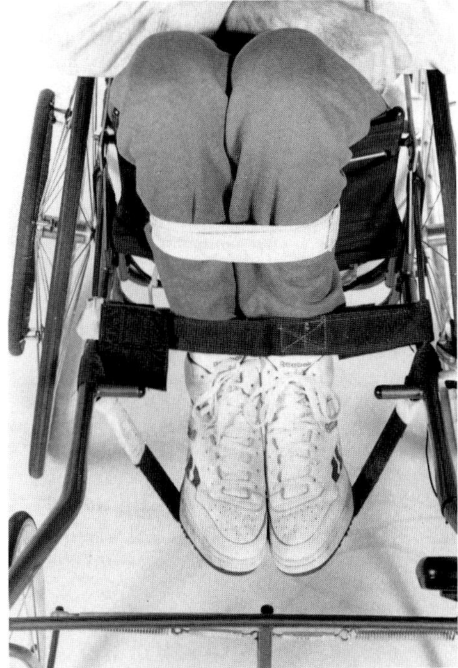

FIG. 41-6. Correct strapping for racing wheelchair. Note position of sacrum and buttocks.

sure spots, cuts, or abrasions. Care and treatment should be initiated immediately upon recognition of the injury and the causal agent identified so that preventative measures can be taken.

In long-distance roadracing, speeds of up to 35 mph can be attained and helmets are recommended—even mandated, in this author's opinion—to prevent head injury. The rules of long-distance roadracing do not allow simultaneous starts with footrunners. Commonly, the wheelchair division will start 5 to 15 minutes before the runners. Competitors who experience a mishap may be assisted in remounting. Assistance must be provided in a manner not to impede other racers, nor impart forward assistance to the participant. In races with footrunners, the ultimate right of way belongs to the runner.

INJURIES TO DISABLED ATHLETES

Athletic injuries in this now very active population have been documented few times in the literature,[2,4,5] yet the number of injuries may be high. In one study, 72% of all athletes responding to a questionnaire had at least one injury since they started participating, with some athletes reporting as many as fourteen. Most information is anecdotal, from trainers, coaches, and physical therapists who assist in training and classifying wheelchair athletes. Many of these athletes do not seek aid from a physician because they have an unsatisfactory experience associated with their original injury.[2] At the 1976 Olympiad, more than 1500 athletes participated and 184 were treated for injury or illness. Common problems were muscle strain, headache, abrasions, burns, upper respiratory infections, and catheter and colostomy changes.[4,5] In one large series, common sports associated with injuries are track, 26% of all injuries; basketball, 24% of all injuries; road racing, 22% of all injuries; tennis, 6% of all injuries; field events, 4% of all injuries; and swimming, 4% of all injuries.

In the same series, 33% of all injuries were soft tissue injuries (sprain, strains, tendonitis, bursitis).[2] The shoulder, elbow, or wrist can be involved. Routine stretching, warm-up, and cool-down for each workout will help prevent chronic overuse injuries (Fig. 41-7).

Improper push techniques, with hyperflexion of the wrist, cause **tendonitis and sprains of the wrist.** The pushing technique for a paraplegic differs from that of a quadriplegic, with loss of wrist extension and triceps power (Figs. 41-3 and 41-8). Rest with a wrist splint, followed by a rehabilitation program and instruction in proper technique, are necessary to treat the injury and prevent recurrence.

Blisters accounted for 18% of the injuries in the same series. The hand and fingers were most commonly involved, though the inner arm from tire friction and irritation of skin at the top of the seat post and on the back of the wheelchair also occur. To prevent these blisters, callous formation is encouraged as initial protection. Taping fingers, wearing gloves, padding over the seat post area, and wrist bands or sleeves on the upper arm should also be used, as needed. Seventeen percent of the injuries in this series were lacerations, abrasions, or cuts, including skin infections.[2] The fingers and thumb in contact with brakes, metal edge on empty arm rest sockets, spokes, or push rims are at risk for injury (Fig. 41-9). To rule out bone, tendon, or ligament damage, immediate treatment and protection is initiated. Removal of hand brakes eliminates the primary hazard. Filing off the sockets of the armrests, camber wheels, protective clothing, and gloves also prevent lacerations. Decubitus sores are caused by shear forces and pressure, mainly in those athletes without sensation over the sacrum and buttocks. Friction from the chair, newer racing wheelchair design with the kneees higher than the buttocks, and sweat are contributing factors. Decubitus sores require prompt treatment by keeping the area clean and dry and avoiding pressure in the area. Ulcers may require reconstructive surgery, with removal of bony prominences and skin flap rotation. To prevent decubitus ulcers, adequate cushioning and padding is needed for the buttocks (Fig. 41-10). Frequent skin checks, shifting weight intermittently, good nutrition and hygiene, and clothing that absorbs moisture help prevent difficult problems.

Carpal tunnel syndrome is caused by median nerve compression at the wrist, from constant trauma and compression of the heel of the hand with each arm stroke on the push rim. Carpal tunnel syndrome has also been reported in tennis. Night pain, paresthesias, decreased grip strength, and lack of digit dexterity are the most common symptoms, in spite of a normal physical examination. Acute cases should be splinted, nonsteroidal antiinflammatory medication can be used, and a carpal tunnel steroid injection considered. If symptoms are not abated after 6 to 10 weeks, or if thenar atrophy is present, operative decompression should be performed if EMGs and nerve conduction studies confirm the di-

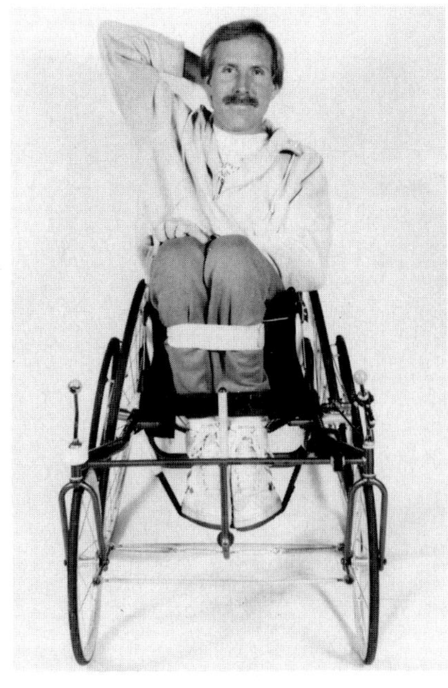

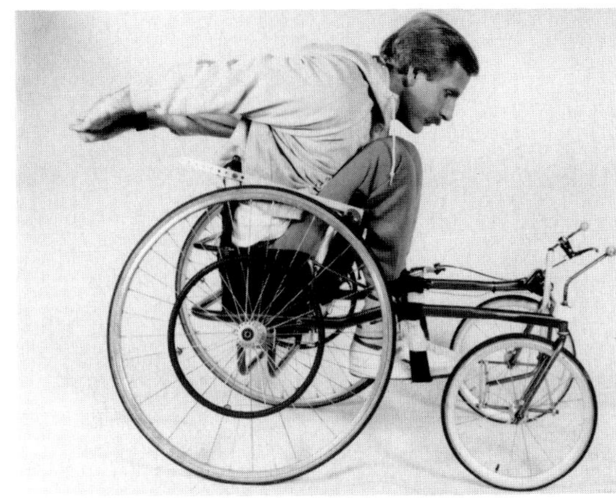

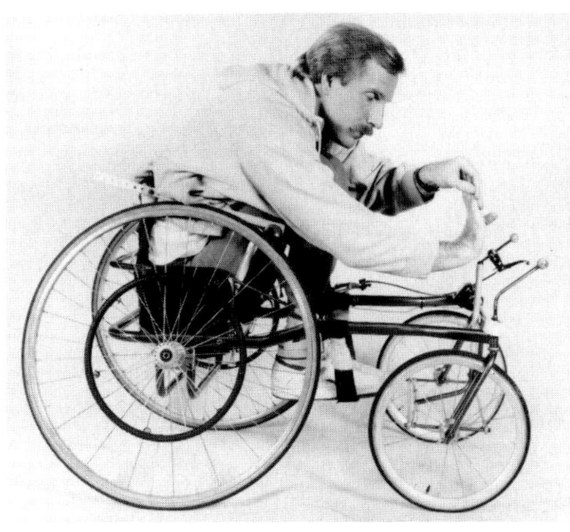

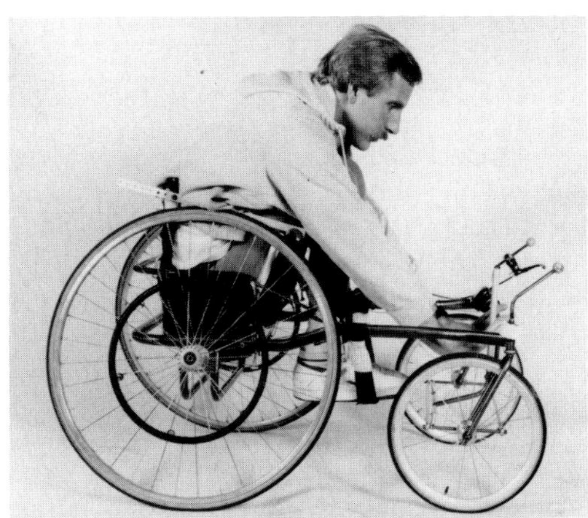

FIG. 41-7. Stretching exercises for the upper extremity with emphasis on shoulders and wrists.

agnosis. Cubital tunnel problems have not been reported.

Temperature regulation disorders, hyperthermia, or hypothermia have occurred in roadracing, track, and field events.[2] Athletes with spinal cord injury may have altered sweating responses, with unpredictable results. In the able-bodied runner, evaporative heat loss is enhanced in the legs as they move back and forth. The wheelchair marathoner has to rely on evaporative heat loss from the arms. Sweating below the level of the spinal cord injury may be deficient.[1] A special problem for paraplegic and quadriplegic marathoners is the vasomotor paralysis and the absence of active muscles to help pump blood past the valves in the veins past the heart. These problems, when associated with dehydration, can lead to hyperthermia. This can lead to heat exhaustion and, rarely, heat stroke. The athlete needs to be rehydrated, moved to shade, and observed. Check the skin under the arms of the athlete and, if it feels cool, the individual is sweating and probably losing heat adequately. If the skin is hot, the individual is not getting rid of enough heat and requires more fluid, fewer clothes, and cooling of the trunk and extremities.[1] To prevent hyperthermia, the athlete must be well hydrated, wear clothing that allows ventilation, and minimize exposure to high temperature, humidity, and sunshine.

Unlike hyperthermia, which usually occurs during a race, hypothermia may become a problem at the end of the race.[1] When the wheelchair marathoner stops, heat production stops, and shivering, which is a natural way to control heat loss, may not occur be-

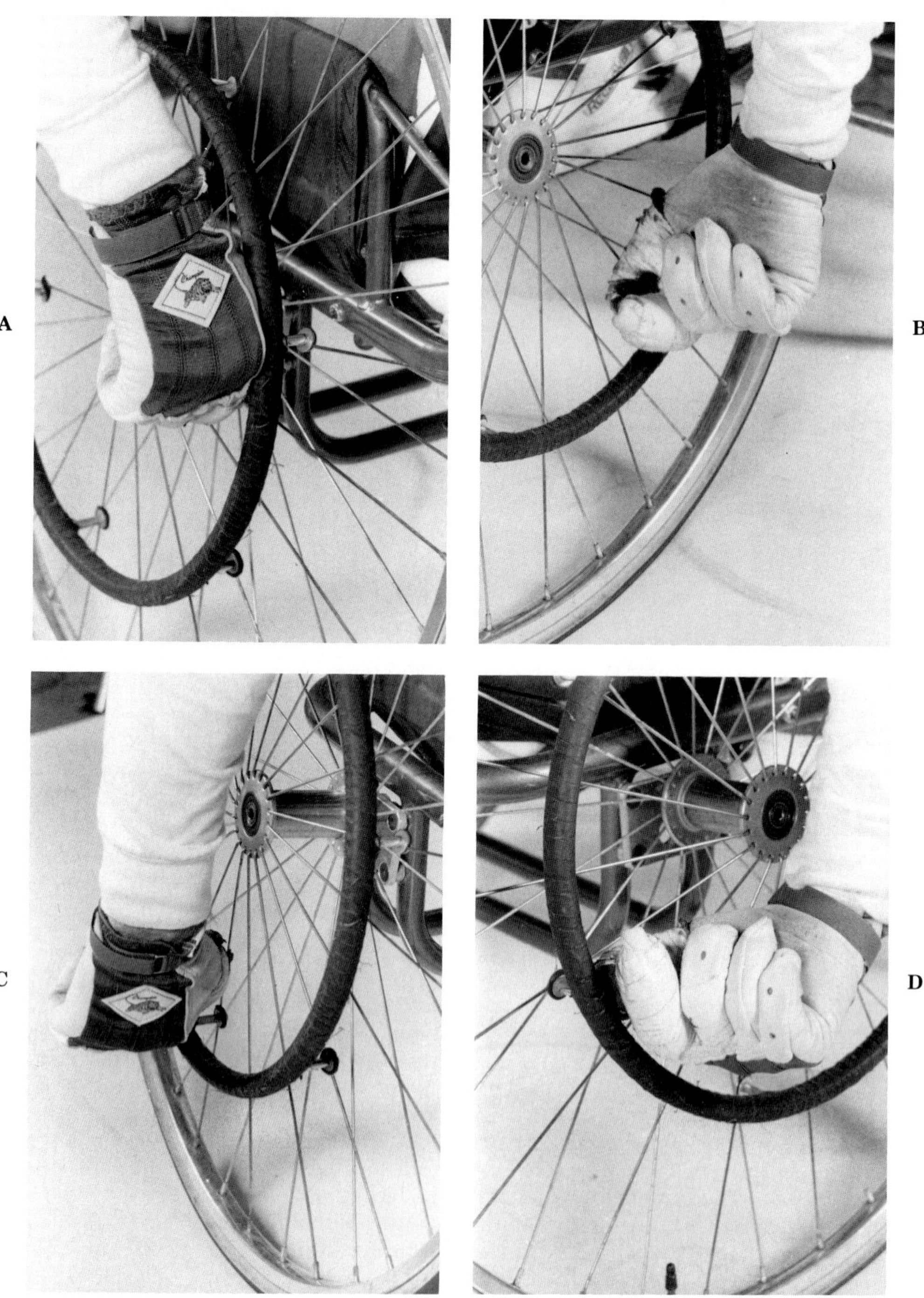

FIG. 41-8. Technique of propelling wheel when wrist extension power is absent. The athlete keeps gloved hand in contact with rim, using biceps power. Propulsion is provided by pistoning motion of shoulders, using trapezius muscle. Front (**A** and **C**) and side (**B** and **D**) views.

A 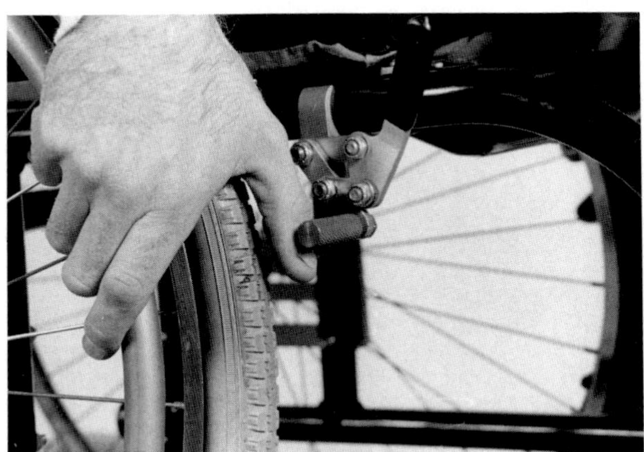

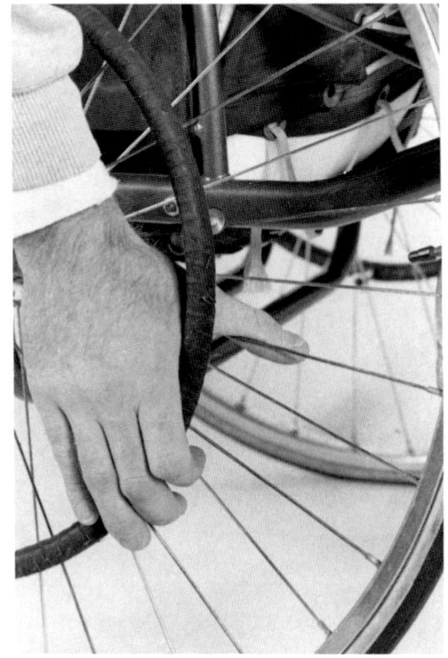 B

FIG. 41-9. A, Exposed brake handles need to be removed to prevent hand injuries. **B,** Thumb injuries can occur if thumb is caught between spokes and frame.

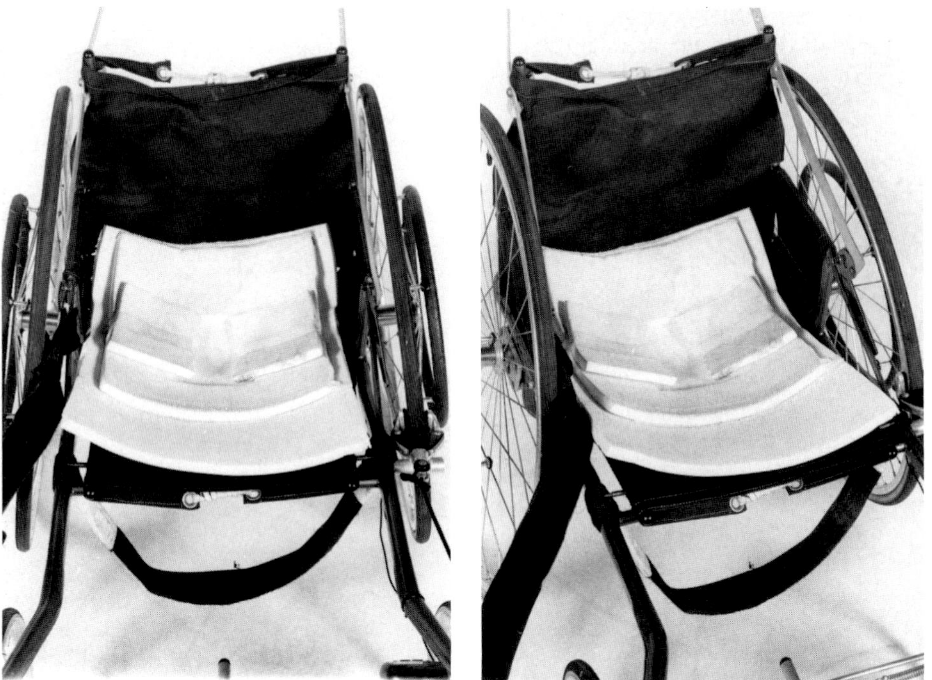

FIG. 41-10. To prevent decubitus sores, special padding is added to the seat of the wheelchair.

cause of the spinal cord injury. The skin remains vasodilated, hyperemic, and saturated with sweat, allowing heat loss to continue at a high rate, leading to hypothermia. In cold, rainy, windy conditions, slower competitors can spend more than 5 hours completing a race. To prevent hypothermia, all wet clothing should be removed and dry warm clothing and blankets applied. Adequate hydration is equally important in treating hypothermia and hyperthermia.

CONCLUSION

In the past four decades, wheelchair athletes have expanded on an international level, to take their place next to nondisabled athletes. The benefits for the athletes are physical and psychologic. Disabled athletes are exercising their right to accept the challenges and risks of able-bodied athletes. They are also experiencing many overuse injuries, similar to those of the able-bodied athlete, and are at risk for certain injuries unique to their sport or disability. Physicians who treat these athletes should be aware of potential problems. Disabled athletes are very independent, make few complaints, and impress observers with their ability, not disability. A keen awareness of these overuse syndromes, and the unique qualities of these athletes with their poor physical image, is mandatory for physicians dealing in these areas.

REFERENCES

1. Concoran PJ et al: Sports medicine and the physiology of wheelchair marathon racing, Orthop Clin North Am 11:4,697-716,1980.
2. Curtis KA: Wheelchair sportsmedicine: Part 4, athletic injuries, Sports n Spokes 8(1):20-24,1982.
3. Guttman L: Textbook of sports for the disabled, Aylesbury, England, 1976, H.M. & M. Publishers.
4. Jackson RW: What did we learn from the Torontolympiad? Can Fam Phys 23:586-589,1977.
5. Jackson RW: Sports for the physically disabled. Am J Sports Med 7:5,293-296,1979.
6. Jackson RW: Sports and recreation for the physically disabled, Orthop Clin North Am 14:2, 401,1983.
7. Jackson RW: Sports for the spinal paralyzed person, Paraplegia 25:301-304,1987.
8. Jordan T: Just 7000 miles to go, Sports n Spokes 12(3):12-15,1986.
9. Krog MH and Messmer DG: Skiing by the physically handicapped, Clin Sports Med 1:2,319-333,1982.
10. Madorsky JGB and Curtis KA: Wheelchair sports medicine, Am J Sports Med 12:2,128-132,1984.
11. Madorsky JGB and Madorsky A: Wheelchair racing: an important modality in acute rehabilitation after paraplegia, Arch Phys Med Rehabil 64:186-187,1983.
12. Molnar G: Rehabilitative benefits of sports for the handicapped, Conn Med 45:9,574-577,1981.
13. Norten B: The best little bass tourney in Texas, Sports n Spokes 13(2):8-10,1987.
14. NWAA: A guide for wheelchair sports training, Colorado Springs, Colo, 1986, NWAA.
15. NWAA: Rules of long distance roadracing, Colorado Springs, Colo, 1987, NWAA.
16. Prietz J: Second annual blade run, Sports n Spokes 13(1):51-52,1987.
17. Taylor AW et al: Skeletal muscle analysis of wheelchair athletes, Paraplegia 17:456-460,1979.
18. Windover R: Canadian ice sports, Sports n Spokes 13(2):45-47,1987.

Index

A

B

C

F

I

J

K

L

N

O

P

Q

R

S

T

X

Y

Z